May, 1983

PATHOLOGY OF SOFT TISSUE TUMORS

"In order to treat malignant tumors of mesenchymal origin one must first learn to recognize them." STOUT, 1964

Steven I. Hajdu, M.D.

Attending Pathologist
Memorial Sloan-Kettering Cancer Center
Associate Professor of Pathology
Cornell University Medical College
New York, New York

Pathology of Soft Tissue Tumors

LEA & FEBIGER PHILADELPHIA

Library of Congress Cataloging in Publication Data

Hajdu, Steven I.
Pathology of soft tissue tumors.

Includes bibliographies and index.
1. Tumors. 2. Histology, Pathological. I. Title.
RC269.H35 616.9′92 79-21735
ISBN 0-8121-0693-8

PRINTED IN THE UNITED STATES OF AMERICA
3 2

To My Wife

preface

Soft tissues, such as muscle, fat, and fibroconnective tissue, constitute more than 50% of the human body but for some unknown reason have received little attention in the medical literature. No book has been devoted solely to the pathology of soft tissue tumors.

The clinical management of a number of soft tissue sarcomas has improved dramatically during the last 10 years as a consequence of combining surgery with irradiation and/or chemotherapy. No longer must the treatment of soft tissue sarcomas be viewed as hopeless. Because successful treatment depends upon the understanding of the natural history and proper classification of these tumors, a comprehensive textbook on their pathology is very much needed.

My objective in writing this text has been to place in the hands of those involved in the diagnosis and treatment of soft tissue tumors—pathologists, surgeons, medical oncologists, and radiation therapists—a book which embodies most of the pertinent information on the morphology, epidemiology, and prognosis of soft tissue neoplasms.

An in-depth discussion of fibrous, tendosynovial, adipose, muscle, vascular, neurogenic, extraskeletal bone, and miscellaneous tumors is presented in separate chapters. Each chapter is treated as a complete unit, from a histogenetic point of view, and begins with a classification of tumors and tumor-like lesions. Chapter 1 is a review of the history of classification and terminology of soft tissue tumors and contains a grading and staging system for primary soft tissue sarcomas. The Appendix summarizes recent trends in the therapy and differential diagnosis of soft tissue neoplasms and has 150 self-assessment questions.

Some topics are considered at greater length, perhaps, than their importance merits. However, after considering recent trends in terminology, classification, grading, and staging of soft tissue sarcomas. I believe that a thorough discussion of the clinicopathologic aspects of certain tumors, e.g., fibrous histiocytomas, is warranted.

In reference to classification I have attempted to coordinate my own thoughts with those of others, and I have retained many of the terms advanced previously. However, a number of new concepts presented are based on observations deduced from studying thousands of soft tissue sarcomas and tumor-like conditions in clinicopathologic and experimental settings.

Although in selecting illustrative material I have tried to maintain a balance between photomicrographs and other illustrations, I have put weight on the light microscopic and differential diagnostic aspects of each tumor.

The references are arranged in chronologic order at the end of each chapter. This arrangement should facilitate easy location of pertinent works and help students follow the course of development of each topic. Review articles have been given preference over case reports, and I regret that many valuable reports could not be listed.

Whether I have accomplished my objective and readers will consider the information presented in this book worthwhile is not for me to determine. I would like to assure every reader that in presenting the facts and theories concerning soft tissue tumors I am completely aware that nobody has the eternal truth.

STEVEN I. HAJDU

New York

acknowledgments

My grateful appreciation is expessed to Myron R. Melamed, M.D., for his continued encouragement, interest, and willingness to listen to my endless discourses.

I am also indebted for suggestions to Philip H. Lieberman, M.D., and members of the attending staff of the Department of Pathology of Memorial Sloan-Kettering Cancer Center, including Robert A. Erlandson, Ph.D., who selected and annotated the ultrastructural illustrations.

Most of the illustrations were prepared in the Medical Illustration Department of Memorial Sloan-Kettering Cancer Center by Mr. Lloyd Edwards, Ms. Lynn McDowell, Ms. Lucille Morgan, and Mr. David Purnell under the able supervision of Mr. John Pedersen. My special thanks to all of them and to Mr. Roy Keppie, Department of Pathology, who skillfully printed the electron microscopic pictures.

I should like to acknowledge the able assistance of Mr. Erich Meyerhoff and his staff at the Samuel J. Wood Library and the staff of the Lee Coombe Memorial Library in locating pertinent references.

For her secretarial assistance and phenomenal typing skills I am particularly indebted to Miss Robin Nager who typed the entire manuscript often by sacrificing her social hours. I also express my appreciation to Miss Gloria H. Bischoff for her accurate record keeping and tireless researching of essential data.

And finally, I wish to thank members of the editorial, illustration and production staff of Lea & Febiger for their professional resourcefulness and artful reproduction of illustrative material. I am particularly appreciative to Mr. R. Kenneth Bussy, Executive Editor, for his continued interest and editorial guidance. I thank Ms. Isabelle L. Clouser, Copy Editor, for making the manuscript readable and Mr. Thomas J. Colaiezzi for his many suggestions and promptness in production.

S.I.H.

contents

chapter 1

History and Classification of Soft Tissue Tumors

THE PERIOD OF GROSS PATHOLOGY
(*From Antiquity to Bichat*)

THE PERIOD OF CELLULAR PATHOLOGY
(*From J. Müller to P. Ehrlich*)

THE PERIOD OF HISTOPATHOLOGY
(*From Ewing to Stout*)

THE PERIOD OF GRADING AND STAGING
(*The 1970's*)

LIKE so many other classifications in medicine, the classification of soft tissue tumors developed by fits and starts. It has been said that "in history there is no beginning." Indeed, in medicine similar ideas have often recurred, sometimes in ignorance of their previous appearances and other times as Starling said, "Every discovery, however important and apparently epoch-making, is but the natural and inevitable outcome of a vast mass of work, involving many failures, by a host of different observers."

This chapter is not an all inclusive account of the history of soft tissue tumors. The role of the historian is to present the facts *that were found* the way they were found. In my search for facts I do not claim to have followed all leads and exhausted all potential reference sources. Although my records may be incomplete, I present what I have found because I believe with E. R. Lang that "nothing gives a better perspective of the subject than an appreciation of the steps by which it has reached its present state."

THE PERIOD OF GROSS PATHOLOGY

(From Antiquity to Bichat)

The earliest description of cancer is in the *Smith Papyrus* which dates prior to 2000 B.C. and may have been written by the famous Egyptian physician Imhotep. It is regarded as the oldest nucleus of scientific medical knowledge and is in the possession of the New York Academy of Medicine (Fig. 1-1). The *Papyrus Ebers*, which is housed in the Library of Leipzig and was written in 1552 B.C., a century before the exodus of the Israelites, is a collection of therapeutic suggestions such as "Cancer is a tumor which is not to be touched" and "If the tumor goes and comes under your finger, trembling even when your hand is still, it is a fatty tumor, and treat it with the knife." The Egyptians are regarded as the founders of Medicine, but without question they included various non-neoplastic swellings in their description of tumors.

The fatalistic view of ancient physicians who believed that "cancer is incurable because it cannot be cured; if curable, it is not cancer" was also the view of Hippocrates (460–375 B.C.) who advised never to operate on an ulcerating cancer. Hippocrates contributed to the literature on soft tissue tumors by giving the first description of nasal angiofibroma.

Celsus (25 B.C.–A.D. 50) in his *De re Medicina,* which is the oldest medical document after the Hippocratic writings, attempted to separate benign neoplasms, e.g., lipoma and ganglion, from malignant growths and described the enlargement of the axillary lymph nodes in association with cancer of the breast.

The better understanding of soft tissue tumors, like that of many other tumors, was held back for centuries by, among other things, misuse and misunderstanding of various names and definitions. For example, etymologically *carcinoma* means "crab-like tumor" (Greek) for which the Latin equivalent is *cancer*; therefore, sarcomas were not regarded as cancers or malignant tumors. Galen's definition of sarcomas as "fleshy excrescence" led to the description of swellings as well as benign tumors as sarcomas or "fungus." Galen (A.D. 130–200) did not entirely neglect surgery, but he considered surgical intervention of secondary value because he believed that most diseases are constitutional and not local affections (Fig. 1-2). The doctrines of Galen were repeated for centuries and celebrated surgeons such as Albucasis of Arabia (A.D. ?–1105) advised: "Refrain from attempting to excise tumors which are of a livid color and of an irregular aspect, for these tumors are cancerous." Arderne (1306–?), celebrated English surgeon of the Hundred Years' War was equally pessimistic. He said, "I have never seen any man who

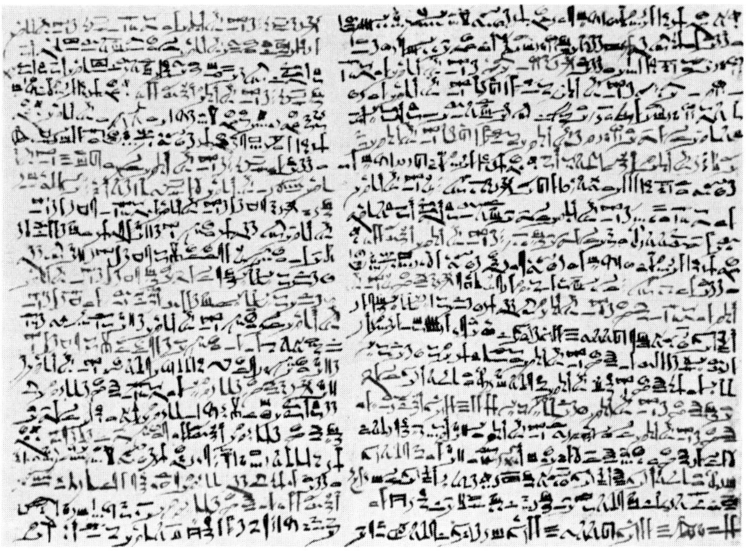

Figure 1-1. *Smith Papyrus,* 2000 B.C. (Courtesy of New York Academy of Medicine Library.)

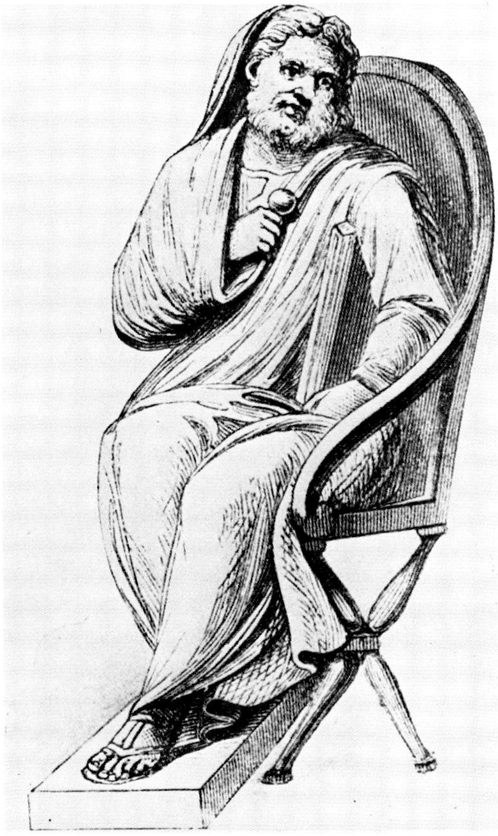

Figure 1-2. Galen (A.D. 130–200).

recovered from cancer but I have known many who died of it and it will only give you disgrace if you operate. There is no cure, and death is at the gate."

A French surgeon, the most eminent authority on surgery in the fourteenth century, Guy de Chauliac (1300–1368), was a man with different views. He believed in excising cancer at an early stage with the knife and recommended, in his book published in 1478 after his death in Lyon, cautery for the fungus (sarcoma) variety.

Soon after the invention of printing by Coster of Haarlem (1440) and Gutenberg of Mainz (1450) the first printed medical book *De Sermonum Proprietate Seu de Universo* written by Rabanus Maurus was published in Strassburg in 1467. It was followed soon by the appearance of the first printed surgical treatise, written by Brunschwig and published in Strassburg in 1497 (Fig. 1-3). From the beginning of the sixteenth century printing was fully utilized to disseminate medical information in the form of text and illustrations. The first picture of an amputation was published by Gersdorff in 1517 (Fig. 1-4).

Progress in medicine was blocked by the lack of knowledge about the composition of the human body. Vesalius (1514–1564), of Brussels, who attended the University of Louvain and Padua, wrote the

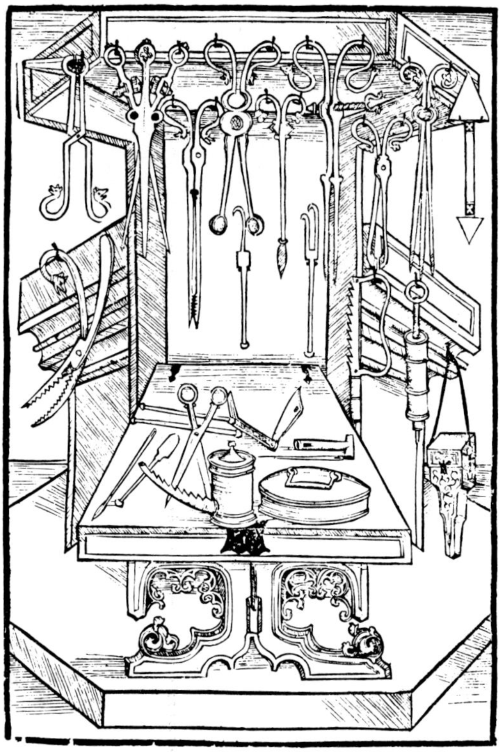

Figure 1-3. Surgical instruments of the 15th century. (From Brunschwig, H.: Dis ist das Buch der Cirurgia Hantwirkckung der Wundartzny von Hyeronimus Brunschwig. Strassburg, Gruninger, 1497.)

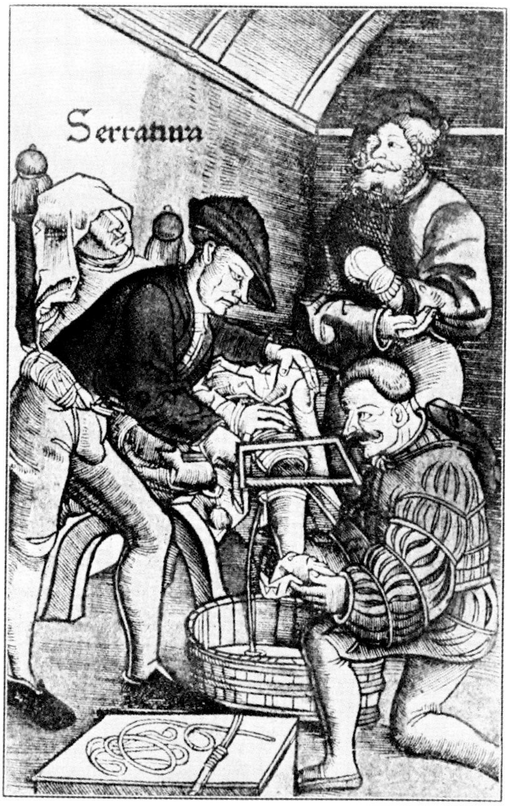

Figure 1-4. The first printed picture of an amputation (From Gersdorff, H.: *Feldtbuch der Wundartzney.* Strassburg, Schott, 1517.

first comprehensive anatomic text, *De Humani Corporis Fabrica* in 1543. The magnificently illustrated work of Vesalius was the greatest event in medical history since the work of Galen. It paved the way for physiologic and morphologic studies and laid the foundation for morbid anatomy (Fig. 1-5).

Fernel (1497–1558) in his *Medicina,* in 1542, called attention to physiology, and was the first to call the subject by that name. He also introduced the term *pathology.* His book went through several editions (Fig. 1-6). He is justly called the first pathologist. He stressed the importance of necropsies and classified diseases as (1) *simple* (when confined to a part of an organ), (2) *compound* (when affecting an entire organ), and (3) *complex* (when affecting a group of organs).

Harvey (1578–1657), one of the greatest names in experimental medicine and the father of modern embryology, published *De Motu Cordis et Sanguinis* in 1628 in which he foresaw the need for microscopic observation (Fig. 1-7). The invention of the microscope opened up a new area for observation. Velsch, in 1670, described brown fat in hibernating animals. Kircher (1602–1680), a Jesuit priest, who was probably the first to employ the microscope in investigating the cause of disease, made unbelievable observations with his primitive microscope, e.g., "every kind of plant is formed of a different and wonderful union of filaments" (Fig. 1-8). Hook (1635–1703) in England published his famous *Micrographia,* in 1665, in which the first illustration of cellular structures and the word *cell* appeared. Malpighi (1628–1694) in his *De Formatione Pulli in Ovo,* in 1673, described the red blood cells. Bartholin (1616–1680) discovered the thoracic duct and the intesti-

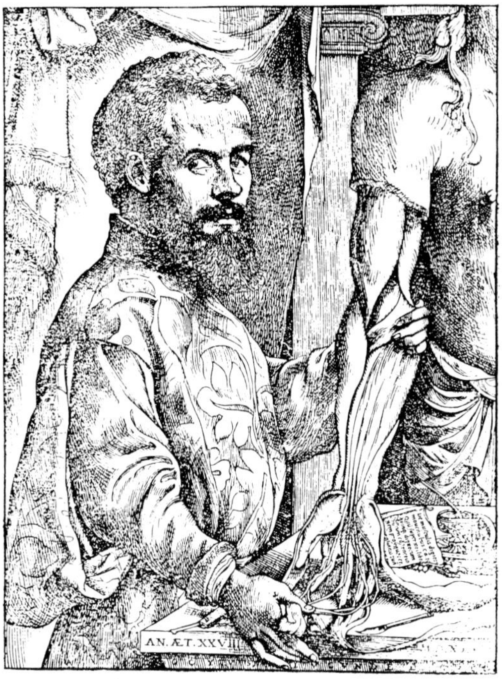

Figure 1-5. Portrait of Vesalius (1514–1564). (From Vesalius, A.: De humani corporis fabrica libri septem. Basileae, I. Oporini, 1543.

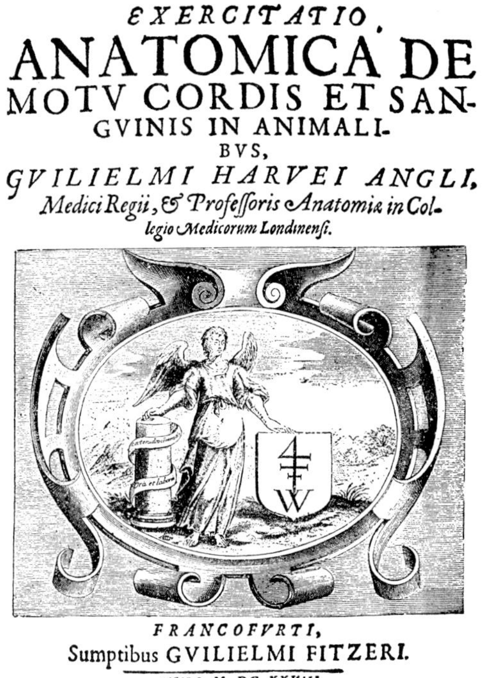

EXERCITATIO
ANATOMICA DE
MOTU CORDIS ET SAN-
GUINIS IN ANIMALI-
BUS,
GUILIELMI HARVEI ANGLI,
*Medici Regii, & Professoris Anatomiæ in Col-
legio Medicorum Londinensi.*

FRANCOFVRTI,
Sumptibus GVILIELMI FITZERI.
ANNO M. DC. XXVIII.

Figure 1-7. Title page of Harvey's *De Motu Cordis et Sanguinis.*

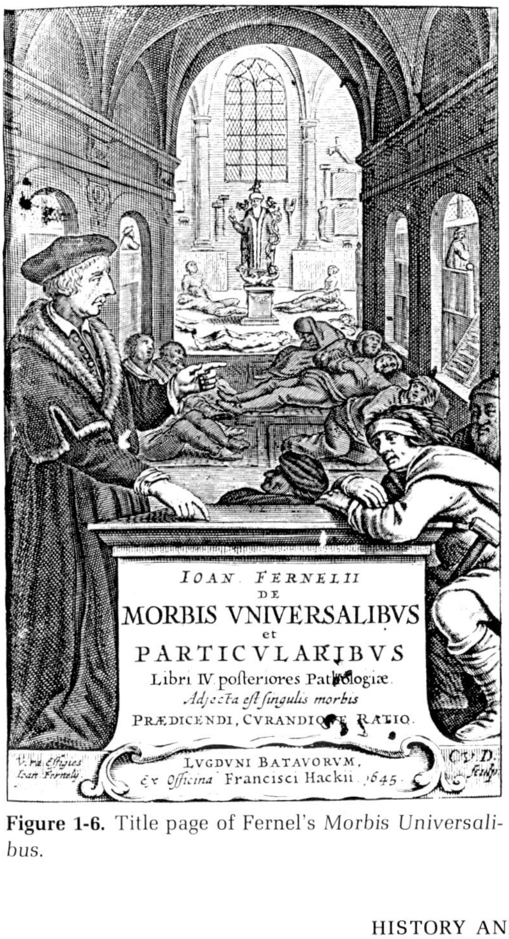

IOAN. FERNELII
DE
MORBIS VNIVERSALIBVS
et
PARTICVLARIBVS
Libri IV posteriores Pathologiæ.
Adjecta est singulis morbis
PRÆDICENDI, CVRANDIQVE RATIO.
LVGDVNI BATAVORVM,
Ex Officina Francisci Hackii, 1645.

Figure 1-6. Title page of Fernel's *Morbis Universalibus.*

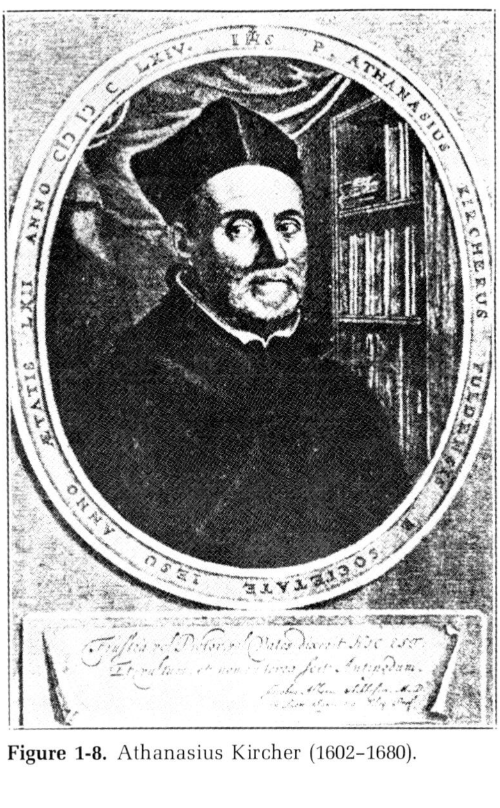

Figure 1-8. Athanasius Kircher (1602–1680).

nal lymphatics, and his book on this subject was published in 1653 (Fig. 1-9).

Sculteti (1595–1645), one of the greatest illustrators of surgical procedures, showed the way to remove cancerous organs. Gendron, in 1701, pleaded in a text devoted to cancers "for use of the knife rather than nostrums." Boneti, in 1700, described a tumor he called "osteoma of the mammary gland." The best illustrations of English surgery of the seventeenth century are found in the *Diary of the Rev. John Ward Extending from 1648 to 1679,* which was published in 1839 and also contained a recommendation to treat torticollis: "cut wry neck, cut three tendons."

Leeuwenhoek (1632–1723) began to publish his letters on microscopic observations in the world-renowned *Philosophical Transactions.* Among other things he is credited with the microscopic description of the striation of voluntary muscle, the sarcolemma, and epithelial cells which he scraped off the trunk of an elephant (Fig. 1-10).

The third edition of *Etmullerus'* book (Fig. 1-11A), published in 1712, contains the first published classification of tumors (Fig. 1-11B), the first reference to the use of the microscope in the diagnosis of disease (Fig. 1-11C), and a list of recommended remedies for the cure of tumors (Fig. 1-11D). Etmullerus explained the formation of tumors by saying, "If the thinner humors force their passage, while thick viscous excrements stick by the way, they gather into a body by degrees, and so cause tumours." On the other hand, his assessment of synovial lesions is fairly accurate: "Sometimes we meet with spongy swellings about the joints, that proceed from the nutritious juice of the membranes mixed with the glutinous matter that bedews the joints and are for the most part very dangerous, by reason of their tendency to cancers."

Helvetius, one of the best known therapists of the time, received 20,000 francs from Louis XIV to publish his secret remedies, including the ones for cure of cancer. They appeared in print in 1731.

Freke, in 1740, described myositis ossificans; Peyronie, in 1743, studied penile fibromatosis; Hody, in 1747, illustrated uterine leiomyoma; and Bonn, in 1763, described the synovial membrane. Despite such original observations, in 1740, de Superville stated, "It is still a dispute, whether the male or the female contributes most towards generation."

Cheselden, in 1741, in the sixth edition of his anatomy book illustrated the feasibility of scapulohumeral amputation and disarticulation (Fig. 1-12). Middletown, in 1769, published the first American contribution to medical history. He and Bard are also known for performing the first autopsy in America for the purpose of

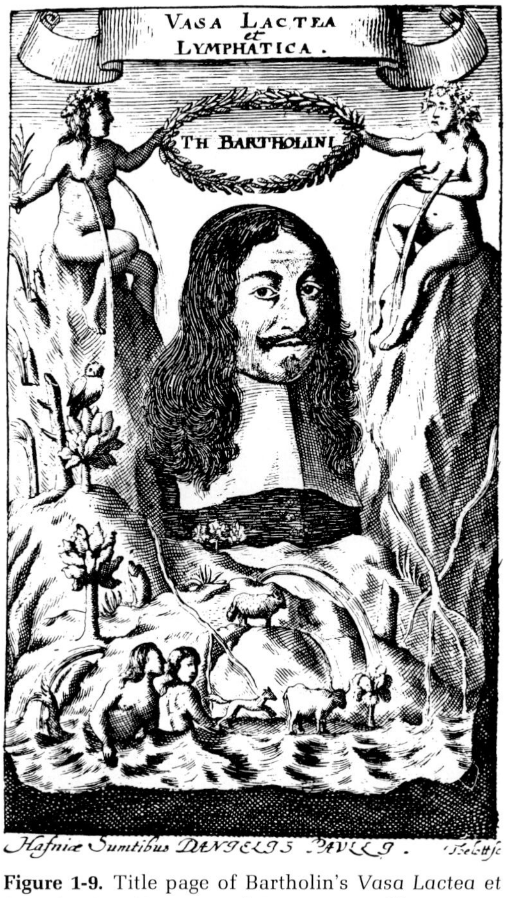

Figure 1-9. Title page of Bartholin's *Vasa Lactea et Lymphatica.* (Courtesy of Dr. J. Rygaard.)

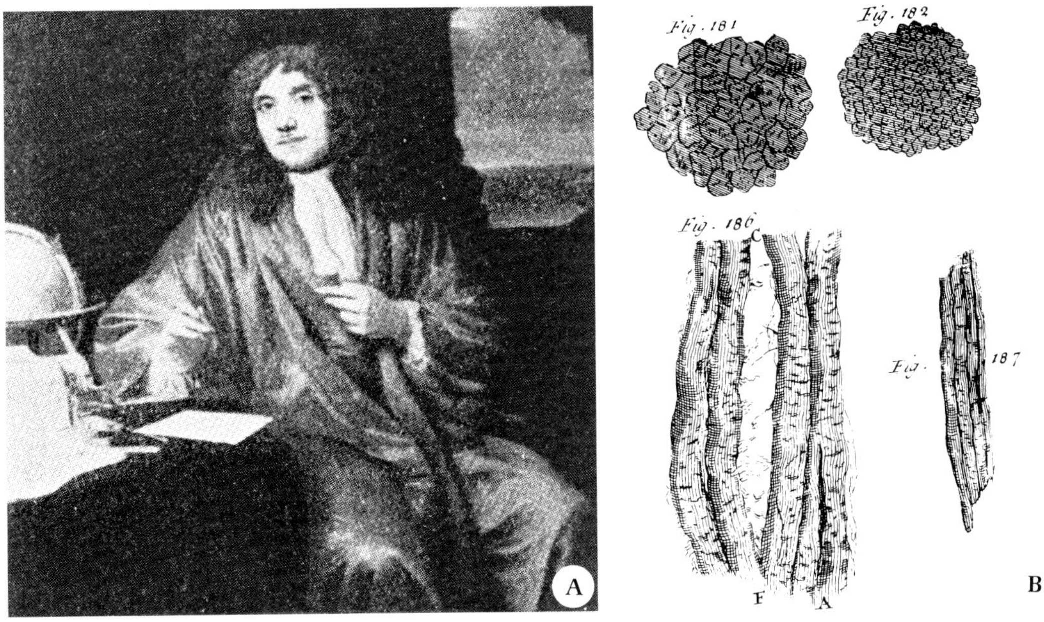

Figure 1-10. **A,** Antonj van Leeuwenhoek (1632–1723). **B,** Leeuwenhoek's illustration of striated muscle. (From Philos. Trans. London, 5:422, 1721.)

Etmullerus Abridg'd :
O R,
A Compleat Syſtem of the Theory and Practice of Phyſic.
BEING A
DESCRIPTION
OF
All Diſeaſes Incident to Men, Women and Children.
WITH
An Account of their *Cauſes*, *Symptoms*, and moſt approved Methods of *Cure*, both *PHYSICAL* and *CHIRURGICAL*.
To which is prefix'd a ſhort View of the Animal and Vital Functions; and the ſeveral Virtues and Claſſes of Medicines.
Tranſlated from the laſt Edition of the Works of *MICHAEL ETMULLERUS*, late Profeſſor of Phyſic in the Univerſity of *Lipſic*.
A BOOK very proper for Families.
The Third Edition, Corrected and much Improv'd.
LONDON:
Printed for *Andrew Bell* at the *Croſs Keys* and *Bible* in *Cornhill*, near *Stocks-Market*; and *Richard Wellington*, at the *Dolphin* and *Crown*, at the Weſt end of St. *Paul's* Church-yard 1712.

A

The general Doctrine of Tumours being thus premis'd, we proceed to the Deſcription of particular Swellings, which we draw up in four Heads. 1. Thoſe that proceed from the Stagnation of Blood. 2. Such as are Critical. 3. Such as ariſe from the Depravation of the Lymph; and 4. Thoſe which relate to the Blood-Veſſels.

B

Having diſpatch'd the general Cure of Ulcers, we ſhall now deſcend to a few Particulars; as, 1. The Ulcers that are attended by a *Caries*, or Rottenneſs of the Bones, which muſt be particularly accounted for before the Ulcer can be cur'd. When a *Caries* begins, the Bone appears fat, oily, and yellowiſh; and when it is perfectly rotten, it becomes black, uneven, and full of little Holes. If the Bone be not expos'd to one's view, either by the naked Eye, or thro' a Microſcope, its Roughneſs and little Pits are diſcover'd by a Probe. If a *Caries* approach to the Joints, or be ſurrounded by many nervous Parts, 'tis not eaſily cur'd. How-

C

5. Cancrous Ulcers. Their Cauſes and Symptoms are accounted for in the Chapter of *Tumours*. As for their Cure; let the Dung of a Cat fed with River-crabs, or the Pouder of a Toad and a Lizard calcin'd together in a new cloſe Veſſel, or mix'd with black Pepper, Salt, dry Soot, and Orpine, be ſprinkl'd upon the Ulcer after 'tis waſh'd with Plantain-water. If theſe prove ſucceſsleſs, apply the Oil of Mans-dung; and for the laſt Refuge Arſenic fix'd with Nitre, and mix'd with Soot and *Rulandus's* Balſam of Sulphur in the form of an Ointment; or the Oil *per deliquium* of the Arſenic thus fix'd, it being dulcify'd with Spirit of Wine. If the Cancer ſtill continue after theſe Applications, 'twill be needful to cut it off, and then burn out its Roots with a hot Iron; for if the leaſt Particle of the Ferment be left, 'twill revive again. *Alliot*

D

Figure 1-11. **A,** Title page of Etmullerus' book. **B,** Classification of tumors by Etmullerus. **C,** Recommendation to use the microscope by Etmullerus. **D,** A summary of "chemotherapy" printed in Etmullerus' book.

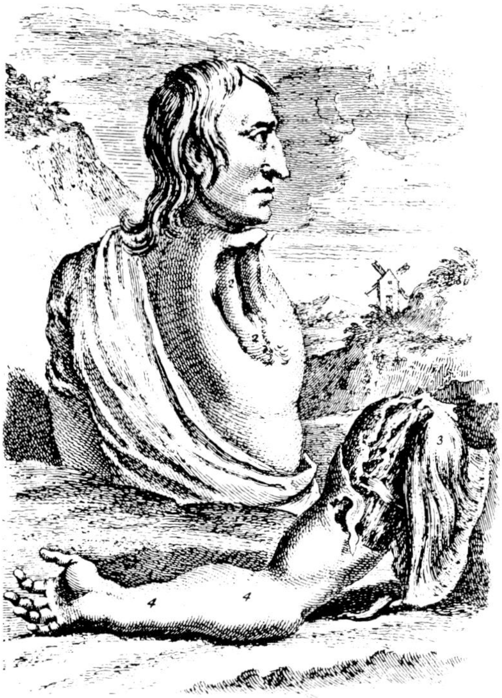

Figure 1-12. Illustration of a "spontaneous scapulohumeral amputation" by the wheel of a windmill (From Cheselden, W.: *The Anatomy of the Human Body,* 6th edition. Londres, Bowyer, 1741).

acquiring medical knowledge. It took place in New York City in 1750.

Peyrilhe, in 1773, was awarded the first prize of the Academy of Science of Lyon for his dissertation on the nature, causes, effects, and better treatment of cancer. His study, which was published in Paris, in 1776, is regarded as the first comprehensive work on cancer. After reviewing published works on cancer, he said that cancer is classified as (1) perfect scirrhous, (2) imperfect scirrhous, (3) benign, (4) malignant, (5) vascular, (6) lymphatic, and (7) occult. Peyrilhe is best known for his injection of a cell suspension of human mammary carcinoma into a dog, but he discontinued the experiment because of his housekeeper's objections.

Bell's book published in Boston in 1791 contained a detailed account on the nature and treatment of ulcers and joint diseases. Unfortunately, microscopists and their discoveries were often ignored and ridiculed like Hooke in Shadwell's *Virtuoso*. In 1784, Weikard, physician to Catherine of Russia, exemplified the cynical views of the eighteenth century physicians. He said, "We kill so much time with such unnecessary literature. As a matter of fact, I have mistrusted much in the deluge of German periodicals. I did not believe in the English, Swedish or Dutch journals. The Viennese I trusted even less; of the French, I believed not a word."

The microscope was not appreciated as a valuable instrument by such giants in morbid anatomy as Morgagni (1682–1771) and Baillie (1761–1823) (Figs. 1-13, 1-14). Morgagni's book, published in 1761, and Baillie's book, whose first edition was published in London in 1793, were the first texts treating pathology as an entity. However, the first atlas in pathology, written by Baillie and published in 1799 as a supplement to his book, contains not even one microscopic picture among more than 100 beautifully executed engravings. He is credited with a number of first observations, including the description of metastatic osteogenic sarcoma. Baillie was a morbid anatomist in the classic sense. He believed as Rokitansky did that "pathology constitutes the groundwork of all

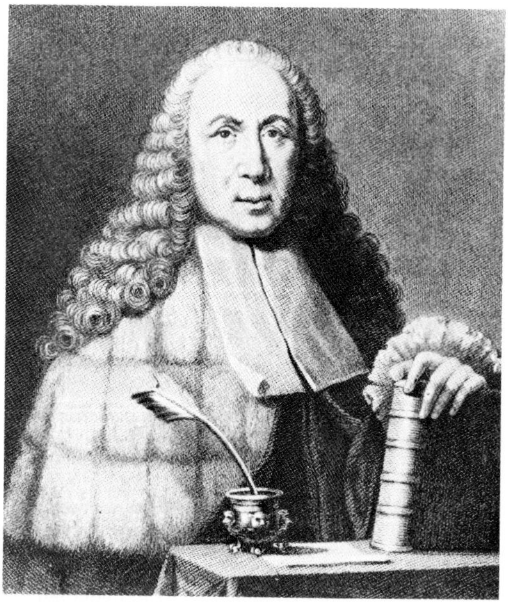

Figure 1-13. Giovanni Battista Morgagni (1682–1771).

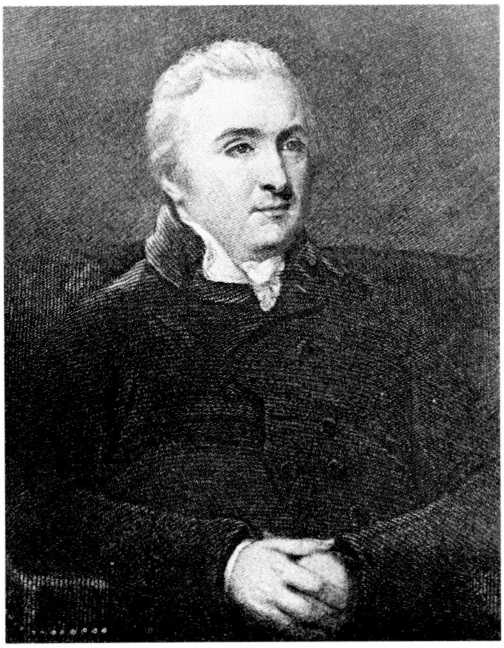

Figure 1-14. Matthew Baillie (1761–1823).

medical knowledge." He said with foresight, "The knowledge of morbid structure does not lead with certainty to the knowledge of morbid actions, although the one is the effect of the other. Yet surely it lays the most solid foundation for prosecuting such enquiries with success. In proportion, therefore, as we shall become acquainted with the changes produced in the structure of parts from diseased actions, we shall be more likely to make some progress toward a knowledge of the actions themselves, although it must be very slowly."

Hunter (1728–1793), the famous English surgeon, believed that a disposition to cancer exists in the surrounding tissues prior to the actual occurrence of the tumor. He proposed that "a surgeon ought not to be contented with removing merely the indurated or actually diseased part, but that he should also take away some portion of the surrounding substance, in which a diseased disproportion may probably have been excited." This is the first recommendation that cancer should not be violated and should be removed with clean surgical margins.

Oncology owes many things to Abernethy (1780–1848), a pupil of Hunter and a leading surgeon in London. He was the first to point out, in *Surgical Observations,* in 1809, the great differences between tumors, which are merely accumulation of blood, pus, or other fluids and should not be considered tumors, and true adventitious new formations. He also suggested that tumors should be named according to their anatomic structure and offered the first classification of sarcomas (Table 1-1). He is credited with the first description of "osseous tumors unconnected with bone or periosteum" and described "fatty tumors growing at the same time in different parts of the body of the same person."

The advent of Bichat (1771–1802) marks the beginning of histology. He introduced the term *tissue* and was able to distinguish 21 different forms of tissues. According to him, "The filament (or cell) is the elementary solid. A fiber (or tissue) consists of a number of filaments (cells) united together; an organ is a compound of several tissues." In his short life he revolutionized morbid anatomy by demonstrating that not only whole organs can be diseased, as Morgagni and Baillie believed, but also individual tissues can be separately affected.

The term *soft cancer* was introduced by Wardrop (1782–1869) an Edinburgh surgeon and ophthalmologist, who studied in Vienna after he escaped from France, in 1803, when Napoleon ordered that English residents in France be arrested. However, full credit for calling

TABLE 1-1. ***Classification of Sarcomas According to Abernethy, in 1811***

Common vascular, or organized sarcoma
Adipose sarcoma
Pancreatic sarcoma
Cystic sarcoma
Mammary sarcoma
Tuberculated sarcoma
Pulpy or medullary sarcoma
Carcinomatous sarcoma

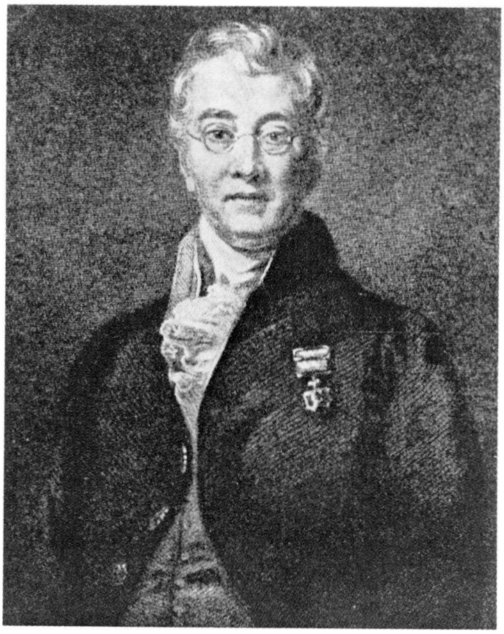

Figure 1-15. Charles Bell (1774–1842).

attention to characteristic features which distinguish "soft cancers" from carcinoma must be given to Bell (1774–1842) (Fig. 1-15), a leading British anatomist who is better known for his contributions to neurophysiology than to soft tissue tumors (Fig. 1-16).

THE PERIOD OF CELLULAR PATHOLOGY

(From J. Müller to P. Ehrlich)

During the first half of the nineteenth century a number of important discoveries took place. Burns, in 1811, described chloroma, at autopsy of a young man. Tumor nodules were found in the lacrimal gland, orbits, skull, and meninges. King, in 1853, gave the name *chloroma* to the neoplasm because of the green color. Cruveilhier and Wilks, in 1859, independently described synovial chondromatosis. In 1832, Dupuytren reported plantar and palmar fibromatosis and McFarlane reported the first case of an abdominal tumor believed now to have been a desmoid tumor. The term *desmoid* was coined later, in 1838, by J. Müller. Stafford, in 1839, reported the first case of rhabdomyosarcoma in a child's prostate. Mohr, in 1840, described "Fröhlich's syndrome" 61 years before Fröhlich. Zappoli, in 1843, coined the name *liposarcoma* and reported a case with illustration (Fig. 1-17). Van Leuw, in 1845, reported a case of macroglossia due, almost certainly, to rhabdomyoma. In 1849, Robin described multinucleated giant cells, or myeloplaxes, in bone marrow and Smith recorded the first cases of multiple cutaneous neuromas, but it was Odier, in 1803, who coined the term *neurom*. Alibert (1768–1837), a prolific writer, first described mycosis fungoides, illustrated a congenital hemangioma in 1806 (Fig. 1-18), and gave the first accurate description of keloid in 1816.

Bichat's "cellular tissue" concept was upheld by Oken (1779–1851), who suggested, in 1805, "All organisms originate from and consist of cells" and the great German comparative anatomist Meckel (1781–1833) who concluded, in 1824, that "the globules (cells) differ in shape, size, and number in different animals and in different parts of the same animal." Donne, in 1836, and Turpin, in 1838, described human cells and their organization into tissue. Hence, the formal announcement of the "cell theory" by Schwann and Schleiden, in 1838, was somewhat of an anticlimax. As a fact, Schwann in his book, in 1839, mentioned that Turpin, in 1837, confirmed the original observation of Donne who said in reference to vaginal epithelium, "Un tissu cellulaire bien organise et compose, comme tous les tissues cellulaires vegetaux." Incidentally, in the same volume Schwann described the nerve sheath that later was named after him.

The cellular tissue concept was advanced and applied in pathology by three French pathologists—Andral (1797–1876), Lebert (1813–1878), and Cruveilhier (1791–1874)—and a German one, Müller (1801–1858). Andral recognized (1829) several

SURGICAL OBSERVATIONS;

BEING A

Quarterly Report

OF

CASES IN SURGERY;

TREATED

IN THE MIDDLESEX HOSPITAL,

IN THE CANCER ESTABLISHMENT,

AND

IN PRIVATE PRACTICE:

EMBRACING

AN ACCOUNT OF THE ANATOMICAL AND PATHOLOGICAL RESEARCHES

IN THE

SCHOOL OF WINDMILL STREET.

BY

CHARLES BELL.

London:

PRINTED FOR LONGMAN, HURST, REES, ORME, AND BROWN,
PATERNOSTER-ROW.

1816.

A

STRUCTURE OF THE SOFT CANCER.

Soft cancer may attack any of the structures of the body. We find it here arising in the bone after bruise or fracture. If it do not arise in the muscles, it very readily attaches to them, and is propagated through their substance, and it certainly arises in the soft substance of the limbs. It often commences in the lymphatic glands, as in the first case, in those of the groin. It attaches to them also in a secondary way, and yet not always in the course of the lymph. For example: the disease of the testicle will be succeeded by the affection of the popliteal glands, as in the seventh case. Of the internal parts, its most frequent seat is in the liver. It affects the lungs also. I have an example of this disease in the eye, and then it readily communicates to the brain. In the eighth case there is an example of this disease in the popliteal nerve; and hereafter we shall have examples of it in the mamma.

In its structure, this tumour has some slight resemblance to the carcinoma; but at the same time there is something which distinguishes it from that disease, and from all other diseased structures.

The soft cancer, which has burst into full maturity, exhibits two distinct portions. The central

B

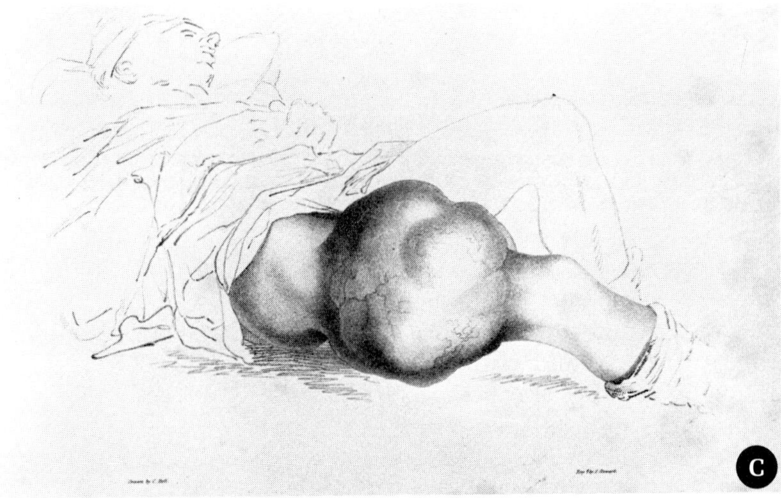

Figure 1-16. A, Title page of Bell's book which contains the first description (B) and illustration (C) of "soft cancer."

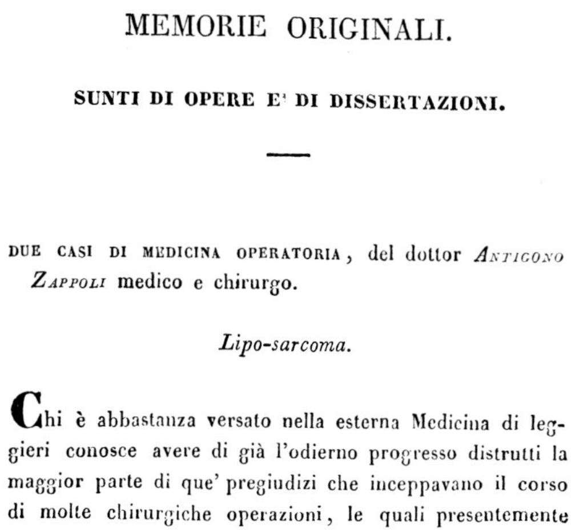
MEMORIE ORIGINALI.

SUNTI DI OPERE E' DI DISSERTAZIONI.

DUE CASI DI MEDICINA OPERATORIA, del dottor *Antigono Zappoli* medico e chirurgo.

Lipo-sarcoma.

Chi è abbastanza versato nella esterna Medicina di leggieri conosce avere di già l'odierno progresso distrutti la maggior parte di que' pregiudizi che inceppavano il corso di molte chirurgiche operazioni, le quali presentemente

A

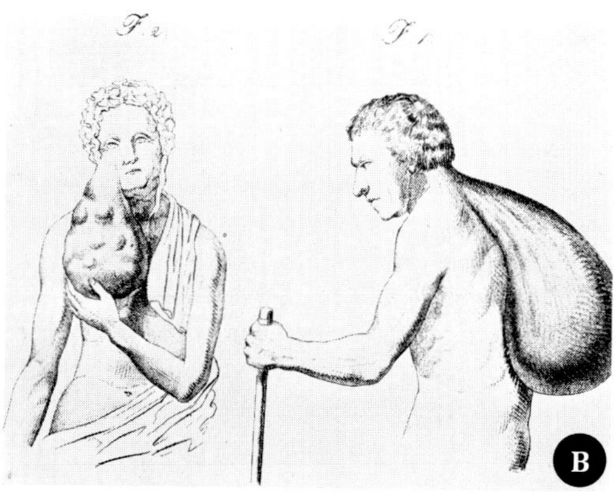

Figure 1-17. A, Article written by A. Zappoli on liposarcoma. (From Bull. Sci. Med. Bologna 3:5, 1843.) **B,** Illustration of liposarcoma from the same article, page 14.

forms of anemia and invented the term *anemia.*

Cooper (1836) and Müller (1838) agreed in principal on the classification of sarcomas. Both held the view that a sarcomatous tumour is one that is chiefly or entirely composed of a fatty, fibrous, medullary, fungous, or other substance of inferior hardness to bone; and both felt that "some kinds of sarcoma are merely new formations, unconnected with any malignant tendency." The direct application of this view led J. Müller, in 1838, to create the term *cystosarcoma phyllodes,* meaning benign tumor of the breast.

Müller realized the necessity of the cell theory for the understanding of the nature and forms of cancer. In his book, published in 1838, he illustrated cells with nuclei and nucleoli (Fig. 1-19). He described and illustrated straightened or serpentine, ramified striae, interlaced to form a mesh or network composed of a substance he called *reticulum.* He laid the foundation for the current nomenclature of tumors and proposed that "the structural elements of every tumor have their analogues in the embryonic or adult tissues of the normal organism." Müller and his students, Schwann, Virchow, Henle, Wagner, Volkmann, Vierordt, Kolliker, Remak, Lieberkuhn, and many others less illustrious, all turned to experimentation when they were unable to explain what they had seen.

Rokitansky (1804–1878) ranks with Morgagni and Baillie as a gross pathologist (Fig. 1-20). The last volume of his book, *Handbuch der pathologischen Anatomie,* published in 1846, included contemporary theories on sarcomas. He wrote, "Sarcomata represent benign new growths. They are always purely local affections. They are curable by complete extirpation; that is, they do not recur at the same spot, and still less do they multiply in other localities," but he added that

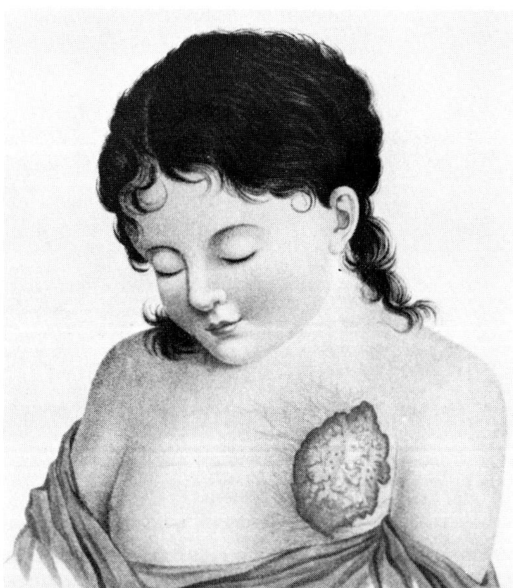

Figure 1-18. Congenital hemangioma, illustrated by Alibert, in 1806.

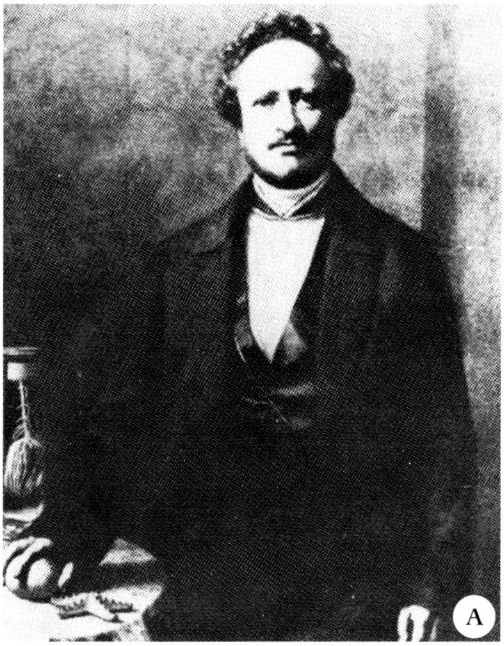

A

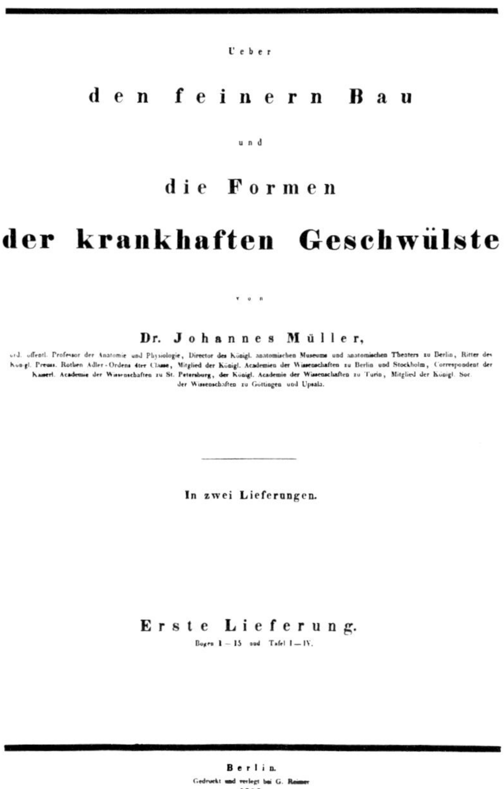

Ueber

den feinern Bau

und

die Formen

der krankhaften Geschwülste

von

Dr. Johannes Müller,

ord. öffentl. Professor der Anatomie und Physiologie, Director des Königl. anatomischen Museums und anatomischen Theaters zu Berlin, Ritter des Königl. Preuss. Rothen Adler-Ordens 4ter Classe, Mitglied der Königl. Academien der Wissenschaften zu Berlin und Stockholm, Correspondent der Kaiserl. Academie der Wissenschaften zu St. Petersburg, der Königl. Academie der Wissenschaften zu Turin, Mitglied der Königl. Soc. der Wissenschaften zu Göttingen und Upsala.

In zwei Lieferungen.

Erste Lieferung.

Bogen 1 – 15 und Tafel I – IV.

Berlin.

Gedruckt und verlegt bei G. Reimer

1838.

B

Figure 1-19. **A,** Johannes Muller (1801–1858). **B,** Title page of J. Muller's book, published in 1838.

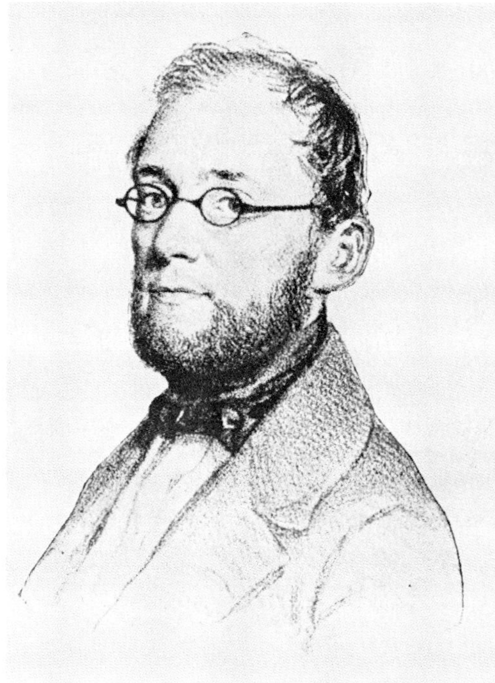

Figure 1-20. Carl Rokitansky (1804–1878).

"we should distinguish two groups of new growths, innocent and malignant. I have selected the term *sarcoma* to designate the innocent growths, the malignant should be called according to their ancient description cancer or carcinoma."

It is difficult to understand how Rokitansky reached the foregoing conclusion when he knew so much about sarcomas that he classified them into four categories (Table 1-2), and said that there are "varieties of fibrous sarcoma, dependent upon the form and arrangement of the fibers." He also knew that "sarcomata affect the areolar tissue, the fibrous membranes, the muscles, inter-muscular tissues, submucous muscular textures, the bones, glandular organs, the mammary, the parotid glands, even the testicle; and in rare in-

TABLE 1-2. ***Classification of Sarcomas by Rokitansky in 1842***

I. Gelatinous sarcoma
II. Albumino-fibrous tumor: fibrous sarcoma
III. Albumen-like fibrous tumor
IV. Cystosarcoma

stances, the brain." He pointed out that "primary cancer may be developed at the peripheral extremity of a nerve, or at any other spot in its course, up to its termination in the nervous centre." He knew that lipoma is composed of fat and he described steatopygia. He described "ganglia" as a collection of serum in synovial sacs and called loose bodies "articular mice."

Henle, a favorite student of Müller, demonstrated in 1840 the existence of smooth muscle in the walls of small arteries. In 1846, another pupil of the great Viennese descriptive pathologist, Kolliker showed that each involuntary muscle is made up of small, spindle-shaped cells.

Lebert, one of the most skillful microscopists of his time, published his *Physiologie Pathologique,* in 1845 (Fig. 1-21). The third volume of this three-volume work is a microscopic atlas of pathology and contains more than 250 illustrations, including several on non-epithelial tumors. Lebert introduced the term *xanthoma* and described "cicatricial neuroma." After his book was published, he was asked how he felt as a pathologist. He said, "I was an exceedingly humble pathologist, and I am now even more humble as a result of the lessons that I have learned." He emphasized that "it is important to examine every pathology specimen under the microscope." In his advice to students in microscopy he reminded them of Pythagoras who required from his students five years of silence before they were permitted to teach his doctrines, and added, "Every observer is his own teacher, in microscopy just like anything else, the most important things are common sense, perseverance and sound judgment." He advised his students not to be afraid to explore unknown territories and to use new techniques, but he warned them that "there are critics of every new technique."

PHYSIOLOGIE

PATHOLOGIQUE

RECHERCHES

CLINIQUES, EXPERIMENTALES ET MICROSCOPIQUES

SUR L'INFLAMMATION, LA TUBERCULISATION, LES TUMEURS, LA FORMATION DU CAL, ETC.

PAR H. LEBERT,

Docteur en médecine et en chirurgie, médecin à Lavey canton de Vaud, en Suisse, Membre titulaire de la Société helvétique d'histoire naturelle, de la Société médicale et de celle d'histoire naturelle de Lausanne, de la Société médicale allemande de Paris, Membre correspondant de la Société philomathique et de la Société anatomique de Paris, de la Société médicale de Genève et de la Société médicale d'émulation de Lyon.

ATLAS DE VINGT-DEUX PLANCHES.

A PARIS,

CHEZ J.-B. BAILLIÈRE,

LIBRAIRE DE L'ACADÉMIE ROYALE DE MÉDECINE.

RUE DE L'ÉCOLE-DE-MÉDECINE, Nº 17.

A LONDRES, CHEZ H. BAILLIÈRE, 219, REGENT-STREET

1845.

Figure 1-21. Title page of Lebert's pathology text, published in 1845.

Bennett (1812–1875), a pupil of Donne, a man regarded by many as the greatest British cellular pathologist, introduced microscopy into England and published his famous treatise *On Cancerous and Cancroid Growths* in 1849 (Fig. 1-22). Bennett denied that cancer was necessarily fatal and said that "cancer is dependent for its power of growth, extension and redevelopment on the cells it contains."

In 1852, Broca published his *Anatomie pathologie du cancer,* and Chassaignac gave the first description of villonodular synovitis. Michon, in 1851, wrote a text on synovial tumors. In 1854, Guersant reported the first case of botryoid sarcoma of the vagina in a young girl and Weber first used the term *rhabdomyosarcoma* in describing a lesion of the tongue. Paget, in 1856, reported the first case of extra-abdominal desmoid tumor and concluded that "tumors seem all purposeless or hurtful."

Virchow (1821–1902), who systematized the works of his predecessors perhaps was

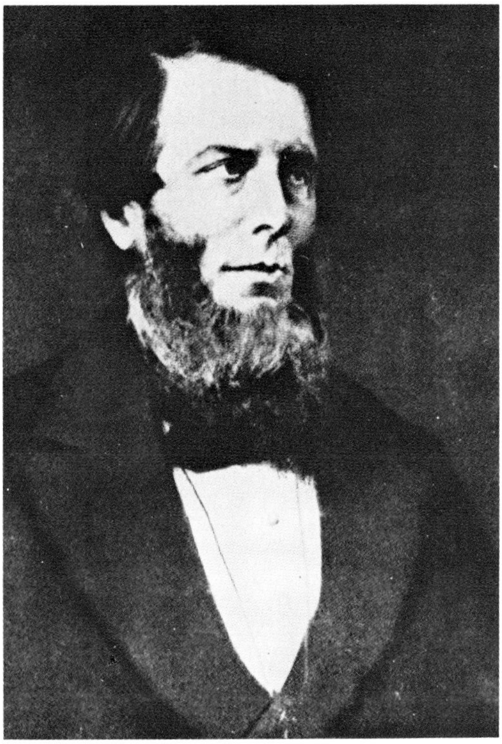

Figure 1-22. John H. Bennett (1812–1875).

not unjustly accused of plagiarizing the thoughts of others and presenting them as his own. In his two books—*Die Cellularpathologie . . .* and *Die krankhaften Geschwülste*, published in 1858 and 1863, respectively—he attempted to explain the appearance of pathologic tissues by theorizing that what he called connective tissue is capable of producing epithelial as well as mesenchymal cells under the influence of morbid excitations (Fig. 1-23). Making such an error did not prevent him from giving the most succinct definition of sarcomas. According to him, sarcomas are "new formation of the connective tissue and are distinguishable from the corresponding fully evolved tissue by their immaturity." Virchow's contribution to pathology is diversified and immense and ranged from the introduction of new terms such as *leukemia* and *myxoma* to *histogenesis*. He felt, for example, that osteoblasts and chondroblasts merely represent modified, differentiated fibroblasts. Later in his life when he was asked to define tumors he said, "No human being can define, even under torture, exactly what a tumor is." As he mellowed he also advised, "Science is large enough to accommodate every worker in its field who does not pretend that his contribution is of exclusive value."

Wilks (1824–1911) discussed tumors in his book published in 1859. He wrote, "In most of the softer structures of the body the main constituents of tumor deposits are cells and fibers of various forms and combinations: the purely cellular structure being analogous to cancer, and malignant; while the fibrous shows a tendency to be less malignant." He divided tumors into three categories: innocent, semimalignant, and malignant (Table 1-3).

Also, in 1859, Delameter's report on the largest lipoma was published in the *Cleveland Medical Gazette* (Fig. 1-24) and Gross' great book *A System of Surgery . . .* was published by H. C. Lea of Philadelphia (Fig. 1-25). Gross was a prolific writer and student of medical history. He wrote the first comprehensive American treatise on pathologic anatomy (*Elements of Pathologic Anatomy*, Boston,

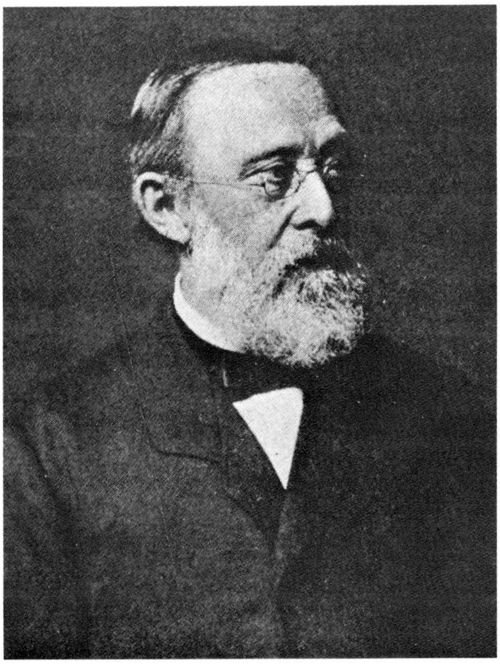

Figure 1-23. Rudolf Virchow (1821–1902).

TABLE 1-3. *Classification of New Growths, According to Wilks in 1859*

SITE	CHARACTER		
	INNOCENT	SEMIMALIGNANT	MALIGNANT
Mamma	Adenocele Cystosarcoma	Fibroplastic, recurrent, or fibroid	Cancer: scirrhous, medullary, colloid
Uterus and prostate	Muscular	Fibroplastic, recurrent, or fibroid	Cancer: scirrhous, medullary, colloid
Epithelial surface	Warts or papilloma	Epithelioma	Epithelioma
Hollow organs	Villous disease	Epithelioma	Epithelioma
Pigment	Melanosis	Epithelioma	Epithelioma
Vessels	Teleangiectasis	Epithelioma	Epithelioma
Bone	Exostosis Enchondroma Myeloid	Osteosarcoma	Osteoid cancer

1839) and published a number of biographies, including ones on Hunter, Richter, and Paré. He gave a concise tabulation of tumors based on teachings of German and American schools. His comparative description of encephaloid and scirrhous tumors is a medical classic. It is the first comparative study of sarcomas and carcinomas. By his own admission, "Encephaloid has various synonyms of which the most common are soft cancer, medullary sarcoma, cerebriform cancer, and fungus hematodes." On the other hand, "The term scirrhous is employed to designate a morbid product which is more dense and firm than any of the natural tissues, excepting tendon, cartilage and bone." He was a skillful surgeon, as well as a microscopist, and was the first to recover cancer cells, presumably endometrial in origin, from vaginal discharge (Table 1-4).

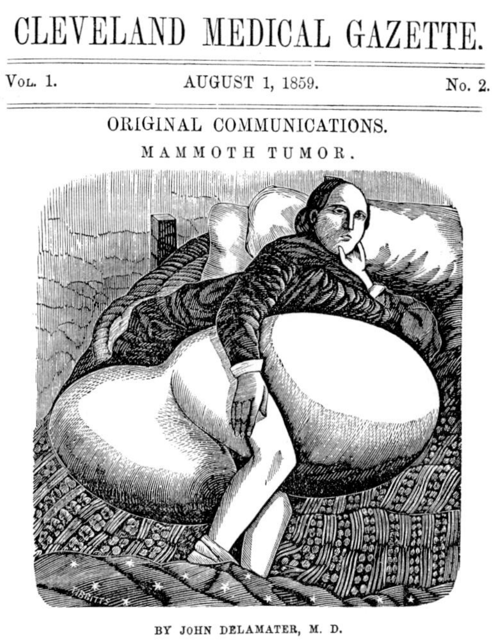

Figure 1-24. The largest lipoma reported in 1859.

During the 1860's a number of important firsts occurred. Broca described giant cell tumor of the tendon sheath, Moore wrote a book on precancerous lesions, Siman reported a synovial sarcoma, Thiersch disproved Virchow's theory of the connective tissue origin of all cancer, Neuman reported a paratesticular "myoma," known today as paratesticular embryonal rhabdomyosarcoma, Aufrecht described a case of leiomyosarcoma of the saphenous vein, Heller reported on "multiple neurome," and Munchmeyer coined the term *myositis ossificans*.

Malhéné, in 1866, wrote the first monograph on fibrous tumors (Fig. 1-26). He wrote that fibroplastic tumors are more common in soft tissues than in bone and affect most commonly, in order of frequency, the upper and lower extremities and the trunk. He classified his so-called

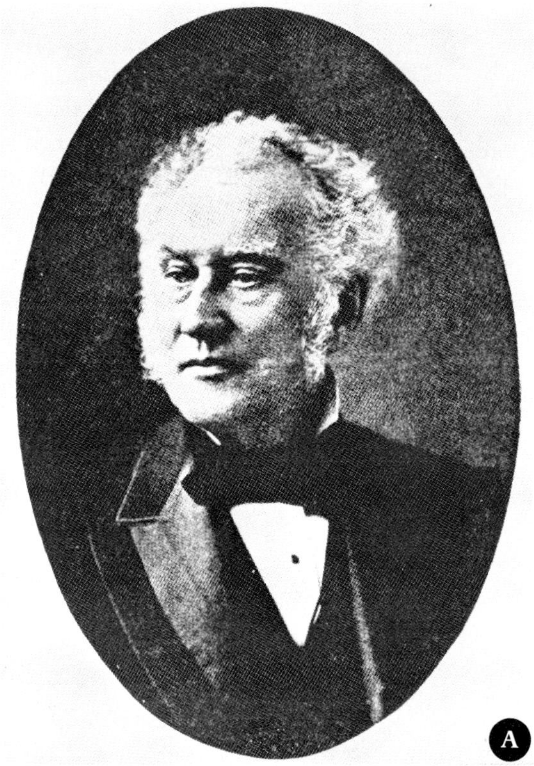

A

ENCEPHALOID.	SCIRRHUS.
1. The tumor is soft and elastic, not uniformly, but more so at some points than at others.	1. Uniformly hard and inelastic, feeling like a marble beneath the skin.
2. It grows rapidly and soon acquires a large bulk, perhaps ultimately attaining the volume of an adult's head.	2. Growth is slow, and bulk comparatively small; the tumor rarely, even in the worst cases, exceeding the volume of a double fist.
3. The pain is slight, and erratic, until ulceration begins, when it becomes more severe and fixed.	3. The pain begins early, is distinctly localized, and is of a sharp, darting, burning, or lancinating character.
4. There is always marked enlargement of the subcutaneous veins.	4. In scirrhus these vessels retain their natural size, or are only slightly enlarged.
5. The ulcer is foul and fungous, with thin, undermined, and livid edges, and is subject to frequent and copious hemorrhage.	5. The ulcer is incrusted with spoiled lymph, and has steep, abrupt edges, looking as if it had been scooped out of the part; bleeding little, and seldom.
6. There is generally early lymphatic involvement.	6. Usually not until late, or just before ulceration is about to occur.
7. Occurs at all periods of life.	7. Seldom before the age of forty-five.
8. Is most frequent in the eye, testicle, mamma, lymphatic ganglions, bones, skin, and cellular tissue.	8. Never occurs in the eye and testicle, and rarely in the bones, skin, and lymphatic ganglions.
9. The disease usually terminates fatally in from nine to twelve months.	9. Seldom sooner than eighteen months or two years.

B

Figure 1-25. **A**, Samuel D. Gross (1805–1884), a native of Easton, Pennsylvania. **B**, Gross' comparative description of "sarcoma" and "carcinoma" in the fourth edition of his book, *A System of Surgery*, H. C. Lea, Philadelphia, 1866.

TABLE 1-4. ***Classification of Tumors by Gross, 1859***

I. BENIGN TUMORS
- Hypertrophic tumors
- Vascular tumors
- Fatty tumors
- Horny tumors
- Fibrous tumors
- Cartilaginous tumors
- Osseous tumors
- Calcareous tumors
- Neuromatous tumors
- Encysted tumors
- Hydatic tumors
- Polypoid tumors
- Myeloid tumors

II. MALIGNANT TUMORS
- Scirrhous
- Encephaloid
- Epithelioma
- Colloid
- Melanosis

ÉTUDE CLINIQUE

SUR LES

TUMEURS FIBRO-PLASTIQUES

PAR ARTHUR MALHÉNÉ

DOCTEUR EN MÉDECINE,

Interne en médecine et en chirurgie des hôpitaux de Paris,
Lauréat de l'Ecole de Médecine de Caen (1er prix 1858 et 1859),
Médaille de bronze des hôpitaux.

PARIS

A. PARENT, IMPRIMEUR DE LA FACULTÉ DE MÉDECINE

31, RUE MONSIEUR-LE-PRINCE, 31

1866

Figure 1-26. Title page of a monograph devoted entirely to "fibroblastic" tumors.

fibroplastic tumors as (1) colloid type, (2) sarcomatous type, and (3) fibroid type. He said that these tumors are composed of fusiform, stellate, and racket-shaped cells.

The 1870's were also full of significant events in the growth of knowledge about soft tissue tumors. Paget first referred to chondroma, Kaposi described Kaposi's sarcoma (Fig. 1-27), Butlin reported the first case of extraskeletal osteogenic sarcoma, Andrée documented a case of a pelvic soft tissue sarcoma which spread along pelvic veins, Morton's neuroma was publicized, Billroth's famous text in surgical pathology appeared, Kolaczek described glomus tumor and coined the term *angio-sarkom,* and Langhans published the first report on a metastatic angiosarcoma.

Ehrlich (1854–1915) was a great pioneer in special cellular pathology. His discovery in 1877 that specific granules in white blood cells could be stained by aniline

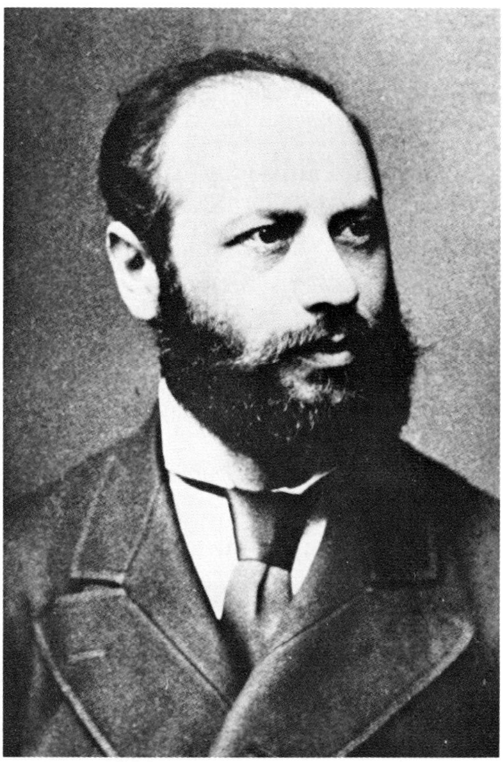

Figure 1-27. Moritz Kaposi (1837–1902). (From Bluefarb, S.: Kaposi's Sarcoma. Springfield, Ill., Charles C Thomas, 1957.)

dyes signaled the beginning of hematology and histochemistry. He discovered the mast cells and introduced methylene blue as an intravital stain.

Cohnheim (1839–1884), an experimental pathologist and a pupil of Virchow and Kölliker, demonstrated that inflammation is caused by the passage of leukocytes through capillary vessels. His book was one of the most influential texts in pathology. Caen, in 1881, described a tumor that may be the first reported case of extraskeletal chondrosarcoma and Mason, in 1883, reported the first leiomyosarcoma of the spermatic cord.

Takacs, a Hungarian physician working in the Institute of Recklinghausen in Strassburg, published his observations on multiple neuromas, in 1879, three years prior to Recklinghausen's article on multiple neurofibromatosis. Chauffard, in 1889, added the café-au-lait spots to the tumors described by Takacs.

In 1888, Chiari described heredofamilial angiomatosis. Salzer coined the term *myxoid lipoma* and Williams published his text on cancer formation.

Hausemann's description of asymmetrical mitoses in neoplastic growths signaled the beginning of further increases in knowledge about soft tissue tumors during the last decade of the nineteenth century. In this decade Taylor described what is thought to be the first case of dermatofibrosarcoma protuberans, Heurteux pointed out that not all giant cell tumors of tendons are benign, Dercum described and illustrated adiposis dolorosa (Fig. 1-28), and Garré called attention to glandlike structures in neuroma (Fig. 1-29). Hamilton summarized his thoughts on the differential diagnosis of sarcomas and carcinomas and illustrated the clinical appearance of multiple neurofibromatosis (Table 1-5; Fig. 1-30). He pointed out that "there is a difference in the malignancy of sarcoma, according to its site." He also reported the first soft tissue sarcoma diag-

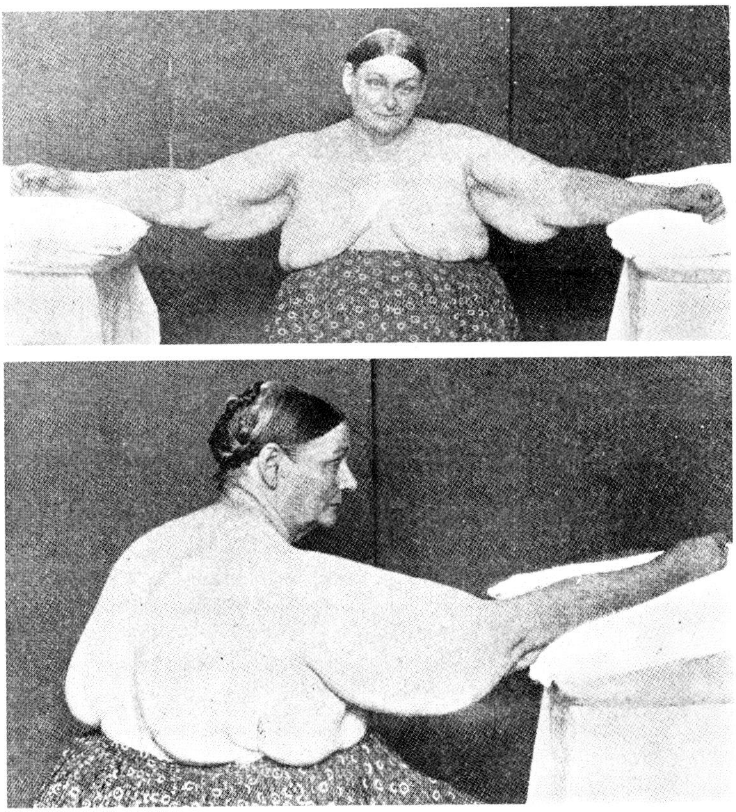

Figure 1-28. Dercum's disease. The first of Dercum's cases was a woman, who died both alcoholic and syphilitic. When she was 48, her arms and shoulders began to enlarge and were painful. (From Am. J. Med. Sci. 104:521, 1892.)

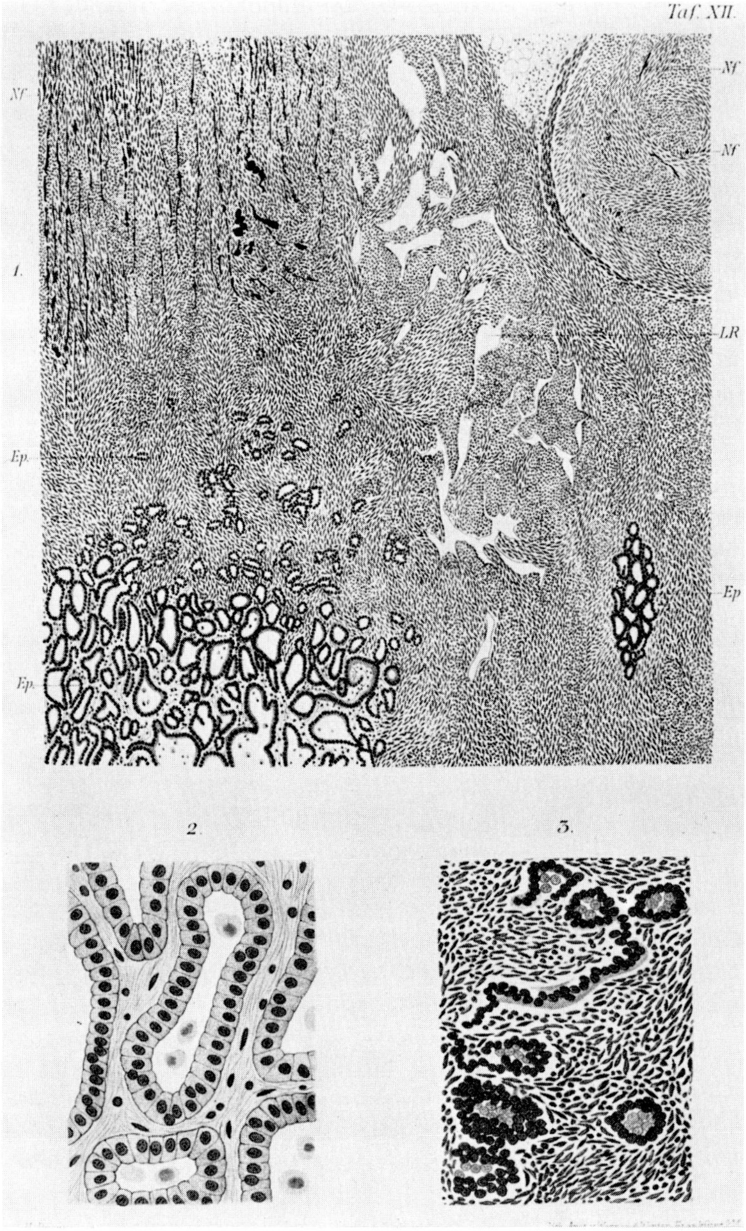

Figure 1-29. Illustration of the first reported case of glandular schwannoma by Garré. (From Beitr. Klin. Chir. 9:465, 1892.)

TABLE 1-5. *Differential Diagnosis of Sarcomas and Carcinomas According to Hamilton, in 1892*

	SARCOMA	CARCINOMA
Origin	Mesoblastic	Meso- and epi- or hypoblastic
Cells	Shape various Granulation tissue or embryonic cells	Shape and size various Epithelial cells Distinct nuclei and nucleoli
Stroma	Intercellular Does not form alveoli	Forms alveoli, which communicate with one another and surround masses of cells
Intercellular substance	Present	Absent or merely fluid
Recurrence	Frequent at site of excision	Not frequent at site of excision
Spread	By blood vessels	By lymphatics, except in the later stages, when they also spread by blood vessels and then very rapidly
Malignancy	Great	Greater

nosed from aspirate by Surgeon General Woodward as round celled sarcoma. The patient died four months later. Berard coined the term *embryonal rhabdomyosarcoma*. Mallory (1862–1941) published his book, *Pathological Technique* (Fig. 1-31), and Targett described the first case of giant cell tumor of soft tissues. Mallory's staining methods made his name familiar in histology laboratories in all quarters of the globe. As Ewing said, "The older pathologist had largely exhausted the possibilities of pathologic anatomy and histology, but it remained for Mallory, Ramon y Cajal and del Rio Hortega to carry histo-

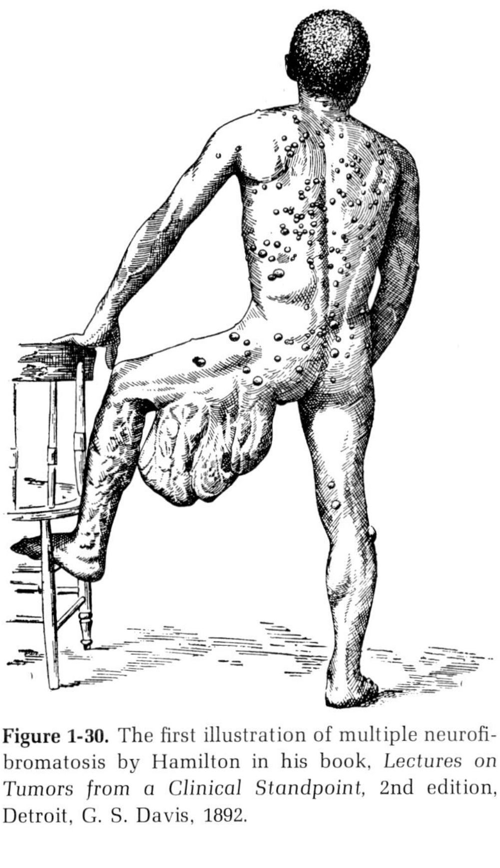

Figure 1-30. The first illustration of multiple neurofibromatosis by Hamilton in his book, *Lectures on Tumors from a Clinical Standpoint*, 2nd edition, Detroit, G. S. Davis, 1892.

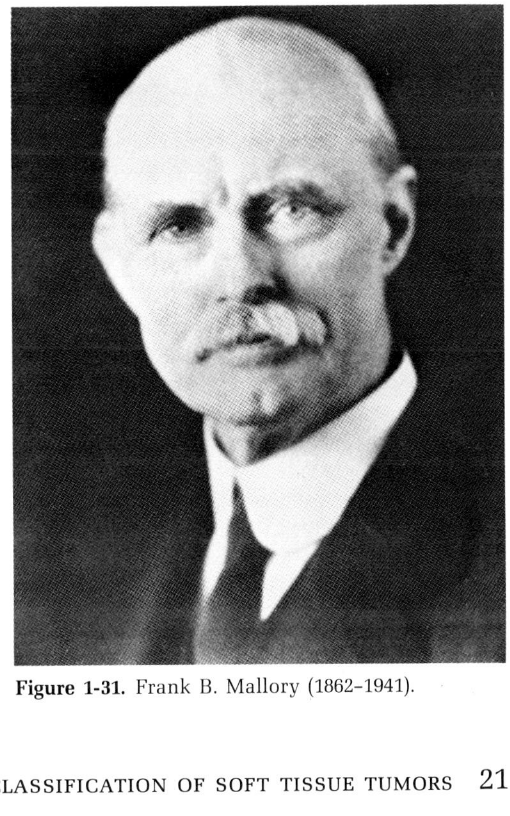

Figure 1-31. Frank B. Mallory (1862–1941).

pathology to its highest development, and to make contributions beyond the reach of other methods."

Adami of McGill University published his *Pathological Notes,* in 1898. He not only gave a detailed description and tabulation of connective tissue tumors (Table 1-6) but also gave an original description of giant cell formation. According to him, "All cells may become giant cells when substances which are absorbed with difficulty are brought into contact with them, because this leads to rapid nuclear division. Possibly too, they are sometimes formed from a fusion of degenerated cells."

It must be acknowledged that in the nineteenth century two new divisions of morphology, histology and histopathology, were born out of cellular pathology. It would be unfair not to mention another branch of medicine, radiology, which evolved from the discovery of x-rays by Röntgen, in 1895 (Fig. 1-32).

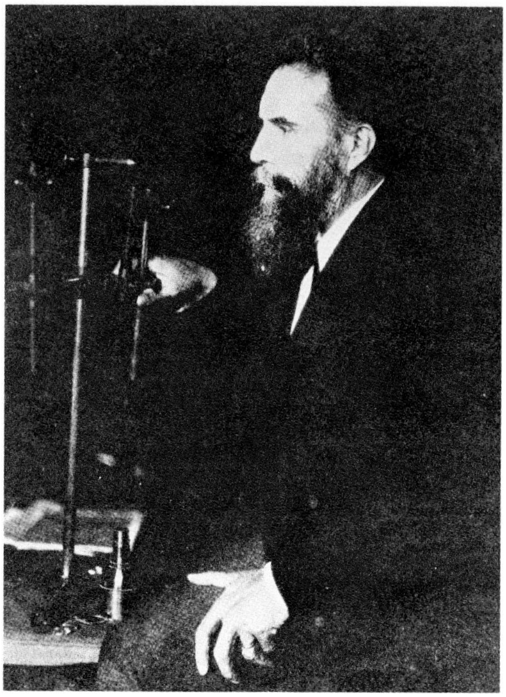

Figure 1-32. William Conrad Röntgen (1845–1923).

TABLE 1-6. ***Classification of Sarcomas According to Adami, in 1898***

I. SIMPLE SARCOMATA
 A. Small round cell sarcoma
 B. Lymphosarcoma
 C. Large round cell sarcoma*
 D. Small spindle-celled sarcoma†
 E. Large spindle-celled sarcoma
 F. Giant cell sarcoma‡
II. ALVEOLAR SARCOMATA
 A. Haemangiosarcoma
  1. Intravascular
  2. Perivascular
 B. Lymphangiosarcoma
 C. Cylindroma
 D. Myxosarcoma
III. DEGENERATIVE SARCOMATA
 A. Melanotic sarcoma
 B. Chloroma
 C. Psammoma
IV. MIXED FORMS OF SARCOMATA
 A. Fibrosarcoma
 B. Osteosarcoma

*Epithelioid type.
†Oat-shaped.
‡Myeloid.

THE PERIOD OF HISTOPATHOLOGY

(From Ewing to Stout)

With the first decade of the twentieth century began the serious application of information obtained from histologic studies to better understanding of tumors. This did not take place without opposition. Senn (1844–1908), in 1900, said, "The value of the microscope as an aid in the diagnosis of tumors has been greatly over-estimated. The greatest blunders in diagnosis and treatment have been committed by surgeons of eminence through placing too great reliance on the microscopic examination of fragments of tumor-tissue." This and similar views failed to impede the use of the microscope. Thomson reported the hereditary nature of neurofibromatosis, Bellamy was preoccupied with the formation of giant cells (Fig. 1-33), Benenati recognized rhabdomyoblasts in a nerve tumor, Albrecht described and defined hamartoma,

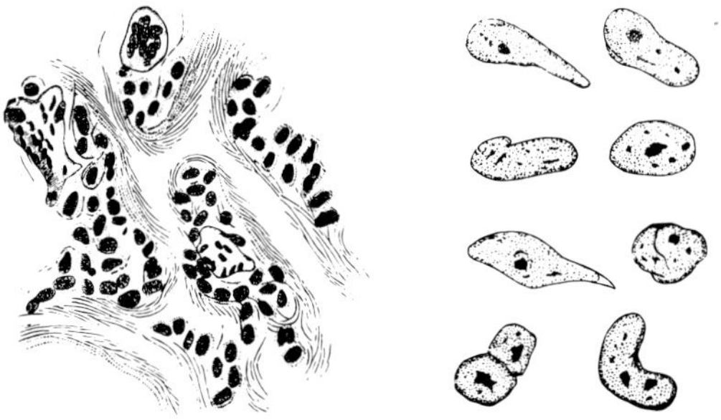

Figure 1-33. Bellamy's illustration of "giant cell tumor of tendon sheath." (From J. Pathol. Bacteriol. 7:465, 1901.)

Benda reported a case of ganglioneuroma of the vagus nerve, Hartzell wrote an article on pyogenic granuloma, and Albarran, in 1905, described Ormond's disease, 43 years prior to the publication of the description by Ormond.

Borst's pathology atlas with hundreds of magnificent color illustrations was published in 1902. It is a summary of what was known concerning the natural history and the pathology of cancer at the end of the nineteenth century (Table 1-7).

Once again the preoccupation with giant cells surfaced. Gordon-Taylor, in 1905, wrote, "If giant cells with many nuclei be found in a growth it is very unlikely to form metastases, while the presence of large cells with few nuclei must be regarded as warranting an unfavorable prognosis." To this Williams added, in 1908, "The nuclei of the cells of malignant tumors are as a rule, larger and richer in chromatin, and they more frequently originate mitoses." And, as a word of caution he added, "Malignancy is a relative term, of which there is no absolute morphologic criterion."

Characterization of tumors at the cellular level induced Mallory, in 1908, the same year in which he devised the term *hemangioendothelioma*, to say, "The fibroblast is a flat cell with flat oval nucleus and delicate cytoplasm spreading out in one plane. It is definitely characterized by the production of two kinds of fibrils: fibroglia fibrils and collagen fibrils." Verocay, in 1908, published a book on nerve tumors and two years later an article on the same topic which includes the original description of "Verocay-bodies." In 1910, Lejars recognized "epthelioid" cells in synovial sarcoma and Wohlgemuth reported a liposarcoma arising in a lipoma. McDonagh, in 1912, gave a sum-

TABLE 1-7. ***Classification of Mesenchymal Tumors by Borst, in 1902***

I. CONNECTIVE TISSUE TUMORS
- Fibroma
  - Fibroma durum
  - Fibroma molle
  - Elephantiasis
  - Keloid
  - Naevi
  - Xanthoma
- Myxoma
- Lipoma
- Chondroma
- Osteoma
- Hemangioma
- Lymphangioma

II. TUMORS OF MUSCLE AND NERVOUS SYSTEM
- Myoma
  - Leiomyoma
  - Rhabdomyoma
- Neuroma
- Glioma

III. ENDOTHELIAL TUMORS
- Lymphangioendothelioma
- Hemangioendothelioma
- Perithelioma
- Cylindroma
- Psammoma
- Cholesteatoma

IV. UNDIFFERENTIATED SARCOMAS
- Round cell sarcoma
- Spindle cell sarcoma
- Giant cell sarcoma

V. DIFFERENTIATED SARCOMAS
- Fibroma sarcomatosum
- Myxoma sarcomatosum
- Lipoma sarcomatosum
- Chondroma sarcomatosum
- Osteoma sarcomatosum
- Melanosarcoma
- Chloroma
- Lymphoma sarcomatosum
- Myeloma multiplex
- Angioma sarcomatosum
- Myoma sarcomatosum
- Neuroma sarcomatosum
- Glioma sarcomatosum

mary on subcutaneous "naevoxanthoendotheliomata." Burgess, in 1914, reported a metastatic "rhabdomyoma" of the thigh with illustration of longitudinal and cross-striations (Fig. 1-34). He wrote, "To such tumors the terms-sarcoma,-alveolar sarcoma, or other indefinite name would probably [be] applied in the ordinary course of routine pathological examination but after a very extended search it was possible to find tumor cells which had reached a sufficient degree of differentiation to enable them to be recognized as striated muscle cells." Coley called attention to the traumatic origin of myositis ossificans and a few years later, in 1919, Jaidka reported an "ossifying sarcoma" of the vastus externus.

At this time as Woglom said, in 1903, "Every one whose experience has been limited to the investigation of human material must have felt dissatisfaction at one time or another with the inconclusiveness of his observations," and he added with foresight, "The value of working with a tumor which can be propagated in animals through many generations is apparent; we can alter at will the conditions under which it is growing, and we can submit it to examination at any period of its growth." This and related ideas were one step closer to realization in 1910, when Harrison introduced the tissue culture technique and Carrel and Burrows succeeded in growing a fowl sarcoma in vitro. They received the sarcoma from

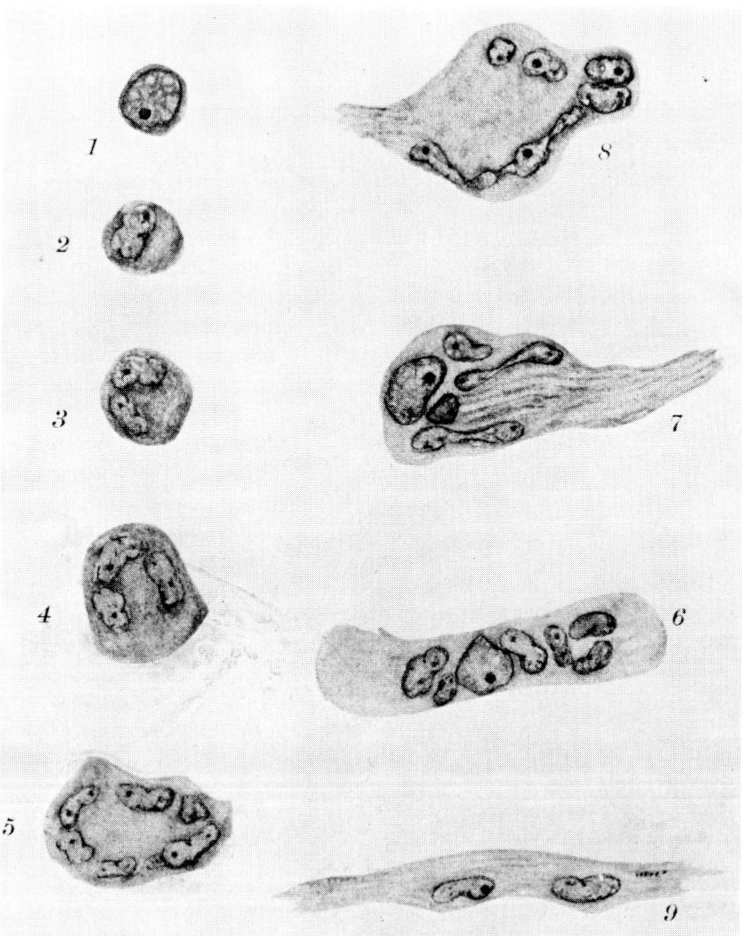

Figure 1-34. Burgess' illustration of tumor cells from a metastatic rhabdomyosarcoma. Note the longitudinal and cross-striated filaments. (From J. Med. Res. 29:447, 1913–14.)

Rous, who, in 1911, performed a remarkable experiment by transferring sarcoma in chickens by inoculation of cell-free filtrate (Fig. 1-35). He received the Nobel prize for his work in 1966.

Rous (Fig. 1-36) prophetically predicted, "It is probable that malignant tumors of the human organism can, in similar manner, be caused to grow outside the body." Fell and Andrews, in 1927, gave a detailed account of the histologic morphology of Jensen's rat sarcoma grown in vitro, and confirmed earlier observations of Lambert and Hanes, in 1911, and Lewis and Gey, in 1923, that in cultures of rat and mouse sarcomas, two fairly distinct cell types, a long spindle-shaped type and a second type, clasmatocytes (resting wandering cells or macrophages) were observed. These attempts led to the in vitro cultivation of a human sarcoma, osteogenic sarcoma, by Losee and Ebeling in 1914 (Fig. 1-37). In 1916, Marinesco and Minea succeeded in growing fat cells in vitro from a patient with Dercum's disease.

At the time these exciting experimental advances were made, pathologists diligently continued to record observations obtained from surgically excised human tumors. Despite discouraging statements like the one by Kettle, in 1916, who said,

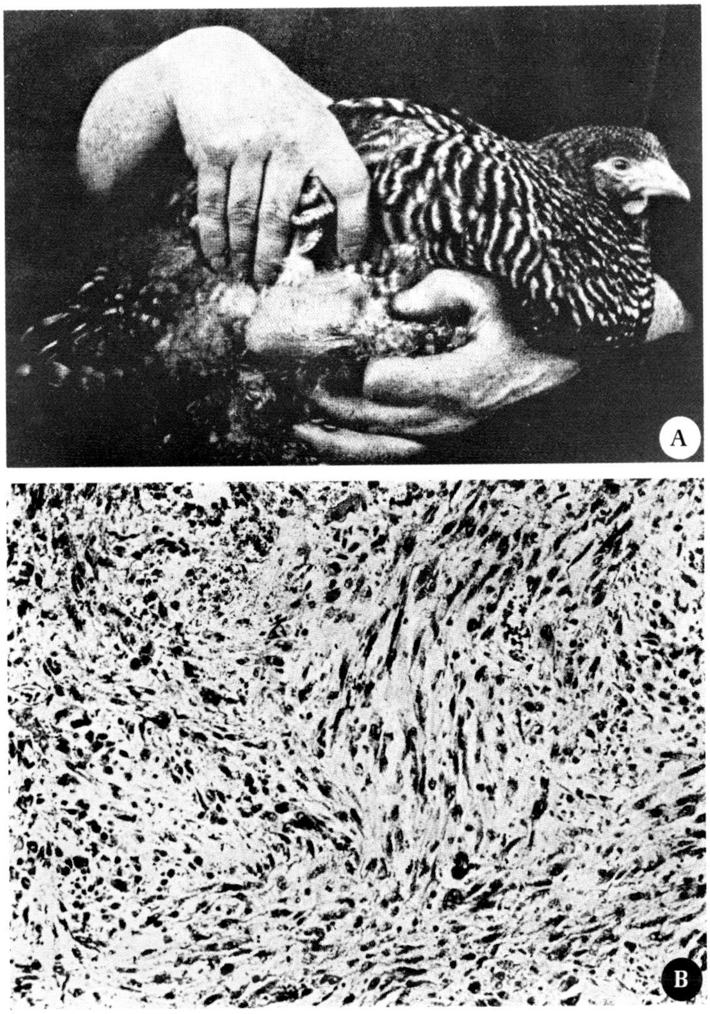

Figure 1-35. Peyton Rous' original illustration of gross (**A**) and microscopic (**B**) appearance of fowl sarcoma which was established from cell-free filtrate of the tumor. (From J. Exp. Med. 12:696, 1910.)

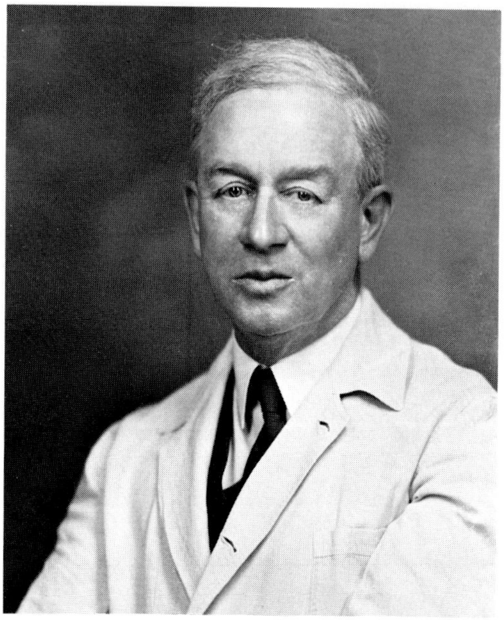

Figure 1-36. Peyton F. Rous (1879–1970). (From the Rockefeller University Archives).

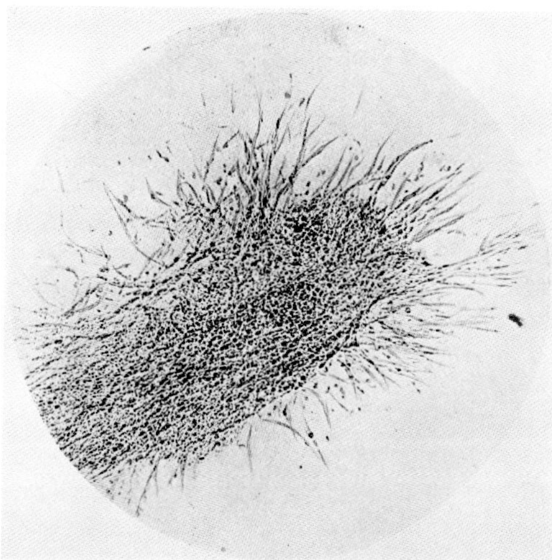

Figure 1-37. The first human sarcoma grown in tissue cultures by Losee and Ebeling. (J. Exp. Med. 20:140, 1914.)

"The study of sarcomata demands a considerable histological experience, and, even then, the diagnosis in individual cases may be purely a matter of opinion," pathologists labored on. Ewing (1866–1943), in 1919, published the first edition of his *Neoplastic Diseases,* in which he laid the foundation of surgical pathology of neoplasms (Figs. 1-38, 1-39). Two years

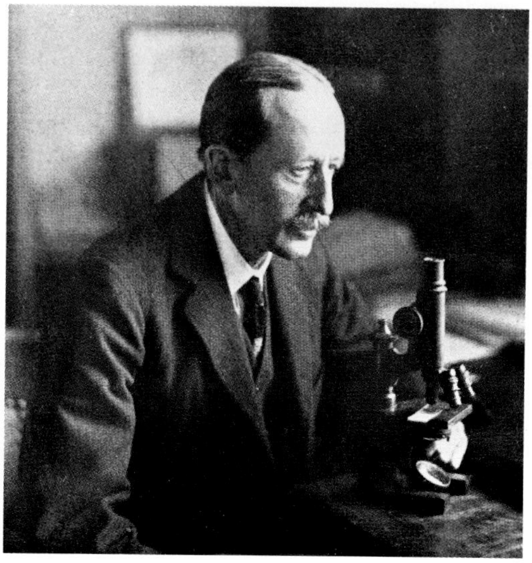

Figure 1-38. James Ewing (1866–1943).

NEOPLASTIC DISEASES

A TEXT-BOOK ON TUMORS

By

JAMES EWING, A. M., M. D., Sc. D.

Professor of Pathology at Cornell University Medical College
New York City

WITH 479 ILLUSTRATIONS

PHILADELPHIA AND LONDON
W. B. SAUNDERS COMPANY
1919

Figure 1-39. Title page of Ewing's book which went through several editions.

later he reported his first account on a neoplasm which less than a decade later became known as Ewing's sarcoma. In the second edition of his book, in 1922, he refined his classification of neoplasms and concluded, "The final classification of tumors must depend chiefly on histogenesis and structure." He also added countless new case reports to his book, including one on papillary endothelial hyperplasia (Table 1-8).

In the 1920's a number of important observations were published. Antoni from Stockholm publicized his observation on the peculiar growth patterns of certain nerve tumors which were soon known as Antoni A and Antoni B patterns (Fig. 1-40). Schmincke described congenital rhabdomyoma of the heart, Sokoloff called attention to hyperchromasia and altered nucleocytoplasmic ratio in cancer cells, Masson observed myofibrils in glomus cells, Darier and Ferrand reported on recurrent dermatofibrosarcoma protuberans, Jura and Sakurane discussed mesenteric and digital fibromatosis, respectively, Levy attempted to distinguish fibroblastic and histiocytic tumors, Fischer observed transformation of fibroblasts to macrophages in vitro, and

TABLE 1-8. ***Histologic Classification of Tumors According to Ewing****

CONNECTIVE TISSUE
- Fibroma (composed of connective tissue)
- Chondroma (composed of cartilage)
- Chordoma (composed of tissue of chorda dorsalis)
- Osteoma (composed of bone)
- Myxoma (composed of mucous tissue)
- Lipoma (composed of fat tissue)
- Angioma (composed of blood vessels)
- Lymphoma (composed of lymphatic tissue)
- Sarcoma (a cellular tumor composed of anaplastic tissue of any of the above types)

MUSCLE TISSUE
- Leiomyoma (composed of smooth muscle)
- Rhabdomyoma (composed of striated muscle)

ELEMENTS OF THE NERVOUS SYSTEM
- Neuroma (composed of nerve fibers)
- Neuroma (composed of nerve fibers and ganglion cells)
- Glioma (composed of glia tissue)
- Neuro-epithelioma (composed of neuroepithelium)

ENDOTHELIUM
- Endothelioma

EPITHELIUM
- Papilloma (a tumor of pavement epithelium, with supporting tissues in normal arrangement)
- Adenoma (a benign tumor of glandular epithelium, with supporting tissue in normal arrangement)
- Epithelioma or epidermoid carcinoma (epithelium in atypical arrangement)
- Carcinoma (a tumor of glandular epithelium in atypical arrangement)

COMPLEX TISSUES
- Simple mixed tumors (composed of more than one type of neoplastic tissue—named according to composition: e.g., chordoepithelioma, adenosarcoma)
- Teratoma (composed of tissues and organs of one, two, or three germinal layers)
- Embryoma (composed of tissues from three germinal layers in more or less orderly imitation of a fetus)

*This classification was introduced by Ewing in 1919 in the first edition of *Neoplastic Diseases*. It was retained in all subsequent editions and was in use until the late 1940's.

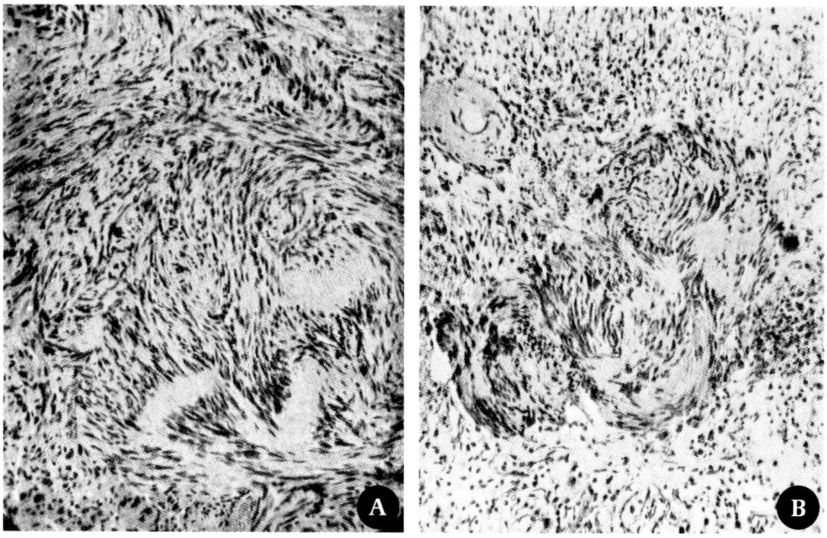

Figure 1-40. Antoni's original illustration of "Antoni's A and B patterns" in neurofibroma. (From Uber Ruckenmarkstumoren und Neurofibroma. Munchen und Wiesbaden, J. F. Bergmann, 1920.)

Abrikossoff reported the first case of granular cell myoblastoma which was actually named as such by Diss a year later, in 1927.

An almost innumerable number of new terms were introduced. The term *pericyte* was coined by Zimmerman. Barre and Mason first used the name *glomus tumor,* Jaffe coined the term *lipoblastoma,* Aschoff introduced the concept of the "reticuloendothelial system," Montpellier suggested the descriptive term *alveolar rhabdomyoma* to mean alveolar rhabdomyosarcoma and referred to "megasarcocytes," giant cells with asteroid bodies. According to Montpellier the term *rhabdomyoma* was first proposed by Zenker, in 1864, and Masson was the first to divide rhabdomyomas into the dysgenetic (embryonic) and adult types.

Recognition of the need for better classification of soft tissue sarcomas is seen in the statement of Gilford, in 1925, that "without biological understanding of cancer we cannot hope for a real and lasting solution of the problem" and of Carrel and Ebeling that "tissue cells, like bacteria, must be defined not only by their morphology but also by their physiological properties." In an attempt to express the biological potentials of soft tissue tumors, Quick and Cutler, in 1927, introduced histologic grading of sarcomas.

In the 1930's the discovery of new entities and the refinement of known concepts continued. Masson continued his investigation of tumors of peripheral nerves and called attention to the diagnostic significance of palisades in schwannomas (Fig. 1-41). And, in reference to their histogenesis he concluded that "the palisades that

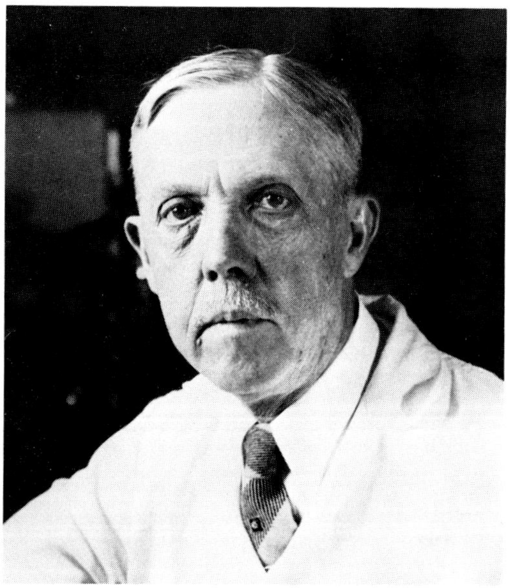

Figure 1-41. Pierre Masson (1880–1959). (Courtesy of Dr. F. Wiglesworth and Dr. T. Seemayer).

are found in schwannomas are derived from the sheath of Schwann."

From Memorial Hospital for Cancer and Allied Diseases, Martin and Ellis popularized the biopsy technique by needle puncture and aspirates, Adair wrote a comprehensive text on the clinical aspect of cancer, Ewing's *Causation, Diagnosis and Treatment of Cancer* was published, Stewart reported the first case of liposarcoma of bone and the term *neurogenic sarcoma* which was first proposed in 1927 by Quick and Cutler, also from Memorial Hospital, was again proposed by Stewart and Copeland. Stewart and Copeland in their article on neurogenic sarcoma described tumors of the deeper nerve trunk "which looked like certain nonpigmented melanomas, yet did not run the clinical course of melanoma." They also described and illustrated neurogenic sarcomas in brothers and sisters. Millar added a case report, in 1932, of a malignant melanotic tumor of ganglion cells.

Ewing wrote in his book, in 1931, that cancer was considered "the master medical problem of the age." In reference to sarcomas he said, "If one reviews the whole scope of variation and subtleties in the form, structure, and course of sarcomas, one must conclude that sarcomas present a wider and more complex field in oncology than do epithelial tumors." He added, "The grade of potential malignancy is very important information."

Woringer and Cellina first used the term *histiocytoma*, in 1931 and 1932, respectively. Klein introduced the term *mesenchymoma*, and Seidelin described and illustrated "chordoma-like cells" in liposarcoma, in 1932 (Fig. 1-42).

In 1934, Sabrazes et al introduced the term *synovial sarcoma* and referred to a certain histologic form as "epitheliosarcoma." Klemperer described the first case of alveolar soft part sarcoma under the name of "myoblastoma of striated muscle." In 1939, Stout coined the term *neurilemoma*, and Ewing defined myxoid liposarcoma and called attention to its radiosensitivity.

In 1936, Bartkowiak introduced the term *leiomyoblastoma*, Geormatigh et al described "lipoblasts" and "lipoblastomatosis," Hudson reported the first case of congenital fibrosarcoma, and Warren and Sommer published a report of the first two cases of postirradiation fibrosarcoma.

Carrel, the cell biologist, and Lindbergh, the aviator, published their book, *The Culture of Organs*, in 1938. Lindbergh's contribution was to design and assemble a pump to carry the nutrients to the tissues in an attempt "to obtain knowledge on the nutrition of each part of the body and to pursue it through the complexity of its unpredictable consequences."

In 1939, Meyer et al isolated hyaluronate from synovial fluid, Potozky and Fried reported the first cases of extraskeletal Ewing's sarcoma, Stout described cutaneous leiomyoma, and Steiner reported the first case of metastasizing leiomyoma of the uterus.

In 1940, Brinkley and Stewart studied the morphogenesis of extraskeletal osteogenic sarcoma, and Wells called attention to the existence of congenital malignant neoplasms. He reviewed the literature on the subject and found 29 sarcomas. Papanicolaou and Traut, in 1941, published their definitive study on the diagnosis of uterine carcinoma by smear technique.

Murray (Fig. 1-43) and Stout, in 1942, published their observations on Schwann cells in tissue culture and stated that "Schwann cells can and do form collagen and reticulin." This study was followed by a report, in 1943, on liposarcomas in tissue culture and, in 1949, on the in vitro morphology of synovial sarcoma and synovial tissue, which apparently led to Murray's attempt to grow all forms of sarcomas in tissue culture.

Stout, in 1942, introduced the term *hemangiopericytoma* and in an article he co-authored with Murray he wrote that these tumors are "composed of capillary blood vessels with one or more layers of rounded cells arranged about them, which cannot be called glomus tumors because

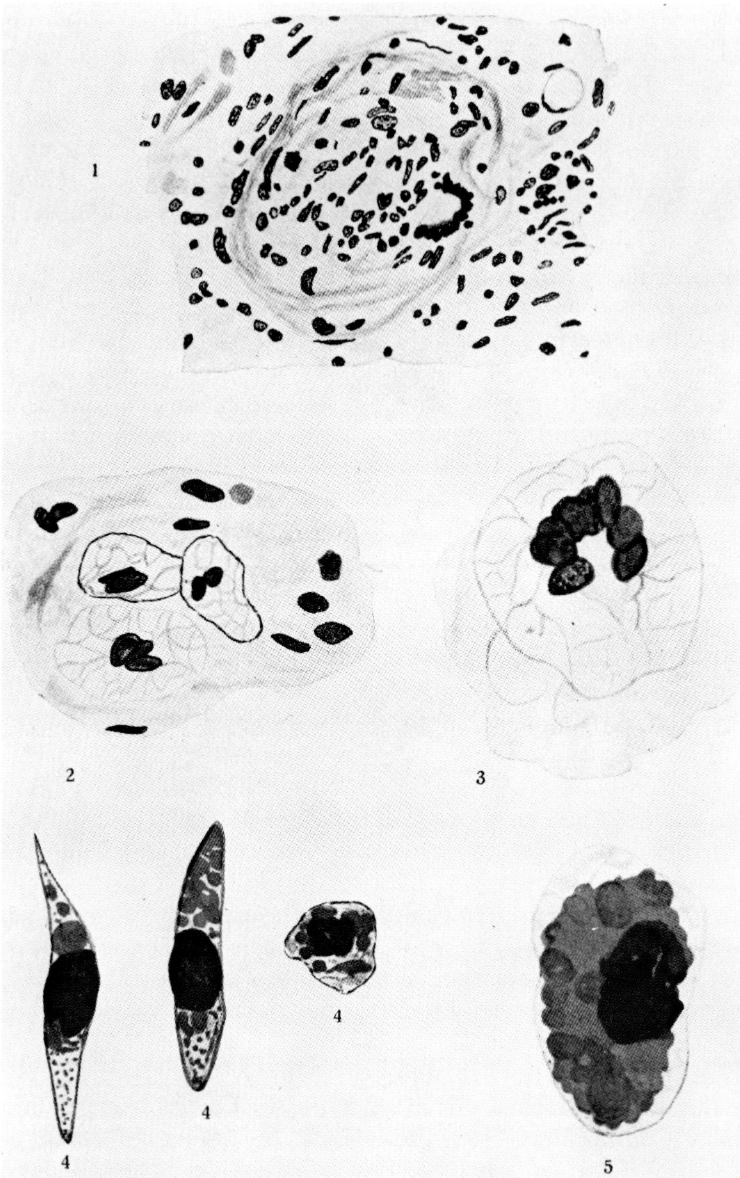

Figure 1-42. Seidelin's illustration of neoplastic fat cells of various shapes and sizes. (From Seidelin, H.: Liposarcoma with chordoma-like cells. Acta Path. Microbiol. Scand. 9:289, 1932.)

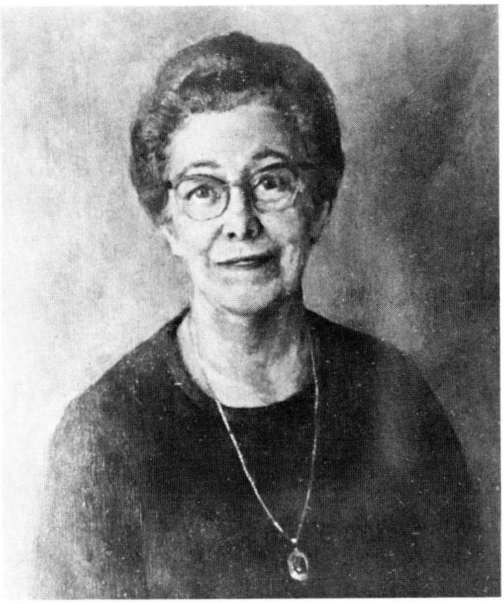

Figure 1-43. Margaret Murray (1901–). (Courtesy of Dr. D. King and Dr. M. King.)

they lack the organoid features of those encapsulated complex neoplasms, yet differ from single capillary hemangiomata because of the presence of their perivascular cells" (Fig. 1-44).

Stout was also the first to subclassify liposarcomas, in 1944, and reported the first article, with Ackerman, on leiomyosarcoma of soft tissue, in 1947. In the same year the first authentic report on sarcomas, as seen with the electron microscope, was published by Porter and Thompson.

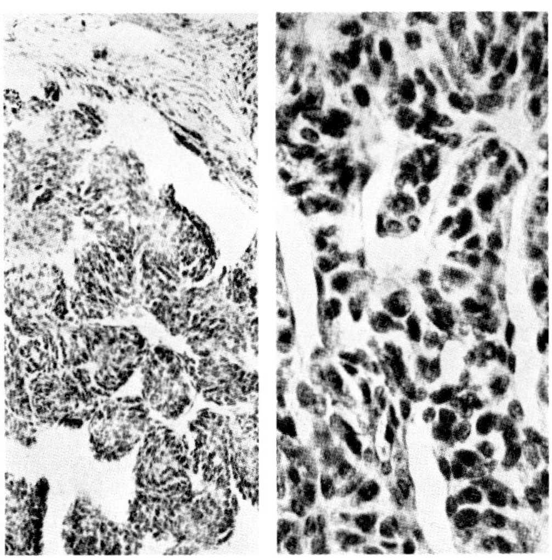

Figure 1-44. First illustration of hemangiopericytoma by Stout and Murray. (From Stout, A. P., and Murray, M. R.: Hemangiopericytoma: A vascular tumor featuring Zimmerman's pericytes. Ann. Surg. 116:26, 1942.)

Stewart and Treves, in 1948, following the best tradition of morphologists by correlating clinical and microscopic findings, reported the first 6 cases of postmastectomy lymphangiosarcoma (Fig. 1-45). This report, from the Memorial Hospital for Cancer and Allied Diseases, was followed by another equally important contribution by Christopherson, Foote, and Stewart in 1952, who reported the first cases of "alveolar soft part sarcoma" (Fig. 1-46). Stewart, in 1948, also coined the term *chordoid sarcoma*.

Koback and Perlow, in 1949, reported on malignant xanthomatous giant cell tumor of soft tissues. Morgan et al first reported on angiomyolipoma of the kidney in 1951, and Grailly et al called attention to the changing morphology of recurrent mesenchymal tumors and reported that "the most aggressive tumors are very cellular, very vascular and very undifferentiated."

In 1953, Bennett and Porter studied muscle with the electron microscope, Gardner and Richards described the first cases of "Gardner's syndrome," Keasbey reported on juvenile aponeurotic fibroma, and the first comprehensive treatise on soft tissue tumors was published by Stout (Fig. 1-47). In the classification and morphology of soft tissue tumors great credit belongs to Stout. He attempted, as early as 1949, at the combined symposium of the National Cancer Institute and the American Cancer Society, in Memphis, Tennessee, to lay down the foundation for classification and subclassification of soft tissue tumors (Table 1-9).

During the following years, Enterline and Roberts published a report on "lymphangiopericytoma," Fischer summarized his thoughts on the histochemistry of alveolar soft part sarcoma, Hicks published the first case of synovial cysts in bone, Reye described the first cases of

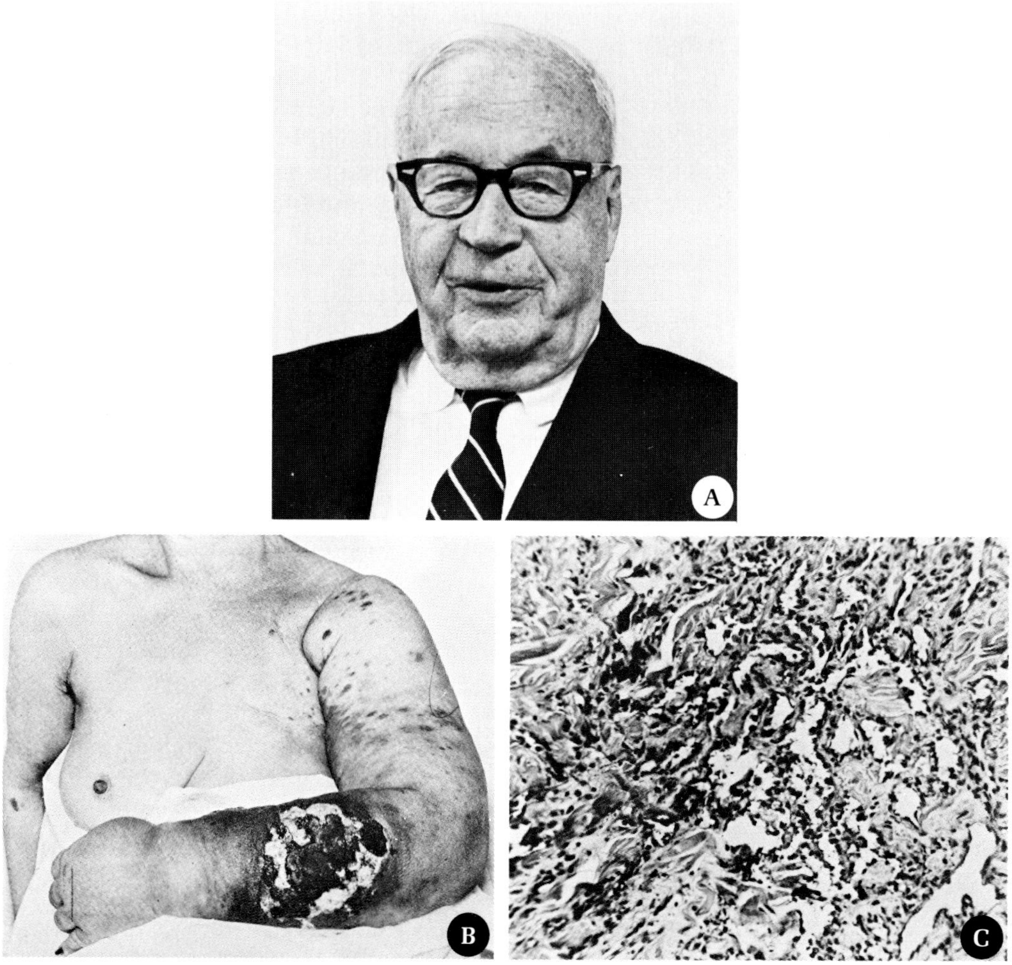

Figure 1-45. A, Fred W. Stewart (1894–). **B, C,** First illustration of postmastectomy lymphangiosarcoma. (From Stewart, F. W., and Treves, N.: Lymphangiosarcoma in post-mastectomy lymphedema. Cancer 1:64, 1948.)

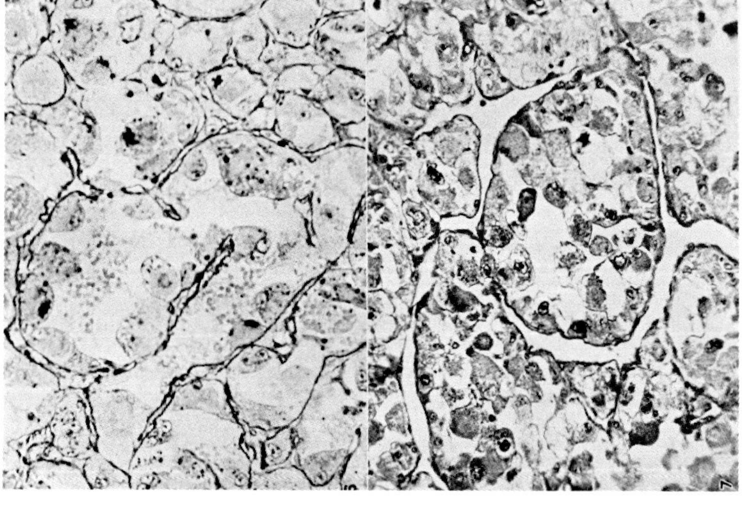

Figure 1-46. Illustration of distribution of reticulin (left); the classic pattern in a metastatic alveolar soft part sarcoma (right). (From Christopherson, W. M., Foote, F. W., and Stewart, F. W.: Alveolar soft part sarcoma: structurally characteristic tumors of uncertain histogenesis. 5:100, 1952.)

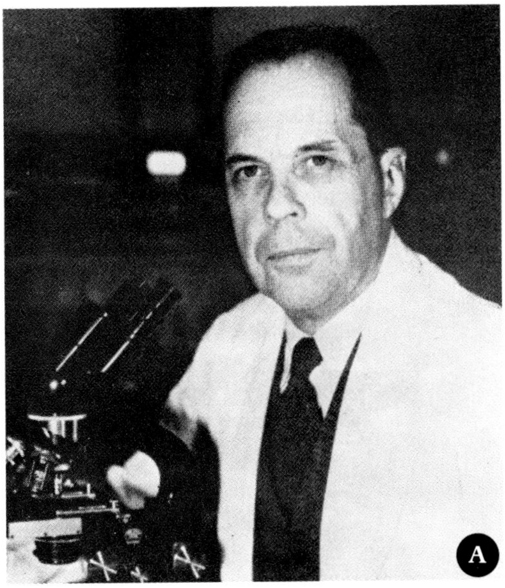

ATLAS OF TUMOR PATHOLOGY

Section II—Fascicle 5

TUMORS OF THE SOFT TISSUES

by

Arthur Purdy Stout, M. D.

Professor of Pathology

Columbia University, College of Physicians and Surgeons

New York City

Published by the

ARMED FORCES INSTITUTE OF PATHOLOGY

Under the Auspices of the

SUBCOMMITTEE ON ONCOLOGY

of the

COMMITTEE ON PATHOLOGY

of the

NATIONAL RESEARCH COUNCIL

Washington, D. C.

1953

B

Figure 1-47. A, Arthur Purdy Stout (1885–1967). **B,** Title page of Stout's AFIP fascicle.

subdermal fibromatosis of infancy, Riopelle and Theriault firmly established the term *alveolar rhabdomyosarcoma,* and Bednar described pigmented and nonpigmented forms of storiform neurofibroma.

Bluefarb, in 1957, published his booklet on Kaposi's sarcoma. Pack and Ariel's clinical treatise, *Tumors of the Soft Somatic Tissue,* appeared in 1958. In the same year Vellios et al popularized the term *lipoblastomatosis,* and Bowden and Booher summarized the state of the art from the surgeon's point of view: "Sarcomas of soft parts are characterized by an absence of true encapsulation, by filamentous extension within muscle fasciculi and along contiguous fascial planes and nerve trunks well beyond visible and palpable tumor. When resection of soft parts is automatically feasible for the removal of a sarcoma, it includes wide ablation of surrounding grossly normal tissue, removal of entire muscle bundles at points of origin and insertion, employment of sharp dissection throughout, minimal handling and massage of the tumor and proximal ligation of major venous tributaries early in the procedure."

In 1959, Lichtenstein and Bernstein reported the first case of mesenchymal chondrosarcoma. In the same year Rich and Myers reported excretion of acid mucopolysaccharides in the urine of patients with certain malignant neoplasms.

In the 1960's, a number of firsts occurred in reference to soft tissue tumors. Kern, in 1960, introduced the term *proliferative myositis* and reported the first 7 cases (Fig. 1-48). Luse reported the first ultrastructural study of a synovial sarcoma. Martin et al reported the first case of gastric leiomyoblastoma and Jarvi and Saxen described "elastofibroma dorsi." Winslow and Enzinger called attention to the presence of hyaluronidase-sensitive acid mucopolysaccharides in liposarcomas, Chaoman et al reported their ultrastructural findings in rhabdomyosarcoma, Ozzello et al studied malignant histiocytomas in tissue culture, and

TABLE 1-9. *Tumors of the Soft Tissues According to Stout, in 1953*

BENIGN TUMORS AND TUMOR-LIKE PROLIFERATIONS

- Fibromatoses
  - Fibroma durum
  - Fibroma molle
  - Nonmetastasizing fibrosarcomas
  - Desmoid tumor
  - Keloid
  - Cicatricial fibromatosis
  - Palmar fibromatosis (fibroma or pseudotumor of Dupuytren's contracture)
  - Plantar fibromatosis
  - Penile fibromatosis (Peyronie's disease)
  - Fibromatosis colli (congenital wry neck)
  - Progressive myositis fibrosa (hereditary polyfibromatosis)
  - Irradiation fibromatosis
- Myxomatoses
  - Ganglion
  - Localized myxedema
- Xanthomatoses
  - Xanthoma diabeticorum
  - Multiple xanthomatous giant cell tumors
  - Xanthelasma
  - Fibrous xanthoma
  - Sclerosing hemangioma
  - Xanthogranuloma
  - Giant cell tumor
  - Eosinophilic granuloma
  - Histiocytoma
- Fat necrosis
- Lipomatoses
  - Lipoma
  - Multiple lipomas
  - Multiple symmetrical lipomatosis
  - Lipoma dolorosa
  - Lipoma arborescens
  - Myelolipoma
  - Myxolipoma, lipomyxoma, myxofibrolipoma, etc.
- Hibernoma
- Benign Tumors of Muscle
  - Leiomyoma
    - Superficial leiomyomas
    - Vascular leiomyomas
  - Rhabdomyoma
  - Granular cell myoblastoma
- Benign Angiomatoses
  - Hemangiomatoses
    - Capillary hemangioma
    - Cavernous hemangioma
    - Capillary hemangioma, granuloma type (granuloma pyogenicum)
    - Venous hemangioma
    - Benign hemangioendothelioma (or infantile hemangioendothelioma)
    - Benign hemangiopericytoma
    - Glomus tumor
    - Cirsoid aneurysm
    - Venous racemose aneurysm
    - Diffuse angiomatosis
  - Lymphangioma
    - Lymphatic Cysts
    - Cystic hygroma (hygroma cysticum colli)
- Other Benign Tumors
  - Benign tumors composed of cartilage or bone
    - Osteoma, osteochondroma, chondroma
    - Solitary myositis ossificans
    - Progressive myositis ossificans
  - Benign synovioma
  - Mixed tumor
  - Benign mesenchymoma
  - Benign mesothelioma
    - Benign mesothelioma of the genital tract
    - Benign solitary fibrous mesothelioma
    - Benign diffuse fibrous mesothelioma
  - Blue Nevus

MALIGNANT TUMORS OF THE SOFT TISSUES

- Fibrosarcoma
  - Dermatofibrosarcoma protuberans of Hoffmann
  - Progressive and recurring dermatofibroma of Darier
- Liposarcoma
  - Differentiated liposarcoma
  - Undifferentiated liposarcoma
- Malignant Tumors of Muscle
  - Leiomyosarcoma
  - Rhabdomyosarcoma
  - Malignant granular cell myoblastoma
- Angiosarcomatoses
  - Malignant hemangioendothelioma
  - Malignant hemangiopericytoma
  - Kaposi's sarcoma
  - Lymphangiosarcoma
- Malignant Lymphoid and Reticuloendothelial Tumors
  - Lymphosarcoma
    - Giant follicle lymphosarcoma
    - Lymphocytic cell lymphosarcoma
    - Reticulum cell lymphosarcoma
  - Reticulum cell sarcoma
  - Mycosis fungoides
  - Plasma cell tumor
- Myxoma
- Other Malignant Tumors
  - Osteogenic sarcoma and chondrosarcoma
  - Synovial sarcoma
  - Malignant mesenchymoma
  - Malignant mesothelioma
  - Melanosarcoma (?)

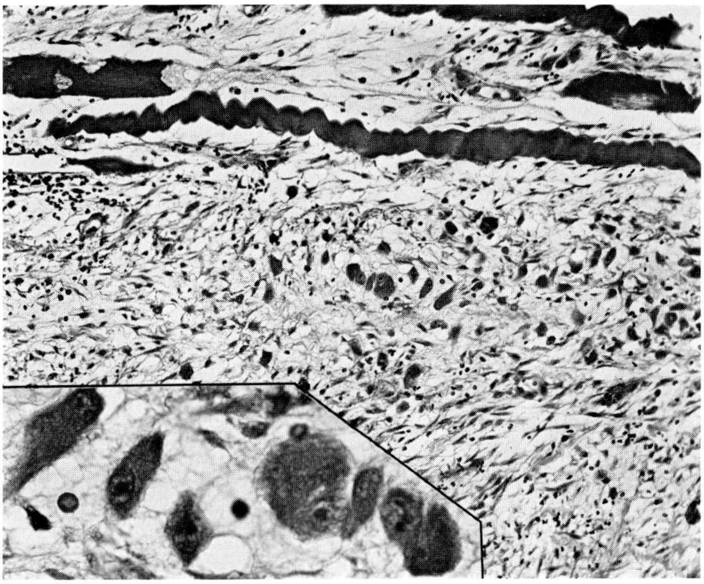

Figure 1-48. Original illustration of proliferative myositis by Kern. (From Kern, W. H.: Proliferative myositis: a pseudosarcomatous reaction to injury. Arch. Pathol. 69:209, 1960. Copyright 1960 by the American Medical Association.)

Helwig introduced the term *atypical fibroxanthoma.*

Baldwin, in 1965, giving credit to Potter's first study, in 1930, called attention to hypoglycemia associated with bulky neoplasms. While searching for a precise histogenesis, Enzinger came across a number of tumors he thought to be clear cell sarcoma of tendons and aponeuroses. It is unfortunate that later, because some of the tumors were proven to contain melanin pigment, he felt that all of the clear cell sarcomas should be regarded as neuroectodermal tumors.

Kawada et al called attention to Kimura's disease, in 1965, and Shelly and Rawnsley, in 1968, introduced the term *piezogenic pedal papules.*

In the 1960's there were a number of important ultrastructural observations. Weibel and Palade described the "bodies" in endothelial cells which were soon named as Weibel-Palade bodies. Shipkey et al discussed crystals in alveolar soft part sarcoma (Fig. 1-49). Stembridge et al felt that electron microscopy permits histogenetic classification of soft tissue sarcomas. Ross and Greenless described the attachment sites between connective tissue cells and Cornog, in 1969, studied the ultrastructure of leiomyoblastoma.

Advances were also attempted in biochemistry and immunology. Gardner wrote *Pathology of Connective Tissue Diseases* in 1965. Welsh and Meyer studied the prepolymerized collagen fibers; Archer and Kao concentrated on the identification and role of actomyosin. Schubert and Hamerman, in 1968, wrote a book on the biochemistry of connective tissue.

Perhaps one of the most important advents of this decade was the formal announcement by Stout and Lattes, in 1967, of the term *fibrous histiocytoma.* They defined fibrous histiocytomas as "embryonal forms of fibroblastic neoplasms." This definition was a direct outgrowth of the description of Broders, who, in 1939, said, "Xanthomas are undifferentiated fibrogenic tumors."

THE PERIOD OF GRADING AND STAGING

(The 1970's)

As the 1970's approached it was felt that Stout was right, in 1964, when he said, "Soft tissue sarcomas vary in prognosis and natural history, depending on cell

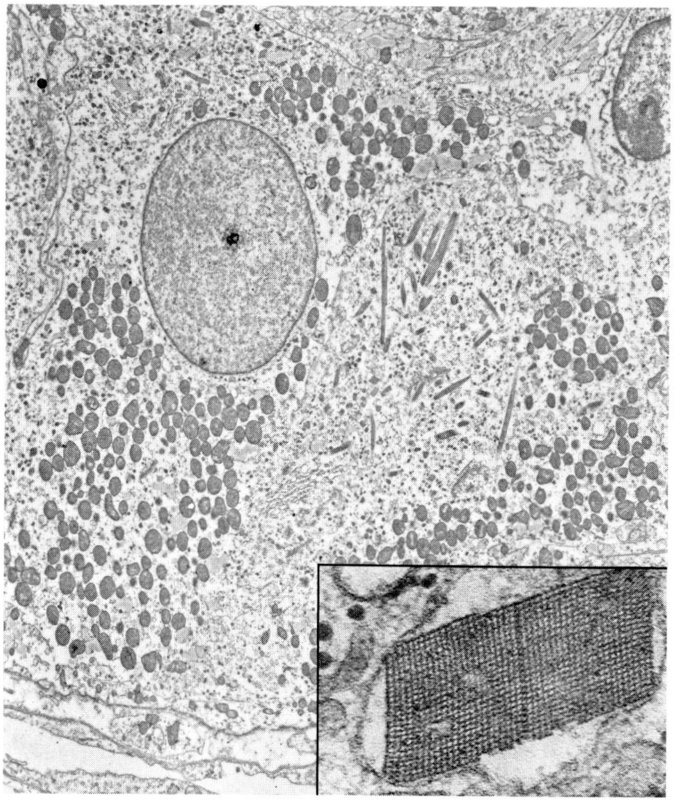

Figure 1-49. First illustration of crystals in alveolar soft part sarcoma by Shipkey et al. (From Shipkey, F. H., Lieberman, P. H., Foote, F. W., and Ashworth, C. T.: Ultrastructure of alveolar soft part sarcoma. Cancer 17:821, 1964.)

type, anatomic site and the patient's age." Enzinger et al, in 1969, published *Histological Typing of Soft Tissue Tumors* under the auspices of the World Health Organization and Mackenzie's book, *Differential Diagnosis of Fibroblastic Disorders*, was printed in which he reclassified and defined fibrous tumors and tumor-like lesions.

Enzinger revived, popularized, and defined the concept of epithelioid sarcoma in 1970 and pointed out the need for careful scrutiny of every subcutaneous granulomatous-looking lesion. Martini et al, in 1971, publicized the existence of primary pulmonary sarcomas and Lavin et al, in 1972, called attention to the fact that leiomyoblastomas can be extragastric in origin and often behave like a fully malignant leiomyosarcoma.

The electron microscope gradually became a useful instrument in differential diagnosis of soft tissue neoplasms. Merkow et al (1971), Mackay (1972), Gyorkey et al (1975), Gonda et al (1976), and Gonzalez-Crussi et al (1978) all felt that careful consideration of ultrastructural features of soft tissue lesions complement observations made with the light microscope. This technique is especially valuable in identification of undifferentiated tumors; e.g., demonstration of primordial sarcomeres in undifferentiated rhabdomyosarcoma or myofilaments with fusiform dense areas in undifferentiated leiomyosarcoma or neurofilaments, neurotubules, and desmosomes in certain neurogenic tumors is essential to proper diagnosis of these tumors (see Appendix Table B-20).

Becker and Nachman's description, in 1973, of contractile proteins in endothelial cells, platelets, and smooth muscle renewed the importance of functional studies. It became clear that if we want to obtain any further information, soft tissue tumors must be studied from the biologic, cytologic, cytochemical, and immunochemical standpoint.

Enzymatic and immunologic techniques have been used to make the diagnosis of soft tissue tumors more precise. Mucopolysaccharides constitute an important part of the ground substance in soft tissues. Most of the biochemically identified mucopolysaccharides are included in the term *heteroglycan* which includes the glycosaminoglycans (keratan sulfate, sialoglycan) and the glycosaminoglucuronoglycans (hyaluronic acid, chondroitin 4- and 6-sulfate, dermatan sulfate, heparin). Heteroglycans can be separated from each by using various techniques (Katenkamp and Stiller, 1975). By using the critical electrolyte concentration technique, Kindblom and Angervall (1975) found that the heteroglycans of the myxoid tumors vary according to the tissue of origin.

Hyaluronidase-sensitive mucopolysaccharides have been demonstrated in myxoid soft tissue tumors, but myxoid chondrosarcomas have been known to contain mostly hyaluronidase-resistant mucosubstances, (Winslow and Enzinger, 1962). PAS-stain was found useful to separate diastase-sensitive glycogen, which is present in rhabdomyosarcoma and Ewing's sarcoma from diastase-stable material, found in alveolar soft part sarcoma.

Histochemical techniques demonstrate the presence of acid phosphatase and ATP-ase and the absence of alkaline phosphatase in tumor cells of Kaposi's sarcoma and are helpful in distinguishing tumor cells and endothelial cells (Becker, 1962).

With antisera and the fluorescein-labeling technique, it is possible to demonstrate the presence of actomyosin and myosin in myosarcomas (Hiramoto et al, 1961; Archer and Kao, 1968; Pertshuk et al, 1975). Otten et al (1971) observed that rapidly growing fibroblasts have low levels of cyclic adenosine monophosphate (cyclic AMP), and cyclic AMP treatment increases cellular growth in tissue culture. The mechanism by which cyclic AMP is able to influence cell growth is unclear but may be related to phosphorylation of certain regulatory and structural proteins such as myosin, actin, and tubulin. Specific inhibition to sarcoma-specific cellular immunity, by sera from patients with growing sarcomas has been reported. This should be considered in the design of various immunotherapeutic protocols (Hellstrom and Hellstrom, 1969; Cohen et al, 1973).

Giraldo et al (1971) found that 12 out of 15 sarcoma cultures contained an antigen (S) demonstrable by indirect immunofluorescence with human sera. Considerable effort is presently being made by a number of investigators to detect sarcoma-associated antigens. Sethi and Hirshaut (1977) reported elevation of the level of circulating antibody to S antigen in patients after surgical removal of the sarcoma.

There is a growing recognition that many cells are directly influenced by macromolecules of the extracellular or intercellular milieu. Perhaps the role of these substances on sarcoma cells and thëir morphologic appearance can be best assessed by studying tumor cells in tissue culture and in heterotransplants (Hajdu and Hajdu, 1976; Sethi et al, 1977; Hajdu and Fogh, 1978). Lindberg and Mitelman (1974) found by studying sarcomas with different karyotypes that the cellular morphology is altered in a nonrandom and possibly predetermined way and is related to the predetermined sequence of chromosomal changes when a malignant tumor undergoes an evolution from a normal karyotype to an abnormal karyotype.

The complexity of the process of differentiation and dedifferentiation perhaps can be best appreciated by remembering the formation of the embryonic mesoderm (Fig. 1-50), which is located between layers of ectoderm and endoderm. Hertwig (1886) introduced the term *mesenchyme* and according to him the mesoderm is not the sole source of mesenchymal cells and both ectoderm and endoderm contribute to its embryogenesis, just as the mesoderm can produce epithelial cells. Cytologically all cells of the individual embryonic layers are at first similar, but soon the cells

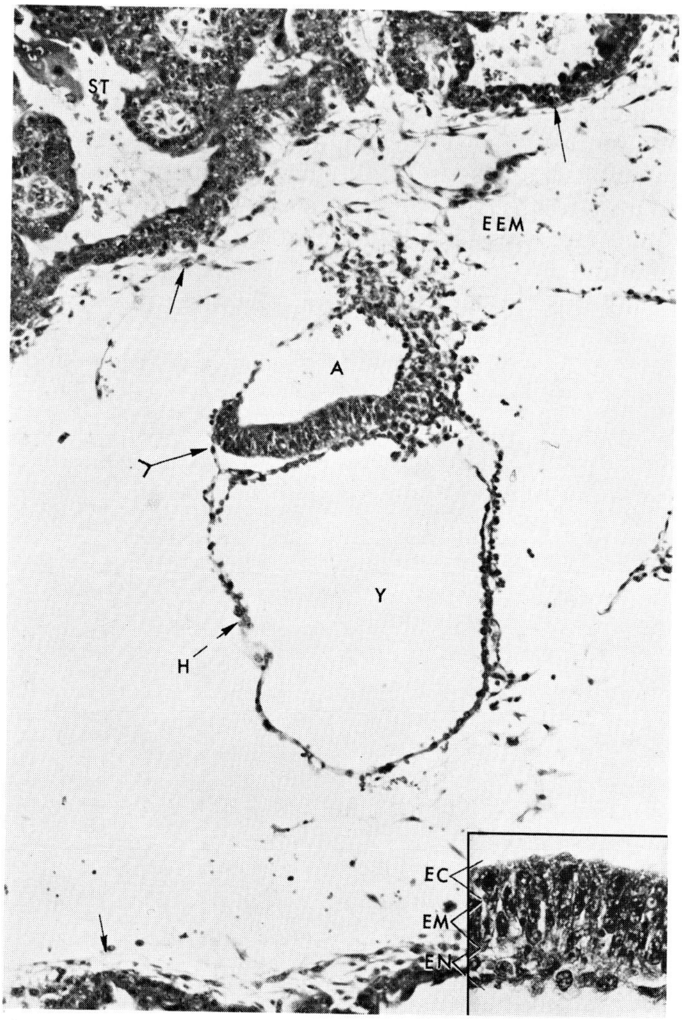

Figure 1-50. Histologic section of an 18-day-old human embryo embedded in the endometrium. The endometrium almost completely surrounds the embryo. The cytotrophoblasts (arrows) form an irregular solid inner lining. Beyond this are irregular lacunae containing syncytiotrophoblasts (ST).

The embryonic side of the cytotrophoblastic lining is covered by extraembryonic mesoderm (EEM), which is condensed on its inner aspect to form Heuser's membrane (H) around the yolk sac (Y). The amniotic cavity (A) is separated from the yolk sac by the embryonic disc (arrow with tails). The embryonic disc is composed of three distinct linings (see inset): ectoderm (EC), embryonic mesoderm (EM), and endoderm (EN). (From Hajdu, S. I., and Hajdu, E. O.: Cytopathology of Sarcomas and Other Nonepithelial Malignant Tumors. Philadelphia, W. B. Saunders, 1976).

are organized into specific tissues and then into organs and organ systems (Figs. 1-51, 1-52).

The basic component of differentiated connective tissue are fibroblasts, tissue histiocytes, adipocytes, myocytes, and cells such as mast cells and plasma cells. The shape and size of connective tissue cells are influenced by their genetic coding, growth potentials, and local tissue conditions. We have found, for example, that simple mobilization of growing spindle cells from the surface of the culture tube by trypsin alters the shape of non-neoplastic as well as neoplastic cells. The detached cells following trypsinization become round or oval, and fibroblastic spindle cells appear histiocytic (Figs. 1-53, 1-54). We have shown that the tumor cells which have been treated with trypsin are

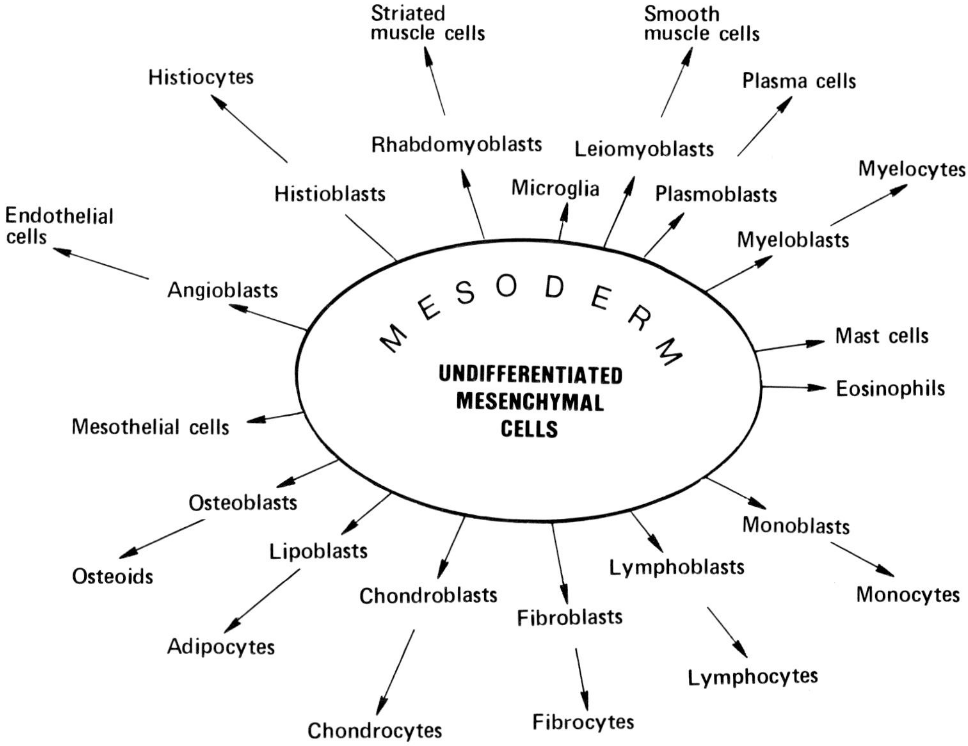

Figure 1-51. Primitive mesenchymal cells may produce any of these forms, and mature cells may dedifferentiate to undifferentiated or poorly differentiated elements.

capable of producing tumor in athymic nude mice identical to that of tumor cells which are transplanted without trypsinization (Hajdu et al, 1974; Helson et al, 1975; Hajdu and Hajdu, 1976; Sethi et al, 1977; Hajdu and Fogh, 1978).

At the present time, despite the well-known fact that mesenchymal cells are multipotential cells and certain differentiated forms such as fibroblasts, tissue histiocytes, pericytes, and Schwann cells retain their multipotential nature, soft tissue tumors are classified according to their dominant cell type and growth pattern (Table 1-10).

Although soft tissue tumors, just like epithelial tumors, can be benign or malignant, in situ soft tissue sarcoma, analogous to carcinoma in situ, is not recognized. Because the in situ or preinvasive form of soft tissue sarcomas is not recognized, grading and staging of these tumors are needed to express their malignant potentials. The first grading system for soft tissue neoplasms was offered by Quick and Cutler in 1927. However, no grading system can be adopted and put into practical use unless there is a clear understanding of the histogenesis and natural history of various tumors.

The exact incidence of soft tissue tumors is unknown, but acording to the American Cancer Society (1979) an estimated 5,000 new cases of soft tissue sarcomas are diagnosed annually in the United States and the estimated deaths are over 2,000. The difficulty in obtaining statistical figures for incidence and mortality is increased by the ambiguity in terminology. The 40 major forms of soft tissue sarcomas (Table 1-10) are known in the literature by more than 300 synonyms.

I believe Abernethy (1809) was the first to show that the various growths constituting tumors ought to be distinguished and characterized by the differences of their structure, and the tendency to characterize tumors according to the most

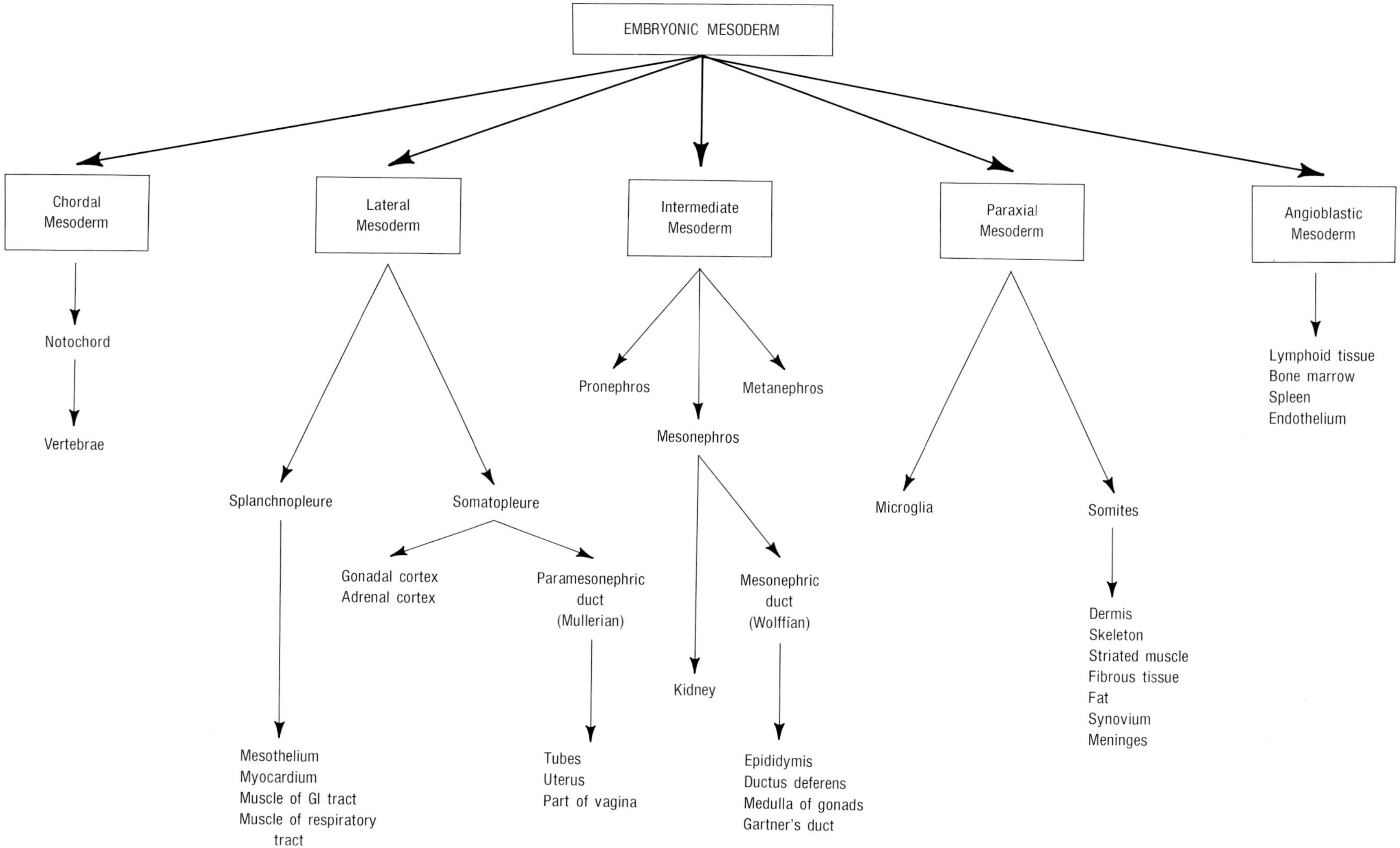

Figure 1-52. Schematic illustration of the origin of various organs and organ systems from the embryonic mesoderm through a series of intermediate structures. Note the role of the *lateral mesoderm* in the development of the mesothelial lining, the smooth muscle, and female genitalia. Practically all soft tissues and the skeleton develop from the *paraxial mesoderm;* the entire lymphoreticular system originates from the *angioblastic mesoderm* (From Hajdu, S. I., and Hajdu, E. O.: Cytopathology of *Sarcomas and Nonepithelial Malignant Tumors.* Philadelphia, W. B. Saunders, 1976.)

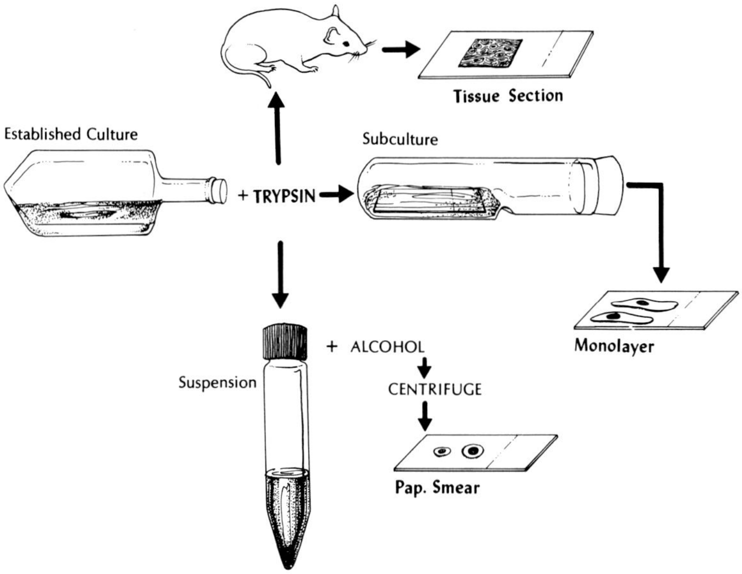

Figure 1-53. Tissue cultures established from human tumors are carried through subpassages and transplanted into athymic "nude" mice.

striking features has continued to this day. Ewing, in 1931, wrote: "The grade of potential malignancy is very important information regarding any tumor. The more carefully the pathologist investigates this field of study, the more apparent it becomes that the course is chiefly determined by its potential malignancy." To this Stout added in 1964 that the potential malignancy of any given tumor varies from site to site. He said, "There is such a great difference in the behavior of tumors bearing the same name, but developing in different parts of the body, that in reporting a case the pathologist should not only give the growth a name but explain how it can be expected to behave in the region where it has arisen. . . . Sarcomas vary in

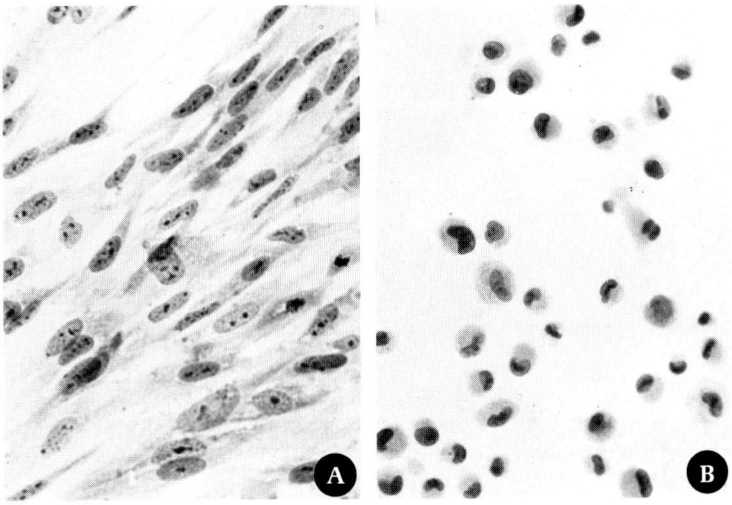

Figure 1-54. A, Human fibroblast (WI 38) in monolayer culture. The fibroblasts are long spindly cells with oval clear nuclei (Papanicolaou ×350).

B, Fibroblast of cell line WI 38 in smear prepared from trypsinized monolayer culture. Here the cells are oval or round with displaced semilunar nuclei resembling histiocytes. (Pananicolaou ×350). (From Hajdu, S. I., and Hajdu, E. O.: Cytopathology of Sarcomas and Other Nonepithelial Malignant Tumors. Philadelphia, W. B. Saunders, 1976.

TABLE 1-10. ***Classification of Soft Tissue Tumors and Tumor-like Lesions****

SITE	NON-NEOPLASTIC LESIONS	BENIGN NEOPLASTIC LESIONS	MALIGNANT NEOPLASTIC LESIONS
TUMORS OF FIBROUS TISSUE (see Chapter 2)	Fasciitis Keloid Elastofibroma Fibromatosis	Benign fibroblastic fibrous histiocytoma Benign histiocytic fibrous histiocytoma Benign pleomorphic fibrous histiocytoma Fibroma Myxoma	Malignant fibroblastic fibrous histiocytoma Malignant histiocytic fibrous histocytoma Malignant pleomorphic fibrous histiocytoma Desmoid tumor Fibroblastic fibrosarcoma Pleomorphic fibrosarcoma
TUMORS OF TENDOSYNOVIAL TISSUE (see Chapter 3)	Tendosynovial cyst Tendosynovitis Synovial chondromatosis	Fibroma Lipoma Villonodular synovitis Benign giant cell tumor	Malignant giant cell tumor Biphasic tendosynovial sarcoma Monophasic spindle cell type tendosynovial sarcoma Monophasic pseudoglandular tendosynovial sarcoma Epithelioid sarcoma Clear cell sarcoma Chordoid sarcoma
TUMORS OF ADIPOSE TISSUE (see Chapter 4)	Fat necrosis Lipogranuloma Lipodystrophia Piezogenic papules Adiposis dolorosa Steatopygia	Well-differentiated lipoma Myxoid lipoma Fibroblastic lipoma Pleomorphic lipoma Angiolipoma Angiomyolipoma Myelolipoma Lipoblastoma Hibernoma	Well-differentiated liposarcoma Myxoid liposarcoma Lipoblastic liposarcoma Fibroblastic liposarcoma Pleomorphic liposarcoma
TUMORS OF MUSCLE (see Chapter 5)	Atrophy Dystrophy Polymyositis Rhabdomyolysis Proliferative myositis Fibromatosis Myositis ossificans	Leiomyoma Angiomyolipoma Rhabdomyoma	Leiomyosarcoma Leiomyoblastoma Embryonal rhabdomyosarcoma Pleomorphic rhabdomyosarcoma Rhabdomyoblastoma
TUMORS OF VESSELS (see Chapter 6)	Pyogenic granuloma Angioblastic lymphoid hyperplasia Hereditary hemorrhagic telangiectasia Arteriovenous fistula	Capillary hemangioma Cavernous hemangioma Venous hemangioma Papillary endothelial hyperplasia Hypertrophic hemangioma Angiomatosis Angiofibroma Angiolipoma Angiomyolipoma Hemangioblastoma Glomus tumor Lymphangioma Lymphangiomyoma	Hemangiopericytoma Hemangiosarcoma Kaposi's sarcoma Lymphangiosarcoma

TABLE 1-10. ***Classification of Soft Tissue Tumors and Tumor-like Lesions* (*Continued*)**

SITE	NON-NEOPLASTIC LESIONS	BENIGN NEOPLASTIC LESIONS	MALIGNANT NEOPLASTIC LESIONS
TUMORS OF PERIPHERAL NERVE (see Chapter 7)	Degeneration Hypertrophy Traumatic neuroma	Neurofibroma Neurofibromatosis Angioneuroma Plexiform neuroma Pacinian neurofibroma Glandular schwannoma Pleomorphic schwannoma Cystic schwannoma Storiform schwannoma Epithelioid schwannoma	Malignant collagenous schwannoma Malignant, non-collagenous schwannoma Primitive neuroectodermal tumor
EXTRASKELETAL BONE TUMORS (see Chapter 8)	Chondroid metaplasia Osteoid-metaplasia Myositis ossificans	Chondroma Osteochondroma Osteoma	Osteogenic sarcoma Chondrosarcoma Ewing's sarcoma
MISCELLANEOUS SOFT TISSUE TUMORS (see Chapter 9)		Benign granular cell tumor Benign mesenchymoma	Malignant granular cell tumor Alveolar soft part sarcoma Malignant lymphoma Granulocytic sarcoma Plasmacytoma Postirradiation sarcoma Malignant mesenchymoma Undifferentiated soft tissue sarcoma

*This classification is followed closely and adhered to as far as possible throughout this book. For synonyms and related terms see individual chapters.

prognosis and natural history, depending on cell type, anatomic site and the patient's age."

During the 1960's as various therapeutic protocols combining surgery, irradiation and chemotherapy were introduced, it became clear that a classification scheme of primary soft tissue sarcomas was much needed. The Soft Tissue Task Force of the American Joint Committee published its grading and staging system in 1977 (Russell et al, 1977). This classification is based on histologic grade and gross size of the tumors with consideration of presence or absence of metastatic tumor (Table 1-11). Members of the Task Force recognized that the proposed staging scheme is far from perfect and certain adjustment is needed.

Anybody attempting to assess the malignant potentials of a soft tissue sarcoma must consider its *histologic type, size, site,* and *degree of differentiation,* but what Bucy and Gustafson said in 1939 must be remembered: "Classification must be regarded as providing merely arbitrary pockets into which we can place tumors in order that they may be more easily considered."

By proposing the following staging system of soft tissue sarcomas, which is a modified form of the staging scheme developed by the Soft Tissue Task Force (Table 1-11), I am aware that I lay myself open to criticism, but I believe that progress is made occasionally only by presenting controversial issues. During the development of the revised staging system I kept in mind what Virchow said at the XI International Congress of Medicine in Rome, in 1894: "Medicine is based on an enormous heap of individual facts which

TABLE 1-11. *Staging of Soft Tissue Sarcomas, According to the Soft Tissue Task Force, 1977**

STAGE	GRADE†	SIZE‡	METASTASIS§	
Stage IA	G_1	T_1	N_0	M_0
Stage IB	G_1	T_2	N_0	M_0
Stage IIA	G_2	T_1	N_0	M_0
Stage IIB	G_2	T_2	N_0	M_0
Stage IIIA	G_3	T_1	N_0	M_0
Stage IIIB	G_3	T_2	N_0	M_0
Stage IIIC	G_1-G_3	T_1-T_2	N_1	M_0
Stage IVA	G_1-G_3	T_3	N_0-N_1	M_0
Stage IVB	G_1-G_3	T_1-T_3	N_0-N_1	M_1

*See Russell et al, 1977.

†G_1 = low grade sarcoma; G_2 = intermediate grade sarcoma; G_3 = high grade sarcoma.

‡T_1 = sarcoma less than 5 cm; T_2 = sarcoma 5 cm or greater; T_3 = sarcoma that grossly invades bone, major vessel, or major nerve.

§N_0 = no histologically verified metastasis to regional lymph nodes; N_1 = histologically verified regional lymph node metastasis; M_0 = no distant metastasis; M_1 = distant metastasis.

appear to confuse the mind of many. But for him who masters the facts on which the new views are founded, an order is revealed, that departing from a general biological principle, permits the facts to be connected according to their mutual relationship."

The staging system I propose is based on the review of the clinicopathologic records and histopathologic material of more than 2,400 patients who were treated for soft tissue sarcoma at Memorial Sloan-Kettering Cancer Center during the period of 1950–1974 (Table 1-12). While designing this grading and staging system I also obtained information from autopsied cases (Table 1-13) and from soft tissue sarcomas grown in tissue culture and athymic "nude" mice.

First of all, the reader is reminded that proper and specific histologic identification of soft tissue neoplasms must be attempted. By doing so it is hoped that one is able to place the tumor in one or another category or grade (Table 1-14). Of course, *in limited material we must be satisfied that we can tell whether the lesion is benign or malignant.*

TABLE 1-12. *2,489 Patients, Treated for Soft Tissue Sarcoma at Memorial Sloan-Kettering Cancer Center from 1950 to 1974*

HISTOLOGIC TYPE	NO. OF CASES
Malignant fibrous histiocytoma	392
Fibrosarcoma (including desmoid)	358
Tendosynovial sarcoma	187
Liposarcoma	416
Embryonal rhabdomyosarcoma	398
Pleomorphic rhabdomyosarcoma	148
Angiosarcoma	212
Neurogenic sarcoma	141
Alveolar soft part sarcoma	51
Miscellaneous sarcoma	186

In addition to histologic type, the size, site, and histologic grade of the tumor are the most important factors to consider in prognosis (Fig. 1-55). Once the size, site, and histologic grade (Fig. 1-56) are defined, the stage of the primary tumor can be estimated (Fig. 1-57). It should be pointed out that the value of counting mitoses in soft tissue sarcomas has been debated from the time mitosis is known. Most writers agree that mitosis counting is subjective and not reliable. Therefore, one

TABLE 1-13. *Soft Tissue Sarcomas at Autopsy (1950–1974)**

HISTOLOGIC TYPE	NO. OF CASES
Embryonal rhabdomyosarcoma	98
Malignant fibrous tumor	34
Tendosynovial sarcoma	30
Liposarcoma	29
Angiosarcoma	27
Pleomorphic rhabdomyosarcoma	27
Miscellaneous sarcoma	20
Malignant schwannoma	14
Leiomyosarcoma	13
	292

*See autopsy findings at the end of individual chapters.

TABLE 1-14. *Listing of Soft Tissue Sarcomas According to Histologic Grade**

LOW GRADE	HIGH GRADE
Dermatofibrosarcoma protuberans	Pleomorphic fibrosarcoma
Desmoid tumor	Tendosynovial sarcoma, monophasic spindle cell type
Chordoid sarcoma	Lipoblastic liposarcoma
Well-differentiated liposarcoma	Pleomorphic liposarcoma
Myxoid liposarcoma	Embryonal rhabdomyosarcoma
Kaposi's sarcoma	Pleomorphic rhabdomyosarcoma
Malignant granular cell tumor	Lymphangiosarcoma
Alveolar soft part sarcoma	Primitive neuroectodermal tumor
	Osteogenic sarcoma
	Ewing's sarcoma
	Granulocytic sarcoma

* Soft tissue sarcomas that are not listed here can be either high grade or low grade (see Figure 1-56).

	GOOD PROGNOSTIC SIGNS	BAD PROGNOSTIC SIGNS
SIZE	Small	Big
SITE	Superficial	Deep
HISTOLOGIC GRADE	Low	High

Figure 1-55. Factors influencing prognosis.

SIZE

SMALL = Less than 5 cm
BIG = More than 5 cm

SITE

SUPERFICIAL = {Not beyond superficial fascia}

DEEP = {Beyond superficial fascia}

HISTOLOGIC GRADE

LOW GRADE	HIGH GRADE
Hypocellular	Hypercellular
Much stroma	Minimal stroma
Minimal necrosis	Much necrosis
Good maturation	Poor maturation
Mitosis $<$ 5/10 HPF	Mitosis $>$ 5/10 HPF

Figure 1-56. Size, site, and histologic grade.

STAGE 0 TUMOR = {3 Good Prognostic Signs}

STAGE 1 TUMOR = {2 Good Prognostic Signs + 1 Bad Prognostic Sign}

STAGE II TUMOR = {1 Good Prognostic Sign + 2 Bad Prognostic Signs}

STAGE III TUMOR = {3 Bad Prognostic Signs}

STAGE IV TUMOR = {Evidence of Metastasis}

Figure 1-57. Stages of primary tumor.

should not depend solely on the mitotic count in the prognostication of soft tissue tumors. Ironically, some of the non-neoplastic lesions, e.g., pyogenic granuloma, may have more mitotic figures than most of the fully malignant sarcomas.

As an aid to remembering, the various prognostic signs can be illustrated in circles, in which the upper light halves indicate good prognostic signs and the lower, dark halves are signs of bad prognosis (Fig. 1-58). From this, for easy reference, the composite illustrated in Figure 1-59 can be put together.

Table 1-15 lists the most common soft tissue sarcomas discussed in this book according to histologic type and stage of

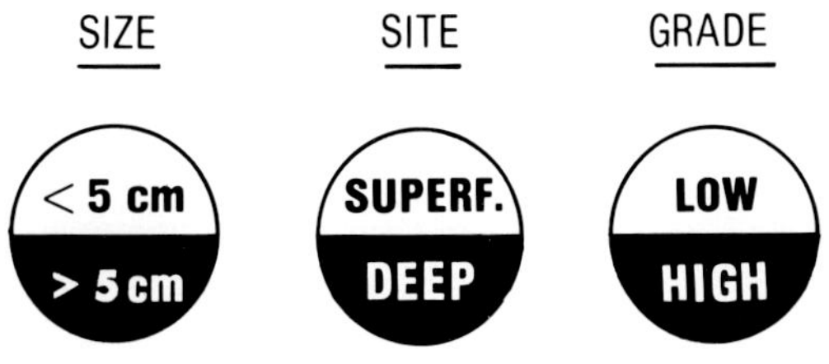

Figure 1-58. Good prognostic signs are shown in the white half of the circles and bad prognostic signs are illustrated by the dark semicircles.

the primary lesion. This staging should serve as a baseline for future studies. To the critics I would like to repeat what Stout used to say: "Pathologists are fallible like everyone else." Let us minimize the impact of our mistakes and above all let us learn from every mistake we make.

The past decade has been a time of reconsideration of tumors according to histogenesis. More progress has been made in understanding the natural history of soft tissue tumors than in any other decade, but we must continue the efforts to find the functional differences between normal and neoplastic mesenchymal cells if we want to make real progress.

Soft tissue tumors have been long neglected and therapy has improved little since Stout said in 1953, "Mesenchymal tumors of the soft tissues are the least understood and probably the most inadequately treated of all tumors." The same view was expressed by Bowden and Booher, two surgeons, in 1958: "No neoplasms are more indifferently treated in contemporary practice than soft tissue sarcomas."

TABLE 1-15. ***Case Fatality Rate of Soft Tissue Sarcomas According to Histologic Type and Stage of Primary Tumor during a Period of 25 Years***

HISTOLOGIC TYPE	TOTAL NO. OF CASES STAGED*	STAGE AND MORTALITY IN (%)*					
		I†	(%)	II†	(%)	III†	(%)
Malignant fibroblastic fibrous histiocytoma‡	130	1/76	(1)	7/42	(16)	11/12	(92)
Malignant histiocytic fibrous histiocytoma§	24	0/8	(0)	1/3	(33)	12/13	(92)
Malignant pleomorphic fibrous histocytoma	125	0/9	(0)	12/32	(38)	60/84	(71)
Desmoid tumor	160	2/58	(3)	15/102	(15)	-	-
Fibrosarcoma‖	114	1/4	(25)	16/42	(38)	52/68	(76)
Tendosynovial sarcoma	120	1/3	(33)	26/66	(39)	48/51	(94)
Liposarcoma	220	1/9	(11)	26/98	(27)	75/113	(66)
Embryonal rhabdomyosarcoma	240	-	-	35/58	(60)	137/182	(75)
Pleomorphic rhabdomyosarcoma	88	-	-	12/21	(57)	62/67	(93)
Hemangiosarcoma¶	30	1/6	(17)	7/8	(88)	15/16	(94)
Neurogenic sarcoma**	80	9/16	(56)	22/29	(76)	33/35	(94)
Total	1331	16/189	(8)	179/501	(36)	505/641	(79)

*Patients who were admitted with metastatic tumor are not included. Also excluded are 17 patients who had stage 0 tumor. Twelve had malignant fibrous histiocytoma and 5 patients had desmoid tumor. All 17 patients who had stage 0 sarcoma are alive and well. See individual chapters for 5-year and 10-year survival figures.

†Numerator: died with disease; denominator: total number of patients.

‡These are all dermatofibrosarcoma protuberans except the 12 Stage III tumors.

§These are all malignant giant cell tumors of soft tissue.

‖Fibrosarcoma other than desmoid.

¶Kaposi's sarcoma is not included.

**Includes malignant collagenous and non-collagenous schwannomas.

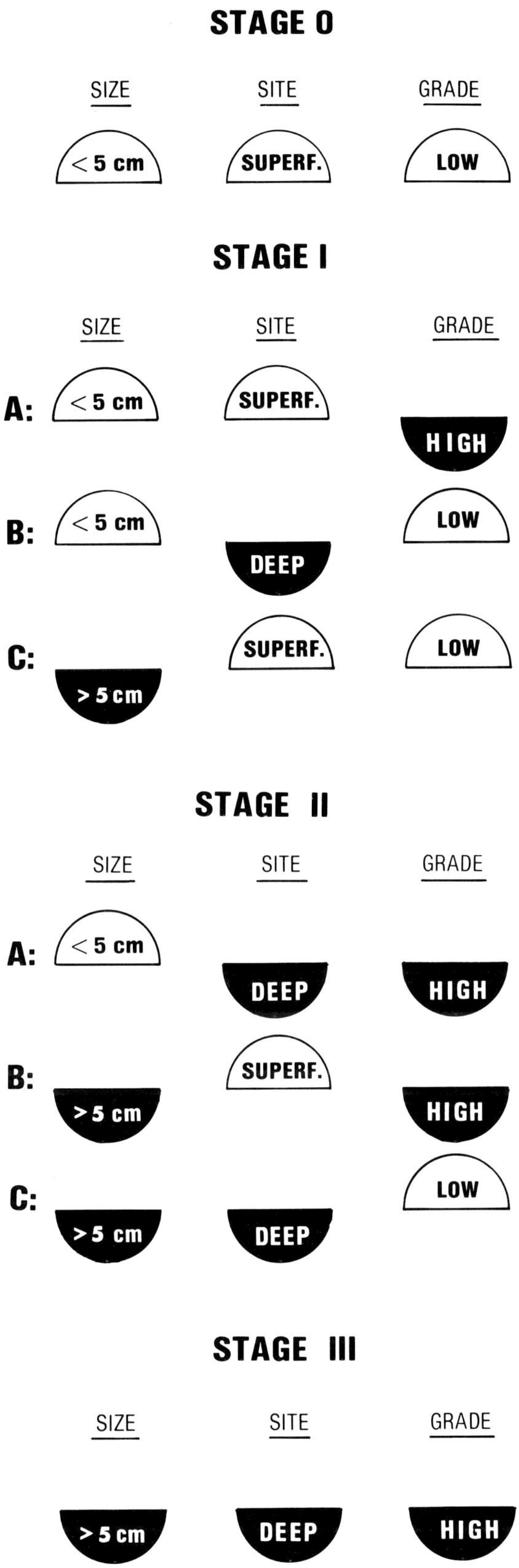

Figure 1-59. Correlation among size, site, histologic grade, and stage of the primary soft tissue sarcomas.

Three good prognostic signs indicate *Stage 0* sarcoma.

Two good prognostic signs and one bad sign indicate *Stage I* sarcoma.

One good prognostic sign and two bad ones are consistent with *Stage II* sarcoma.

Three bad prognostic signs indicate *Stage III* neoplasm.

Metastatic soft tissue sarcomas should be considered *Stage IV* lesions. (*Stage IV A* indicates regional metastasis; *Stage IV B* denotes distant metastasis.)

The radiologist's ability to evaluate soft tissue tumors by plain film examination is limited. However, angiography, radiography density measurement coupled with computerized transaxial tomography (CT), and the use of radioactive isotopes offer new potentials in diagnosis (Samuels, 1972; Martel and Abel, 1973).

Irradiation therapy, the way it is given at most institutions, except in cases of embryonal rhabdomyosarcoma and myxoid liposarcoma has no proven and long lasting beneficial effect on soft tissue sarcomas in the majority of cases. Many patients undoubtedly could benefit from medical oncologic treatment provided it is administered under controlled conditions before the far advanced stages of the disease.

Future studies are needed to add to our basic knowledge concerning the morphology and therapy of soft tissue tumors. It is the duty of the pathologist to inform the clinician about the diagnosis, differential diagnosis, and the natural history of any given tumor, but it is also the duty of the pathologist to study the tumor cells with all available techniques in an attempt to show the way to new and improved modalities of therapy.

REFERENCES

Maurus, R.: De Sermonum Proprietate, Seu de Universo. Strassburg, A. Rusch, 1467.

Guy de Chauliac: La Pratique en chirurgie du maistre Guidon de Chauliac. Lyon, B. Buyer, 1478.

Fernel, I.: Medicina. Physiologia, Pathologia, Therapeutica. Wechelum, Lutetiae Parisiorum, 1554.

Kircher, A.: Ars Magna lucis et umbrae. Rome, 1646.

Harvey, W.: Exercitatio Anatomica de Motu Cordis et Sangvinis in Animalibus. Francofurt, Fitzer, 1628.

Fernel, I.: Morbis Universalibus et Particularibus. Batavorum, Hacki, 1645.

Bartholin, Th.: Vasa Lactea and Lymphatica. Hafniae, P. Hakins, 1656.

Sculteti, I.: Armamentarium Chirurgiae. Amsterdam, Someron, 1672.

Boneti, T.: De ventris tumore, in Sepulchretum, sive anatomia practica excadaveribus morbo denatis, Vol. 3. Geneva, Cramer and Perachon, 1700, p. 522.

Gendron, C. D.: Enquiries into the Nature, Knowledge and Cure of Cancers. (English Translation), London, 1701.

Etmullerus, M.: A Compleat System of the Theory and Practice of Physic. London, A. Bell, 1712.

Leeuwenhoek, A.: Observations on the fibers of the muscles. Philos. Trans. 5:390, 1721.

Helvetius, J. A.: Traite des Maladies les plus fequentes . . . Accompagne de sa lettre sur la nature et la guerison du cancer. Bruxelles, 1731.

De la Croix, F. S.: Pathologia Methodica. Monspeli, Martil, 1739.

Freke, J.: A case of extraordinary exostosis. Philos. Trans. 456, London, 1740.

Peyronie, F.: Sur quelques obstacles qui s'opposent a l'ejaculation naturelle de la semence. Mem. Acad. Roy. Chir. Paris 1:425, 1743.

Hody, E.: An account of a large boney-structure found in the womb. Philos. Trans. 9:191, 1747.

Morgagni, J. B.: De Sedibus, et causis Morborum. Venetiis, Remondiniana, 1761.

Bonn: De Continuationibus Membranarum. Amsterdam, 1763.

Rouppe, L.: De Morbis Navigantium, liber unus. Accedit Observatio de Effectu Extracti Cicutae Storkiano in Cancro. Lugd. Bat., 1764.

Middletown, P.: A Medical Discourse, or an Historical Inquirey into the Ancient and Present State of Medicine. New York, H. Gaine, 1769.

Peyrilhe, B.: Dissertation Academique sur le Cancer. Paris, Ruault, 1776.

Bell, B.: A Treatise on the Theory and Management of Ulcers: With a Dissertation of White Swellings of the Joints. Boston, Thomas and Andrews, 1791.

Baillie, M.: The Morbid Anatomy of Some of the Most Important Parts of the Human Body. Albany, Barber and Southwick, 1795.

Bichat, M. F. X.: Anatomie generale, appliquee a la physiologie et a la medecine. Paris, Brosson, Gabon & Cie, 1801.

Odier, L.: Manuel de Medecine Pratique. Geneve, 1803.

Oken, L.: Die Zeugung. Bambert und Wurzburg, Goebhardt, 1805.

Alibert, J. L. M.: Description des maladies de la peau. Paris, 1806.

Abernethy, J.: Surgical Observations. London, Longman, 1809.

Wardrop, J.: Observations on Fungus Haematodes or Soft Cancer. Edinburgh, Constable, 1809.

Burns, A.: Observation on the Surgical Anatomy of the Head and Neck. Edinburgh, Bryce, 1811.

Bell, C.: Surgical Observations. London, Longman, 1816.

Meckel, J. F.: System der vergleichenden Anatomie. Halle, Renger, 1821–1831.

Andral, G.: Prècis d'Anatomie Pathologique. Paris, Gabon, 1829.

Cruveilhier, J.: Anatomie pathologique du corps humain. Paris, Bailliere, 1829–1835.

Dupuytren, G.: Leçons orales de clinique chirurgicale faites a l'Hotel-Dieu de Paris. Vol. 1, Chap. 1, 1832.

McFarlane, J.: *In* Clinical Reports of the Surgical Practice of the Glasgow Royal Infirmary. Edited by Robertson, 1832, p. 63.

Cooper, S.: The First Lines of the Practice of Surgery. London, Longman, 1836.

Donne, A.: Animalcules observes dans les matieres purulentes et le produit des secretions des organes genitaux de l'homme et de la femme. C. R. Acad. Sci. 3:385, 1836.

Müller, J.: Jahresbericht uber die Fortschritte der anatomischphysiologischen Wissenschaften in Jahre 1835. Arch. Anat. Physiol. Med. 3:175, 1836.

Turpin, P. J.: Observations sur l'organisation tissulaire des secretions produites aux surfaces des membranes muqueuses animales, comparees aux secretions muqueuses productrices et reparatrices des vegetaux. Ann. Sci. Nat. 7:207, 1837.

Velpaeu, A.: Traite complet d'anatomie chirurgical. Paris, 1837.

Müller, J.: Ueber den feinern Bau and die Formen der krankhaften Geschwulste. Berlin, G. Reimer, 1838.

Schwann, T., and Schleiden, M. J.: Mikroskopische Untersuchungen uber die Uebereinstimmung in der struktur und dem Wachstum der Thiere und Pflanzen. Muller's Arch., p. 137, 1838.

Diary of the Rev. John Ward, Extending from 1648 to 1679. Edited and published by Cr. Severn, London, 1839.

Schwann, T.: Mikroskopische Untersuchungen. Berlin, Sander, 1839.

Stafford, R. A.: A case of enlargement from melanoid tumor of the prostate gland in a child five years of age. Med. Chir. Tr. 22:218, 1839.

Mohr, B.: Hypertrophie der Hypophysis cerebri und dadurch bedingter Druck auf die Hirngrundflache, imsbesondere auf die Sehnerven, das Chiasma derselben und den liknseitigen Hirnschenkel. Wschr. ges. Heilk. 6:565, 1840.

Rokitansky, C.: Handbuch der pathologischen Anatomie. Wien, Braumuller u. Seidel, 1842–46.

Zappoli, A.: Lipo-sarcoma. Bull. Soc. Med. Bologna 3:5, 1843.

Lebert, H.: Physologie Pathologique. Paris, Bailliere, 1845.

van Leuw: De macroglossia seu linguae prolapsu. Berol., 1845.

Bennett, J. H.: On Cancerous and Cancroid Growths. Edinburgh, Sutherland and Knox, 1849.

Cruveilhier, J.: Traite d'Anatomie Pathologique Generale. Paris, Bailliere, 1849.

Robin, M. C.: Sur l'existence de deux especes nouvelles d'elements anatomique qui se trouvent dans le canal medullaire de os. C. R. Soc. Biol. 1:149, 1849.

Smith, R. W.: A Treatise on the Pathology, Diagnosis and Treatment of Neuroma. Dublin, Hodges and Smith, 1849.

Kolliker, A.: Mikroskopische Anatomie. Leipzig, Engelmann, 1850.

Michon, L. M.: Des Tumeurs Synoviales. Paris, Germer-Bailliere, 1851.

Broca, M.: Anatomie pathologie du cancer. Mem. Acad. Med. Paris, 1852.

Chassaignac, M.: Tumeur des gaines tendineuses. Gaz. Hôp. Chir. Mil. 47:185, 1852.

King, A.: Case of chloroma. Monthly J. Med. Sci. 7:97, 1853.

Guersant, M. P.: Polypes du vagin chez une petite fille de treize mois. Monit. Hopit. 2:187, 1854.

Rokitansky, C.: A Manual of Pathological Anatomy. London, Sydenham Society, 1954.

Weber, C. O.: Anatomische Untersuchung einer hypertrophische Zunge nebst Besnerkungen uber die Neubildung quergestreifter Muskelfasern. Virchows Arch. [Pathol. Anat.] 7:115, 1854.

Paget, J.: Fibro-nucleated tumor of the abdomen of fourteen years growth: removal. Lancet 1:625, 1856.

Virchow, R.: Die Cellularpathologie in ihrer Begrundung auf physiologische und pathologische Geweblehre. Berlin, A. Hirschwald, 1858.

Virchow, R.: Das wahre Neurom. Arch. Pathol. Anat. Physiol. 13:256, 1858.

Delameter, J.: Mammoth tumor. Cleveland Medical Gazette 1:31, 1859.

Gross, S. D.: A System of Surgery: Pathological, Diagnostic, Therapeutic and Operative. Philadelphia, H. C. Lea, 1859.

Wilks, S.: Lectures on Pathological Anatomy. London, Longman, 1859.

Broca, M.: Tumeur a myeloplaxes de la main. Bull. Soc. Chir. 1:342, 1860.

Virchow, R.: Die krankhaften Geschwulste. Berlin, Hirschwald, 1863.

Moore, C. H.: The antecedents of cancer. Br. Med. J., Aug, 1865.

Simon, G.: Exstirpation einer sehr grossen, mit dicken Stiele angewachsenen Kneigelenkmaus mit gluklichem Erfolge. Arch. Klin. Chir. 6:573, 1865.

Thiersch, C.: Der Epithelialkrebs namentlich der Haut. Leipzig, Engelmann, 1865.

Waldeyer, W.: Grosses Lipo-myxom des Mesenteriums mit secondaren sarcomatosen Heerden in der Leber und Lunge. Virchows Arch. [Pathol. Anat.] 32:543, 1865.

Malhéné, A.: Etude clinique sur la Tumeurs Fibro-Plastiques. Paris, A. Parent, 1866.

Neuman, E.: Ein Fall von Myoma striocellular am Hoden. Virchows Arch. [Pathol. Anat.] 30:497, 1866.

Aufrecht, E.: Ein myom der vena saphena. Virchows Arch. [Pathol. Anat.] 44:133, 1868.

Heller, A.: Multiple Neurome. Virchows Arch. [Pathol. Anat.] 44, 1868.

Munchmeyer, E.: Ueber myositis ossificans progressiva. Z. rat. Med. 34:9, 1869.

Paget, J.: Lectures on Surgical Pathology. London, Longmans and Green and Company, 1870.

Kaposi, M.: Idiopathisches multiples pigment-sarkom der Haut. Arch. Dermatol. Syphil. 4:265, 1872.

Butlin, H. T.: Recurrent ossifying spindlecelled sarcoma from the subcutaneous tissue of the thigh. Trans. Path. Soc. London, 24:211, 1873.

Andrée, C.: Beitrag Zur Lehre von der Entstehung des Geschwulstmetastasen auf embolischem Wege. Virchows Arch. [Pathol. Anat.] 61:383, 1874.

Morton, T. C.: A peculiar and painful affection of the fourth metatarsophalangeal articulation. Am. J. Med. Sci. 71:37, 1876.

Billroth, T.: Lectures on Surgical Pathology and Therapeutics. London, Sydenham Society, 1877–1878.

Cohnheim, J. F.: Vorlesungen uber allgemeine Pathologie. Berlin, Hirschwald, 1877–80.

Ehrlich, P.: Beitrag Zur Kenntnis der Anilinfarbungen und ihrer Verwendung in der mikroskopischen Technik. Arch. Mikr. Anat. 13:263, 1877.

Kolaczek, T.: Uber das Angio-Sarkom. Deutsch. Z. Chir. 9:1; 889, 1878.

Langhans, T.: Pulsirende cavernose Geschwulst der Milz mit metastatischen Knoten

in der leber. Virchows Arch. [Pathol. Anat.] 75:273, 1879.
Takacs, A.: Ueber multiple Neurome. Arch. Path. Anat. Physiol. Klin. Med. 75:431, 1879.
Caen, E.: Chondroosteosarkom der weiblichen Brustdruse. Deutsche Z. Chir. 15:247, 1881.
von Recklinghausen, F.E.: Ueber die multiple Fibrome der Haut und ihre Bezeihung zu den multiplen Neuromen. Berlin, Hirschwald, 1882.
Mason, G. W.: Sarcoma of the spermatic cord with hernia of the vermiform appendix. Med. News 42:554, 1883.
Hertwig, W. A. O.: Lehrbuch der Entwinklungsgeschichte des Menschen und der Wirbelthiere. Jena, G. Fischer, 1886.
Chiari, O.: Erfahrungen auf dem Gebiete der Hals-und-Nasen-Krankheiten. Vienna, Toepflitz und Deuticke, 1887.
Salzer, F.: Myxoma lipomatodes capsulae adiposae renis. Wien Klin. Wochenschr. 1:199, 1888.
Williams, W. R.: The Principle of Cancer and Tumour Formation. London, 1888.
Chauffard, A. M. E.: Xanthelasma dissemine et symmetrique, sans insuffisance hepatique. Bull. Mem. Soc. Med. Hosp. 6:412, 1889.
Hansemann, D.: Ueber asymmetrische Zellteilung in Epithelkrebsen und deren biologische Bedeutung. Virchows Arch. [Pathol. Anat.] 119:229, 1890.
Taylor, R. W.: Sarcomatous tumors resembling in some respects keloid. J. Cutan. Genito-Urin. Dis. 8:384, 1890.
Heurteux, A.: Myelome des gaines tendineuses. Arch. Gen. Med. 28:40; 160, 1891.
Dercum, F. X.: Three cases of hitherto unclassified affection resembling in its grosser aspects obesity, but associated with special nervous symptoms; adiposis dolorosa. Am. J. Med. Sci. 104:521, 1892.
Garré, C.: Uber sekundar maligne Neurome. Beitr. Z. Klin. Chir. 9:465, 1892.
Hamilton, J. B.: Lectures on Tumors from a Clinical Standpoint, 2nd edition. Detroit, G. S. Davis, 1892.
Berard, M.: Tumeur embryonnaire du muscle striae. Lyon Med. 77:52, 1894.
Röntgen, W. C.: Ueber eine neue Art von Strahlen. Sb. Phys.-Med. Ges. Würzburg. 132, 1895.
Mallory, F. B.: Pathological Technique. Philadelphia, W. B. Saunders Company, 1897.
Targett, J. H.: Giant-celled tumeurs of the integuments. Trans. Path. Soc. London 48:230, 1897.
Adami, J. G.: Pathological Notes. Montreal, Lovell and Son, 1898.
Osler, W.: Lectures on the Diagnosis of Abdominal Tumours. New York, Appleton and Company, 1898.
Senn, N.: The Pathology and Surgical Treatment of Tumors. Philadelphia, W. B. Saunders Company, 1900.
Thomson, R.: On Neuroma and Neurofibromatosis. Edinburgh, Turnbull and Spears, 1900.
Bellamy, H.: The myeloid tumour of tendon sheaths. J. Pathol. Bacteriol. 7:405, 1901.
Borst, M.: Die Lehre von den Geschwulsten mit einem mikroskopischen Atlas. Wiesbaden, Bergmann, 1902.
Benenati, U.: Uber einen fall von Rhabdomyom in einen verlagerten Hoden. Virchows Arch. [Pathol. Anat.] 171:418, 1903.
Woglom, W.H.: The Study of Experimental Cancer. New York, Columbia University Press, 1903.
Albrecht, D.: Uber Hamartome. Verh. Dtsch. Ges. Pathol. 7:153, 1904.
Benda, C.: Ganglioneurome des N. vagus. Verh. Dtsch. Ges. Pathol. 7:266, 1904.
Hartzell, M. B.: Granuloma pyogenicum. J. Cutan. Dis. 22:520, 1904.
Walker, C. E.: On the cytology of malignant growths. Trans. Path. Soc. 4:449, 1904.
Albarran, J. M.: Retention renale par periureterite. Assoc. Fr. Urol. 9:511, 1905.
Gordon-Taylor, G.: Giant cells in sarcoma. Arch. Msex. Hosp. 5:223, 1905.
Mallory, F. B.: The results of the application of special histological methods to the study of tumors. J. Exp. Med. 10:575, 1908.
Verocay, J.: Multiple Geschwulste als Systemerkrankung am nervosen Apparate. Wien, W. Braumuller, 1908.
Williams, W. R.: The Natural History of Cancer, New York, W. Wood and Company, 1908.
Carrel, A., and Burrows, M. T.: Cultivation of sarcoma outside of the body. JAMA 55:1554, 1910.
Harrison, R. G.: The outgrowth of the nerve fiber as a mode of protoplasmic movement. J. Exp. Zool. 9:787, 1910.
Lejars, F. and Rubens-Duval, H.: Les sarcomes primitifs des synoviales articulaires. Rev. Chir. 41:751, 1910.
Rous, F. P.: A transmissible avian neoplasm (sarcoma of the common fowl). J. Exp. Med. 12:696, 1910.
Verocay, J.: Zur Kenntnis der "Neurofibrome." Beitr. Pathol. Anat. Allg. Path. 48:1, 1910.
Wohlgemuth, H.: Demonstration eines Myxosarkome aus einen Lipom enstanden. Verh. Berl. Med. Gesellsch. 40:22, 1910.
Lambert, R. A., and Hanes, F. M.: Growth *in vitro* of the transplantable sarcomas of rats and mice. JAMA 7:33, 1911.
McDonagh, J. E. R.: A contribution to our knowledge of the naevoxanthoendotheliomata. Br. J. Dermatol. 24:85, 1912.
Coley, W. B.: Myositis ossificans traumatica. Ann. Surg. 57:305, 1913.

Burgess, A. M.: Malignant rhabdomyoma with multiple metastases. J. Med. Res. 29:447, 1913–1914.

Losee, J. R., and Ebeling, A. H.: The cultivation of human sarcomatous tissue *in vitro.* J. Exp. Med. 20:140, 1914.

Mallory, F. B.: The Principles of Pathologic Histology. Philadelphia, W. B. Saunders Company, 1914.

Kettle, E. H.: The Pathology of Tumors. New York, P. B. Hoebner, 1916.

Marinesco, G., and Minea, J.: Deux cas de maladie de Dercum avec culture des tumeurs "in vitro." C. R. Soc. Biol. 79:866, 1916.

Jaidka, K. C.: Ossifying sarcoma of vastus externus. Brit. Med. J. 2:379, 1919.

Antoni, N. R. E.: Uber Ruckenmarkstumoren und Neurofibrome. Munchen und Wiesbaden, J. F. Bergmann, 1920.

Ewing, J.: Diffuse endothelioma of bone. Proc. N.Y. Path. Soc. 21:17, 1921.

Ewing, J.: Neoplastic Diseases, 2nd edition. Philadelphia, W. B. Saunders Company, 1922.

Schmincke, A.: Kongenitale Herzhypertrophie, bedingt durch diffuse Rhabdomyombildung. Beitr. Pathol. 70:513, 1922.

Sokoloff, B.: The nucleo-cytoplasmic ratio and cancer. J. Cancer Res. 7:395, 1922.

Lewis, W. H., and Gey, G. O.: Clasmatocytes and tumor cells in cultures of mouse sarcoma. Bull. Johns Hopkins Hosp. November, 369, 1923.

Zimmerman, K. W.: Der Feinerg Bau der Blutkapillaren Ertwichlungesch. Zr. Anat. 68:20, 1923.

Aschoff, K. A. L.: Das reticulo-endotheliale System. Ergeb. Inn. Med. 26:1, 1924.

Barre, J. A., and Masson, P.: Etude anatomoclinique de certaines tumeurs sousunguealles douloureuses. Bull. Soc. Franc. Dermat. Syphil. 31:148, 1924.

Darier, J., and Ferrand, M.: Dermatofibromes progressifs et recidivants ou fibrosarcomes de la peau. Ann. Dermatol. Syphil. 5:545, 1924.

Jura, V.: Sulla mesenterite retrattile e sclerosante. Policlinico 31:575, 1924.

Sakurane, K. A.: A case of fibroma durum multiplex of the fingers and toes of an infant. Jap. J. Dermatol. 24:8, 1924.

Fischer, A.: Observations on the division of sarcoma cells in vitro. J. Cancer Res. 9:71, 1925.

Gilford, H.: Tumors and Cancers. A Biological Study. London, Selwyn and Blount, 1925.

Levy, G.: Xanthelasma et xanthome. Ann. Anat. pathol. 2:247, 1925.

Abrikossoff, A. L.: Uber Myome, ausgehend von der quergestreiften willkurlichen Muskulatur. Virchows Arch. [Pathol. Anat.] 260:215, 1926.

Christopher, F.: Giant cell sarcoma apparently arising from the aponeurosis of the forearm. JAMA 87:167, 1926.

Fischer, A.: Umvandlung von Fibroblasten zu Makrophagen in vitro. Arch. Exp. Zellfr. 3:345, 1926–27.

Jaffe, R. H.: Recurrent lipomatous tumours of the groin. Liposarcoma and lipoma pseudomyxomatodes. Arch. Pathol. 1:381, 1926.

Diss, A.: Un nouveau type de tumeur musculaire; le rhabdomyome granulocellulaire. Bull. Assoc. Franc. Cancer 16:862, 1927.

Fell, H. B., and Andrews, J. A.: A cytological study of cultures in vitro of Jensen's rat sarcoma. Br. J. Exp. Pathol. 8:413, 1927.

Quick, D., and Cutler, M.: Neurogenic sarcoma: a clinical and pathological study. Ann. Surg. 86:810, 1927.

Montpellier, J.: Les rhabdomyomes. Caracteres genereux et varietes anatomo-clinique. Bull. Assoc. Franc. Cancer 18:538, 1929.

Martin, H. E., and Ellis, E. B.: Biopsy by needle puncture and aspirates. Ann. Surg. 92:119, 1930.

Potter, R. P.: Intrathoracic tumors: Case report. Radiology 14:60, 1930.

Masson, P.: Experimental and spontaneous schwannomas. Am. J. Pathol. 8:367, 1932.

Adair, F. E.: Cancer. Philadelphia, J. B. Lippincott Company, 1931.

Ewing, J.: Causation, Diagnosis and Treatment of Cancer. Baltimore, Wiliams & Wilkins Company, 1931.

Phemister, D. E.: Undifferentiated round-cell sarcomas. Ann. Surg. 93:125, 1931.

Stewart, F. W.: Primary liposarcoma of the bone. Am. J. Pathol. 7:87, 1931.

Stewart, F. W., and Copeland, M. M.: Neurogenic sarcoma. Am. J. Cancer 15:1235, 1931.

Woringer, F.: Histiocytoma of the leg. Bull. Soc. Franc. Dermat. Syphil. 38:1401, 1931.

Cellina, M.: Il reticolo-endotelioma (istiocitoma) primitivo del fegato. Arch. It. Anat. Histol. Path. 3:421, 1932.

Klein, W.: Mesenchymoma. J. Med. Soc. N.J. 29:774, 1932.

Millar, W. G.: A malignant melanotic tumor of ganglion cells arising from a thoracic sympathetic ganglion. J. Pathol. Bacteriol. 35:351, 1932.

Seidelin, H.: Liposarcoma with chordoma-like cells. Acta Pathol. microbiol. Scand. 9:289, 1932.

Klemperer, P.: Myoblastoma of striated muscle. Am. J. Cancer 20:324, 1934.

Sabrazes, J., Loubat, E., DeGrailly, R., and Magendie, J.: Synovial-sarcomes. Gaz. Hebd. Sci. Méd. Bordeaux 55:754, 1934.

Bartkowiak, Z.: Ein Fall von Sarcoma leiomyoblasticum der Haut. Zentralb. Allg. Pathol. 65:179, 1936.

Geormatigh, N., Venderlinden, P., and Puysselier, R.: Lypocytomes et lipocytoses (lipoblastomes et lipoblastoses). Cancer 13:3, 1936.

Hudson, O. C.: Intra-uterine fibrosarcoma of the foot. Am. J. Cancer 26:568, 1936.

Warren, S., and Sommer, G. N. J.: Fibrosarcoma of soft parts; with special reference to recurrence and metastasis. Arch. Surg. 32:425, 1936.

Carrell, A., and Lindbergh, C. A.: The Culture of Organs. New York, P. B. Hoeber, 1938.

Bucy, P.C., and Gustafson, W. A.: Structure, nature and classification of cerebellar astrocytomas. Am. J. Cancer 35:327, 1939.

Meyer, K., Smyth, E. M., and Dawson, M. H.: The isolation of a mucopolysaccharide from synovial fluid. J. Biol. Chem. 128:319, 1939.

Potozky, H., and Fried, J. R.: Ewing's tumor simulating sarcoma of soft-tissue origin. Am. J. Cancer 36:1, 1939.

Steiner, P.: Metastasizing fibroleiomyoma of the uterus. Am. J. Pathol. 15:89, 1939.

Stout, A. P.: Solitary cutaneous and subcutaneous leiomyoma. Am. J. Cancer 29:435, 1939.

Brinkley, J. S., and Stewart, F. W.: Morphogenesis of extraskeletal osteogenic sarcoma and pseudo-osteosarcoma. Arch. Pathol. 29:42, 1940.

Wells, H. G.: Occurrence and significance of congenital malignant neoplasms. Arch. Pathol. 30:535, 1940.

Papanicolaou, G. N., and Traut, H. F.: The diagnostic value of vaginal smears in carcinoma of the uterus. Am. J. Obstet. Gynecol. 42:193, 1941.

Murray, M. R., and Stout, A. P.: Demonstration and formation of reticulin by schwannian tumor cells in vitro. Am. J. Pathol. 18:585, 1942.

Murray, M. R., and Stout, A. P.: The glomus tumor: Investigation of its distribution and behavior and the identity of its "epitheloid" cell. Am. J. Pathol. 18:183, 1942.

Stout, A. P., and Murray, M. R.: Hemangiopericytoma: A vascular tumor featuring Zimmerman's pericytes. Ann. Surg. 116:26, 1942.

Ackerman, L. V., and Stout, A. P.: Leiomyosarcoma of arm. J. Missouri Med. Assoc. 44:592, 1947.

Porter, K. K., and Thompson, H. P.: Some morphological features of cultured rat sarcoma cells as revealed by the electron microscope. Cancer Res. 7:431, 1947.

Stewart, F.W.: Case #24. Division of Lab. and Res., Albany, New York, 1948.

Stewart, F. W., and Treves, N.: Lymphangiosarcoma in post-mastectomy lymphedema: A report of six cases in elephantiasis chirurgica. Cancer 1:64, 1948.

Koback, M. W., and Perlow, S.: Xanthomatous giant cell tumors arising in soft tissue. Report of an instance of malignant growth. Arch. Surg. 59:909, 1949.

Murray, M. R., Stout, A. P., and Pogogeff, I. A.: Synovial sarcoma and normal synovial tissue cultivated in vitro. Ann. Surg. 31A:619, 1949.

Morgan, G. S., Straumfjord, J. V., and Hall, E. J.: Angiomyolipoma of the kidney. J. Urol. 65:525, 1951.

Christopherson, W. M., Foote, F. W., and Stewart, F. W.: Alveolar soft part sarcoma; structurally characteristic tumors of uncertain histogenesis. Cancer 5:100, 1952.

Grailly, R., Leger, H., and Biraben, J.: Contribution a l'étude histologique du potential de recidive de certaines tumeurs d'origine mesenchymateuse. Bull. Assoc. Franc. 39:306, 1952.

Bennett, H. S., and Porter, K. R.: An electron microscope study of sectioned breast muscle of the domestic fowl. Am. J. Anat. 93:61, 1953.

Gardner, E. J., and Richards, R. C.: Multiple cutaneous and subcutaneous lesions occurring simultaneously with hereditary polyposis and osteomatosis. Am. J. Human Genetics 5:139, 1953.

Keasbey, L. E.: Juvenile aponeurotic fibroma (calcifying fibroma). A distinctive tumor arising in the palms and soles of young children. Cancer 6:338, 1953.

Stout, A. P.: Tumors of the Soft Tissues. Washington, D.C., Armed Forces Institute of Pathology, 1953.

Enterline, H. T., and Roberts, B.: Lymphangiopericytoma. Cancer 8:582, 1955.

Fischer, E. R.: Histochemical observations on an alveolar soft part sarcoma with reference to histogenesis. Am. J. Pathol. 32:721, 1956.

Hicks, J. D.: Synovial cysts in bone. Aust. N.Z. J. Surg. 26:138, 1956.

Reye, R. K.: A consideration of certain subdermal "fibromatous tumours" of infancy. J. Pathol. Bacteriol. 72:149, 1956.

Riopelle, J. I., and Theriault, J. P.: Sur une forme meconnue de sarcome des parties molles: le rhabdomyosarcome alveolaire. Ann. Anat. Pathol. 1:88, 1956.

Bednar, B.: Storiform neurofibromas of the skin, pigmented and nonpigmented. Cancer 10:368, 1957.

Bluefarb, S.: Kaposi's Sarcoma. Springfield, Illinois, Charles C Thomas Company, 1957.

Bowden, L., and Booher, R. J.: The principles and technique of resection of soft parts for sarcoma. Surgery 44:963, 1958.

Pack, G. T., and Ariel, I. M.: Tumors of the Soft Somatic Tissues. A Clinical Treatise. New York, Paul B. Hoeber, Inc., 1958.

Vellios, F., Baez, J., and Shumacker, H. B.: Lipoblastomatosis: A tumor of fetal fat different from hibernoma. Am. J. Pathol. 34:1149, 1958.

Lichtenstein, L., and Bernstein, D.: Unusual benign and malignant chondroid tumors of bone. Cancer 12:1142, 1959.

Rich, C., and Myers, W. P. L.: Excretion of acid mucopolysaccharides in the urine of patients with malignant neoplastic diseases. J. Lab. Clin. Med. 54:223, 1959.

Kern, W. H.: Proliferative myositis: a pseudosarcomatous reaction to injury. Arch. Pathol. 69:209, 1960.

Luse, S. A.: A synovial sarcoma studied by electron microscopy. Cancer 13:312, 1960.

Martin, J. F., Bazin, P., Feroldi, J., and Cabanne, F.: Tumeurs myoides intra-murales de l'estomac. Ann. Anat. Pathol. 5:484, 1960.

Hiramoto, R., Jurandowski, J., Bernecky, J., and Pressman, D.: Immunochemical differentiation of rhabdomyosarcomas. Cancer Res. 21:383, 1961.

Jarvi, O., and Saxen, E.: Elastofibroma dorsi. Acta Pathol. Microbiol. Scand. 51 (suppl); 83, 1961.

Becker, B. J. P.: The histogenesis of Kaposi's sarcoma. Int. J. Cancer 18:447, 1962.

Winslow, D. J., and Enzinger, F. M.: Hyaluronidase-sensitive acid mucopolysaccharides in liposarcomas. Am. J. Pathol. 37:497, 1962.

Chaoman, G. B., Jones, K. S., and Spelsberg, W. W.: An electron microscopic study of rhabdomyosarcoma. Invest. Ophthalmol. 2:538, 1963.

Helwig, E. B.: Atypical fibroxanthoma. Tex. Med. 59:604, 1963.

Ozzello, L., Stout, A. P., and Murray, M. R.: Cultural characteristics of malignant histiocytoma and fibrous xanthoma. Cancer 16:331, 1963.

Shipkey, F. H., Lieberman, P. H., Foote, F. W., and Stewart, F. W.: Ultrastructure of alveolar soft part sarcoma. Cancer 17:821, 1964.

Stembridge, V. A., Luibel, F. J., and Ashworth, C. T.: Soft tissue sarcomas: Electron microscopic approach to histogenetic classification. South. Med. J. 57:772, 1964.

Stout, A. P.: Pathological aspects of soft part sarcomas. Ann. N.Y. Acad. Sci. 114:1041, 1964.

Weibel, E. R., and Palade, G. E.: New cytoplasmic components in arterial endothelia. J. Cell. Biol. 23:101, 1964.

Baldwin, R. S.: Hypoglycemia with neoplasia (Doege-Potter syndrome). Wisc. Med. J. 64:185, 1965.

Enzinger, F. M.: Clear cell sarcoma of tendons and aponeuroses. An analysis of 21 cases. Cancer 18:1163, 1965.

Gardner, D. L.: Pathology of Connective Tissue Diseases. London, E. Arnold, 1965.

Kawada, A. K., Takahashi, H., and Anzai, T.: Eosinophilic folliculosis of the skin (Kimura's disease). Jpn. J. Dermatol. 76:61, 1965.

Ross, R., and Greenless, T. K.: Electron microscopy: Attachment sites between connective tissue cells. Science 153:997, 1966.

Stout, A. P., and Lattes, R.: Tumors of the soft tissue. In Atlas of Tumor Pathology, 2nd series. Washington, D.C., Armed Forces Institute of Pathology, 1967.

Welsh, R. A., and Meyer, A. T.: Intracellular collagen fibers. Arch. Pathol. 84:354, 1967.

Archer, F. L., and Kao, V. C. Y.: Immunohistochemical identification of actomyosin in myoepithelium of human tissues. Lab. Invest. 18:669, 1968.

Schubert, M., and Hamerman, D.: A Primer of Connective Tissue Biochemistry. London, H. Kimpton, 1968.

Shelly, W. B., and Rawnsley, H. M.: Painful feet due to herniations of fat. JAMA 205:308, 1968.

Cornog, J. L.: The ultrastructure of leiomyoblastoma. Arch. Pathol. 87:404, 1969.

Enzinger, F. M., Lattes, R., and Torloni, H.: Histological Typing of Soft Tissue Tumors. Geneva, World Health Organization, 1969.

Fine, G., and Horn, R.: Soft tissue tumors: Aids in differential diagnosis. *In* Pathology Annual. Edited by S. C. Sommers. New York, Appleton-Century-Crofts, 1969.

Hajdu, S. I., and Koss, L. G.: Diagnosis of metastatic myosarcomas. Acta Cytol. 13:545, 1969.

Hellstrom, I., and Hellstrom, K. E.: Studies on cellular immunity and its serum mediated inhibition in Moloney-virus-induced mouse sarcomas. Internat. J. Cancer 4:587, 1969.

Enzinger, F. M.: Epithelioid sarcoma. A sarcoma simulating a granuloma or a carcinoma. Cancer 26:1029, 1970.

Mackenzie, D. H.: The Differential Diagnosis of Fibroblastic Disorders. Oxford, Blackwell, 1970.

Giraldo, G., Beth, E., Hirshaut, Y., Aoki, T., Old, L. J., Boyse, E., and Chopra, H. C.: Human sarcomas in culture. Foci of altered cells and a common antigen; Induction of foci and antigen in human fibroblast cultures by filtrates. J. Exp. Med. 133:454, 1971.

Martini, N., Hajdu, S. I., and Beattie, E. J.: Primary sarcoma of the lung. J. Thorac. Cardiovasc. Surg. 61:33, 1971.

Merkow, L. P., Frich, J. C., Slifkin, M., Kyreages, C. G., and Pardo, M.: Ultrastructure of a fibroxanthosarcoma. Cancer 28:372, 1971.

Otten, J., Johnson, G., and Pastan, I.: Cyclic AMP levels in fibroblasts: Relationship to growth rate and contact inhibition of growth. Biochem. Biophys. Res. Comm. 44:1192, 1971.

Lavin, P., Hajdu, S. I., and Foote, F. W.: Gastric and extra-gastric leiomyoblastoma. Cancer 29:305, 1972.

Mackay, B.: Electron microscopy and tumor diagnosis. Cancer Bull. 24:42, 1972.

Samuels, L. D.: Detection and localization of extra-skeletal malignant neoplasms of children with Strontium 87m. Am. J. Roentgenol. Rad. Ther. Nucl. Med. 115:777, 1972.

Whaley, W. G., Dauwalder, M., and Kephart, J. E.: Golgi apparatus: Influence on cell surfaces. Science 175:596, 1972.

Becker, C. G., and Nachman, R. L.: Contractile proteins of endothelial cells, platelets and smooth muscle. Am. J. Pathol. 70:1, 1973.

Cohen, A. M., Ketcham, A. S., and Morton, D. L.: Specific inhibition of sarcoma-specific cellular immunity by sera from patients with growing sarcomas. Internat. J. Cancer 11:273, 1973.

Hajdu, S. I., and Melamed, M. R.: The diagnostic value of aspiration smears. Am. J. Clin. Pathol. 59:350, 1973.

Martel, W., and Abell, M. R.: Radiologic evaluation of soft tissue tumors. Cancer 32:352, 1973.

Wanebo, H., Shah, J., Knapper, W., Hajdu, S. I., and Booher, R.: Reappraisal of surgical management of sarcoma of the buttock. Cancer 31:97, 1973.

Creech, J. L., and Johnson, M. N.: Angiosarcoma of liver in the manufacture of polyvinyl chloride. J. Occup. Med. 16:150, 1974.

Hajdu, S. I., Bean, M. A., Hajdu, E., and Ricci, A.: Papanicolaou smears of cultured human tumor cells. Acta Cytol. 18:327, 1974.

Laurent, J. X., and Jeanpierre, R. E.: Endocrinologically active mesenchymal tumors. Ann. N.Y. Acad. Sci. 230:391, 1974.

Lindberg, L. G., and Mittelman, F.: Morphometric analysis of sarcomas with different karyotypes. Lab. Invest. 31:90, 1974.

Ghavimi, F., Exelby, P. R., D'Angio, G. J., Cham, W., Lieberman, P. H., Tan, C., Mike, V., and Murphy, L.: Multidisciplinary treatment of embryonal rhabdomyosarcoma in children. Cancer 35:677, 1975.

Gyorkey, F., Min, K. W., Krisko, I., and Gyorkey, P.: The usefulness of electron microscopy in the diagnosis of human tumors. Hum. Pathol. 6:421, 1975.

Helson, L., Das, D. K., and Hajdu, S. I.: Human neuroblastoma in nude mice. Cancer Res. 35:2594, 1975.

Katenkamp, D., and Stiller, D.: Structural patterns and histological behaviour of experimental sarcomas. I. General consideration, histology and histochemistry. Exp. Pathol. 11:182, 1975.

Katenkamp, D., and Stiller, D.: Structural patterns and histological behaviour of experimental sarcomas. II. Ultrastructural cytology. Exp. Pathol. 11:190, 1975.

Kindblom, L. G., and Angervall, L.: Histochemical characterization of mucosubstances in bone and soft tissue tumors. Cancer 36:985, 1975.

Li, F. P., Cassady, J. R., and Jaffe, N.: Risk of second tumors in survivors of childhood cancer. Cancer 35:1230, 1975.

Pertshuk, L. P. Immunofluorescence of soft tissue tumors with anti-skeletal muscle antibodies. Am. J. Clin. Pathol. 63:322, 1975.

Shiu, M., Castro, E. B., Hajdu, S. I., and Fortner, J. G.: Surgical treatment of 297 soft tissue sarcomas of the lower extremity. Ann. Surg. 182:597, 1975.

Suit, H. D., Russell, W. O., and Martin, R. G.: Sarcoma of soft tissue: Clinical and histopathologic parameters and response to treatment. Cancer 35:1478, 1975.

Berlin, S. J.: Soft Somatic Tumors of the Foot. Diagnosis and Surgical Management. Mt. Kisco, New York, Futura, 1976.

Gonda, M. A., Aaronson, S. A., Ellmore, M., Zeve, V. H., and Nagashima, K.: Ultrastructural studies of surface features of human normal and tumor cells in tissue culture by scanning and transmission electron microscopy. J. Natl. Cancer Inst. 56:245, 1976.

Hajdu, S. I., and Hajdu, E. O.: Cytopathology of Sarcomas and Other Nonepithelial Malignant Tumors. Philadelphia, W. B. Saunders, 1976.

Morton, D. L., Eilber, F. R., Townsend, C. M., Grant, T. T., Mirra, J., and Weisenburger, T. H.: Limb salvage from a multidisciplinary treatment approach for skeletal and soft tissue sarcomas of the extremity. Ann. Surg. 184:268, 1976.

Sethi, J., and Hirshaut, Y.: Complement-fixing antigen of human sarcomas. J. Natl. Cancer Inst. 57:489, 1977.

Hajdu, S. I.: Cytology from antiquity to Papanicolaou. Acta. Cytol. 21:668, 1977.

Pritchard, D. J., Miller, G. C., Ritts, R. E., and Ivins, J. C.: Thymus-dependent and non-thymus-dependent lymphocytes in patients with sarcomas. Cancer 40:803, 1977.

Rockoff, S. D.: The evolving role of computerized tomography in radiation oncology. Cancer 39:694, 1977.

Rosen, G.: Beginnings of surgical biopsy. Am. J. Surg. Pathol. 1:361, 1977.

Russell, W., Cohen, J., Enzinger, F., Hajdu, S. I., Heise, H., Martin, R. G., Meissner, W., Miller, W. T., Schmitz, R. L., and Suit, D.: A clinical and pathological staging system for soft tissue sarcomas. Cancer 40:1562, 1977.

Sethi, J., Hirshaut, Y., Hajdu, S. I., and Clements, L. G.: Growing human sarcomas in culture. Cancer 40:744, 1977.

Suit, H. D., and Russell, W. O.: Soft part tumors. Cancer 39:830, 1977.

Asbury, A. K., and Johnson, P. C.: Pathology of Peripheral Nerve. Philadelphia, W. B. Saunders, 1978.

Gonzalez-Crussi, F., Hull, M. T., and Mirkin, D. L.: Intranuclear filaments in a soft tissue sarcoma. Hum. Pathol. 9:189, 1978.

Hajdu, S. I., and Fogh, J.: The Nude Mouse as a Diagnostic Tool in Human Tumor Research. *In* The Nude Mouse Experimental and Clinical Research. Edited by J. Fogh and B. Giovanella. New York, Academic Press, 1978, pp. 235–266.

Cancer Facts and Figures. American Cancer Society, New York, 1979.

Hajdu, S. I., Lemos, L. B. Kozakewich, H., Helson, L., and Beattie, E. J.: Growth pattern and differentiation of human soft tissue sarcomas in nude mice. Cancer 47:90, 1981.

chapter 2

Tumors of Fibrous Tissue

NON-NEOPLASTIC LESIONS
- ***Fasciitis***
- ***Keloid***
- ***Elastofibroma***
- ***Fibromatosis***

NEOPLASTIC LESIONS

Non-collagenous Fibrous Tumors
- ***Fibroblastic Fibrous Histiocytoma***
  - Sclerosing Hemangioma
  - Myxoma
  - Dermatofibrosarcoma Protuberans
- ***Histiocytic Fibrous Histiocytoma***
  - Histiocytoma
  - Giant Cell Tumor of Tendon Sheath
  - Giant Cell Tumor of Soft Tissues
- ***Pleomorphic Fibrous Histiocytoma***
  - Xanthoma
  - Atypical Fibroxanthoma
  - Xanthosarcoma

Collagenous Fibrous Tumors
- ***Fibroma***
- ***Ganglion***
- ***Fibrolipoma***
- ***Angiofibroma***
- ***Neurofibroma***
- ***Desmoid Tumor***
- ***Fibroblastic Fibrosarcoma***
- ***Pleomorphic Fibrosarcoma***

THE search for a specific progenitor of the fibroblast was begun in 1867 by Cohnheim, who suggested that inflammatory exudates and, possibly, connective tissues originate in blood cells. After tissue culture studies, Maximow, in 1924, suggested that the nongranulated leukocytes have latent mesenchymal potentialities, which under the proper circumstances can differentiate into macrophages, fibroblasts, and other components of connective tissue. Petrakis et al, in 1961, showed by studying human leukocytes in a subcutaneous diffusion chamber that mononuclear leukocytes underwent differentiation into *macrophages, "polyblasts," histiocytes,* and *fibroblasts.*

The issue of cell of origin of the fibroblast is far from settled, but most investigators believe that *fibroblasts derive from primitive pluripotential mesenchymal cells.* These cells in the course of differentiation become more specialized and assume the cytologic characteristics of fibroblasts, chondroblasts, osteoblasts, and lipoblasts according to the functional status and type of tissue where they are found (see Chapter 1).

Wiener et al, in 1976, by studying the activation of DNA synthesis in fibroblasts and endothelial cells, came to the conclusion that neutropenia and amonocytosis have no effect on DNA synthesis of fibroblasts. This is considered further evidence that fibroblasts do not arise from hematogenous precursors.

Connective tissue in the form of adult fibrous tissue is widely distributed throughout the body. Proper understanding of this tissue is lacking, since despite the advice of Carrel and Ebeling, in 1926, that "Tissue cells, like bacteria, must be defined not only by their morphology but also by their physiological properties," connective tissue cells and tumors have scarcely been studied from any other point of view than pure morphology.

F. B. Mallory, in 1908, defined the fibroblast as "a flat cell with a flat oval nucleus and delicate cytoplasm spreading out in one plane. It is definitely characterized by the production of two kinds of fibrils: fibroglia fibrils and collagen fibrils." Without doubt he was referring to the fine *reticulum fibers* and the thick *collagen fibers.* Since the fundamental work of Mall, in 1891, histologists have busied themselves with reticulin. Mallory and Parker, in 1927, were the first to point out that reticulin does not differ essentially from collagen and the transition from reticulin to collagen is gradual and continuous.

Collagen is a polypeptide and varies according to the number and kind of the constituent amino acids, the manner of union of the radicals, and the polymerization of the molecules. Three steps of collagen synthesis must be completed within the fibroblast for the fourth to take place extracellularly: (1) protocollagen synthesis on ribosomes, (2) release of protocollagen from the ribosomes with subsequent hydroxylation of certain proline and lysine residues, and (3) glycosylation of selected hydroxylysine residues possibly at the cell membrane. After the precursor polypeptides are secreted from the cell, the collagen fibers are formed through molecular cross-links. The association of collagen fibers into bundles is related to the biosynthetic activity of the fibroblasts which determines their architectural and mechanical properties. For example, tendons are made of trichrome positive, polymeric type I, thick collagen fibers; the thin, type III collagen fibers, which are positive with reticulin stain, are found in vessel walls; and the polymeric type II collagens are found in cartilage.

During the formation of fibrous tumors the proportion of the collagen molecules may shift from type III, non-trichrome-positive fibers (the ones seen, e.g., in fibrous histiocytomas) to type I, trichrome-positive fibers (commonly seen in fibrosarcomas). Luse et al, in 1960, were the first to notice cross-banded interstitial collagen fibers exhibiting a periodicity of 900 to 1500 Å. These long-spacing collagen fibers have been encountered close to mature collagen and basement membrane, and development of such structures from long-spacing collagen was suggested by the recognition of transitional forms.

The fibers are related to basement membrane and it has been suggested that under certain circumstances the mucopolysaccharide of the membrane may provoke their formation. Pappas, in 1960, reported that the addition of chondroitin sulfate to tissue cultures of fibroblasts has also been observed to result in the formation of such long-spacing collagen fibers.

According to Im et al, in 1976, glycolytic enzymes, especially phosphofructokinase, are the most important sources of energy for fibroblasts during collagen synthesis. It is believed that fibroblasts while synthesizing intracytoplasmic new collagen are capable of lysing preformed extracellular collagen.

Connective tissue in the form of adult fibrous tissue is widely distributed throughout the body, but it is certain that collagen has not a uniform composition in the body. Although fibroblasts play the principal part in its formation, many other cells are capable of producing collagen. It seems probable that the function of the fibroblast, whether producing collagen or not, and which type, depends upon the requirements of the environment. Narayanan et al (1978) reported that the collagen obtained from inflamed fibroblasts differs phenotypically from that of non-inflamed fibroblasts.

The mechanism of collagen production is complex and is believed to be carried out in fibroblasts simultaneously with the synthesis of polysaccharides, but not all fibroblasts possess these two specialized functions. Green and Hamerman, in 1964, studying fibroblasts in tissue culture, noted that some fibroblasts are able to synthesize collagen but not hyaluronate.

The exact chemical nature of the *intercellular ground substance* is not known, but it is believed that dysfunction of fibroblasts or plasma abnormalities play an important role in alterations of the ground substance. This view is supported by the fact that in many of the collagen diseases the major abnormalities are in the composition of the ground substance. For example, in Hurler's syndrome, according to Renteria and Ferrans, in 1976, high urinary excretion of dermatan sulfate and heparin sulfate is coupled with abnormally high synthesis and intracytoplasmic polymerization of collagen.

In addition, motion in the connective tissue appears to inhibit the formation of intermolecular cross-links of collagen by stimulating the synthesis of glycosaminoglycans (hyaluronic acid, chondroitin sulfate, and dermatan sulfate). Immobilization, on the other hand, plays a role in the maturation of collagen fibers by eliminating the lubricating and plasticizing functions of glycosaminoglycans. Belton et al, in 1977, studied the structural abnormalities of the collagen fibrils in emphysema and came to the conclusion that disorientation of the collagen fibers in the alveolar septae occurs according to the degree of the emphysema.

Motion also appears to be important as a determinant for the orientation of new collagen fibers. Parallel arrangement of fibroblasts in tissue culture, according to Elsdaler (1968), is maintained because this configuration allows the maximum mobility to fibroblasts.

Gabbiani et al, in 1971, and Ryan et al, in 1974, found in fibroblasts in granulation tissue, contractile fibers which resemble morphologically, chemically, and antigenically those seen in smooth muscle cells. They named these cells "myofibroblasts" because of their structural and functional resemblance to both fibroblasts and myoblasts. The fibroblastic origin of myofibroblasts is supported by the fact that fibroblasts in tissue culture develop intracytoplasmic fibers identical to those observed in vivo.

Churg and Kahn, in 1977, found large numbers of myofibroblasts in tumor cells of fibrosarcoma and malignant fibrous histiocytoma and concluded that such cells may blur the distinction between fibrous and smooth muscle tumors. Myofibroblasts were also identified in desmoid tumors and fibromatosis. According to Becker and Nachmann (1973) and Weber and Groeschel-Stewart (1974) such filaments, so-called attachment filaments or contractile elements, are composed of actin and myosin and can be identified by immunofluorescence techniques in the cytoplasms and cell walls not only in fibroblasts but also in endothelial cells, macrophages, and thrombocytes.

Under what influence fibroblasts become neoplastic is not known. Pack and Ariel, in 1952, attempted to develop the concept that tumors and tumor-like conditions of fibrous tissue represent, in certain instances, a desmoplastic diathesis of the connective tissue.

Rokitansky as early as 1846 recognized that "varieties of fibrous sarcoma are dependent upon the form and arrangement of the fibers." Today, it is well recognized that the shapes and sizes of neoplastic cells and their fibers are influenced by their genetic coding as well as by structural characteristics of the environment in which the tumor cells are found.

Students of soft tissue neoplasms are familiar with the treacherous mimicry of fibrous tumors. Stout, in 1953, stated that "It is doubtful whether a true benign neoplasm of fibroblasts exists." This view was seconded by Mackenzie, in 1964, who said that "Fibroblastic tumors have a wide range of differentiation and behavior, but even the more differentiated ones should be regarded as fibrosarcomas." And in 1970 he added, "It is quite impossible for any pathologist however experienced to know whether or not a well-differentiated fibroblastic growth is capable of metastatic spread."

The history of soft tissue sarcomas shows that some of these statements are perhaps unwarranted, but they point out the narrow margin that separates benign and malignant fibrous growths. In the light of this, and because of the overlapping morphology of many of the fibrous tumors, the wisdom of any classification is debatable.

Fibroblastic lesions can be divided, from the clinicopathologic point of view, into three categories: (1) *non-neoplastic tumor-like lesions,* (2) *neoplastic non-collagenous lesions* (fibrous histiocytomas), and (3) *neoplastic collagenous lesions* (e.g., fibrosarcomas). Such a distinction is facilitated by using Mallory's trichrome stain and considering overall cellularity, growth pattern, and cytomorphology of these lesions. Since fibrous histiocytomas are embryonal forms of fibroblastic neoplasms, they contain various amounts of collagen type III, or reticulin fibers, stainable with silver stains, and do not possess significant numbers of tumor cell-related collagen type I fibers which stain an intensive blue with trichrome stain.

It is hoped that this classification will eliminate some of the confusion in definition and nomenclature, especially that which surrounds fibrous histiocytomas. However, it must be understood that fibrous histiocytomas, or so-called non-collagenous fibrous neoplasms, regardless of their dominant cell component, are not entirely different lesions because each form represents a spectrum of neoplastic fibroblasts and histiocytes. It is hoped that the scheme of dividing them into *fibroblastic, histiocytic,* and *pleomorphic* forms not only will be tolerable but also may appear logical (see Fig. 2-14C).

NON-NEOPLASTIC LESIONS

FASCIITIS *

Fasciitis may be characterized as a self-limited, non-neoplastic proliferation

* *Synonyms and related terms:* nodular fasciitis, infiltrative fasciitis, proliferative fasciitis, subcutaneous pseudosarcomatous fibromatosis, pseudosarcomatous fasciitis, parosteal fasciitis.

of subcutaneous or deep fascial fibroconnective tissues with a distinct microscopic pattern. Credit for the recognition of this lesion as a non-malignant proliferative disease in 1941 goes to F. W. Stewart of Memorial Hospital for Cancer and Allied Diseases. However, it was Konwaler and his associates, in 1955, who reported the first cases. Stout, in 1961, summarized his experience, and Price et al, also in 1961, reviewed the clinicopathology of 65 cases. These reports were followed by detailed studies by Soule, in 1962, and Hutter and his co-workers, in 1962 (Table 2-1). A series of 53 cases was reported by Chung and Enzinger, in 1975.

In more than 50% of reported cases the lesions were located in the upper extremities, particularly in the forearm. Fasciitis is found as an ill-defined proliferative process or as a nodular infiltrate in subcutaneous tissues, but not uncommonly it can be deeply situated or intramuscular. Scleroderma-like skin changes, arthralgia, myositis, and eosinophilia associated with fasciitis have been reported (Mehregan, 1966).

The majority of patients are in the third and fourth decades of life and give a history of a few months' duration. Nearly one third of the patients noticed the lesions because of pain and tenderness. It is suspected, because of the superficial location of most of the lesions, that trauma may play an important role in the onset of fasciitis (Miller et al, 1975).

Grossly, these lesions are usually freely movable, plaque-like, subcutaneous, firm nodules without fixation to the skin. The average size ranges from 0.5 to 4.0 cm. They are often gray to gray-white with yellowish-brown finger-like extensions into the surrounding connective tissues.

Histologically, fasciitis is composed of haphazardly arrayed proliferating fibroblasts and blood vessels in a loosely arranged myxoid stroma. The dominant cells are large vesicular fibroblasts with a meshwork of interdigitating fibrils imitating monolayer tissue culture (Fig. 2-1A). The cytoplasms of the spindle cells stain reddish-brown with trichrome stain. The myxoid material stains strongly blue with alcian blue stain, which may be removed by hyaluronidase.

The cellularity may vary from one microscopic field to another, but the presence of numerous lymphocytes, histiocytes, and other inflammatory cells is a constant finding almost throughout the lesion. The presence of a varying number of histiocytic giant cells, scattered mitotic figures, and hypertrophic blood vessels may appear worrisome, especially when they are found in deep fascia, muscle, or near periosteum (Hutter et al, 1962) (see Fig. 2-1B).

In fasciitis, the stroma is not collagenous, and the ubiquitous inflammatory cell infiltrate helps to differentiate it from *cicatrix*, *fibromatosis*, *desmoid tumor*, and *fibrosarcoma*. The mixed cellularity, the infiltrative and reticular arrangement, and the presence of proliferating vessels

TABLE 2-1. ***Anatomic Sites of Fasciitis***

	STOUT (1961)	PRICE ET AL (1961)	SOULE (1962)	HUTTER ET AL (1962)	TOTAL
Head and neck	12	4	2	4	22
Upper arm	16	17	8	7	48
Forearm and hand	40	15	28	27	110
Trunk	24	21	7	10	62
Thigh	18	8	4	9	39
Leg and foot	7	—	6	5	18
Total	117	65	55	62	299

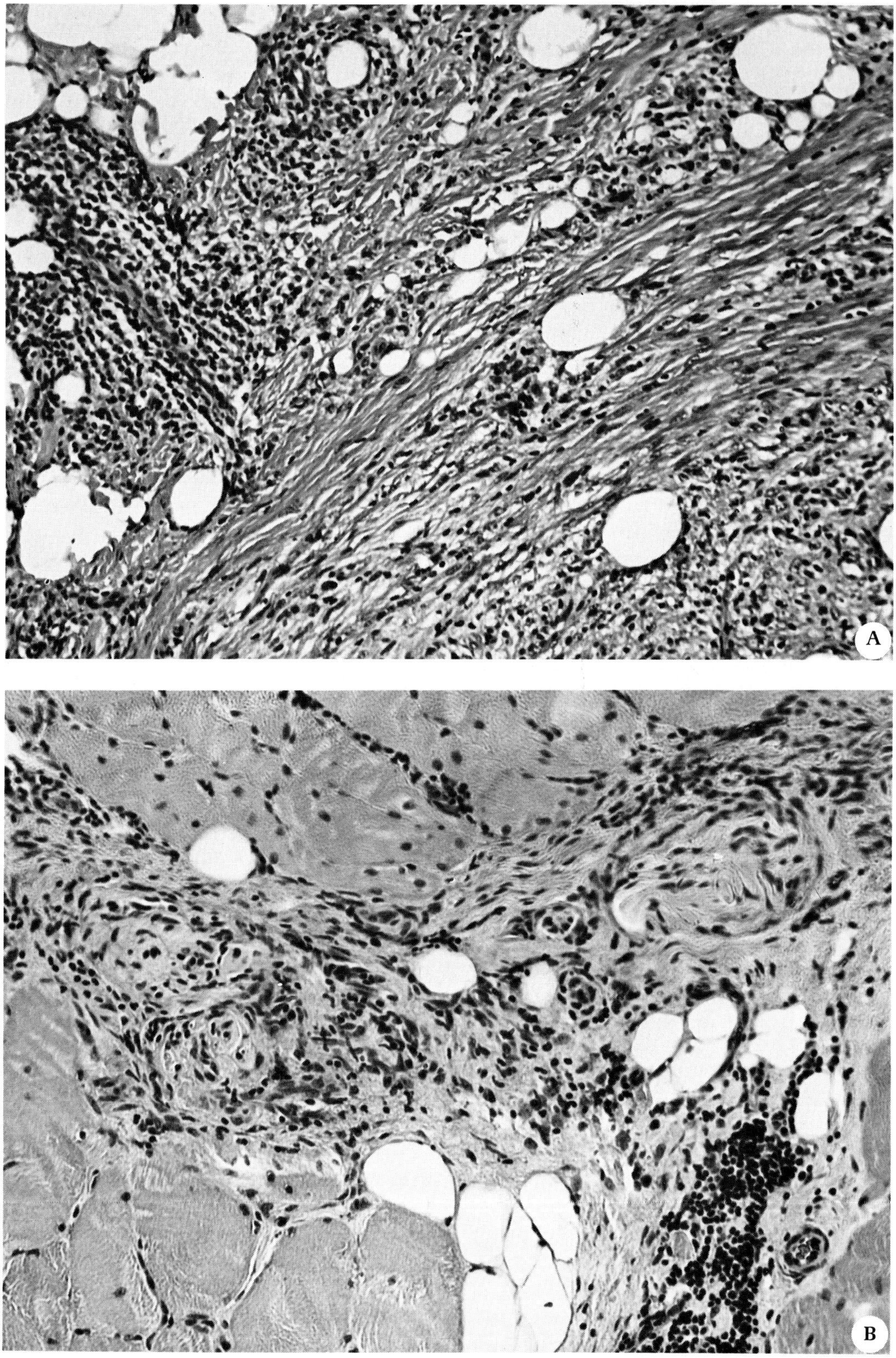

Figure 2-1. Fasciitis is composed of slender fibroblasts which are arranged in tight bundles, slim cords, and occasionally in heavy fascicles. **A,** The cellularity of fasciitis may vary according to anatomic site and duration of the lesion, but a generous complement of inflammatory cells is almost always present (H & E, ×140). **B,** Proliferating fibroblasts usually follow the fibrovascular partitions of affected tissues, e.g., inter- and intramuscular fascial bands (H & E, ×140).

help to distinguish nodules of fasciitis from *myxoid fibrous histiocytoma, myxofibrosarcoma,* and *myxoid liposarcoma.*

The treatment of choice is surgery. It is most unlikely that fasciitis will recur following wide excision with a clean surgical margin.

KELOID*

The name *keloid* is derived from the Greek meaning "claw." Alibert first described keloid in 1814 erroneously as a cancerous growth. An excellent review of the literature and of the various theories in connection with keloids has been reported by Garb and Stone in 1942.

Keloid is a non-neoplastic proliferation of dermal and subcutaneous fibrous tissues, developing more in dark-skinned people than in white. The estimated ratio of keloids in colored to white patients is about 12 to 1.

Although keloids most commonly follow injuries such as vaccination, injection, surgical incision, mosquito bite, scratching, and burning, the primary reason for these growths is still unknown. There is a striking congenital predisposition to keloids, and a few instances of congenital keloids have been reported.

Although keloids may appear at all ages, they are found most commonly in patients between the ages of 10 and 25 years. They may range in size from a couple of centimeters to several inches. They may be single or multiple and usually take months or years to attain their maximum size. No part of the body is exempt from keloids, but they have a predilection for the back, sternum, neck, and ear lobes (Fig. 2-2).

Histologically, the bulk of the keloid is composed of an overgrowth of almost acellular collagenous tissue. The collagenous bundles are densely packed and appear to run in various directions with finger-like processes extending into fibroadipose

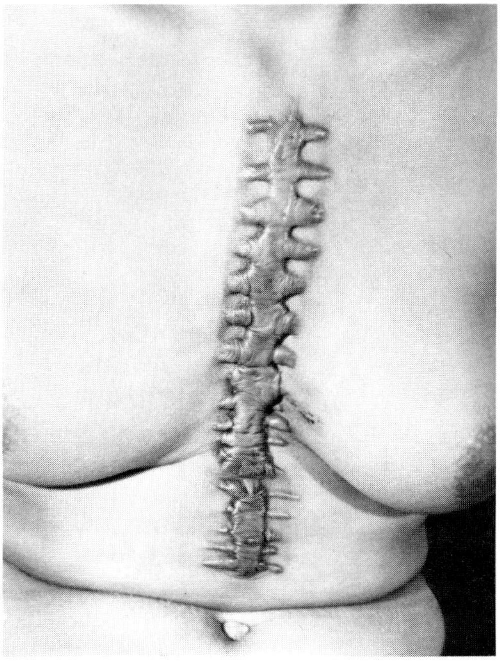

Figure 2-2. Keloid following midline sternotomy. (From Gläser, A.: Klinische Pathologie der Geschwülste. Stuttgart, Gustav Fischer, 1974.)

subcutaneous tissues. In keloids, elastic fibers are absent and blood vessels are usually scanty. The overlying epidermis is either slightly acanthotic or atrophic (Fig. 2-3).

Both keloids and *hypertrophic scars* are due to trauma and have their origin in the dermis, but hypertrophic scars do not have the propensity of growth of keloids and do not extend beyond the boundaries of an injury. Subcutaneous *fibromas* are usually solitary, small, and well-defined nodules composed of cellular bundles of fibrotic tissue.

Spontaneous involution of keloids may occur, but in most cases ablation by irradiation or surgical excision is required. The results of surgical excision are often disappointing because the surgeon may not appreciate how widely the tumor extends beyond its palpable margins and the excision is followed by rapid and excessive recurrence. On the other hand, according to reports, radiation therapists may also achieve only temporary and unpredictable success.

Synonyms and related terms: keloid fibroma, Alibert's keloid, cheloid, congenital keloid, folliculitis keloidalis.

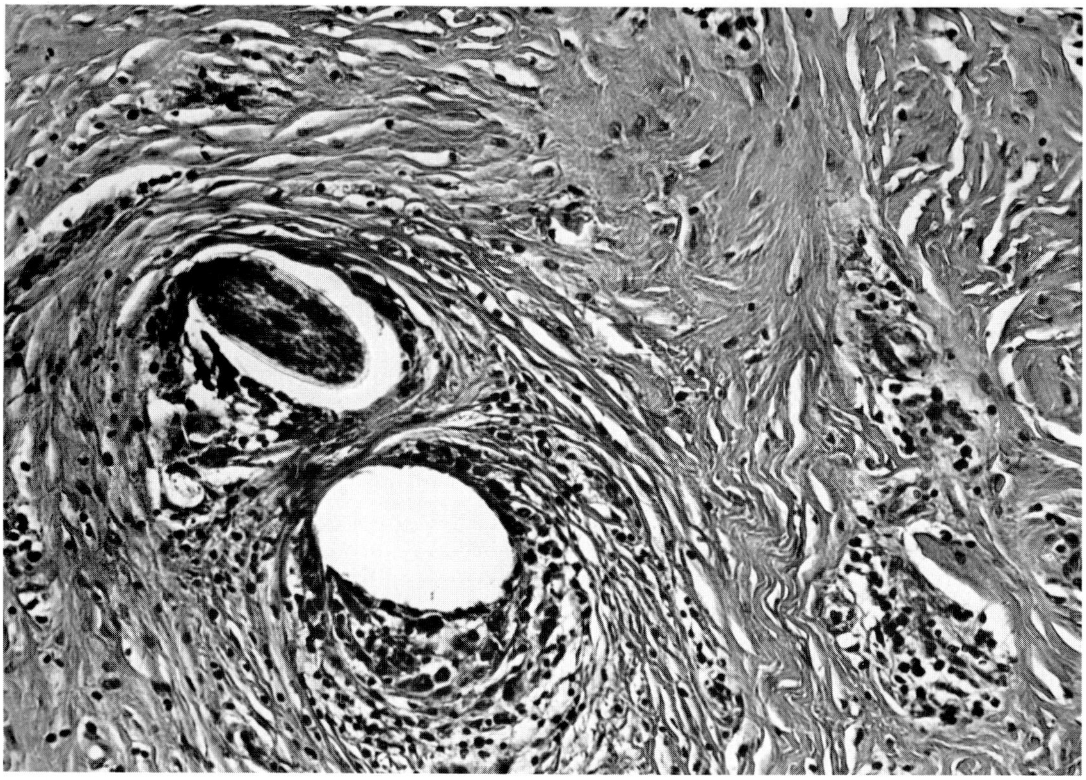

Figure 2-3. Folliculitis keloidalis shows a combination of dense collagenous, mostly acellular, bundles and inflamed hair follicles (H & E, ×140).

ELASTOFIBROMA*

Elastofibroma is a rare non-neoplastic connective tissue lesion first reported by Jarvi and Saxen in 1961. Since then more than 30 additional cases have been reported. The ultrastructure of elastofibroma has been studied by several investigators, including Waisman and Smith, in 1968, Winkelmann and Sams, in 1969, and most recently by Akhtar and Miller in 1977. With one exception, all of the reported lesions occurred at the lower angle of the scapula, hence the term *elastofibroma dorsi.*

Elastofibromas occur most commonly during the fifth and sixth decades of life. The pathogenesis of these lesions is obscure, but they are most likely the product of either a degenerative or a reparative process, or of both.

**Synonyms and related terms:* elastofibroma dorsi, elastodysplasia.

These lesions usually range in size from 5 to 10 cm. They are ill-defined and nonencapsulated, lobulated semisolid masses. Microscopically, elastofibromas are characterized by the presence of broad bands of almost acellular fibrous connective tissue in the background of numerous branching eosinophilic and refractile fibers. In addition, one may find conglomerates of globular and granular structures with the same staining characteristics dispersed throughout the lesion. The true nature of these fibers and granules is unclear, but they strongly stain with elastic tissue stains. Ultrastructural studies suggest that this abnormal elastic material is derived from excessive production of young elastic tissue by fibroblasts.

Elastofibroma must be distinguished from *collagenoma,* a rare inherited abnormality, characterized by multinodular accumulation of subcutaneous collagen fibers and fragmentation of elastic fibers.

Wide local excision with clean margins is the treatment of choice. None of the reported cases recurred after surgical excision.

FIBROMATOSIS*

Fibromatosis is a term that refers to a group of non-neoplastic proliferative connective tissue lesions that tend to infiltrate surrounding tissues and often recur after surgical excision. This definition is not too different from that of Stout and Lattes (1967): "The term fibromatosis is applied to a group of benign fibroblastic proliferative lesions of the soft tissues that are distinguished from the self-limiting scar." The concept of fibromatosis is a useful one, although, even today, the term is often misused and abused.

Stout, in 1954, was the first to call attention to these lesions by reporting a series of 44 cases under the title "juvenile fibromatoses." He observed that fibromatoses most frequently affect infants and children and as a group have many features in common. Although there are various forms of fibromatoses, the subdivision results more from clinical than from histopathologic differences (Table 2-2). These lesions can occur at any age and anywhere in the body, but certain forms have a particular affinity to certain anatomic sites and tend to appear at certain ages (Fig. 2-4; Table 2-3).

Fibromatoses are customarily subdivided into "juvenile" and "adult" forms. Since specific forms of these lesions do not afflict juveniles or adults exclusively, classification based on age of the patient can be misleading.

Many hypotheses have been proposed about the etiology, but none have proved reliable. The fact that many fibromatoses are congenital seems to indicate that a congenital anomaly of connective tissue development is responsible for such lesions. Kauffman and Stout, in 1965, found 37 fibromatoses among the 120 congenital

TABLE 2-2. ***Fibromatoses***

	SYNONYMS AND RELATED TERMS
Subdermal fibromatosis	Fibrous hamartoma of infancy; subdermal fibromatous tumor of infancy; Reye's disease
Fibromatosis colli	Torticollis, wry neck; fibrous sternomastoid tumor of infancy; congenital muscular torticollis; congenital sternocleidomastoid tumor
Digital fibromatosis	Recurring digital fibrous tumor of infancy; infantile dermal fibromatosis
Fascial fibromatosis	Congenital localized fibromatosis; myositis fibrosa; diffuse infantile fibromatosis
Multifocal fibromatosis	Congenital generalized fibromatosis; aggressive infantile fibromatosis
Gingival fibromatosis	Hereditary gingival fibromatosis
Plantar fibromatosis	Ledderhose's disease
Aponeurotic fibromatosis	Juvenile aponeurotic fibroma; calcifying fibroma of Keasbey
Mesenteric fibromatosis	Sclerosing mesenteritis; retractile mesenteritis; sclerosing lipogranulomatosis; subperitoneal sclerosis
Palmar fibromatosis	Dupuytren's contracture; fibroplasia of palmar fascia
Penile fibromatosis	Peyronie's disease
Mediastinal fibromatosis	Chronic mediastinitis; idiopathic mediastinitis; fibrous mediastinitis
Retroperitoneal fibromatosis	Ormond's disease; periureteral fibromatosis; periureteritis; periureteritis plastica; pelvic fibrosis; idiopathic retroperitoneal fibrosis

**Synonyms and related terms:* See Table 2-2.

TABLE 2-3. *Incidence of Fibromatoses According to Age of Patients*

	INFANTS	CHILDREN	ADULTS
Subdermal	+++	++	−
Colli	+++	−	−
Digital	+++	−	−
Fascial	+++	++	+
Multifocal	+++	++	−
Gingival	−	+++	−
Plantar	+	+++	++
Aponeurotic	++	+++	+
Mesenteric	−	+++	++
Palmar	−	−	+++
Penile	−	−	+++
Mediastinal	−	−	+++
Retroperitoneal	−	−	+++

+++ = most common; ++ = common; + = uncommon; − = very uncommon.

mesenchymal tumors studied by them. Touraine and Ruel, in 1945, suggested that some underlying hereditary factor links many of these lesions together and proposed a common name for all—hereditary polyfibromatosis.

Fibromatoses may be multiple and familial and may be complicated by contractures and other deformities. They are painless, subcutaneous or submucosal, poorly circumscribed, firm nodules without adherence to the skin. Despite the apparent diversity and individual peculiarity, fibromatoses have many features in common. *They are all composed of fibrous tissue of varying cellularity infiltrating fat, muscle, and other soft tissues.* The dominant cells are well-differentiated, uniform fibroblasts with vesicular nuclei and moderately collagenous cytoplasmic processes. Many of the cells are oriented in one direction; however, haphazard arrangement of the fusiform and elongated cells is not uncommon. The strands of fibroblasts may extend to a considerable distance between muscle cells and trabeculae of fat cells. Giant cells, inflammatory cells, and cells in mitoses are quite rare. Similarly, calcification and ossification are uncommon findings.

Although many fibromatoses are self-limited growths, they appear histologically invasive and have a tendency to recur after incomplete excision. Certain forms of fibromatoses, especially in infants and young children, may exhibit great cellularity, aggressive infiltrative growth, and poor differentiation without any particular aggressive clinical behavior. The cellularity is also influenced by

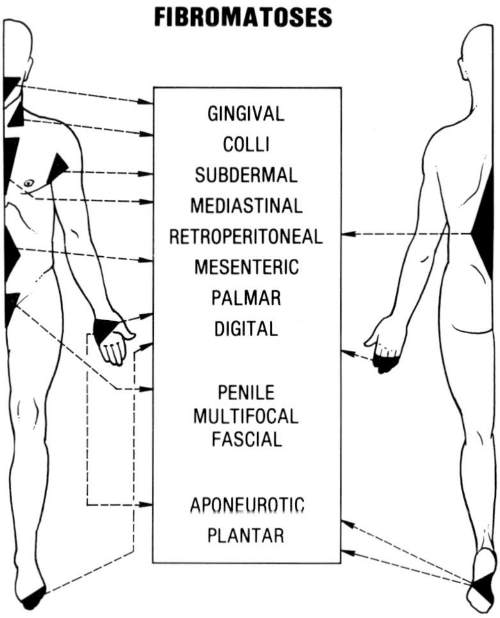

Figure 2-4. Subclassification of fibromatoses according to anatomic sites shows that these lesions occur most commonly in the distal parts of the extremities, axilla, midline of the body, and the head and neck areas (see also Table 2-2).

the duration of the lesion and is analogous to the stromal changes in gynecomastia described by Banayan and Hajdu in 1972.

Fibromatosis is a relatively uncommon disorder (see Table 2-4). Partly because of this, the accurate diagnosis of fibromatoses is perhaps one of the most challenging undertakings in diagnostic pathology. The reader should also be aware that the term *fibromatosis* is often used indiscriminately for fibroblastic lesions which are either fibromas, benign fibrous histiocytomas, or low-grade fibrosarcomas of the desmoid type. Despite numerous common features of various fibromatoses there are certain, mostly clinical, features that allow us to distinguish individual forms.

Subdermal Fibromatosis. The first description of subdermal fibromatosis was that of Reye, in 1956, who described 6 cases of "subdermal fibromatous tumors of infancy." More than a dozen case reports appeared in the literature during the last two decades, and Enzinger, in 1965, reported 30 cases. He coined the term *fibrous hamartoma of infancy*. Although it affects predominantly male infants, to define it as a disease exclusively of infants is misleading, since it may occur in children. It appears most commonly in the region of the shoulder, axilla, and upper arm as a small circumscribed subcutaneous node, but multiple examples have been noted. Histologically, subdermal fibromatosis is composed of a mixture of proliferating fibroblastic, adipose, vasoformative, and muscle components with some resemblance to angiomyolipoma (Fig. 2-5 and see Chapter 4). The interlacing fibrous trabeculae may resemble the nerve bundles of a neuroma, but they stain negative with the Bodian stain and positive with trichrome stain for collagen. Ultrastructural and immunofluorescent studies show that these lesions are partly composed of cells showing characteristics of both fibroblasts and smooth muscle cells suggesting that it is perhaps a disease of myofibroblasts (Benjamin et al, 1977). Local excision is considered curative.

Fibromatosis Colli* or *Torticollis. This is a rare, one in 150,000 births, congenital abnormality characterized by localized fibrous replacement of the muscle fibers of the sternocleidomastoid muscle. The first references to torticollis were made by Aquapendente (1538–1619) who developed an apparatus for correcting it and by Minnius who performed the first tenotomy for torticollis in 1685. According to Severn who published and edited the "Diary of the Rev. John Ward Extending from 1648 to 1679," in London in 1839, there is reference to the treatment of torticollis: "To cut wry neck, cut three tendons in the child's neck."

Fibromatosis colli appears as a small intramuscular mass usually during the first two weeks after birth. In most cases the mass gradually enlarges and then regresses in 5 to 6 months, but because of the fibrous shortening and thickening of the muscle, the torticollis develops in a few months but may remain undetected for years. The principal location of the lesion is the lower third of the sternomastoid muscle. Torticollis affects the right and the left sides almost equally.

The pathogenesis is unknown, but

TABLE 2-4. ***Reported Series of Various Fibromatoses with Follow-up Information***

	NUMBER OF PATIENTS	RECURRENCE (%)	DIED WITH DISEASE (%)
Stout (1954)	44	30	10
Luck (1959)	154	31	—
Enzinger (1965)	71	23	1
Mitchinson (1970)	40	35	—
Dehner and Askin (1976)	17	18	—

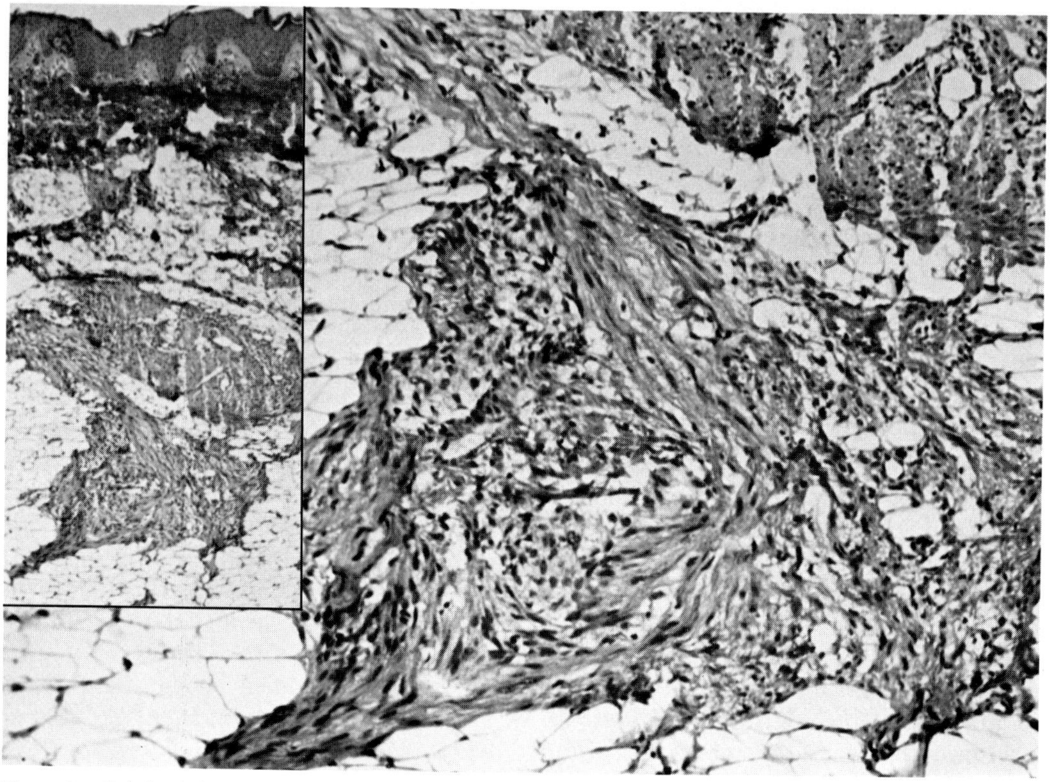

Figure 2-5. Subdermal fibromatosis is composed of slender finely collagenous or reticular fibroblasts arranged in multidirectional narrow bundles and positioned between fat lobules or around blood vessels (H & E, ×140; inset ×35).

many theories of etiology have been proposed, ranging from intrauterine malposition to trauma during labor, none of which is satisfactory. It has been reported that patients with torticollis have a high (14%) incidence of ipsilateral dislocation of the hip. The natural history of these lesions has been studied in large numbers of cases by Middleton, in 1930, and Chandler, in 1948.

Histologically, fibromatosis colli is characterized by proliferating fibrous tissue separating muscle bundles. The muscle fibers may undergo partial or complete degeneration.

The treatment of torticollis varies with the severity of the deformity. Most authors advocate excision of the diseased muscle prior to age two or three. In most instances, surgical excision results in complete restoration of muscle function.

Digital Fibromatosis. The first series of 18 cases of digital fibromatosis was reported by Reye in 1965; however, Sakurane, in 1924, is credited with the first description of these lesions. Additional cases were reported by Enzinger in 1965, Allen in 1972, and Mehregan et al, also in 1972.

The lesions of digital fibromatosis are prone to appear in the extensor surfaces of the distal phalanges of the fingers and toes of male infants predominantly or very young children, but Prior and Sisson reported 3 cases in persons older than 40 years of age. These small, usually less than 1 cm, subcutaneous nodules may be firmly attached to the skin or underlying fibroconnective tissues and bone. Recurrence is almost certain unless removal is complete, even if this requires digital amputation (Fig. 2-6).

Histologically, these growths are composed of uniformly arranged bundles of mature fibroblasts. In the cytoplasm of a few fibroblasts structures like inclusion

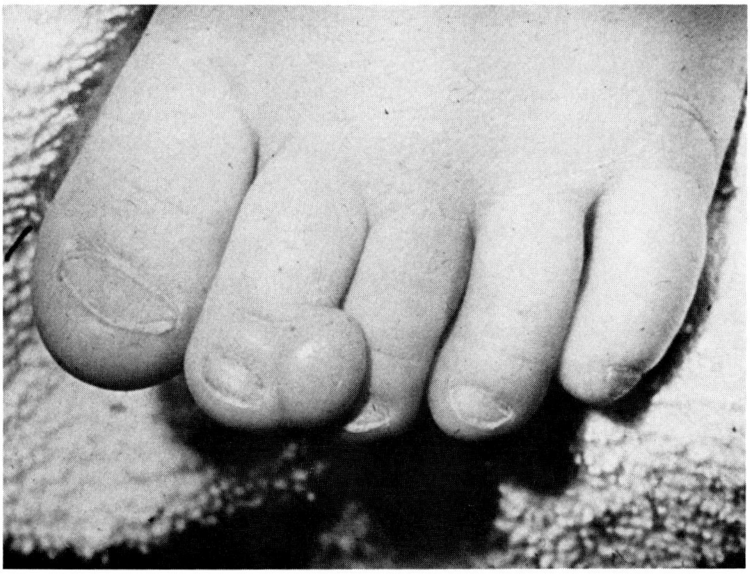

Figure 2-6. Digital fibromatosis of an infant. (Courtesy of Dr. L. Lemos).

bodies can be seen occasionally. Attempts to establish the viral nature of these structures have failed (Battifora and Hines, 1971). In all probability they are imperfectly polymerized tropocollagen particles or accumulated lipoprotein granules (Fig. 2-7).

Fascial* or *Congenital Localized Fibromatosis. This type is similar to fibromatosis colli; however, this is not limited to any particular muscle group but most commonly is found in the arm and thigh. It is usually discovered soon after birth. Grossly, it has an alarming appearance because of its considerable size and location, usually in deep muscle (Fig. 2-8). Microscopically, it may also resemble fibromatosis colli; however, it is usually more cellular and less fibrous than the excised lesions in torticollis (Fig. 2-9). Excision of the muscle with a clean surgical margin is the treatment of choice to prevent recurrence.

Multifocal Fibromatosis. This form was called congenital generalized fibromatosis by Stout, in 1954. It is an aggressive and deadly form of fibromatoses. Afflicted babies are usually born with multiple subcutaneous fibrous nodules. Histologically identical fibroconnective nodules also may be found in bones, muscles, walls of intestines, kidneys, and the heart. Several examples of this mostly congenital disease have been reported. Shnitka et al, in 1958, summarized their experience with these lesions. Since mesenchymal tissues other than fibroblasts are also involved and because this is almost invariably a progressive and lethal disease, one may wonder whether it belongs to the fibromatoses.

Gingival Fibromatosis. Ramon et al, in 1967, described a case of gingival fibromatosis combined with cherubism and reviewed the clinical pathology of this entity. It is often inherited and usually appears when the permanent teeth erupt. Other anomalies such as hypertrichosis and neurofibromatosis were reported in association with gingival fibromatosis. It presents as a small gingival nodule with ill-defined margins (Fig. 2-10). The proliferating submucosal fibroblasts with their collagenous cytoplasmic processes usually extend beyond the clinically appreciable margins. Surgical excision with clean margins is the best assurance against recurrence.

Plantar Fibromatosis. Although it was Dupuytren, in 1832, who first described

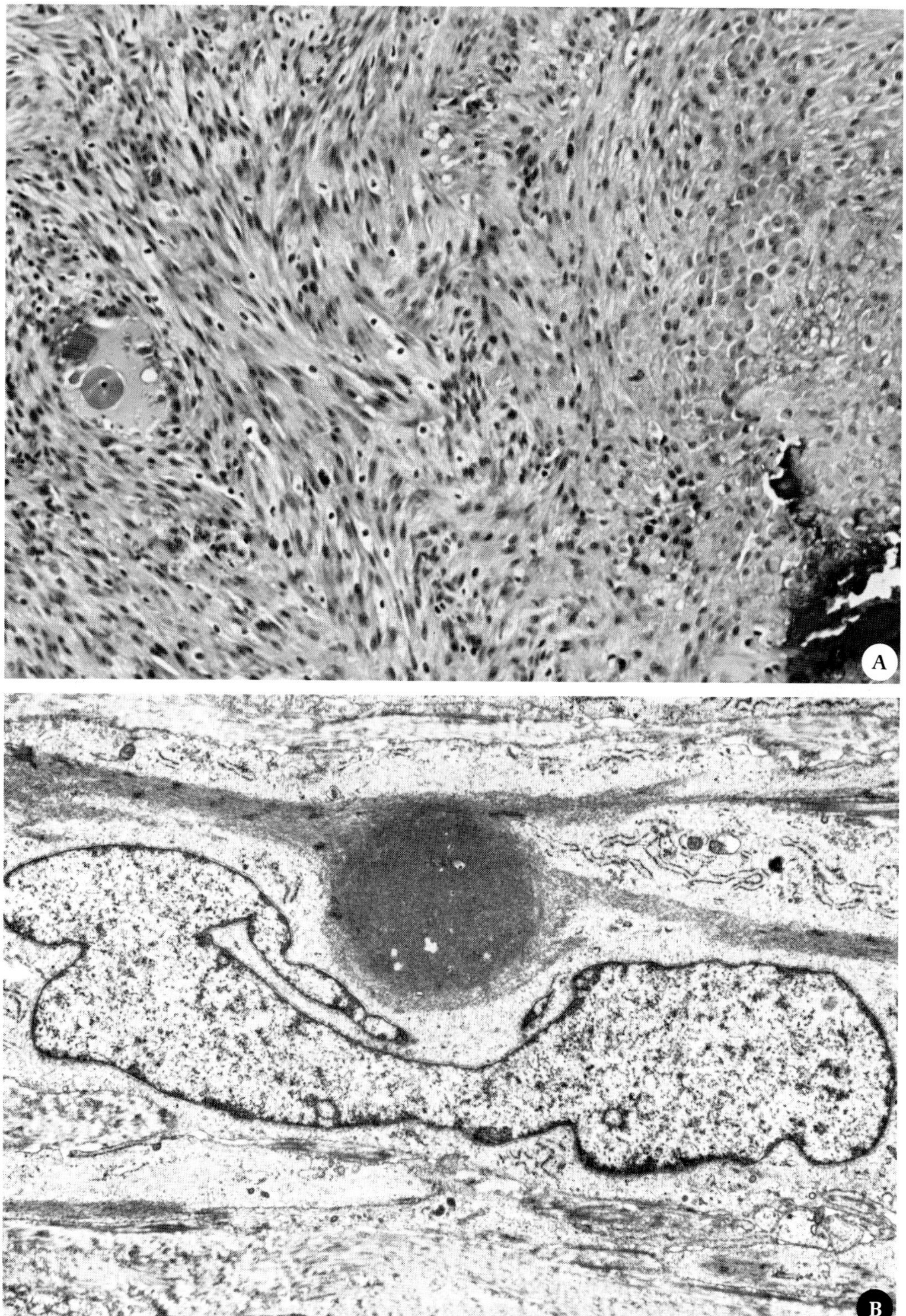

Figure 2-7. A, Histologically, digital fibromatosis may be more cellular than fibromatosis of other sites, and areas of calcification may be found (H & E, ×140).

B, Part of a cell in digital fibromatosis containing a rounded "inclusion body" which impinges onto the nucleus. Three bundles of filaments with dense bodies radiate from it (×8,500). (From Bhawan, J., Bocchetta, C., Joris, I., and Majno, G.: et al: A myofibroblastic tumor: Infantile digital fibroma (digital tumor of childhood). Am. J. Pathol. 94:19, 1979.)

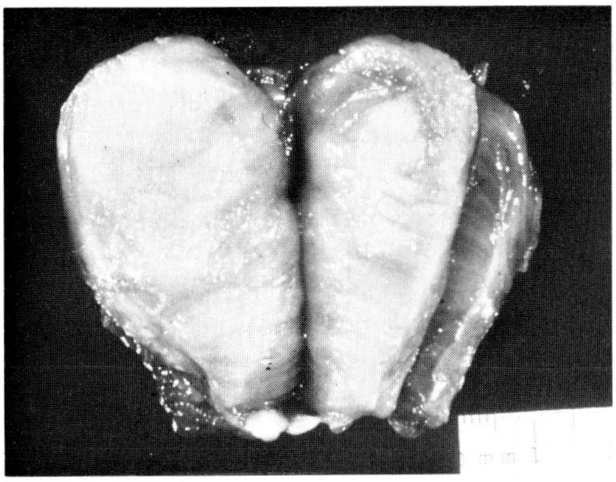

Figure 2-8. Fascial fibromatosis excised in toto with adjacent skeletal muscles from the thigh of an eight-month-old baby. There is no evidence of recurrence three years after the excision.

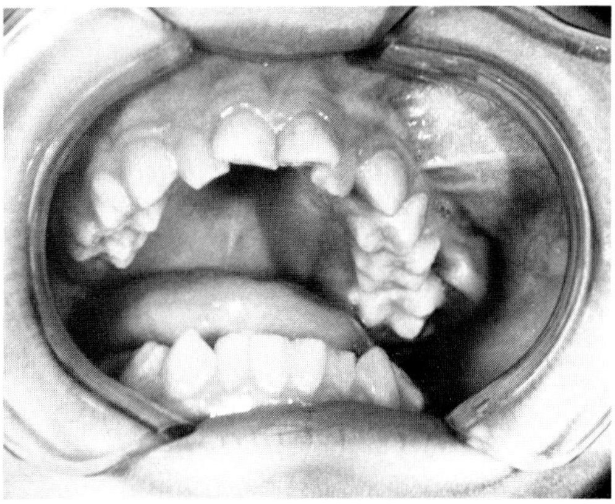

Figure 2-10. Gingival fibromatosis of a 12-year-old child. Note the swelling of the gingiva and part of the palate. (Courtesy Dr. L. Eisenbud, Long Island Jewish Hospital.)

plantar fibromatosis in his classic text on contractures of the hand and fingers, Ledderhose is credited with reporting the first case in 1897. Until the report of 18 cases by Pickren et al in 1951, however, not much has been written about these lesions.

The exact etiology of plantar fibromatosis remains unknown, but according to Meyerding the etiology seems to be a

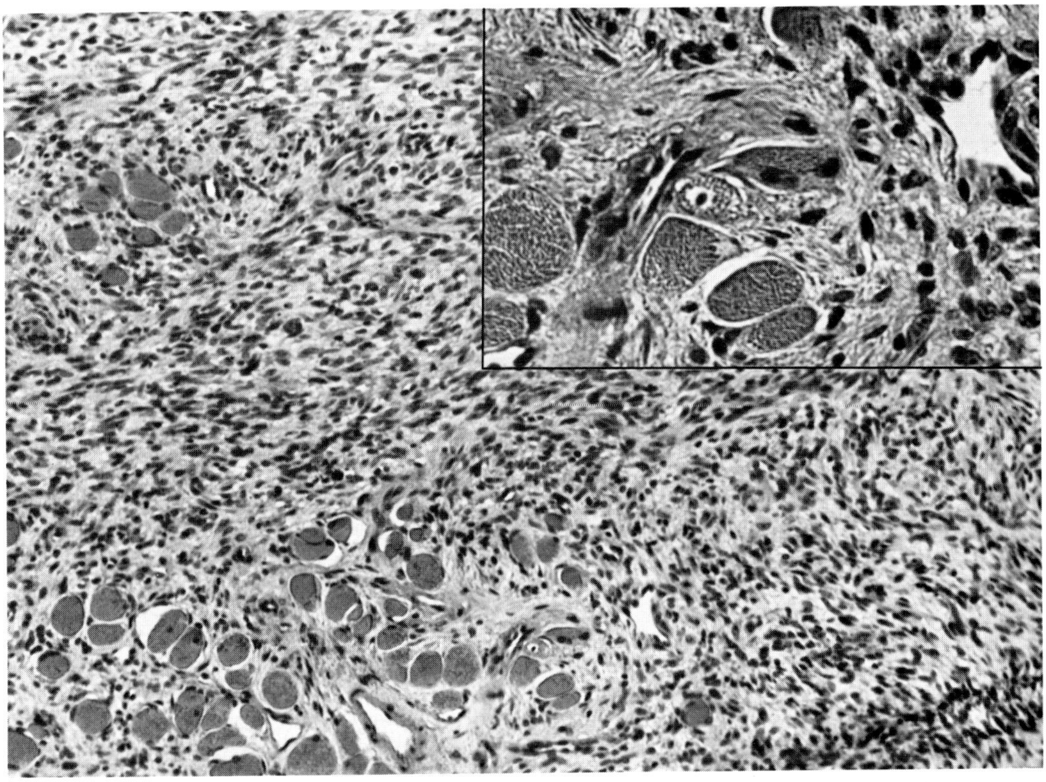

Figure 2-9. Histologically fascial fibromatosis (see Figure 2-8), especially in the very young may show extreme cellularity, and mitotic figures are not uncommon. Note the multidirectional infiltrate of fibroblasts, partition, and destruction of skeletal muscle fibers, also capillary hyperplasia (see inset) (H & E, ×140; inset ×350).

combination of chronic inflammation aggravated by trauma. It is difficult to assess how common plantar fibromatosis may be because, unlike palmar fibromatosis, it rarely produces flexion deformity and in many instances remains unnoticed unless the fibroblastic proliferation produces visible tumor. It has a predilection for males, and most cases occur in persons under 30 years of age.

Plantar fibromatosis is usually asymptomatic, and in one third of the cases it is bilateral and affects most commonly the medial portion of the plantar aponeurosis and may extend toward the dorsum of the foot. It is a multinodular and an irregular thickening of the plantar fascia composed of strands and whirls of young fibroblasts. Commonly, there is considerable loss of cell polarity and pleomorphism, but the overall histopathologic appearance is that of other fibromatoses. Plantar fibromatosis is often associated with other connective tissue disorders, e.g., Dupuytren's contracture, arthritis, and Peyronie's disease. In spite of complete excision and meticulous surgical dissection of the plantar tissues, a high rate of local recurrence has been reported, but it is doubtful if it ever develops into a neoplasm.

Aponeurotic Fibromatosis. Keasbey, in 1953, reported for the first time, aponeurotic fibromatosis, a tumor-like proliferation of fibroconnective tissue cells with foci of calcification and ossification and areas of cartilagenous differentiation. Most commonly it affects the palms and soles of small children and young adults and one cannot escape comparing it with palmar and plantar fibromatoses which usually appear in somewhat older people. The etiology is unknown, but aponeurotic fibromatosis may represent some type of reactive connective tissue process with a tendency to form metaplastic bone and cartilage. It is an uncommon lesion and there are no more than two dozen well-documented cases in the literature. The best review articles are by Allen and Enzinger in 1970 and Goldman also in 1970; however, none of these writers could add too much to the original description by Keasbey in 1953. She wrote that aponeurotic fibroma is characterized by "(1) its high cellularity; (2) the appearance microscopically of wide infiltration, with distinctive overgrowth and replacement of voluntary muscle, fat, blood vessels, nerves and skin adnexa; (3) its stubborn tendency to recur after limited surgical excision; (4) its natively benign character; and (5) its controllability, in the end, by conservative surgery."

Mesenteric Fibromatosis. This non-neoplastic tumor-like lesion was first described by Jura, in 1924. Yannopoulos and Stout, in 1963, reported 12 cases of mesenteric fibromatosis, and Simpson et al, in 1964, described 7 cases, and reviewed 15 additional cases from the literature, of mesenteric fibromatosis associated with *Gardner's syndrome.* Gardner's syndrome consists of several stigmata that are inherited as an autosomal dominant trait: intestinal polyposis, osteomas, lipomatosis, cutaneous cysts, and fibromatosis. Weary et al (1964) in their review article state that all 118 reported cases had polyps, 45% had adenomas, 50% had osteomas, 65% had cutaneous cysts, and 45% had fibromatosis. The most frequently used terms for this lesion are listed in Table 2-2. It is usually found in people older than 40 years of age and has no apparent sex predilection. The etiology is obscure, but numerous possible factors, e.g., trauma, vasculitis, and abnormal fat metabolism, among others, have been implicated in the etiology of mesenteric fibromatosis.

Recent investigations suggest that fibroblastic abnormalities, detectable in tissue culture, exist in individuals with Gardner's syndrome, familial polyposis coli, and Peutz-Jeghers syndrome (Kopelovich et al, 1979).

Most of the lesions have been described to be confined to the mesentery of the small intestine, but sometimes concomitant involvement of the omentum, mesocolon, and retroperitoneum has been reported. The largest mesenteric lesion,

3,185 gm, was reported by Simpson et al, in 1964. These lesions are composed of chronically inflamed fibroadipose tissue with myxomatous and solid collagenous areas (Fig. 2-11). There is general agreement that surgery should be limited to debulking and relief of mechanical obstruction.

Palmar Fibromatosis. This has been known for more than a century because of the lucid description of Dupuytren, in 1832. However, it is believed that it was perhaps Plater, in 1614, who first called attention to this peculiar flexion deformity of hand and fingers.

Palmar fibromatosis is the nodular thickening and flexion contracture of a portion of the superficial palmar aponeurosis. Males are affected much more frequently than females, and it is almost exclusively a disease of whites. Because it affects most commonly middle-aged adults, trauma may play an important role in the etiology of this disease. Conway, in 1954, compiled reports from the literature and correlated the history of manual labor with the incidence of palmar fibromatosis. His study revealed that of the nearly 5,000 patients with Dupuytren's contracture, 73% were engaged in continuous heavy manual labor. Many investigators also believe that hereditary factors may also play an important role in the appearance of this disease. Palmar fibromatosis is often bilateral and not uncommonly is associated with non-contractile plantar fibromatosis and Peyronie's disease.

Luck, in 1959, reporting his surgical experience with 206 lesions of 154 patients, pointed out that the disease process has three stages: the *proliferative stage*, the *contracting stage*, and the *residual stage*. He added that the selection and extent of surgical therapy should be based on the stage of the disease but should not be short of excision of the involved fascia.

Histologically, palmar fibromatosis is similar to plantar fibromatosis. It begins as a localized fibroblastic overgrowth of the palmar fascia with gradual involvement of the entire palmar aponeurosis and extension to the subcutaneous fat and the skin. It is not uncommon to find giant pacinian corpuscles in the excised fibrous tissue (Fig. 2-12).

Penile Fibromatosis. This fibroproliferative disease of the corpora cavernosa of the penis was described in detail by Peyronie, in 1743, but it is believed that it was first described by Ephemerides in 1687. The exact etiology is unknown, but trauma may be a significant etiologic factor as reported by Burford et al in 1951. It affects middle-aged adults and may be found in association with other fibromatoses such as Dupuytren's contracture and plantar fibromatosis. Clinically it is a palpable induration of rubbery consistency of the dorsum or lateral aspects of the penis which results in considerable deformities. Smith, in 1954, studied 26 cases histologically and found that the initial phase of the disease consists of perivascular chronic inflammatory infiltrate and endothelial cell hyperplasia which is followed by proliferation of fibroconnective tissue with ossification and subsequent destruction of muscle fibers.

The advocated treatments have been as numerous as the suggested etiologic factors. There is no one sure modality of treatment. Surgical excision, irradiation therapy, and various vitamin and steroid injections have been reported to result in only partial success.

Mediastinal Fibromatosis. The etiology of mediastinal fibromatosis, like that of many of the other fibromatoses, is unknown. The disease is often detected by signs of obstruction of the superior vena cava. A comprehensive review of this condition was published by Barrett in 1958. It affects middle-aged males as well as females and the fibrous tissue is usually found over the aortic arch, trachea, bronchi, and the heart. Microscopically, the fibrous tissue is not encapsulated and is composed of dense collagenous tissue with variable numbers of lymphocytes, plasma cells, and other inflammatory elements.

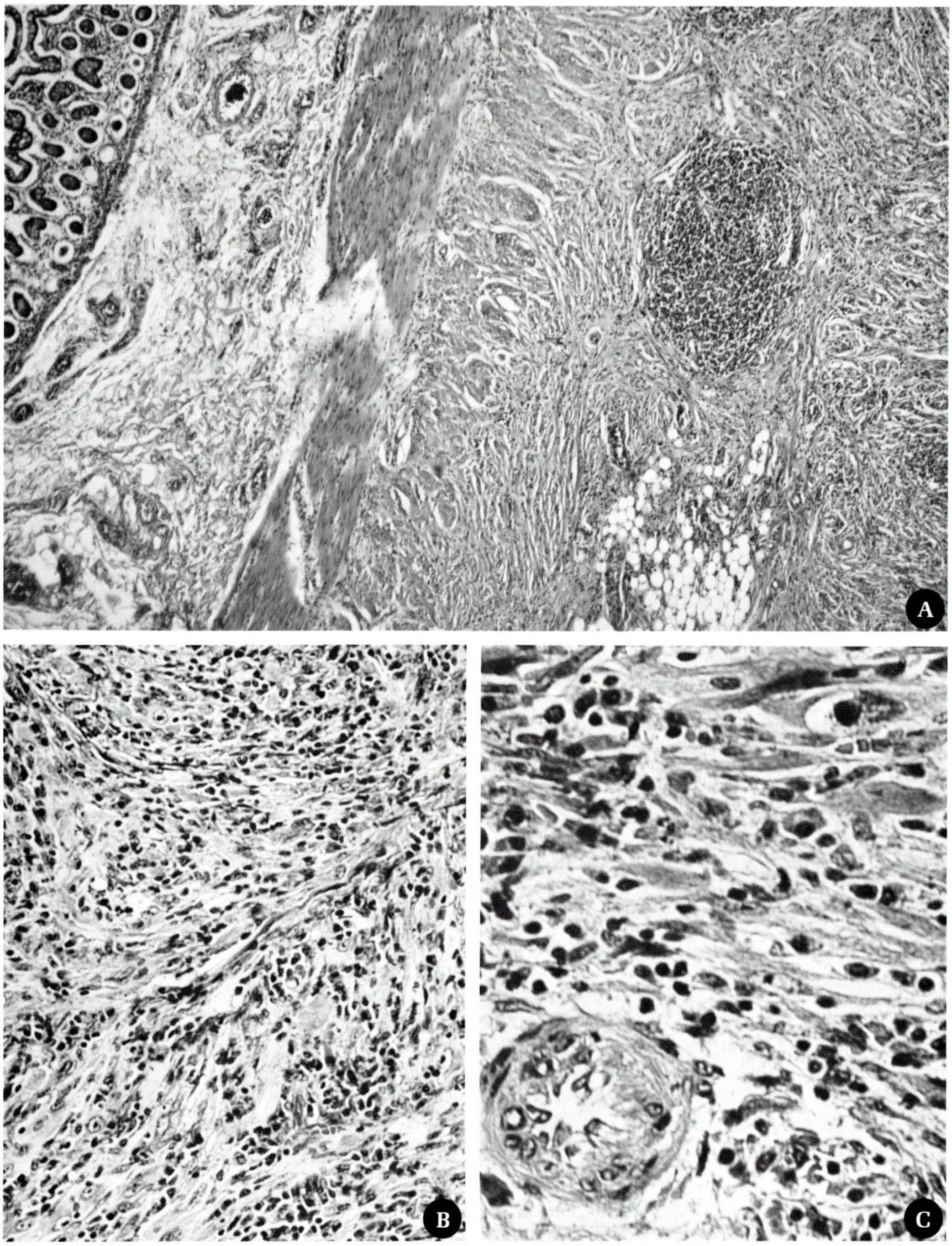

Figure 2-11. Mesenteric fibromatosis with extension into the wall of the small intestine. Slender reticular or partly collagenous fibroblasts are forming multidirectional cords or bundles. There are more than the usual number of inflammatory cells positioned between fibroblasts and adipocytes. Some of the lymphocytes attempt to form aggregates or lymphoid nodules. Note the capillary endothelial hyperplasia in C (**A,** H & E, ×35; **B,** H & E, ×85; **C,** H & E, ×140).

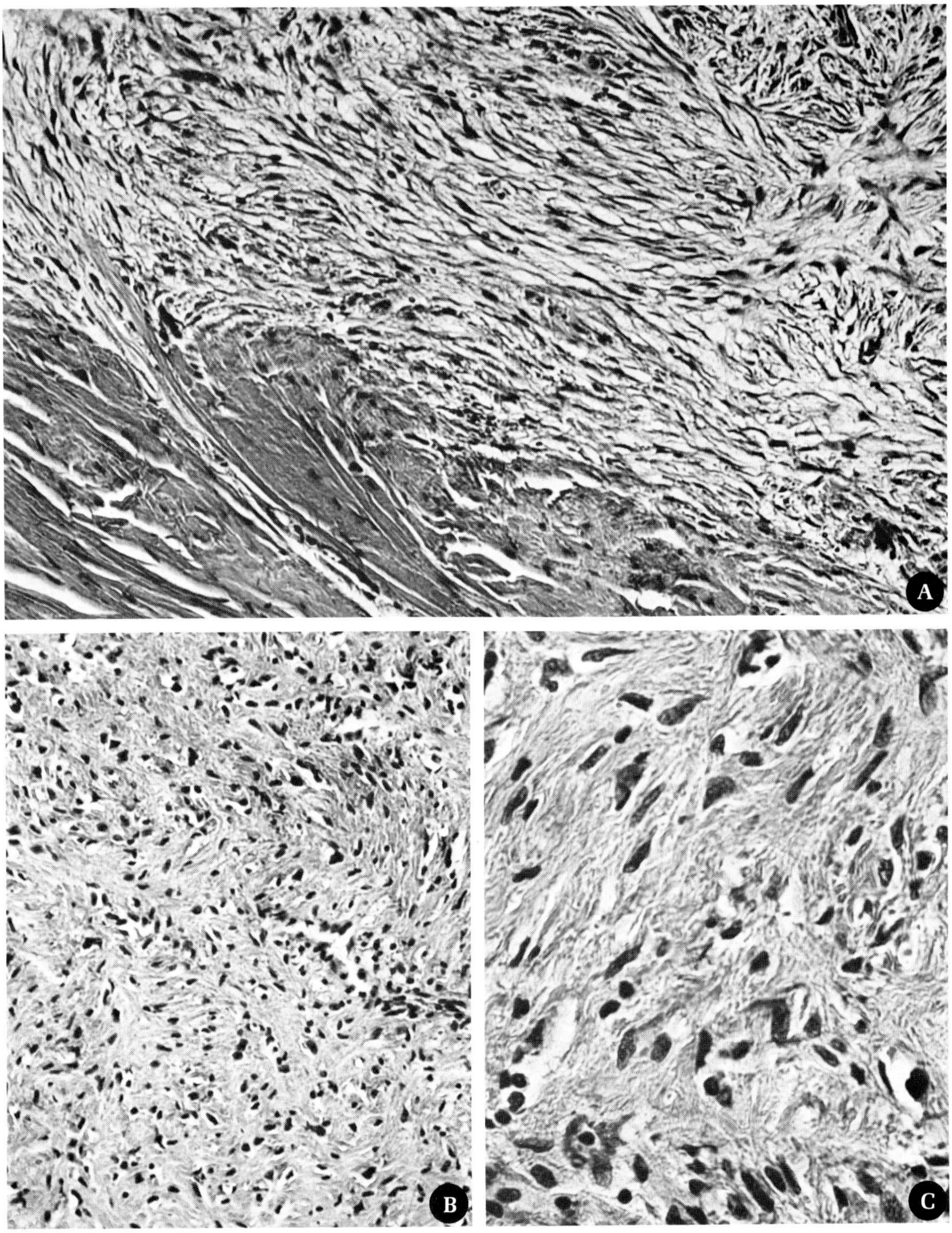

Figure 2-12. Palmar fibromatosis. **A,** Typical fascicular or bundle arrangement of slender fibroblasts. Note an abortive spiral nebula at the left upper corner (H & E, ×85).

B and **C,** An area of palmar fibromatosis showing heavy collagenous fibroblasts. Stromal deposits of collagen give a sclerosing appearance to this lesion (**B,** H & E, ×85; **C,** H & E, ×140).

The cellularity of this lesion largely depends on the age of the process. Treatment should be aimed at relieving the obstruction of vital structures. Morgan et al, in 1966, reported a case of combined mediastinal and retroperitoneal fibromatosis.

Retroperitoneal Fibromatosis. Many writers suggested that mediastinal and retroperitoneal fibromatosis, Riedel's thyroiditis, and sclerosing cholangitis might be manifestations of the same disease process affecting interstitial and perivascular fibroconnective tissues. The first description of a case of retroperitoneal fibromatosis under the title of periureteritis was reported by Albarran, in 1905; however, it remained for Ormond, in 1948, to popularize the disease with his case reports in the English-language literature. It is a disease characterized by proliferation of collagenous fibrous tissue around retroperitoneal and pelvic organs with obstruction of the ureters, vena cava, and aorta. The cause of retroperitoneal fibrosis is unknown in most cases, but thrombophlebitis, trauma, cholecystitis, pyelitis, ureteritis, and serotonin- and kinin-producing tumors such as carcinoids have been suggested along with many other factors in the etiology of this disease. Graham, in 1967, reported cardiac and pulmonary fibrosis during methysergide therapy, and Iversen et al, in 1975, reported retroperitoneal fibrosis following treatment with methyldopa (Table 2-5).

Retroperitoneal fibromatosis is predominantly a disease of males in the fourth to sixth decades. Some studies suggested the role of autoimmune processes and genetic predisposition in the development of retroperitoneal fibrosis. A comprehensive study of the clinicopathology of retroperitoneal fibrosis, based on the review of 481 cases published in the literature, has been published by Koep and Zuidema, in 1977. Microscopically, as stated by Mitchinson, in 1970, in his review of 40 cases, the fibrous tissue is relatively avascular, acellular, and often calcified. The collagenous tissue may be pleomorphic and may be interspersed with large numbers of lymphocytes, eosinophils, and plasma cells. The fibrotic process commonly extends from the retroperitoneum into adjacent skeletal muscles. It has been reported that malignant neoplasms were found in about 8% of patients with retroperitoneal fibromatosis (Fig. 2-13).

TABLE 2-5. ***Associated Findings in 491 Patients with Retroperitoneal Fibromatosis****

FINDINGS	%
Methysergide therapy	12
Malignant neoplasms	8
Mediastinal fibromatosis	3
Other fibromatosis	3
Arteritis	2
Sclerosing cholangitis	2

*No associated findings were detected in 68% of the cases.

Modified from Koep, L., and Zuidema, G. D.: The clinical significance of retroperitoneal fibrosis. Surgery 81:250, 1977.

Therapy should be directed at relief of ureteral and vascular obstructions. The prognosis in fibromatosis is considered fair and the reported mortality is less than 10%.

Differential Diagnosis

In the differential diagnosis of fibromatoses a number of lesions must be considered.

Fasciitis has a distinctly mixed fibrovascular and inflammatory element often arranged in a pallisading pattern.

Progressive fibrosing myositis is another lesion which may simulate microscopically fibromatosis. However, the progressive clinical course with involvement of an entire muscle group or a whole extremity distinguishes it from fibromatosis (see Chapter 5).

Postirradiation fibrosis is a homogeneous hyalinization of subcutaneous tissues without evidence of proliferation. The finding of bizarre mono- or multinuclear fibroblasts is not uncommon (see Chapter 9).

The infiltrative pattern of growth dis-

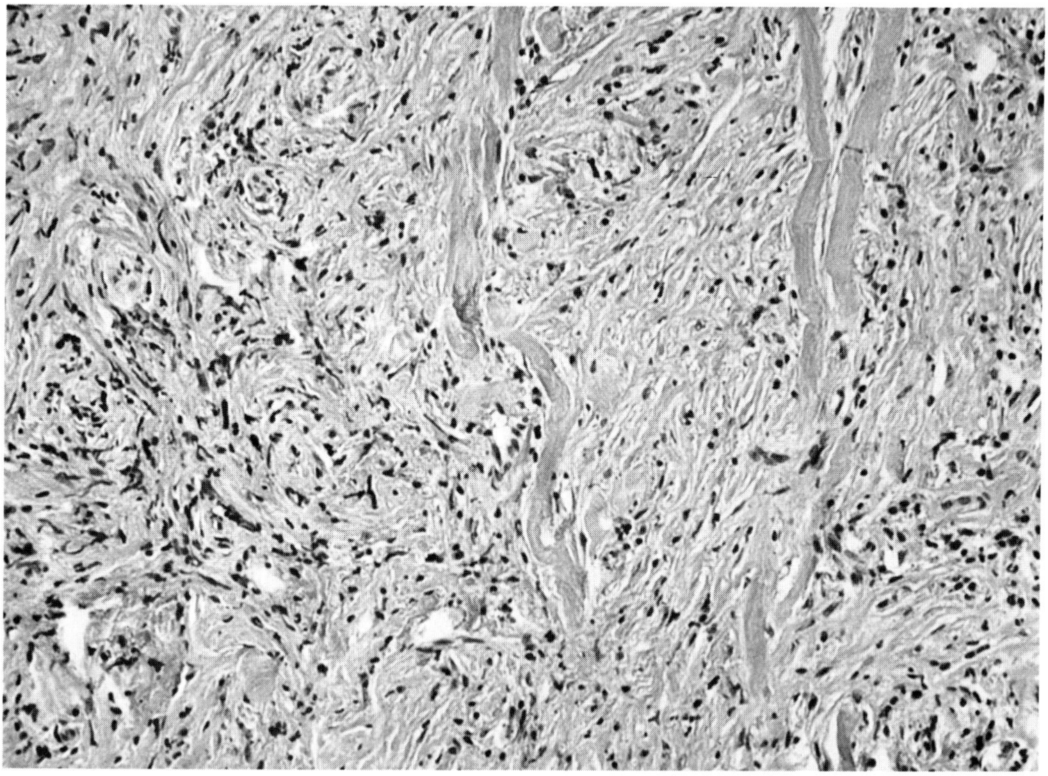

Figure 2-13. A fairly typical photomicrograph from a case of retroperitoneal fibromatosis. Note sparse cellularity, haphazardly positioned fibroblasts, and extreme build-up of intra- and extracellular collagen (H & E, ×85).

tinguishes fibromatosis from *keloid* and fibroma.

Schwannoma is less collagenous than fibromatosis and the tumor cells have slender, cigar-shaped nuclei (see Chapter 7).

Fibrous histiocytomas are usually noncollagenous, less fibrillar, and more cellular lesions than fibromatoses. The characteristic round cells, foamy histiocytes, giant cells, and storiform pattern of undifferentiated fibroblasts are other distinguishing features.

The spectrum of cellular fibromatoses merges imperceptibly into well-differentiated fibrosarcomas of the *desmoid* type. Fibromatoses and desmoids have overlapping histopathologic features that sometimes make distinction difficult. In most cases, however, if adequate material is available for histopathologic examination, the differential diagnosis is not too difficult. Desmoid tumors are more homogeneous and collagenous fibrous lesions than fibromatoses. Characteristically, they are deeply seated, bulky neoplasms of young adults without involvement of the skin (Table 2-6).

NEOPLASTIC LESIONS

The primitive mesenchymal cells are multipotential cells. The differentiated mesenchymal cells may appear morphologically as histioblasts or fibroblasts and may assume morphologically as well as functionally the identity of histiocytes or fibroblasts. Differentiation is almost certainly coupled with dedifferentiation in many instances (Fig. 2-14A).

If we accept that tissue histiocytes do not form heavy band collagen (collagen type I) and that fibroblasts may (see Table 2-10), it seems logical that neoplasms that

TABLE 2-6. *Distinguishing Features of Fibromatoses and Desmoid Tumors*

	FIBROMATOSES	DESMOID TUMORS
Average age of patient	Younger than 20 years	Older than 20 years
Most common anatomic sites	Hand, foot, and digits	Trunk, head, and neck
Average size	Less than 5 cm	More than 5 cm
Location	Superficial	Deep
Growth pattern	Non-encapsulated, proliferative, and inflammatory	Pseudoencapsulated, infiltrative, and destructive
Histopathology	Partly collagenous, cellular, myxoid, and haphazardly arranged	Collagenous, hypercellular, sclerosing, and uniformly arranged
Rate of recurrence	Low	High

are predominantly composed of non-collagenous fibrous histiocytic cells should be separated from the ones that are predominantly collagenous neoplasms (Figs. 2-14, 2-32, 2-72).

Once the *non-collagenous fibrous neoplasms* have been separated from the *collagenous fibrous neoplasms,* it is appropriate to concentrate on the morphology of individual tumor cells and their pattern of growth. Both of these groups of neoplasms have tumors predominantly composed of slender *reticular fibroblasts* and both may form tumors composed of *pleomorphic* cells. On the other hand, neoplasms predominantly composed of cells we identify today as either *histiocytes* or *facultative fibroblasts* belong to the non-collagenous group, and neoplasms composed of well-differentiated collagenous fibroblasts and fibrocytes should be, of course, listed with the collagenous neoplasms (Fig. 2-14B).

Many readers may find such subclassification of a complex group of neoplasms simplistic and perhaps less than scientific. I believe that the classification and labeling of certain neoplasms according to the scheme presented in Figure 2-14C not only may eventually prove to be practical from the clinical point of view but also will lead to better understanding of the natural history and cellular composition of many of these neoplasms.

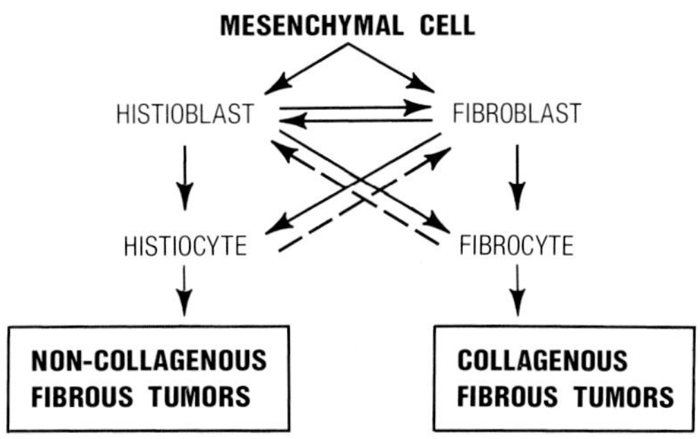

Figure 2-14. A, Schematic illustration of theoretical pathways of differentiation and dedifferentiation of fibrous-histiocytic cells.

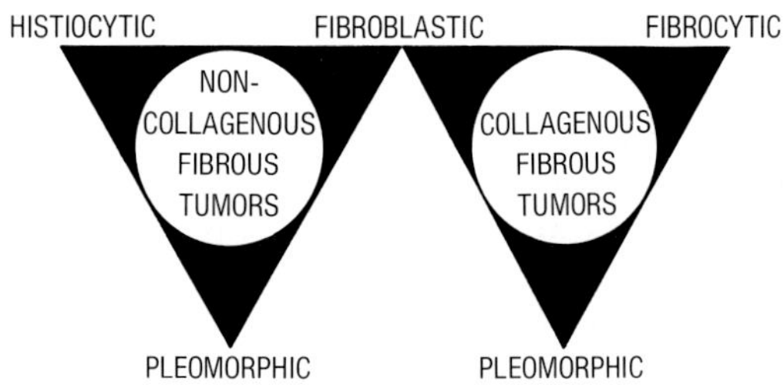

Figure 2-14. (continued) **B,** Two groups of fibrous tumors with their related cellular elements.

Non-Collagenous Fibrous Tumors*

FIBROBLASTIC FIBROUS HISTIOCYTOMAS

Fibroblastic fibrous histiocytomas will be discussed according to the traditional subdivisions: sclerosing hemangioma, myxoma, and dermatofibrosarcoma pro-

* *Synonyms and related terms:* fibrous histiocytoma (Fig. 2-32).

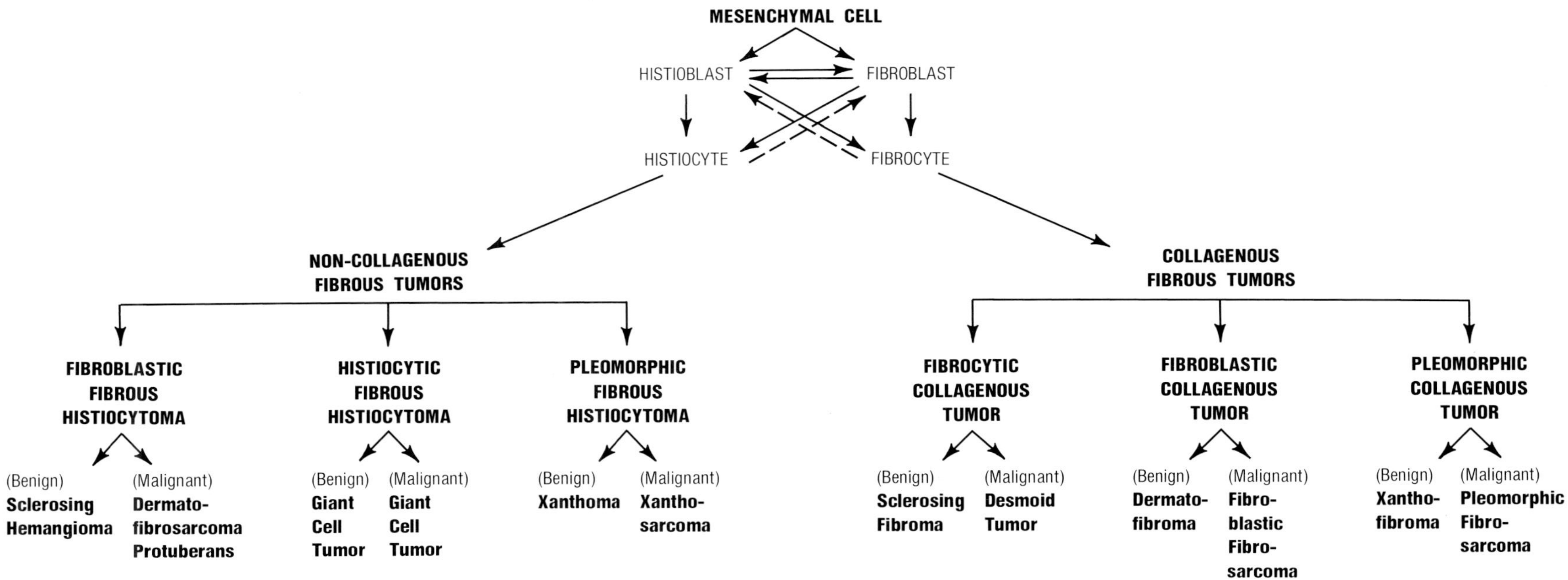

Figure 2-14. (continued) **C,** Classification scheme of fibrous tumors. Noncollagenous fibrous tumors are the so-called fibrous histiocytomas. Collagenous fibrous tumors are tumors which are composed of collagenous fibroblasts and fibrocytes and stain positive with trichrome stain.

tuberans. From the histogenetic point of view, however, these three entities, as well as the so-called myxoid fibrous histiocytoma, are forms of fibroblastic fibrous histiocytoma.

Sclerosing Hemangioma.* This benign neoplasm rarely appears before adolescence or adulthood. These lesions are usually found on the extremities and are seldom larger than one centimeter in diameter.

The etiology of these neoplasms is unknown. The vascular origin for sclerosing hemangioma was first considered by Wolbach in 1912 and restated by Gross and Wolbach in 1943. Carstens and Schrodt, in 1974, studied 9 cases of sclerosing hemangiomas with the electron microscope and after demonstrating the Weibel-Palade bodies came to the conclusion that sclerosing hemangiomas are endothelial in origin.

At present, proponents of the histiocytic or fibroblastic origin of these neoplasms outnumber the believers in the endothelial origin. Perhaps both of these groups are right, since endothelial cells and pericytes may act as facultative fibroblasts and may assume the role of histiocytes. On the other hand, it is possible that the sclerosing process is imitated by the proliferation of perivascular fibroblasts and histiocytes, and the capillary vessels, which are eventually obliterated and destroyed, are merely trapped in such a process.

Histologically, sclerosing hemangiomas are composed of thin-walled capillary vessels surrounded by stellate fibroblasts and hemosiderin-containing histiocytes. The cellularity of these lesions and the amount of various cellular elements may vary from case to case. They are usually ill-defined lesions that blend into the surrounding tissue (Fig. 2-15A). The fibrillar cytoplasmic processes stain strongly with reticulum stain and weakly with trichrome stain.

* *Synonyms and related terms:* dermatofibroma, histiocytoma, myxofibroma, myxoma, benign fibrous histiocytoma.

These neoplasms rarely undergo myxoid changes which are reflected by the typical gross and microscopic appearance of the tumors. Grossly they become soft and translucent; histologically the stellate or spindle-shaped fibroblasts will be distributed in a loose myxoid stroma that stains faintly positive with mucicarmine and alcian blue stains.

On rare occasions benign fibroblastic fibrous histiocytomas, especially those of the non-sclerosing, myxoid variety, may occur in muscle and other deeper soft parts. They are commonly called myxomas.

Simple surgical excision will permanently eliminate most of these lesions.

Myxoma. According to Kettle, myxomas are tumors composed of embryonic connective tissue similar to that present in the umbilical cord. They are extremely rare, and their existence has been questioned by many authors. It must be admitted that the majority of the reported myxomas are, in reality, myxoid lipomas, ganglions, myxoid liposarcomas, or other forms of soft tissue growths with extreme mucoid degeneration. The term *myxoma* was introduced by Virchow in the first edition of *Die krankhaften Geschwulste* in 1863.

While I question the existence of myxosarcoma, I believe there is a place in our terminology for myxoma. Primitive and undifferentiated mesenchymal cells, as well as fibroblasts, are capable of biosynthesis of mucopolysaccharides (Baitsell, 1925). When this mucinous substance is abundant in a sparsely cellular and sparsely vascular, well-encapsulated, subcutaneous or intramuscular innocuous lesion of long duration, the growth can be classified as myxoma. From another point of view, if mesenchymal tumor cells fail to develop into histiocytes, fibroblasts, or lipoblasts and remain in the embryonal mucinous stage, they may produce myxoma. Mallory said in 1908, "The only difference between a fibroblast and a myxoma cell is that in the latter the collagen fibrils are more or less separated from each other by a varying amount of fluid containing mucin."

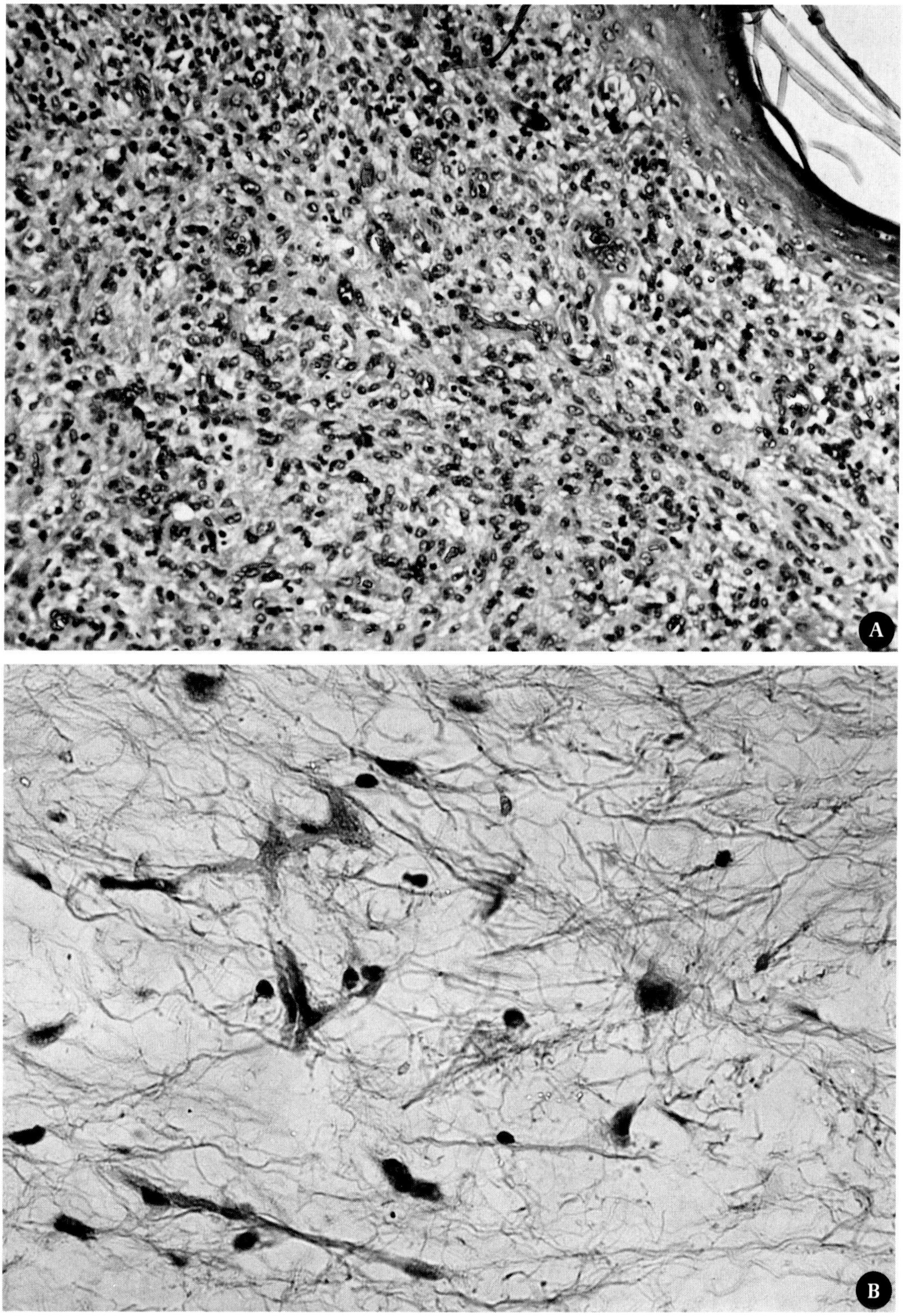

Figure 2-15. A, So-called sclerosing hemangioma or benign fibroblastic fibrous histiocytoma is composed of short spindle and oval cells. Tumor cells are clustering about capillary vessels (H & E, ×140).

B, Intramuscular myxoma shows scant cellularity and a stroma rich in mucopolysaccharides. Note the fine spiderweb-like network of reticular filaments in the background of positioned slim cells (H & E, ×140).

A number of reports on myxomas have been published during the last 65 years: Leitao (1913), Stout (1948), Attar (1958), Glazunov and Puckhov (1960), Kauffman and Stout (1961), Enzinger (1965), and Mori et al (1975). Stout (1948) found over 100 myxomas reported in the literature (exclusive of those of the heart; see Feldman et al 1977) and added 49 additional cases from his laboratory. Enzinger, in 1965, reported 34 cases of intramuscular myxomas from his files of almost 200 myxomas.

Myxomas vary in size from small subcutaneous tumors to large retroperitoneal masses. *Histologically*, the tumor cells are inconspicuous and have pyknotic round or elongated nuclei and drawn-out fibrillar cytoplasm which stains positive with reticulum stain. These fibrillar processes, despite sparse vascularity, have a tendency to parallel wavy rows. The ground substance stains faintly positive with mucicarmine and alcian blue stains, and most of the mucinous material can be removed by prior treatment with hyaluronidase. There is no mitotic activity or appreciable pleomorphism of the tumor cells (Fig. 2-15B).

Myxomas have been reported to recur after local excision. There are references in the literature to rare and inadequately documented instances when myxomas lost their innocent myxomatous character and assumed sarcomatous features.

Dermatofibrosarcoma Protuberans.* At an early stage dermatofibrosarcoma protuberans is regarded by many investigators as an outgrowth of a pre-existing sclerosing hemangioma. This tumor is perhaps one of the most typical and best-known forms of the group of malignant neoplasms I call fibroblastic fibrous histiocytomas (Figs. 2-14C, 2-32).

The first description of dermatofibrosarcoma protuberans was published by Taylor, in 1890. Despite sporadic case reports, it was not until Darier and Ferrand published their article in 1924 that this tumor became established as a clinicopathologic entity. Hoffman, in 1925, reviewed 15 published case reports and added 3 cases of his own and coined the term *dermatofibrosarcoma protuberans*. Following these two articles, dermatofibrosarcoma as a specific entity was generally accepted. Hertzler, in 1926, illustrated the characteristic "cartwheel pattern" of the fibroblasts, and Bezency, in 1933, reported metastatic spread of a dermatofibrosarcoma protuberans.

The first series of 39 cases reported by Pack and Tabah, in 1951, was followed by the series of Taylor and Helwig, in 1962; Burkhardt et al, in 1966; and McPeak et al,

* *Synonyms and related terms:* progressive recurring dermatofibroma, fibrosarcoma of the skin, sarcomatoid fibroma of the skin, hypertrophic morphea, superficial and nodular fibrous histiocytoma, Darier's tumor.

TABLE 2-7. ***Series of Dermatofibrosarcoma Protuberans***

	NUMBER OF CASES					
	TOTAL	MALE	FEMALE	RECURRENCE %	METASTASIS	DIED WITH DISEASE
Pack and Tabah (1951)	39	24	15	20%	3	2
Taylor and Helwig (1962)	115	—	—	49%	—	—
Burkhardt et al (1966)	56	32	24	55%	2	2
McPeak et al (1967)	82	48	34	20%	5	5
Hajdu (unpublished data)	119	76	43	53%	10	9

in 1967. Brenner et al, in 1975, reviewed the literature and found 402 reported cases of dermatofibrosarcoma protuberans, 23 of which metastasized (Table 2-7).

Our experience at Memorial Sloan-Kettering Cancer Center with 119 cases of dermatofibrosarcoma protuberans is summarized in Figures 2-16 through 2-19. The ages of the 119 patients ranged from 4 to 78 years at the time of diagnosis. Seventy-six were male and 43 were female (Fig. 2-16).

The majority of the tumors were located on either the trunk or the shoulder. Eight tumors were situated below the knee, and two below the elbow. Grossly the tumors were firm and multinodular or polypoid in appearance and were fixed to the skin. They had grown slowly, most of them for several years, and started to enlarge suddenly (Fig. 2-17).

All of the 119 tumors were treated by wide excision. Sixty-four (53%) of the tumors recurred, most of them within one year following excision. Nine of the 10 patients who had metastatic tumor died with pulmonary metastasis. Regional lymph node involvement was not observed in any of the patients (Figs. 2-18, 2-19).

Trauma has frequently been mentioned in the etiology of dermatofibrosarcoma protuberans. Injury as an etiologic factor played no significant role in our series. As noted by many authors, dermatofibrosarcoma has a predilection for the trunk.

Grossly, these tumors may vary from a couple of centimeters to several inches in the greatest diameter. They are usually bosselated or polypoid nodules, gray-white in color and firm in consistency (Figs. 2-20, 2-21, 2-22). But, the color and firmness may vary according to the presence or absence of highly vascular myxomatous areas in the tumor. Erosion or ulceration of the skin surface is not uncommon and repeated recurrence may necessitate amputation (Fig. 2-23).

Microscopically, dermatofibrosarcoma protuberans exhibits a fairly uniform proliferation of non-collagenous fibroblasts. The fibroblasts are arranged in whorls or bundles around central acellular zones or blood vessels producing the cartwheel or storiform pattern characteristic of superficial fibroblastic fibrous histiocytomas, e.g., dermatofibrosarcoma, as well as deeper fibroblastic fibrous histiocytomas. This pattern, which is also described as a twisted strip, spiral nebula, whirled, or rosette-like pattern, is considered pathognomonic but not always apparent, and often adequate study of multiple tissue blocks is required for the demonstration of these structures (Fig. 2-24). The Latin word *storia* or *storea* means "straw-mat" or a "mat made of ropes." The most cellular portion of the tumor is the peripheral, most actively growing part, and the less cellular and more fibrous portion is the central, older areas. Usually the central parts of the tumors become hard and sclerotic and show the presence of broad bands of collagenous fibers with trichrome stain. As a rule, the amounts of collagen and reticulum fibers are inversely proportional to the cellularity and one should not expect to find other than reticulum fibers in most areas of dermatofibrosarcoma protuberans. On microscopic examination there is often a relatively uninvolved zone immediately beneath the epidermis.

The individual cells are plump fibroblasts which tend to be rounded or histiocytic in appearance in some of the cellular areas. However, histiocytic cells with foamy vesicular cytoplasms in small aggregates are rare findings. Mono- or multinucleated giant cells are not a feature of these tumors, but perivascular or peripheral deposits of inflammatory cells are commonly seen. In regard to mitoses in fibroblastic fibrous histiocytomas, it is claimed that five or more mitoses per ten high-power fields is an ominous sign, but a low mitotic rate does not preclude the possibility of aggressive behavior (Fig. 2-25).

Dermatofibrosarcoma protuberans is a clinicopathologic entity. It is a multinodular and superficial fibroblastic fibrous

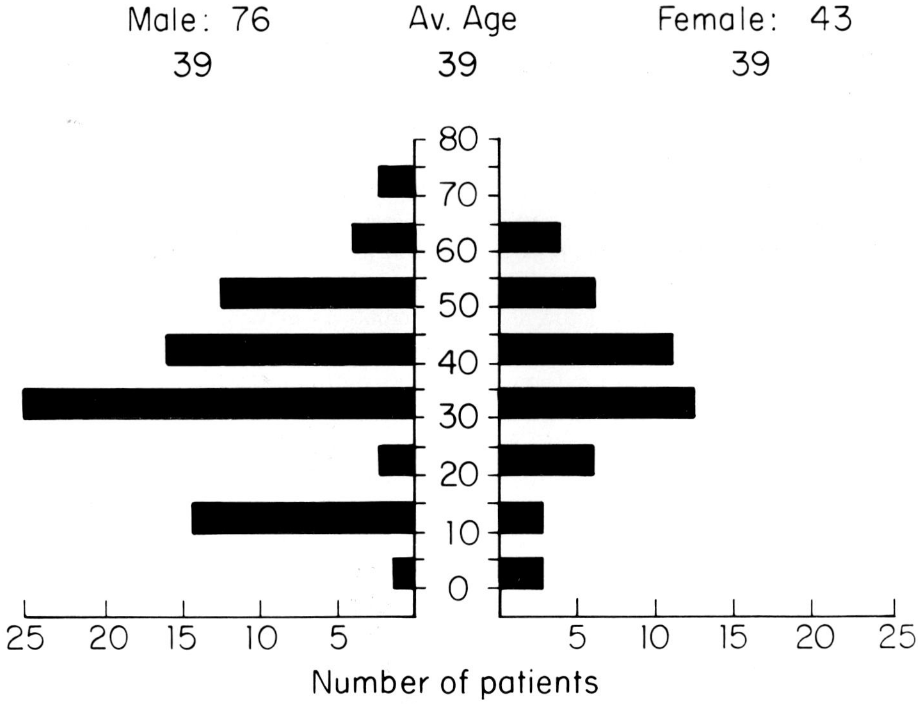

Figure 2-16. Age and sex distribution of 119 patients who were treated for dermatofibrosarcoma protuberans or malignant fibroblastic fibrous histiocytoma at Memorial Sloan-Kettering Cancer Center.

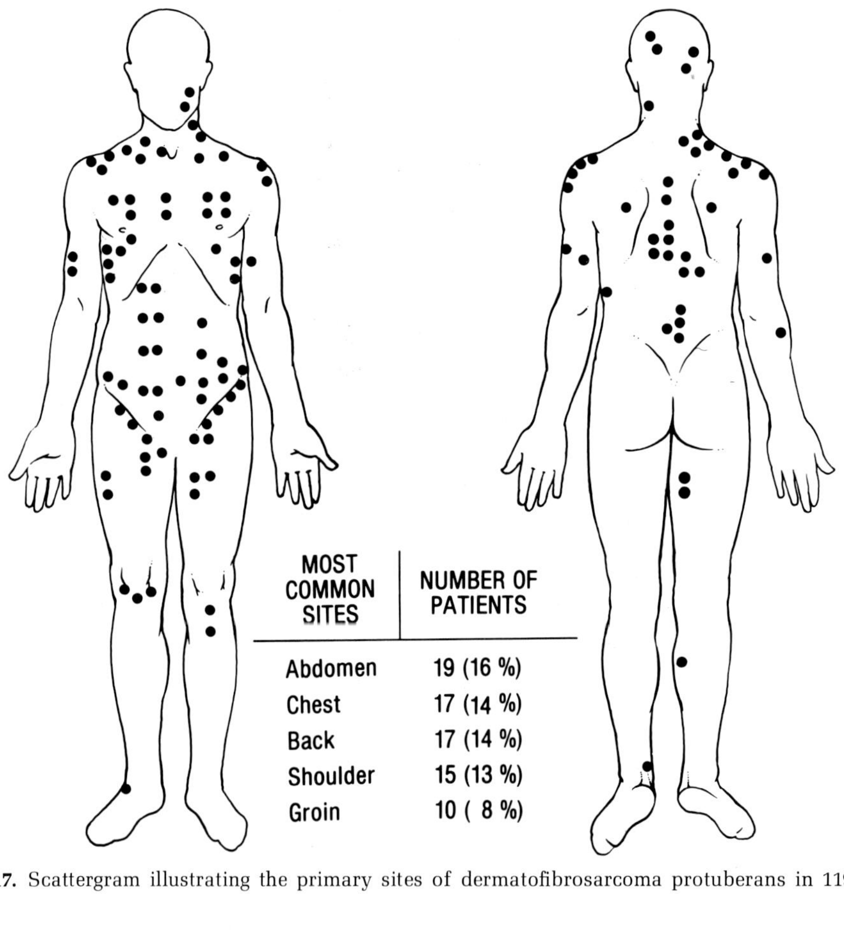

Figure 2-17. Scattergram illustrating the primary sites of dermatofibrosarcoma protuberans in 119 patients.

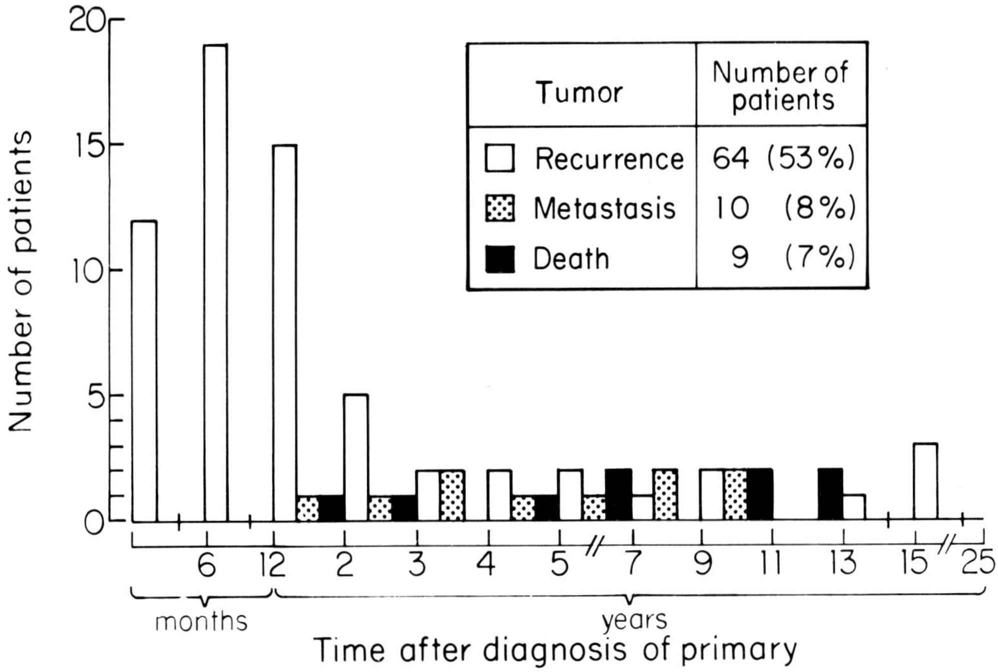

Figure 2-18. Listing of recurrences, metastases, and mortality associated with dermatofibrosarcoma protuberans.

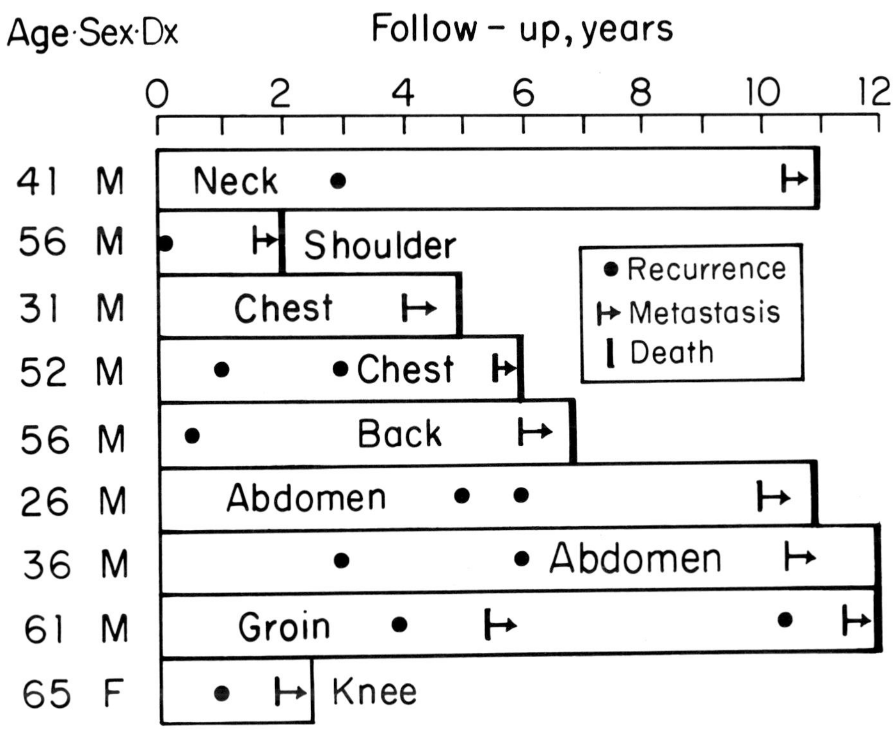

Figure 2-19. Nine patients died with metastatic dermatofibrosarcoma protuberans. Most tumors recurred prior to metastasis and in most cases several years elapsed between primary diagnosis and time of death.

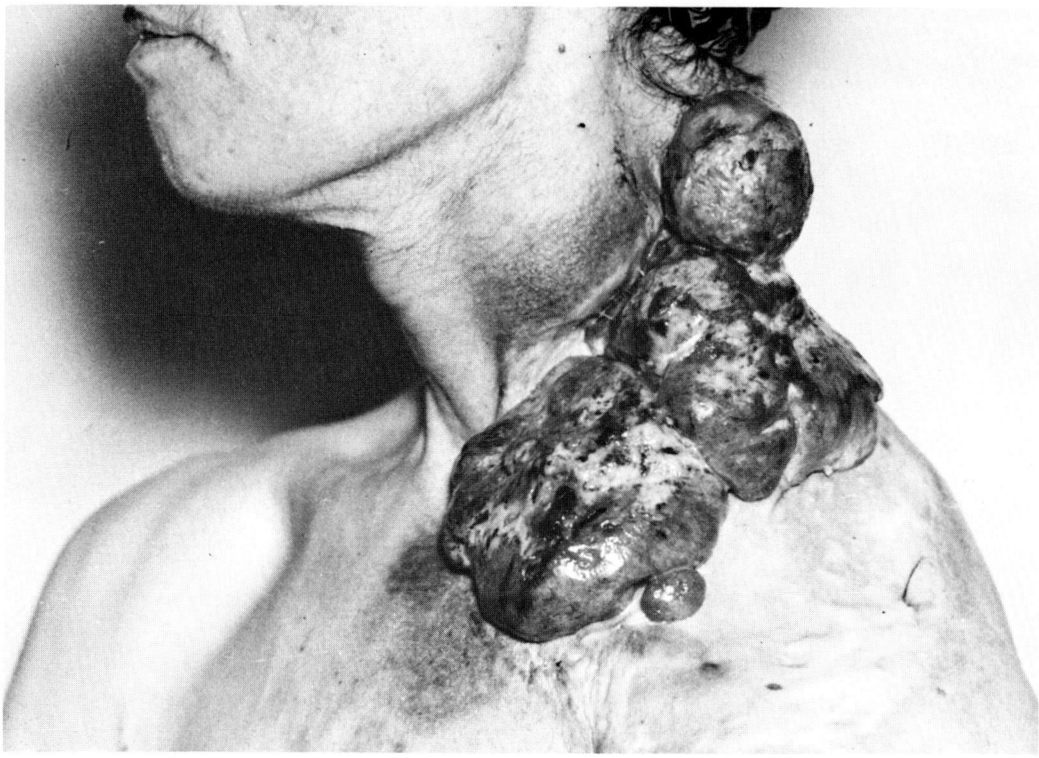

Figure 2-20. Recurrent and neglected dermatofibrosarcoma protuberans.

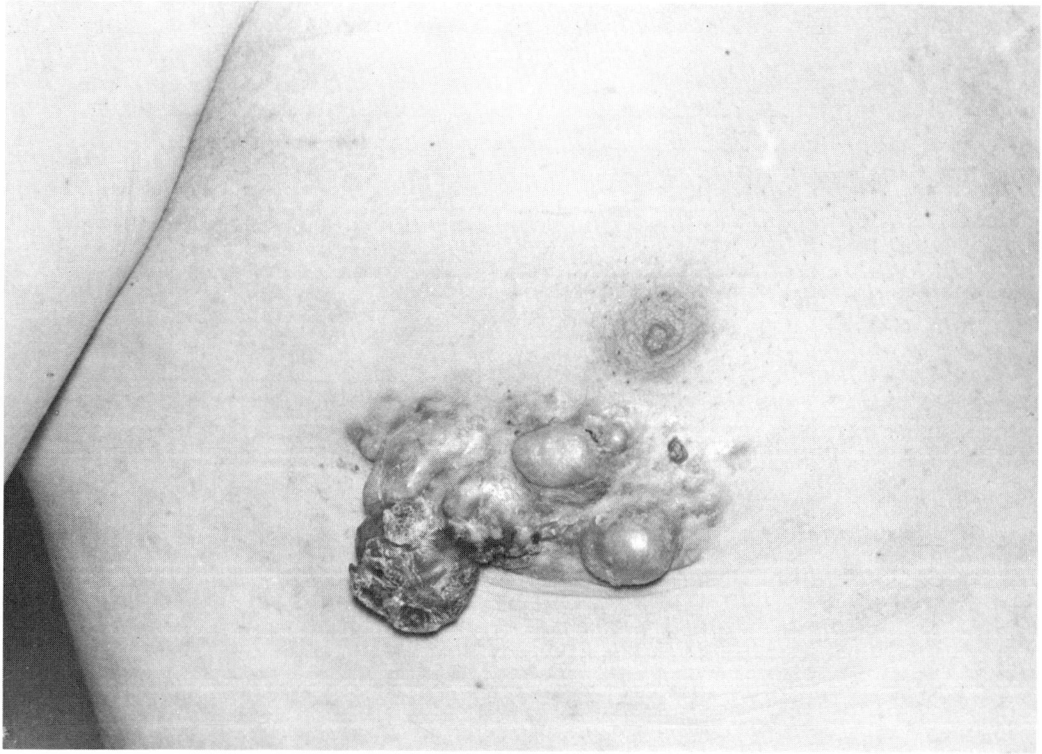

Figure 2-21. Primary dermatofibrosarcoma protuberans prior to complete excision.

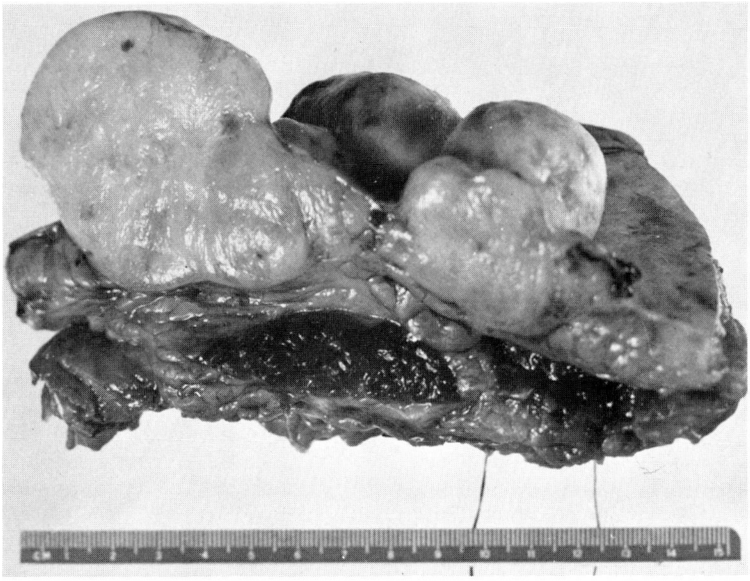

Figure 2-22. Recurrent multinodular dermatofibrosarcoma of the neck (see Figure 2-20) after excision. Note the solid, noncystic, tumor nodules.

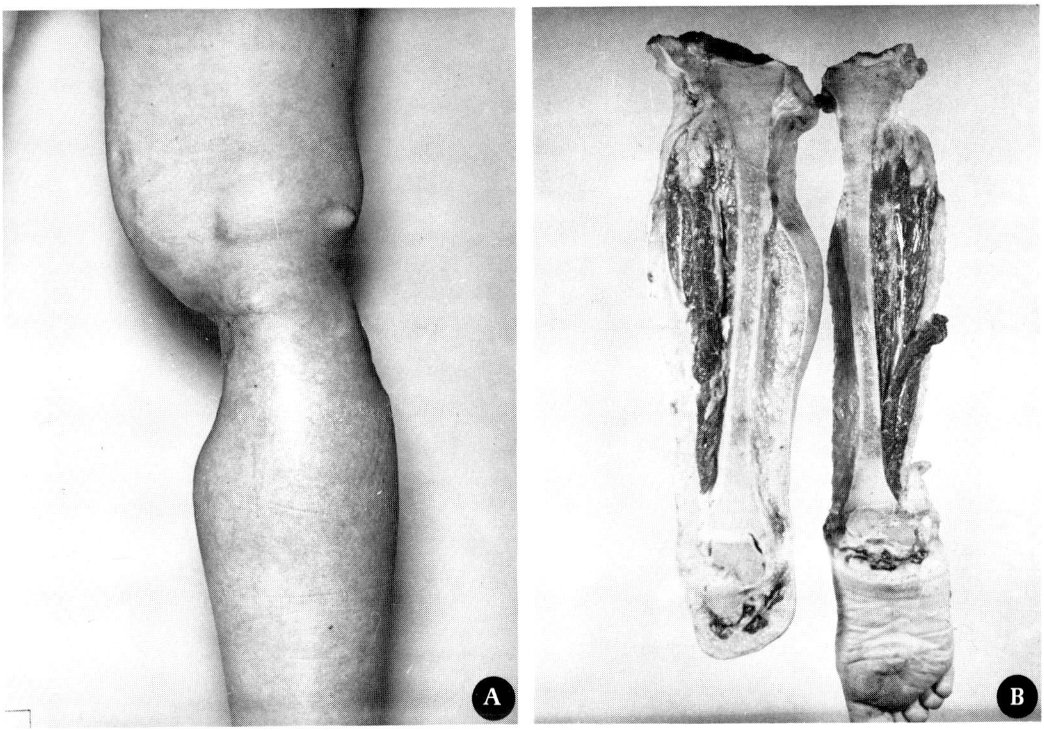

Figure 2-23. Dermatofibrosarcoma of the right leg. This 65-year-old female had several recurrences and excisions. Two years after the first recurrence, and one year prior to the evidence of metastases, amputation was performed. Note multiple tumor nodules, one of which is involving the proximal tibia.

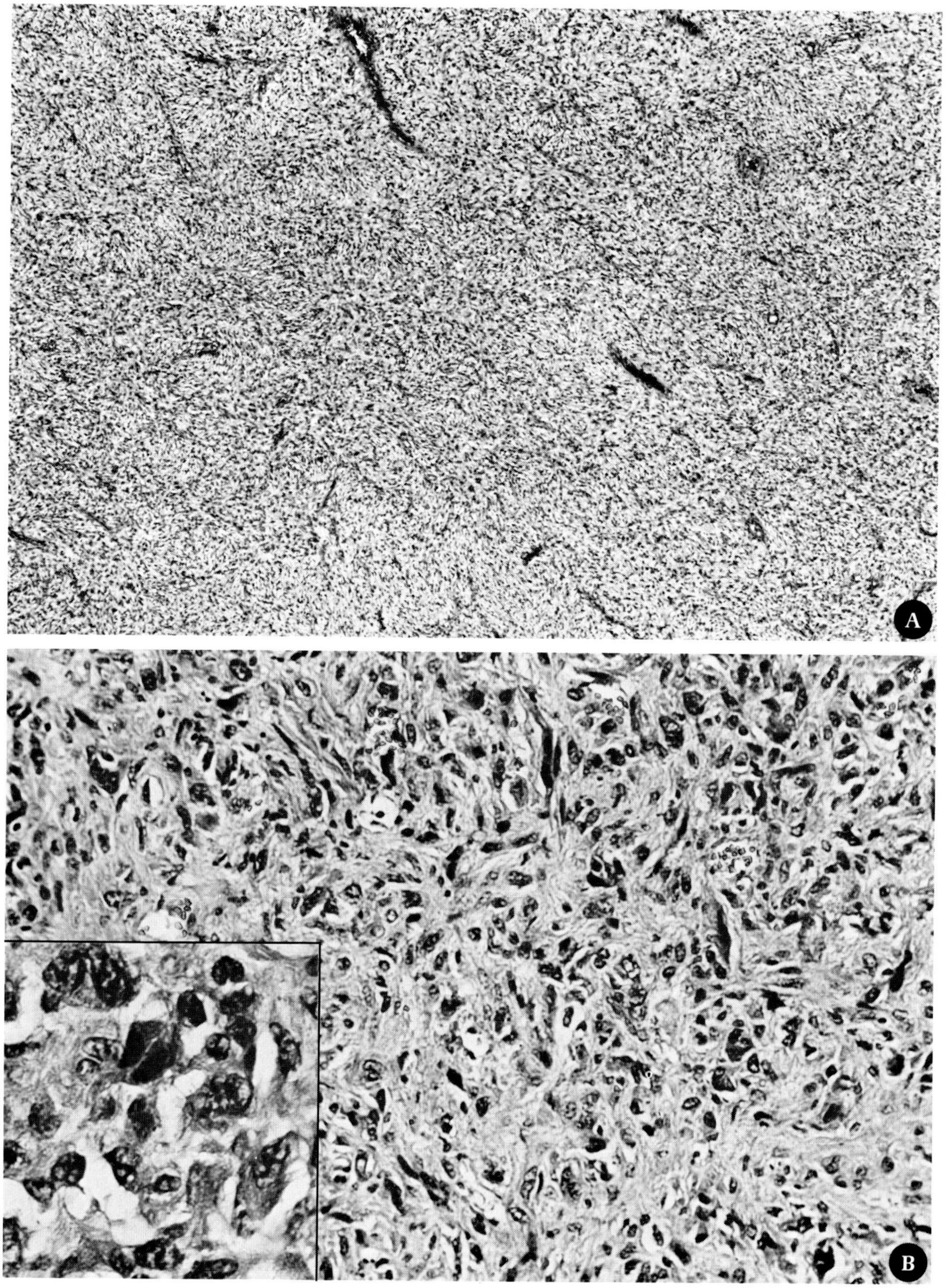

Figure 2-24. Microscopic appearance of dermatofibrosarcoma protuberans (see classification, Figure 2-14C). Short spindle or oval cells possessing finely reticular cytoplasmic filaments arranged in nests and clusters. Note a number of stellate, or small storiform units of neoplastic cells. Some of the cells are bizarre elongated forms with pyknotic nuclei; also there are occasional small binucleated forms (see inset). (**A,** H & E, ×35; **B,** H & E, ×140; inset ×350). (See also Figure 2-50.)

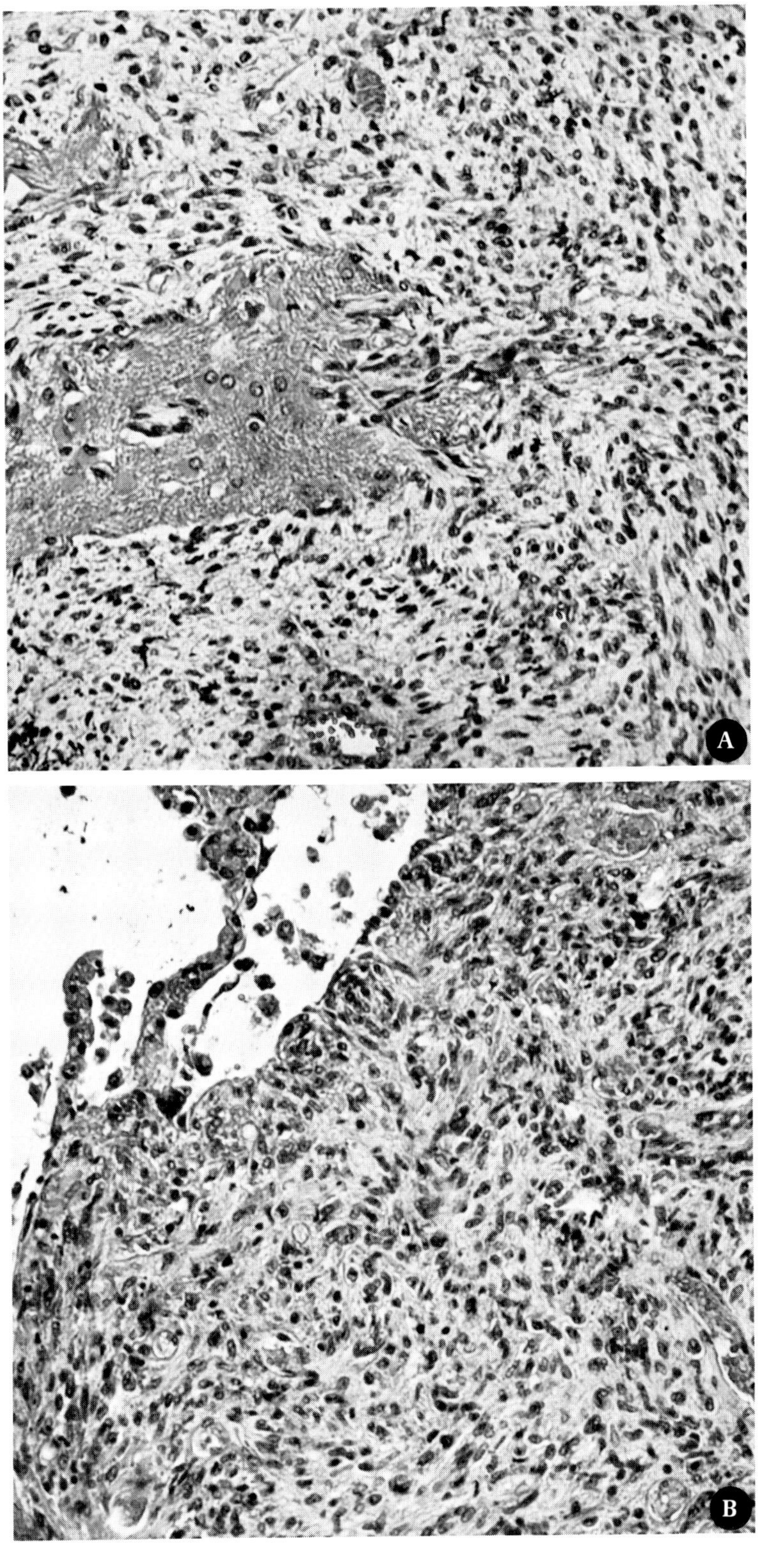

Figure 2-25. Dermatofibrosarcoma protuberans metastatic to the brain, **A,** and metastatic to the lung, **B.** Notice the precise reproduction of the typical stellate pattern commonly seen in primary tumors (H & E, ×140).

histiocytoma of low-grade malignancy (see Table 2-7). However, *neoplasms composed of similar, non-collagenous fibroblasts arranged in typical storiform pattern can be seen in deeper soft parts as well as in the retroperitoneum.* The gross and microscopic appearance of these neoplasms is so strikingly similar to the well-known appearance of dermatofibrosarcoma protuberans that one may think of displaced or metastatic dermatofibrosarcoma. Contrary to the low-grade malignancy of dermatofibrosarcoma, lesions of the deeper soft parts, which are deeper than the superficial fascial plane, are fully malignant neoplasms and should be treated accordingly (Fig. 2-26; see also Fig. 1-59 and Table 1-15).

Many fibroblastic fibrous histiocytomas, regardless of whether their location is superficial or deep, are highly vascular with many myxoid components. The myxoid changes can be so dominant that one may be justified in using the term *myxoid fibrous histiocytoma*. However, this term, coined by Weiss and Enzinger, in 1977, should be reserved for tumors which, after generous sampling, show no significant solid components and it must be understood that they are a variety of fibroblastic fibrous histiocytoma. It is apparent that many of the myxomas and myxosarcomas of earlier reports may belong to this category, but according to Lagace et al (1979) there are no specific ultrastructural features of these neoplasms that would permit their differentiation (Fig. 2-27).

Accumulation of various inflammatory cells with or without necrosis is not uncommon in fibroblastic fibrous histiocytoma, especially in tumors of the deeper soft parts. These lesions, called by some authors "inflammatory fibrous histiocytomas" carry poorer prognoses than many other fibrous histiocytomas not because of their inflammatory component but because of their size, anatomic location, and infiltrative nature (Fig. 2-28). A rare association between fibrous histiocytomas and leukemoid blood has been reported by Roques et al in 1979.

The fact that tumors with histologic patterns identical to that of dermatofibrosarcoma protuberans occur in deep soft tissues indicates that the term *dermatofibrosarcoma* is inappropriate. Unfortunately, the name *dermatofibrosarcoma*, just like cystosarcoma phyllodes, is so well established that elimination of the term is impossible, but it should be used only for malignant fibroblastic fibrous histiocytomas that are superficial in location.

Fisher and Hellstrom, in 1966, reported two metastatic dermatofibrosarcoma protuberans in which the metastatic deposits appeared morphologically indistinguishable from Hodgkin's disease and histiocytic lymphoma. Our experience with metastatic dermatofibrosarcoma protuberans (Fig. 2-29; see also Fig. 2-25) and other metastatic fibroblastic fibrous histiocytomas has supported the observation of Fisher and Hellstrom. In 4 of 9 metastatic tumors the metastatic foci were composed predominantly of monomorphic, round, histiocytic forms. We observed similar "rounding-out" of fibroblastic cells in tissue cultures and heterotransplants of fibroblastic fibrous histiocytomas (Hajdu and Hajdu, 1976; Sethi et al, 1977; and Hajdu and Fogh, 1978). The bimorphic appearance of these neoplastic cells indicate a close histogenetic relationship between histiocytes and fibroblasts. After studying cell cultures of dermatofibrosarcoma protuberans with the electron microscope, Ozzello and Hamels, in 1976, came to the conclusion that the fibroblast-like cells were histiocytes that secondarily acquired fibroblastic features (Fig. 2-30). Alguacil-Garcia et al (1978) felt that dermatofibrosarcoma protuberans is composed of primitive fibroblastic cells resembling perineurial cells. It seems to me the discussion of the histogenesis of dermatofibrosarcoma is an exercise in futility. As Bednar (1957) pointed out, "dermatofibrosarcoma protuberans is not a histogenetic entity." Dermatofibrosarcoma, along with other fibroblastic fibrous histiocytomas, is a morphologic entity with a characteristic growth pattern of undifferentiated fibro-

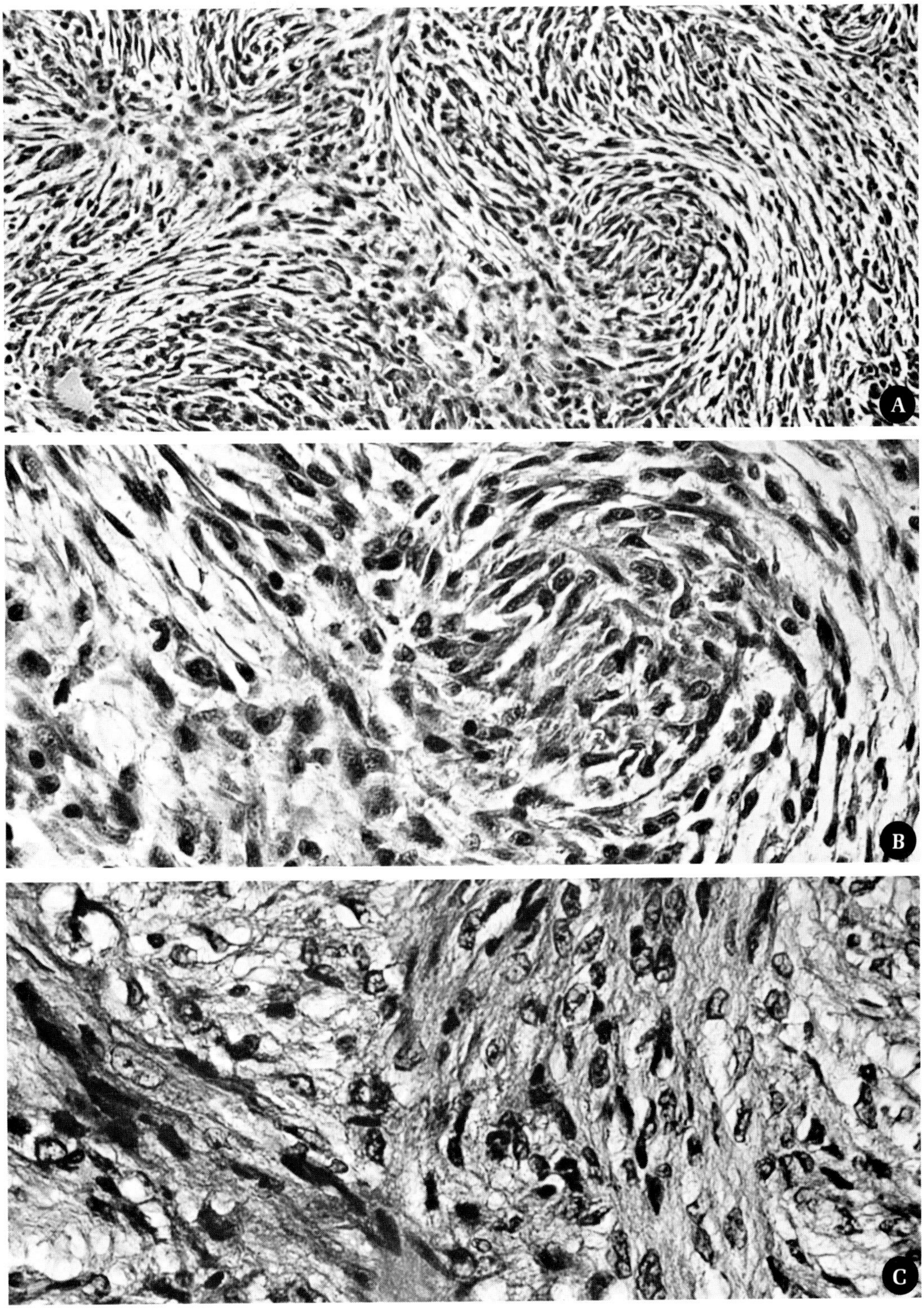

Figure 2-26. Malignant fibroblastic fibrous histiocytoma of deeper soft tissues shows striking resemblance microscopically to dermatofibrosarcoma protuberans. **A,** This sarcoma is composed of slender reticular fibroblasts arranged in storiform pattern.

B and **C,** The tumor cells are fairly uniform and packed together in loosely composed bundles (**A,** H & E, ×140; **B,** H & E, ×350; **C,** H & E, ×420).

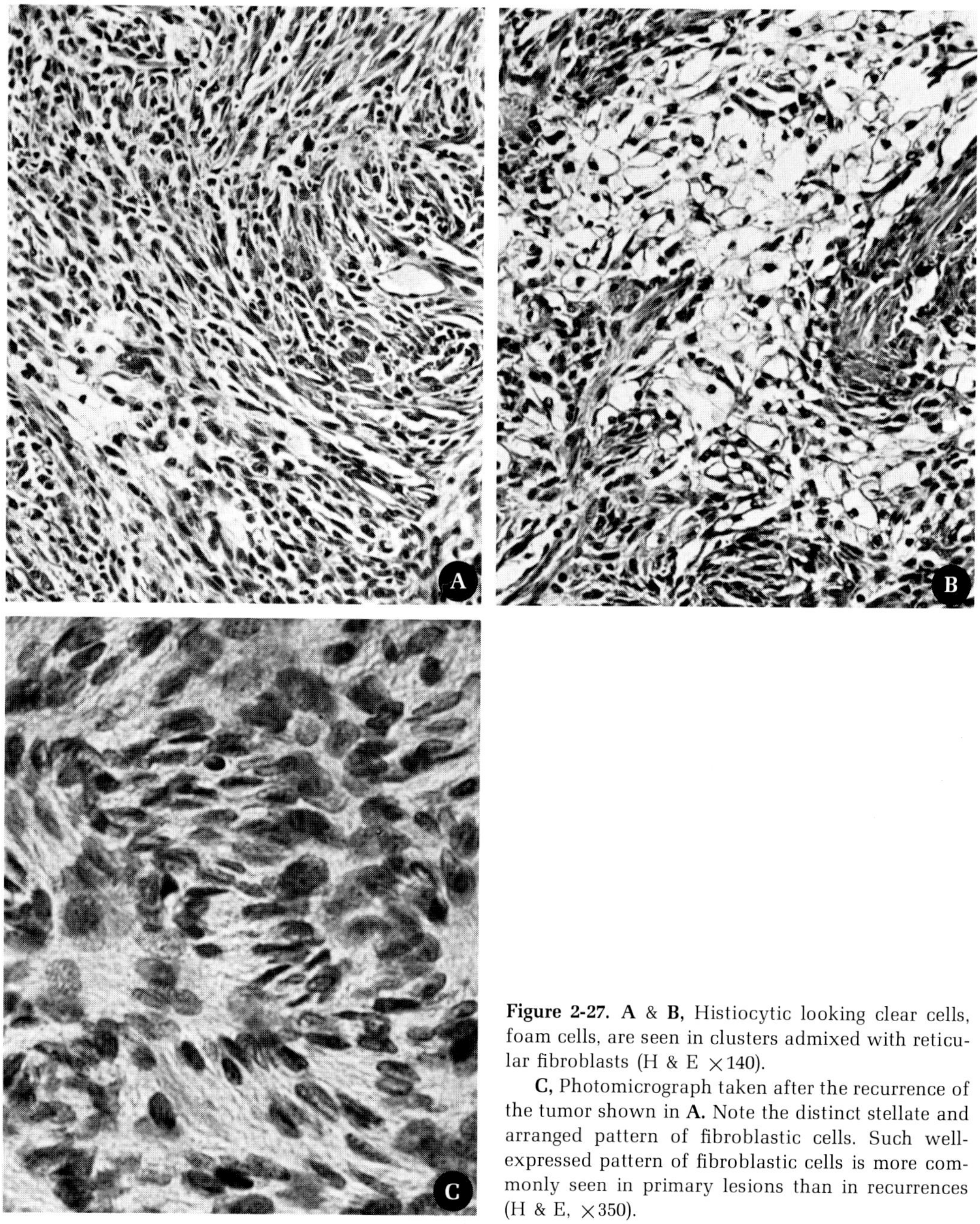

Figure 2-27. A & **B,** Histiocytic looking clear cells, foam cells, are seen in clusters admixed with reticular fibroblasts (H & E ×140).

C, Photomicrograph taken after the recurrence of the tumor shown in **A.** Note the distinct stellate and arranged pattern of fibroblastic cells. Such well-expressed pattern of fibroblastic cells is more commonly seen in primary lesions than in recurrences (H & E, ×350).

blastic cells which may derive histogenetically from primitive mesenchymal cells, histiocytes, dedifferentiated fibroblasts, pericytes, Schwann cells, or perineurial cells (Fig. 2-31).

The primary treatment of dermatofibrosarcoma should be surgical resection with a clean and generous surgical margin which almost always requires removal of the underlying deep fascia. Adequate resection of deep fibroblastic fibrous histiocytomas may require muscle group resection or more mutilating surgical intervention.

Differential Diagnosis

In the differential diagnosis of fibroblastic fibrous histiocytomas, including

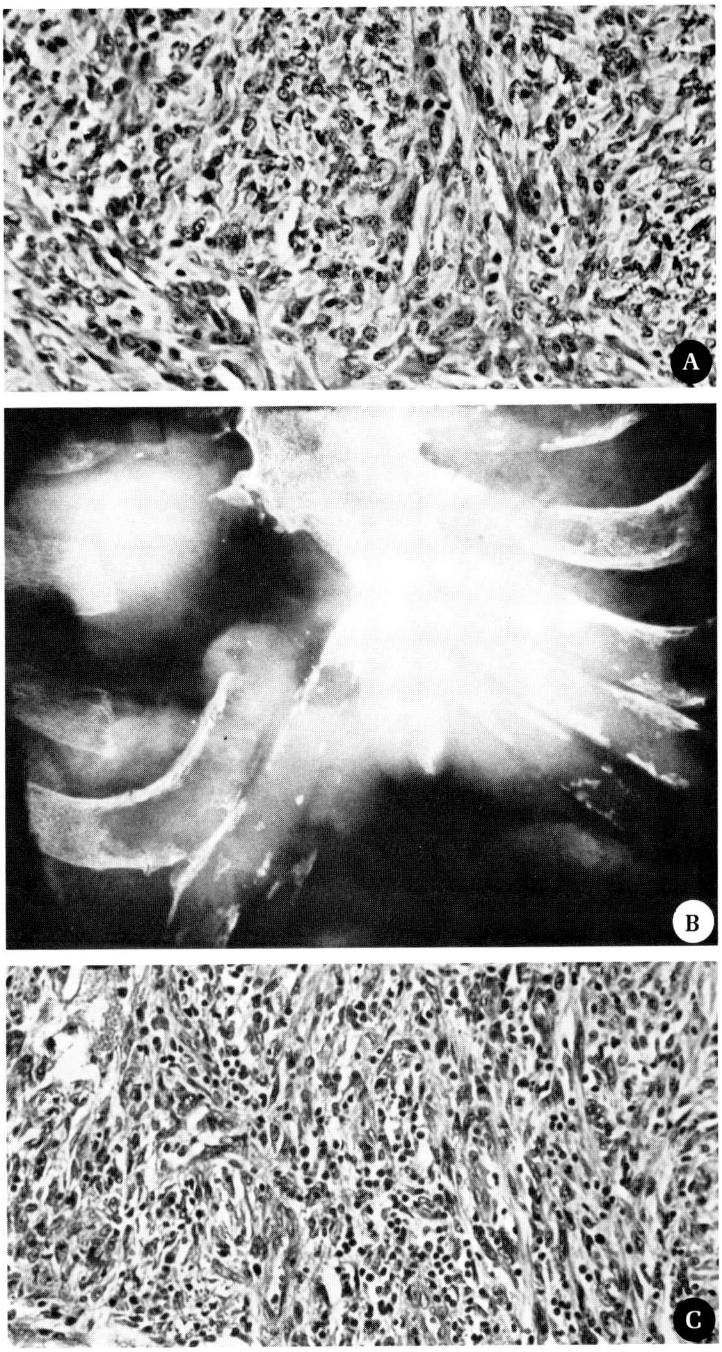

Figure 2-28. A, A primary fibroblastic fibrous histiocytoma of the chest wall (H & E, ×140).

B, A specimen radiograph showing the recurrent tumor with destruction of several ribs and part of the sternum.

C, A histologic section of the recurrent tumor. Note the numerous inflammatory cells between neoplastic cells away from a necrotic area (H & E, ×140).

dermatofibrosarcoma protuberans, the following tumors should be considered.

Fibroblastic fibrosarcoma may appear histologically similar to dermatofibrosarcoma protuberans. However, fibrosarcomas are usually composed of less slender and more collagenous fibroblasts and do not have prominent cartwheel or storiform arrangement of fibroblasts.

Superficial, subcutaneous *leiomyosarcoma* is rare, and the tumor cells are more slender and less arranged than those in dermatofibrosarcoma (see Chapter 5).

Benign schwannomas are neoplasms of

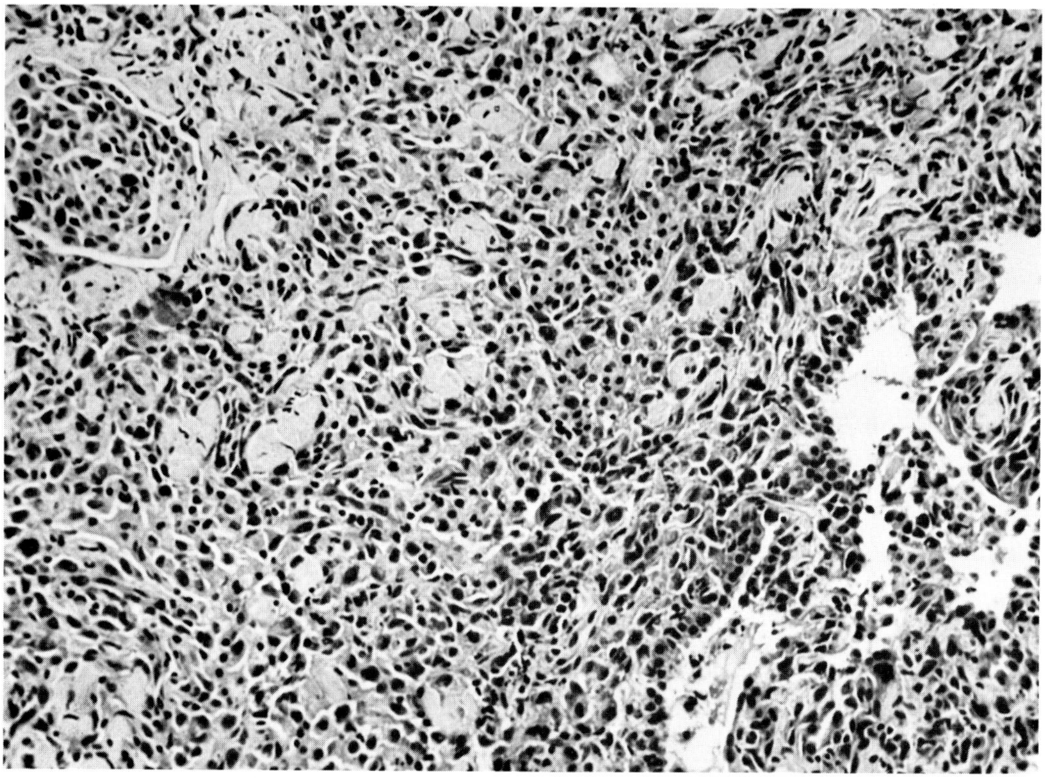

Figure 2-29. Fibroblastic fibrous histiocytoma of the thigh metastatic to the lung. Note that slender elongated cells are not present. Most of the tumor cells are either round or oval histiocytic forms (H & E, ×140). (Compare with Figure 2-39A.)

elongated cells with narrow nuclei and long cytoplasmic processes. Malignant schwannomas, as well as other neurogenic sarcomas, on the other hand, may lose their schwannian features, and morphologically their growth pattern may be identical with the growth pattern of fibroblastic fibrous histiocytomas (see Chapter 7).

HISTIOCYTIC FIBROUS HISTIOCYTOMA* AND PLEOMORPHIC FIBROUS HISTIOCYTOMA†

Morphologically, histiocytic fibrous histiocytomas and pleomorphic fibrous histiocytomas often blend into each other so well that sharp distinction is impossible. More importantly, it is often difficult to distinguish, purely on histopathologic ground, the benign neoplasms from the corresponding malignant forms (Fig. 2-32).

Histologically, these neoplasms have been reported under various names (see footnotes and Table 2-8). A subcutaneous form of histiocytic fibrous histiocytoma was first described by McDonagh in 1912. Credit for the first distinction between histiocytic and fibroblastic tumors is due Levy (1925). Carrel, in 1926, was perhaps the first to come to the conclusion that *fibroblasts may transform to histiocytes.* Christopher, in 1926, and Fry, in 1927, reported the first cases of *giant cell tumors of soft tissues.* Phemister, in 1931, described 5 cases of round-cell sarcomas in which cures lasting from 5 to 10 years were obtained "although all had a very cellular structure and almost devoid of

Synonyms and related terms:

* Giant cell tumor of tendon sheath, histiocytoma, osteoclastoma, reticulum cell sarcoma of soft tissues, giant cell tumor of soft tissues, round-cell sarcomas, reticulohistiocytic granuloma, pseudosarcomatous reticulohistiocytoma, nevoxanthoendothelioma.

† Histiocytoma cutis, xanthoma, juvenile xanthoma, xanthogranuloma, malignant xanthoma, xanthosarcoma, pseudosarcoma, atypical fibroxanthoma.

stroma." And, also in 1931 Woringer introduced the term *histiocytoma* and pointed out that the cells of these lesions were capable of phagocytizing fat. Oberling, in 1935, used the term *xanthogranuloma* in describing certain retroperitoneal tumors, and Senear and Caro, in 1936, coined two new names: *histiocytoma cutis* and *nevoxanthoendothelioma*.

Broders et al, in 1939, described a group of tumors "composed of plump, spindle-shaped, or polyhedral cells often with abundant acidophilic cytoplasm and very little intercellular substance." They added that "tumors of this nature probably represent highly malignant, undifferentiated fibrogenic or spindle-cell tumors." Bloom et al, in 1942, called attention to hereditary xanthomatosis, and Arnold and Tilden, in 1943, came to the conclusion by studying 23 cases of histiocytic skin lesions that histiocytoma cutis is a variant of xanthoma. Foster, in 1947, recognized the similarities between giant cell tumor of tendon sheath and sclerosing hemangioma, and Stewart, in 1948, by studying the morphology of giant cell tumors, recognized the relation between giant cell tumors of tendon sheath and xanthomas. Up to that time it was believed that most of these lesions were benign or atypical neoplasms. Kobak and Perlow, in 1949, were the first to report a case of malignant xanthomatous giant cell tumor. Purvis and Helwig, in 1954, emphasized difficulty in histologic diagnosis whether "reticulohistiocytic" lesions are benign or malignant and referred to many of these tumors as "atypical." In 1963, Schmaman reported a case of giant cell tumor of soft tissues and cited 4 earlier case reports; Ozzello et al (1963) studied the morphologic characteristics of malignant histio-

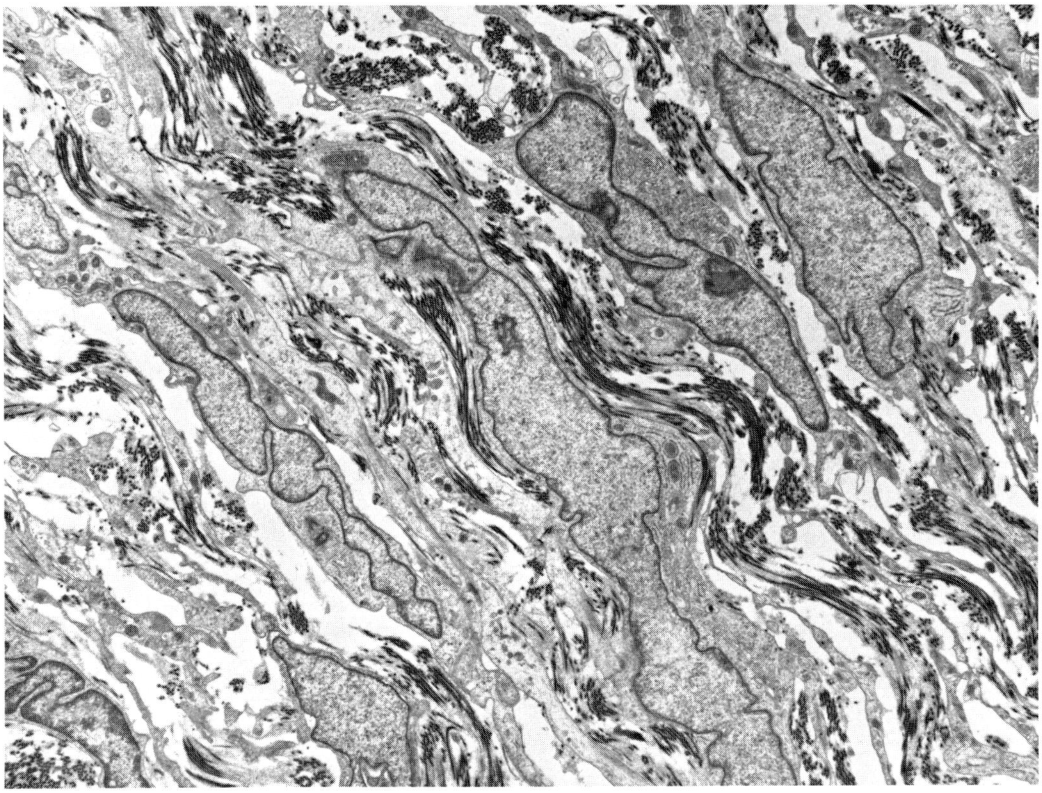

Figure 2-30. Ultrastructure of dermatofibrosarcoma protuberans. The tumor consists of long, thin, and tightly arranged fibroblast-like cells. Note the long, attenuated bipolar cell process and nuclear invaginations. Some of the tumor cells are in sparsely collagenous stroma (×4,800).

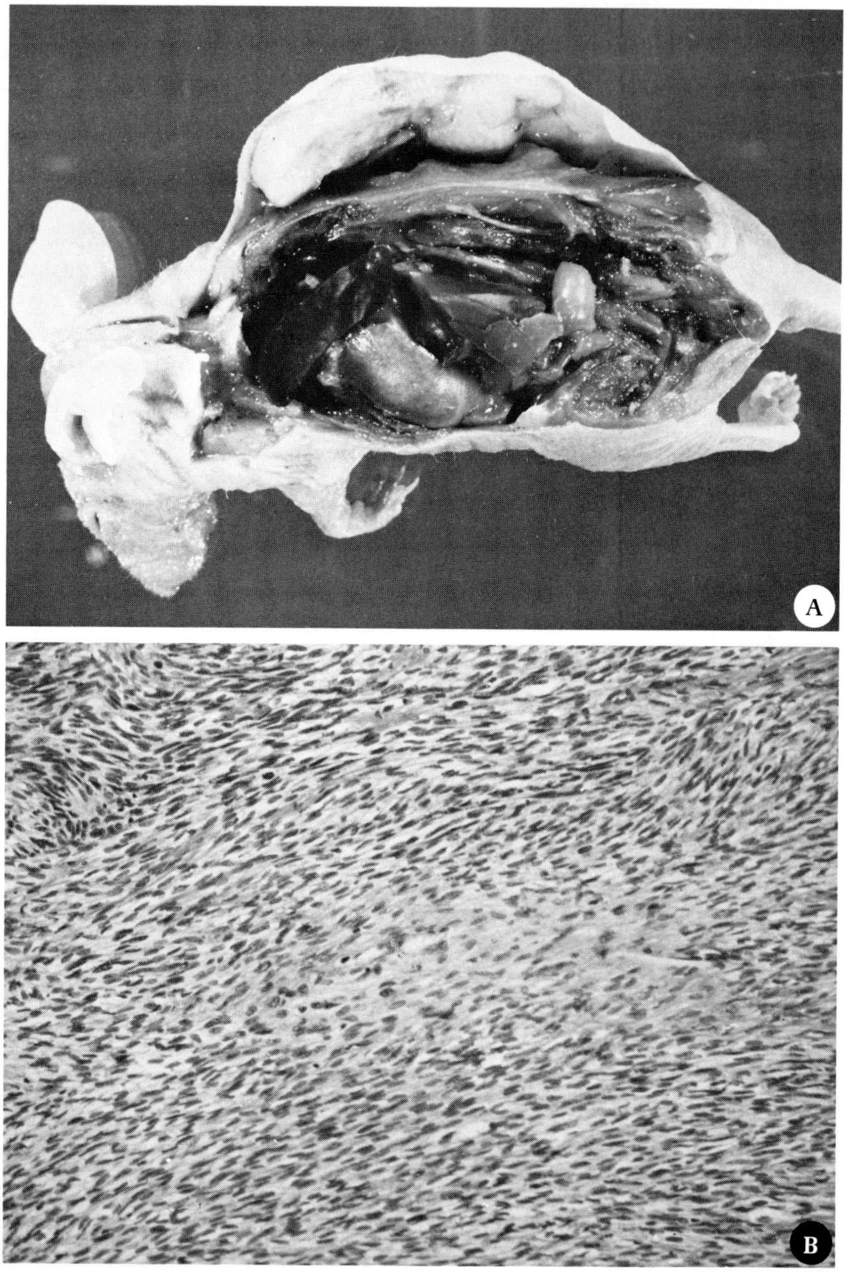

Figure 2-31. A, Fibroblastic fibrous histiocytoma (dermatofibrosarcoma protuberans) in nude mouse 5 weeks after subcutaneous injection of cell suspension prepared from a surgically excised tumor of a patient.

B, Microscopically, the tumor in nude mouse is composed of fairly uniform reticular fibroblasts. Note (left upper corner) the attempt of the cells to form a storiform pattern (H & E, ×85).

cytoma and fibrous xanthoma in tissue culture. Further emphasizing the diagnostic difficulties, Gordon, in 1964, proposed the term *pseudosarcomatous reticulohistiocytoma.* O'Brien and Stout, in 1964, in an attempt to define the co-existence of fibroblast-like spindle cells and xanthomatous elements coined the term *fibrous xanthoma,* which was soon replaced by a more appropriate term *fibrous histiocytoma,* first publicized by Stout and Lattes in 1967. The first ultrastructural study of fibrous histiocytomas was published by Merkow et al in 1971.

In 1972, the reports of Guccion and Enzinger and Salm and Sissons on giant cell tumors of soft tissues were published. Also, Kouri and Ancheta reported transformation of macrophages into fibroblasts, and Kempson and Kyriakos concluded that fibroxanthosarcoma is a variant of malignant fibrous histiocytoma. We studied the cytomorphology of various fibrous histiocytomas by in vitro and in vivo techniques (Hajdu and Hajdu, 1976) and came to the same conclusion that these neoplasms are composed of two elements—fibroblastic and histiocytic—with potential to change in shape from elongated to round and in size from mononuclear to multinucleated forms.

The pathophysiology of the development of fibrous histiocytomas is far from settled. Some of the investigators suggested that these tumors arise from the tissue histiocytes which have the ability to undergo transformation to facultative fibroblasts. Maximow and Bloom (1930), who were proponents of this theory, said that fibroblasts are highly specialized cells incapable, unlike multipotential tissue histiocytes, of changing their structure and function. Civatte, quoted by Senear and Caro (1936), suggested that the *histiocyte should be regarded as the parent cell of the fibroblast and histiocytoma might therefore be regarded as fibroma arrested in an early stage of development.* Petrakis et al (1961) observed *in vivo* differentiation of leukocytes into histiocytes, fibroblasts, and fat cells in subcutaneous diffusion chambers. Ozzello et al (1963) studied fibrous histiocytomas in tissue culture and stated that the histiocyte functioned as a facultative fibroblast and represented the stem cell of these neoplasms. In 1976, after studying tissue cultures of dermatofibrosarcoma protuberans with the electron microscope, they added that the fibroblast-like cells are histiocytes with some secondarily acquired fibroblastic features. Sutton (1967) studied the ultrastructural aspects of *in vitro* development of monocytes into macrophages, multinucleated giant cells, and so-called epithelioid cells. Kouri and Ancheta, in 1972, went one step further by demonstrating the transformation of macrophages into fibroblasts (Fig. 2-14).

It has also been suggested (Fischer,

TABLE 2-8. ***Classification of Fibrous Histiocytomas***

	BENIGN	MALIGNANT
Fibroblastic fibrous histiocytoma	Sclerosing hemangioma Dermatofibroma Fibrous xanthoma Xanthofibroma Storiform fibrous xanthoma Myxoma	Dermatofibrosarcoma protuberans Fibrous xanthoma Myxoid fibrous histiocytoma
Histiocytic fibrous histiocytoma	Giant cell tumor of tendon sheath Reticulohistiocytic granuloma Xanthogranuloma Pigmented nodular synovitis Nevoid xanthoma	Malignant histiocytoma Malignant giant cell tumor of soft tissues Round cell sarcoma Pseudosarcomatous reticulohistiocytosis Xanthomatous giant cell tumor Nevoxanthoendothelioma
Pleomorphic fibrous histiocytoma	Atypical fibroxanthoma Xanthoma Xanthogranuloma Histiocytic xanthoma	Malignant xanthoma Fibroxanthosarcoma Xanthosarcoma Histiocytic xanthoma

1925; Stout, 1953; Mackenzie, 1970; Ross et al, 1970) that the *histiocyte* may not be a specific cell type but rather a functional and morphologic state which can be achieved by different cells—endothelial, schwannian, mesothelial, synovial, pericytic, and lipoblastic—and is capable of appearing as a facultative fibroblast. Our studies (Hajdu et al, 1974; Hajdu and Hajdu, 1976; Sethi, et al, 1977; Hajdu and Fogh, 1978) of fibroblasts and fibrous tumors in tissue cultures support these observations but also give credit to the observation of Carrel and Ebeling (1926) who first concluded that fibroblasts may also transform to histiocytes. It is important to remember that our definitions of *histiocyte* and *fibroblast* are vague and in most instances are based on morphologic rather than functional differences. Yet, they are practical and can be applied to a better understanding of neoplasms. The nomenclature of fibrous histiocytic lesions is not entirely standardized, but there is far less confusion than a decade ago. However, *it would be wrong to assume that all of the poorly differentiated soft tissue sarcomas that fail to develop specific structures perceptible with the light microscope should be considered fibrous histiocytoma rather than, e.g., fibrosarcoma or rhabdomyosarcoma.*

Fibrous histiocytomas often are difficult to diagnose and classify because of the diversity of clinical presentation and histologic pattern, but if we adhere to the definition of Stout and Lattes (1967), who said that "Fibrous histiocytomas are embryonal forms of fibroblastic neoplasms," it will become clear that differentiated fibrous tumors, e.g., fibrosarcomas, are mostly collagenous and stain positive with trichrome stain, but undifferentiated fibrous tumors such as fibrous histiocytomas are mostly non-collagenous and do not take the trichrome stain. Although most of these lesions are superficial, subcutaneous, benign lesions, some occur deep in soft tissues and are infiltrative, bulky, and malignant (Fig. 2-33).

They occur at any age, but the majority occur during the middle years of life. The male-to-female ratio is, according to reports, 2 to 1.

These neoplasms have no typical gross appearance. They are usually asymptomatic or slightly painful lesions, most often of the extremities, buttocks, and shoulders (Fig. 2-34). They tend to be softer than the collagenous fibrous tumors and the fibroblastic fibrous histiocytomas. The sizes of histiocytic fibrous histiocytomas and pleomorphic fibrous histiocytomas vary but the deeper tumors tend to be

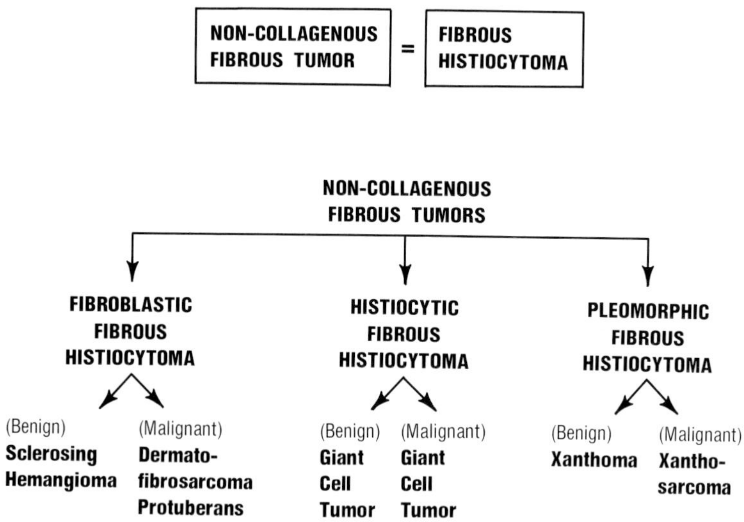

Figure 2-32. Subclassification of fibrous histiocytomas or noncollagenous fibrous tumors (see also Figures 2-14 and 2-72).

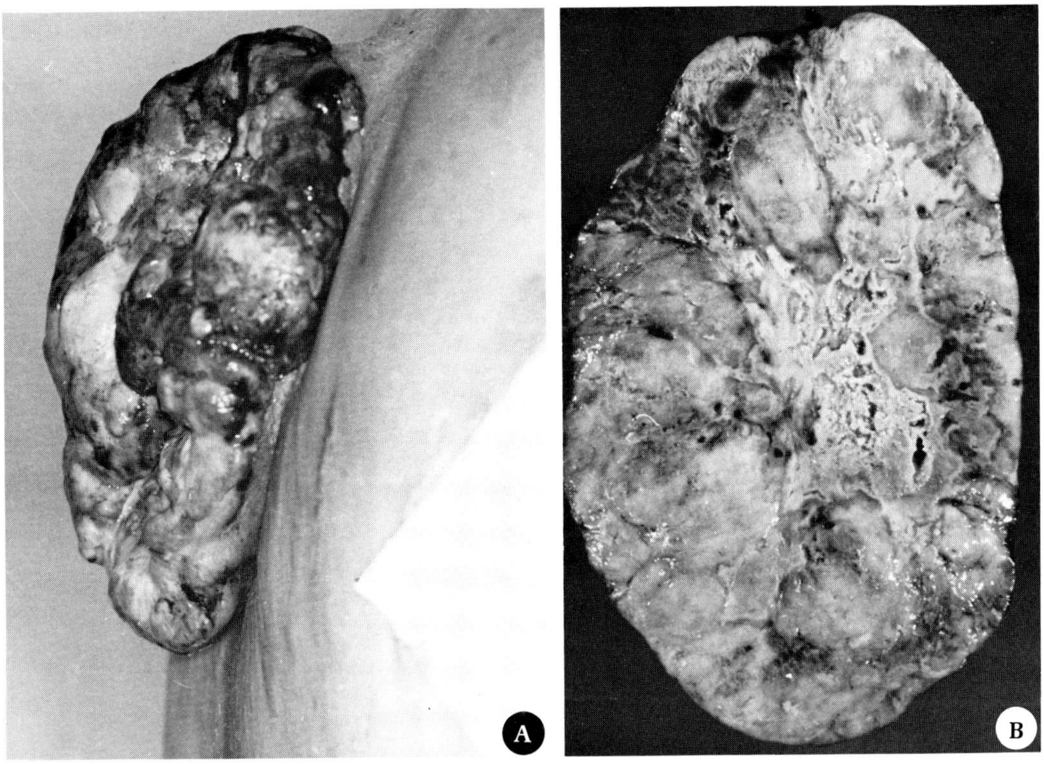

Figure 2-33. A and B, So-called malignant giant cell tumor or malignant histiocytic fibrous histiocytoma of soft tissues before and after excision.

larger than the superficial ones. Many of these tumors appear demarcated but not truly encapsulated. They are made up of fleshy, indurated tissue of pale yellowish-gray color which appears trabeculated or occasionally cystic on cut section. The malignant ones, as well as many of the benign or atypical forms, infiltrate the surrounding soft tissue, especially muscles and tendons, and blend into them (Figs. 2-35, 2-36).

Most of the difficulties in understanding the nature of many of these tumors apparently stem from the improper classification and misuse of various terms. Histiocytic fibrous histiocytomas are known by a score of names (see page 94 and Table 2-8), and many of them were classified in the past as histiocytic lymphoma (reticulum cell sarcoma), histiocytosis-X, or some sort of granulomatous disease. The first reference to these rare neoplasms is the article published by Phemister in 1931.

It is admittedly difficult to appreciate

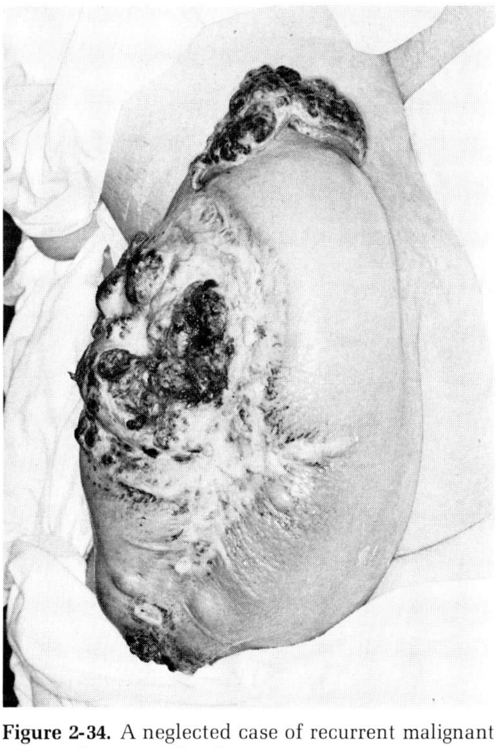

Figure 2-34. A neglected case of recurrent malignant giant cell tumor of soft tissues.

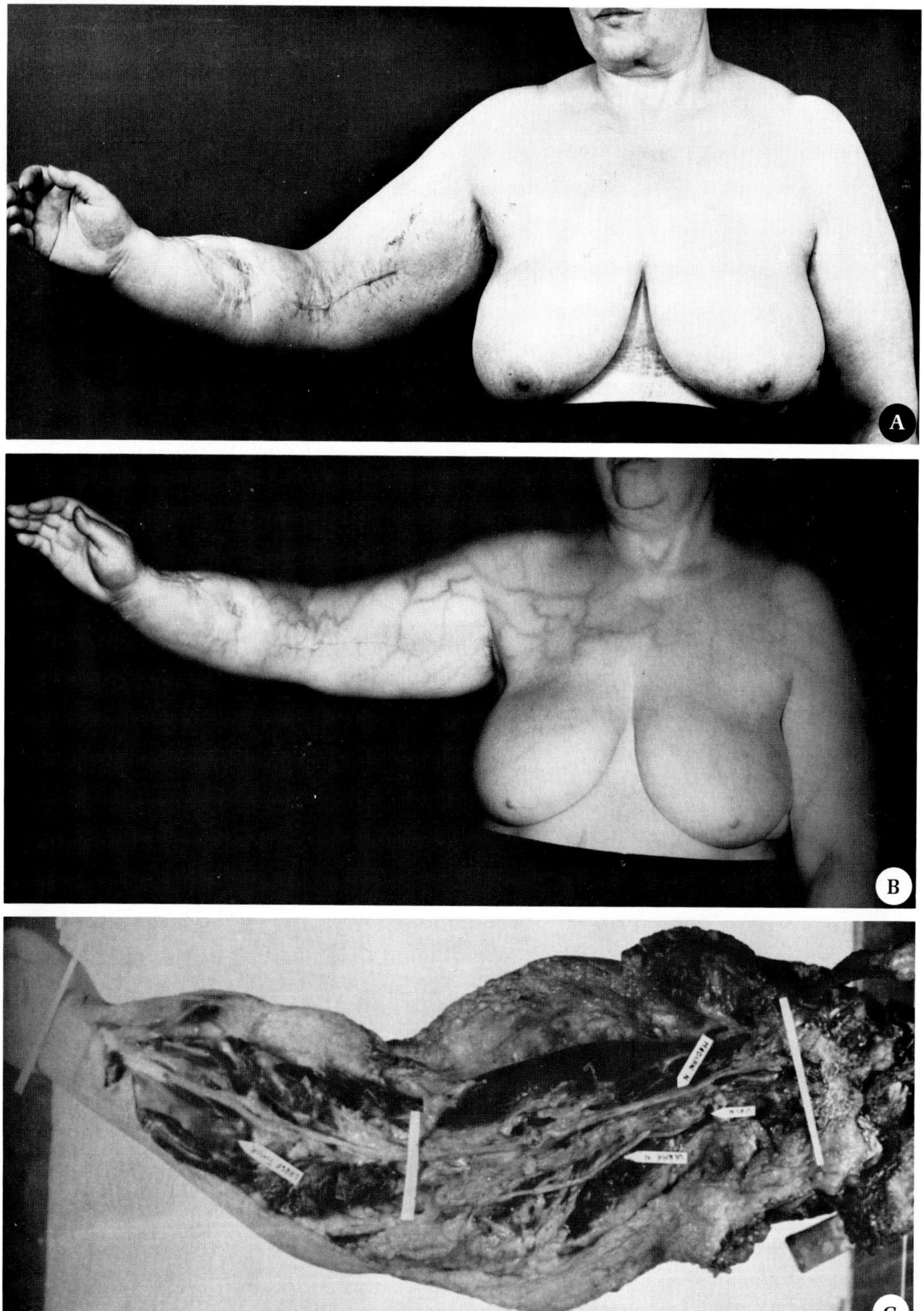

Figure 2-35. A, Recurrent malignant pleomorphic fibrous histiocytoma of the right arm.
B, Hypervascularity of the arm after the patient developed lymphedema demonstrated by infrared light.
C, The surgical specimen after amputation. Multiple tumor nodules were found in the entire length of the arm.

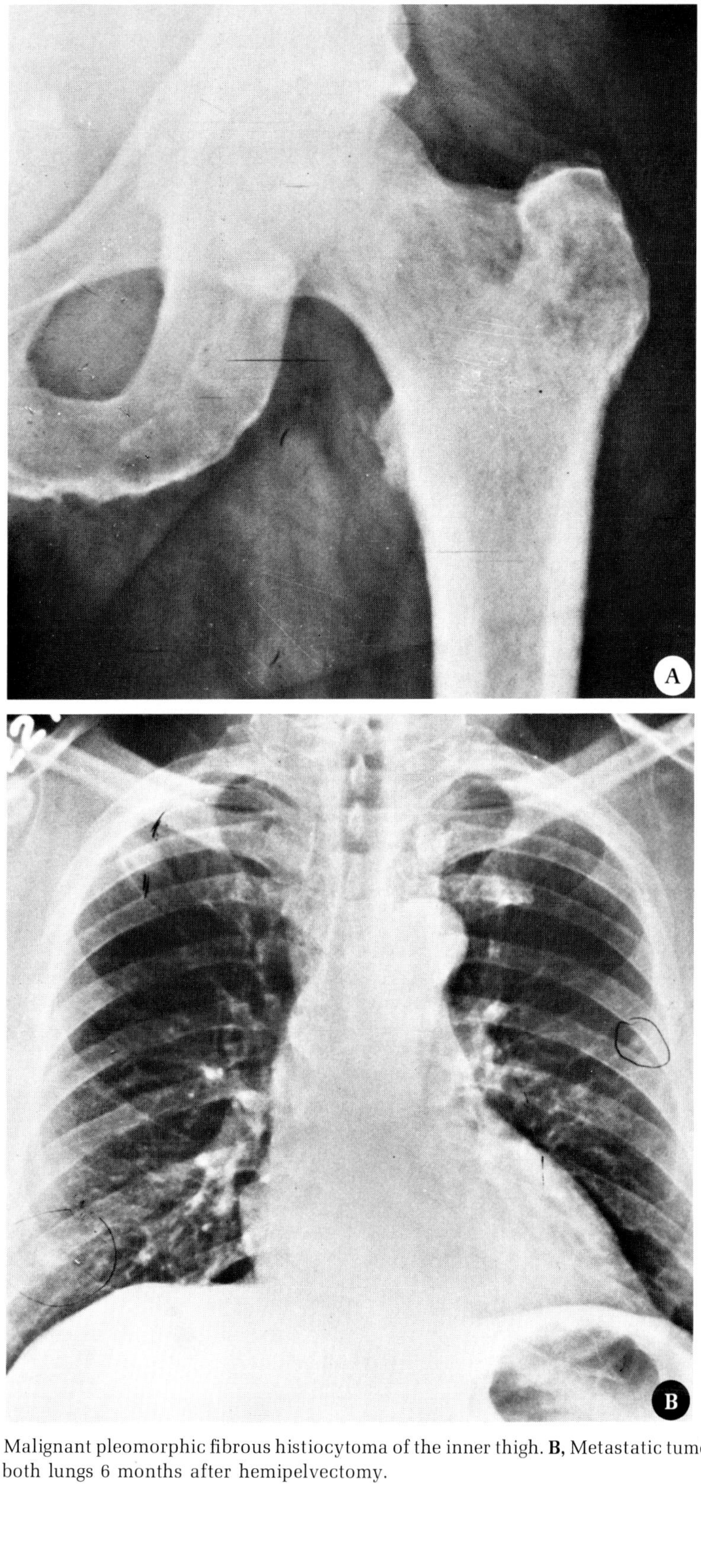

Figure 2-36. A, Malignant pleomorphic fibrous histiocytoma of the inner thigh. **B,** Metastatic tumor nodules were discovered in both lungs 6 months after hemipelvectomy.

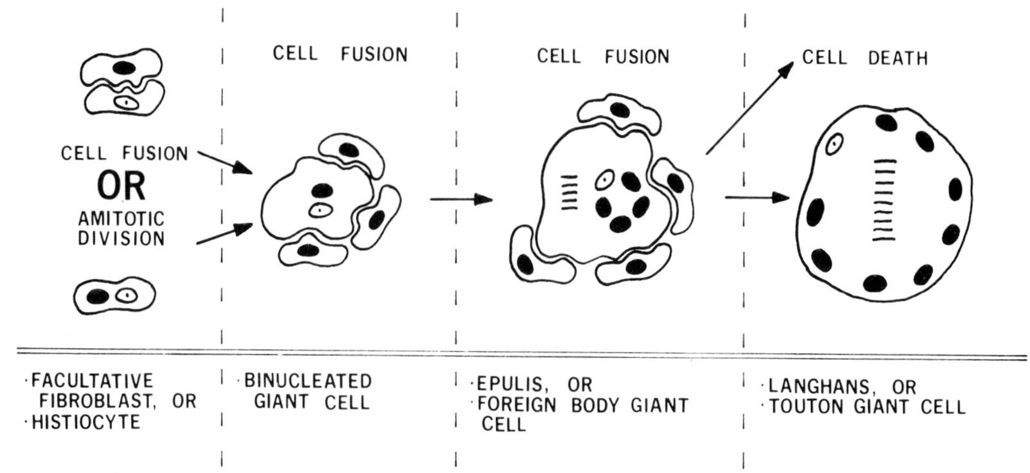

Figure 2-37. Schematic illustration of the formation of multinucleated giant cells by cell fusion.

the proper nature of many of these tumors from limited biopsy material, especially the ones without multinucleated tumor giant cells. However, careful gross and microscopic examination will almost invariably disclose their soft tissue origin. These tumors blend intimately with the subcutaneous and deeper soft tissues, and the monotonous histiocytic appearance is often interrupted by numerous foamy histiocytes and granulomatous areas. Myxoid areas with short spindle cells and occasional binucleate histiocytes resembling Reed-Sternberg cells, in a highly vascular background, are other features characteristic of these tumors (Figs. 2-37, 2-38, Chapter 3).

It is almost certain that after generous sampling of such tumors one will find microscopic areas containing fibroblasts, arranged in the typical cartwheel pattern characteristic of fibroblastic fibrous histiocytomas, and epulis-type multinucleated giant cells (Fig. 2-39). It is difficult to find any good description of these rare monomorphic forms of histiocytic fibrous histiocytomas. Without doubt, most of the reported xanthomas, xanthogranulomas, and xanthosarcomas short of the characteristic Touton giant cells belong to this category. *The clinical behavior of these neoplasms cannot be predicted purely on the basis of histologic examination.* Our experience with these neoplasms shows

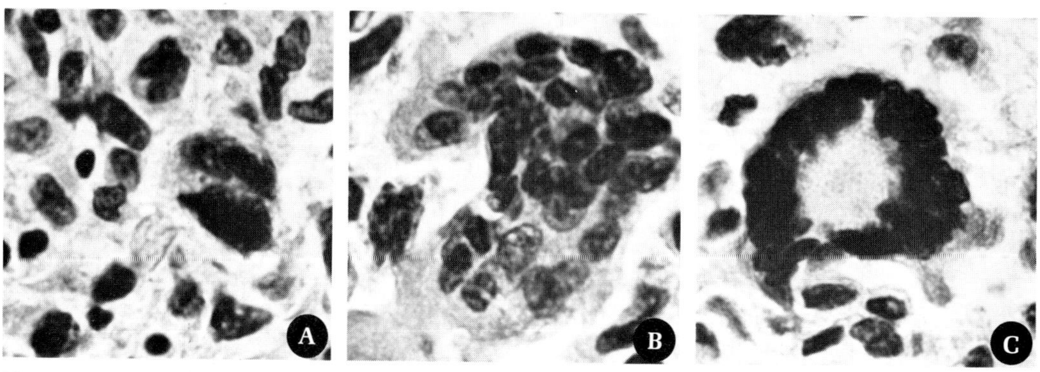

Figure 2-38. A, Binucleated histiocytic form (H & E, ×350).

B, Multinucleated epulis type of giant cell. Note cytoplasmic extensions and adherence of nearby mononuclear forms (H & E, ×350).

C, Multinucleated Touton-type giant cells with nuclei arranged in a ring shape at the edge of the cytoplasm. Note cytoplasmic extensions and surrounding mononuclear cells.

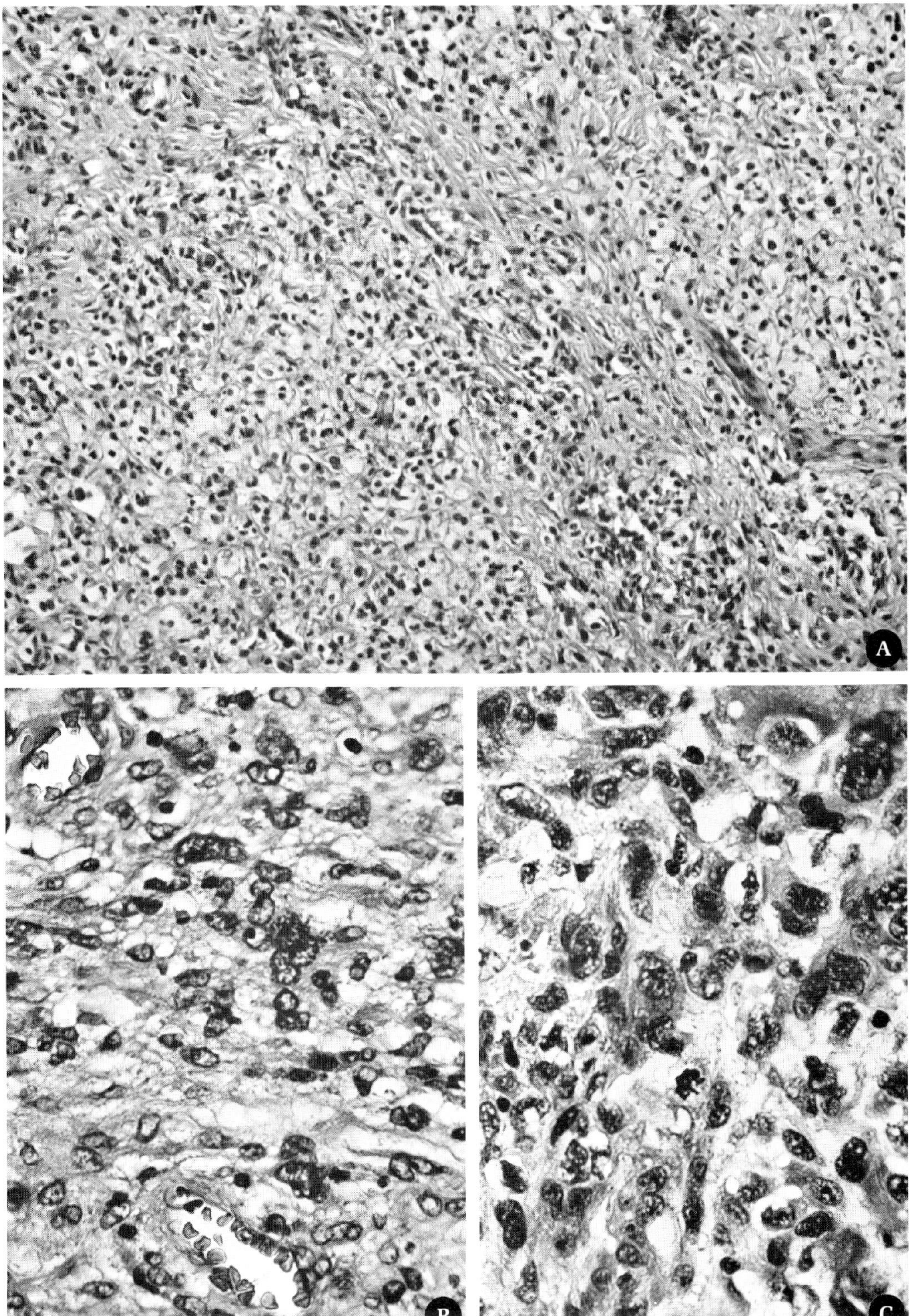

Figure 2-39. A, Malignant histiocytic fibrous histiocytoma without giant cells is composed of round cells with well-defined cytoplasmic membrane and clear or granular cytoplasm; **B** and **C,** short spindle or polygonal cells with finely reticular cell process in other areas (**A,** H & E, ×140; **B** & **C,** H & E, ×350). (See also Figure 2-41.)

TABLE 2-9. *Malignant Giant Cell Tumors of Soft Tissues*

	NO. OF CASES	NUMBER OF PATIENTS		
		RECURRENCE	METASTASIS	DIED
Salm and Sissons (1972)	10	0	0	0
Guccion and Enzinger (1972)	32	17	16	14
Hajdu (unpublished data)	24	18	14	13

that the superficial and subcutaneous lesions are benign neoplasms, whereas the ones in the retroperitoneum and deeper soft tissues should be regarded as malignant neoplasms (see Fig. 1-59; Table 1-15).

A special form of histiocytic fibrous histiocytoma is the so-called giant cell tumor of soft tissues. The benign giant cell tumors, the lesions commonly referred to in the literature as giant cell tumors of tendon sheath or villonodular synovitis, are discussed in Chapter 3 because of their close association with synovial, bursal, and tendinous tissues. The history of these tumors dates back to Christopher who reported the first case in 1926.

There is considerable controversy about the malignant nature of giant cell tumors of soft tissues, and the two reported series help little to diminish the confusion surrounding these neoplasms. None of the 10 tumors reported by Salm and Sissons, in 1972, recurred or metastasized, but 14 of the 32 patients reported by Guccion and Enzinger, in 1972, died with metastatic disease. Our experience with these tumors corresponds to that of Guccion and Enzinger (Table 2-9).

The size of giant cell tumors of soft tissues varies considerably. Their size may range from a few centimeters to several inches. In general, the deeper ones tend to be much larger than the subcutaneous ones. The extremities, especially the leg and the thigh, are the most common sites affected.

There is fairly convincing histologic and ultrastructural evidence that these rare neoplasms belong to the fibrous histiocytomas and, more specifically, should be regarded as histiocytic fibrous histiocytoma (Fig. 2-32). Microscopically, giant cell tumors of soft parts are identical with giant cell tumors of bone and are composed of mononuclear histiocytes, multinucleated epulis-type giant cells, and fibroblasts (Fig. 2-40).

The mononuclear histiocytic forms are similar to those seen in the monomorphic histiocytic fibrous histiocytomas (Fig. 2-39) and in pleomorphic fibrous histiocytomas (Fig. 2-50). These are mostly plump, mononuclear cells closely resembling reactive histiocytes. The nuclei of these neoplastic histiocytes are vesicular and contain prominent nucleoli. The cytoplasms are foamy or vacuolated with round or polyhedral contour. Binucleated or trinucleated cells showing similar cytologic features may be seen occasionally.

The most characteristic feature of these neoplasms is, however, the large number of multinucleated, epulis-type giant cells. These giant cells vary in size and may contain numerous equally sized nuclei usually grouped at the center of the cytoplasms. The giant cells have an intimate association with the much smaller histiocytic-looking mononuclear cells and spindly fibroblasts.

The combination of mononuclear cells and multinucleated giant cells showing phagocytic activity and resembling reactive histiocytes seems to support the histiocytic origin of these neoplasms. With the electron microscope, intracytoplasmic collagen has been noted in some of the histiocytic cells which may explain the occasional finding of *asteroid bodies*, fragmented intracytoplasmic collagen fibrils, in multinucleated epulis-type giant cells. In addition, intercellular proteoglycan, fine elastic fibrils, and fibrillar tropocollagen have been observed in some of these tumors. The epulis-type of giant cells may also occur in other soft tissue lesions such as, fat necrosis, pyogenic granuloma, reparative granuloma, foreign body granuloma, various benign and malignant fibrous histiocytomas, and occasionally malignant neoplasms such as liposarcomas and myosarcomas. However, the giant cells in most of these lesions are not numerous, and the supportive stroma is different from that of giant cell tumors of soft tissues (Table 2-10).

The bimorphic pattern of giant cell tumors of soft parts, the most common form cf histiocytic fibrous histiocytoma, is accentuated by the presence of plump or short fusiform fibroblasts. These cells often form dense cellular clusters fused together by fine reticular or collagenous filaments.

Classification of giant cell tumors, whether they are benign or malignant, is based on the fibroblastic stromal cells and the size and location of the lesion. In the malignant forms more polymorphic and atypical stromal cells can be seen than in the benign ones. The number of abnormal mitotic figures is not a good guide in prognosis, but far more atypical mitoses have been observed in large, deeply situated malignant tumors than in considerably smaller superficial lesions (Figs. 2-41, 2-42, 2-43).

Our experience with 24 giant cell tumors of soft parts shows that subcutaneous tumors of less than 5 cm (8 cases) may recur after incomplete excision but do not metastasize. On the other hand, giant cell tumors of deep soft parts larger than 5 cm (16 cases) carry a grave prognosis due to metastatic spread to the lung (Table 2-9). It is of interest that both recurrent and metastatic tumors closely resemble histiologically the primary lesion.

Pleomorphic fibrous histiocytomas are most commonly referred to as xanthomas, atypical xanthomas, or malignant xanthomas according to their clinical behavior. (See Synonyms, page 94 and Fig. 2-32.) This group of neoplasms, like the histiocytic forms, cannot be evaluated purely on the basis of microscopic appearance. O'Brien and Stout's statement, in 1964, "In fibrous xanthomas there may be no really reliable histological evidence to indicate malignancy," has been restated by many investigators. Bizarre tumor giant cells by themselves are not necessarily indicative

TABLE 2-10. ***Characteristics of Histiocytes and Fibroblasts of Fibrous Histiocytoma***

HISTIOCYTES	FIBROBLASTS
Oval or round cytoplasm	Oval or spindly cytoplasm
Oval or round nucleus	Oval or spindly nucleus
Ruffled cell membrane	Smooth cell membrane
Filopodia	Elongated cytoplasmic processes
Sparse rough endoplasmic reticulum	Abundant rough endoplasmic reticulum
Few mitochondria	Many mitochondria
Lamellated cytoplasmic dense bodies	Longitudinal microfilaments
Many free ribosomes	Many attached ribosomes
Extensive smooth endoplasmic reticulum	Inconspicuous smooth endoplasmic reticulum
Numerous phagosomes	Desmosome-like structures
Glycogen deposits	Capable of biosynthesis of proteins, lipoproteins, polysaccharides, and lipids
Lipid droplets	
Contain non-specific esterases and acid phosphatase	

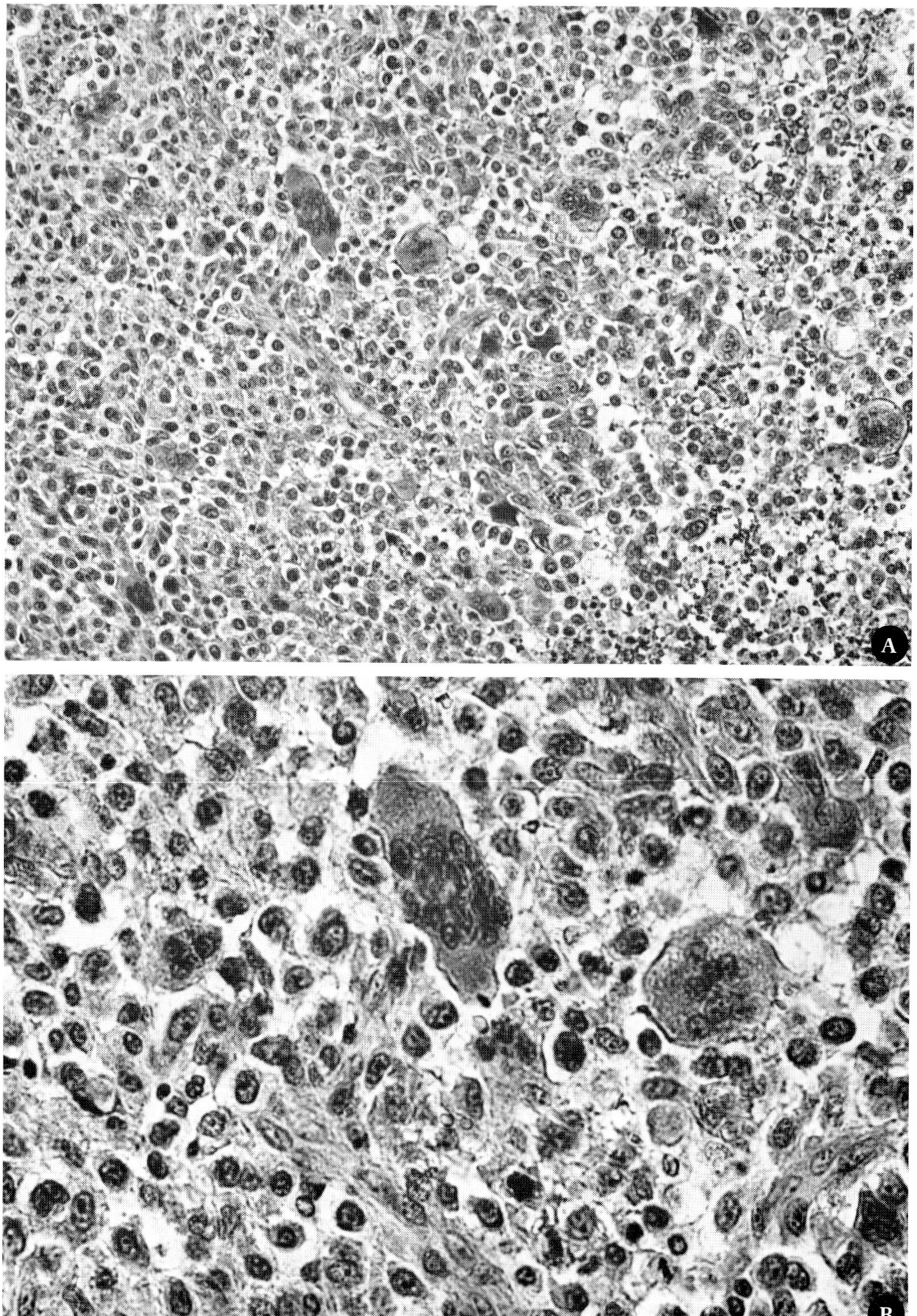

Figure 2-40. So-called benign giant cell tumor or benign histiocytic fibrous histiocytoma of soft tissues. Note the uniform round or oval histiocytic stromal cells and the numerous multinucleated epulis type of giant cells (**A**, H & E, ×140; **B**, H & E, ×350).

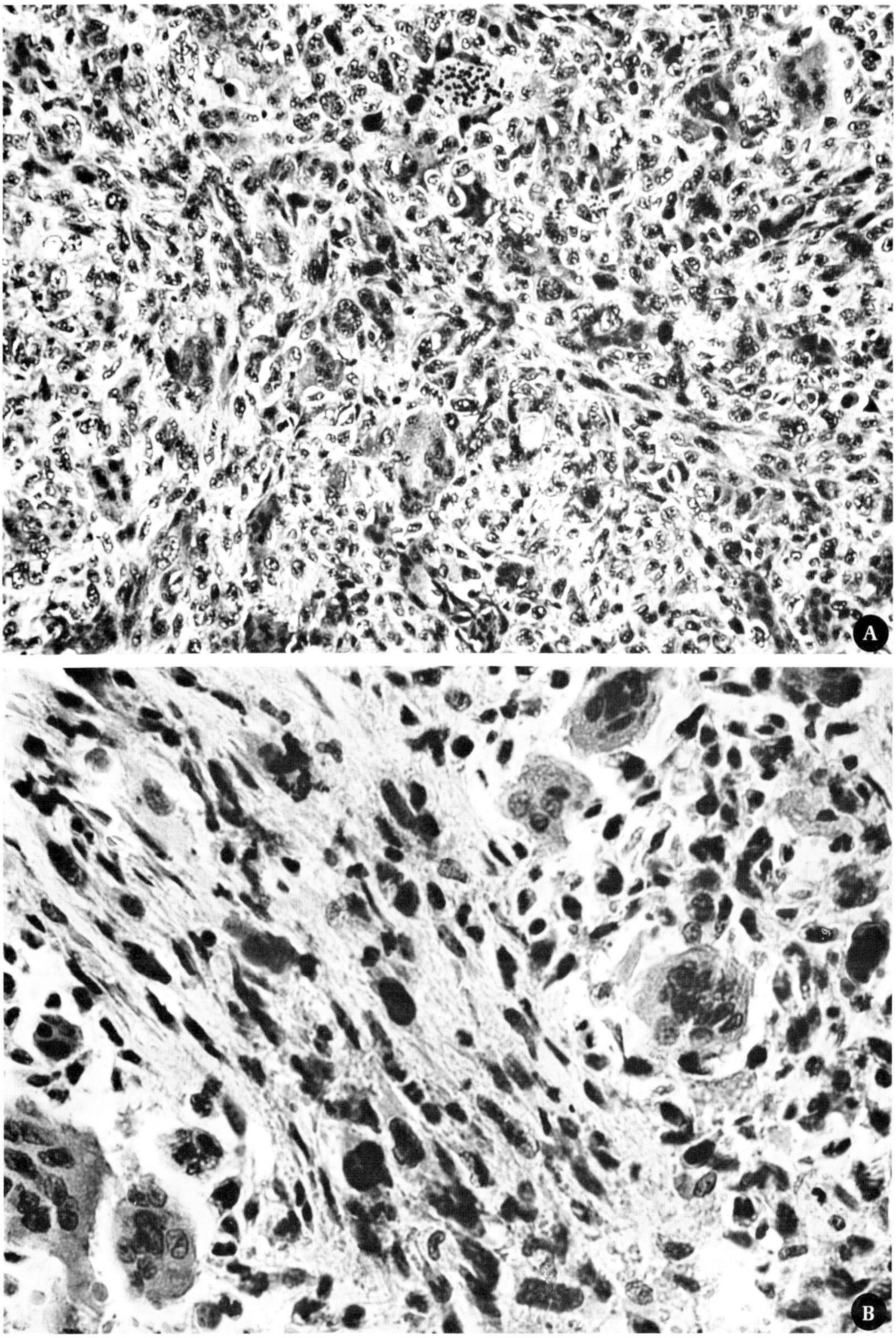

Figure 2-41. So-called malignant giant cell tumor or malignant histiocytic fibrous histiocytoma of soft tissues. The stroma is cellular and occupied by spindle and polygonal, often tightly packed, neoplastic cells. There are epulis type of giant cells throughout the tissue, but their presence is overshadowed by the sarcomatous stroma (**A,** H & E, ×140; **B,** H & E, ×350). (See also Figure 2-39.)

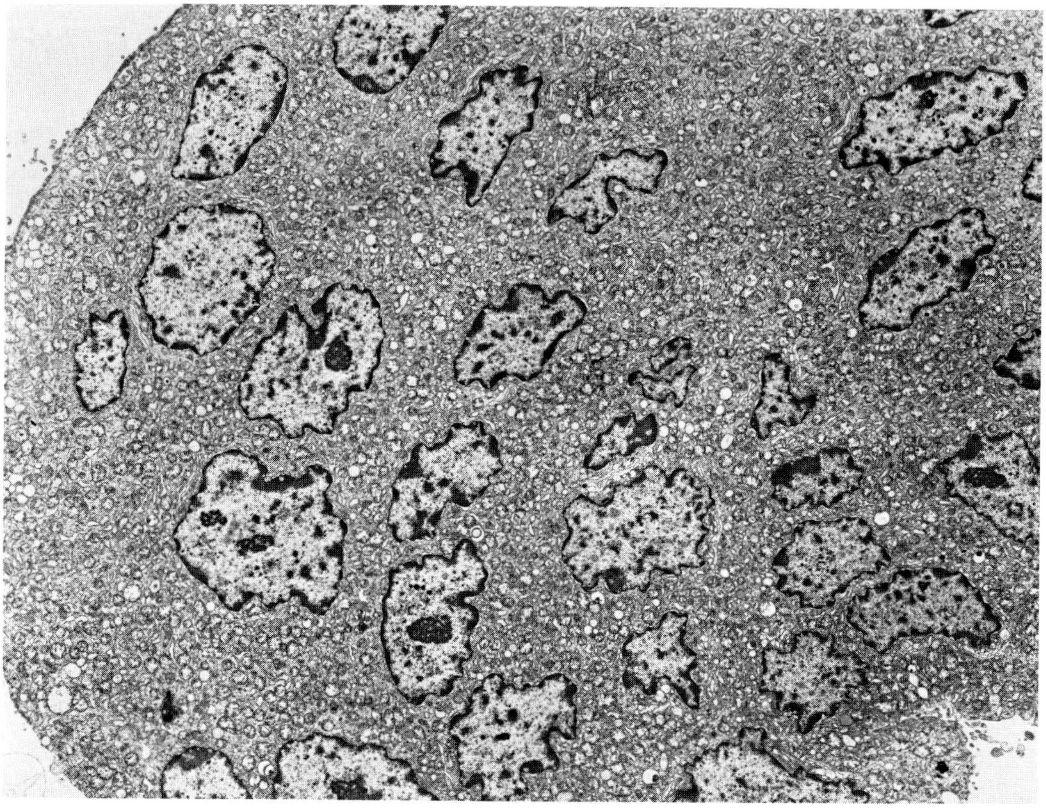

Figure 2-42. Portion of a multinucleated epulis-type giant cell from a benign giant cell tumor as seen with the electron microscope. Note the abundant cytoplasmic organelles (×3,000).

of malignancy, nor can one rely on the number of atypical mitotic figures.

Historically, McDonagh's report in 1912 began the accumulation of information about these neoplasms (Chapter 1). To the present day, however, nobody has succeeded in assigning microscopic criteria that definitely separate these pleomorphic tumors into benign and malignant groups. There is conclusive evidence that the malignant form exists, but because it is histopathologically difficult or impossible to distinguish benign from malignant forms, *all pleomorphic fibrous histiocytomas should be regarded as potentially malignant lesions until proven otherwise.*

Superficial, subcutaneous, or submucosal tumors are commonly called *atypical fibrous xanthomas,* a term first used by Helwig in 1963, to describe a sarcomalike proliferation of histiocytes, fibroblasts, and multinucleated giant cells. They are most commonly found in sun-exposed areas of the head, neck, and arm, at sites of prior trauma or irradiation, in elderly persons. They are curable by local excision (Fig. 2-44). More than 300 cases of subcutaneous pleomorphic fibrous histiocytomas (atypical fibroxanthoma of the skin) are recorded in the literature. The clinical course has almost always been benign; however, recurrences have been described and 5 cases of metastasis have been reported (Table 2-11).

Light and electron microscopic findings suggest a considerable morphologic spectrum in these lesions. Most of the tumors consist of bizarre elongated fibroblasts, as well as mononuclear and multinucleated cells which appear histiocytic. The characteristic Touton type of multinucleated giant cells is a round cell with uniform nuclei arranged in a peripheral ring in a foamy and vacuolated cytoplasm (Fig. 2-38C). Mitotic figures are common and may

TABLE 2-11. ***Reported Series of Atypical Subcutaneous Fibrous Histiocytoma****

	NUMBER OF PATIENTS				
	TOTAL NUMBER	HISTORY OF TRAUMA	HISTORY OF IRRADIATION	RECURRENCE	METASTASIS
Kempson and McGavran (1964)	21	3	3	2	—
Reed (1967)	17	3	2	3	—
Kroe and Pitcock (1969)	10	—	2	1	—
Hudson and Winkelmann (1972)	19	—	11	1	—
Vargas-Cortes et al (1973)	19	—	1	4	—
Fretzin and Helwig (1973)	140	5	6	9	1
Dahl (1976)	57	2	—	1	1
	283	13	25	21	2

*All reported as atypical fibroxanthoma of the skin.

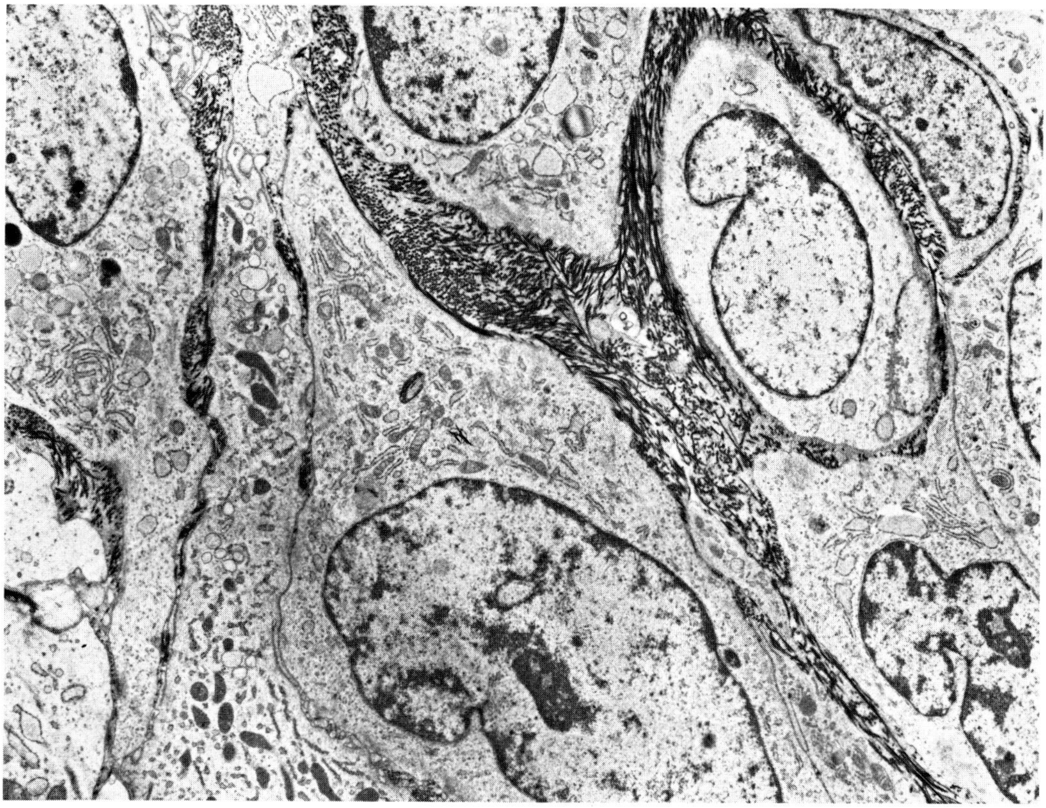

Figure 2-43. Ultrastructure of mononuclear stromal components of a malignant giant cell tumor. The neoplastic cells closely resemble neoplastic fibroblasts. Note collagen fibrils between cells in intercellular spaces (×5,300).

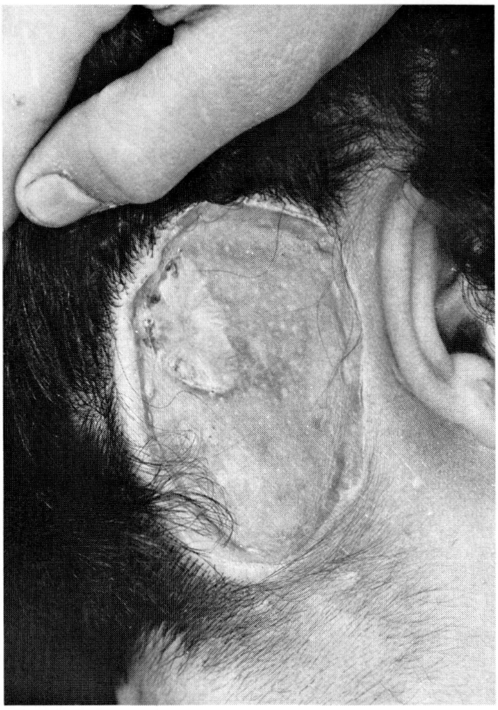

Figure 2-44. Site of recurrence of an atypical fibrous histiocytoma or so-called subcutaneous xanthoma (see Figure 2-32).

be abnormal. Nucleoli of the tumor cells are prominent and stain eosinophilic with hematoxylin and eosin. The stroma is sparsely vascular, loosely arranged, and often myxoid (Figs. 2-45, 2-46). At the time of microscopic evaluation of such pleomorphic histiocytomas the observer must know the anatomic site of the lesion and the age of the patient in order to prevent unwarranted diagnosis.

Without doubt, several lesions other than pleomorphic fibrous histiocytoma may be included in some of the reported studies. The possibility of incorrect classification further complicates evaluation of reported observations.

Our experience with 133 cases of *malignant pleomorphic histiocytomas* is summarized in Figures 2-47, 2-48, and 2-49 and Table 2-12. These tumors occur mostly in adults after the age of 40. The most common anatomic sites of the primary lesion are the thigh, the buttock, and the upper arm. They are tumors of considerable size, on the average larger than 10 cm in diameter, and are situated in deep soft tissues. Grossly these tumors do not possess distinctive features that would allow separation from other fibrous histiocytomas. About one third of the tumors recur after local excision and more than half of the tumors metastasize predominantly to the lung.

The studies reported by O'Brien and Stout, in 1964; Kempson and Kyriakos, in 1972; and Soule and Enriquez, in 1972 contribute to the understanding of the natural history of these tumors. Our findings are somewhat in variance with some of the reported series but are comparable

TABLE 2-12. *Series of Malignant Pleomorphic Fibrous Histiocytomas**

	NUMBER OF PATIENTS				
	TOTAL CASES	MEAN AGE	RECURRENCE	METASTASIS	DIED
O'Brien and Stout (1964)	53	47	32	16	13 (25%)
Kempson and Kyriakos (1972)	30	52	9	3	2 (7%)
Soule and Enriquez (1972)	40	58	10	14	16 (40%)
Hajdu (unpublished data)	133†	51	46	74	72 (54%)

*Variation in survival figures is partly due to the inclusion of other than pleomorphic fibrous histiocytomas in some of the studies.

†All pleomorphic fibrous histiocytoma.

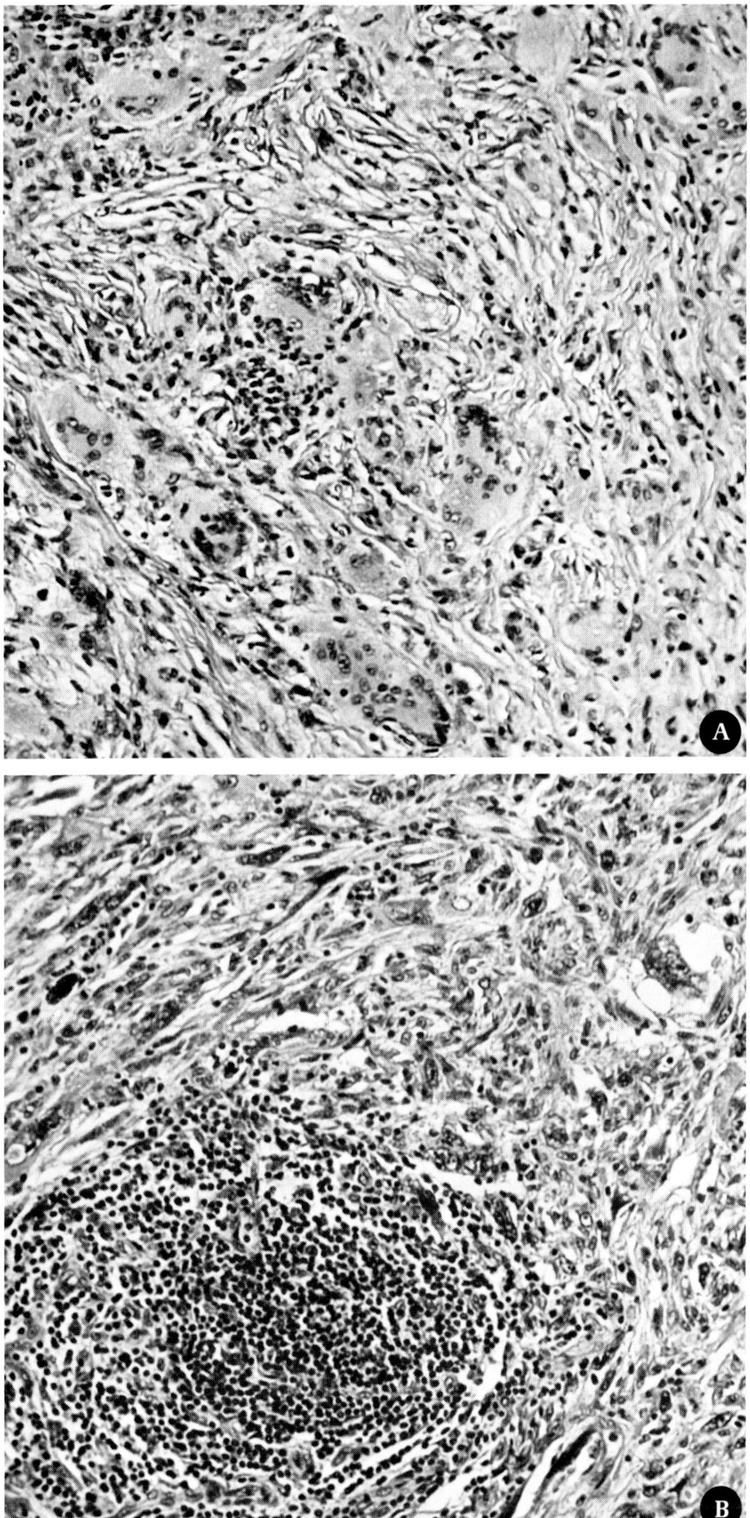

Figure 2-45. Atypical subcutaneous fibrous histiocytoma or benign histiocytic fibrous histiocytoma is composed of fusiform and round, often foamy, mononuclear cells and Touton or foreign body type of multinucleated giant cells. Inflammatory cells such as lymphocytes are not uncommon (H & E, ×140).

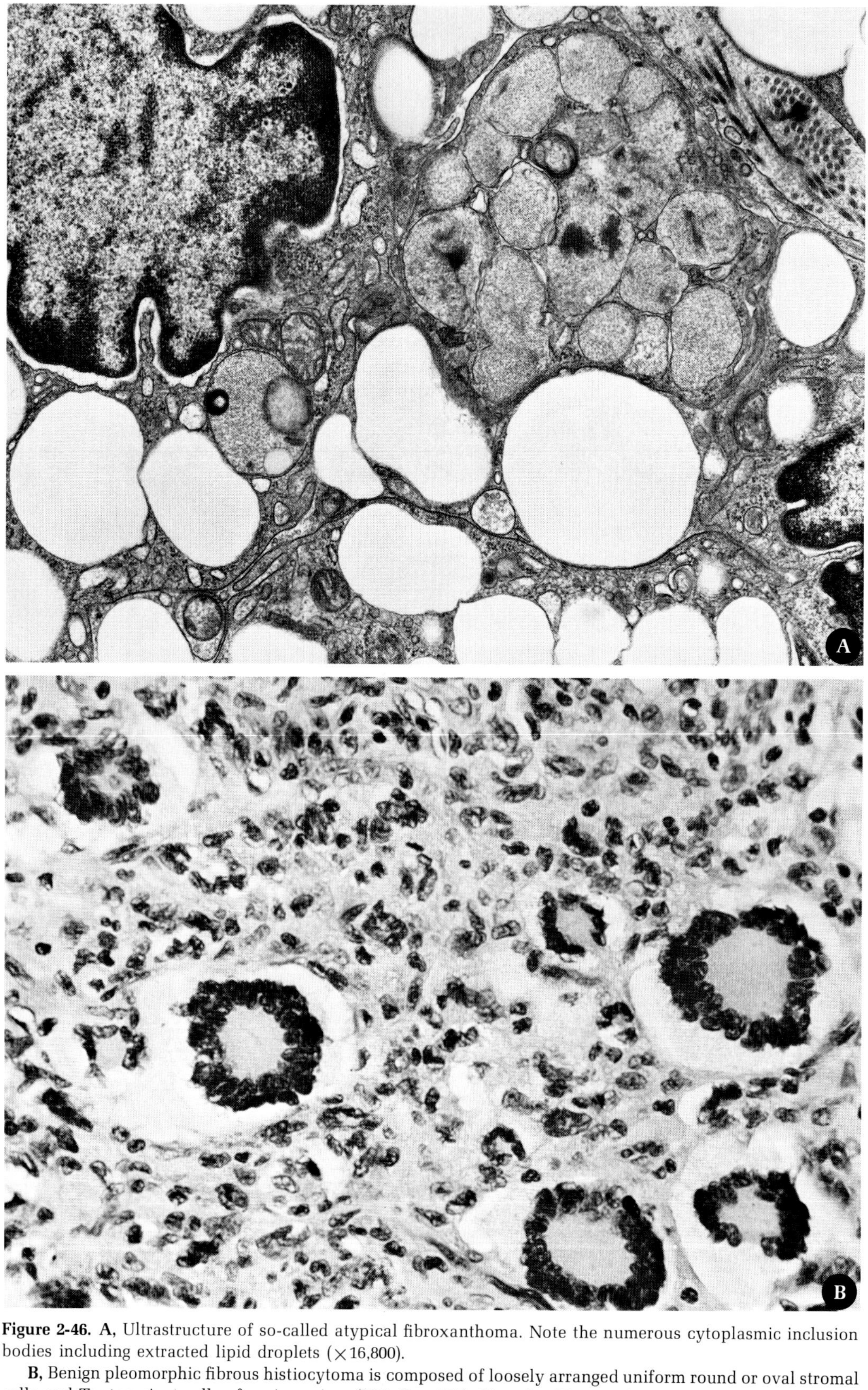

Figure 2-46. A, Ultrastructure of so-called atypical fibroxanthoma. Note the numerous cytoplasmic inclusion bodies including extracted lipid droplets (×16,800).

B, Benign pleomorphic fibrous histiocytoma is composed of loosely arranged uniform round or oval stromal cells and Touton giant cells of various sizes (H & E, ×350). (See also Fig. 2-37.)

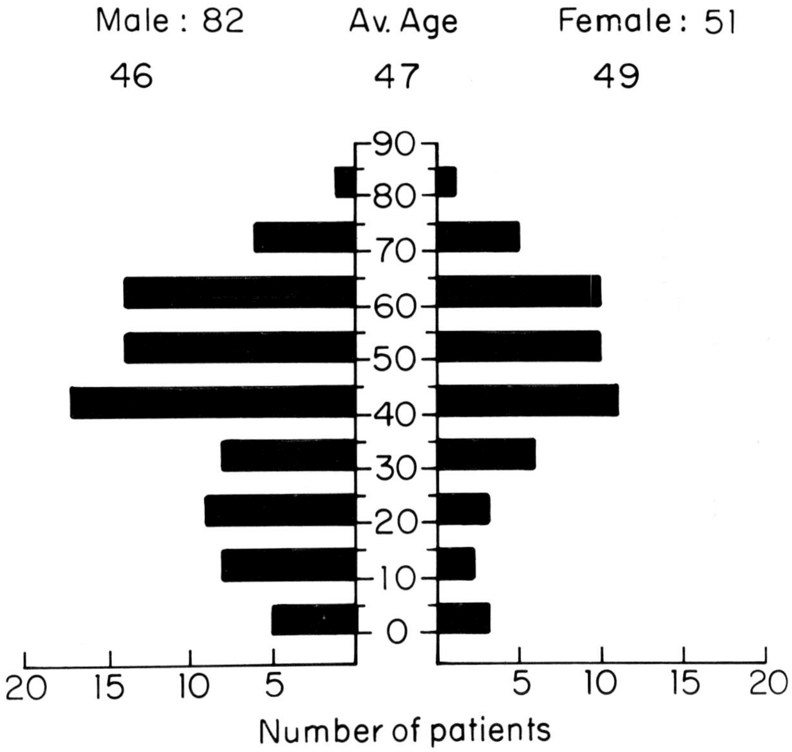

Figure 2-47. Age and sex distribution of 133 patients who were treated at Memorial Sloan-Kettering Cancer Center for malignant pleomorphic fibrous histiocytoma (see Figure 2-32 and Table 2-9).

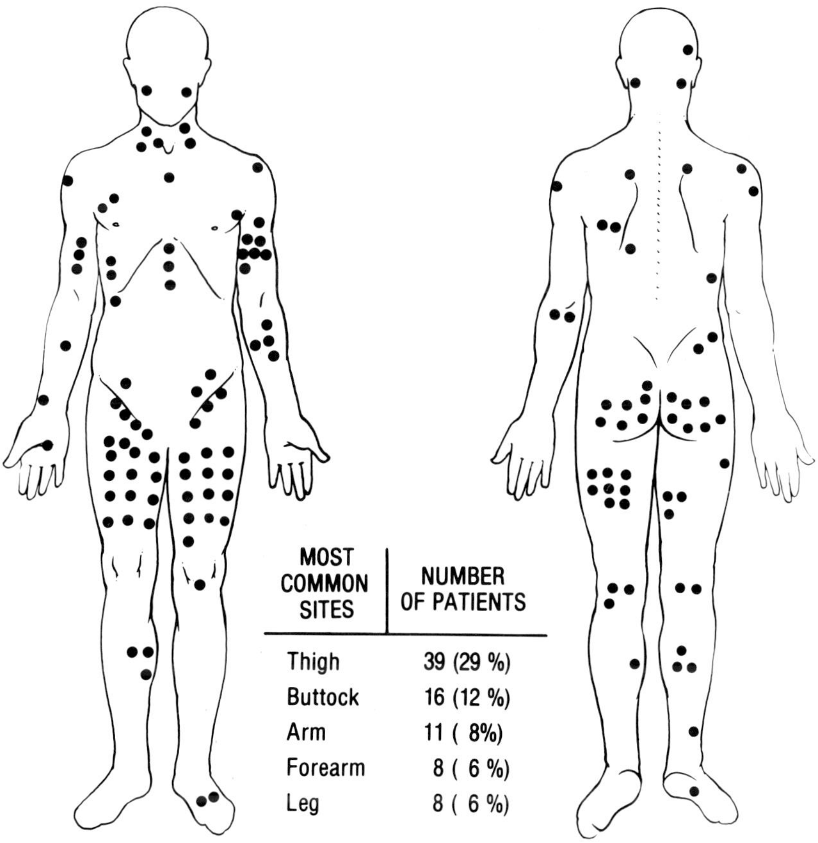

Figure 2-48. Anatomic distribution of 133 malignant pleomorphic fibrous histiocytomas.

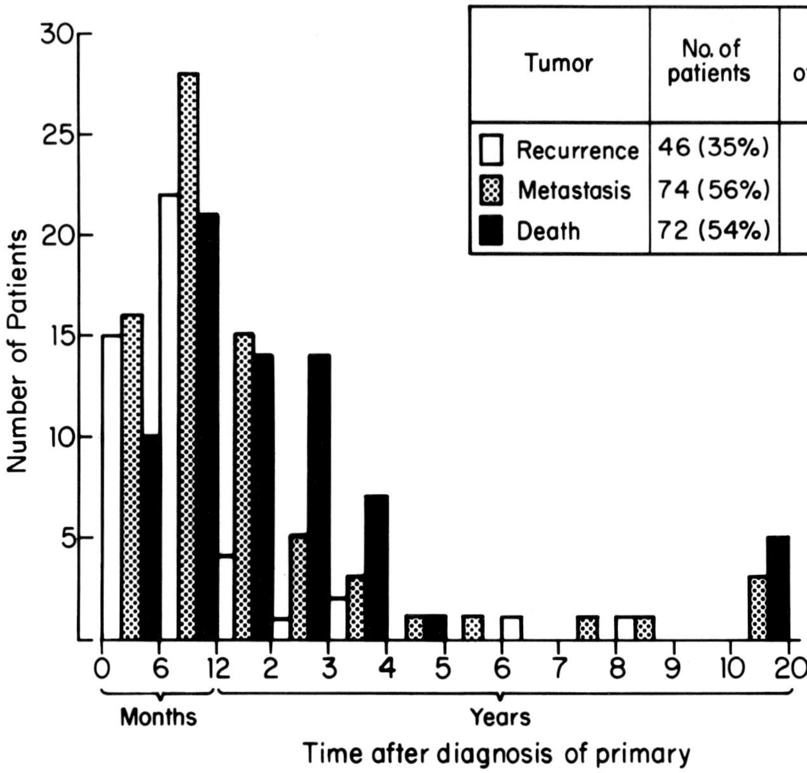

Figure 2-49. Rate of recurrence and metastasis of malignant pleomorphic fibrous histiocytomas. Note that 72 (54%) of the 133 patients treated at Memorial Sloan-Kettering Cancer Center died of their disease.

with the findings of Soule and Enriquez (Table 2-12).

The difficulty of predicting the metastatic potentials or recurrence of pleomorphic fibrous histiocytomas on the basis of histologic criteria is emphasized in many studies. However, certain microscopic features, in addition to large size and certain anatomic site, should be considered as signs of malignancy. The microscopic appearance of malignant pleomorphic fibrous histiocytomas (malignant xanthomas or xanthosarcomas) (Fig. 2-32) varies according to the combination of five basic components: *mononuclear histiocytic round cells, multinucleated Touton-type giant cells, plump or elongated fibroblasts, bizarre polymorphic tumor giant cells, and stromal elements* (Fig. 2-50, color). By definition the fibrous tissue elements, reticulum and collagen fibers, are minimal in fibrous histiocytomas; however, in the malignant ones occasionally there is a considerable amount of fibrillar material stainable with reticulin stain. The neoplastic fibroblasts are often anaplastic with irregular hyperchromatic nuclei and large nucleoli and are arranged in broad fascicles (Fig. 2-51). Bizarre tumor giant cells with polymorphic and branching cytoplasmic processes similar to those seen in pleomorphic fibrosarcoma are constant findings in malignant pleomorphic fibrous histiocytomas (Fig. 2-52).

The histiocytic cells tend to be less vacuolated and less foamy than those in the atypical or benign histiocytomas (Fig. 2-45). The mononuclear, as well as the multinucleated, forms appear anaplastic. The nuclei contain giant nucleoli and the cytoplasm is glassy and acidophilic.

A prominent and branching vascular network serves as a background to the tumor cells. Many of the mononuclear cells, histiocytes, and fibroblasts are arranged around blood vessels (Fig. 2-53).

Myxoid areas in malignant neoplasms

are usually inconspicuous, but in some tumors there are ill-defined myxomatous areas adjacent to necrotic or inflamed areas. Occasionally the infiltrating edges of these tumors contain large numbers of lymphocytes, neutrophils, plasma cells, and eosinophils and give the impression of a reactive or granulomatous process rather than neoplastic proliferation. Similarly, deposits of inflammatory cells are commonly accompanied by tumor cells in recurrent and metastatic lesions. Recurrent and metastatic tumors, however, do not necessarily resemble the primary lesion. As a rule, metastatic nodules usually show fewer histiocytic and more fibroblastic forms (Fig. 2-54).

Special stains are of little value in the diagnosis of malignant fibrous histiocytomas. Most of the tumors show scant reticulin with reticulin stain. Fine intracytoplasmic lipid granules are demonstrable by staining with oil-red O or Sudan black dyes. However, no appreciable quantity of trichrome-positive collagen can be found in cellular areas. According to Klaus and Winkelmann, 1966, fibrous histiocytomas stain consistently positive for acid phosphatase and leucine amino-peptidase (Table 2-13).

Despite the fact that there are no valid ultrastructural criteria for predicting malignancy, electron microscopic studies help to clarify the nature of fibrous histiocytomas and play an important role in the differential diagnosis of these tumors. The bimorphic pattern of fibrous histiocytomas is clearly demonstrable by ultrastructural and tissue culture studies (Hajdu and Hajdu, 1976). The ubiquitous fibroblasts are plump cells containing many free polyribosomes, Golgi complexes, an extensive network of rough endoplasmic reticulum, and occasionally a zone of fine filaments adjacent to the cell membrane (see Appendix).

The histiocytes or xanthoma cells contain within the cytoplasm vacuoles, glycogen-like particles, dense bodies, and abundant lysosomes. Many of the cells possess numerous cytoplasmic processes or filopodia, on their surfaces, indicating pinocytotic activity. Search for transitional forms exhibiting features of both

TABLE 2-13. *Comparison of Microscopic Features of Fibrous Histiocytomas*

	FIBROBLASTIC FIBROUS HISTIOCYTOMA	HISTIOCYTIC FIBROUS HISTIOCYTOMA	PLEOMORPHIC FIBROUS HISTIOCYTOMA
Storiform pattern	+++	+−	+−
Plump fibroblasts	+++	++	+
Vacuolated fibroblasts	+−	+++	++
Foam cells	+−	++	+
Epulis-type giant cells	+−	+++	+−
Touton giant cells	−	+−	+++
Pleomorphic tumor giant cells	−	+−	+++
Inflammatory cells	+−	++	+++
Reticulum fibers	+++	+−	+
Intracytoplasmic lipids	−	+++	++
Cytoplasmic acid phosphatase	−	++	+++
Cytoplasmic leucine aminopeptidase	−	++	+++
Erythrophagocytosis	−	++	+++
Tumor necrosis	−	++	+++
Bimorphic cells in tissue culture	+−	++	+++
Bimorphic cells in cytologic preparation	+−	++	+++
Bimorphic ultrastructural features	+−	++	+++

+++ = most common; ++ = common; + = uncommon; +− = may be present; − = absent.

Figure 2-50. A, Malignant fibroblastic fibrous histiocytoma (dermatofibrosarcoma protuberans) is a low grade malignant neoplasm. The tumor cells are mononuclear slender oval or short spindle cells. The nuclei are somewhat pyknotic and usually positioned at the center of the cytoplasm. The cytoplasm is tapering off into long reticular filaments which are often tangled.

Not all, but numerous, tumor cells are arranged in the typical storiform or cartwheel pattern. At the center of twisted nebulae the overlapping and fused cytoplasmic processes of the neoplastic fibroblasts are clearly visible.

Tumors such as this one may show only trace elements of trichrome positive collagen (collagen type I), but they are richly positive with any conventional reticulum stain for collagen type III.

Note the monotonous mononucleated, often ambiguous, appearance of this tumor and compare it with **B** and **C** and also with some of the schwannomas illustrated in Chapter 8 (H & E, ×350).

B, Malignant histiocytic fibrous histiocytoma (malignant giant cell tumors of soft tissue) can be low grade or high grade histologically.

This is a low-grade bimorphic tumor with a delicate blending of spindle cells and multinucleated epulis-type giant cells. There are numerous recognizable transitional forms between these two extremes of the morphologic spectrum.

Alone, on the basis of the area where the giant cells are clustered (left lower corner) without considering the right upper half of the picture, one would call this lesion benign. However, the distinctly fibrosarcomatous area indicates the true malignant nature of this neoplasm. Whether a histiocytic fibrous histiocytoma of this type is benign or malignant must be decided by considering the stromal spindle cell components. When the sarcomatous area is dominant and appears malignant and fibroblastic fibrous histiocytoma-like (**A**) or looks like a fibrosarcoma, histiocytic fibrous histiocytomas behave like a malignant neoplasm (H & E, ×350).

C, Malignant pleomorphic fibrous histiocytoma (xanthosarcoma) is potentially a high-grade malignant neoplasm. This neoplasm is composed of numerous bizarre and polymorphic cells. The cells range in size and shape from mononuclear histiocytic forms to multinucleated Touton giant cells and enormous pleomorphic cells.

Although it is difficult to recognize any particular growth pattern or arrangement of the tumor cells, there is a definite contact between the neoplastic cells by fibrillar cell processes.

The almost complete absence of Touton and foreign body giant cells, which are dominant in benign pleomorphic fibrous histiocytomas, and the presence of a cellular and vascular neoplastic stroma, rich in abnormal mitotic figures, which appear more fibroblastic than histiocytic, warrant the classification as malignant (H & E, ×350).

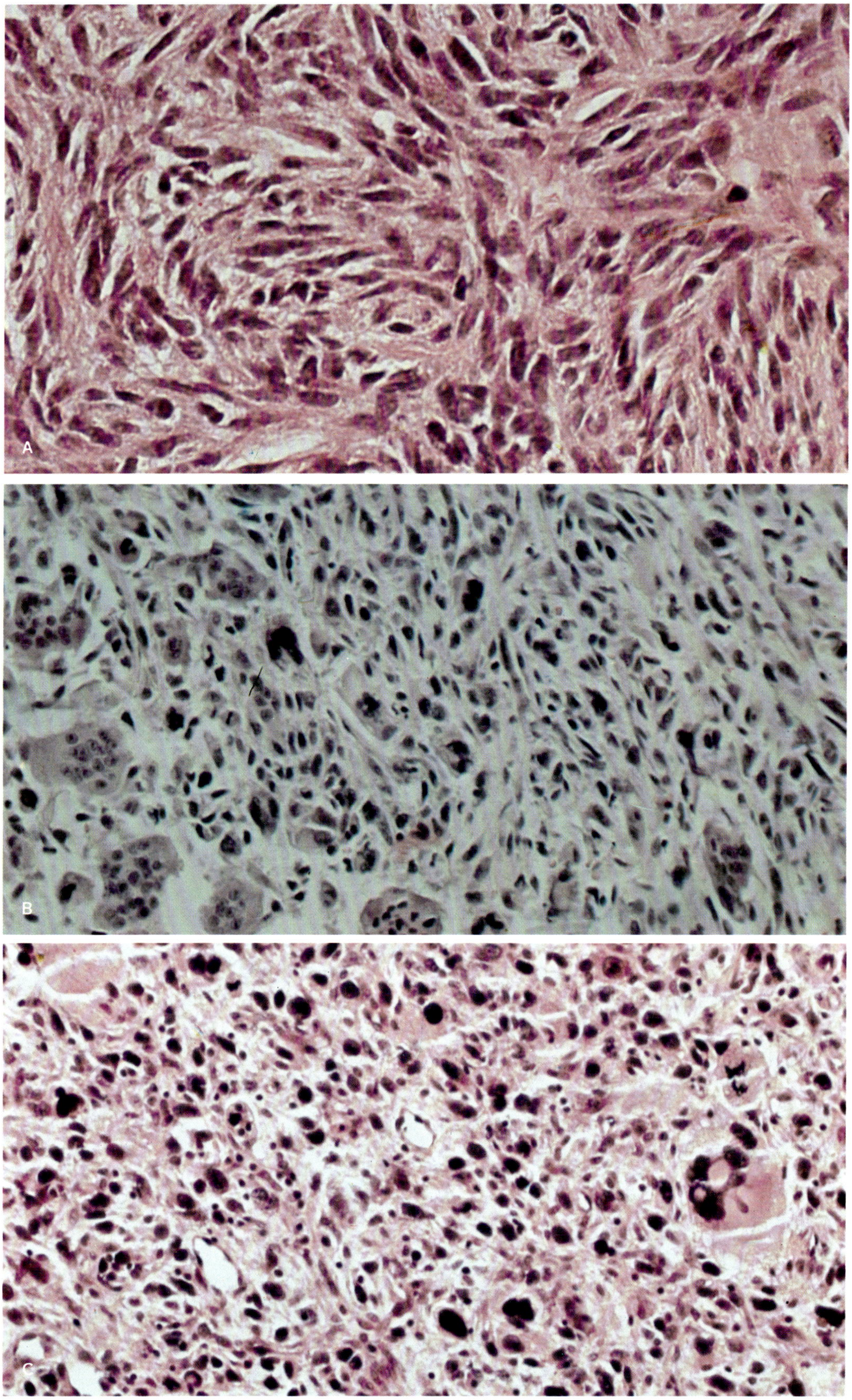

Figure 2-50.

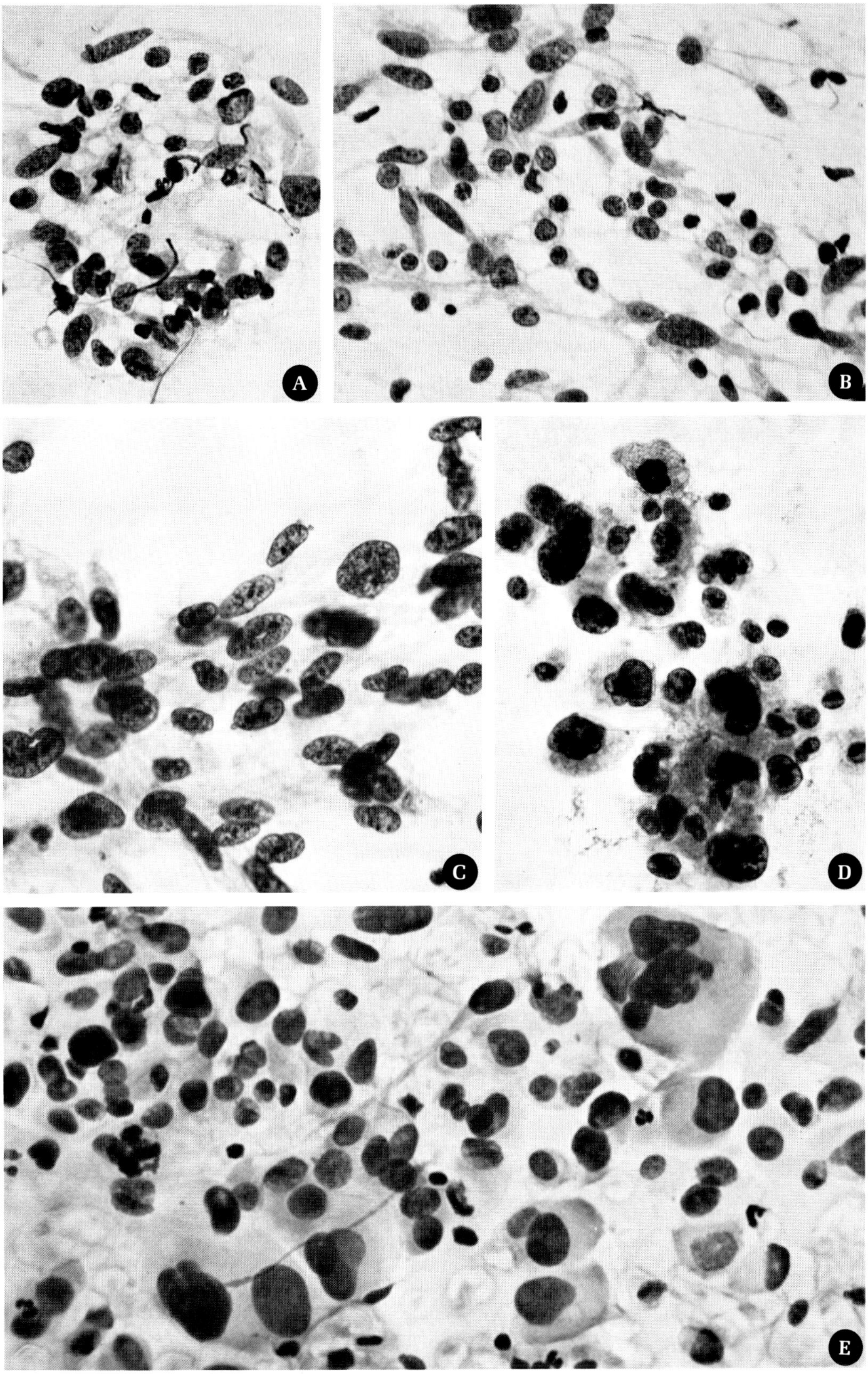

Figure 2-51. Tumor cells of malignant pleomorphic fibrous histiocytomas in smear preparations.

A and **B**, Exfoliated tumor cells in pleural effusion. Slender elongated cells with cigar-shaped and solitary nuclei. Note the numerous round histiocytic forms (Papanicolaou, ×450).

C and **D**, Smears prepared from pleural effusion of malignant pleomorphic fibrous histiocytoma show plump oval and round nuclei and pale filamentous or granular cytoplasm. There is evidence of cytoplasmic cohesion and tendency to form clusters (Papanicolaou, ×450).

E, Pleomorphic neoplastic cells in a smear prepared from percutaneous aspirate of a gluteal malignant pleomorphic fibrous histiocytoma. Note the extreme variation in size of the tumor cells (H & E, ×450).

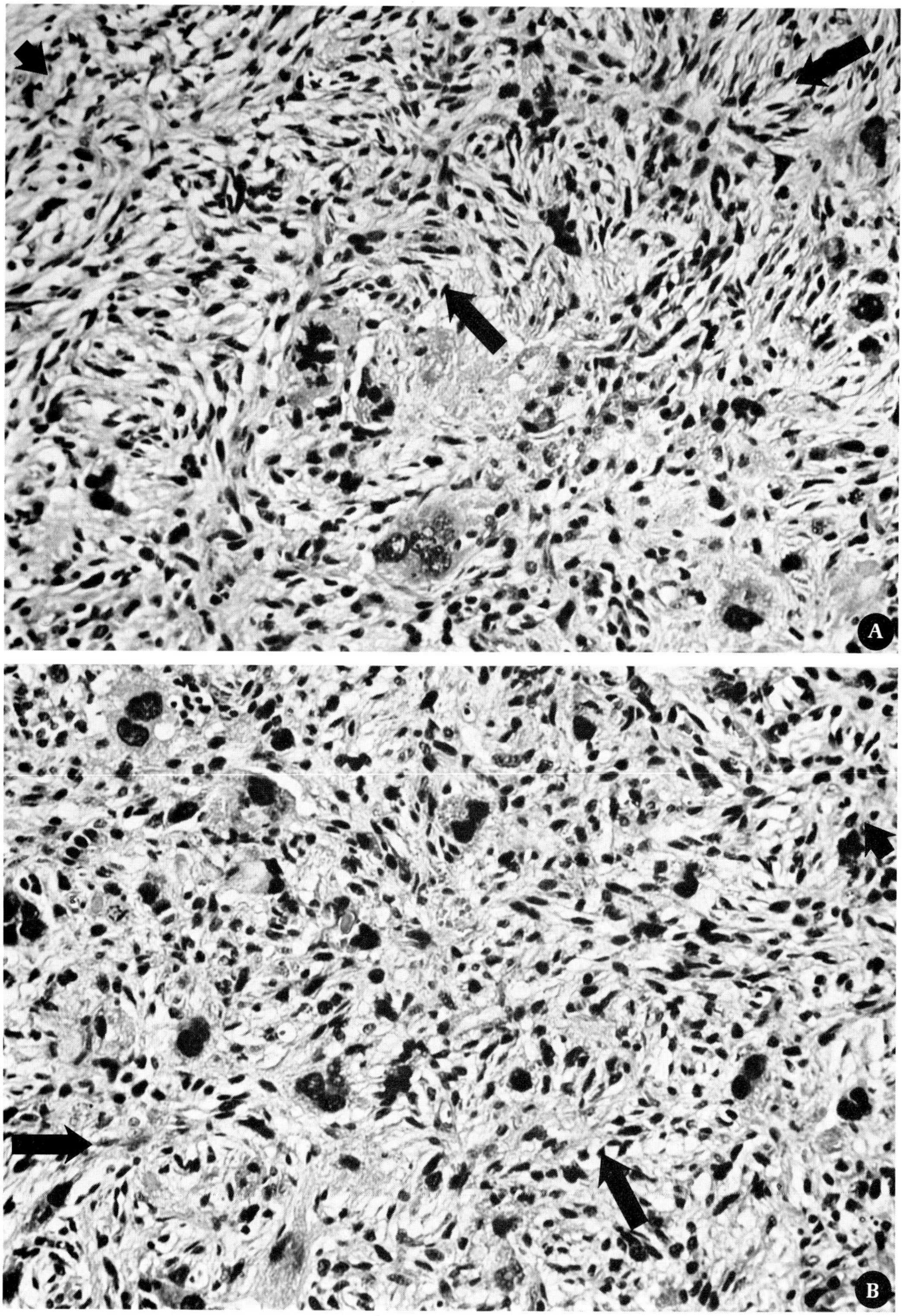

Figure 2-52. Malignant pleomorphic fibrous histiocytoma. This tumor is composed of reticular stromal cells of the type commonly seen in malignant fibroblastic fibrous histiocytoma (see Figure 2-26). Even the storiform arrangement is reproduced by the neoplastic stromal cells (arrows). The giant cells are bizarre multinucleated forms in tight contact with the fibrous histiocytic stromal cells unlike those in benign pleomorphic fibrous histiocytoma (see Figure 2-46) (H & E, ×350).

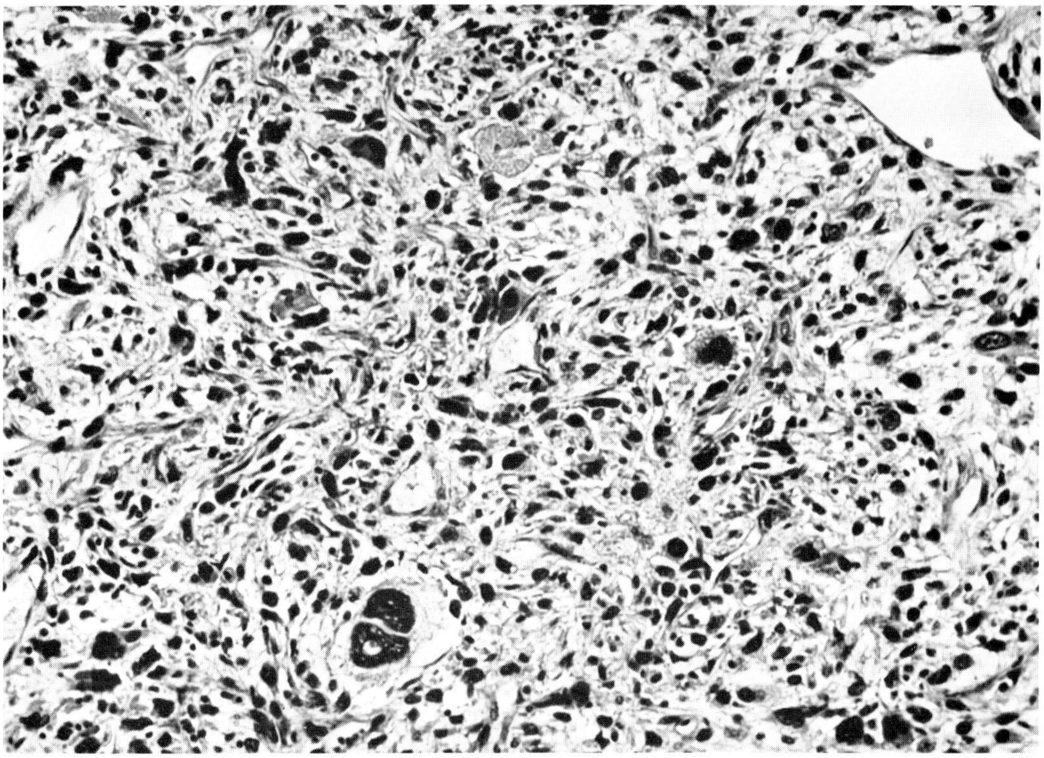

Figure 2-53. Malignant pleomorphic fibrous histiocytoma showing pleomorphic neoplastic stromal cells and occasional inflammatory cells. Note the numerous bizarre tumor giant cells and absence of collagenous material (H & E, ×350).

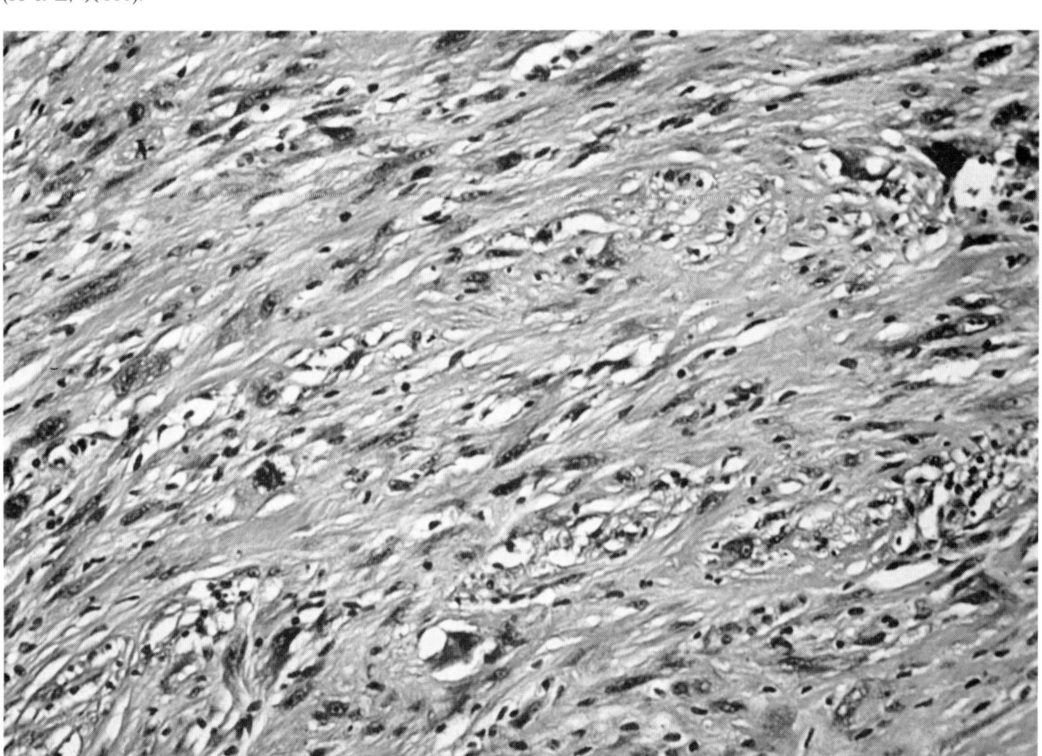

Figure 2-54. Recurrent malignant pleomorphic fibrous histiocytoma (the primary tumor illustrated in Figure 2-53) treated by irradiation prior to excision. The tumor is a clearly malignant tumor and looks like a pleomorphic, collagenous tumor rather than a noncollagenous fibrous histiocytoma (H & E, ×350). (See Figure 2-72.)

fibroblasts and histiocytes is almost always rewarding (Taxy and Battifora, 1977).

Malignant pleomorphic fibrous histiocytoma is a fully malignant neoplasm and should be treated accordingly. Our limited experience with irradiation and chemotherapy of these tumors does not allow any definite conclusion about the prognosis (see Fig. 1-59 and Table 1-15).

Subcutaneous benign or atypical fibrous histiocytoma of the pleomorphic type has been reported following irradiation therapy, and I have seen 4 cases of fibrous histiocytoma which developed 5, 9, 20, and 25 years after irradiation therapy. The capacity of the skin to develop atypical tumor-like proliferation of fibrous tissue and fibrosarcoma after irradiation is well documented (Chapter 9). It seems that irradiation may be a predisposing factor in the development of certain fibrous histiocytomas as well as in fibrosarcomas.

It is not uncommon to see in children fibrous histiocytomas, commonly called *juvenile xanthomas, xanthogranulomas,* or *atypical juvenile fibrous histiocytomas.* In children most of these lesions are regarded as harmless, although many recur after excision. Kauffman and Stout, in 1961, reviewed the literature and reported 39 cases. Twenty-four of the tumors were classified as fibroblastic and 15 were called histiocytic. Only 3 of the 39 patients died with metastatic disease.

Primary fibrous histiocytoma of the head and neck areas is rare. There are about three dozen well-documented cases in the literature. There is an apparent male-to-female predominance of 3:1 and the average age of patients is 42 years. Most of these lesions are locally infiltrative, atypical, histiocytic, or pleomorphic, and excision with clean margins should be considered as adequate treatment.

Fibrous histiocytomas of the retroperitoneum, mediastinum and mesentery are commonly referred to as xanthogranulomas. Despite the large size and heavy inflammatory infiltrate, none of the so-called xanthogranulomas reported metastasized. They are, however, troublesome lesions because of their location.

A primary case of atypical fibrous histiocytoma of the *vulva* was reported by Hensley and Friedrich in 1973.

Differential Diagnosis

Apart from the difficulty of distinguishing benign histiocytic and pleomorphic fibrous histiocytomas from the malignant ones, at least a dozen benign and malignant neoplasms must be considered in the differential diagnosis.

Fibromatosis is characteristically composed of well-differentiated collagenous fibroblasts and there are no significant numbers of histiocytes and giant cells.

Fibroblastic fibrosarcoma consists of well-differentiated partially collagenous and uniform fibroblasts arranged in the characteristic herringbone pattern. Vacuolated and foamy histiocytes, as well as the multinucleated giant cells of histiocytic and pleomorphic fibrous histiocytomas, are absent.

Pleomorphic fibrosarcoma basically is composed of mononuclear and multinucleated collagenous fibroblasts without significant numbers of mononuclear or multinucleated histiocytic cells, except in areas of necrosis.

Lipoblastic liposarcoma contains numerous round, monomorphic and vacuolated lipoblasts which may closely resemble the round cells of histiocytic fibrous histiocytoma. However, the multinucleated epulis-type or Touton giant cells are absent or few (Chapter 4).

Pleomorphic liposarcoma is an admixture of pleomorphic lipoblasts and lipocytes in a highly vascular stroma. It may be extremely difficult indeed to distinguish it from pleomorphic fibrous histiocytoma in limited material; however, the ubiquitous presence of bimorphic cells and Touton giant cells in pleomorphic fibrous histiocytomas makes the distinction relatively easy (Chapter 4).

Benign or malignant schwannoma may resemble fibroblastic fibrous histiocytoma. The presence of slender, extremely long tumor cells in a palisading pattern is characteristic for neurogenic tumors (Chapter 7).

Another tumor that occasionally can have extremely spindly cells is the *leiomyosarcoma*. The site of origin and the invariable presence of longitudinal myofilaments help to distinguish smooth muscle tumors from fibrous histiocytomas (Chapter 5).

The *pleomorphic rhabdomyosarcoma* may resemble pleomorphic fibrous histiocytoma, but careful search for cross-striated and small embryonal rhabdomyoblasts is rewarding, in most cases (see Chapter 5).

The malignant histiocytic fibrous histiocytoma may appear similar to *histiocytic lymphoma* in limited material. However, the distinctly monomorphic presentation and high fibrillar reticulin content are suggestive of histiocytic lymphoma rather than fibrous histiocytoma (Chapter 9).

What makes specific identification of fibrous histiocytomas often difficult is the fact that fibroblasts and histiocytes are ubiquitous in the human body and may contribute to the composition of several other neoplasms than the ones called fibrous histiocytomas. In addition, many mesenchymal neoplasms in dedifferentiated or embryonal form, e.g., at time of recurrence and metastasis, may assume fibrous histiocytic features (Fig. 2-32; Table 2-8).

Collagenous Fibrous Tumors

FIBROMA*

Fibromas are non-metastasizing, self-limiting lesions of proliferating fibroblasts. A peculiarity of fibromas is that they occur with extreme rarity in the soft tissues where fibrous tissue is most abundant.

Fibromas are usually subcutaneous in location and may appear from infancy to old age. Their consistency may vary considerably; some are extremely *firm* (fibroma durum, sclerosing fibroma, or calcifying fibroma), others are *soft* (fibroma molle or xanthofibroma), and others are *semisolid* (fibromyxoma or dermatofibroma). The cut surface shows variation according to the consistency of the tumor. The soft fibromas are often edematous and myxomatous in appearance. Firm fibromas, on the other hand, exhibit a glistening and whirled appearance. The cellularity of fibromas ranges from the acellular hyalinized forms to the loosely arranged cellular myxoid fibromas (Figs. 2-55, 2-56).

Tendosynovial fibromas are relatively uncommon neoplasms. Whether these lesions are true fibromas or metaplastic lesions of synovial cells is difficult to ascertain. Not uncommonly they contain a hamartomatous vascular component.

Vulvar fibromas are not uncommon and most frequently arise from the labia majora.

Periungual fibromas usually appear after puberty. According to reports, these lesions are associated with tuberous sclerosis in one third of the patients. They are found more commonly on the toes than on the fingers.

The treatment is surgical excision. They usually do not recur after excision with clean margins.

GANGLION

(See Chapter 3, Tumors of Tendosynovial Tissue.)

FIBROLIPOMA

(See Chapter 4, Tumors of Adipose Tissue.)

ANGIOFIBROMA

(See Chapter 6, Tumors of Vessels.)

NEUROFIBROMA

(See Chapter 7, Tumors of Peripheral Nerves.)

**Synonyms and related terms:* sclerosing fibroma, fibromyxoma, desmoma, desmoid fibroma, fibromyoma, adenofibroma, fibroma durum, fibroma molle, nodular subepidermal fibrosis, fibroma simplex, dermatofibroma, xanthofibroma, juvenile aponeurotic fibroma.

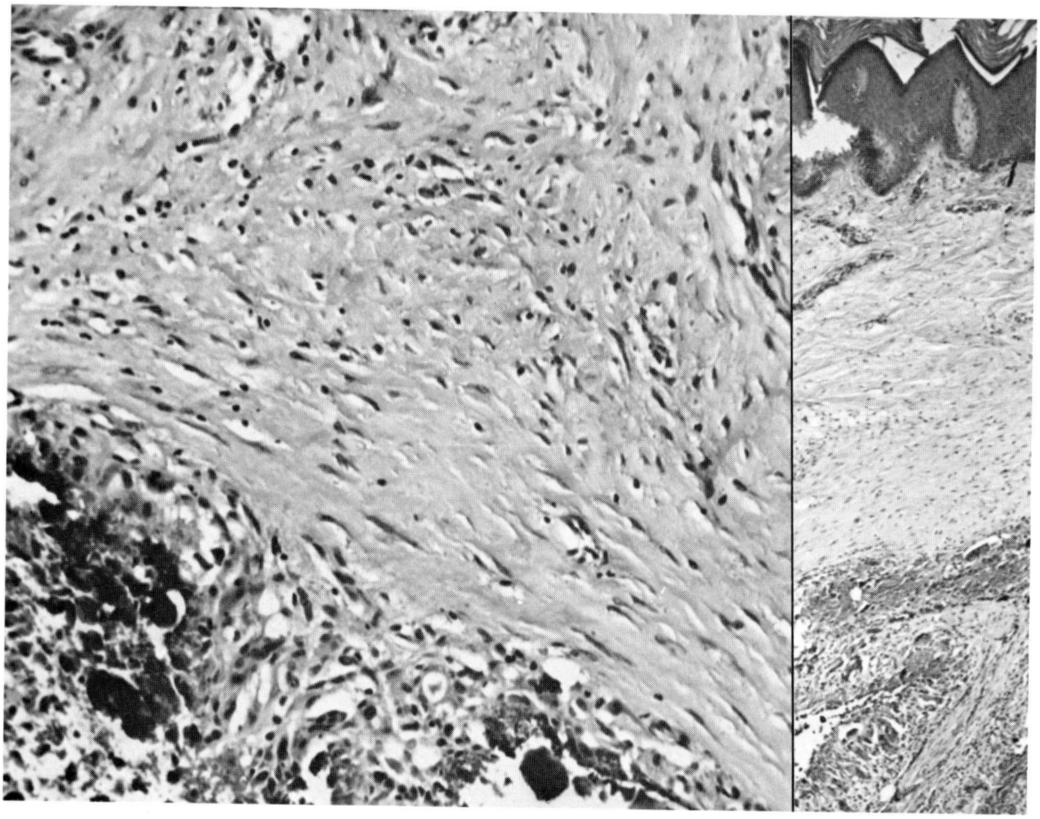

Figure 2-55. Calcifying fibroma of the foot. The lesion is in the dermis and subcutaneous tissues. The dominant tissue is sparsely cellular collagenous fibrous tissue. Note areas of calcification (H & E, ×140; inset, ×35).

DESMOID TUMOR*

At Memorial Sloan-Kettering Cancer Center desmoid tumors are considered as low-grade fibrosarcomas. However, because of their unique natural history and the controversy about them, we are discussing them apart from fully malignant fibrosarcomas.

The name *desmoid* derives from the Greek *desmos* which means "band or tendon." The term *desmoid tumor* was coined by Muller in 1838, but Macfarlane (1832) of Glasgow is credited with the first report of desmoid tumors occurring in the anterior abdominal wall. The first microscopic description of desmoid tumors was given by Rokitansky in 1846 and Bennett in 1849. Bennett called these tumors "fibronucleated cancroid growths." Paget, in 1856, reported the first case of extra-abdominal desmoid tumor and recognized "a very near affinity" between abdominal and extra-abdominal desmoids. Both Bennett and Paget stressed the high incidence of local recurrence. Wilks, in 1859, referring to these tumors stated, "the fibrous and fibronucleated tumors are innocent, but the recurrent fibroids are of a semi-malignant character." And, he added, "they were formerly classed with the cancers, but they are found merely to recur at the same spot after removal, unless, indeed, they have existed for a long time, when they may be propagated throughout the body like a cancer, and are therefore sometimes styled malignant fibroid. In appearance they resemble somewhat the cancers, but are firmer, give out only a serous instead of a milky juice, have a

** Synonyms and related terms:* desmoid fibromatosis, musculo-aponeurotic fibromatosis, desmoid, aggressive fibromatosis, infiltrative fibromatosis, desmoma, fibroma, recurring fibroid tumor, desmoid fibroblastoma, malignant fibrocytic tumor (Fig. 2-4).

fibrous structure when torn, and display nucleated fiber by the microscope."

Sanger, in 1884, was the first author to call attention to the predilection of desmoid tumors to the abdominal wall, and Temoin, in 1893, was the first to describe a desmoid tumor of the abdominal wall in a child. Hartman and Nichols, in 1923, were independently the first to report a series of desmoids, and Nichols defined the extra-abdominal desmoid tumors. Despite this report, the concept that desmoid tumor was a disease of the abdominal wall prevailed for many years.

Prior to the report by Musgrove and McDonald, in 1948, in which they called desmoid tumors benign neoplasms, the clinicopathology of these tumors was analyzed in several studies. All observers, with the exception of Mason, in 1930, concluded that desmoid tumors should be classified as low-grade fibrosarcomas. It is of interest to note that Musgrove and McDonald reached their conclusion despite the fact that 21 of the 34 cases in their series had no follow-up or were followed for less than 5 years. Ewing (1935) regarded desmoid tumors as low-grade fibrosarcomas. He stated that he had seen no metastasis from desmoids but locally they could cause such grievance that the term of choice, *low-grade fibrosarcoma,* was justified. He felt that desmoid tumor should be named after its clinical rather than its histologic trait. Stout, in 1953, expressing his doubt about the malignant potentials of desmoid tumors, coined the term *desmoid fibromatosis.* This attempt, designed to make unnecessary the distinction between fibromatoses and desmoids, led to considerable confusion. However, Mackenzie, in 1970, restated the views of earlier investigators: "It is the natural history of the disease, and not the

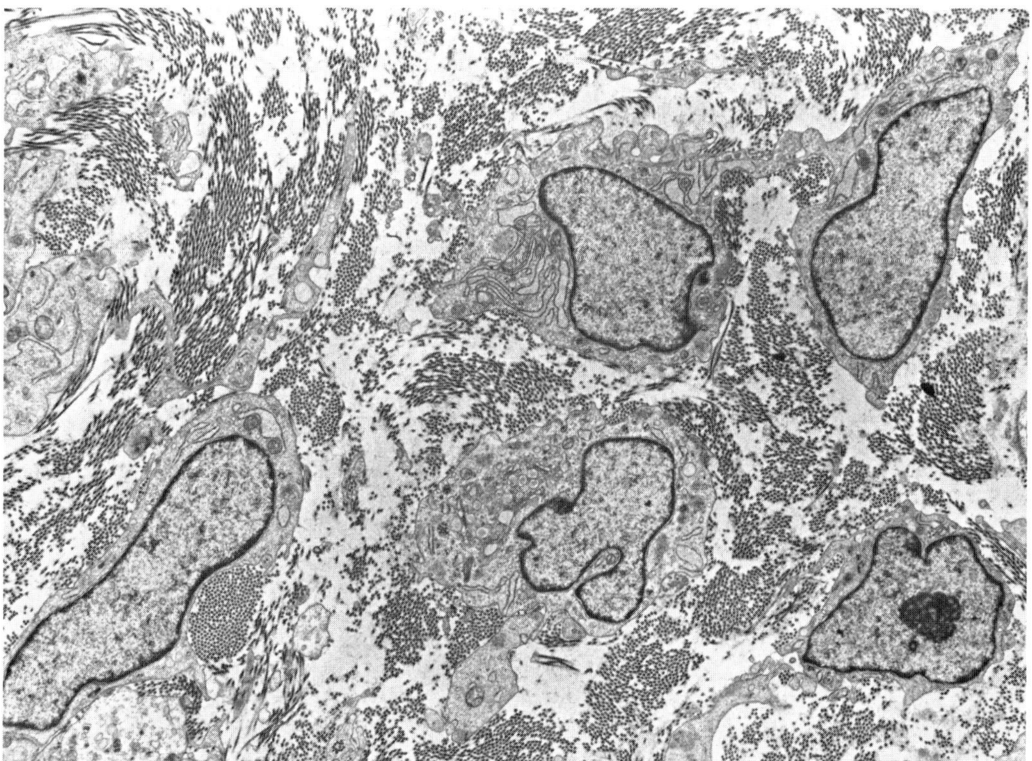

Figure 2-56. Ultrastructure of dermatofibroma. The tumor is composed of small fibroblasts containing prominent rough endoplasmic reticulum and is surrounded by numerous collagen fibrils (×5,000). (See also Figure 2-72.)

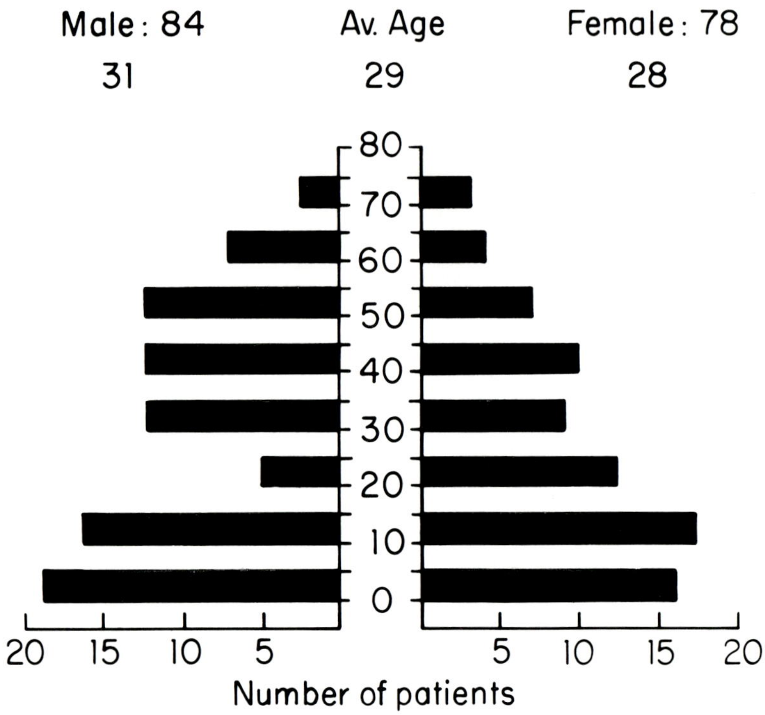

Figure 2-57. Age distribution of 162 patients treated at Memorial Sloan-Kettering Cancer Center for desmoid tumor.

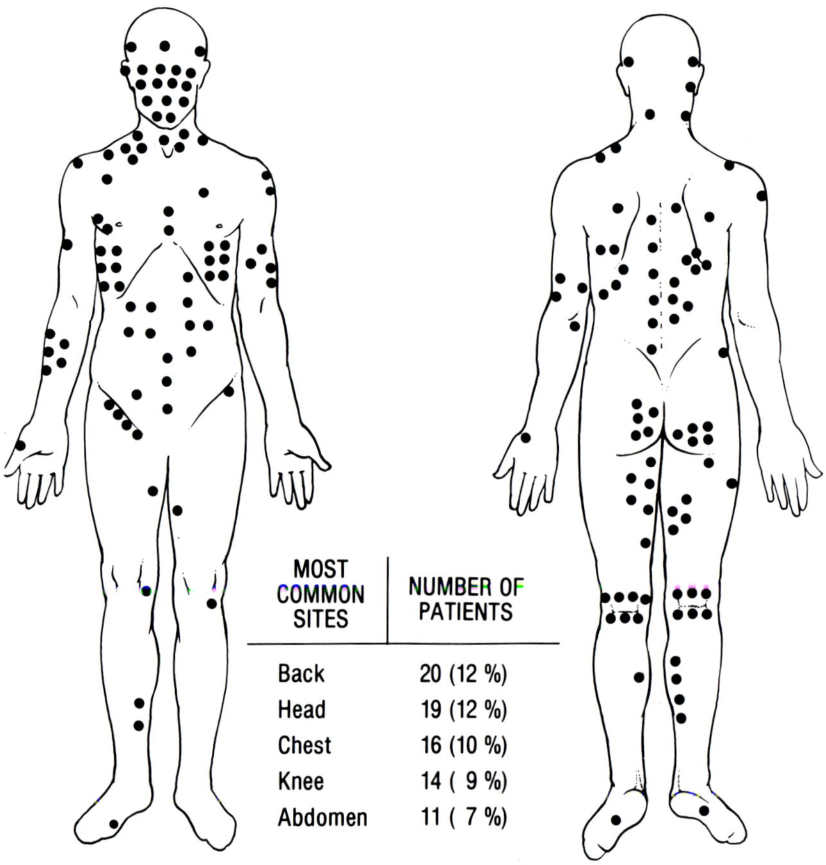

Figure 2-58. Anatomic distribution of the sites of 162 desmoid tumors.

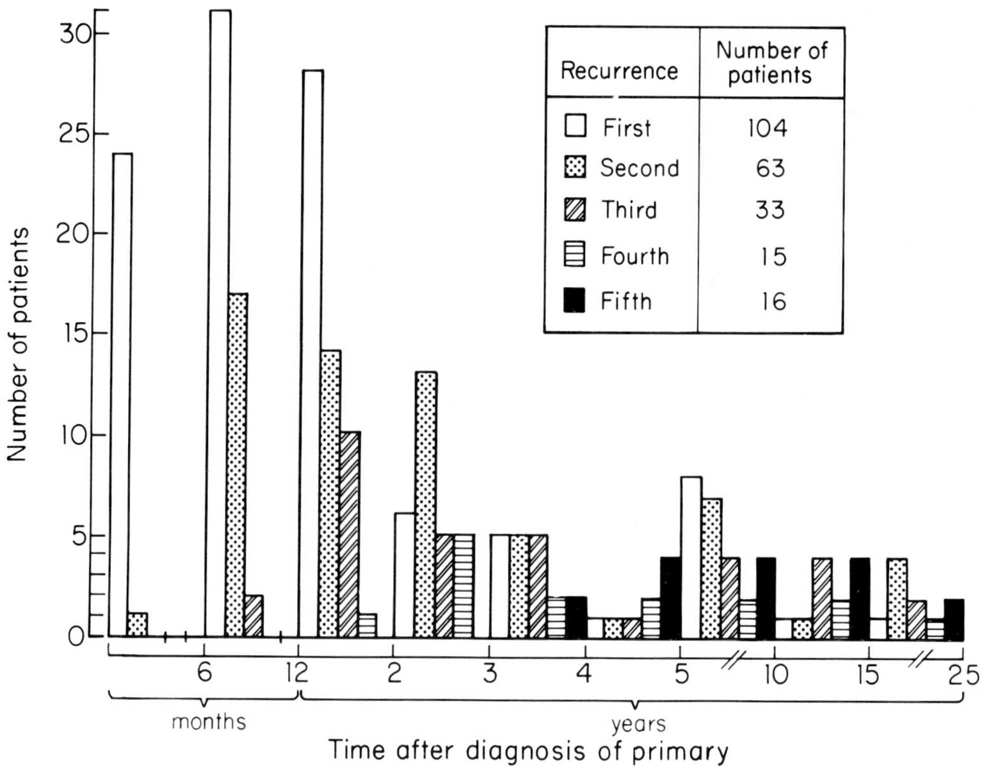

Figure 2-59. Of the 162 desmoid tumors studied, 104 recurred at least once. Several recurred more than once.

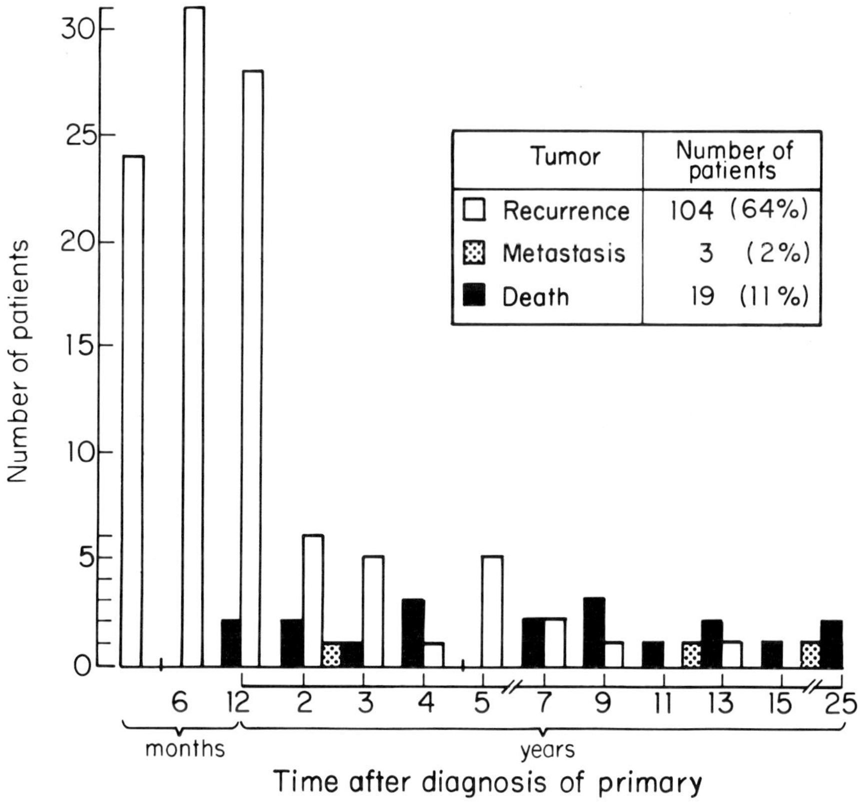

Figure 2-60. Rate of local recurrence and metastasis of 162 desmoid tumors. Note the mortality of 11%.

morphology which should determine the attitude of pathologists and surgeons" (Table 2-14).

Our experience with desmoid tumors shows (Figs. 2-57 through 2-60) that labels such as musculoaponeurotic fibromatosis, aggressive fibromatosis, benign desmoid, and others, with the assurance they carry, are never justified for an unencapsulated or pseudoencapsulated infiltrating fibrous tumor, of fascial or aponeurotic origin, located in deep soft tissues, bigger than 5 cm, and appearing at an age and an anatomic site other than that where fibromatoses are customarily found (Fig. 2-4). It is true that on the basis of histologic appearance alone many of the desmoids are not malignant. On the basis of clinical course, however, many of these neoplasms show that the ultimate result justifies their classification as low-grade malignant neoplasms.

Etiologic factors responsible for desmoids are difficult to assess. Numerous theories have been advanced in an attempt to explain the origin and to clarify the unpredictable nature of desmoid tumors. Among the etiologic factors most commonly listed are trauma (e.g., abdominal desmoid in female patients following pregnancy), hormonal disturbances (supported by the evidence that desmoid-like tumors in experimental animals are hormone dependent), and possible genetic or hereditary factors. Desmoid tumors in association with Gardner's syndrome have been reported, and Smith in 1959, suggested the existence of a genetically controlled *fibromatogenic factor* in patients with familial polyposis.

Desmoid tumors of the anterior abdominal wall are much less common than would appear from the number of case reports in the literature. Pack and Ehrlich, in 1944, found only 17 desmoid tumors of the abdominal wall in a series of 50,346 cases of neoplastic disease. During the years 1931 through 1966 Brasfield and Das Gupta (1969) were able to find, on the average, one patient a year admitted to Memorial Sloan-Kettering Cancer Center, with abdominal desmoid (Table 2-15, Fig. 2-61).

Extra-abdominal desmoid tumors may occur at any age but are commonest, according to reported studies, in the third and fourth decades. Our experience shows that desmoid tumor is not uncommon in children and teenagers (Fig. 2-62). It may also present as a congenital neo-

TABLE 2-14. ***The Changing Definition of Desmoid Tumor through History***

LOW GRADE MALIGNANT NEOPLASM		BENIGN LESION
Wilks	1859	
	1904	Peiffer
	1923	Nichols
	1930	Mason
Warren and Sommer	1936	
Broders et al	1939	
Ewing	1940	
Stout	1948	
Stewart	1948	Musgrove and McDonald
	1954	Stout
Mackenzie	1964	
Butler	1965	
Enzinger	1965	
	1967	Enzinger and Shiraki
	1970	Mackenzie
Soft Tissue Task Force (Russell, et al, 1977)	1977	

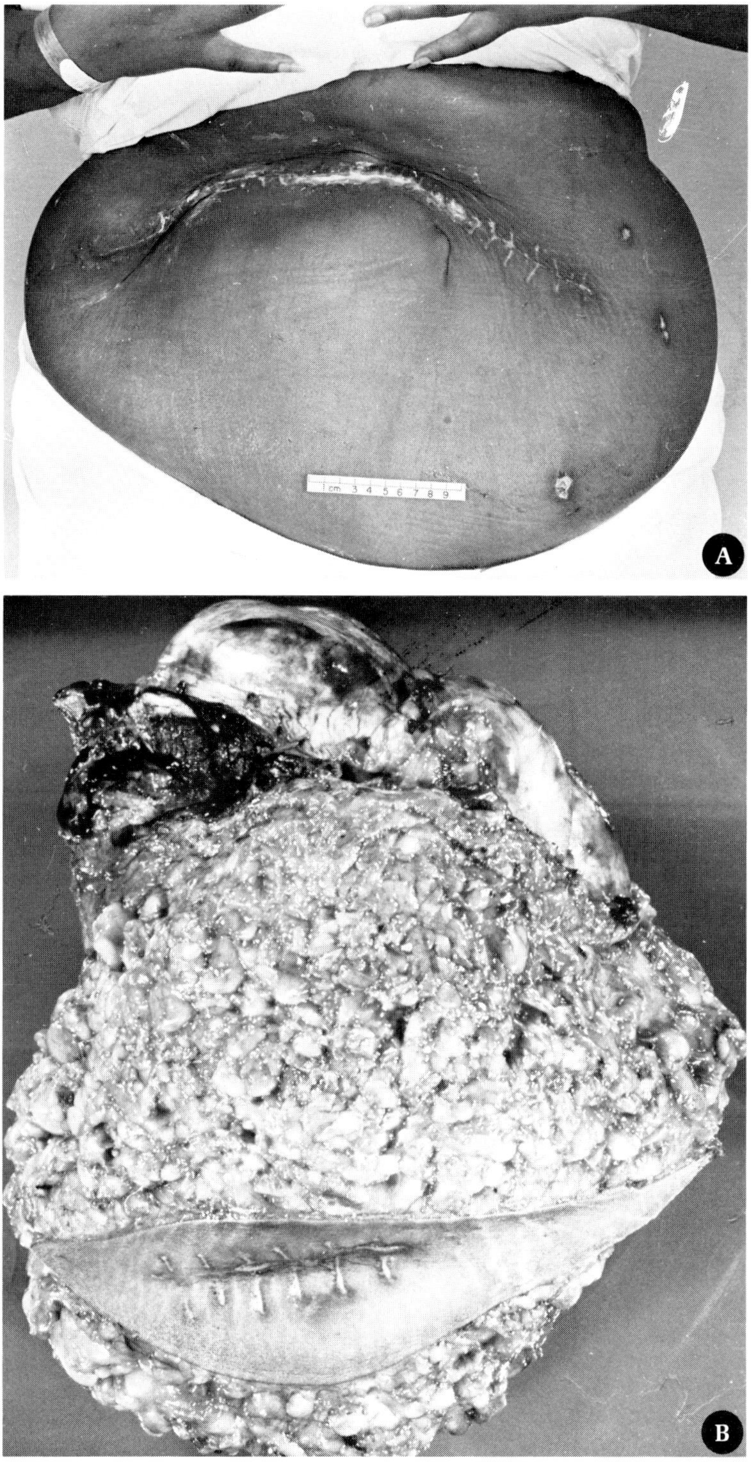

Figure 2-61. **A,** Recurrent desmoid tumor of the abdominal wall prior to excision. **B,** The surgical specimen.

TABLE 2-15. ***Relation of Abdominal Desmoids to Abdominal Wall Muscle****

MUSCLE	NUMBER OF PATIENTS
Rectus abdominis	18
Linea alba	8
External oblique	4
Internal oblique	2
Transversus abdominis	2

*Modified from Brasfield, R. D., and Das Gupta, T. K.: Desmoid tumors of the anterior abdominal wall. Surgery 65:241, 1969.

plasm. Exelby and his colleagues, in 1973, published a series of 22 cases of desmoid tumors in children. In their series the youngest patient was 18 months old, but 80% of the children were older than 6 years.

Although both sexes are affected, abdominal desmoids predominate in females, especially in females in childbearing age. Extra-abdominal ones have a male preponderance (Fig. 2-57).

The back, the chest wall, and the head and neck areas, as well as the lower extremity, are the most common sites of origin of these tumors. A few instances of multicentric sites of origin are recorded in the literature (Figs. 2-63, 2-64). The majority of patients complain of a painless mass of several months' or years' duration (Fig. 2-58).

There is no question that the extra-abdominal desmoid is identical, grossly and microscopically, with that of the anterior abdominal wall. *The most remarkable feature of these neoplasms is their tendency to recur usually at the site of prior surgical excision* (Table 2-16; Figs. 2-59, 2-60).

Desmoid tumors are in general solitary well-defined neoplasms. The size may vary from a few centimeters to several inches in diameter. Growth generally is progressive and may reach hugh proportions. The largest tumor recorded in the literature by Rokitansky weighed 17 kg. They have a hard, rubbery consistency and may appear pseudoencapsulated. On gross examination, the cut surface is glistening and grayish-white with interlacing or trabeculated bundles of collagenous fibrous tissue. The long axes of these fibers are usually oriented parallel with the fibers of adjacent muscle bundles.

Histologically, the desmoid tumor is composed of well-differentiated and uniform collagenous fibroblasts and fibrocytes. The tumor cells are plump, with elongated normochromatic and vesicular nuclei which are dispersed between well-formed collagen fibers. In general, the tumor cells in desmoid tumors are shorter, less pyknotic, and more vesicular than those in higher grade fibrosarcomas (Fig. 2-65). The degree of cellularity is variable from area to area, and from tumor to tumor, and there is no evidence of mitotic activity. The tumor cells are commonly arranged in interdigitating fasciculi. Areas of the stroma may be myxomatous and hypocellular, but cystic degeneration or necrosis is almost unseen in desmoid (Fig. 2-66). Allegra and Broderick (1973) studied the ultrastructure of a tumor they called "desmoid fibroblas-

TABLE 2-16. ***Series of Extra-abdominal Desmoid Tumors***

SERIES	NO. OF CASES	RECURRENCE	METASTASIS	DEATH
Musgrove and McDonald (1948)	34	20	—	—
Masson and Soule (1966)	34	21	—	3
Enzinger and Shiraki (1967)	30	17	—	—
Das Gupta et al (1969)	72	58	—	2
Mackenzie (1970)	44	20	?3	4
Hajdu et al (unpublished data)	162	104	3	19
Total	376	240	?6	28

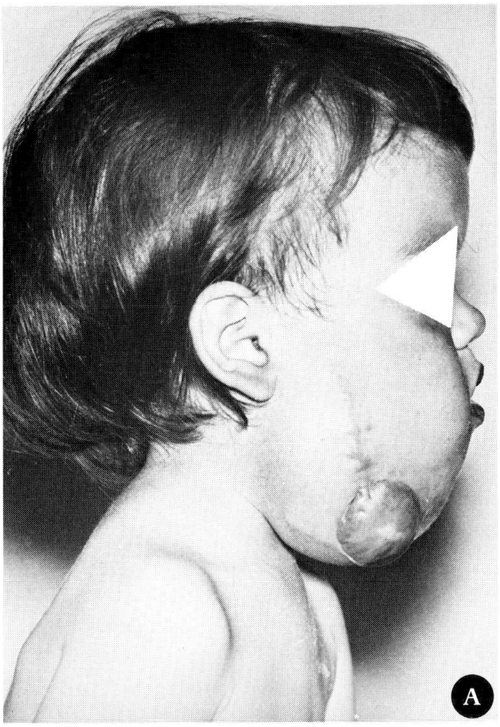

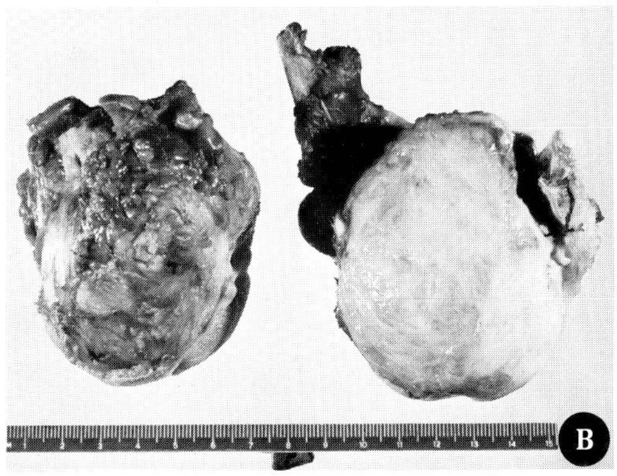

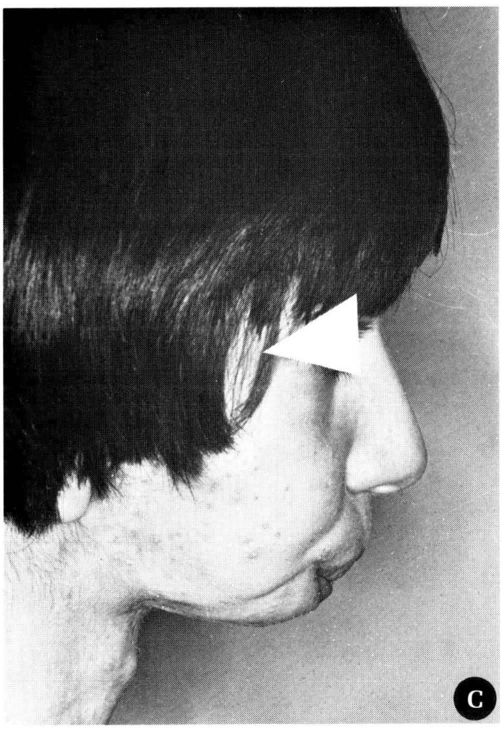

Figure 2-62. Desmoid tumor.

A, This 3-year-old girl presented with a recurrent mass of the face.

B, Hemimandibulectomy was performed and the tumor was removed with clean surgical margins.

C, The patient 11 years later is alive without evidence of the disease.

toma." They illustrated the intracytoplasmic collagenosynthesis and concluded that there is evidence that fibroblasts are capable, perhaps through the functions of the Golgi apparatus, of lysing preformed pericellular collagen while synthesizing new collagen (Fig. 2-67). Desmoids commonly compress or invade muscles, vessels, nerves, tendons, periosteum, bones, and lymph nodes with subsequent de-

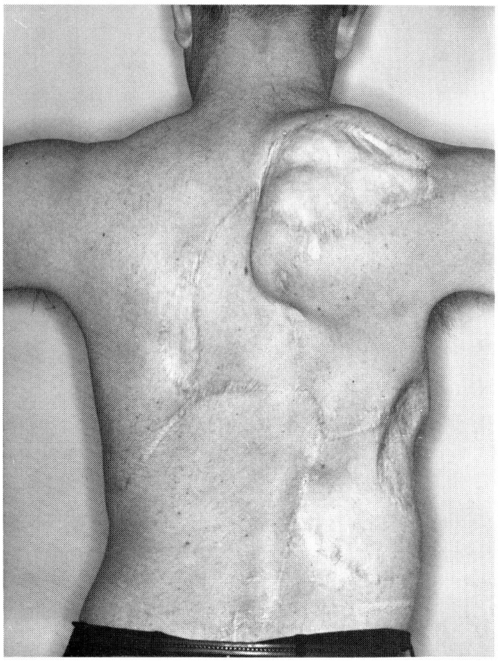

Figure 2-63. A rare, multifocal presentation of desmoid tumor. Desmoid tumors were removed from six different body sites.

struction of many of these structures (Fig. 2-68), but it is generally believed that desmoid tumors do not infiltrate the skin. At the periphery of desmoid tumors, or around myxomatous areas, one may see lymphocytes, histiocytes, or a few eosinophils infiltrating the tumor. Most of the blood vessels are thin-walled capillary vessels, but thick-walled hamartomatous vascular channels can be seen within the tumor.

Desmoid tumors can be defined as *pseudoencapsulated infiltrative growths of well-differentiated collagenous fibroblasts and fibrocytes arising either in fascia or musculoaponeurotic structures.* It must be remembered that the innocuous histologic appearance does not correlate well with the clinical behavior. Willis pointed out in 1960 that it is bizarre that "a seeming benign fibromatous structure is compatible with malignant growth properties."

The primary consideration in treatment of desmoid tumors should be prevention of local recurrence. In most instances, this

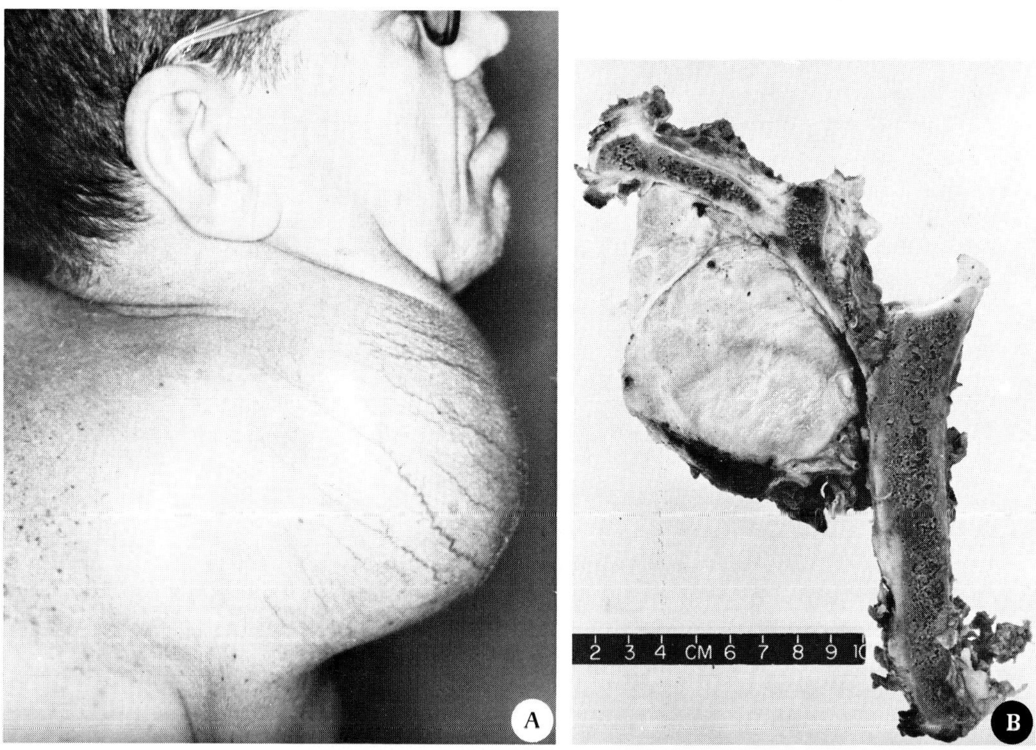

Figure 2-64. Desmoid tumor of the neck (**A**) with extension into parasternal and subclavian areas (**B**).

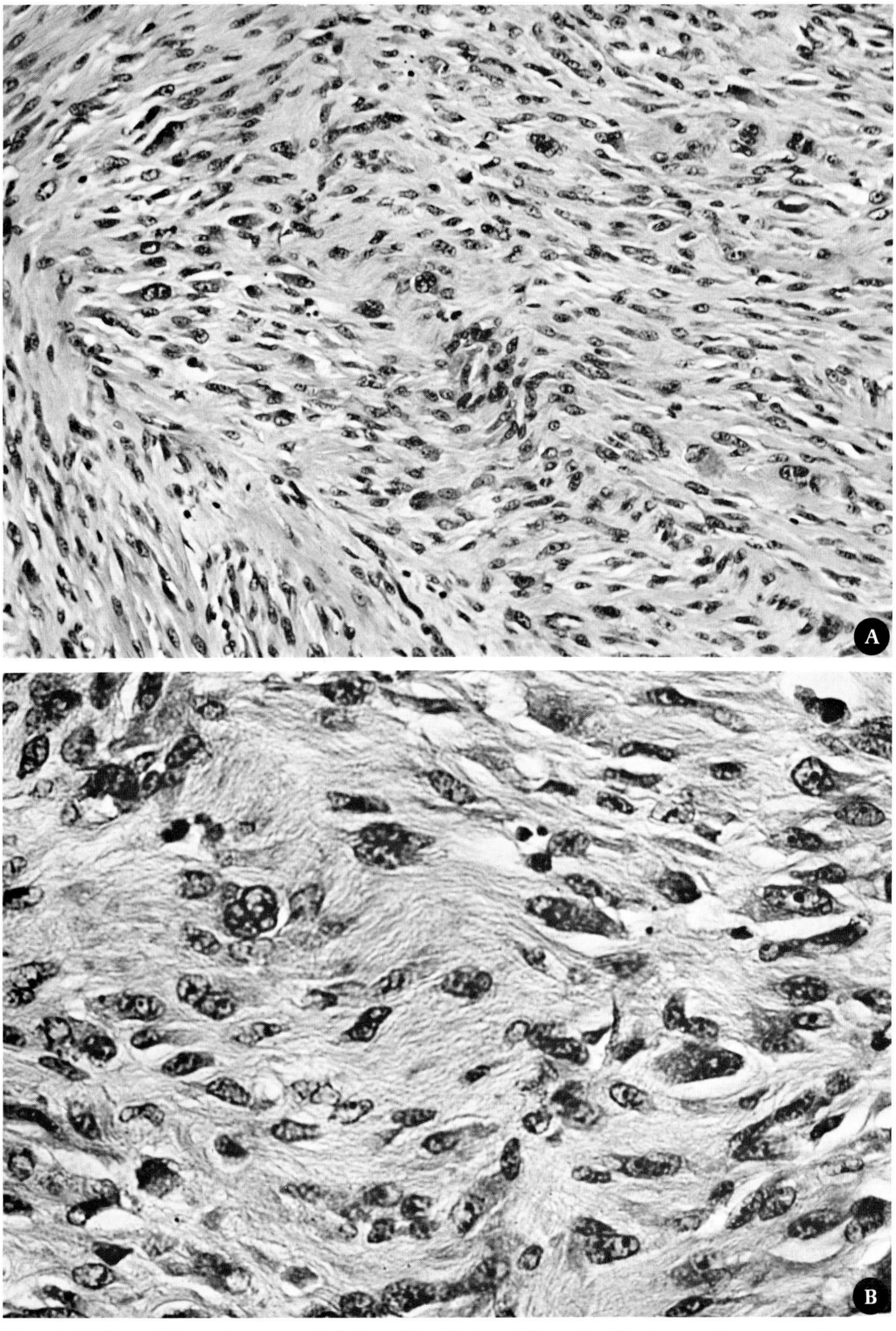

Figure 2-65. Desmoid tumor is composed of plump fibroblasts and fibrocytes. The tumor cells possess collagenous cytoplasmic extensions and the stroma is filled by collagenous material. The tumor cells "run" in the same direction and same dimension. It is almost an avascular tumor and there are no myxomatous or foamy areas (**A,** H & E, ×140; **B,** H & E, ×350). (See also Figure 2-4 and 2-12.)

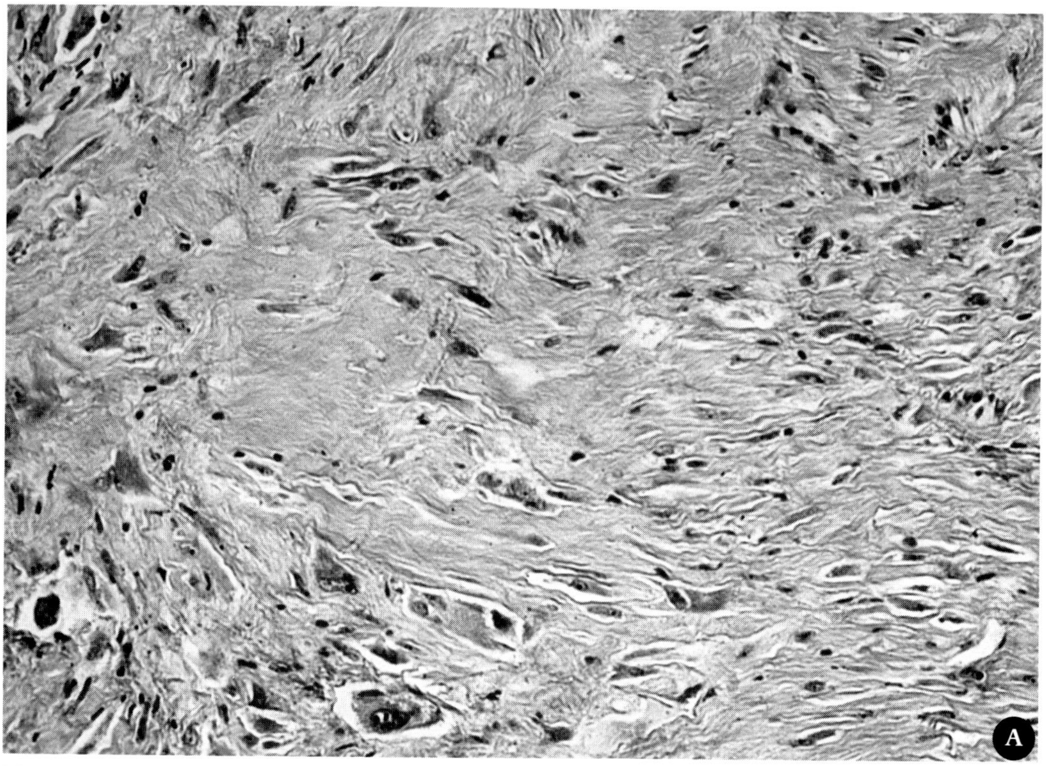

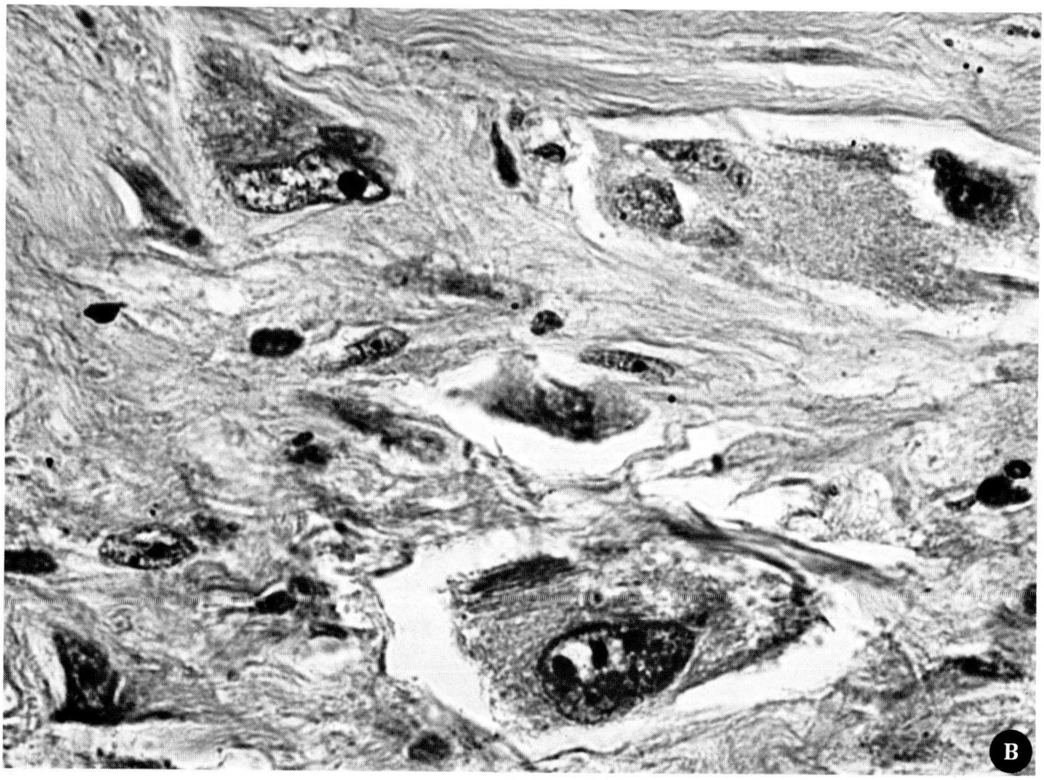

Figure 2-66. **A,** The monotonous tranquility of desmoid tumor is interrupted by large fields of acellular collagenous areas and occasional large bizarre neoplastic fibroblasts.

B, These "monster cells" are embedded in a heavily collagenous stroma and their cytoplasm itself is filled with fibrillar or collagenous substance (**A,** H & E, ×140; **B,** H & E, ×570).

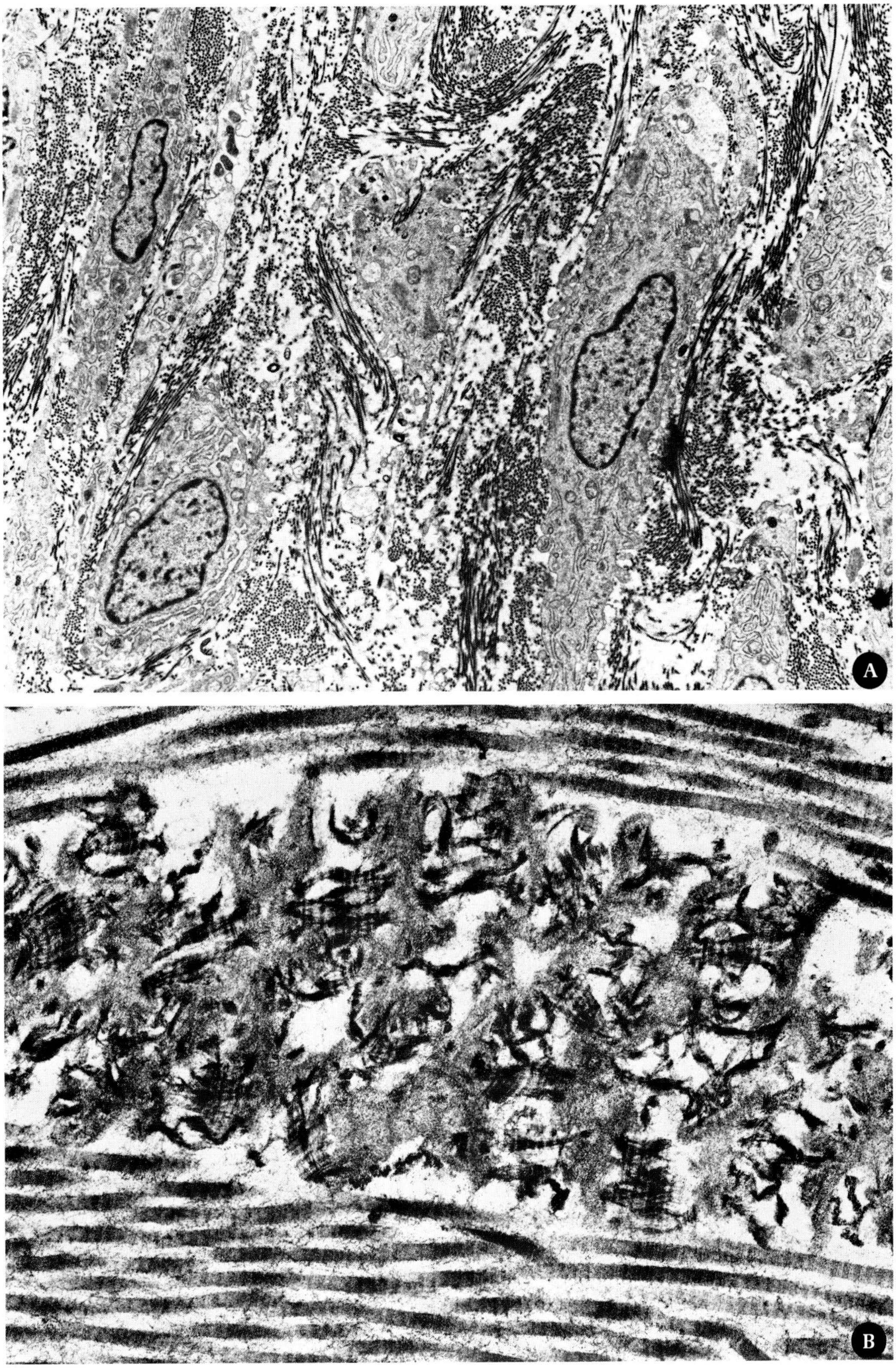

Figure 2-67. A, Ultrastructure of a desmoid tumor of the left shoulder. The tumor is composed of neoplastic fibroblasts surrounded by dense collagen.

B, Fibrillogranular complex found by Allegra and Broderick in tumor they called "desmoid fibroblastoma." According to them, these aggregates are found dispersed throughout the collagen matrix and are believed to represent imperfectly cross-linked tropocollagen (×18,500) (Courtesy of Allegra, S. A., and Broderick, P. A.: Desmoid fibroblastoma. Intracytoplasmic collagenosynthesis in a peculiar fibroblastic tumor. Hum. Pathol. 4:419, 1973.)

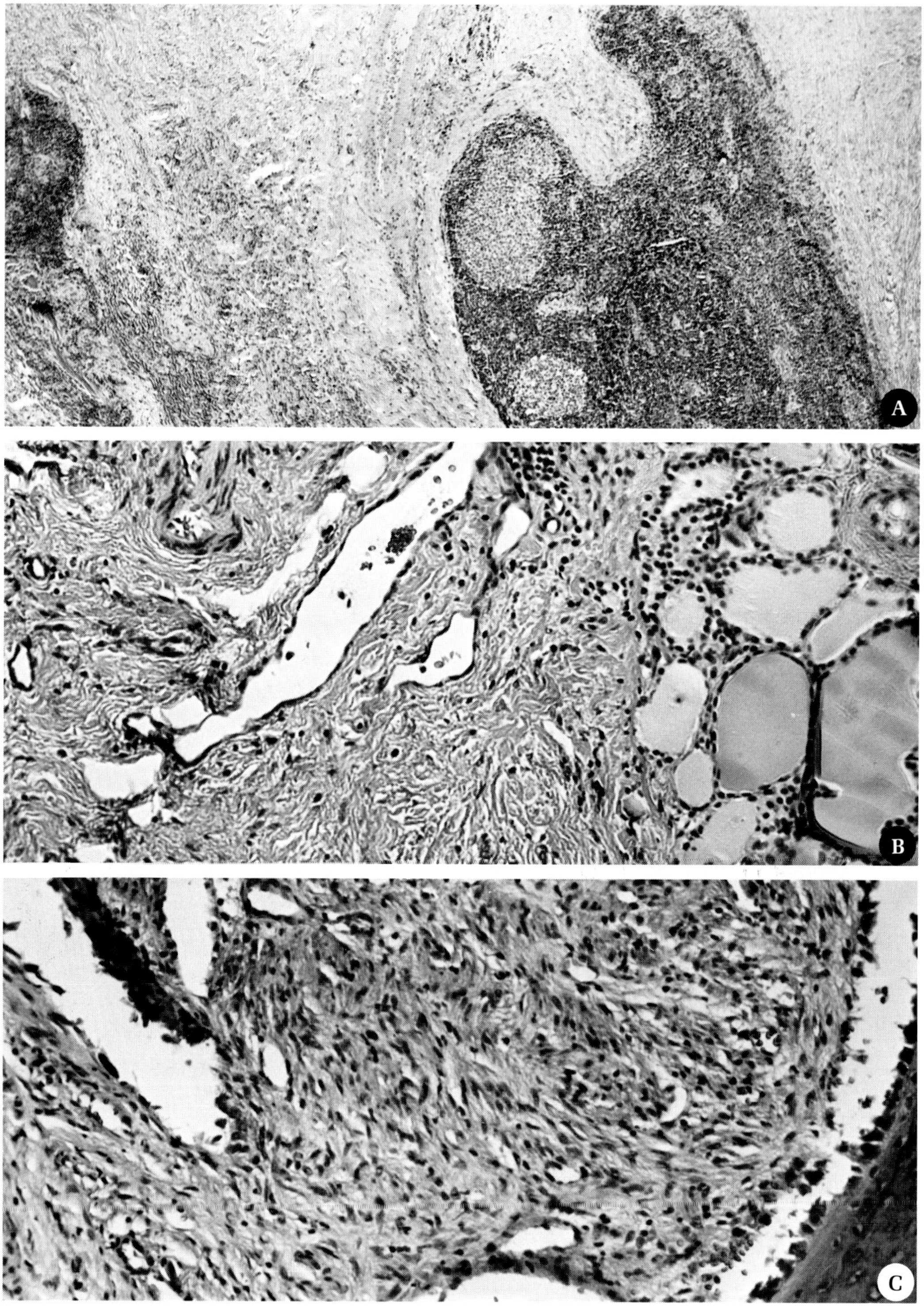

Figure 2-68. A, Desmoid tumor invading and surrounding a lymph node. Note the circular compression of the lymph node (H & E, ×35).

B, Desmoid tumor invading the thyroid gland (H & E, ×85).

C, Desmoid tumor invading and destroying the iliac bone (H & E, ×85).

can be achieved by wide local excision or muscle group resection. A close cooperation between pathologist and surgeon is mandatory. *By proper gross and histopathologic evaluation of margins of the surgical specimen the danger of inadequate or overly radical surgery can be avoided* (Fig. 2-69). It is not always easy to draw the lines between the extremes; as Mackenzie said, in 1964, "The treatment of fibroblastic lesions is a matter of experience and fine judgment." The guide in management of patients with desmoid tumor should be the understanding of the natural history of these neoplasms. Recurrences must be excised, with clean surgical margins. Although most authors recommend surgical excision as the treatment of choice, a number of patients will ultimately require amputation in an attempt to control the disease (Fig. 2-70). There is no clear evidence that irradiation or any of the current chemotherapeutic agents are effective in controlling desmoid tumors (see Table 1-15).

Death from local extension of primary or recurrent tumor into vital structures is rare. Malignant transformation of desmoid without metastasis has been reported by Donald and Caylor in 1929, and Soule and Scanlon in 1962. Although the tumor may extend directly into adjacent lymph nodes (Fig. 2-68A), no nodal metastasis has been reported.

Histologically proven metastasis from desmoid tumor, to my knowledge, has not been reported in the literature; however, Mackenzie, in 1970, in his monograph on fibrous tumors referred to 3 cases with clinical evidence of metastases. Recently we found (Hajdu et al, in press) in our series of 162 cases of desmoid tumors, 3 cases of metastatic desmoids. All three patients died with pulmonary metastases (Table 2-16; Figs. 2-70, 2-71, 2-78).

Differential Diagnosis

In most instances the histologic appearance of desmoid tumors is characteristic enough to separate it from *fully malignant fibrosarcoma*. Fully malignant fibrosarcomas are usually highly cellular pleomorphic neoplasms with numerous tumor giant cells and abnormal mitotic figures. The difficulty in differentiating these two neoplasms occurs most often in infants and children.

Various forms of *fibromatoses* may simulate desmoid tumor, and the diagnosis is one of the most difficult decisions a pathologist has to make. Admittedly, the differences often result more from clinical presentation than from histologic morphology. Although fibromatoses are mostly situated subcutaneously, desmoid tumors invariably have their origin in deep tissues. Also, fibromatoses show less tendency to recur after excision.

The infiltrative growth pattern separates desmoid tumor from self-limited *keloid* and *fibroma*. *Benign fibrous histiocytoma* or *dermatofibroma* is usually a subcutaneous or dermal nodule less than a centimeter in size.

FIBROSARCOMA*

Fully malignant or true fibrosarcomas are collagenous malignant neoplasms, which arise from fibroblasts, have an invasive growth pattern, are capable of metastasizing, and show various degrees of pleomorphism and mitotic activity (Fig. 2-72). Virchow and Billroth employed the term *fibrosarcoma* as early as 1863 and 1877, respectively, and published some of the earliest cases. The identification and study of these neoplasms have been difficult because the literature contains many neoplasms that were indiscriminately classified as fibrosarcoma. In the past a variety of lesions both benign and malignant have been labeled as fibrosarcoma.

There are various reasons for this confusion. The historical reason is the traditionally vague definition and misunderstanding of the term *sarcoma* and the inability to distinguish between benign and malignant fibrous growths. This misunderstanding was compounded

* *Synonyms and related terms:* fibrosarcoma, spindle and giant cell sarcoma, recurrent fibroids, spindle cell sarcoma, myxofibrosarcoma, myxosarcoma, malignant myxoma, neurofibrosarcoma.

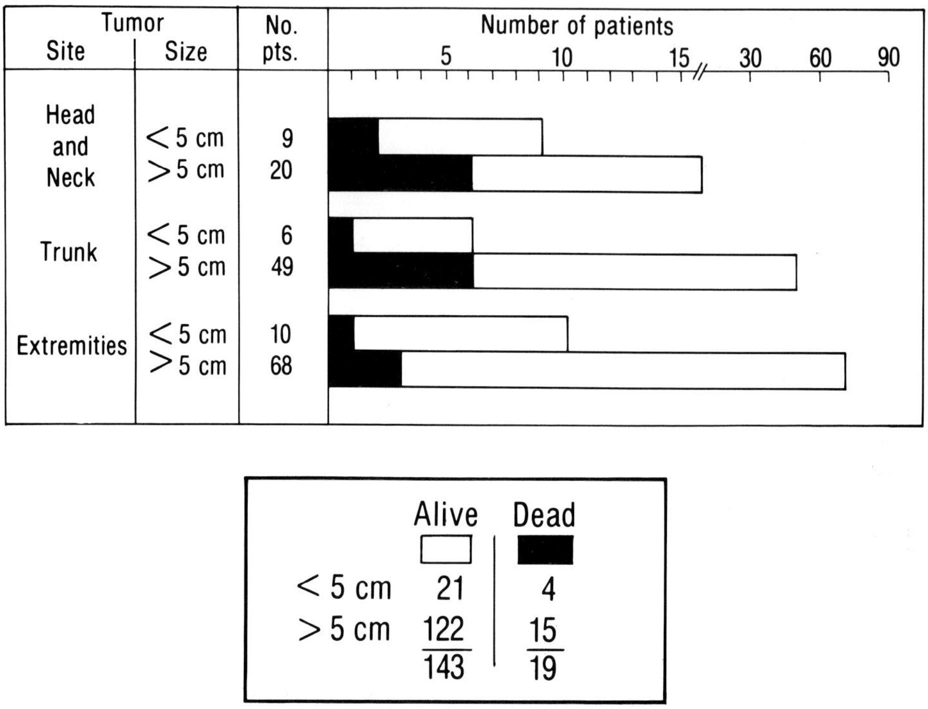

Figure 2-69. Mortality of patients treated for desmoid tumors at Memorial Sloan-Kettering Cancer Center during the last 25 years. Two major factors influencing prognosis are size and anatomic site of the tumor.

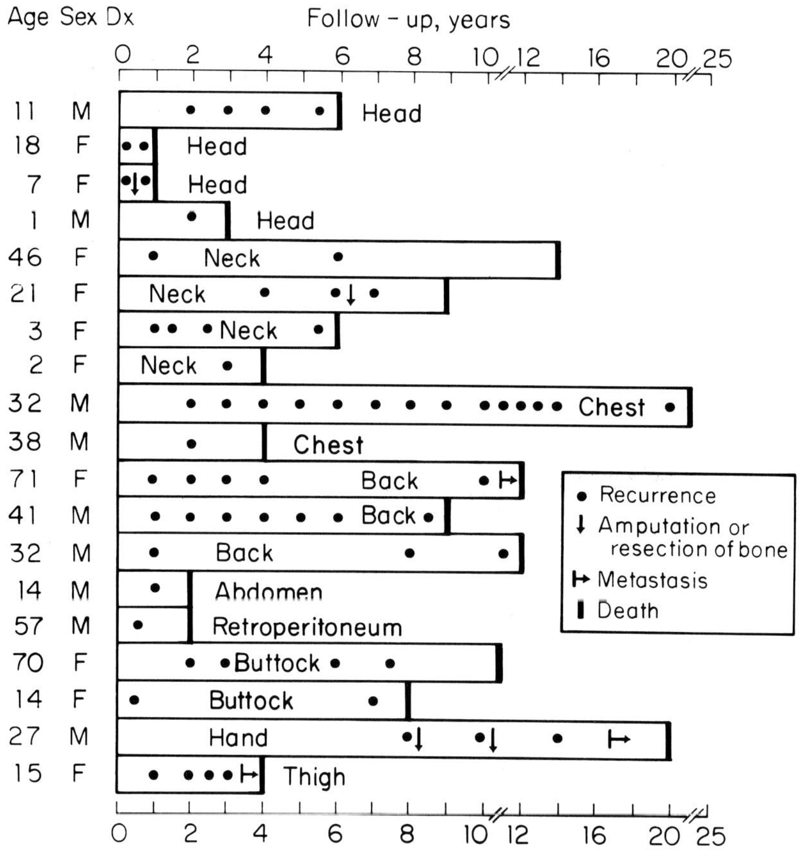

Figure 2-70. Nineteen of the 162 patients treated at Memorial Sloan-Kettering Cancer Center for desmoid tumor died because of the disease. Note that 3 patients died with metastatic disease. In all three the tumor metastasized to the lung; however, autopsies were done on only two of the three.

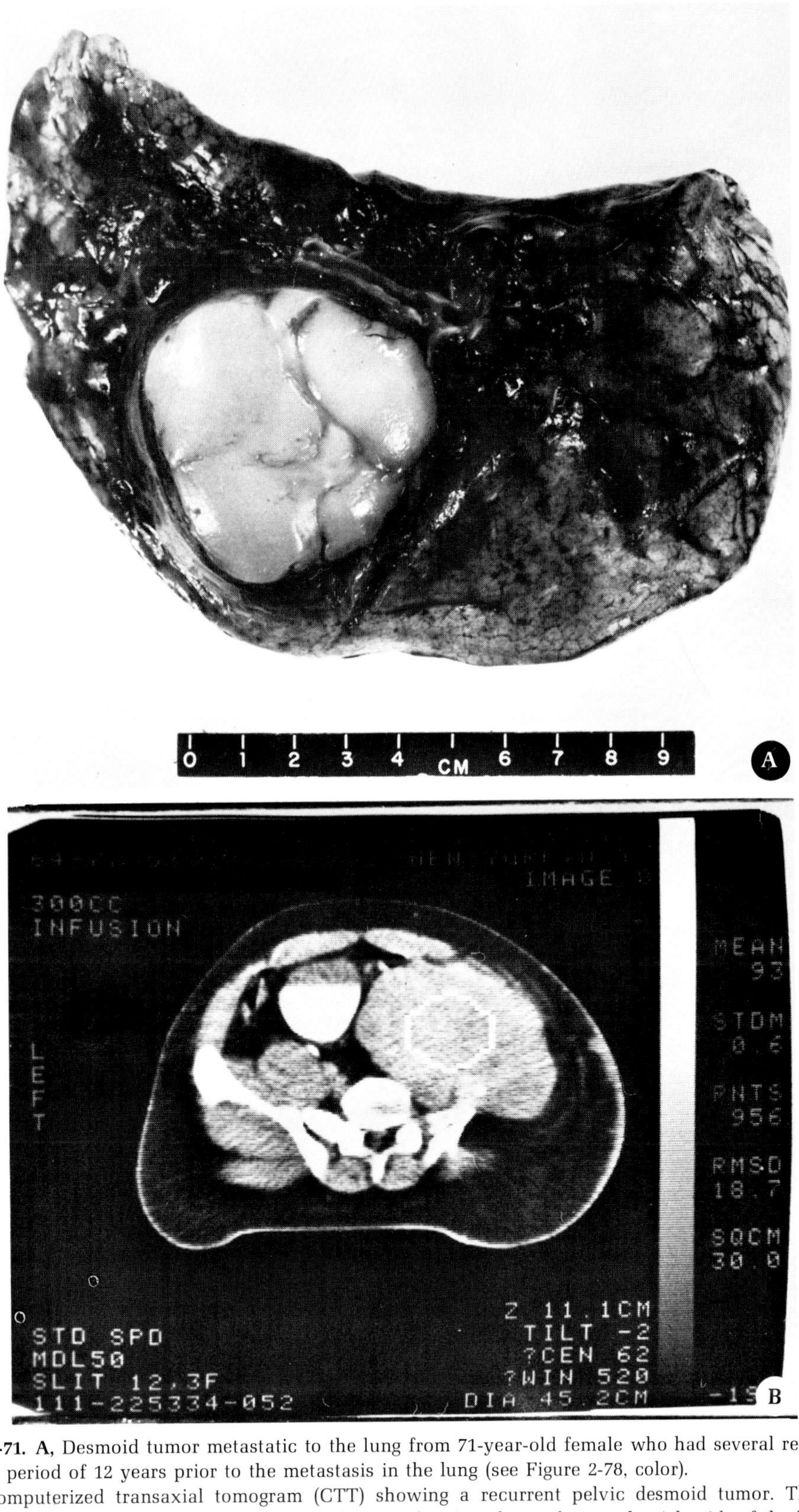

Figure 2-71. A, Desmoid tumor metastatic to the lung from 71-year-old female who had several recurrences during a period of 12 years prior to the metastasis in the lung (see Figure 2-78, color).

B, Computerized transaxial tomogram (CTT) showing a recurrent pelvic desmoid tumor. The tumor surrounds the right iliac bone and has a mean density of 93 (see the readout at the right side of the figure and compare it with Figure 4-18C). (Courtesy Dr. R. Watson, Memorial Sloan-Kettering Cancer Center.)

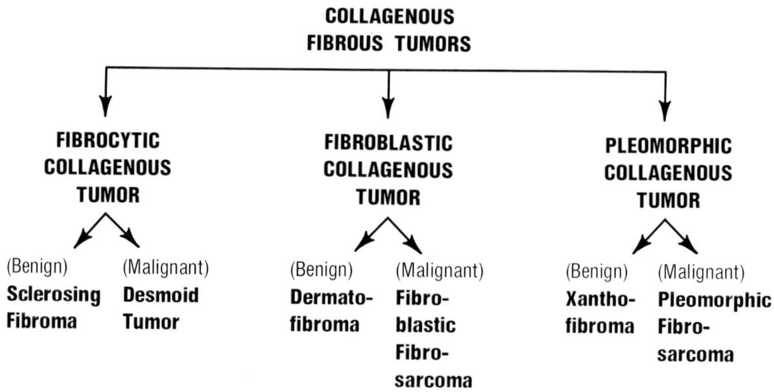

Figure 2-72. Subclassification scheme of collagenous fibrous tumors (see also Figures 2-14 and 2-32).

by reports which included neurogenic sarcomas, mesotheliomas, metaplastic carcinomas, and various "spindle cell sarcomas" under the name of fibrosarcoma. It was not recognized for almost 100 years that sarcomas such as liposarcoma, rhabdomyosarcoma, synovial sarcoma, and many other soft tissue sarcomas may have areas that seem to be fibroblastic in origin. According to Stout and Lattes (1967), "One should try to restrict the term *fibrosarcoma* to growths that are composed of cells and fibers derived from fibrocytes and exclude all the fibrous growths derived from other types of cells acting as facultative fibroblasts."

Ewing (1935) was a leading proponent of the opinion that fibrosarcomas originated in the nervous system and coined the term *neurogenic sarcoma*. Stout (1948) opposed this view, and at the First National Cancer Congress in the USA, in 1949, it was the consensus of the Panel on Soft Tissue Tumors, chaired by Stout, that the term *neurogenic sarcoma* should not be used.

The history of fibrosarcoma is the history of the grading of soft tissue neoplasms. The fundamental principle of grading of cell differentiation of fibrosarcoma is basically the same as that developed by Broders for grading carcinomas.

Quick and Cutler, in 1927, at Memorial Hospital for Cancer and Allied Diseases, were the first to introduce grading of sarcomas. They divided soft tissue sarcomas to indicate their relative grade of malignancy. Hargrave was the first to develop grading for fibrosarcomas and described it in his thesis from the University of Minnesota, in 1934. Geschickter and Lewis, who published their article on grading of fibrosarcomas in 1935, divided fibrosarcomas into differentiated and undifferentiated types. The differentiated sarcomas were composed of malignant fibroblasts and collagen and were named fibromas; the undifferentiated tumors were composed of tightly packed cells with few intercellular structures.

Meyerding et al, in 1936, discussed the etiology, clinical features, prognosis, and treatment of fibrosarcomas of the soft tissues of the extremities on the basis of a series of 152 cases. Three years later, in 1939, Broders et al discussed the same cases in greater detail and presented the grading of malignancy by microscopic examination. The tumors were divided into groups according to the number of mitotic figures and tumor giant cells and the relative proportion of collagen fibers and tumor cells. Employing this system they distinguished: (1) fibrous tumors, (2) fibrocellular tumors, and (3) cellular and fibrous tumors.

Ivins et al, in 1950, Castro et al, in 1973, and Pritchard et al, in 1974, used a four-grade classification in which the most differentiated tumors are grade I and the most anaplastic ones are grade IV. Stout, in 1948, used two grades only according to whether the tumors showed good or poor differentiation, but in his report, in 1962,

TABLE 2-17. ***Histologic Appearance of Fibrosarcomas***

	DESMOID TUMOR	FIBROBLASTIC FIBROSARCOMA	PLEOMORPHIC FIBROSARCOMA
Cellularity	Sparse	Moderate or high	Moderate
Stroma	Collagenous	Partly collagenous	Collagenous
Pattern	Uniform monomorphic	Uniform "herringbone" appearance	Pleomorphic
Tumor giant cells	None or few	None or few	Many
Mitotic figures	None	Few	Many

on fibrosarcomas in infants and children he used a three-grade system.

Our present system of two grades is based on the histopathology of the tumor. *Low-grade fibrosarcomas,* including desmoid tumors, are monomorphic, fibroblastic neoplasms with abundant collagenous stromal tissue and almost complete absence of mitotic figures and tumor giant cells. *High-grade fibrosarcomas* (fibroblastic fibrosarcomas and pleomorphic fibrosarcomas) are more cellular and less collagenous than low-grade tumors. The tumor cells are often arranged in herringbone pattern, and isolated tumor giant cells or cells in mitosis are not uncommon (Table 2-17).

Our experience (Castro et al, 1973) with fully malignant, grade II and grade III fibrosarcomas confirms the findings of Mackenzie, in 1964, and Pritchard et al, in 1974, that the 5-year survival figures are clearly related to the histologic grade. However, let us not forget during histologic grading of fibroblastic neoplasms that *good differentiation is not always indicative of good behavior* (Table 2-18).

Fibrosarcomas usually develop with no apparent relationship to any etiologic agent. *Trauma,* according to reports, plays a definite but apparently an infrequent role in the development of fibrosarcomas. Meyerding, in 1936, reported a history of trauma to the site of development of the sarcoma in 11% of his cases.

In our studies we could not establish a relationship between trauma and the formation of fibrosarcoma. However, fibrosarcoma has been described as having appeared in burn scars, injection sites, and various ulcers. Also, a number of recorded cases of fibrosarcoma developed in tissues that were irradiated (see Chapter 9). It was apparently Warren and Sommer, in 1936, and Gricouroff, in 1937, who reported the first cases of postirradiation fibrosarcomas. According to medical historians, Ouidin, as early as 1897, scarcely two years after Roentgen's publication of his discovery, warned the profession of

TABLE 2-18. ***Survival of Patients with Fibrosarcoma According to Histologic Grade of the Tumor***

	NO. OF PATIENTS	GRADE 1 %	GRADE 2 %	GRADES 3 & 4 %
Broders et al (1939)	70	46	37	17
Mackenzie (1964)	205	83	55	35
Castro et al* (1973)	75	88	72	46
American Soft Tissue Task Force* (Russell et al, 1977)	128	73	33	30

*5-year survival.

See also Chapter 1 (Fig. 1-59 and Table 1-15).

the possible dangers attached to the use of x-rays. It is noteworthy to remember that Porter published his first paper on roentgen carcinoma in 1907.

Fibroblastic and pleomorphic fibrosarcomas are essentially a disease of adults (Fig. 2-73). The majority of these neoplasms occur in patients between the ages of 35 and 55 years. The incidence is higher in males, and the males are apparently somewhat older than the females when the disease occurs.

Fibrosarcomas occur most frequently on the extremities, especially on the thigh and upper arm, but may appear anywhere in the body where fibrous tissue is found (Fig. 2-74; Table 2-19).

Fibrosarcoma of the lung (Martini et al, 1971), trachea and larynx has been reported. A case report of bilateral fibrosarcoma of the epididymis has been reported by McCormack, in 1975, and Tanimura et al reported a case of penile fibrosarcoma also in 1975.

Fibrosarcoma of major blood vessels has been reported, but many of these neoplasms, just like the retroperitoneal ones, are suspected to be leiomyosarcomas. Several examples of fibrosarcoma of the head and neck regions (Lewis, 1969; Farr, 1971; Fu and Perzin, 1976) have been reported. Also, instances of anal (Espinosa and Quan, 1975) and hepatic (Alrenga, 1975) fibrosarcomas have been recorded in the literature.

Perhaps one of the most complex of malignant fibrous neoplasms is that called *congenital fibrosarcoma*. It is almost certain that many examples of congenital fibrosarcomas or so-called juvenile fibrosarcomas have been included in reports on fibromatosis, fibromas, and desmoid tumors. Hudson, in 1936, reported the first case of congenital fibrosarcoma. Wells, in 1940, by reviewing the literature of congenital malignant neoplasms, found only one case of fibrosarcoma among the 29 reported cases. Kauffman and Stout, in 1961, in review of 120 congenital mesenchymal tumors, classified only three as fibrosarcomas.

Subsequent studies (Balsaver et al,

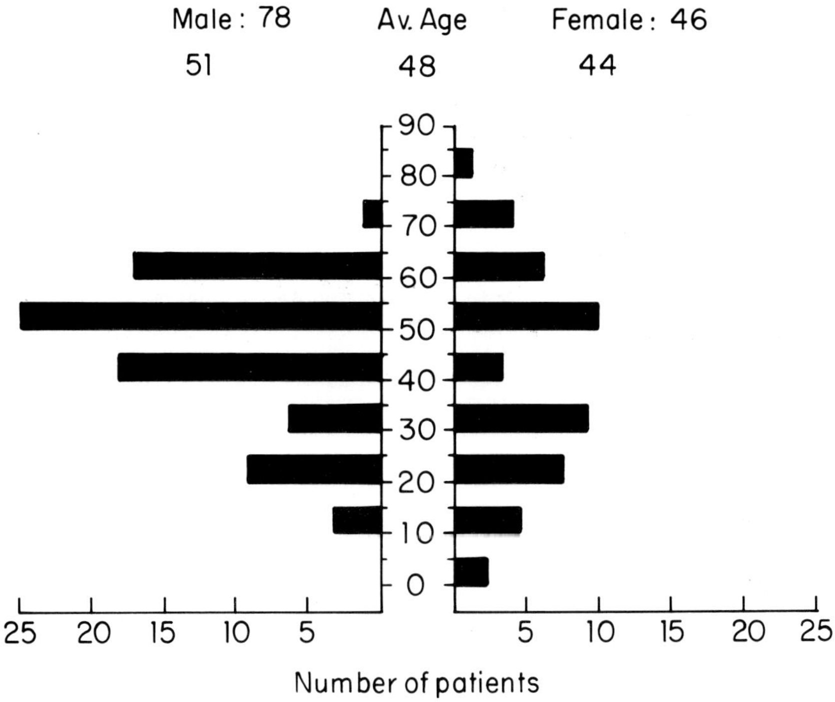

Figure 2-73. Age and sex distribution of 124 patients treated at Memorial Sloan-Kettering Cancer Center for fibroblastic and pleomorphic fibrosarcoma.

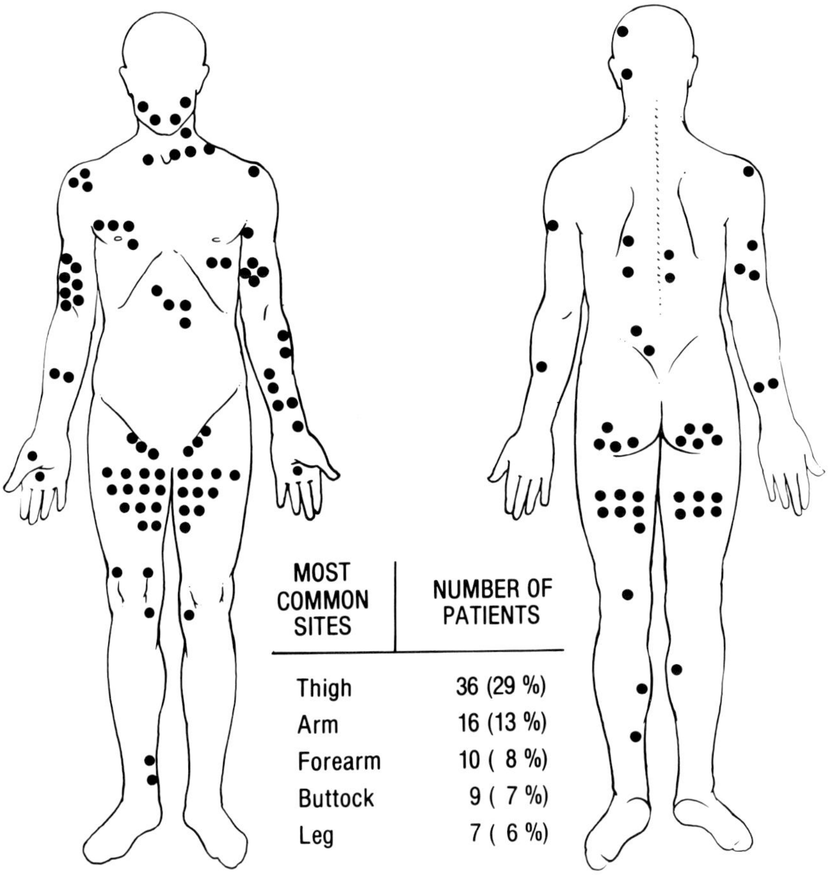

Figure 2-74. Scattergram illustrates the anatomic distribution of 124 fibrosarcomas.

1967; Pingitore and Bachechi, 1975; Chung and Enzinger, 1976; Soule and Pritchard, 1977) emphasized the gross and microscopic similarity of congenital and infantile fibrosarcomas to those in the adults (Table 2-20). These are rather large, bulky and moderately well-circumscribed neoplasms. Most of the tumors are detected at birth. There is an apparent predilection for males, and the commonest sites are the extremities. Most of the tumors are deeply embedded in skeletal muscle with infiltrating edges extending into surrounding fascia and other soft parts.

TABLE 2-19. ***The Most Common Anatomic Sites of Fibroblastic and Pleomorphic Fibrosarcomas According to Sex****

NUMBER OF PATIENTS			
MALE: 78		FEMALE: 46	
Thigh	25 (32%)	Thigh	11 (24%)
Arm	11 (14%)	Arm	5 (11%)
Forearm	8 (10%)	Head	4 (9%)
Back	6 (8%)	Neck	4 (9%)
Buttock	6 (8%)	Chest	4 (9%)

*Hajdu, unpublished study.

Microscopically congenital fibrosarcomas are comprised of spindly fibroblasts (fibroblastic fibrosarcoma) arranged in sinuous intertwining fascicles. They are generally cellular with conspicuous collagenous fibers which can be demonstrated with trichrome stain. They closely resemble adult fibroblastic fibrosarcoma. Mitotic figures are common, but their number varies from area to area in the same tumor. Most observers agree that even tumors with frequent mitoses have much better prognoses than similar lesions in adults (Fig. 2-75).

TABLE 2-20. ***Congenital Fibrosarcoma***

	PATIENTS			AVG. AGE AT DIAGNOSIS	MOST COMMON SITES	RECURRENCE	DIED WITH DISEASE
	TOTAL	MALE	FEMALE				
Stout (1962)	2	2	—	Birth	Lower extremities	2	1
Balsaver et al. (1967)	5	3	2	Birth	Upper extremities	2	0
Pingitore and Bachechi (1975)	25	18	7	2 mo.	Extremities Head & Neck	11	5
Chung and Enzinger (1976)	34	22	12	1 mo.	Extremities	—	3
Soule and Pritchard (1977)	12	3	9	2 wk.	Lower extremities	4	1

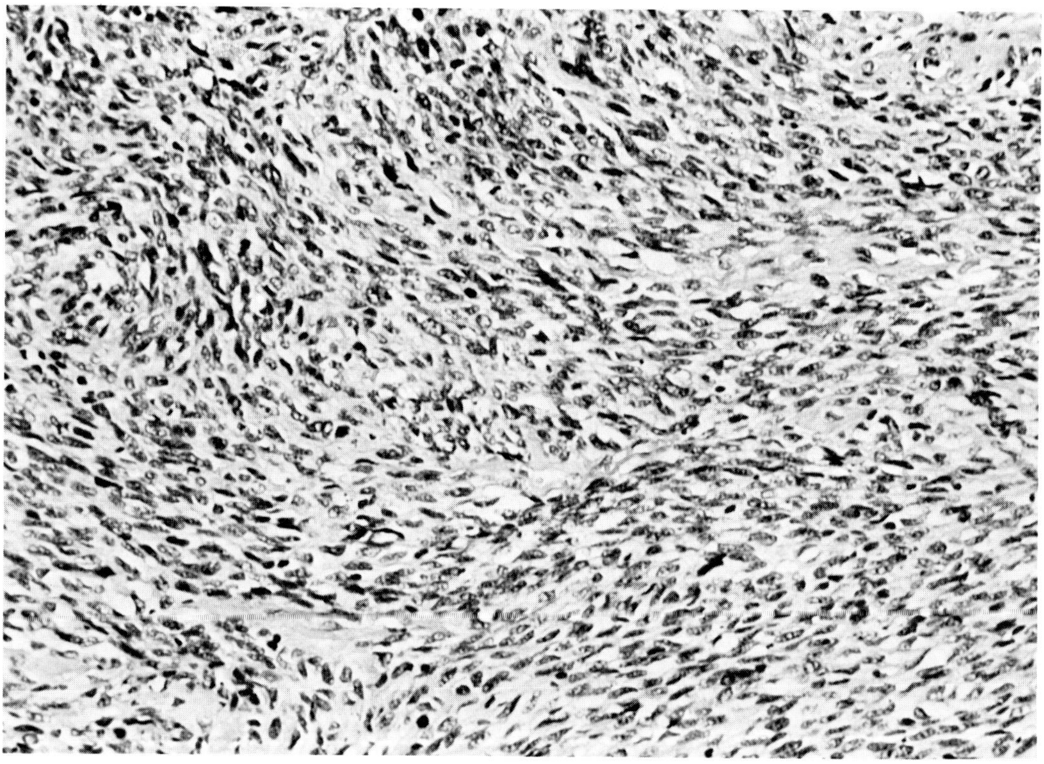

Figure 2-75. Congenital fibrosarcoma excised by wide excision from the thigh of a young baby. The tumor is composed of partly collagenous fairly uniform fibroblasts arranged in a fairly well-constructed herringbone pattern. There are numerous mitotic figures and no evidence of inflammatory or other reactive cells (H & E, ×140). (See also Figure 2-78.)

There is general agreement in the literature that the prognosis for congenital or infantile fibrosarcomas is much more favorable than that for the adult type of fibrosarcoma. It is believed that most of the congenital and infantile fibrosarcomas should be treated initially by excision of the lesion without sacrificing significant function of the part involved.

Grossly, fully malignant fibrosarcomas are not too different from low-grade desmoid type of fibrosarcomas. They are usually rubbery and firm movable tumors and may reach considerable size. Most patients give a history of long duration and show enlargement of a painless nodule. Most of these neoplasms appear to be encapsulated and have rounded or lobulated edges. They may be fungating with eroded or ulcerated skin (Fig. 2-76).

The cut surface is usually grayish-pink, hard, or soft and friable, depending on the amount of collagenous tissue which they contain. Anastomosing branches of dense collagen and trabeculae of more delicate fibrous tissue are easily identifiable with the naked eye on the bulging cut surface. Myxomatous or cystic areas may be seen in the so-called fibromyxosarcomas (Fig. 2-77).

In recent years the term *fibrous histiocytoma* has overshadowed the term *fibrosarcoma.* One perhaps is justified in asking whether there is any distinguishing histopathologic feature by which a fibrosarcoma may be recognized. Fibrosarcomas are tumors composed of collagen-forming neoplastic fibroblasts and fibrocytes. The fibroblasts are almost invariably spindle-shaped with elongated pointed nuclei. The collagen fibers are thin and slender (reticulin or collagen type III fibers which

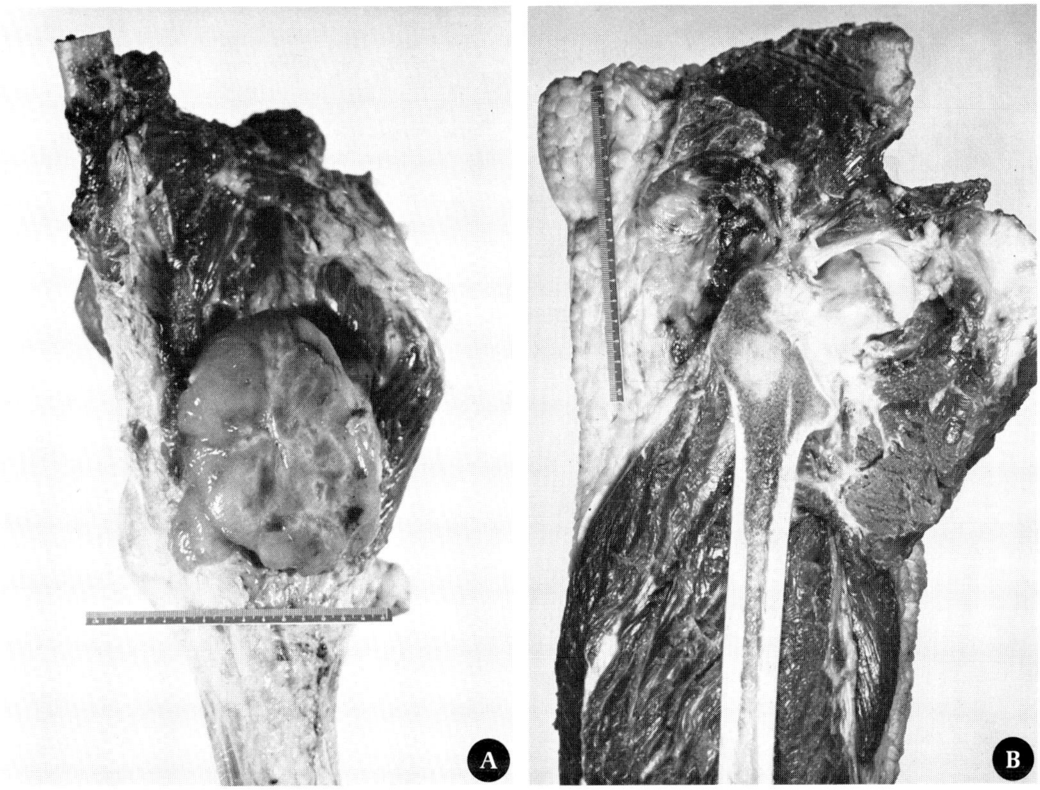

Figure 2-76. A, Fibroblastic fibrosarcoma of the popliteal space. There was gross as well as microscopic evidence of erosion of the tibia. The patient died with metastatic disease in less than 3 years.

B, Recurrent pleomorphic fibrosarcoma of the thigh with extension into the proximal femur.

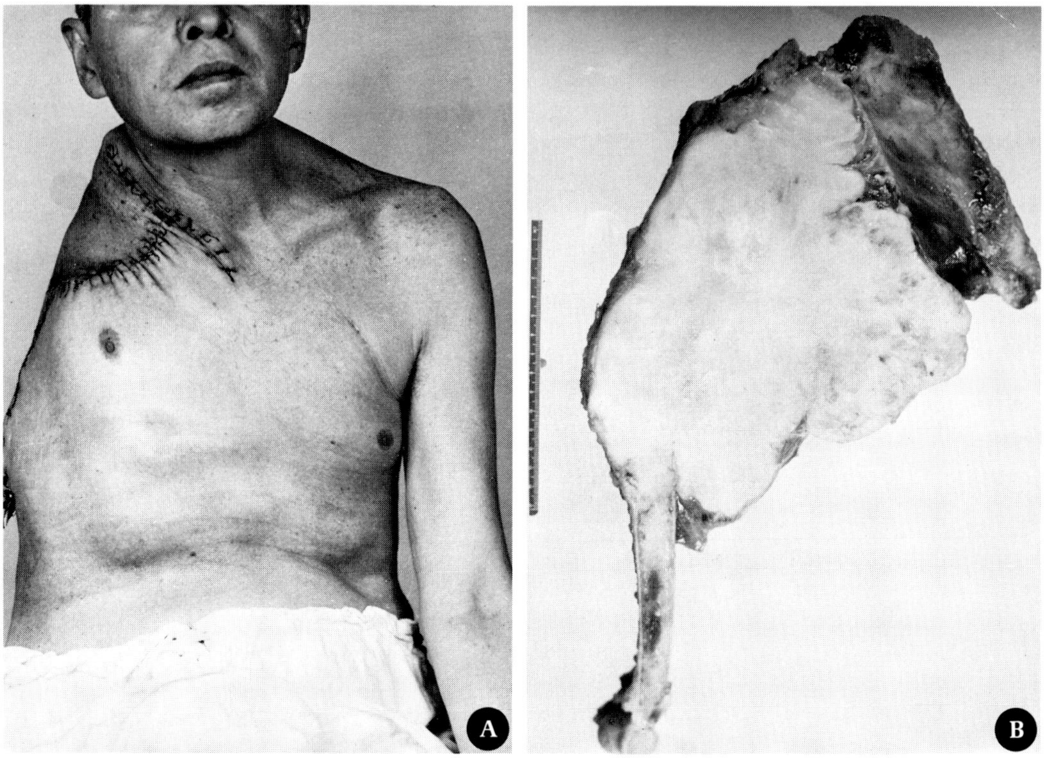

Figure 2-77. This patient had nothing more in treatment than excision for more than 3 years. He died with metastatic fibrosarcoma a year after interscapulothoracic amputation was performed.

stain black with reticulin stain) or thick and broad (collagen type I fibers which stain blue with trichrome stain) and are wrapped around the cells and infiltrate the surrounding tissues to a much greater extent than can be appreciated at gross examination (Fig. 2-78, color). Turren and Seeling, in 1933, believed that the variety and appearance of the collagen fibers that will be formed in a given tumor are influenced by local tissue conditions and site in the body. To this it must be added that age, sex, and perhaps a host of other factors may determine whether a neoplasm becomes collagenous fibroblastic (fibrosarcoma) or will remain more primitive non-collagenous fibrous histiocytic (fibrous histiocytoma).

In fibroblastic fibrosarcoma and to a certain extent also in pleomorphic fibrosarcoma the fibroblasts and their fibers are arranged in interlaced bands (Figs. 2-79, 2-80). The pattern of growth may vary, however, and some of the tumors may show bands of parallel fibers only.

Pleomorphic fibrosarcomas may contain, in addition to the usual fibroblastic neoplastic elements, bizarre mononuclear or multinuclear giant cells. In general in these tumors, the tumor cells may show considerable variation in size and the amount of collagen may also vary from area to area (Figs. 2-81, 2-82).

Histopathologically, the degree of malignancy is determined by the cellularity, pleomorphism, number of mitotic figures, and the quantity of collagenous fibers. In fibrous tumors of low-grade malignancy, desmoid tumors, the fibroblasts show a moderate degree of variation in size and shape, and there is a large amount of dense collagen (see Desmoid Tumors).

As the tumors ascend in the scale of malignancy, the tumors become more cellular and less collagenous (fibroblastic fibrosarcoma) and the tumor cells show considerable variation in size and shape (pleomorphic fibrosarcoma) (Fig. 2-83; Table 2-17). Most of the time the three distinct (desmoid, fibroblastic, and pleomorphic) histopathologic forms can be easily distinguished, but occasionally all gradations are found among various forms. Occasionally, in a uniformly low grade malignant tumor a very malignant focus can be seen. Without additional evidence, it seems that upgrading the tumor is not justified (see Fig. 1-59 and Table 1-15).

Whether the so-called myxosarcoma is a variant of fibrosarcoma or liposarcoma is uncertain (see Chapter 4, Lesions of Adipose Tissue and Myxoma, this chapter). As Mallory stated in 1908, "There seems to be little reason for putting the myxoma and myxosarcoma in a class by themselves." Despite the fact that many soft tissue tumors show areas of loose structure composed of stellate and spindle cells in a mucinous background, a number of publications attest to the existence of believers in myxomas and myxosarcomas as distinct entities (Dixon and Vadheim, 1944; Dutz and Stout, 1961; Leak et al, 1967).

Although I question the existence of pure myxoma and myxosarcoma, gelatinous or edematous areas as the result of vascular occlusion, stasis, or degeneration may produce myxomatous changes in fibrosarcomas and fibrous histiocytomas which perhaps deserve separate classification as *myxofibrosarcoma* or *myxoid fibrous histiocytoma*. If it is understood that these are variants of malignant fibrous tumors owing their appearance to an increased amount of intercellular myxoid substance and that they should be treated as neoplasms according to histologic grade of the cellular elements, separate classification will indeed become unnecessary.

Necrosis, calcification, or ossification, first described in a fibrosarcoma by Butlin in 1873, are uncommon in fibroblastic and pleomorphic fibrosarcomas. The edges of fibrosarcomas are usually more cellular than other parts of the tumor. The mixture of crowded tumor cells and inflammatory cells representing the advancing edge of the tumor may give the impression of a capsule or pseudocapsule at gross examination (Fig. 2-76A). It is important to recognize this illusion to prevent unwarranted conservatism in the management of these neoplasms.

Fibroblastic and pleomorphic fibrosarcomas are fully malignant neoplasms irrespective of the number of mitotic figures. However, the relative malignancy can be approximately estimated by the number of cells in mitosis. In general, the number of mitotic figures decreases in inverse proportion to the number of collagenous fibers.

Fibrosarcomas must be excised with clean surgical margins when they are first encountered. Amputation should be the treatment of choice if there is any possibility that excision or muscle group resection will fail.

Following excision, these tumors frequently recur (Table 2-21). Our experience with fibroblastic and pleomorphic fibrosarcomas shows that 46% recurred, some second or third times, after excision and 64% metastasized. Regional lymph node involvement is rare. In Broder's series of 152 patients, in 1939, only 5 had positive lymph nodes. In our series of patients, histologically positive regional lymph nodes were found in 6 patients (Fig. 2-84).

Postmortem findings in 27 patients revealed that fibrosarcomas metastasize most commonly in the lungs, bones, and liver (Fig. 2-85). Death from fibrosarcoma usually occurs during the first 5 years after the diagnosis, but late dissemination is not uncommon (Fig. 2-84). Death and metastatic rates from tumors of the lower extremities and deeper structures such as the retroperitoneum are higher than for other areas.

The cytomorphology of neoplastic fibroblasts in smear preparations is influenced by the type of specimen and the

Figure 2-78. A, Desmoid tumor (low grade fibrosarcoma).

This tumor is composed of monomorphic oval or plump spindle fibroblasts and fibrocytes with heavy collagenous cytoplasmic processes. The tumor cells are fused together and the cell boundaries blend into the collagenous stroma. The nuclei are vesicular, range in shape from round to oval, and contain small dark nucleoli.

There is a monotonous tranquility in appearance of this tumor and the tumor cells have a one-directional spread. The blood vessel at the upper left corner is infiltrated and compressed by the tumor cells; ultimately it will be completely obliterated (H & E, ×140).

B, Desmoid tumor metastatic to the lung. The primary lesion of this case is illustrated in **A.** Collagenous fibroblasts and fibrocytes infiltrate the lung parenchyma. The tumor cells possess heavy collagenous cytoplasmic processes and slender pyknotic nuclei. The lung parenchyma is almost completely replaced by the tumor; however, remnants of a partly destroyed bronchus are visible in the lower left corner, and there is a collection of pulmonary histiocytes in the lumen of compressed alveoli. (H & E, ×35).

C, Fibrosarcoma. The tumor cells are arranged in the classic herringbone pattern. The tumor cells are fibroblasts and fibrocytes with reticular and partly collagenous cytoplasm.

It is of interest that despite the fact that most of the cells are positioned opposite each other or are running tangentially the appearance of this tumor is orderly and uninterrupted.

Notice the sparse vascularity and absence of necrosis. This pattern should be recognized and considered as that of a high-grade neoplasm (H & E, ×140).

D, Pleomorphic fibrosarcoma. This is a fully malignant and high-grade neoplasm. The tumor cells vary in size and shape and contain considerable amounts of collagen. The cell borders of the elongated fibroblasts and fibrocytes blend with deposited stromal collagen and form a solid indivisible stroma which stains strongly positive with trichrome stain. Note fibrillar and wavy appearance of the collagen fibers; also notice areas of pseudocross-striation which is due to cross-links between heavy collagen fibers.

Multinucleated and odd-shaped tumor giant cells are seen at the lower edge of the tumor (H & E, ×350).

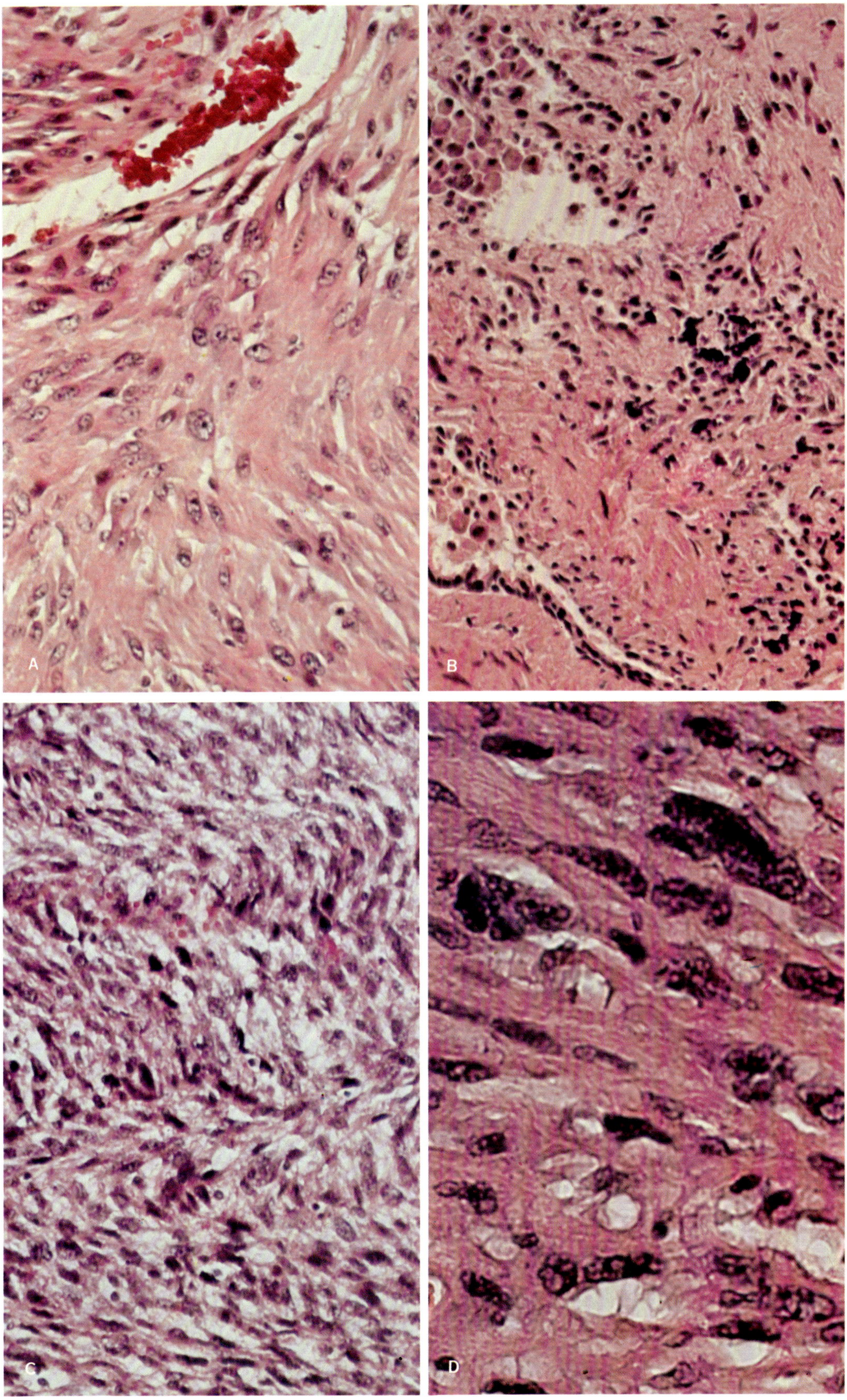

Figure 2-78.

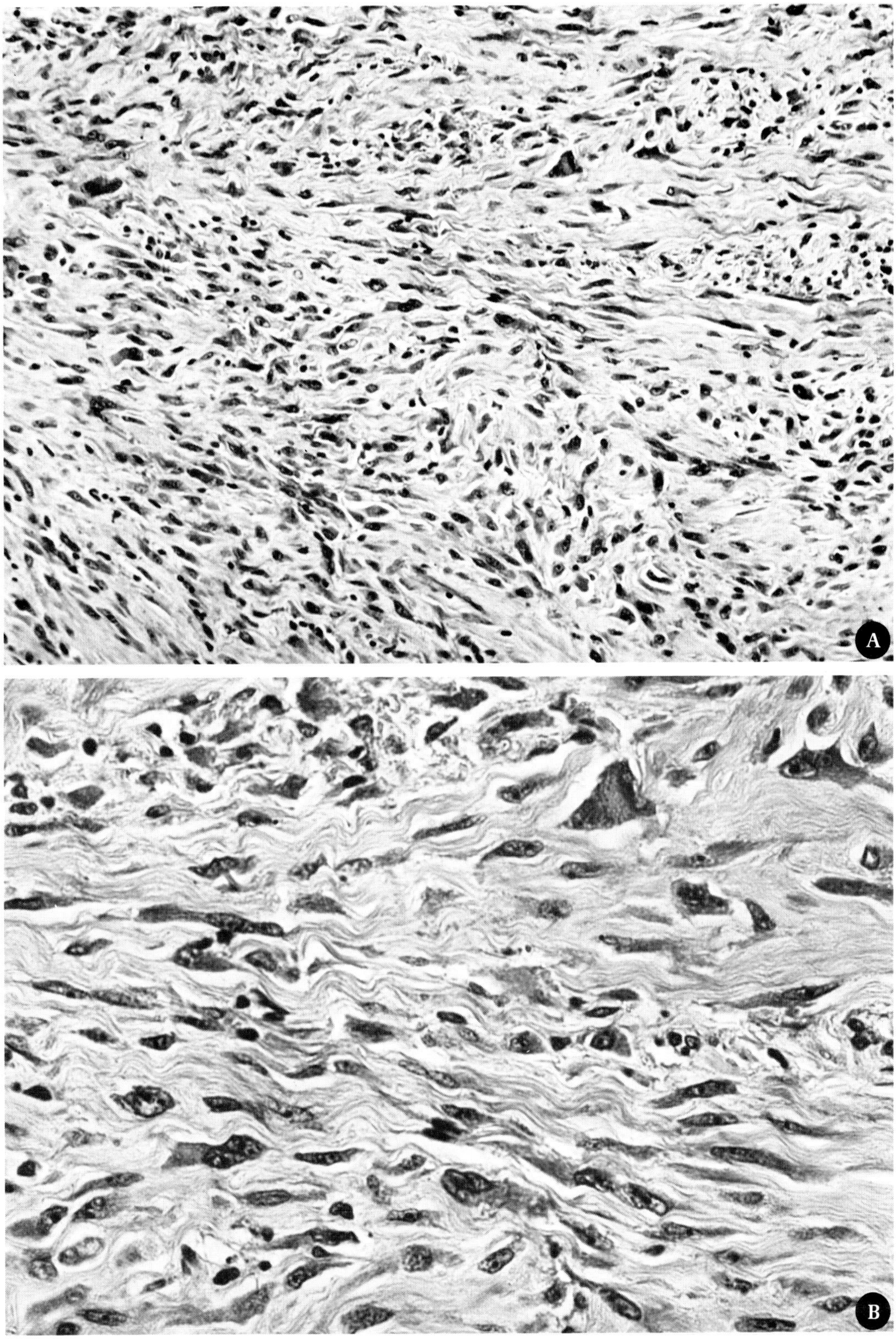

Figure 2-79. Fibroblastic fibrosarcoma is composed of collagenous fibroblasts. The tumor cells are joined in broad collagenous bundles by their cytoplasmic process. Occasional mitotic figures and a few enlarged tumor cells are apparent (**A,** H & E, ×140; **B,** H & E, ×350). (See also Figure 2-78.)

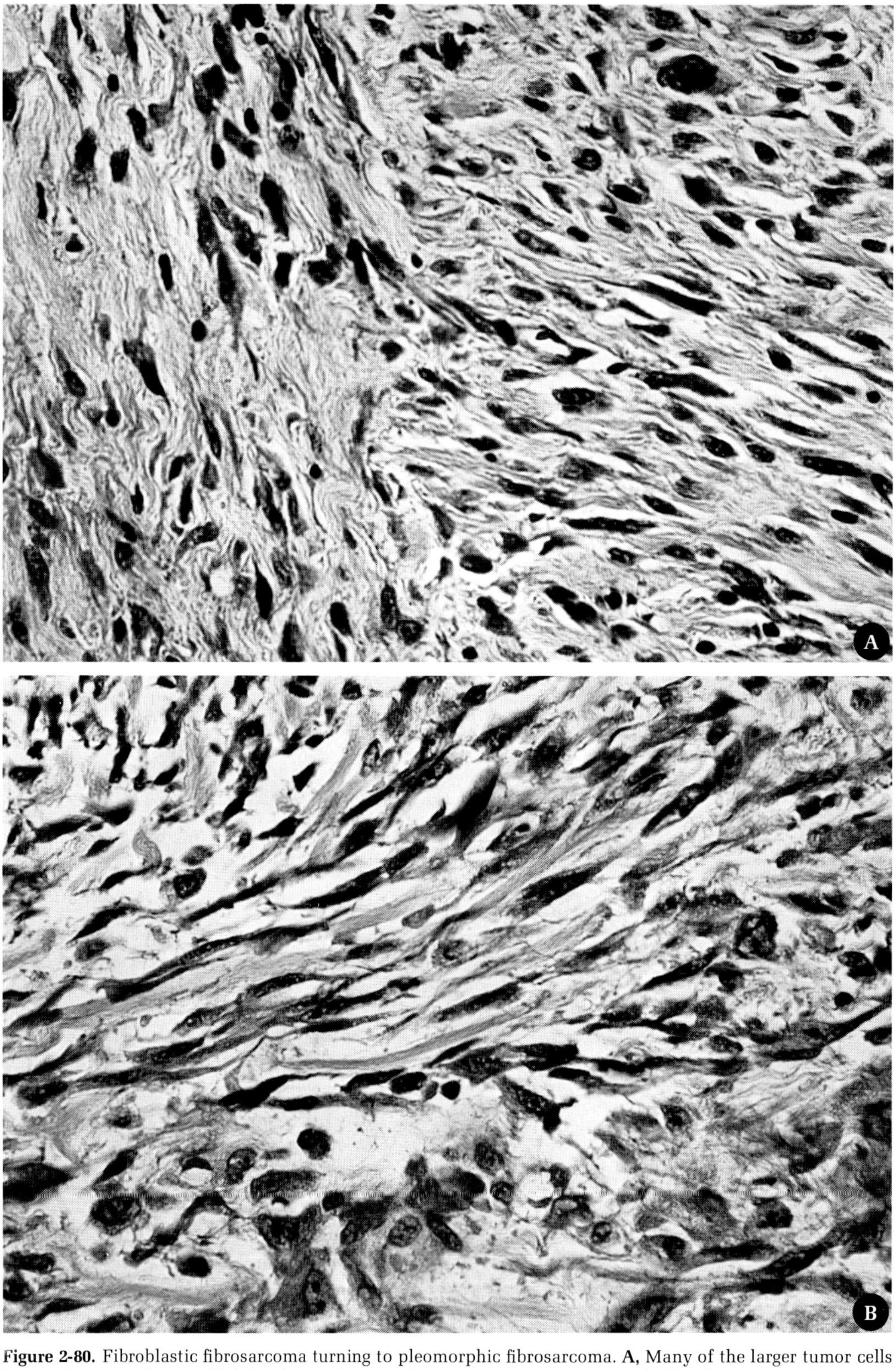

Figure 2-80. Fibroblastic fibrosarcoma turning to pleomorphic fibrosarcoma. **A,** Many of the larger tumor cells have pyknotic nuclei and ill-defined granular cytoplasm. **B,** Note the peculiar snakelike elongated nuclei and the fibrillar collagenous cords between the tumor cells (H & E, ×350).

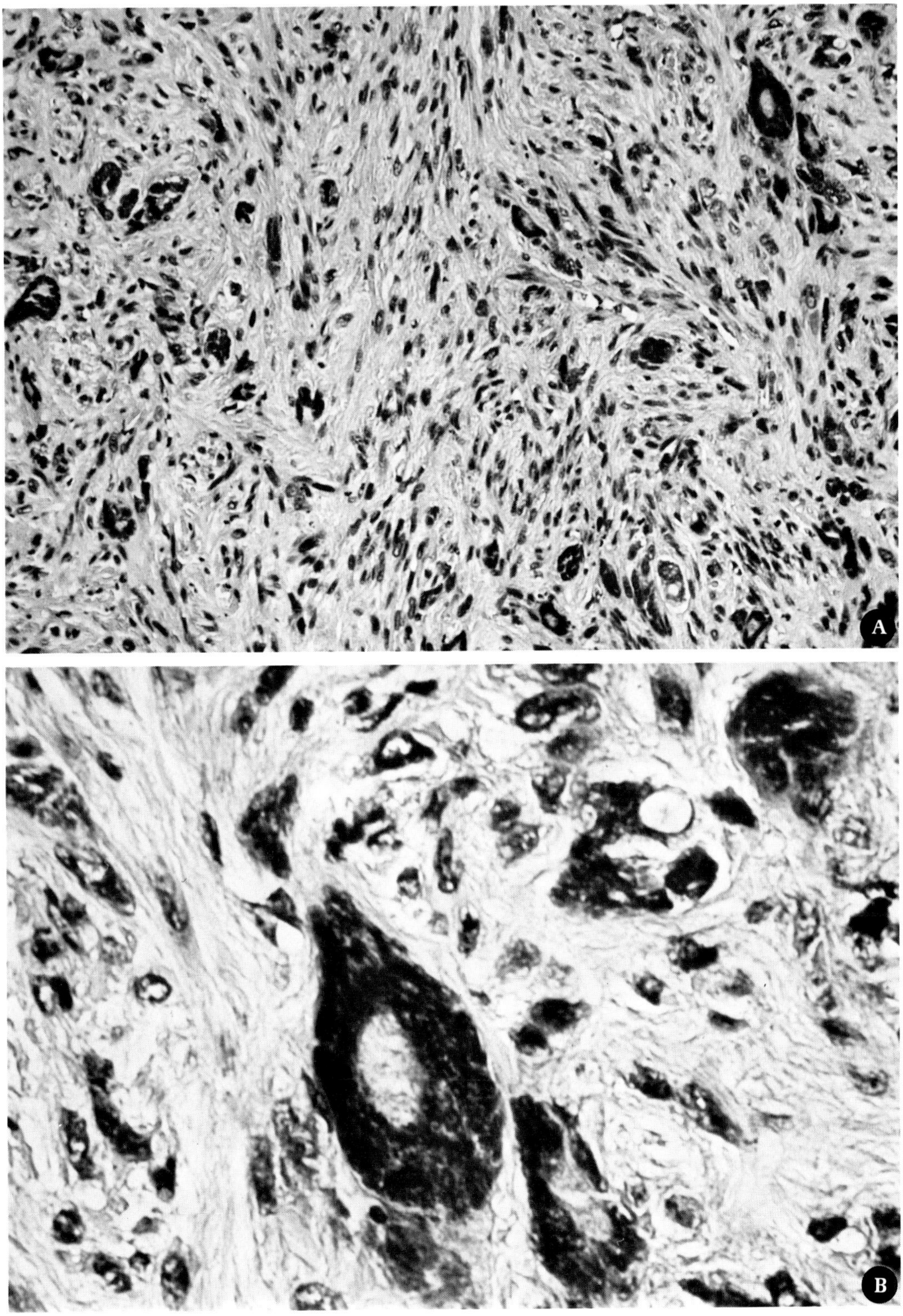

Figure 2-81. Pleomorphic fibrosarcoma. The pleomorphism of this tumor is due mainly to the bizarre multinucleated neoplastic fibroblasts. **A,** Note the sparsely cellular and haphazardly arranged mononuclear fibroblasts between the giant cells.

B, The giant cells have pyknotic fused nuclei, and the shape and size of these bizarre forms may show striking variations (**A,** H & E, ×140; **B,** H & E, ×350).

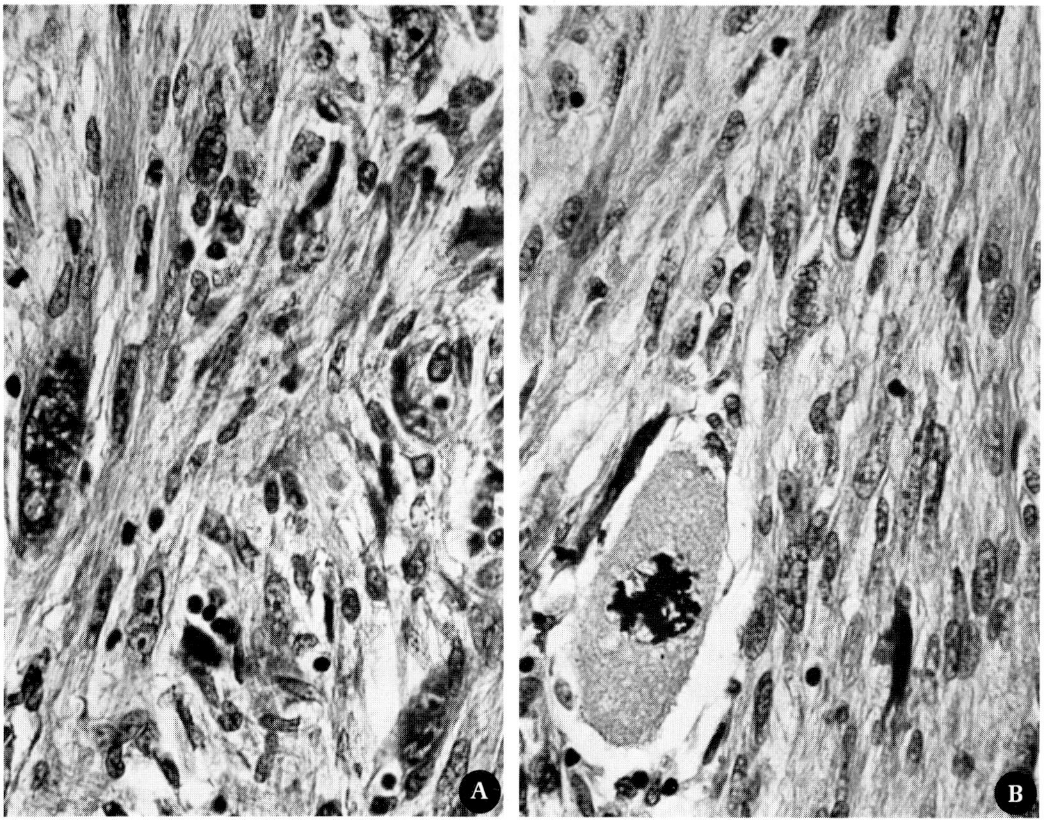

Figure 2-82. Pleomorphic fibrosarcoma showing combination of mononuclear collagenous fibroblasts and granular cytoplasmic tumor giant cells (H & E, ×350).

cytologic technique. The morphology of tumors is also influenced by local tissue factors. Like most other sarcomas, fibrosarcomas are less differentiated in tissue cultures and in heterotransplants than in patients (Figs. 2-86, 2-87, 2-88).

Differential Diagnosis

In differential diagnosis the following should be considered: various forms of *fibromatosis* may be difficult to distinguish histologically from low-grade fibrosarcoma of the desmoid type or fibrosarcoma of children. However, fully malignant fibrosarcomas are distinctly different from fibromatosis by virtue of their uniformly aggressive look histologically and by their pseudoencapsulated bulky nature.

Fibroblastic fibrous histiocytoma (desmatofibrosarcoma protuberans) and *pleomorphic fibrous histiocytoma* are non-collagenous malignant neoplasms. The tumor cells are slender fibroblasts and foamy mono- or multinucleated histiocytic forms. Identification of these elements in arranged, storiform pattern make the differentiation relatively easy.

Schwannoma, benign or malignant, is composed of much more delicate and slender neoplastic cells than fibrosarcoma. The presence of palisading long fibrillar cells should be considered characteristic for neurogenic tumors (see Chapter 7).

Leiomyosarcoma is distinguished by non-collagenous cytoplasmic processes and plump non-pointed nuclei. There are almost always a few ill-defined areas which stain positive with trichrome stain, but most parts of the tumor show features of muscle origin (Chapter 5).

Pleomorphic rhabdomyosarcoma is

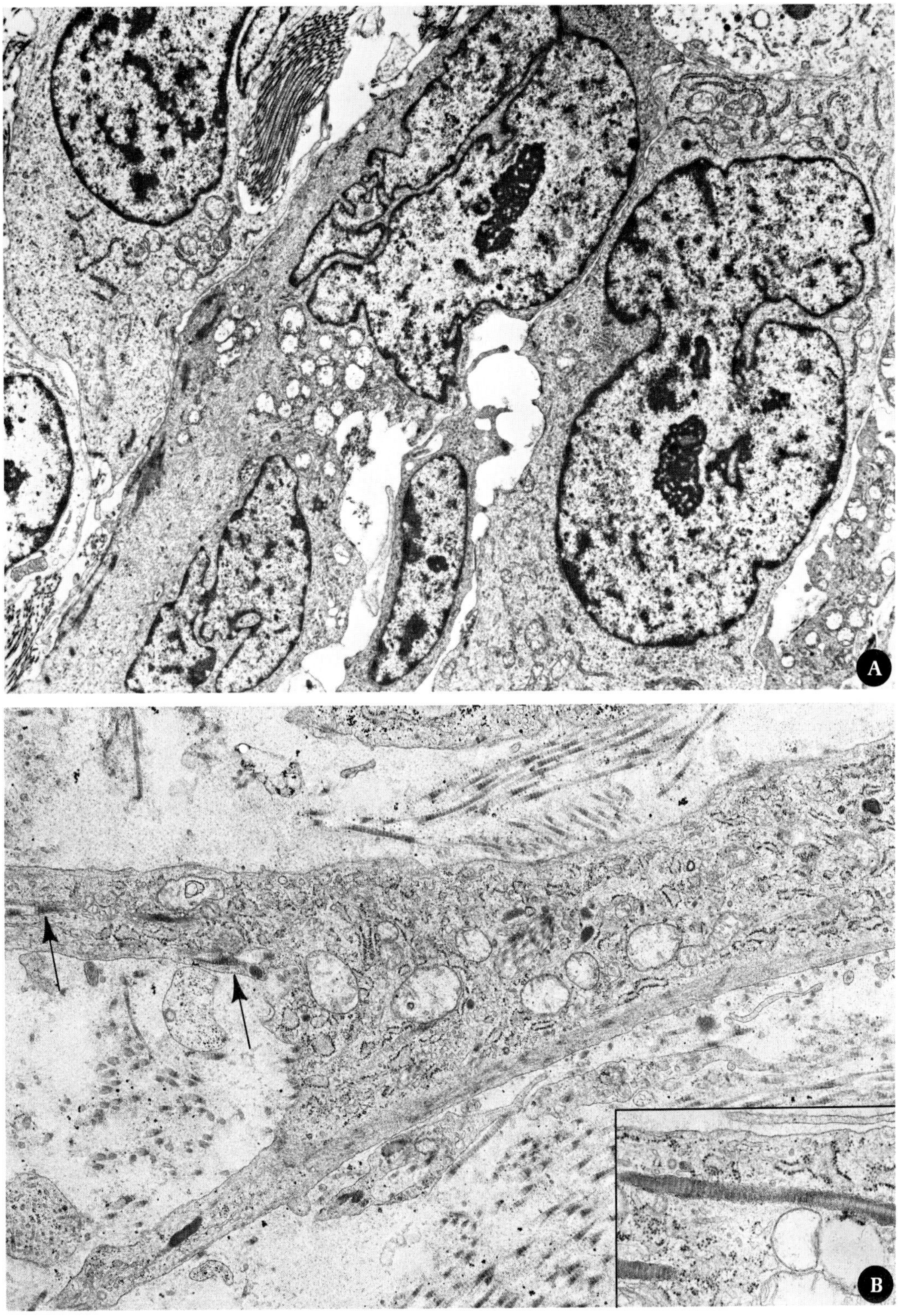

Figure 2-83. A, Pleomorphic fibrosarcoma possess no specific ultrastructural features beyond pleomorphism of the tumor cells and collagenous deposits in the stroma (×5,500).

B, Myofibroblast in a fibrosarcoma showing myofilament bundles in the peripheral part of the cytoplasm (arrows). The intercellular space contains numerous collagen fibers (×13,000).

Inset, High power view of an intracytoplasmic myofilament showing characteristic 46 nm periodicity (×26,000) (Courtesy Churg, A. M., and Kahn, L. B.: Myofibroblasts and related cells in malignant fibrous and fibrohistiocytic tumors. Hum. Pathol. 8:205, 1977).

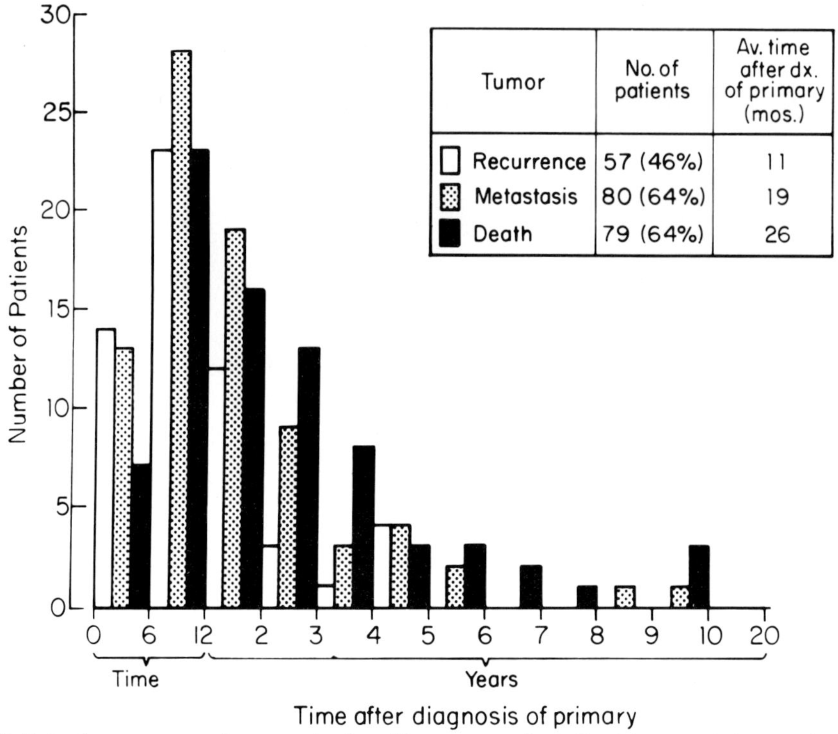

Tumor	No. of patients	Av. time after dx. of primary (mos.)
Recurrence	57 (46%)	11
Metastasis	80 (64%)	19
Death	79 (64%)	26

Figure 2-84. Rate of recurrence and metastasis of 124 fibrosarcomas both fibroblastic and pleomorphic. Note the mortality of 64% (see Figure 2-69).

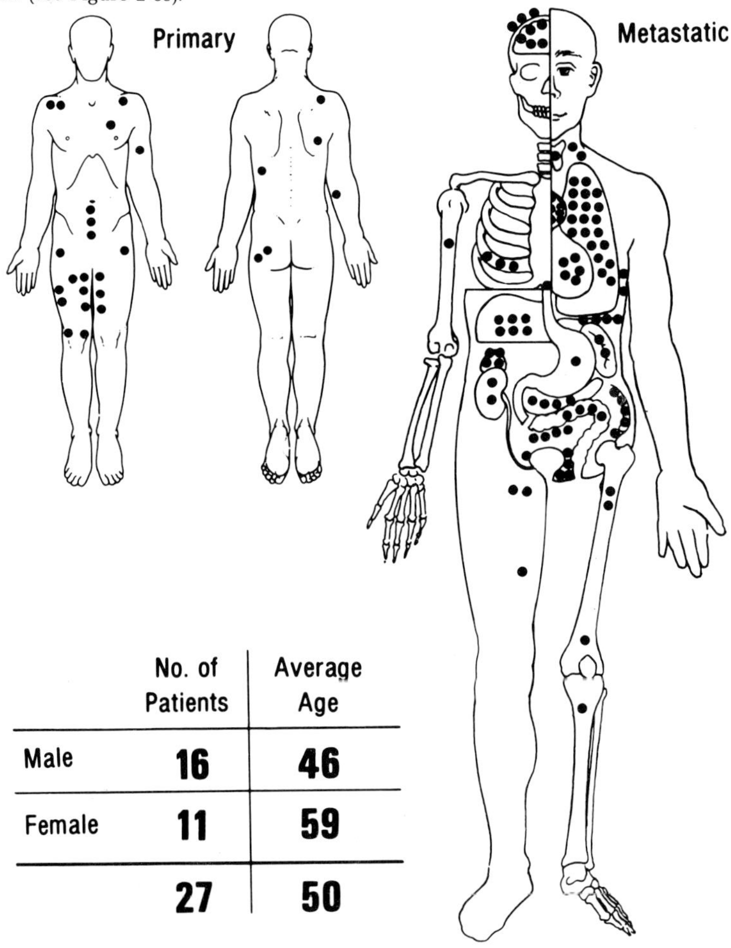

	No. of Patients	Average Age
Male	16	46
Female	11	59
	27	50

Figure 2-85. Anatomic distribution of metastatic sites of fibrosarcomas as seen at autopsy of 27 patients. Metastasis to parenchymal organs such as lung and liver are common, but it is of interest that five of the tumors metastasized to the brain, heart, and also to the iliac bone (see Appendix).

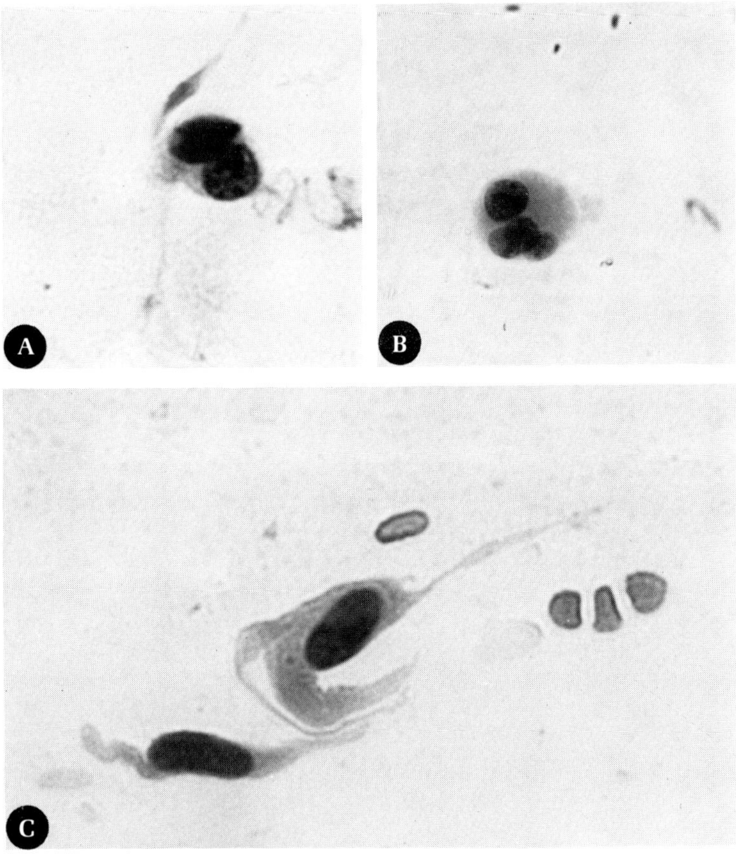

Figure 2-86. A & B, Tumor cells of metastatic fibrosarcoma in pleural effusion. In body cavity fluids tumor cells of spindle cell tumors commonly appear as oval or round cells (Pap stain, ×450).

C, Aspiration smear of fibrosarcoma. The elongated fibrillar cytoplasm is well preserved, but no nuclear detail can be seen in the poorly preserved nuclei (H & E, ×450).

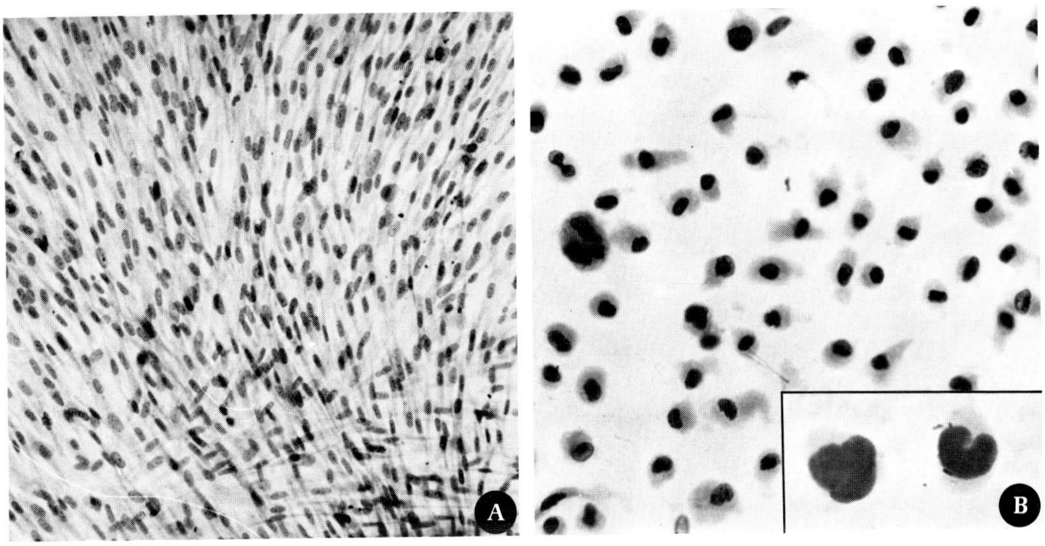

Figure 2-87. Tissue culture of human fibrosarcoma.

A, Monolayer culture shows a nonspecific growth pattern of neoplastic fibroblasts (Pap stain, ×140).

B, Smear of neoplastic fibroblasts prepared from trypsinized monolayer culture illustrated in **A.** Here the fibroblasts appear neoplastic. Note the numerous lobulated nuclei and the multinucleated forms (Pap stain, ×250; inset, ×450). (For technique see Hajdu et al: Acta Cytol. 18:327, 1974.)

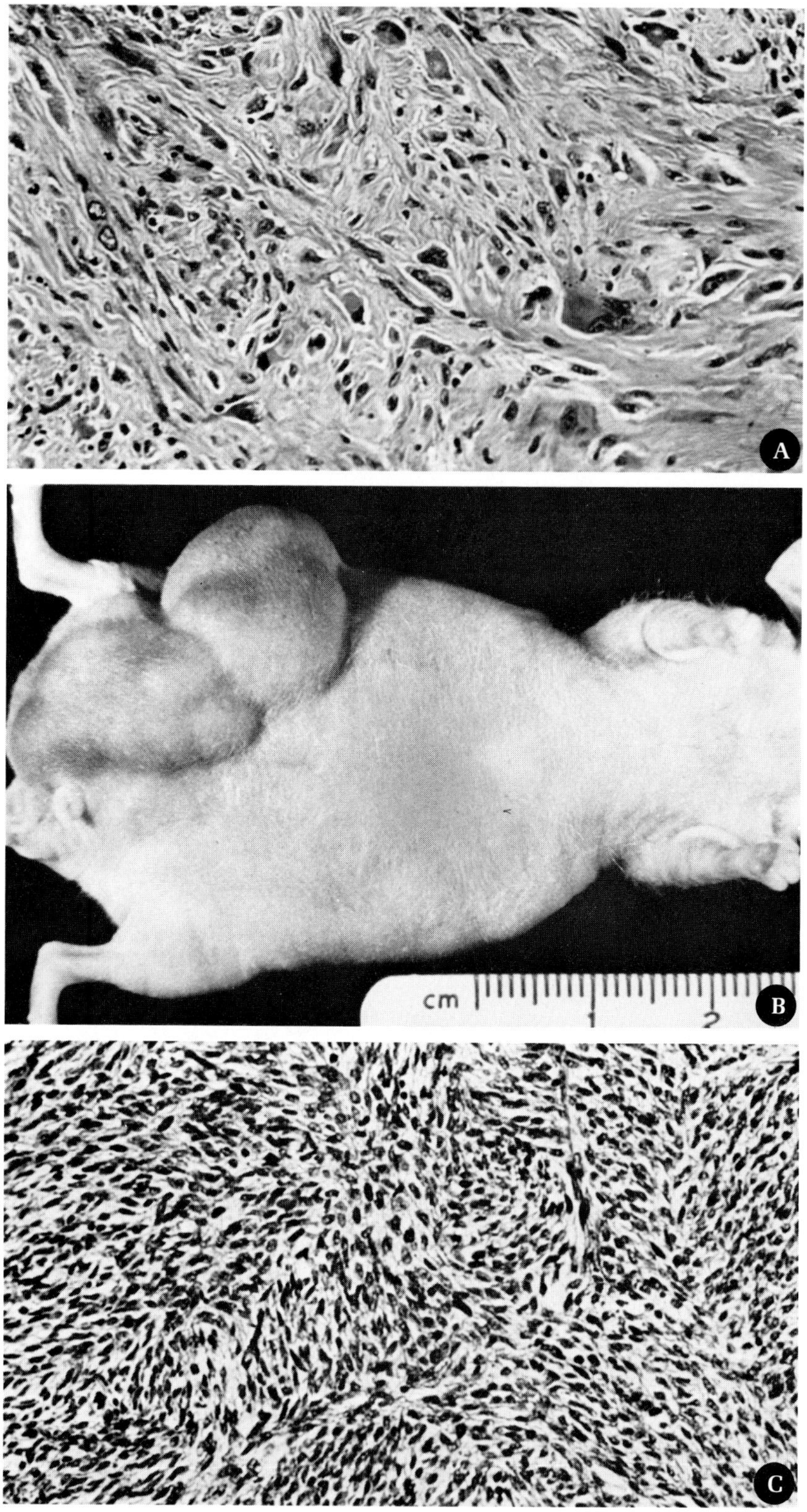

Figure 2-88. A, Fully malignant pleomorphic fibrosarcoma excised from the patient. Cell suspension of this tumor was injected into an athymic nude mouse (H & E, ×140).

B, Two tumor nodules at the site of subcutaneous injection grow to the size illustrated in four weeks.

C, Histologic appearance of the subcutaneous tumor excised from the nude mouse. Note the loss of pleomorphism, as well as the collagen of the primary tumor (see **A**). Also, note growth of the tumor, in the animal, as poorly differentiated reticular fibroblastic neoplasm closely resembling in cellularity and pattern of growth a fibroblastic fibrous histiocytoma (H & E, ×140) (See Figure 2-26). (See Hajdu et al 1979.)

TABLE 2-21. ***Reported Series of Fibrosarcomas***

		NO. OF CASES	RECURRENCE %	SURVIVAL %
Warren and Sommer	1936	118	40	30
Meyerding et al	1936	132	—	21
Wilson	1945	111	—	30
Stout	1948	145	60	45
Ivins et al	1950	63	—	36
Mackenzie*	1964	134	—	54*
Werf-Messing and Unnik	1965	139	56	—
Castro et al*	1973	75	28	70*
Pritchard et al*	1974	199	42	41*
Hajdu	(unpublished)	124	46	36

*5-year survival.
See Chapter 1 (Fig. 1-59; Table 1-15) for reference to grade and stage.

composed of large polymorphous tumor giant cells having bizarre-shaped nuclei and granular, violaceous cytoplasm. Careful and prolonged search may be necessary to identify longitudinal or cross-striated cytoplasmic processes. Admittedly, it is difficult at times to distinguish pleomorphic rhabdomyosarcoma and fibrosarcoma (Chapter 5).

Liposarcoma, either fibroblastic or pleomorphic, should be suspected when there are numerous vacuolated tumor cells with eccentrically displaced, bizarre nuclei. Liposarcomas are usually more loosely textured and less collagenous than fibrosarcomas (Chapter 4).

Desmoplastic or metaplastic changes, mimicking the appearance of fibroblastic fibrosarcoma, may occur in *malignant epithelial tumors* and in *malignant melanoma*. In most cases, diligent search for specific structures with special stains and the electron microscope should prove to be rewarding.

REFERENCES

References are listed in chronological order in each category.

INTRODUCTION

Rokitansky, C.: Handbuch der pathologischen Anatomie. Wien, Braumuller u. Seider, 1842–46.

Malhéné, A.: Etude clinique sur la Tumeurs Fibro-Plastiques. Paris, A. Parent, 1866.

Cohnheim, J.: Ueber Entzundung und Eitenung. Virchows Arch. Pathol. Anat. 40:1, 1867.

Mall, F.: Das reticulierte Gewebe und seine Beziehungen zu den Bindegewebsfibrillen. Abh. d. math-phys. cl. d. Konigl. Wiss. 17:299, 1891.

Mallory, F. B.: The results of the application of special histological methods to the study of tumors. J. Exp. Med. 10:575, 1908.

Maximow, A.: Relation of blood cells to connective tissues and endothelium. Physiol. Rev. 4:533, 1924.

Fischer, A.: Sur la transformation in vitro des gros leukocytes mononucleaires en fibroblastes. C. R. Soc. Biol. 92:109, 1925.

Carrel, A., and Ebeling, A. H.: Fundamental properties of fibroblast and macrophage. J. Exp. Med. 44:261, 1926.

Fischer, A.: Umwandlung von Fibroblasten zu Makrophagen in vitro. Arch. Exp. Zellforsch. 3:345, 1926–27.

Mallory, F. B., and Parker, F.: Reticulum. Am. J. Pathol. 3:515, 1927.

Weidman, F. D., and Boston, L. N.: Generalized xanthoma tuberosum with xanthomatous changes in fresh scars of intercurrent zoster. Arch. Intern. Med. 59:793, 1937.

Stout, A. P.: Myxoma—the tumor of primitive mesenchyme. Ann. Surg. 127:706, 1948.

Pack, G. T., and Ariel, I. M.: Fibrosarcoma of the soft somatic tissue. Surgery 31:443, 1952.

Stout, A. P.: Tumors of the Soft Tissues. Washington, D.C., Armed Forces Institute of Pathology, 1953.

Luse, S. A.: Electron microscopic studies of brain tumors. Neurology 10:881, 1960.

Pappas, G. D.: *In* Glaucoma. Edited by

A. Newell. New York, J. Macy Foundation, 1960, p. 54.
Holmstrand, K., Lougaire, J. J., and De Stefano, G. A.: The ultrastructure of collagen in skin, scars and keloids. Plast. Reconstr. Surg. 27:597, 1961.
Petrakis, N., Davis, M., and Lucia, S. P.: The *in vivo* differentiation of human leukocytes into histiocytes, fibroblasts and fat cells in subcutaneous diffusion chambers. Blood 17:109, 1961.
Chapman, J. A.: Fibroblasts and collagen. Br. Med. Bull. 18:233, 1962.
Delaunay, A., and Bazin, S.: Mucopolysaccharides, collagen and nonfibrillar proteins in inflammation. Int. Rev. Connect. Tissue Res. 2:301, 1964.
Green, H., and Hamerman, D.: Production of hyaluronate and collagen by fibroblast clones in tissue culture. Nature 20:710, 1964.
Ross, R., and Greenlee, T. K.: Electron microscopy: attachment sites between connective tissue cells. Science 153:997, 1966.
Stout, A. P., and Lattes, R.: Tumors of the soft tissues. *In* Atlas of Tumor Pathology, 2nd series. Washington, D.C., Armed Forces Institute of Pathology, 1967.
Elsdaler, T. R.: Parallel orientation of fibroblasts *in vitro*. Exp. Cell Res. 51:439, 1968.
Kaye, G. I., Lane, N., and Pascal, R. R.: The colonic pericryptal fibroblast sheath—Replication, migration and cytodifferentiation of a mesenchymal cell system in adult tissue. Gastroenterology 54:852, 1968.
Kaye, G. I., Siegel, L. F., and Pascal, R. R.: Cell replication of mesenchymal elements in adult tissues. Bull. N.Y. Acad. Med. 45:487, 1969.
Mackenzie, D. H.: The Differential Diagnosis of Fibroblastic Disorders. Oxford and Edinburgh, Blackwell, 1970.
Miles, C. P., and O'Neill, F.: Time-lapse studies of mitosis and sex chromatin in human fibroblasts. Acta Cytol. 14:468, 1970.
Perez-Tamayo, R.: Collagen resorption in carrageenin granulomas. II. Ultrastructure of collagen resorption. Lab. Invest. 22:142, 1970.
Ross, R., Everett, N. B., and Tyler, R.: Wound healing and collagen formation. The origin of the wound fibroblast studied in parabiosis. J. Cell Biol. 44:645, 1970.
Gabbiani, G., Ryan, G. B., and Majno, G.: Presence of modified fibroblasts in granulation tissue and their possible role in wound contraction. Experientia 27:549, 1971.
Trelstad, R. L., and Coulombre, A. J.: Morphogenesis of the collagenous stroma in the chick cornea. J. Cell Biol. 50: 840, 1971.
Wheatley, D. N.: Cilia in cell-cultured fibroblasts. J. Anat. 113:85, 1972.
Becker, C. G., and Nachmann, R. L.: Contractile proteins of endothelial cells, platelets and smooth muscle. Am. J. Pathol. 71:1, 1973.
Hay, E. D., and Dodson, J. W.: Secretion of collagen by corneal epithelium. Morphology of the collagenous products produced by isolated epithelia grown on frozen killed hens. J. Cell Biol. 57:190, 1973.
Ryan, G. B., Cliff, W. J., Gabbiani, G., Irle, C., Montandon, D., Statkov, P. R., and Majno, G.: Myofibroblasts in human granulation tissue. Hum. Pathol. 5:55, 1974.
Vaheri, A., and Ruoslahti, E.: Disappearance of a major cell type specific surface glycoprotein antigen (SF) after transformation of fibroblasts by Rous sarcoma virus. Int. J. Cancer 13:579, 1974.
Weber, K., and Groeschel-Stewart, U.: Antibody to myosin: The specific visualization of myosin containing filaments in nonmuscle cells. Proc. Natl. Acad. Sci. 71:4561, 1974.
Cervos-Navarro, J., and Matakas, F.: The ultrastructure of reticulin. Acta Neuropathol. Suppl. 6:173, 1975.
Kuusela, P., Ruoslahti, E., and Vaheri, A.: Polypeptides of a glycoprotein antigen (SF) present in serum and surface of normal but not of transformed chicken fibroblasts. Biochim. Biophys. Acta 379:295, 1975.
Mackenzie, D. H.: Miscellaneous Soft Tissue Sarcomas. *In* Recent Advances in Pathology. Edited by C. V. Harrison and K. Weinbren. London, Churchill Livingston Press, 1975.
Battifora, H.: Spindle cell carcinoma. Ultrastructural evidence of squamous origin and collagen production of the tumor cells. Cancer 37:2275, 1976.
Filipe, M. I., and Mackenzie, D. H.: Histochemical characteristics of mucosubstances in three soft-tissue tumours. J Pathol. 118:17, 1976.
Im, M. J. C., Freshwater, M. F., and Hoopes, J. E.: Enzyme activities in granulation tissue: Energy for collagen synthesis. J. Surg. Res. 20:121, 1976.
Renteria, V. G., and Ferrans, V. J.: Intracellular collagen fibrils in cardiac valves of patients with the Hurler Syndrome. Lab. Invest. 34:263, 1976.
Wiener, S. L., Urivetzky, M., Isenberg, H. D., Havier, R., Wiener, R., Belenko, M., Hajdu, E., and Meilman, E.: Fibroblast DNA synthesis activation in sponge induced granulation tissue. Connect. Tissue Res. 4:223, 1976.
Belton, J. C., Crise, N., McLaughlin, R. F., and Tueller, E. E.: Ultrastructural alterations in collagen associated with microscopic foci

of human emphysema. Hum. Pathol. 8:669, 1977.
Churg, A. M., and Kahn, L. B.: Myofibroblasts and related cells in malignant fibrous and fibrohistiocytic tumors. Hum. Pathol. 8:205, 1977.
Lapiere, C. M., Nusgens, B., and Pierard, G. E.: Interaction between collagen type I and type III in conditioning bundles organization. Connect. Tissue Res. 5:21, 1977.
Russell, W. O., Cohen, J., Enzinger, F., Hajdu, S. I., Heise, H., Martin, R. G., Meissner, W., Miller, W. T., Schmitz, R. L., and Suit, H. D.: A clinical and pathological staging system for soft tissue sarcomas. Cancer 40:1562, 1977.
Sethi, J., Hirshaut, Y., Hajdu, S. I., and Clements, L. G.: Growing human sarcomas in culture. Cancer 40:744, 1977.
Hajdu, S. I., and Fogh, J.: The nude mouse as a diagnostic tool in human tumor cell research. *In* The Nude Mouse in Experimental and Clinical Research. Edited by J. Fogh and B. C. Giovanella. New York, Academic Press, 1978.
Narayanan, A. S., Page, R. C., and Kuzan, F.: Collagens synthesized in vitro by diploid fibroblasts obtained from chronically inflamed human connective tissue. Lab. Invest. 39:61, 1978.

NON-NEOPLASTIC LESIONS

Peyronie, F.: Sur quelques obstacles qui s'opposent a l'ejaculation naturelle de la semence. Memoires Acad Roy Chir. Paris 1:425, 1743.
Alibert, J. L. M.: Note sur la keloide. J. Univ. Sci. Med. 2:207, 1816.
Dupuytren, G.: Leçons orales de clinique chirugicale faites a l'Hotel-Dieu de Paris, Vol. 1, Chap. 1, 1832.
Van Buren, W. H., and Keyes, E. L.: On the Genitourinary Organs. London, Churchill, 1875.
Ledderhose, G.: Zur Pathologie der Aponeurose des Fusses und der Hand. Arch. Klin. Chir. 55:694, 1897.
Albarran, J.: Retention renale par periureterite. Liberation extern de l'ureter. Assoc. Fr. Urol. 9:511, 1905.
Albarran, J., and Dominques, J. M.: Medecine Operatoire des Voies Urinaires. Paris, Masson et Cie, 1909.
Kettle, H.: The Pathology of Tumors. New York, P. B. Hocher, 1916.
Jura, V.: Sulla mesenterite retrattile e sclerosante. Policlinico 31:575, 1924.
Sakurane, K.: A case of fibroma durum multiplex of the fingers and toes of an infant. Jpn. J. Dermatol. 24:8, 1924.
Know, L. C.: Chronic mediastinitis. Am. J. Med. Sci. 169:807, 1925.
Middleton, D. S.: Pathology of congenital muscular torticollis. Br. J. Surg. 18:188, 1930.
Summers, J. E.: Solid pure fibroma of the mesentery in children. Surg. Gynecol. Obstet. 55:244, 1932.
Mason, M. L.: Tumors of the hand. Surg. Gynecol. Obstet. 64:129, 1937.
Wells, H. G.: Occurrence and significance of congenital malignant neoplasms. Arch. Pathol. 30:535, 1940.
Garb, J., and Stone, M.: Keloids: review of literature and report of 80 cases. Am. J. Surg. 58:315, 1942.
Clay, R. C.: Dupuytren's contracture: fibroma of the palmar fascia. Ann. Surg. 120:224, 1944.
Touraine, A., and Ruel, H.: La polyfibromatose hereditaire. Ann. Dermatol. Syph. 5:1, 1945.
Chandler, A.: Muscular torticollis. J. Bone Joint Surg. 30A:566, 1948.
Ormond, J. K.: Bilateral ureteral obstruction due to envelopment and compression by an inflammatory retroperitoneal process. J. Urol. 59:1072, 1948.
Burford, E. H., Glenn, J. E., and Burford, C. E.: Therapy of Peyronie's disease. Urol. Cutan. Rev. 55:337, 1951.
Gruhn, J., and Hurwitt, E. S.: Fibrous sternomastoid tumor of infancy. Pediatrics 8:522, 1951.
Pickren, J. W., Smith, A. G., Stevenson, T. W., and Stout, A. P.: Fibromatosis of the plantar fascia. Cancer 4:846, 1951.
Waller, J. I., and Dreese, W. C.: Peyronie's disease associated with Dupuytren's contracture. J. Urol. 68:623, 1952.
Chandler, F. A.: Congenital muscular torticollis. Bull. Hosp. Joint Dis. 14:158, 1953.
Gardner, E. J., and Richards, R. C.: Multiple cutaneous and subcutaneous lesions occurring simultaneously with hereditary polyposis and osteomatosis. Am. J. Hum. Genet. 5:139, 1953.
Horton, C. E., Crawford, J., and Oakey, R. S.: Malignant change in keloids. Plast. Reconstr. Surg. 12:86, 1953.
Keasbey, L. E.: Juvenile aponeurotic fibroma (calcifying fibroma). A distinctive tumor arising in the palms and soles of young children. Cancer 6:338, 1953.
Vest, S. A., and Barelane, R.: Peri-ureteritis plastica. J. Urol. 70:38, 1953.
Conway, H.: Dupuytren's contracture. Am. J. Surg. 87:101, 1954.
Prior, J. T., and Sisson, B. J.: Dermal and infant fibromatoses. Ann. Surg. 139:453, 1954.
Stout, A. P.: Juvenile fibromatoses. Cancer 7:953, 1954.
Konwaler, B. E., Keasbey, L., and Kaplan, L.:

Subcutaneous pseudosarcomatous fibromatosis (Fasciitis). Am. J. Clin. Pathol. 25:241, 1955.

Reye, R. K.: A consideration of certain subdermal "Fibromatous Tumours" of infancy. J. Pathol. Bacteriol. 72:149, 1956.

Barrett, N. R.: Idiopathic mediastinal fibrosis. Br. J. Surg. 46:207, 1958.

Shnitka, T. K., Asp, D. M., and Horner, R. H.: Congenital generalized fibromatosis. Cancer 11:627, 1958.

Booher, R. J., and McPeak, C. J.: Juvenile aponeurotic fibromas. Surgery 46:924, 1959.

Luck, J. V.: Dupuytren's contracture. J. Bone Joint Surg. 41A:635, 1959.

Cosman, B., Crikelair, G. F., Ju, D. M. C., Gaulin, J. C., and Lattes, R.: Surgical treatment of keloids. Plast. Reconstr. Surg. 27:335, 1961.

Jarvi, O., and Saxen, E.: Elastofibroma dorsi. Acta Pathol. Microbiol. Scand. 51 (suppl):83, 1961.

Price, E. B., Silliphant, W. M., and Shuman, R.: Nodular fasciitis: a clinicopathologic analysis of 65 cases. Am. J. Clin. Pathol. 34:122, 1961.

Stout, A. P.: Pseudosarcomatous fasciitis in children. Cancer 14:216, 1961.

Betty, E. C.: Congenital generalized fibromatosis in infancy. Am. J. Dis. Child. 103:620, 1962.

Hutter, R. V. P., Foote, F. W., Francis, K. C., and Higinbotham, N. L.: Parosteal fasciitis. Am. J. Surg. 104:800, 1962.

Hutter, R. V. P., Stewart, F. W., and Foote, F. W.: Fasciitis. Cancer 15:992, 1962.

Soule, E. H.: Proliferative nodular fasciitis. Arch. Pathol. 73:437, 1962.

Yannopoulos, K., and Stout, A. P.: Primary solid tumors of the mesentery. Cancer 16:914, 1963.

Lichtenstein, L., and Goldman, R. L.: Cartilage tumors in soft tissues, particularly in the hand and foot. Cancer 17:1203, 1964.

Seel, D. J., Booher, R. J., and Joel, R. V.: Fibrous tumors of musculoaponeurotic origin. Surgery 56:497, 1964.

Simpson, R. D., Hanson, E. G., and Mayo, C. W.: Mesenteric fibromatosis in familial polyposis. Cancer 17:526, 1964.

Weary, P. E., Linthicum, A., Cawley, E. P., Coleman, C. C., and Graham, G. F.: Gardner's syndrome, a family group study and review. Arch. Dermatol. 90:20, 1964.

Enzinger, F. M.: Fibrous tumors of infancy. *In* Tumors of Bone and Soft Tissue. Chicago, Year Book Medical Publishers, 1965.

Enzinger, F. M.: Fibrous hamartoma of infancy. Cancer 18:241, 1965.

Kauffman, S. L., and Stout, A. P.: Congenital mesenchymal tumors. Cancer 18:460, 1965.

Reye, R. D. K.: Recurring digital fibrous tumors of childhood. Arch. Pathol. 80:228, 1965.

Rios-Dalenz, J. L., Kim, J. S., and McDowell, F. W.: The so-called juvenile aponeurotic fibroma. Am. J. Clin. Pathol. 44:632, 1965.

Utz, D. C., Rookie, E. D., Spittell, J. A., and Bartholomew, L. G.: Retroperitoneal fibrosis in patients taking methysergide. JAMA 191:983, 1965.

Barr, J. R.: Elastofibroma. Am. J. Clin. Pathol. 45:679, 1966.

Comings, D. E., Skubi, K. B., and Van Eyes, J.: Familial multifocal fibrosclerosis. Ann. Intern. Med. 66:884, 1966.

Conley, J., Healey, W. V., and Stout, A. P.: Fibromatosis of the head and neck. Am. J. Surg. 112:609, 1966.

Mehregan, A. H.: Nodular fasciitis. Arch. Dermatol. 93:204, 1966.

Morgan, A. D., Loughridge, L. W., and Calne, R. Y.: Combined mediastinal and retroperitoneal fibrosis. Lancet 1:67, 1966.

Smith, B. H.: Peyronie's disease. Am. J. Clin. Pathol. 45:670, 1966.

Stout, A. P., and Lattes, R.: Tumors of the soft tissues. *In* Atlas of Tumor Pathology, 2nd series. Washington, D.C., Armed Forces Institute of Pathology, 1967.

Graham, J. R.: Cardiac and pulmonary fibrosis during methysergide therapy for headache. Am. J. Med. Sci. 254:1, 1967.

Ramon, Y., Berman, W., and Bubis, J. J.: Gingival fibromatosis combined with cherubism. Oral Surg. 24:435, 1967.

Malvaney, W. P., Gordon, L. Z., and Gritti, E. J.: Another look at periureteral fibrosis. J. Urol. 99:417, 1968.

Waisman, J., and Smith, D. W.: Fine structure of an elastofibroma. Cancer 22:671, 1968.

Freilich, J., and Bendix, R. M.: Elastofibroma. Geriatrics 24:65, 1969.

Jarvi, O. H., Saxen, A. E., Hopsu-Havu, V. K., Wartiovaara, J. J., and Varisalo, V. T.: Elastofibroma: degenerative pseudotumour. Cancer 23:42, 1969.

Shapiro, L.: Infantile digital fibromatosis and aponeurotic fibroma. Arch. Dermatol. 99:37, 1969.

Winkelmann, R. K., and Sams, W. M.: Elastofibroma: report of a case with special histochemical and electron-microscopic studies. Cancer 23:406, 1969.

Allen, P. W., and Enzinger, F. M.: Juvenile aponeurotic fibroma. Cancer 26:857, 1970.

Goldman, R. L.: The cartilage analogue of fibromatosis (aponeurotic fibroma). Cancer 26:1325, 1970.

Mitchinson, M. J.: The pathology of idiopathic retroperitoneal fibrosis. J. Clin. Pathol. 23:681, 1970.

Battifora, H., and Hines, J. R.: Recurrent digital

fibromas of childhood: Electron microscope study. Cancer 27:1530, 1971.
Allen, P. W.: Recurring digital fibrous tumors of childhood. Pathology 4:215, 1972.
Banayan, G. A., and Hajdu, S. I.: Gynecomastia: Clinicopathologic study of 351 cases. Am. J. Clin. Pathol. 57:431, 1972.
Gabbiani, G., and Majno, G.: Dupuytren's contracture: fibroblast contraction? An ultrastructural study. Am. J. Pathol. 66:131, 1972.
Mackenzie, D. H.: The fibromatoses: A clinicopathologic concept. Br. Med. J. 4:777, 1972.
Mehregan, A. H., Nabai, H., and Matthews, J. E.: Recurring digital fibrous tumor of childhood. Arch. Dermatol. 106:375, 1972.
Chung, E. B., and Enzinger, F. M.: Proliferative fasciitis. Cancer 36:1450, 1975.
Iversen, B. M., Johannesen, J. W., and Nordahl, E.: Retroperitoneal fibrosis during treatment with methyldopa. Lancet 2:302, 1975.
Miller, R., Cheris, L., and Stratigos, G. T.: Nodular fasciitis. Oral Surg. 40:399, 1975.
Reske, M., and Namiki, H.: Sclerosing mesenteritis. Am. J. Clin. Pathol. 64:661, 1975.
Case Records of the Massachusetts General Hospital, N. Engl. J. Med. 294:712, 1976.
Dehner, L. P., and Askin, F. B.: Tumors of fibrous tissue origin in childhood. A clinicopathologic study of cutaneous and soft tissue neoplasms in 66 children. Cancer 38:888, 1976.
Kaplan, E. N., and Henjyoji, E. Y.: Pseudoxanthoma elasticum. Plast. Reconstr. Surg. 58:595, 1976.
Wirman, J. A.: Nodular fasciitis: an ultrastructural study. Cancer 38:2378, 1976.
Akhtar, M., and Miller, R. M.: Ultrastructure of elastofibroma. Cancer 40:728, 1977.
Benjamin, S. P., Mercer, R. D., and Hawk, W. A.: Myofibroblastic contraction in spontaneous regression of multiple congenital mesenchymal hamartomas. Cancer 40:2343, 1977.
Koep, L., and Zuidema, G. D.: The clinical significance of retroperitoneal fibrosis. Surgery 81:250, 1977.
Rosen, Y., Papasozomenos, S. Ch., and Gardner, B.: Fibromatosis of the heart. Cancer 41:1409, 1978.
Bhawan, J., Bacchetta, C., Joris, I., and Majno, G.: A myofibroblastic tumor. Am. J. Pathol. 94:19, 1979.
Kopelovich, L., Pfeffer, L. M., and Bias, N.: Growth characteristics of human skin fibroblasts *in vitro*. Cancer 43:218, 1979.

NON-COLLAGENOUS FIBROUS TUMORS

Taylor, R. W.: Sarcomatous tumors resembling in some respects keloid. J. Cutan. Genito-Urin. Dis. 8:384, 1890.
Mallory, F. B.: The results of the application of special histological methods to the study of tumors. J. Exp. Med. 10:575, 1908.
Wolbach, S. B.: A new type of cell inclusion, not parasitic, associated with disseminated granulomatous lesions. J. Med. Res. 24:244, 1911.
McDonagh, J. E. R.: A contribution to our knowledge of the naevoxanthoendotheliomata. Br. J. Dermatol. 24:85, 1912.
Wolbach, S. B.: Hemangio-endothelioma giving the histological appearance of giant cell xanthoma. Ztschr. Krebsforsch. 12:440, 1912–13.
Leitao, M.: A case of congenital myxoma of the feet. Am. J. Dis. Child. 5:374, 1913.
Darier, J., and Ferrand, M.: Dermatofibromes progressifs et recidivants ou fibrosarcomes de la peau. Ann. Dermatol. Syph. 5:545, 1924.
Baitsell, G. A.: On the origin of the connective-tissue ground-substance in the chick embryo. Qt. J. Microbiol. Sci. 69:571, 1925.
Fischer, A.: Sur la transformation in vitro des gros leukocytes mononucleaires en fibroblasts. C. R. Soc. Biol. 92:109, 1925.
Hoffman, E.: Uber das knollentreibende Fibrosarkom der Haut (Dermatofibrosarkoma protuberans). Dermatol. Zr. 43:1, 1925.
Levy, G.: Xanthelasma et xanthome. Ann. Anat. Pathol. 2:247, 1925.
Christopher, F.: Giant cell sarcoma apparently arising from the aponeurosis of the forearm. JAMA 87:167, 1926.
Fry, H. J. B.: Osteoclastoma (myeloid stroma) of the human female breast. J. Pathol. Bact. 30:529, 1927.
Ratcliff, H. L.: Tumors in captive primates with a description of a giant-cell tumor in a chacma baboon. J. Cancer Res. 14:453, 1930.
Phemister, D. E.: Undifferentiated round-cell sarcomas. Ann. Surg. 93:125, 1931.
Woringer, F.: Histiocytoma of the leg. Bull. Soc. Franc. Dermat. Syph. 38:1401, 1931.
Traub, E. F., and Monash, S.: Dermatofibroma. Arch. Dermatol. Syph. 26:250, 1932.
Oberling, C.: Retroperitoneal xanthogranuloma. Am. J. Cancer 23:477, 1935.
Senear, F. E., and Caro, M. R.: Histiocytoma cutis. Arch. Dermatol. Syph. 33:209, 1936.
Senear, F. E. and Caro, M. R.: Nevoxanthoendothelioma or juvenile xanthoma. Arch. Dermat. Syph. 34:195–206, 1936.
Danks, A. G. and Olafson, P.: Giant cell sarcoma. Cornell Vet. 29:68, 1939.
Stecker, J. F. and Robinson, W. L.: Dermatofibroma. Arch. Dermat. Syph. 43:498, 1941.
Bloom, D., Kaufman, S. R. and Stevens, R. A.: Hereditary xanthomatosis. Arch. Dermat. Syph. 45:1, 1942.
Arnold, H. L., and Tilden, I. L.: Histiocytoma

cutis: A variant of xanthoma. Histologic and clinical studies of twenty-seven lesions in twenty-three cases. Arch. Dermatol. Syph. 47:498, 1943.

Gross, R. E., and Wolbach, S. B.: Sclerosing hemangiomas; their relationship to dermatofibroma, histiocytoma, xanthoma and to certain pigmented lesions of the skin. Am. J. Pathol. 19:533, 1943.

Foster, L. N.: The benign giant cell tumor of tendon sheaths. Am. J. Pathol. 23:567, 1947.

Stout, A. P.: Myxoma, the tumor of primitive mesenchyme. Ann. Surg. 127:706, 1948.

Koback, M. W., and Perlow, S.: Xanthomatous giant cell tumors arising in soft tissue. Report of an instance of malignant growth. Arch. Surg. 59:909, 1949.

Pack, G. T., and Tabah, E. J.: Dermatofibrosarcoma protuberans. Arch. Surg. 62:391, 1951.

Penner, D. W.: Metastasizing dermatofibrosarcoma protuberans; case report. Cancer 4:1083, 1951.

Stout, A. P.: Tumors of the Soft Tissues, Washington, D.C., Armed Forces Institute of Pathology, 1953.

Purvis, W. E., and Helwig, E. B.: Reticulohistiocytic granuloma. Am. J. Clin. Pathol. 24:1005, 1954.

Bednar, B.: Storiform neurofibromas of skin, pigmented and nonpigmented. Cancer 10:368, 1957.

Attar, S.: Myxoma, a clinicopathologic study. Am. J. Surg. 91:755, 1958.

Weimar, V.: Activation of corneal stromal cells to take-up vital dye neutral red. Exp. Cell Res. 18:1, 1959.

Glazunov, M. F., and Puckhov, J. G.: Human muscular myxoma and intracellular inclusions. Vopr. Onkol. 6:11, 1960.

Kauffman, S. L., and Stout, A. P.: Histiocytic tumors (fibrous xanthoma and histiocytoma) in children. Cancer 14:469, 1961.

Petrakis, N. L., Davis, M., and Lucia, S. P.: The *in vivo* differentiation of human leukocytes into histiocytes, fibroblasts and fat cells in subcutaneous diffusion chambers. Blood 17:109, 1961.

Taylor, H. H., and Helwig, E. B.: Dermatofibrosarcoma protuberans. Cancer 15:717, 1962.

Helwig, E. B.: Atypical fibroxanthoma. Tex. Med. 59;604, 1963.

Levan, N. E., Hirsch, P., and Kwong, M. Q.: Pseudosarcomatous dermatofibroma. Arch. Dermatol. 88:908, 1963.

Ozzello, L., Stout, A. P., and Murray, M. R.: Cultural characteristics of malignant histiocytoma and fibrous xanthoma. Cancer 16:331, 1963.

Schmaman, A., Penn, I., and Sorour, V.: Giant-cell tumors of the soft tissues. S. Afr. Med. J. 37:819, 1963.

Gordon, H. W.: Pseudosarcomatous reticulohistiocytoma. Arch. Dermatol. 90:319, 1964.

Kempson, R. L., and McGavran, M. H.: Atypical fibroxanthomas of the skin. Cancer 17:1463, 1964.

O'Brien, J. E., and Stout, A. P.: Malignant fibrous xanthomas. Cancer 17:1445, 1964.

Enzinger, F. M.: Intramuscular myxoma. Am. J. Clin. Pathol. 43:104, 1965.

Volkman, A., and Gowans, J. L.: The origin of macrophages from bone marrow in the rat. Br. J. Exp. Pathol. 46:62, 1965.

Burkhardt, B. R., Soule, E. H., Winkelmann, R. K., and Ivins, J. C.: Dermatofibrosarcoma protuberans. Study of 56 cases. Am. J. Surg. 111:638, 1966.

Fisher, E. R., and Hellstrom, H. R.: Dermatofibrosarcoma with metastases simulating Hodgkin's disease and reticulum cell sarcoma. Cancer 19:1165, 1966.

Klaus, S. N., and Winkelmann, R. K.: The enzyme histochemistry of nodular subepidermal fibrosis. Br. J. Dermatol. 78:398, 1966.

Reed, R. J.: Atypical fibroxanthomas and spindle cell carcinomas of the skin. Bull. Tulane Med. Fac. 26:75, 1967.

Stout, A. P., and Lattes, R.: Tumors of the soft tissue. *In* Atlas of Tumor Pathology, 2nd series. Washington, D.C., Armed Forces Institute of Pathology, 1967.

McPeak, C. J., Druz, T., and Nicastri, A. D.: Dermatofibrosarcoma protuberans—an analysis of 86 cases—five with metastasis. Ann. Surg. 166:803, 1967.

Sutton, J. S.: Ultrastructural aspects of *in vitro* development of monocytes into macrophages, epithelioid cells, and multinucleated giant cells. Natl. Cancer Inst. Monogr. 28:71, 1967.

Elizalde, A., and Korman, S.: Cytochemical studies of glycogen neutral mucopolysaccharides and fat in malignant tissues. Cancer 21:1061, 1968.

Reid, J. D., Hajdu, S. I., and Attah, E.: Infantile cardiomyopathy: a previously unrecognized type with histiocytoid reaction. J. Pediatr. 73:335, 1968.

Kroe, D. J., and Pitcock, J. A.: Atypical fibroxanthoma of the skin. Am. J. Clin. Pathol. 51:487, 1969.

Spector, W. G., and Ryan, G. B.: New evidence for the existence of long lived macrophages. Nature 221:860, 1969.

Mackenzie, D. H.: The Differential Diagnosis of Fibroblastic Disorders. Oxford, Blackwell, 1970.

Ross, R., Everett, N. B., and Tyler, R.: Wound healing and collagen formation. The origin of the wound fibroblast studied in parabiosis. J. Cell Biol. 44:645, 1970.

Soule, E. H., and Enriquez, P.: Atypical fibrous histiocytoma—malignant fibrous histiocy-

toma, malignant histiocytoma and epithelioid sarcoma: A comparative study of sixty-five tumors. Cancer 30:128, 1972.
Merkow, L. P., Frich, J. C., Slifkin, M., Kyreages, C. G., and Pardo, M.: Ultrastructure of a fibroxanthosarcoma (malignant fibroxanthoma). Cancer 28:372, 1971.
Wirth, W. A., Leavitt, D., and Enzinger, F. M.: Multiple intramuscular myxomas. Another extraskeletal manifestation of fibrous dysplasia. Cancer 27:1167, 1971.
Guccion, J. G., and Enzinger, F. M.: Malignant giant cell tumor of soft part. Cancer 29:1518, 1972.
Kempson, R. L., and Kyriakos, M.: Fibroxanthosarcoma of the soft tissues: A type of malignant fibrous histiocytoma. Cancer 29:961, 1972.
Kouri, J., and Ancheta, O.: Transformation of macrophages into fibroblasts. Exp. Cell Res. 71:168, 1972.
Salm, R., and Sissons, R. A.: Giant-cell tumors of soft tissue. J. Pathol. 107:27, 1972.
Wolfowitz, B. L., and Jaffe, A.: Fibrous histiocytoma of the pharynx. S. Afr. Med. J. 46:134, 1972.
Hudson, A. W., and Winkelmann, R. K.: Atypical fibroxanthoma of the skin. Cancer 29:413, 1972.
Fretzin, D. F., and Helwig, E. B.: Atypical fibroxanthoma of the skin—A clinicopathologic study of 144 cases. Cancer 31:1541, 1973.
Vargas-Cortes, F., Winkelmann, R. K., and Soule, E. H.: Atypical fibroxanthomas of the skin. Mayo Clin. Proc. 48:211, 1973.
Hensley, G., and Friedrich, E. G.: Malignant fibroxanthoma: A sarcoma of the vulva. Am. J. Obstet. Gynecol. 116:289, 1973.
Ireland, D. C., Soule, E. H., and Ivins, J. C.: Myoma of somatic soft tissues. Mayo Clin. Proc. 48:401, 1973.
Kahn, L. B.: Retroperitoneal xanthogranuloma and xanthosarcoma (malignant fibrous xanthoma). Cancer 31:411, 1973.
Wanebo, H. J., Shah, J., Knapper, W., Hajdu, S. I., and Booher, R.: Reappraisal of surgical management of sarcoma of the buttock. Cancer 31:97, 1973.
Carstens, P. H. B., and Schrodt, G. R.: Ultrastructure of sclerosing hemangioma. Am. J. Pathol. 77:377, 1974.
Groeschel-Stewart, U., and Groeschel, D.: Immunological evidence for the presence of smooth muscle-type contractile fibers in mouse macrophages. Experientia 30:1152, 1974.
Hajdu, S. I., Bean, M. A., Fogh, J., Hajdu, E. O., and Ricci, A.: Papanicolaou smear of cultured human tumor cells. Acta Cytol. 18:327, 1974.
Pradhan, S. N., Chung, E. B., Ghosh, B., Paul, B. D., and Kapadia, G. J.: Carcinogenicity of some plant extract and their tannin-containing fractions in rats. J. Natl. Cancer Inst. 52:1579, 1974.
Brenner, W., Shoefler, K., Chlabra, H., and Postel, A.: Dermatofibrosarcoma protuberans metastatic to a regional lymph node—report of a case and review. Cancer 36:1897, 1975.
Bridger, M. W. M.: Multifocal malignant histiocytoma. J. Clin. Pathol. 28:825, 1975.
Fu, Y. S., Gabbiani, G., Kaye, G. I., and Lattes, R.: Malignant soft tissue tumors of probable histiocytic origin (malignant fibrous histiocytomas): general considerations and electron microscopic and tissue culture studies. Cancer 35:176, 1975.
Hakimi, M., Pai, R. P., Fine, G., and Davila, J. C.: Fibrous histiocytoma of the trachea. Chest 68:367, 1975.
Mori, M., Murakami, M., Hirose, I., and Shimozato, T.: Histochemical studies of myxoma of the jaw. J. Oral Surg. 33:529, 1975.
Ribari, O., Elemer, G., and Balint, A.: Laryngeal giant cell tumor. J. Laryngol. 89:857, 1975.
Dahl, I.: Atypical fibroxanthoma of the skin. Acta Path. Microbiol. Scand. 84:183, 1976.
Gonzalez-Vitale, J. C., Slavin, R. E., and McQueen, J. D.: Radiation induced intracranial malignant fibrous histiocytoma. Cancer 37:2960, 1976.
Hajdu, S. I., and Hajdu, E. O.: Cytopathology of Sarcomas and Other Nonepithelial Malignant Tumors. Philadelphia, W. B. Saunders, 1976.
Kyriakos, M., and Kempson, R. L.: Inflammatory fibrous histiocytoma. An aggressive and lethal lesion. Cancer 37:1584, 1976.
Ozzello, L., and Hamels, J.: The histiocytic nature of dermatofibrosarcoma protuberans. Tissue culture and electron microscopic study. Am. J. Clin. Pathol. 65:136, 1976.
Alguacil-Garcia, A., Unni, K. K., and Goellner, J. R.: Malignant giant cell tumor of soft parts. An ultrastructural study of four cases. Cancer 20:244, 1977.
Barr, R. J., Wuerker, R. B., and Graham, J. H.: Ultrastructure of atypical fibroxanthoma. Cancer 40:736, 1977.
Churg, A. M., and Kahn, L. B.: Myofibroblasts and related cells in malignant fibrous and fibrohistiocytic tumors. Hum. Pathol. 8:205, 1977.
Feldman, P. S., Horvath, E., and Kovacs, K.: An ultrastructural study of seven cardiac myxomas. Cancer 40:2216, 1977.
Johnson, J. T., and Powshter, D. L.: Fibrous histiocytoma of the subglottic larynx. Ann. Otol. Rhino. Laryngol. 86:243, 1977.

Sethi, J., Hirshaut, Y., Hajdu, S. I., and Clements, L. G.: Growing human sarcomas in culture. Cancer 40:744, 1977.
Russell, W., Cohen, J., Enzinger, F., Hajdu, S. I., Heise, H., Martin, R. G., Meissner, W., Miller, W. T., Schmitz, R. L., and Frich, D.: A clinical and pathological staging system for soft tissue sarcomas. Cancer 40:1562, 1977.
Simstein, N. L., Tuthill, R., Sperber, E. E., Kovaleik, P. J., and Mullen, J. T.: Dermatofibrosarcoma protuberans. South. Med. J. 70:487, 1977.
Taxy, J. B., and Battifora, H.: Malignant fibrous histiocytomas. An electron microscopic study. Cancer 40:254, 1977.
Weiss, S. W., and Enzinger, F. M.: Myxoid variant of malignant fibrous histiocytoma. Cancer 39:1672, 1977.
Alguacil-Garcia, A., Unni, K. K., and Goellner, J. R.: Histogenesis of dermatofibrosarcoma protuberans. Am. J. Clin. Pathol. 69:427, 1978.
Cozzutto, C., DeBernardi, B., Guarino, M., Cornelli, A., and Soave, F.: Retroperitoneal fibrohistiocytic tumors in children. Report of five cases. Cancer 41:1350, 1978.
Sandstrom, R. E., Proppe, K. H., and Trelstad, R.: Fibrous histiocytoma of the trachea. Am. J. Clin. Pathol. 70:429, 1978.
Weiss, S. W., and Enzinger, F. M.: Malignant fibrous histiocytoma. Cancer 41:2250, 1978.
Hajdu, S. I., and Fogh, J.: The nude mouse as a diagnostic tool in human tumor research. *In* The Nude Mouse in Experimental and Clinical Research. Edited by J. Fogh and B. C. Giovanella. New York, Academic Press, 1978.
Lagace, R., Delage, C., and Seemayer, T. A.: Myxoid variant of malignant fibrous histiocytoma. Ultrastructural observations. Cancer 43:526, 1979.
Roques, A. W. W., Horton, L. W. L., Leslie, J., and Buxton-Thomas, M. S.: Inflammatory fibrous histiocytoma in the left upper abdomen with a leukemoid blood picture. Cancer 43:1800, 1979.

COLLAGENOUS FIBROUS TUMORS

Macfarlane, J.: *In* Clinical Reports of the Surgical Practice of the Glasgow Royal Infirmary. Edited by D. Robertson, 1832, p. 63.
Muller, J.: Uber den feinern Bau and die Formen der Krankhaften Geschwulste. Berlin, G. Reimer, 1838.
Rokitansky, C.: Handbuch der pathologischen Anatomie. Wien, Braumuller u. Seidel, 1842–46.
Bennett, J. H.: On Cancerous and Cancroid Growths. Edinburgh, Sutherland and Knox, 1849.
Bennett, J. H.: Review on cancerous and cancroid growth. Lancet 2:428, 1849.
Paget, J.: Fibro-nucleated tumor of the abdomen of fourteen years' growth: removal. Lancet 1:625, 1856.
Wilks, S.: Lectures on Pathological Anatomy. London, Longman, 1859, p. 467.
Virchow, R.: Die krankhaften Geschwulste, Volume 2. Berlin, A. Hirschwald, 1863, p. 324.
Butlin, H. T.: Recurrent ossifying spindle-celled sarcoma from the subcutaneous tissue of the thigh. Trans. Path. Soc. London 24:211, 1873.
Billroth, T.: Lectures on Surgical Pathology and Therapeutics. London, The New Sydenham Society, 1877–1878.
Sanger, M.: Uber desmoide Geschwulste der Bauchwand und deren operation mit Resection des peritoneum parietale. Arch. Gynaekol. 24:1, 1884.
Temoin, D.: Tumeur fibreause de la paroi abdominale chez l'enfant. Ann. Gynec. 39:516, 1893.
Peiffer, C.: Die Desmoide der Bauchdecken und ihre Prognose. Beitr. Klin. Chir. 44:334, 1904.
Mallory, F. B.: The results of the application of special histological methods to the study of tumors. J. Exp. Med. 10:575, 1908.
Porter, C. A.: Surgical treatment of x-ray carcinoma and other severe x-ray lesions based upon an analysis of 47 cases. J. Med. Res. 21:357, 1909.
Hartman, J. P.: Causistic reports on tumors in the abdominal wall. Acta Obstet. Gynecol. Scand. 2:284, 1923.
Nichols, R. W.: Desmoid tumors. A report of 31 cases. Arch. Surg. 7:277, 1923.
Hertzler, A. E.: Fibrosarcomatous tumors of skin of trunk: characterized by attenuated dermal surfaces. Ann. Surg. 83:489, 1926.
Quick, D., and Cutler, M.: Neurogenic sarcoma: a clinical and pathological study. Ann. Surg. 86:810, 1927.
Lamb, H. D.: Myxoma of the orbit, with case report and anatomical findings. Arch. Ophthalmol. 57:425, 1928.
Donald, J. M., and Caylor, H. D.: Fibrosarcoma developing in a desmoid. Ann. Surg. 89:631, 1929.
Grynfeltt, E.: Trame collagene et fibrillogenese dans les sarcomes du tissu conjonctif. Bull. Assoc. Franc. Cancer 18:360, 1929.
Grynfeltt, E.: Myxome vesical a evolution rapidement fatale chez un enfant de neuf mois. Bull. Assoc. Franc. Cancer 18:488, 1929.
Mason, J. B.: Desmoid tumors. Ann. Surg. 92:444, 1930.
French, R. E.: End results in a series of 16 cases of fibrosarcoma. N. Engl. J. Med. 206;393, 1932.
Mankin, Z. W.: Desmoid und Sarkome der

Bauchwandung. Arch. Klin. Chir. 169:688, 1932.

Turren, L. K., and Seeling, M. G.: Reticulum in tumors. Arch. Pathol. 15:498, 1933.

Bick, E. M.: Fibrosarcoma of the extremities. Ann. Surg. 101:759, 1935.

Ewing, J.: Fascial sarcoma and intermuscular myxoliposarcoma. Arch. Surg. 31:507, 1935.

Geschickter, C. F., and Lewis, D.: Tumors of connective tissue. Am. J. Cancer 25:630, 1935.

Hudson, O. C.: Intra-uterine fibrosarcoma of the foot: a case report. Am. J. Cancer 26:568, 1936.

Meyerding, H. W., Broders, A. C., and Hargrave, R. L.: Clinical aspects of fibrosarcoma of soft tissue of extremities. Surg. Gynecol. Obstet. 62:1010, 1936.

Warren, S., and Sommer, G. N. J.: Fibrosarcoma of soft parts; with special reference to recurrence and metastasis. Arch. Surg. 32:425, 1936.

Gricouroff, G.: Sarcome fusocellulaire apres radiumpuncture pour tumeur epitheliale de la langue (deux cas). Bull. Assoc. Franc. Cancer 26:378, 1937.

Hargrave, R.: Fibrosarcoma of the soft tissues of the extremities. Tex. State J. Med. 32:815, 1937.

Nathanson, I. T., and Welch, C. E.: Life expectancy and incidence of malignant disease. Malignant lymphoma, fibrosarcoma, malignant melanoma and osteogenic sarcoma. Am. J. Cancer 31:598, 1937.

Broders, A. C., Hargrave, R., and Meyerding, H. W.: Pathological features of soft tissue fibrosarcoma; with special reference to the grading of its malignancy. Surg. Gynecol. Obstet. 69:267, 1939.

Meade, W. H., and Brewster, W. R.: Tumefactions of the abdominal wall. Am. J. Surg. 45:419, 1939.

Collins, N. C., and Anspach, W. E.: Fibrosarcoma of plantar tissues. Am. J. Cancer 40:465, 1940.

Wells, H. G.: Occurrence and significance of congenital malignant neoplasms. Arch. Pathol. 30:535, 1940.

Perman, R. O., and Mayo, C. W.: Desmoid tumors; a clinical and pathological study. Ann. Surg. 115:114, 1942.

Dixon, C. F., and Vadheim, J. L.: Recurring retroperitonal fibromyxosarcoma. Minn. Med. 27:203, 1944.

Pack, G. T., and Ehrlich, H. E.: Neoplasms of the anterior abdominal wall with special consideration of desmoid tumors. Int. Abstr. Surg. 79:177, 1944.

Wilson, D. A.: Tumors of the subcutaneous tissue and fascia; with special reference to fibrosarcoma. A clinical study. Surg. Gynecol. Obstet. 80:500, 1945.

Musgrove, J. E., and McDonald, J. R.: Extra-abdominal desmoid tumors. Their differential diagnosis and treatment. Arch. Pathol. 45:513, 1948.

Stewart, F. W.: Case #24. Division of Laboratory and Research, Albany, New York, 1948.

Stout, A. P.: Fibrosarcoma, the malignant tumor of fibroblasts. Cancer 1:30, 1948.

Dreyfuss, M. L.: Congenital sarcoma. J. Pediatr. 34:583, 1949.

Heller, E. L., and Sieber, W. K.: Fibrosarcoma—a clinical and pathological study of sixty cases. Surgery 27:539, 1950.

Ivins, J. C., Dockerty, M. B., and Ghormley, R. K.: Fibrosarcoma of the soft tissues of the extremities. Surgery 28:495, 1950.

Williams, J. O., and Schrum, D.: Congenital fibrosarcoma; report of a case in a newborn infant. Arch. Pathol. 51:548, 1951.

Pack, G. T., and Ariel, I. M.: Fibrosarcoma of the soft somatic tissue. Surgery 31:443, 1952.

Stout, A. P.: Juvenile fibromatoses. Cancer 7:953, 1954.

Brindley, H. H., Phillips, C., and Fernandez, J. N.: Fibrosarcoma of the extremities—Review of forty-five cases. J. Bone Joint Surg. 37A:602, 1955.

Jadrijvic, D., Marones, E., and Lipschutz, A.: Antifibromatogenic activity of 19-norethinyltestosterone in the guinea pig. Proc. Soc. Exp. Biol. Med. 91:38, 1956.

Smith, W. G.: Desmoid tumors in familial multiple polyposis. Proc. Mayo Clinic 34:31, 1959.

Dutz, W., and Stout, A. P.: The myxoma in childhood. Cancer 14:629, 1961.

Soule, E. H., and Scanlon, P. W.: Fibrosarcoma arising in an extra-abdominal desmoid tumor—Report of a case. Proc. Mayo Clinic 37:443, 1962.

Stout, A. P.: Fibrosarcoma in infants and children. Cancer 15:1029, 1962.

Phelan, J. T., and Nigogosyan, G.: Fibrosarcoma of superficial soft tissue origin. Arch. Surg. 86:118, 1963.

Mackenzie, D. H.: Fibroma: A dangerous diagnosis. Br. J. Surg. 51:607, 1964.

Butler, J. J.: Fibrous tissue tumors: Nodular fasciitis, dermatofibrosarcoma protuberans and fibrosarcoma, grade I, desmoid type. *In* Tumors of Bone and Soft Tissue. Chicago, Year Book Medical Publishers, 1965.

Enzinger, F. M.: Clear cell sarcoma of tendons and aponeuroses. An analysis of 21 cases. Cancer 18:1163, 1965.

Van der Werf-Messing, B., and van Unnik, J. A. M.: Fibrosarcoma of the soft tissues—A clinicopathologic study. Cancer 18:1113, 1965.

Masson, J. K., and Soule, E. H.: Desmoid tumors of the head and neck. Am. J. Surg. 112:615, 1966.

Welsh, R. A.: Intracytoplasmic collagen formation in desmoid fibromatosis. Am. J. Path. 49:515, 1966.

Balsaver, A. M., Butler, J. J., and Martin, R. G.: Congenital fibrosarcoma. Cancer 20:1607, 1967.

Enzinger, F. M., and Shiraki, M.: Musculo-aponeurotic fibromatosis of the shoulder girdle (Extra-abdominal desmoid). Cancer 20:113, 1967.

Leak, L. V., Caulfield, J. B., Burke, J. F., and McKhann, C. F.: Electron microscopic studies of a human fibromyxosarcoma. Cancer Research 27:261, 1967.

Stout, A. P., and Lattes, R.: Tumors of the soft tissues. *In* Atlas of Tumor Pathology, 2nd series. Washington, D.C., Armed Forces Institute of Pathology, 1967.

Soule, E. H., Mahour, G. H., Mills, S. D., and Lynn, H. B.: Soft tissue sarcoma of infants and children: A clinicopathologic study of 135 cases. Mayo Clin. Proc. 43:313, 1968.

Brasfield, R. D., and Das Gupta, T. K.: Desmoid tumors of the anterior abdominal wall. Surgery 65:241, 1969.

Cole, N. M., and Guiss, L. W.: Extra-abdominal desmoid tumors. Arch. Surg. 98:530, 1969.

Das Gupta, T. K., Brasfield, R. D., and O'Hara, J.: Extra-abdominal desmoids. Ann. Surg. 170:109, 1969.

Lewis, J. S.: Sarcoma of the nasal cavity and paranasal sinuses. Ann. Otol. Rhinol. Laryngol. 78:778, 1969.

Mackenzie, D. H.: The Differential Diagnosis of Fibroblastic Disorders. Oxford, Blackwell, 1970.

Gonzales-Crussi, F.: Ultrastructure of congenital fibrosarcoma. Cancer 26:1289, 1970.

Farr, H. W.: Soft part sarcomas of the head and neck. Am. J. Surg. 122:714, 1971.

Martini, N., Hajdu, S. I., and Beattie, E. J.: Primary sarcoma of the lung. J. Thorac. Cardiovasc. Surg. 61:33, 1971.

Goellner, J. R., Devine, K. D., and Weiland, L. H.: Pseudosarcoma of the larynx. Am. J. Clin. Pathol. 59:312, 1972.

Allegra, S. R., and Broderick, P. A.: Desmoid fibroblastoma. Intracytoplasmic collagenosynthesis in a peculiar fibroblastic tumor: Light and ultrastructural study of a case. Hum. Pathol. 4:419, 1973.

Castro, E. B., Hajdu, S. I., and Fortner, J. G.: Surgical therapy of fibrosarcoma of extremities. Arch. Surg. 107:284, 1973.

Exelby, P. R., Knapper, W. H., Huvos, A. G., and Beattie, E. J.: Soft-tissue fibrosarcoma in children. J. Pediatr. Surg. 8:415, 1973.

Wanebo, H. J., Shah, J., Knapper, W., Hajdu, S. I., and Booher, R.: Reappraisal of surgical management of sarcoma of the buttock. Cancer 31:97, 1973.

Lazarides, E., and Weber, K.: Actin antibody: The specific visualization of actin filaments in nonmuscle cells. Proc. Natl. Acad. Sci. 71:2268, 1974.

Pritchard, D. J., Soule, E. H., Taylor, W. F., and Ivins, J. C.: Fibrosarcoma: clinicopathologic and statistical study of 199 tumors of soft tissues of extremities and trunk. Cancer 33:888, 1974.

Alrenga, D. P.: Primary fibrosarcoma of the liver. Cancer 36:446, 1975.

Espinosa, M. H., and Quan, S. H. Q.: Anal fibrosarcoma. Report of a case and review of the literature. Dis. Colon Rectum 18:522, 1975.

McCormack, M.: Bilateral fibrosarcoma of the epididymis. J. Clin. Pathol. 28:576, 1975.

Pingitore, R., and Bachechi, P.: Congenital fibrosarcoma. Tumori 61:351, 1975.

Shiu, M. H., Castro, E. B., Hajdu, S. I., and Fortner, J. G.: Surgical treatment of 297 soft tissue sarcoma of the lower extremity. Ann. Surg. 182:597, 1975.

Stiller, D., and Katenkamp, D.: Cellular features in desmoid fibromatosis and well-differentiated fibrosarcomas. An electron microscopic study. Virchows Arch. (Pathol. Anat.) 369:155, 1975.

Tanimura, A., Shigematsu, S., Adachi, K., and Kobayashi, H.: Fibrosarcoma of glans penis—case report and review of the literature. Jpn. J. Cancer Clin. 21:432, 1975.

Chung, E. R., and Enzinger, F. M.: Infantile fibrosarcoma. Cancer 38:729, 1976.

Fu, Y. S., and Perzin, K. H.: Nonepithelial tumors of the nasal cavity, paranasal sinuses and nasopharynx. Cancer 37:2912, 1976.

Soule, E. H., and Pritchard, D. J.: Fibrosarcoma in infants and children. Cancer 40:1711, 1977.

Hajdu, S. I., Shiu, M. H., and Fortner, J. G.: Desmoid tumors. A clinicopathologic study of 162 cases. Cancer (In press).

Mena, H., and Garcia, J. H.: Primary brain sarcomas. Cancer 42:1298, 1978.

Hajdu, S. I., Lemos, L. B., Kozakewich, H., Helson, L., and Beattie, E. J.: Growth pattern and differentiation of human soft tissue sarcomas in nude mice. Cancer 47:90, 1981.

Shiu, M. H., Flanebaum, L., Hajdu, S. I., and Fortner, J. G.: Malignant soft tissue tumors of the anterior abdominal wall. Arch. Surg. (In press).

chapter 3

Tumors of Tendosynovial Tissue

KNOWLEDGE of the morphology and the role of tendosynovial tissue has lagged behind that of other tissues. Only since the 1940's has there been general acceptance of the fact that joint spaces consist of a specialized free connective tissue surface, the cells of which are modified connective tissue cells. This surface is not covered by epithelial or mesothelial lining cells. The synovial membrane, therefore, is not a true membrane. It merges imperceptibly with the fibroconnective tissue forming the walls of articular spaces, bursae, and tendon sheaths. Functionally, tendosynovial tissue not only joins the bones together but also represents the junction between bones and muscles.

Bonn, in 1763, named the synovial membrane and until the second half of the eighteenth century, according to Winslow (1782), it was considered a glandular organ which secretes the synovial fluid. Bichat, in 1800, was the first to consider the synovial membrane a non-glandular structure and believed that the synovial fluid is a transudate from the blood. Velpeau (1837) accepted the existence of synovial membrane in the true sense of the word and believed that it is formed by cellular connective tissue. One historical view is that mucin is present in the synovial fluid and is a secretory product of serous lining cells. Von Kolliker (1850) advanced the theory that the synovial membrane is formed by two linings, an inner epithelial and an outer connective tissue. The papillary or villous nature of the synovial membrane was recognized by Henle in 1865. Using silver nitrate impregnation, Hueter, in 1876, came to the conclusion that the synovial membrane is composed of connective tissue cells and the synovial fluid is formed by the inner connective tissue lining cells. Soubbotine (1880) also believed that the synovial fluid was secreted by synovial epithelial cells and concluded erroneously that tendons and ligaments are not covered by synovial membrane.

From the time of the early 1900's attention was focused on the better understanding of the histopathology and the nature of tendosynovial lesions. The developing new nomenclature was based on embryologic and histologic observations. Vaubel, in 1932, studied the form and function of synovial cells in tissue culture and came to the conclusion that synovial cells differ entirely from other mesenchymal cells. He said, "The peculiarity of a synovial growth rests in part on the polymorphism of the cells, the contour of which ranges from round and spindle to polygonal and epithelioid, and especially on their tendency to form membranes composed of syncytial elements."

In tissue sections, synovial cells of joints, bursae, and tendon sheath are similar to fibroblasts, but they may appear oat-shaped, ovoid, or elongated. The form of the cells is at least partly influenced by the anatomic site and cell-to-cell relationship.

As seen with the electron microscope the normal synovium is composed of *two cell types* (Lever and Ford, 1958; Barland et al, 1962; Ball et al, 1964; Ghadially and Roy, 1969; Hirohata, 1974). The first is a histiocytic type of cell—the *A cell*—which has phagocytic capacity and contains many vacuoles as well as filopodia but has sparse rough-surfaced endoplasmic reticulum. While the A cells are found mostly in or near the inner lining, the second type of cells—*B cells*—are found deeper, towards the surrounding tissue. The B cells are fibroblast-like cells with prominent rough endoplasmic reticulum and large numbers of mitochondria and glycogen granules (Table 3-1).

It should be pointed out, however, that both type A and B cells are histogenetically identical cells at different stages of maturation. The fact that in pathologic conditions phagocytized hemosiderin is often found in type B, fibroblast-like cells is an indication that *B cells are differentiated forms of histiocytic A cells.* Ball et al (1964) confirmed this by injection of ferric dextran into the joint cavity. They found that iron accumulates

TABLE 3-1. *Comparison of Certain Ultrastructural Features of Synovial Cells*

TYPE A CELLS	TYPE B CELLS
Sparse rough endoplasmic reticulum	Well-developed, rough endoplasmic reticulum
Numerous lysosomes	Giant cells
Siderosomes	Large numbers of mitochondria
Filopodia	Golgi bodies
Prominent Golgi	Glycogen particles

first in the A cells and is later found in B cells.

The lining tissue of synovial bursae and tendon sheaths is homologous with the synovial membrane of the joints. The innermost layer, mostly A cells, is from one to three cells in depth. The adjacent or external cells, mostly B cells, are thought to be, among other things, involved in production of *hyaluronate.*

At present there is no evidence to suggest that synovial cells form synovial fluid or possess more secretory activity than other types of connective tissue cells. The exact composition of the ground substance is not known, but attempts have been made to classify the mucopolysaccharides and hyaluronate that have been identified between cells (King, 1935; Shaw and Martin, 1962; Blau et al, 1965; Hahn and Hahn, 1971). From the biochemical point of view it appears to be settled that most of the proteins of synovial fluid arise from the plasma.

The synovial fluid was named by Paracelsus. The synovial mucin or hyaluronate or hyaluronic acid was first isolated by Meyer et al, in 1939, and was so named because of the similarity to mucin obtained from vitreous fluid. It is a sulphate-free polymerized mucopolysaccharide, but it is not yet known whether it is free in the synovial fluid or bound to protein. Blau et al, in 1965, observed bright fluorescent staining, indicating the presence of hyaluronate protein in the lining of cells of the synovial membrane following application of rabbit antiserum to hyaluronate protein and a fluorescein-labeled antiserum to rabbit gammaglobulin. They concluded that the protein moiety of hyaluronate protein is not a serum protein and that it is presumably synthesized with the hyaluronate in the synovial lining cells. *Hyaluronidase,* an enzyme, is capable of degrading hyaluronate and thus reducing viscosity.

By radioactive labeling and tissue culture techniques, Castor in 1957 demonstrated the production of hyaluronate by synovial cells. However, the specific cell-producing hyaluronate is not yet identified, but it has been suggested that the inner lining cells—type A cells—as well as external cells—type B cells—are the most likely sources of synthesis.

Normal synovial fluid contains an average of 60 cells per milliliter. *Most of the cells are synovial lining cells, lymphocytes, monocytes, and polymorphonuclear leukocytes.* However, more than 2% of polymorphonuclear leukocytes should be considered abnormal. In addition to cellular elements, amorphous particles, probably arising from articular cartilage, are common findings. The synovial fluid appears to be true dialysate of blood in which mucin and some cells are deposited. The concentration of chloride, bicarbonate, calcium, acid, and alkaline phosphate is slightly higher than in normal serum, but the concentration of nonprotein nitrogen, uric acid, and glucose is equal in synovial fluid and serum (Table 3-3).

The synovial tissue, in addition to its unique physiologic role to produce mucin and to regulate the exchange of substances between the blood, lymph, and synovial fluid, has certain peculiar structural properties. It is rich in blood and lymphatic vessels and poor in stromal connective tissue. The lymphatic vessels have a branching polygonal pattern with numerous large lacunae which drain to the regional lymph nodes. The propensity of synovial cells is to form clefts and villi. *The synovial cells have no basement membrane* and are embedded in a loose matrix whose apparent role is to regulate diffusion of plasma solutes across the synovial membrane.

The synovial tissue of articular surfaces, bursae, and tendon sheaths are being constantly traumatized either from outside or by constant wear and tear of motion. It is further damaged by inflammatory and degenerative diseases. The susceptibility of synovial cells to trauma, inflammation, and infection may produce a host of histologic and functional changes. It is not surprising, therefore, that non-neoplastic, as well as neoplastic, lesions of the synovial tissue defied satisfactory classification and even today there is uncertainty about the origin, pathophysiology, and the nature of many of the synovial lesions (Fig. 3-1).

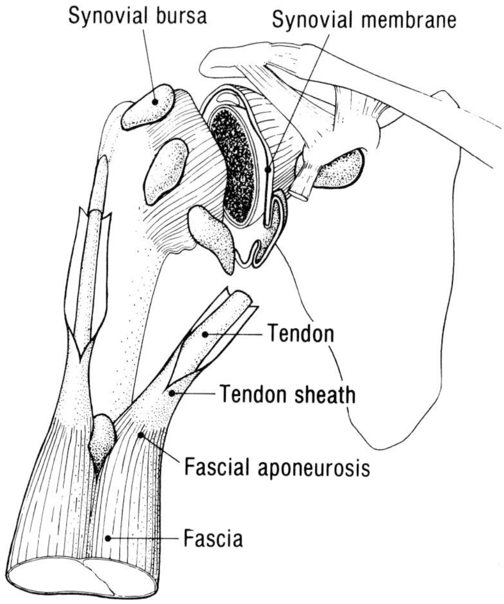

Figure 3-1. The tendosynovial tissue is almost ubiquitous in the human body. Benign or malignant tendosynovial lesions may arise from any of the structures (see also Figure 3-6).

NON-NEOPLASTIC LESIONS

TENDOSYNOVIAL CYST*

The tendosynovial cyst or ganglion is a thin-walled, tumor-like cystic lesion found almost always in direct continuity with the joint capsule, bursa, or tendon sheath. The lumen is filled with colorless viscous fluid. This cyst has a predilection to hands, wrists, and feet. The first reference in writings to synovial cysts is credited to Hippocrates: "certain flabby ganglionic tumors . . . containing only a mucoid flesh." They are called either ganglions or synovial cysts except the popliteal ones which are commonly referred to as *Baker's cyst* (Gristma and Wilson, 1964).

Theories about the etiology range from retention cyst and herniation of tendosynovial tissue to trauma. The exact nature of synovial cyst remains obscure. However, one of the most popular theories is that *any condition capable of producing synovial effusion can produce synovial cyst* by permitting protrusion of synovial tissue (Bowerman and Muhletaler, 1973). Jayson and Dixon (1970) demonstrated by arthrography with radiopaque dyes that the synovial fluid is able to exit from the joint or tendon sheath through a valvular mechanism into the cyst and not return. Taylor and Rana (1973) came to the same conclusion. This "valve" theory seems to be supported by the fact that some of the synovial cysts increase in size on joint motion and diminish if the joint is immobilized for a while.

Clark, in 1908, was the first to study the pathogenesis of synovial cysts. Carp and Stout, in 1928, collected reports of 255 cases and came to the conclusion that these cysts are caused by mucinous degeneration of connective tissue in close

**Synonyms and related terms:* synovial cyst, ganglion, Baker's cyst, bursal cyst, cyst of joint capsule, cyst of tendon sheath, mucinous cyst, myxomatous synovitis, cystic myxoma, mucinous tumor.

proximity to joints and tendon sheaths. Others believe that synovial cysts are the product of proliferation rather than degeneration.

The wall of the cyst is almost invariably composed of an outer dense fibrous layer and an inner myxoid layer forming clefts and acellular villi. It is not uncommon to find microscopic areas of neoplastic chondroid and osteoid tissues or nests of calcification.

Synovial cysts may occur at almost any location, but the distal parts of the extremities are the most common sites. On the hand, they occur most commonly either dorsocarpally or in the volar surface of the wrist. Among the more than 720 ganglion cysts reported there were only 150 in a lower extremity and only 30 in a foot.

The synovial cyst is a disease of the middle-aged, and females outnumber males approximately two to one. According to Dao (1964) 35% of the patients give a history of previous trauma. The size of the average cyst is 2 cm, but the size may fluctuate and the cyst may completely disappear temporarily. It is usually an encapsulated, globoid mass with smaller adjacent cysts.

The synovial cyst may produce osseous deformity by erosion of the cortical bone with subsequent appearance of a homogeneous, well-defined *intraosseous cystic* lesion. Hicks, in 1956, is credited with the first 3 case reports of this peculiar cystic lesion in bone. Since then, 28 cases of intraosseous synovial cysts have been reported. Sim and Dahlin (1971) added 6 new cases and suggested considering this lesion when one is confronted with any solitary cyst of bone. The common feature of intraosseous cysts is their close proximity to adjacent joints and their subchondral locations. The majority of the reported lesions occurred in the distal tibia (13 cases) and talus (3 cases), but other bones such as the malleolus, distal ulna, and carpal bones are also cited in reports (Table 3-2; Fig. 3-2A-D).

The treatment of both intra- and extraosseous synovial cysts should be conservative surgery. Prognosis is favorable and they do not tend to recur after surgical excision. According to reports, more than half of the synovial cysts of soft parts resolve spontaneously without therapy.

In differential diagnosis one should consider *myxoma* (see Chapter 2), *fibroblastic lipoma* (see Chapter 4), *neuroma* (see Chapter 7) and *epidermal inclusion cyst*. If there is erosion into bone or an intraosseous presentation, the lesion may look more alarming on the radiograph than on tissue section. Of course, in these situations genuine *bone cysts* and *chondroblastoma* should also be considered in the differential diagnosis.

TENDOSYNOVITIS*

The term *synovitis* is applied to a number of reactive processes involving the

* *Synonyms and related terms:* tenosynovitis, synovitis, tendonitis.

TABLE 3-2. ***Certain Characteristics of Tendosynovial Lesions***

	AVG. AGE	PREDOMINANCE	MOST COMMON SITES
Tendosynovial cyst	48	Female	Dorsum of wrist
Synovial osteo-chondromatosis	32	Male	Knee Elbow
Giant cell tumor of tendon sheath	37	Female	Digits Ankle
Tendosynovial sarcoma	33	Male	Thigh Foot

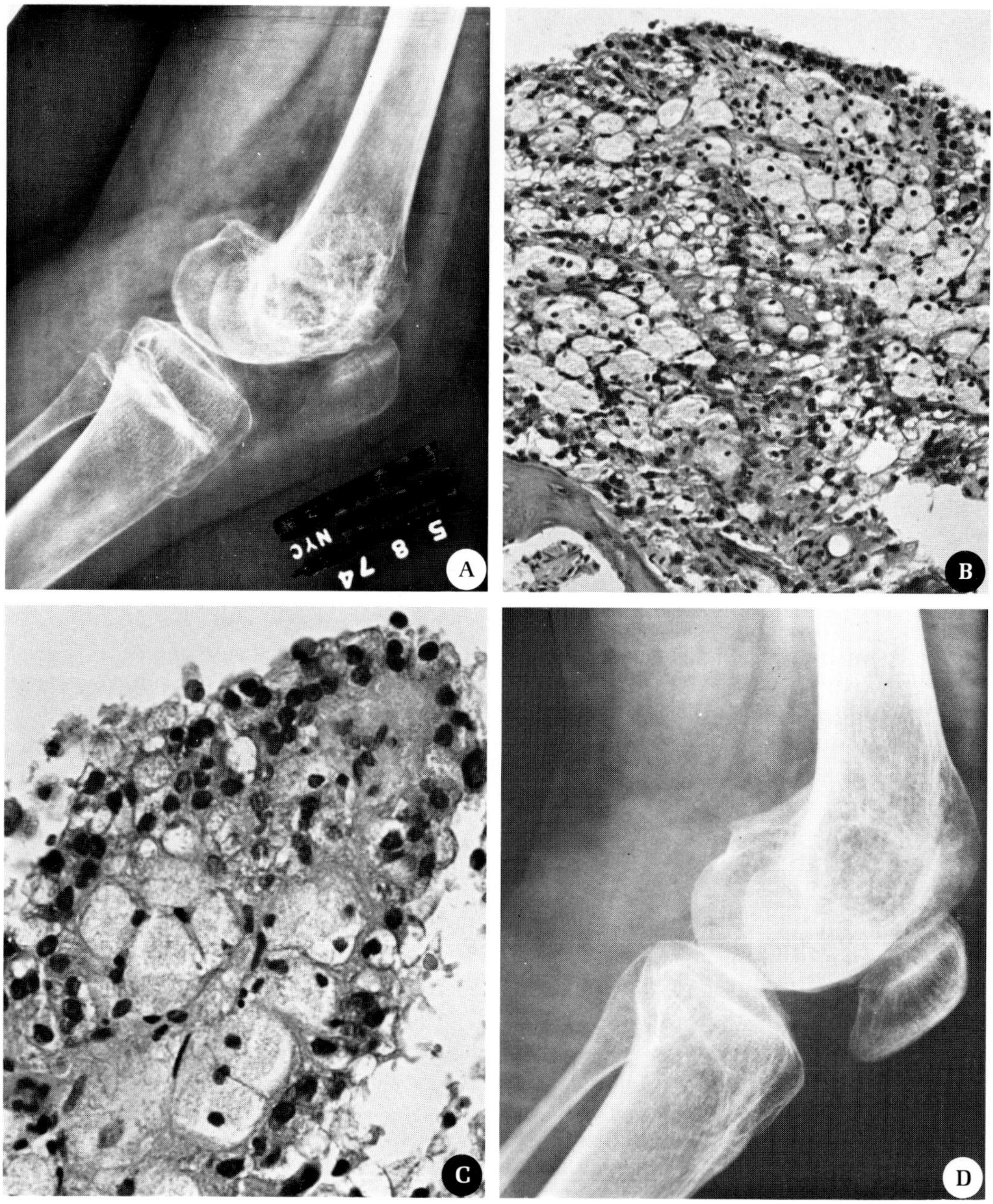

Figure 3-2. Intraosseous synovial cyst.

A, A poorly defined cystic lesion was found in the right distal femur of a 14-year-old girl who had pain in the right knee.

B, C, The lesion was curetted and histologically it was composed of clear foam cells in sheets and papillary structures. Small cuboidal or round cells form a distinct lining about the papillae and sheets which communicate with intraosseous cystic cavities (**A,** H & E, ×140; **B,** H & E, ×350).

D, Four years after initial diagnosis and curettage only slight sclerosis is seen at the site of the cyst.

synovial membrane, tendon sheath, and bursae. It may result from traumatic injury, infection, or reactive and degenerative processes. Jones and Carter showed in 1957 that proliferative synovitis can be induced in guinea pigs by the injection of bacterial polysaccharides. Page-Thomas et al, in 1960, injected a number of polysaccharides into the femorotibial joints of rabbits and found that the maximum proliferation of synovial cells was obtained by injection of carrageenin and agaropectin. These injections produced a spectrum of functional and morphologic alteration as well as changes of the color, consistency, and composition of the synovial fluid.

Reactive synovial cells are much larger than the normal ones and are embedded in richly mucinous stroma. In suppurative processes the synovial tissue is partly replaced by inflammatory cells and granulation tissue.

Malinin et al (1966) observed an increased number of intracytoplasmic sudanophilic vacuoles in polymorphonuclear leukocytes of synovial fluid obtained from patients with joint diseases of various etiologies but especially in effusions of inflammatory nature. Barthel et al (1972) observed by histochemical techniques that the site of increased enzyme activity in synovial fluid in infection was the synovial lining cells. The cytologic morphology of synovial fluid has been studied by, among others, Naib (1973) and Broderich et al (1976) (Table 3-3).

The biochemical events in joint diseases were summarized by Hamerman et al in 1963. In the last two decades voluminous information has accumulated from studies on joint components using biochemical, cytochemical, immunologic, histologic, and ultrastructural techniques.

In *rheumatoid arthritis*, for example, excessive proliferation of lining cells is associated with disorderly arrangement of hypertrophic villi and formation of follicle-free lymphoid nodules. It is also possible to demonstrate with the electron microscope a number of changes, e.g., abnormal mitochondria, dense granules, large cytoplasmic vacuoles, and small Golgi sacs. Admittedly none of the observed morphologic changes can be accepted as specific for rheumatoid arthritis. As Sherman (1951) said, "Every feature of the morbid anatomy of rheumatoid arthritis may be demonstrated in joints which are not involved by rheumatoid arthritis." On the other hand, demonstration of *rheumatoid factor* in the synovial membrane by fluorescent technique is considered a specific test for the diagnosis of rheumatoid arthritis. Dryll et al (1977) went one step further and found that there is a difference in the distribution of immunoglobulins (IgG and IgM) in normal and rheumatoid synovial membrane. They were able to demonstrate IgM in intravascular spaces only in control biopsies, but in rheumatoid synovitis immunoglobulins were present in both intravascular and extravascular spaces.

In *gouty arthritis* the synovial membrane, bursae, and occasionally the tendons are the sites of uric-acid deposits. The first description of urate crystals in a tophus is credited to Leeuwenhoek in 1679. The urate crystals are demonstrable by polarizing microscopy and electron microscopy. Tissue sections, however, should be placed in absolute alcohol rather than in formalin to prevent dissolving of the urate crystals. Lenz et al (1976) refined these techniques and were able to distinguish gout and pseudogout by distinguishing urate and calcium phosphate crystals (Table 3-3; Fig. 3-2, E, F, G, H, and I).

Granulomatous synovitis may be caused by acid-fast bacilli and various fungi. Sporotrichosis is rarely considered in the diagnosis of granulomatous synovitis. Marrocco et al (1975) reported two cases and emphasized that the organisms are difficult to demonstrate in direct smear and tissue sections, but they grow readily on routine culture media.

SYNOVIAL CHONDROMATOSIS*

Synovial chondromatosis is a rare monoarticular arthropathy of unknown etiology. It is characterized by multiple cartilaginous and osteocartilaginous nodules of the synovium and loose bodies in the joint.

Cruveilhier, in 1829, was apparently the first to describe a case of synovial

* *Synonyms and related terms:* synovial chondrometaplasia, osteochondritis dissecans, synovial chondrosis, loose bodies, articular chondrosis, osteochondromatosis.

TABLE 3-3. ***Cytology of Synovial Fluid***

	APPEARANCE	VOLUME	VISCOSITY	FIBRIN CLOT	MUCIN CLOT	NO. OF POLYS (%)	SYNOVIAL CELLS	CRYSTALS	DIFFERENCE BETWEEN SERUM & FLUID SUGAR CONCENTRATION (mg/100 ml)
Normal	Clear	Scanty	235	0	Normal	7	Sparse	0	<10
Traumatic arthritis	Hemorrhagic	Variable	Increased	+	Positive	5	Variable	0	5
Rheumatoid arthritis	Yellow	Variable	Decreased	+++	Poor	65	Sparse	Choles- terol	25
Osteoar- thritis	Yellow	Scanty	Normal	+	Normal	15	Numerous	0	10
Gouty arthritis	Yellow	Variable	Variable	+++	Poor	70	Sparse	Urate	10
Septic arthritis	Purulent	Increased	Decreased	++	Poor	60	Sparse	0	60
Pigmented villonodular synovitis	Brown	Variable	Variable	++	Variable	10	Aggregates	0	25

+++ = most common; ++ = common; + = uncommon.

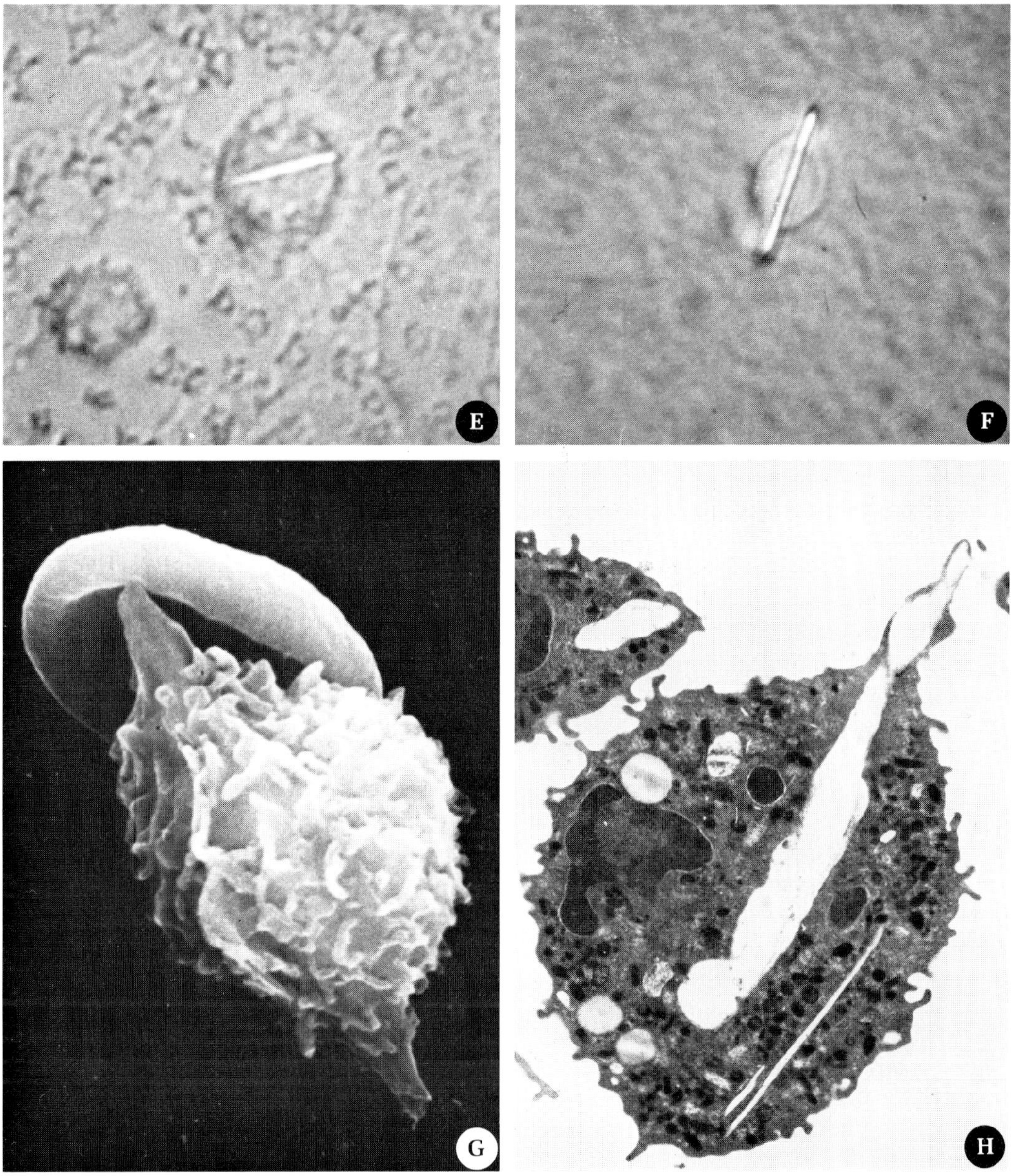

Figure 3-2 (cont.). Urate **(E)** and pyrophosphate crystals **(F)** piercing the cells, so-called stick in olive phenomenon (×600).

G, Pyrophosphate crystal piercing a cell in synovial fluid sediment (×9,500).

H, Leukocytes of synovial fluid sediment in gout with needle-shaped crystal clefts (×6,800). (Courtesy of Gustav Fischer Verlag, Stuttgart, from Lenz, W., et al: Beitr. Pathol. Bd. 157:161, 1976.)

chondromatosis. Wilks, in 1859, gave the first concise description of this condition: "Inside of joints under inflammation present fringe-like processes hanging down into it; some of these become very large and pedunculated. Their structure is fibro-cartilage and may contain bony deposit."

Synovial chondromatosis or osteochondromatosis is the subject of numerous case reports. The largest single series of 136 cases was reported by Villacin et al in 1979. According to Trias and Quintana (1976) there were 137 reported cases in the world literature up to 1974 to which they added 18 cases from the Canadian literature.

Knee, elbow, and hip of middle-aged and young adults are the most commonly involved sites, but involvement of other joints has been reported. According to Akhtar et al (1977) only 8 cases have been reported in the temporomandibular joint. It has a male predominance and pain is the most common symptom.

There is no agreement as to the cause of synovial chondromatosis. Osteochondromatosis may be seen in a wide variety of disturbances of the synovial membrane of joints and bursae. Infection, trauma, and metaplastic transformation of synovial tissues are considered most commonly in the etiology. The radiologic appearance of the joint is suggestive, but histologic proof of cartilage production is necessary to confirm the diagnosis. Villacin et al (1979) subclassified, on the basis of microscopic appearance, 136 cases of synovial chondromatosis and concluded that the so-called primary lesions (10 cases) were locally aggressive and 6 recurred after excision. Secondary lesions (126 cases), on the other hand, were nonaggressive.

Synovial osteochondromatosis progresses through various stages of activity. The process of formation begins with the appearance of collagenous plaques in hypertrophic synovial tissue. These plaques serve as ground to metaplastic cartilaginous transformation. Subsequently calcium salts are deposited. These deposits are followed by the ingrowth of capillaries and conversion of mesenchymal cells to osteoblasts by endochondral ossification. Another possible way is perhaps calcification and ossification of fibrin or excessive mucinous material.

Once the basic structure, the fibrocartilaginous core, is formed, finger-like projections protrude into the articular cavity and may detach. The joint may contain hundreds of small grayish-blue, pearl-shaped chondroid particles some of which are attached to or embedded in the synovial membrane (Fig. 3-2J and K).

On one occasion Robineau (1919) counted up to 1,200 loose bodies in one joint. The loose bodies have a clear center and a shell of calcification and may appear in the typical attached, grape-like formation. Secondary osteoarthritis and severe synovitis may result from the presence of loose bodies.

Although a few isolated cases of malignant transformation to chondrosarcoma have been reported (Reimann and Kienbock, 1931; Nixon et al, 1960; Goldman and Lichtenstein, 1964), it is doubted whether the chondrosarcoma actually originated in chondromatosis. Murphy et al (1962) studied 32 patients and Villacin et al (1979) reviewed the records of 136 patients with synovial chondromatosis, none of whom showed malignant changes on long-term follow-up (see Chapter 8).

The treatment should be conservative synovectomy with removal of all diseased tissues, including the loose bodies.

NEOPLASTIC LESIONS

FIBROMA AND LIPOMA

Fibroma and lipoma are rare benign tumors that may arise from a tendon, tendon sheath, joint capsule, or bursa. They are occasionally multiple and may pose a considerable problem in diagnosis. Fibromas, and not uncommonly lipomas, appear in the distal part of the extremities, especially the fingers, wrist, and forearm (see Chapter 2). Lipomas may be the arborescent type with numerous villi (see Chapter 4). Simple surgical excision with a clean margin is adequate therapy in most instances.

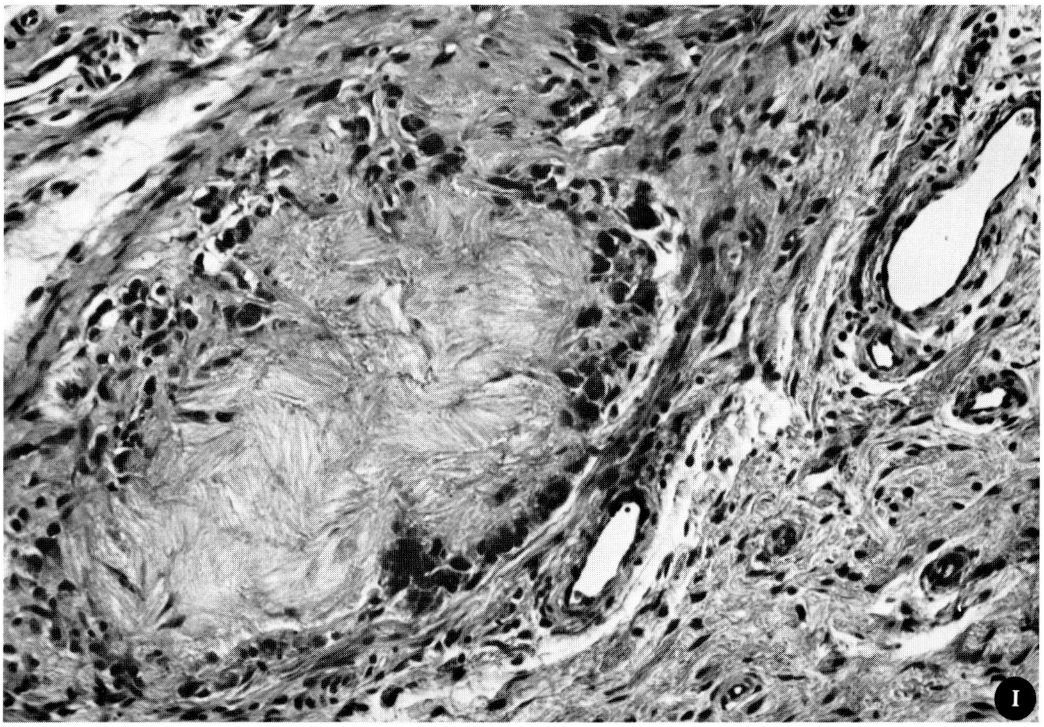

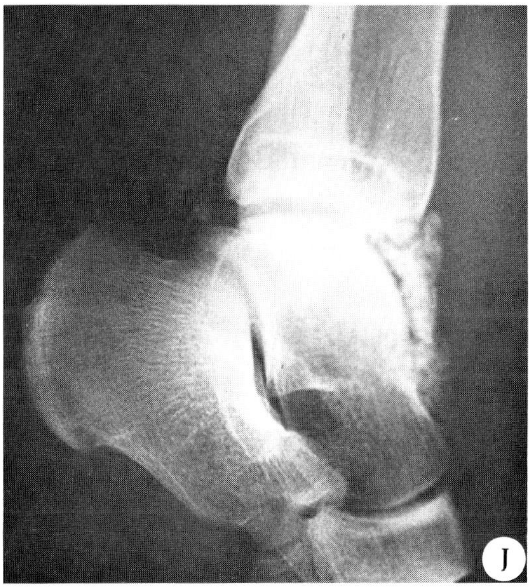

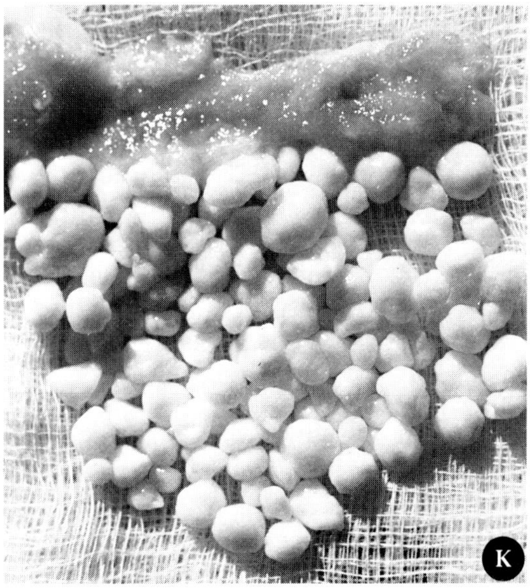

Fig 3-2 (cont.). I, This multinodular mass of inflamed tissues and conglomerate of urate crystals was excised from the elbow of an elderly male with a long history of gout (H & E, ×140).

J, Radiopaque loose bodies demonstrable in a lateral roentgenogram of the ankle two months following initial injury.

K, Gross pathologic specimen consisting of hypertrophied synovium, synovial ectopic chondroid formation, and multiple cartilaginous loose bodies. Primary synovial chondromatosis of the ankle. (Courtesy Holm, C. L.: J. Bone Joint Surg. 58A:878, 1976.)

VILLONODULAR SYNOVITIS AND GIANT CELL TUMOR*

The first reference to villonodular synovitis or giant cell tumor of the tendon sheath is attributed to Chassaignac (1852). The first microscopic description given by Wells (1857) and Wilks (1859) called attention to "fringe-like" processes inside joints.

The first good description of multinucleated epulis-type giant cells, fusiform mononuclear cells, and pigment in a "fibrosarcoma" excised from the tendon sheath of a finger of a 20-year-old woman was given by Czerny in 1869. It was Robin in 1849, who discovered the *myeloplaxes* or *multinucleated giant cells* in the bone marrow. Whether he referred to epulis-type giant cells or actually had seen megakaryocytes cannot be stated with certainty, but it is a historical fact that Rustizky, in 1874, emphasized the role of giant cells in resorption of bone (*osteoclasts*).

Because the cellular elements in these soft tissue lesions resemble components of bone marrow, Broca (1860) named these tumors *tumeur a myeloplaxes* (giant cell tumor). Following this example Gross (1878) reported a case of "myeloid sarcoma" of the left hand of a 17-year-old girl which he described microscopically as "sarcome globo-cellular." Heurtaux (1891), who called all tumors containing giant cells myelome, is credited with the first review of reported cases of giant cell tumors. He pointed out that not all neoplasms containing giant cells are sarcomas, contrary to the belief of Paget who said that "myeloid tumors are the ones in which many nucleated corpuscles are a constant and essential constituent and belong to the *genus sarcoma*."

**Synonyms and related terms:* benign synovioma, pigmented villonodular synovitis, giant cell tumor of tendon sheath, benign giant cell tumor, synovial xanthoma, synovial xanthogranuloma, fibrous histiocytoma, pseudoxanthoma, synovial histiocytoma, myeloplaxoma, polymorphocellular tumor, myeloxanthoma.

The term *myeloplaxe tumor* was adopted by the French writers one after the other (Bonjour, 1897; Venot, 1898) and Dor, in 1898, called attention to a possible relationship between giant cell tumors and xanthomas. He believed that the presence of both xanthomatous (foam cells) and giant cells in the same tumor resulted from different morphologic development of originally identical cells. About the same time another French writer, Bonjour (1897) came to the conclusion that giant cell tumors should be divided into two categories: *fibrous or tendinous origin and osseous origin,* but he concluded erroneously that the mother cell of these distinct lesions originated in the medullary tissues of bones. Despite his error, bone pathologists today should remember his study when they conclude that giant cell tumors of bone and aneurysmal bone cysts are not similar to giant cell tumors of tendon sheaths and pigmented villonodular synovitis. Buxton (1923) felt that *giant cell tumors of tendons are the same as those found in long bones.* It is of historical interest that studying of these tumors up to the turn of the century was undertaken almost exclusively by French pathologists. Later the German authors became interested in these tumors without accepting the French terms *myeloma* and *myeloplax.* They advanced the names *xanthoma, xanthosarcoma* and *giant-celled sarcoma,* not knowing that it was a French pathologist, Lebert, in 1845, who first introduced the term *xanthoma* and another Frenchman Tomaselli (1901) who described a tumor of the foot he called *giant cell sarcoma.*

In 1918 a case of giant cell tumor of the peroneal tendon associated with, but not connected with, giant cell tumor of the distal end of the fibula was reported by Ely. Levy (1925) suggested that giant cell tumors are variants of xanthomas (histiocytomas), and Thannhauser and Magendantz (1938) thought it was warranted to group together tendon sheath tumors and xanthomas. Krogins (1922) suggested the name of *xanthosarcoma* and expressed the opinion that although growths on the fingers are benign, those on the forearm and feet are apt to be malignant.

The confusion about these lesions is evidenced by the variety of names given to them. Jaffe et al, in 1941, in an attempt to simplify the terminology, adopted the term *villonodular* coined by Henle in 1865, and proposed the names *pigmented villonodular synovitis, tenosynovitis,* and *bursitis.* They felt it is further warranted to subdivide each group for either *diffuse* or *nodular* form. Needless to say, this classification added to the already existing confusion and resulted in the situation which exists today in reference to classification and understanding of villonodular and giant cell lesions.

At present there are two different interpretations of the nature of these lesions: one classifies them as neoplasms; another considers them inflammatory or reactive lesions. My view is that *villonodular synovitis and giant cell tumor of the tendon sheath are different morphologic stages of the same process,* analogous to the well-known progression of certain epithelial hyperplasia to papilloma, adenoma, or even carcinoma.

All clinical and morphologic evidence suggests that the earliest phase of the giant cell tumor of tendon sheaths is a villous, nodular, and vascular proliferative growth. Later certain cells will act like facultative fibroblasts and phagocytize lipid and hemosiderin while others will fuse with each other to form multinucleated giant cells (Fig. 2-37). At certain anatomic sites this transition, from villous to giant cell form, is made more readily than at other sites. The facts that in most cases there is no evidence of infection, polymorphonuclear leukocytes, or systemic disease, that no known inflammatory disease induces similar changes, that occasionally (10%) these lesions recur after local excision, and that malignant transformation may take place support their neoplastic nature. Among the numerous proponents of the neoplastic theory can be listed Broders, 1919; Buxton, 1923; Berger, 1938; Ewing, 1942; Stewart, 1948; Spencer and Whimster, 1950; Wright, 1951; Phalen et al, 1959; Jones et al, 1969; Salm and Sissons, 1972 and Patchefsky et al, 1977. Foster (1947) compared giant cell tumor of the tendon sheath with sclerosing hemangioma (see Chapter 2) and Berger as early as 1938 stressed that giant cell lesions are the result of the *histiocytic potentialities of synovial tissue.*

I believe that there are distinct similarities between the nodular lesions of the so-called pigmented villonodular synovitis and giant cell tumor of the tendon sheath. In fact, if one has the opportunity to study an adequate number of cases from each of these lesions, so many features in common will be revealed that the similarity of growth cannot be questioned. The apparent morphologic differences can be readily explained by dissimilarities in the anatomic structures in which the lesions develop; e.g., villonodular synovitis is found most commonly in joints and bursae and giant cell tumors in tendon sheath. In conclusion, *pigmented villonodular synovitis and giant cell tumor of the tendon sheath are but slightly different manifestations of the same neoplastic process* and can be considered together.

Despite the fact that the term *pigmented villonodular synovitis* is misleading and inappropriate because it implies inflammatory origin, perhaps it should be retained for giant cell tumors that spread over a broad surface and have an unusually heavy complement of inflammatory and foam cells at the expense of multinucleated giant cells and be considered as a precursor of giant cell tumor just as dysplasia or epithelial hyperplasia is often the precursor of intraepithelial neoplasia. It seems that the histologic distinction between pigmented villonodular synovitis and giant cell tumor is empirical (Table 3-4).

There is no known etiology of these lesions. Adults in the third and fifth decades are affected most often. The lesions seldom occur in persons under the age of

TABLE 3-4. *Some Reported Series of Villonodular Synovitis and Giant Cell Tumor of Tendon Sheath*

AUTHORS	NUMBER OF CASES	MOST COMMON SITES	RECURRENCE %	BONE INVOLVEMENT %
Galloway et al (1940)	270	Finger Hand	12	—
Foster (1947)	42	Finger	8	—
Stewart (1948)	40	Finger Foot	—	—
Phalen et al (1959)	56	Finger Hand	20	—
Byers et al (1968)	126	Knee Finger	—	15
Gehweiler and Wilson (1969)	300	Knee Hip Ankle	—	—
Jones et al (1969)	118	Finger Knee Hand	18	11

10 years or over the age of 60. Most of the review articles state an equal incidence in males and females. It is a rare monoarthritic disease, but according to estimates it is the second most common tumor of the synovium. Benign giant cell tumors with ganglia comprise the majority of subcutaneous tumors of the hands and feet. In the digits, they may occur on both flexor and extensor aspects, but the index and middle fingers are involved more often than any other fingers. Of the larger joints, the knee, hip, ankle, and elbow are the most commonly affected sites. A number of typical villonodular or giant cell tumors of the temporomandibular joint have been reported (Byers et al, 1968; Lapayowker et al, 1973; Miyamoto et al, 1977). Arthaud (1972) reported 11 cases in *nonarticular locations*. They are usually slowly growing, painless, but tender lesions often associated with considerable swelling.

The gross size of giant cell tumors is frequently determined by their location. In the fingers they rarely grow bigger than 1 or 2 cm, but more proximally they may be as big as 10 or 15 cm. They have an expansile growth pattern and usually appear gray or yellowish in color. The cut sections may show a distinct nodular or villous distribution of solid semifirm areas with irregular patches of hemorrhagic soft areas (Fig. 3-3).

On radiographic examination one may see a soft nonspecific density and possibly erosion or a cyst in adjacent bones. It has been stated (Gehweiler and Wilson, 1969) that about 50% of the giant cell tumors will show bony changes in the form of one or more discrete intraosseous cystic lesions with sclerotic margins most commonly subchondrally and juxta-articularly. The surrounding bone is of normal density and the joint space is preserved in most cases.

Snook (1963) reported two cases with bony involvement and stated that until 1963 only 16 cases of villonodular synovitis with bony invasion had been reported. Most authors consider this number an understatement. For example, Smith and Pugh (1962), reporting their experience with 50 cases of villonodular synovitis, stated that about 50% of the cases studied showed some degree of bone destruction.

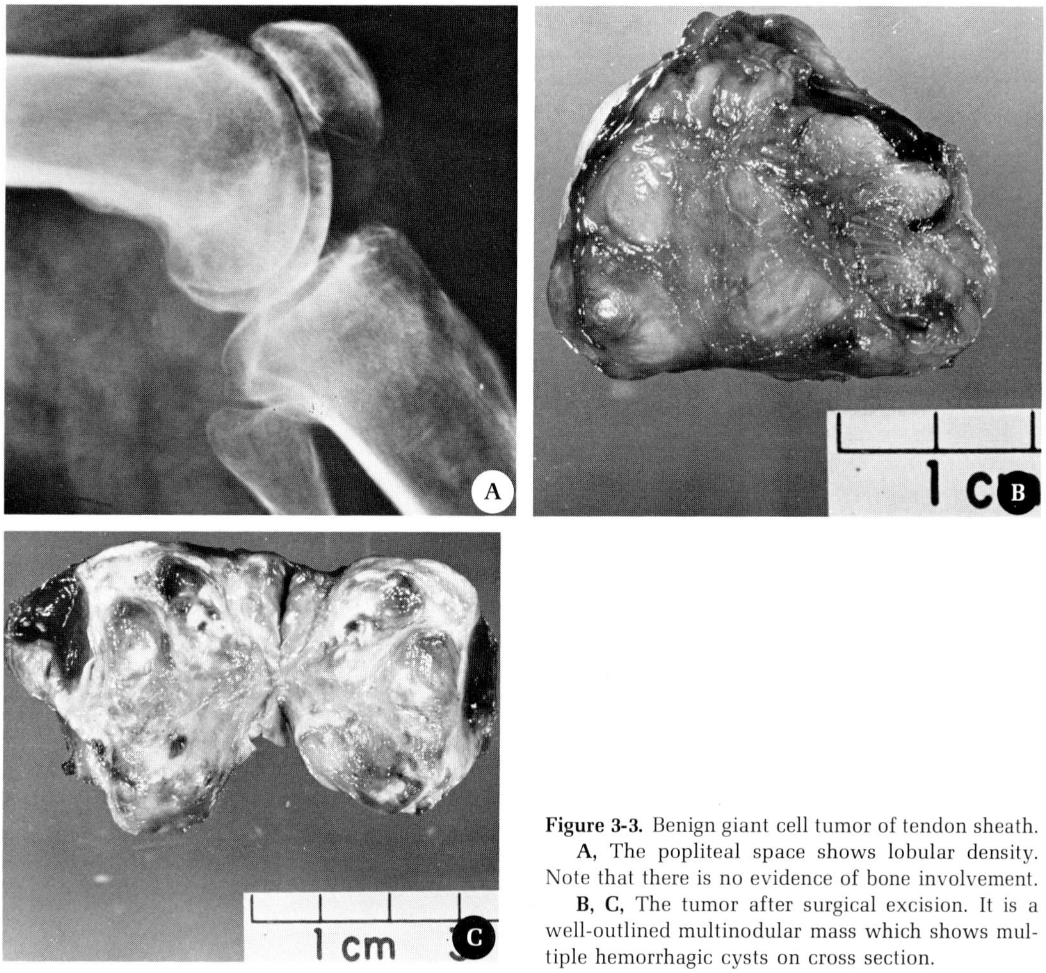

Figure 3-3. Benign giant cell tumor of tendon sheath. **A,** The popliteal space shows lobular density. Note that there is no evidence of bone involvement. **B, C,** The tumor after surgical excision. It is a well-outlined multinodular mass which shows multiple hemorrhagic cysts on cross section.

In the Latin American Register of Bone Pathology, Schajowicz and Blumenfeld (1968) found reports of 52 cases of villonodular synovitis with invasion of one or more bones.

It seems the ability of villonodular synovitis and giant cell tumor to erode bone by pressure is well established, but only rare instances of complete destruction of a phalanx or other small bone have been reported (Feinstein and Rubin, 1973). Since the first report of Suter in 1905, a digital tumor for which the distal phalanx was amputated because of erosion of bone by the tumor, more than 120 cases of villonodular synovitis and giant cell tumor with bone invasion have been reported. Among the many theories proposed to explain how these lesions affect bone, the most attractive ones are direct pressure erosion and invasion through vascular foramina.

Hicks, in 1956, is credited with the first reporting of 3 cases of synovial cysts in bone without any evidence of related lesion in the adjacent soft parts. According to Sim and Dahlin (1971) 28 cases of intraosseous synovial cysts have been reported to which they added their own six cases (see Fig. 3-2).

Microscopically these lesions are characterized by matted villous hyperplasia and development of multilayers of epithelioid cells of the synovial lining which may cover slit-like cavities and synovial clefts to give a lobular or nodular appearance to many of these lesions. Additional characteristics are the appearance of foam cells and multinucleated giant cells. During the early stage of growth and at certain locations, there are more villi and fewer giant cells than in long-standing lesions. The villous or cystic form can be monolocular with solitary papillary projection or diffuse with most of the synovial membrane covered by villonodular outgrowths. The linings of the villi are usually several layers thick and are formed by connective tissue cells of the stroma. Many of the foam cells may contain pigment and possibly lipids in the form of cholesterol esters. Stromal cells, as well as giant cells, may also contain intracytoplasmic phagocytized hemosiderin resulting from the breakdown of erythrocytes. Rarely, one may see intra- or extracellular cholesterol clefts. To refer to foam cells as "xanthoma cells" or "xanthomatous cells" is unfortunate. *Xanthoma* means a specific neoplasm of such cells. Many different types of cells—histiocytes, fibroblasts, endothelial cells, adipocytes, glial cells, as well as epithelial cells—are capable of accumulating lipids in various conditions.

There is a wide variation in the proportion of the three main cell types—spindle and polygonal stromal cells, multinucleated epulis giant cells, and lipid-laden foam cells—from lesion to lesion. The spindle cells or oval cells may appear as a fine meshwork with interlacing plump or round foam cells. As many as 50 multinucleated epulis-type giant cells can be seen occasionally in a single low-power microscopic field. Some of these cells may contain up to 50 or 100 nuclei. At times the nuclei may be arranged in the form of a crescent at one end; at other times they may be in an annulus or ring at the periphery of the cell; at others they occupy the central part of the cell (Figs. 3-4, 3-5). The presence of epulis-type giant cells can be easily demonstrated in air-dried and H & E stained imprint smears prepared from the cut surface of the lesion (Hajdu and Hajdu, 1976).

Broders (1919) and Ewing (1922) sug-

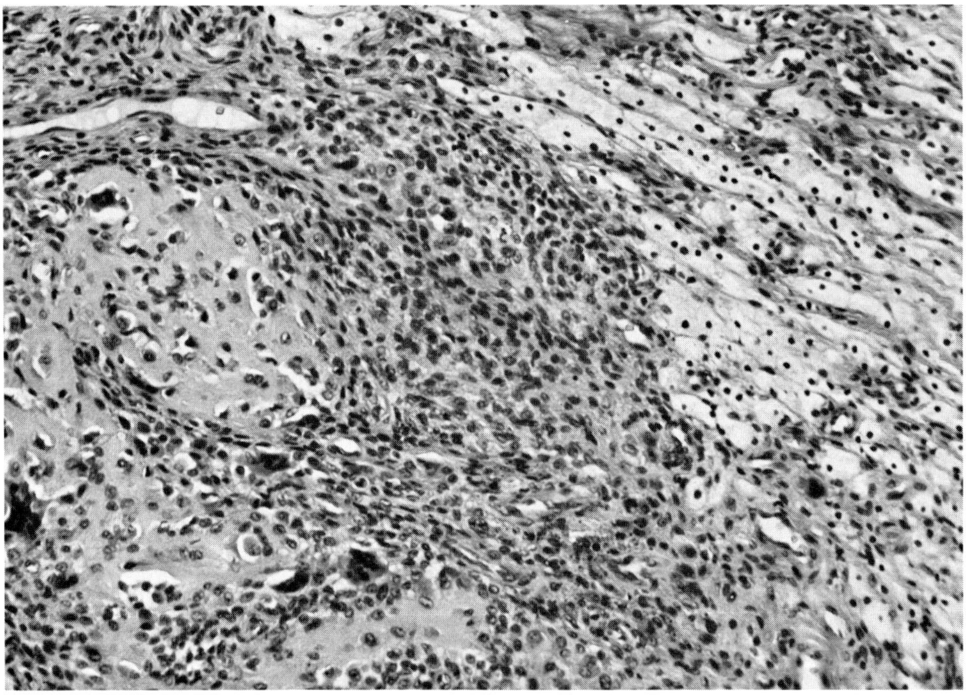

Figure 3-4. Section from the inner or stromal part of a papillary projection of so-called villonodular synovitis. Note the intimate blending of histiocytic foam cells, stromal round cells and small inflammatory cells. Also notice a few epulis type giant cells in an area of chondroid metaplasia (left lower corner) (H & E, $\times 140$).

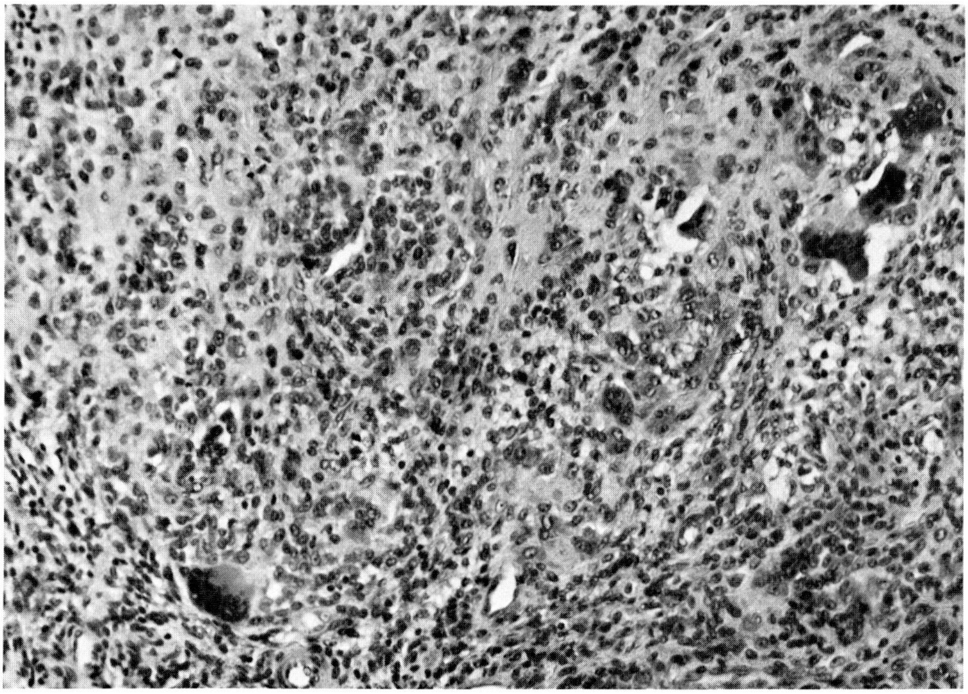

Figure 3-5. Benign giant cell tumor of the right knee. Most of the cells are small round or oval "stromal" histiocytic forms. Numerous well-formed or abortive epulis type giant cells are scattered throughout the tumor. Note the striking similarity to Figures 3-4 and 2-40 (H & E ×140).

gested that the purpose of the giant cells is to phagocytize foreign material. They spoke of the cells' morphologic resemblance to the osteoclasts and pointed out the similarity of these giant cells to those found in giant cell tumors of bones and gums and those associated with granulomatous diseases. Close resemblance of giant cell tumors of tendon sheaths and soft tissues to giant cell tumors of bone is indeed so striking that one immediately thinks of an identical histogenesis.

Multinucleated giant cells are found in numerous benign and malignant neoplasms (see Chapter 2). There is now substantial evidence that *multinucleated cells are the result of fusion of mononuclear cells* and are not produced by amitotic division or endoreduplication of nuclear material. Endoreduplication or amitotic division would require the presence of pairs of centrioles close to each of the nuclei within multinucleated cells at all times. According to Sapp (1976), further mitotic activity is unlikely because the centrioles in fused cells move to a common centrosphere and the nuclei aggregate in another area (see Fig. 2-37).

The mechanism for the clustering of centrioles is unknown; however, Holmes and Choppin (1968), using time-lapse cinematography, were able to show, in tissue culture of virus-infected tissues, that microtubules and spindle fibers play a prominent role in the establishment of various nuclear arrangements seen in multinucleated cells. In giant cells of the epulis type, one giant centrosphere with multiple centrioles is usually located in the nucleus-free area of the cytoplasm. In the so-called foreign body giant cells, according to Sapp (1976), the centrosphere is close to foreign material, and in Langhans' giant cells the centrosphere is constantly in the nucleus-free central zone.

Mariano and Spector, in 1974, studied the formation of giant cells by autoradiography, cytogenetic, and diffusion chamber techniques. They concluded that fusion of cells is the most important process in giant cell formation. Black and Epstein (1974) produced mesenchymal giant cells by injection of zirconium and beryllium and concluded that certain cells can produce a "giant cell factor" which recruits mononuclear cells, perhaps defective or abnormal cells, to fuse with each other in an attempt to eliminate or get rid of them. The fact that giant cells are short-lived may indeed suggest that the formation of giant cells is an efficient disposal system for unwanted cells—cells that may be potentially dangerous or harmful to the host.

The exact factor facilitating fusion of cells is not known, but it is suspected that abnormalities in the plasma membrane and production of certain liposomal enzymes may facilitate adhesion and subsequent fusion of cells. This is further facilitated by intertwining of long cytoplasmic villi of adjacent cells with subsequently less plasma membranes (see Fig. 2-37).

Giant cells of the foreign body and epulis types tend to form earlier than giant cells of the Langhans' or Touton type, and it is possible that the Langhans' cells are formed by maturation of foreign body giant cells (see Chapter 2). According to Mariano and Spector (1974), colchicine inhibits the formation of Langhans' cells; therefore, they are dependent on the activity of intracytoplasmic microtubules.

After studying the ultrastructure of giant cell tumors, Eisenstein (1968) and Alguacil-Garcia et al (1978) concluded that these neoplasms are derived from the synovial lining cells because both type A (histiocytic) and type B (fibroblastic) cells were found in addition to foam cells and giant cells. They also found so-called intermediate forms, an indication that foam cells derive from synovial cells which have accumulated lipids. Eisenstein also felt that the giant cells are formed by fusion of type A cells and pointed out that foreign body giant cells and epulis-type giant cells contain fewer cytoplasmic organelles than Langhans' giant cells.

In some areas giant cell tumors may resemble clear cell sarcoma of tendon. In addition to the changing cellular morphology, malignant giant cell tumors differ from their benign counterparts by the presence of abundant intercellular acid mucopolysaccharide substance and almost complete absence of foam cells.

Giant cell sarcomas arising from tendon sheath have been known from the late 1800's. According to Tourneux (1913), Bilroth, in 1868, reported a case of malignant giant cell tumor which metastasized within a year and caused the death of the patient shortly after. Ten reported cases with follow-up information compiled from the literature plus four personal cases are tabulated in Table 3-5.

Giant cell tumors may recur, and recurrent tumors as a rule are more aggressive in their growth and cellularity. *When a giant cell tumor has fewer epulis-type giant cells and more mononuclear polyhedral stromal cells, the lesion should be considered atypical. When the tumor is predominantly composed of mononuclear spindle and oval cells, the type commonly seen in fibroblastic fibrous histiocytoma* (see Chapter 2) *and fibroblastic fibrosarcoma* (see Chapter 2), *it is a malignant neoplasm.* Occasionally the epulis giant cells are replaced by bizarre Touton giant cells, and the mononuclear cells show obvious pleomorphism. The mitotic index is high (1 or 2 mitoses/high-power field) and almost invariably there is evidence of invasion of surrounding soft tissues by budding or infiltrative tumor nests. However, pressure in underlying bone does not necessarily indicate a malignant tumor. It is apparent that malignant giant cell tumor of tendon sheath, despite its relatively small size, is a highly malignant neoplasm. In general, the treatment should be that usually reserved for tendosynovial sarcomas (see Fig. 2-41).

Treatment of benign giant cell tumors, however, should be conservative. Local or complete synovectomy is considered to be the best primary treatment. If bone is involved, the lesion should be curetted and the bone defect should be packed with bone chips. If a benign giant cell tumor or so-called villonodular synovitis does not

TABLE 3-5. *Malignant Giant Cell Tumor of Tendon Sheath*

AUTHORS	NO. OF CASES	AGE	SEX	SITE	RECURRENCE	THERAPY	FOLLOW-UP
DeSanto	3	25	M	Knee	yes	Exc	DcMD, 30 mo.
et al		48	M	Knee	4 mo.	Exc	Alive, 24 mo.
(1941)		46	M	Knee	12 mo.	Exc	Alive, 12 mo.
Kobak and Perlow (1949)	1	60	M	Elbow	5 mo.	Exc	DcMD, 12 mo.
Wright (1949)	1	32	M	Hand	2 mo.	Amp	Alive, 12 mo.
Bliss and Reed	3	—	—	Hand	—	Exc	DcMD, 6 mo.
(1968)		—	—	Hand	8 mo.	Amp	DcMD
		—	—	Foot	—	Amp	DcMD, 24 mo.
Gravanis	2	—	—	Hand	2 mo.	Amp	DcMD
(1968)		—	—	Arm	—	Exc	DcMD
Kahn (1973)	1	78	M	Hand	12 mo.	Amp	DcMD, 17 mo.
Hajdu	4	42	M	Hand	4 mo.	Exc	Alive, 48 mo.
(unpublished)		49	F	Wrist	—	Amp	DcMD, 24 mo.
		31	M	Foot	2 mo.	Amp	DcMD, 10 mo.
		37	F	Elbow	6 mo.	Amp	Alive, 120 mo.

Exc = excision; amp = amputation; met = metastasis; DcMD = died with metastatic disease.

recur within 5 years after surgery, the case may be classified as a cure.

The *differential diagnosis* of benign giant cell tumor of tendon sheath and villonodular synovitis is relatively simple because of their unique clinical, gross, and microscopic appearance. In case of atypical presentation *giant cell reparative granuloma, parathyroid hyperplasia,* and *giant cell tumor of soft parts* (see Chapter 2) should be ruled out.

TENDOSYNOVIAL SARCOMA*

Since the first report of a sarcoma apparently arising from the synovial membrane was published by Simon in 1865, numerous case reports and review articles on synovial sarcomas have appeared in the literature. The largest series of cases were the following: Haagensen and Stout, 1944; Bennett, 1947; Pack and Ariel, 1950; Cadman et al, 1965; Mackenzie, 1966, Hajdu et al, 1977.

Although Sabrazes et al, in 1934 are credited with the first use of the term *synovial sarcoma,* the tendosynovial origin of these neoplasms was mentioned in several earlier reports (Marsh, 1898; Lejars and Rubens-Duval, 1910; Smirnoff, 1912; Spiess, 1913; Tourneux, 1913; Bolognesi, 1916; Buxton, 1923; Faccini, 1923; Pryn, 1930; Wagner, 1930; Diez, 1931). As a fact, the term *synoviomata* was coined by Smith, in 1927. *Synovial sarcoma* was used in the English literature for the first time by Knox, in 1936, and the first series of 15 cases were published by Coley and Pierson in 1937.

Phemister, in 1931, described five tumors he called "undifferentiated round-cell sarcomas." By reading his article, illustrated with excellent photomicrographs, one concludes that the tumors are tendosynovial clear cell sarcomas. Simi-

* *Synonyms and related terms:* synovial sarcoma, biphasic synovial sarcoma, monophasic synovial sarcoma, epithelioid sarcoma, clear cell sarcoma, chordoid sarcoma, parachordoma, reticulohistioendotheliosarcoma, malignant synovioma, synovial sarcoendothelioma, epitheliosarcoma, synovial endothelioma, sarcomatous perithelioma, round cell sarcoma.

larly, Seidelin's tumor, "liposarcoma with chordoma-like cells," reported in 1932, would be diagnosed today as chordoid sarcoma.

The *diverse morphologic appearance* of sarcomas of tendons, bursae, and joint capsules was pointed out by Berger, in 1938; DeSanto et al, in 1941 and Harkness, in 1952. King, in 1952, deducted from embryologic, anatomic, histologic, and histochemical observations what was already implied by earlier investigators, that is, that *tumors with look-alike morphology may arise from the aponeurotic fascia, tendon, tendon sheath, synovial bursae, and synovial membrane* due to common mesenchymal origin, histologic composition, and to a certain extent, similar functional role. He classified synovial tumors in two categories—undifferentiated spindle cell type and differentiated synovial tissue type—on the basis of recognizable histologic components. Subsequently, the differentiated forms were subdivided for mucoid, epithelial, glandular, and cleft forming. He emphasized the close relation and intermingling of various forms and felt that *they can transform into each other*.

In our report (Hajdu et al, 1977) we emphasized that despite various names, terms, and definitions, all available information obtained by clinical, cytologic, histologic, histochemical, ultrastructural, and tissue culture techniques indicates a common, tendosynovial origin of a group of neoplasms known today by six different names: *biphasic synovial sarcoma, monophasic synovial sarcoma, pseudoglandular synovial sarcoma, epithelioid sarcoma, clear cell sarcoma,* and *chordoid sarcoma* (Fig. 3-6). Most of these tu-

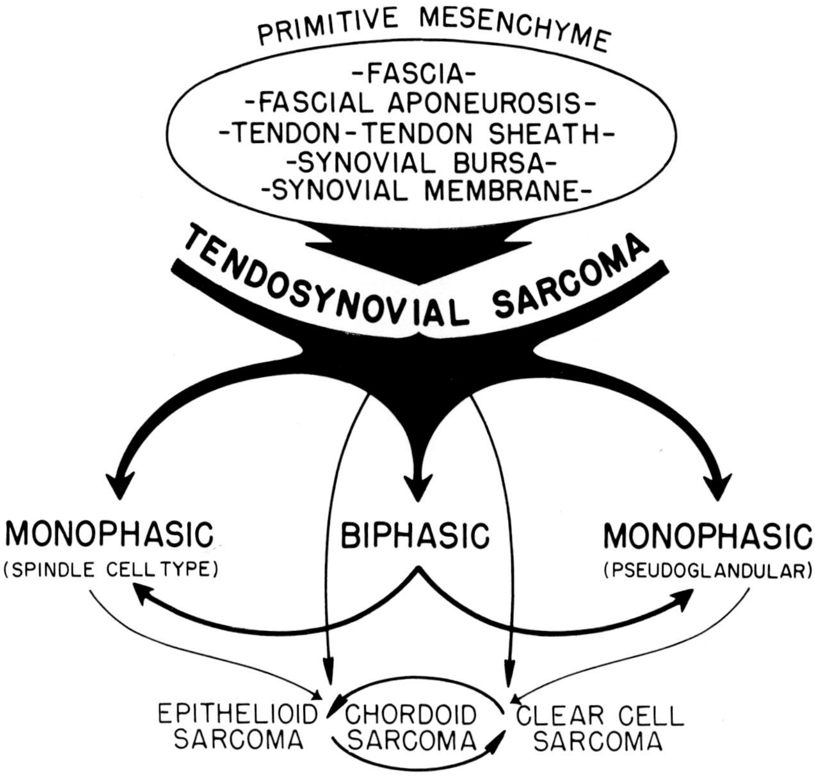

Figure 3-6. The common histogenesis and similar morphology of fascial-aponeurotic and tendon-synovial tissues are also expressed in the tumors which may arise from these structures. This schematic illustration is designed to show possible theoretical pathways of differentiation between various morphologic forms of tendosynovial sarcoma. (From Hajdu, S. I., Shiu, M. H., and Fortner, J. G.: Tendosynovial sarcoma. A clinicopathologic study of 136 cases. Cancer 39:1201, 1977.) (See also Figure 3-1.)

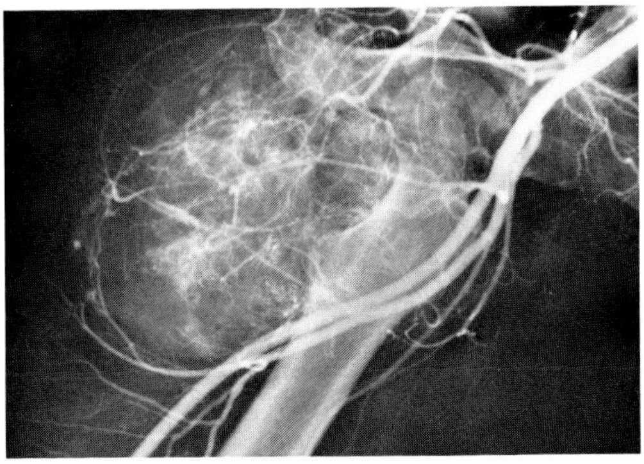

Figure 3-7. Arteriographic demonstration of tendosynovial sarcoma of the right shoulder.

mors can be traced to a common, special type of connective tissue, the synovial tissue, which is almost ubiquitous in the human body and an essential component of tendons, joint membranes, and bursae.

It is of interest that synovial tumors, regardless of the topographic presentation, imitate the morphologic character of normal synovial membrane. Therefore, it seems justified to use *synovial* as an adjective in combination with *tendon* to express with one term the histogenesis, as well as the most common structural origin, of these neoplasms from tendon, tendon sheath, and synovial membrane.

The etiology of tendosynovial sarcomas is not known, and no specific symptom characterizes these neoplasms. On radiographs tumors which are close to bone may induce periosteal reactions. Bones adjacent to the tumor may also show signs of osteoporosis.

The finding of *calcified areas*, especially in the biphasic form, is not uncommon. Vascularity and septate or lobular appearance is nonspecific and can be mimicked by many other neoplasms. However, according to Farmer and Viamonte (1972), angiography may reveal the size of the tumor and may also give information about the vessels that supply the lesion (Fig. 3-7).

Tendosynovial sarcomas are relatively uncommon neoplasms. It is estimated that less than 8% of all malignant soft tissue neoplasms are tendosynovial in origin (see Chapter 1).

The predominance of tendosynovial sarcomas during the third and fourth decades of life is referred to in many studies. Tillotson et al, 1951, are the only authors to report a congenital case in the foot of a baby girl. The tumor was treated by excision, and the patient was known to be alive 20 years later. By reviewing the clinicopathologic records of 136 patients treated for tendosynovial sarcoma at Memorial Sloan-Kettering Cancer Center during a period of 22 years, from 1948 to 1970 inclusive, we found (Hajdu et al 1977) that the age of the patients at the time of diagnosis of the primary tumor ranged from 4 years to 78 years, with the average age being 33 years (Fig. 3-8). More than half of the patients (52%) were between 16 and 36 years of age at the time of diagnosis.

Age may have an important bearing on survival. Our findings show that the chance of survival of the very young and the elderly is better, 59% and 48%, respectively, than the average 5-year survival of 40% of the whole series. Tendosynovial sarcomas occur rarely in children. We summarized our experience with 24 such tumors in patients under age 15 in 1974 (Lee et al, 1974). The tumors occurred predominantly in the extremities. It is of interest that the histologic type of the tumor was biphasic in 8 of 11 patients who are alive. The primary tumors that have proved fatal were predominantly of the monophasic, spindle cell type (Fig. 3-9).

Tendosynovial sarcomas occur more commonly in males than in females. In our study we found male dominance in every decade except during the first and seventh plus decades. Our findings indicate that females in general have a better (45%) chance to survive than males (36%). Considering sex, however, without reference to anatomic sites of the tumors could be misleading, since a significant number of the sarcomas in females were in anatomic areas—foot, ankle, forearm, wrist, and neck—that can be considered *exposed areas* and perhaps the tumors were detected at an earlier stage of the disease.

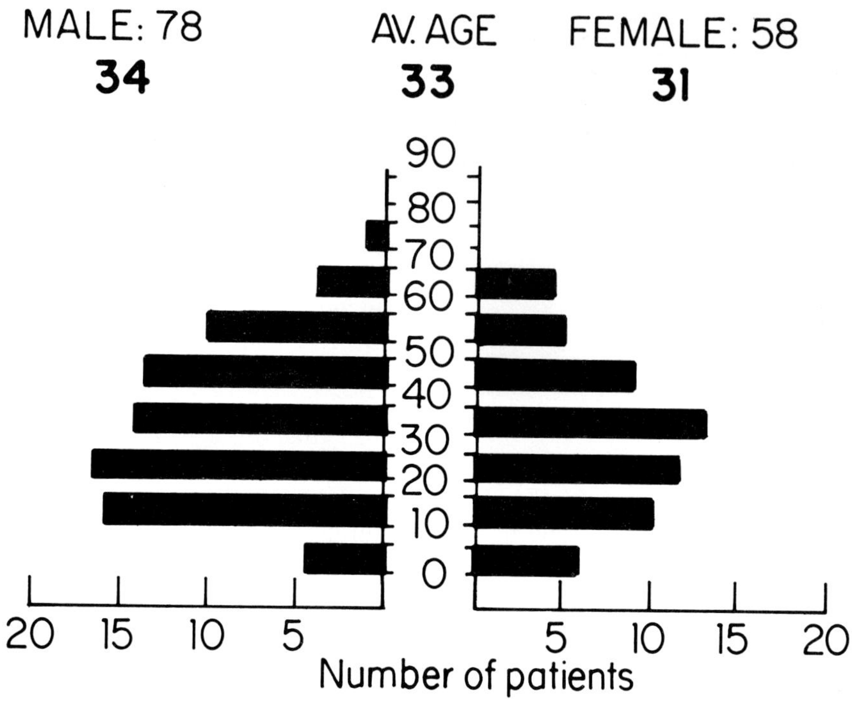

Figure 3-8. Age and sex distribution of 136 patients treated for tendosynovial sarcoma at Memorial Sloan-Kettering Cancer Center.

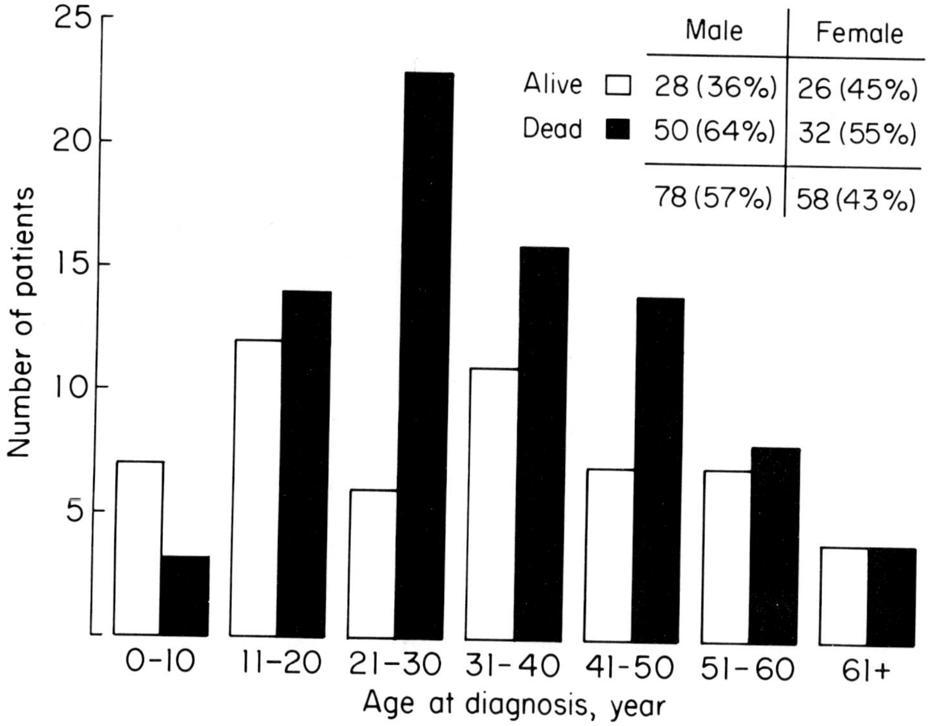

Figure 3-9. Prognosis of patients with tendosynovial sarcoma according to age and sex of the patient.

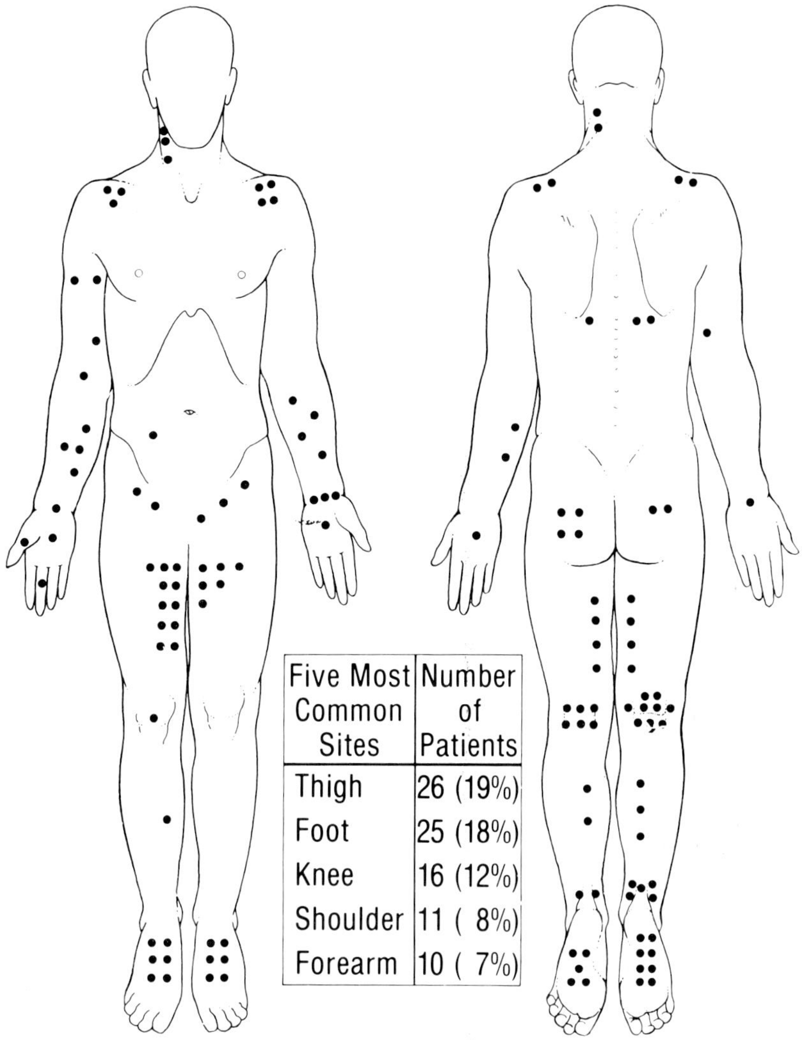

Five Most Common Sites	Number of Patients
Thigh	26 (19%)
Foot	25 (18%)
Knee	16 (12%)
Shoulder	11 (8%)
Forearm	10 (7%)

Figure 3-10. Scattergram illustrating the primary sites of 136 tendosynovial sarcomas. (From Hajdu, S. I., Shiu, M. H., and Fortner, J. G.: Tendosynovial sarcoma. A clinicopathologic study of 136 cases. Cancer 39:1201, 1977.)

It is indeed of interest that about one third of the sarcomas in females are located in the foot and ankle; in males they are in the thigh and knee (Table 3-6).

The lower extremity (namely, the thigh, foot, and knee regions) is the most common primary site of tendosynovial sarcomas. We found that 67% of the tumors were in the lower extremity, 26% in the upper extremity, and only 7% were located in other anatomic sites (Fig. 3-10). The majority of the tumors of the extremities are on the flexor surfaces, but there is a general consensus that they do not necessarily arise from synovial membrane.

The average 5-year survival rate for patients with tendosynovial sarcomas is 40%. We found (Hajdu et al, 1977) that the 5-year survival (19%) of patients with primary thigh tumors is below the average but that the rates for patients with primary tumors of the knee (62%) and foot (52%) are above the average.

Tendosynovial sarcomas of other anatomic sites than the extremities are rare, and few cases are included in any review articles. Published reports on tendosynovial sarcomas at anatomic sites such as the *abdominal wall* and *trunk* (Murphy and Margarit, 1968; Hale and Calder, 1970)

TABLE 3-6. ***The Five Most Common Anatomic Sites of Tendosynovial Sarcomas According to Sex***

NUMBER OF PATIENTS			
MALE: 78		FEMALE: 58	
Thigh	17 (22%)	Foot	15 (26%)
Foot	10 (13%)	Thigh	9 (16%)
Knee	10 (13%)	Knee	6 (10%)
Shoulder	7 (9%)	Forearm	6 (10%)
Groin	5 (6%)	Ankle	5 (9%)

and *tongue* (Moussavi and Ghodsi, 1974) are few. However, there are numerous published accounts of *head and neck primary lesions* (Jernstrom, 1954; Batsakis et al, 1967; Attie et al, 1970; Roth et al, 1975; Mitcherling et al, 1976; and Massarellie et al, 1978). Mitcherling et al in 1976 reviewed 14 cases of head and neck synovial sarcomas from the English literature and added one new case. They found that 3 of the 6 patients with adequate follow-up information were alive for 5 years. Jernstrom in 1954 is credited with the first description of a *cervical synovial sarcoma*. The single largest series of 24 patients with synovial sarcoma of the neck was reported by Roth et al, 1975. They found that this is a disease predominantly of young males (average age 19 years) and the presenting symptoms are hoarseness or difficulty in breathing or swallowing. The primary sites are almost always the retro- and hypopharyngeal regions. In their series 57% of the patients died with pulmonary metastasis. In our series of 136 patients, 3 out of 5 patients with cervical primary tumors survived longer than 5 years (Fig. 3-11). Many tendosynovial sarcomas of unusual sites are included in reported series (Table 3-7).

The *size* of tendosynovial sarcomas may vary according to histologic type and

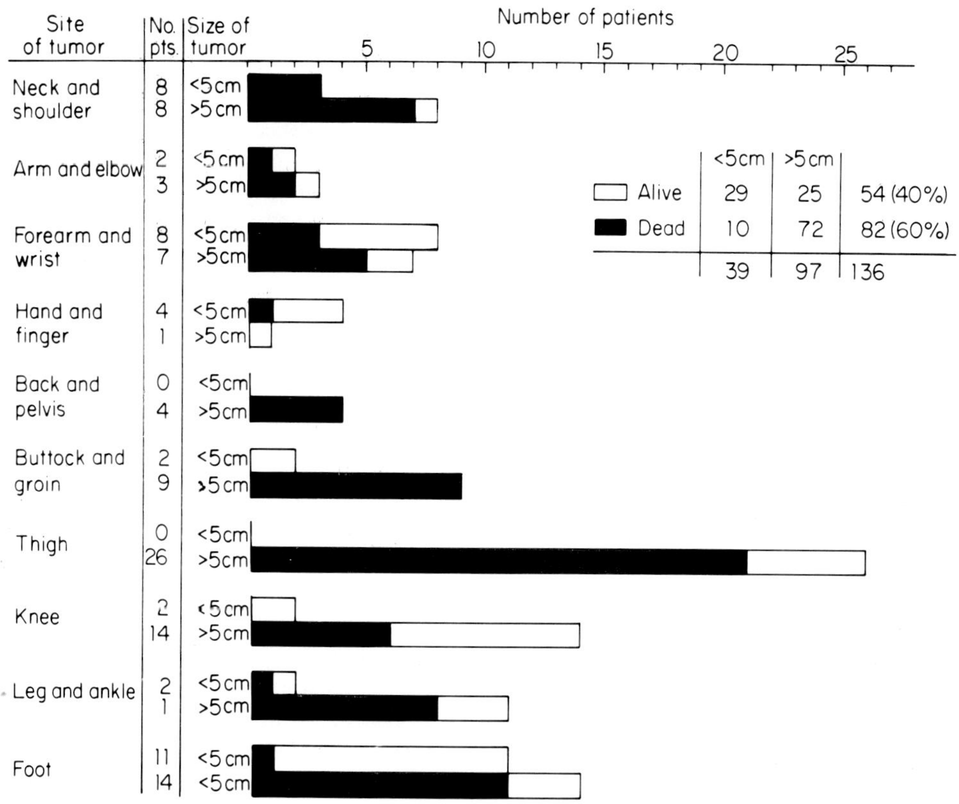

Figure 3-11. Size and location of the tendosynovial sarcoma significantly influenced the prognosis. (See also Figure 1-59 and Table 1-15.)

TABLE 3-7. ***Reported Series of Tendosynovial Sarcomas with Follow-up Information***

AUTHORS	NO. OF CASES	AVG. AGE	MOST COMMON SITES	RECURRENCE %	5-YEAR SURVIVAL %	NOTE
Pack and Ariel (1950)	60	36	Knee Foot	63	19	Memorial Hospital
Wright (1952)	47	—	Knee Foot	—	26	British series
Cade (1962)	100	—	Thigh Leg	50	56	Westminster Hospital
Cadman et al (1965)	107	33	Thigh Knee	—	25	Mayo Clinic
Mackenzie (1966)	58	—	Knee Foot	28	51	British series
Hampole and Jackson (1968)	25	42	Forearm Foot	44	44	Canadian series
Moberger et al (1968)	90	37	Foot Knee	49	37	Swedish Cancer Registry
Enzinger (1970)	62	26	Hand Forearm	85	78	All epithelioid sarcoma, AFIP
Lee et al (1974)	24	12	Foot Thigh	33	78	All pediatric cases, Memorial Hosp.
Hajdu et al (1977)	136	33	Thigh Foot	60	40	Memorial Sloan-Kettering Cancer Center

anatomic site of the tumor, but these tumors are usually not larger than 7 or 8 cm. There are no gross features that are pathognomonic for tendosynovial sarcomas (Fig. 3-12). Most of the tumors appear either encapsulated or circumscribed, but it is not uncommon to see diffuse and infiltrating multinuclear growths, especially along tendons and tendon sheaths. The cross section of the tumors may show cystic cavities, areas of calcification, hemorrhagic areas, and fiber-like strands in an otherwise semisolid, nodular, or lobular grayish tumor.

Small size of tumors other than tendosynovial sarcomas is frequently mentioned in the literature as a sign of favorable prognosis. We found the same principle can be applied to tendosynovial sarcomas. *Small tumors* (5 cm or less) *regardless of anatomic site have far better prognosis* (75%, 5-year survival) *than large tumors* (more than 5 cm) *of the same locations* (26%, 5-year survival) (Fig. 3-13). These figures become even more meaningful when size and site of the tumor are considered together. Seventy-nine percent of the patients who had small tumors in "exposed" areas such as foot, ankle, hand, and wrist survived at least 5 years; only 33% of the patients who had large tumors in the same sites survived for 5 years. At the same time, 80% of the patients with small and 15% of the ones with large tumors of "unexposed" areas such as thigh, groin, buttock, back, and shoulder survived for 5 years. Finally if the size of the tumor is not considered, 53% of the patients with tumors of "exposed" areas and 21% of those "unexposed" areas survived for 5 years (Table 3-8). (See Fig. 1-59 and Table 1-15.)

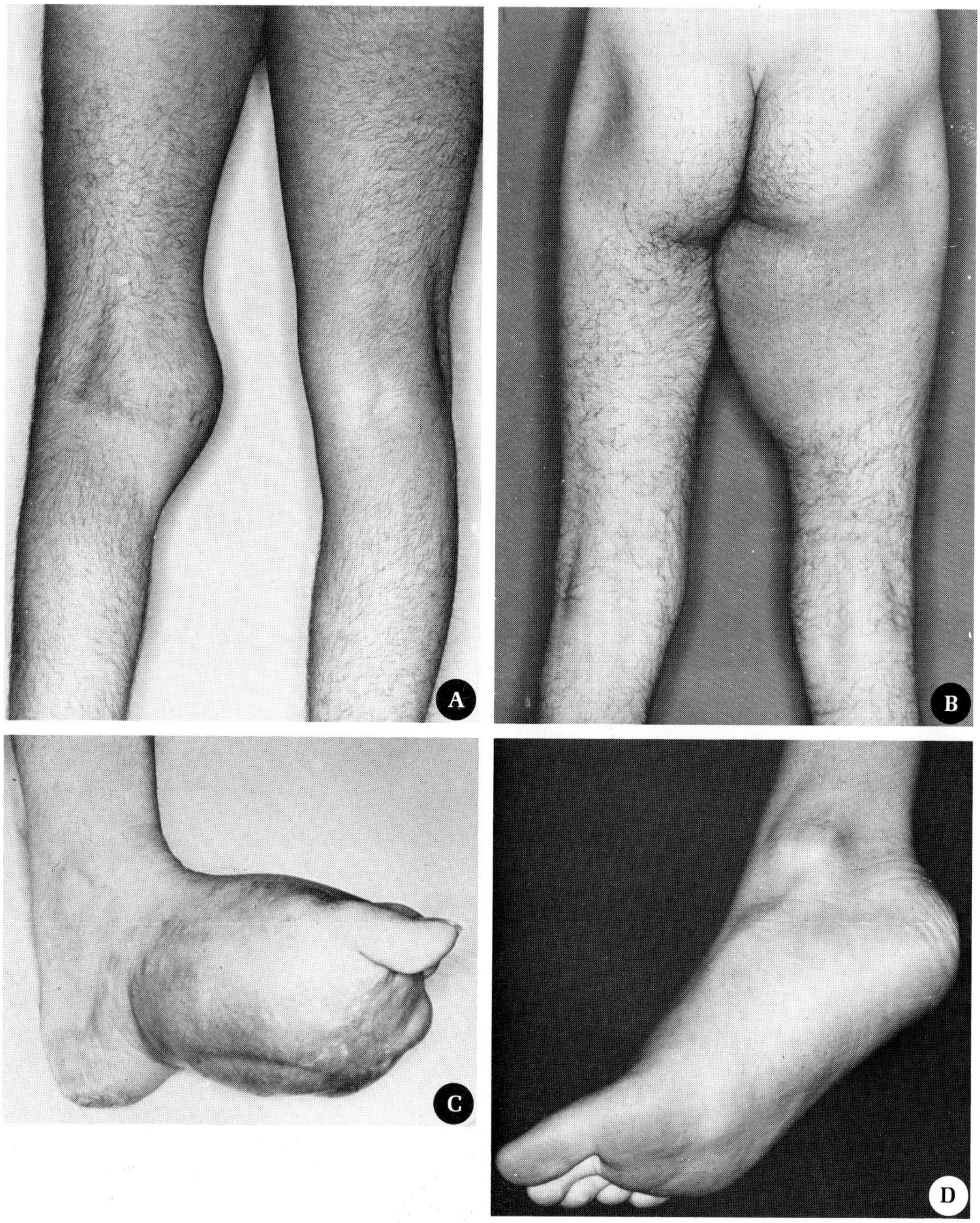

Figure 3-12. A, B, Clinically, tendosynovial sarcomas may range in size from a few centimeters to a bulky mass. **C, D,** Tendosynovial sarcoma of the foot, if neglected, may be extremely large, but in most instances the tumor appears as an ill-defined subcutaneous nodule.

Tendosynovial sarcomas often present a diagnostic and therapeutic challenge because of their histopathologic diversity and nonspecific, often misleading, clinical presentation. The histogenesis of tendosynovial sarcomas is fairly well established. Based on observation obtained from cell culture and cytologic studies (Murray et al, 1949; Hajdu et al, 1977; Koivuniemi and Nickels, 1978) and ultrastructural examinations (Luse, 1960; Gabbiani et al, 1972; Frable et al, 1973;

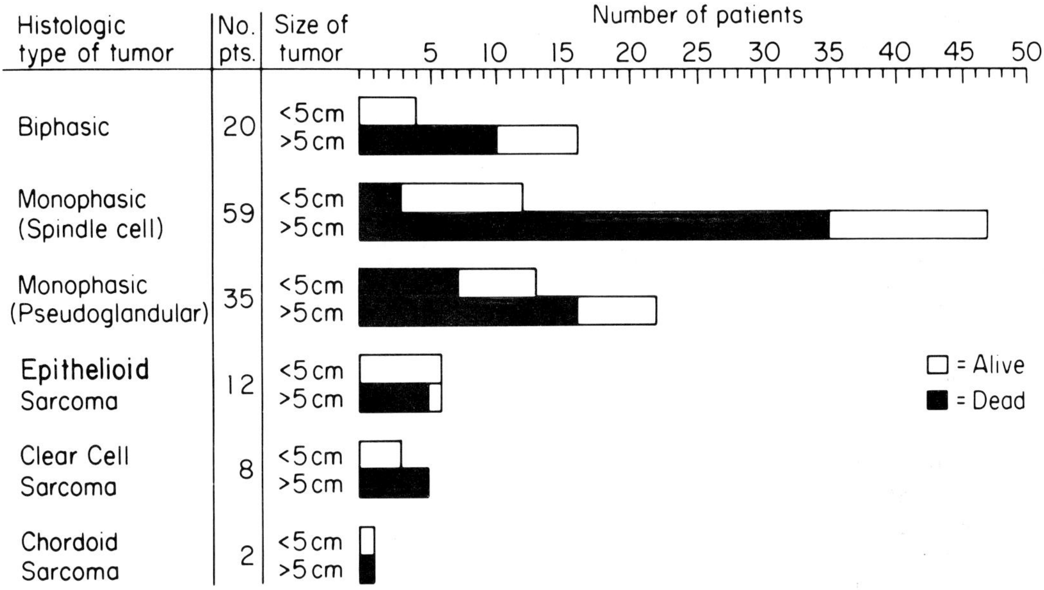

Figure 3-13. Mortality of 136 patients treated for tendosynovial sarcoma according to histologic type and size of the primary tumor.

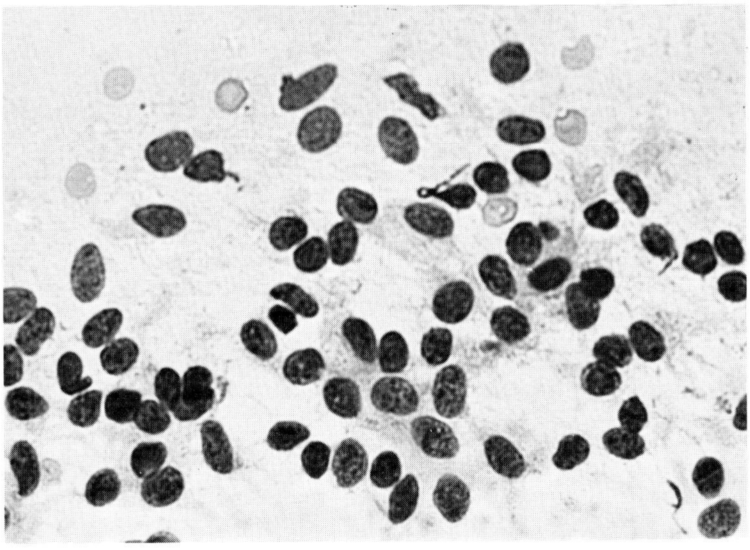

Figure 3-14. Air-dried aspiration smear of tendosynovial sarcoma monophasic spindle cell type. The nuclei have finely granular nuclear chromatin and minute punctate nucleoli. The delicate cytoplasmic processes are seen to form junctions between the tumor cells (H & E, ×450).

Patchefsky et al, 1977) it is certain that although the histologic spectrums of the tumors may vary, they are *all composed of cytologically monomorphic, non-collangenous, oval or short, spindle-shaped cells* (Fig. 3-14).

The variable histologic pattern of tendosynovial sarcomas is reflected by frequent variation in the microscopic appearance of primary, recurrent, and metastatic tumors (Tables 3-9 and 3-10). The majority of the recurrent and metastatic tumors are less differentiated than the corresponding primary tumors. Most of the recurrent and

TABLE 3-8. *Survival of Patients with Small vs. Large Tumor According to Anatomic Site of the Primary Lesion**

	NUMBER OF PATIENTS					
PRIMARY SITE	TOTAL	5-YR. SURVIVAL (%)	TUMOR SIZE <5 cm	5-YR. SURVIVAL (%)	TUMOR SIZE >5 cm	5-YR. SURVIVAL (%)
"Exposed" area	57	53	24	79	33	33
"Unexposed" area	52	21	5	80	47	15
Total	109	38	29	79	80	22

*In reference to grading and staging see Fig. 1-59 and Table 1-15.

metastatic biphasic, epithelioid, and clear cell sarcomas lose their epithelioid and pseudoglandular features and appear as monophasic spindle cell type.

The so-called epithelioid cells which were first recognized by Lejars, in 1910, are somewhat altered mesenchymal cells capable of producing a rich reticular network, demonstrable with silver stain, and viscous fluid, rich in mucopolysaccharides. These mucinous materials may appear as stromal ground substance, e.g., in clear cell sarcoma and chordoid sarcoma, or as deposits in the form of mucicarmine-, PAS-, and alcian blue-positive, not completely, diastase sensitive granular material in the lumen of gland-like and tubular structures, e.g., in biphasic and pseudoglandular forms (Massarelli, 1978). It is of interest that mucin droplets, which are unquestionably intracellular, have never been noted in tendosynovial sarcomas (Fig. 3-15, color).

Biphasic Tendosynovial Sarcoma. Biphasic or bimorphic or so-called synoviocytic tendosynovial sarcomas are composed of slender and monomorphic tumor cells arranged in two distinct patterns. In these tumors the uniform neoplastic cells with minute cytoplasms are arranged in

TABLE 3-9. *Histologic Type of Primary vs. Recurrent Tumors*

		HISTOLOGIC TYPE OF RECURRENT TUMOR					
			MONOPHASIC				
HISTOLOGIC TYPE OF PRIMARY TUMOR	TOTAL NO. OF TUMORS STUDIED	BIPHASIC	SPINDLE CELL TYPE	PSEUDO-GLANDULAR	EPITHELIOID SARCOMA	CLEAR CELL SARCOMA	CHORDOID SARCOMA
Biphasic	5	2	2	0	0	1	0
Monophasic (Spindle cell type)	14	0	9	1	3	1	0
Monophasic (Pseudo-glandular)	8	0	2	4	1	1	0
Epithelioid sarcoma	6	0	2	1	2	1	0
Clear cell sarcoma	2	0	1	0	1	0	0
	35	2	16	6	7	4	0

TABLE 3-10. ***Histologic Type of Primary vs. Metastatic Tumors***

HISTOLOGIC TYPE OF PRIMARY TUMOR	TOTAL NO. OF TUMORS STUDIED	HISTOLOGIC TYPE OF METASTATIC TUMOR					
			MONOPHASIC				
		BIPHASIC	SPINDLE CELL TYPE	PSEUDO-GLANDULAR	EPITHELIOID SARCOMA	CLEAR CELL SARCOMA	CHORDOID SARCOMA
Biphasic	7	2	4	1	0	0	0
Monophasic (Spindle cell type)	14	0	12	2	0	0	0
Monophasic (Pseudo-glandular)	12	0	7	4	0	1	0
Epithelioid sarcoma	3	0	1	1	0	1	0
Clear cell sarcoma	2	0	1	1	0	0	0
Chordoid sarcoma	1	0	1	0	0	0	0
	39	2	26	9	0	2	0

clusters, cords, or cellular sheets. The epithelioid tendosynovial cells (synoviocytes) which line the gland-like structures often resemble genuine epithelial cells; however, there is no evidence of basement membrane. The synovial pseudoglandular spaces were first described by King, in 1935. He believed that these structures are preceded by an accumulation or condensation of synovial cells along a definite line, followed by cleavage and cleft or gland-like formation.

Giant cells and cells in mitosis are few or completely absent. The ratio of "stromal" spindle cells (synovioblasts) and epithelioid cells varies from case to case, but in most cases the spindle cell stromal component is far more abundant than the pseudoglandular areas. Although the epithelioid and stromal cells may appear different, the only true difference between the two components is that cells lining the gland-like spaces are shorter because of their nuclear alignment. It is common to find lumenless epithelioid or clear cell nests at the edges of biphasic tumors. Many of these epithelioid nests with round, clear cytoplasmic cells containing prominent nuclei and nucleoli are the "precursors" of clearly gland-like structures. It is often rewarding to obtain additional sections from such areas, because the pseudoglandular or biphasic pattern can be clearly demonstrated. Occasionally the two components, epithelioid round cells and spindle cells, form parallel cords or rows of cells with intermediate forms positioned haphazardly along the clear epithelioid and darker spindle cells. It is not uncommon to find villi with papillary projections in slit-like or cystic spaces. Amorphous calcium depositions may be seen anywhere in the tumor but are most commonly found in nests of epithelioid cells (Figs. 3-16, 3-17, 3-18).

According to our experience, biphasic tendosynovial sarcomas are found most commonly in areas of the knee, thigh, groin, and shoulder. Despite the bulky, gross appearance, 44% of the patients survive for 5 years (Figs. 3-13, 3-19).

Monophasic Spindle Cell Type of Tendosynovial Sarcoma. This type of tendosynovial sarcoma is more common than any other histologic form. These tumors are predominantly composed of slender spin-

Figure 3-15A. Tendosynovial sarcoma, monophasic spindle cell type, is a high grade malignant neoplasm. It is composed of uniform, nongiant-cell-forming spindle cells in tightly packed sheets. The tumor cells are short spindle or oval cells with finely reticular and short cytoplasmic processes which stain positive with reticulum stain.

The tumor cells are forming clusters, tightly arranged cords, and papillary projections. The tip of a cellular papillary structure is protruding into a slit or tissue space. Note the pileup of the tumor cells near the edge of the slit (H & E, ×140).

B, Biphasic tendosynovial sarcoma, well-differentiated and histologically low grade neoplasm. This tumor is predominantly composed of short oval or cuboidal cells arranged in pseudoglandular formation. The stromal spindle cells are few and intimately adherent to the lining cells of glandlike spaces.

In the lumen of the glandlike structures cell debris and condensed mucopolysaccharide substance can be seen which stains positive with mucicarmine stain (H & E, ×140).

C, Clear cell sarcoma of tendosynovium is a neoplasm which shows two distinct cell components: (a) clear round cells with vesicular nuclei, prominent nucleoli, and prominent, well-defined cytoplasm containing granular material; (b) dark pyknotic cells which are interpositioned between the clear cells. These are small cells with small and ill-defined cytoplasm.

Binucleated forms are seen at the center of the figure; however, there is no evidence of multinucleated forms or giant cells (H & E, ×350).

D, Chordoid sarcoma. This is an extremely rare form of low-grade malignant neoplasm.

It is composed of fairly uniform stellate cells in a myxomatous background. The tumor cells have small round pyknotic nuclei. The cytoplasm is granular and extends into multidirectional short filaments. The tumor cells are separated by the richly mucinous stroma which stains positive with alcian blue, PAS, and almost completely digestible by hyaluronidase (H & E, ×140).

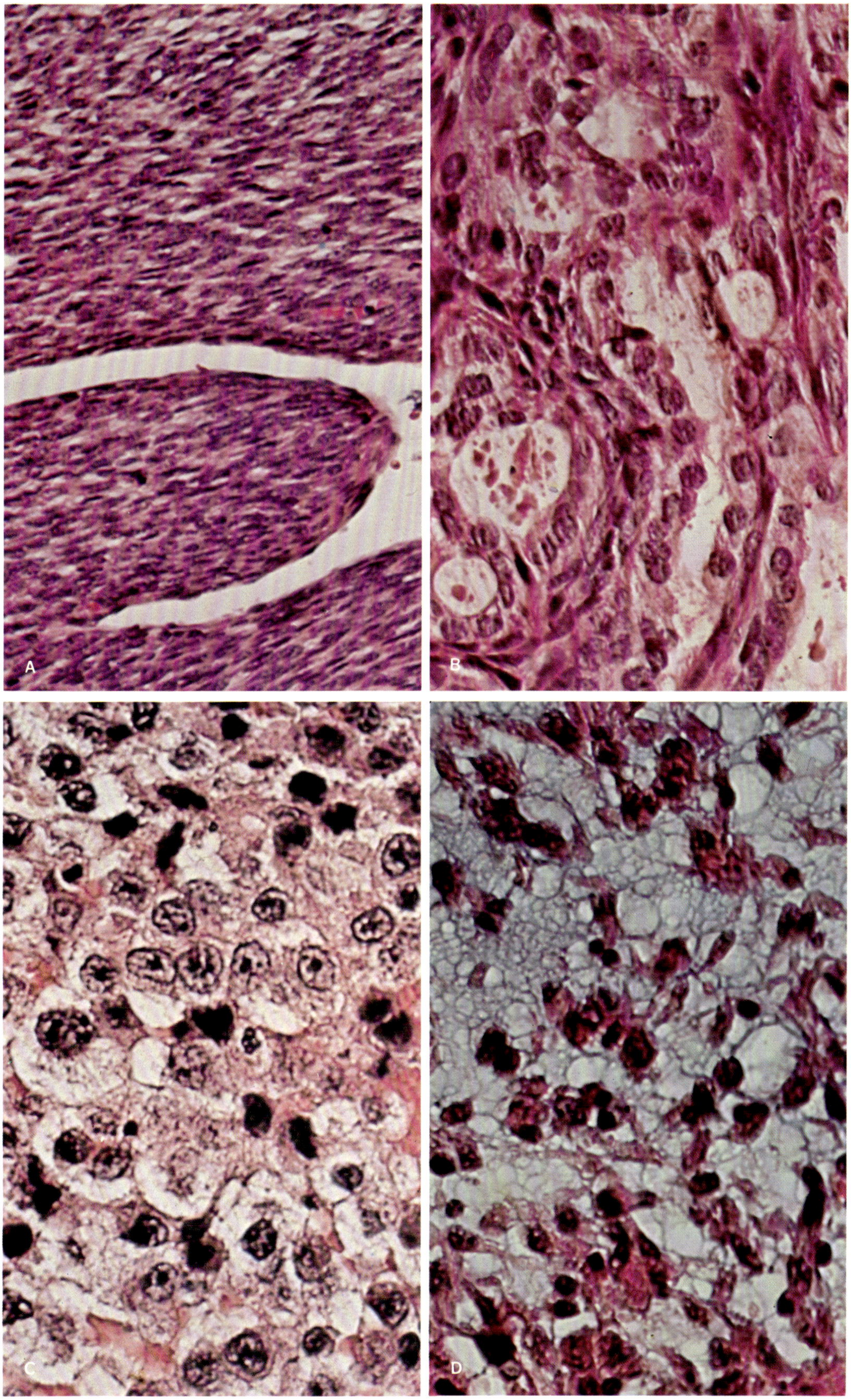

Figure 3-15.

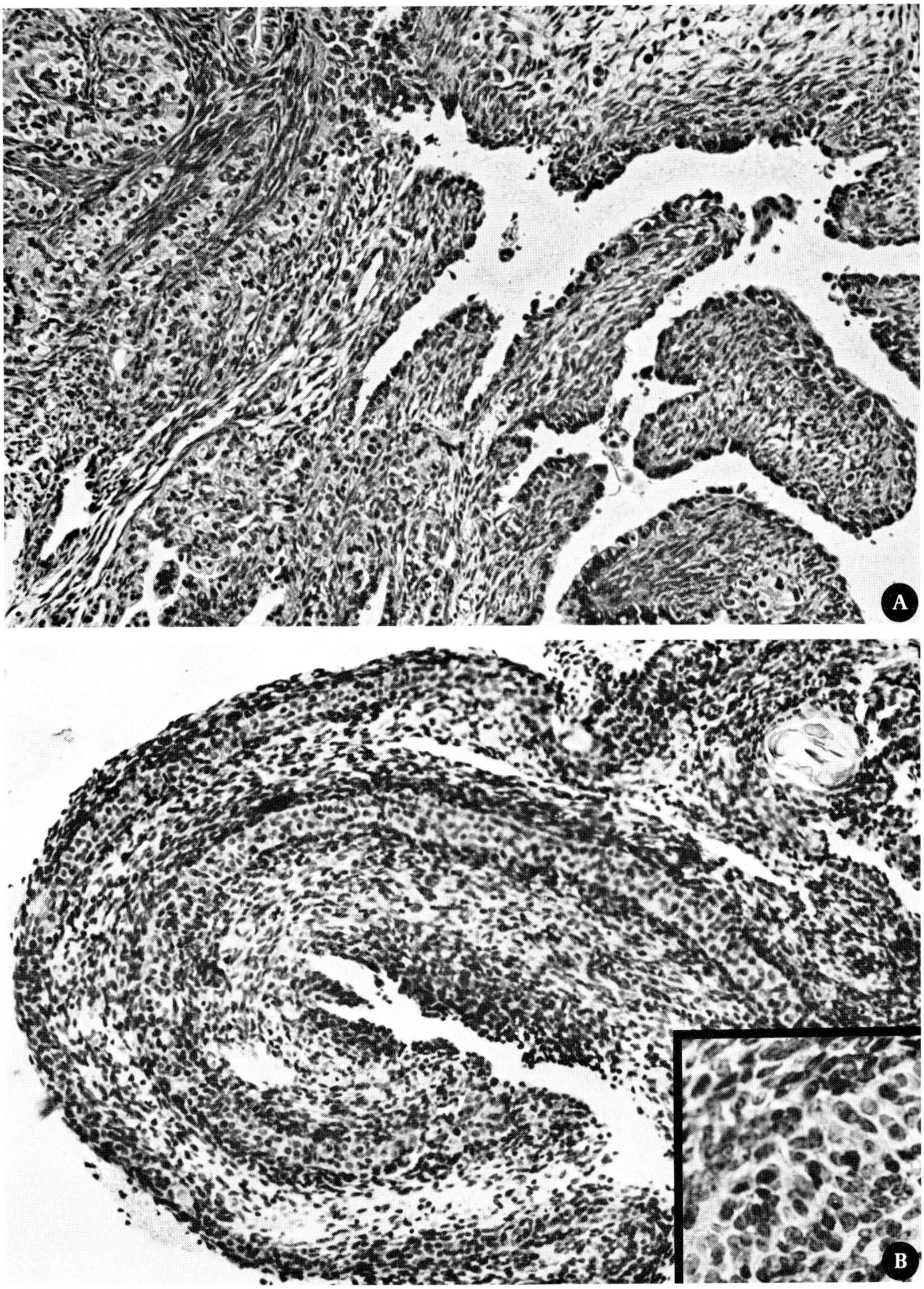

Figure 3-16. Tendosynovial sarcoma, biphasic type. The tumor is composed of small cuboidal and short spindle cells. Despite somewhat diverse morphology, both epithelioid (cuboidal) and stromal (spindle) cells are histogenetically related.

The tumor cells have a tendency to form clefts, slits, cords, and tubules. Note the intimate relationship between stromal and epithelioid cells in **B.** (**A,** H & E, ×140; **B,** H & E, ×140; inset, ×350).

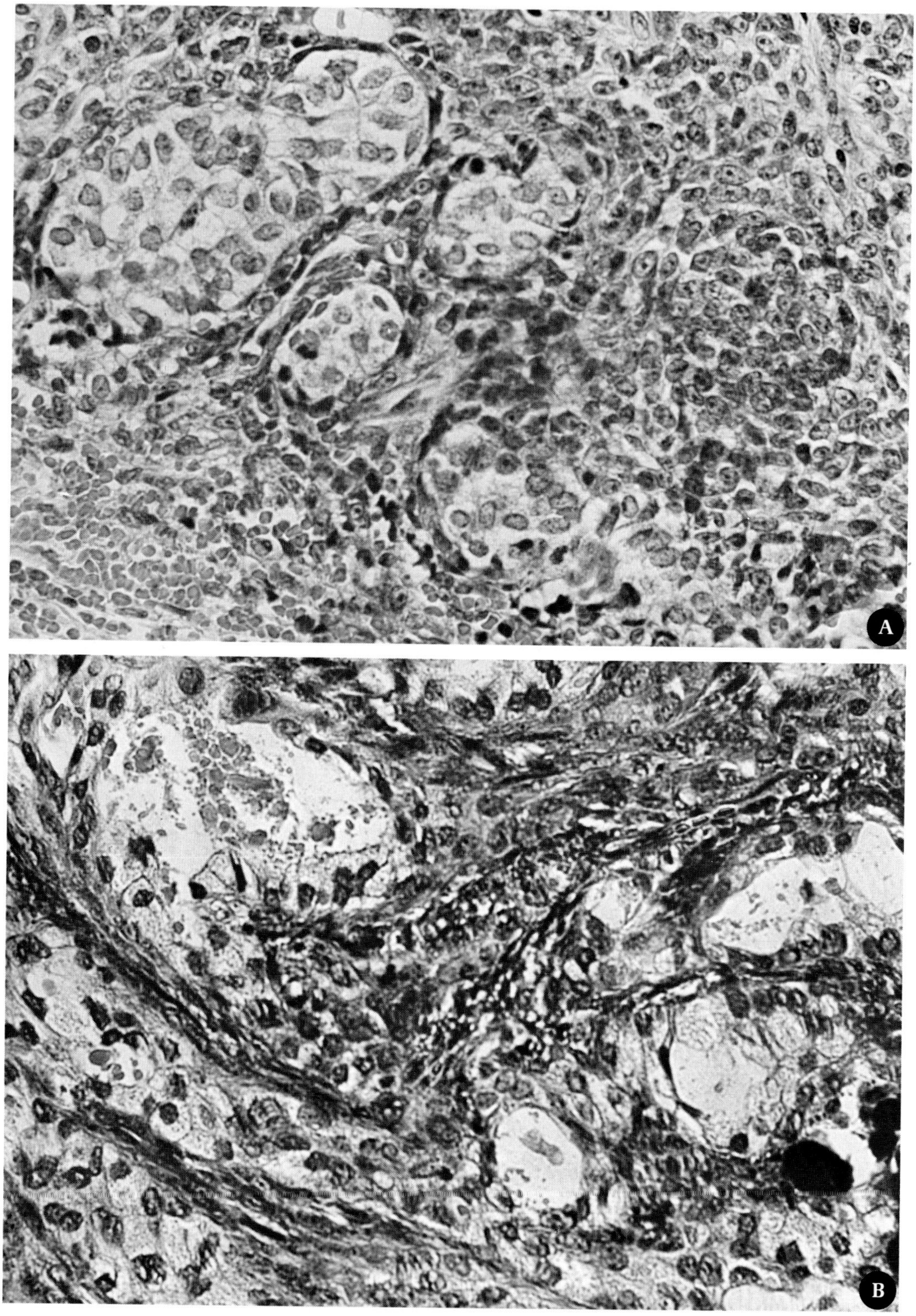

Figure 3-17. Tendosynovial sarcoma, biphasic type.

A, The basic units in this tumor are the epithelioid nests which are surrounded by somewhat darker staining stromal cells (H & E, ×350).

B, It is not unusual to see accumulation of mucicarminophilic or calcified material in the tissue spaces lined by epithelioid cells. Note blending of the epithelioid cells of the pseudoglandular structures with the spindly stromal cells and the absence of giant cells (see also Figure 3-15).

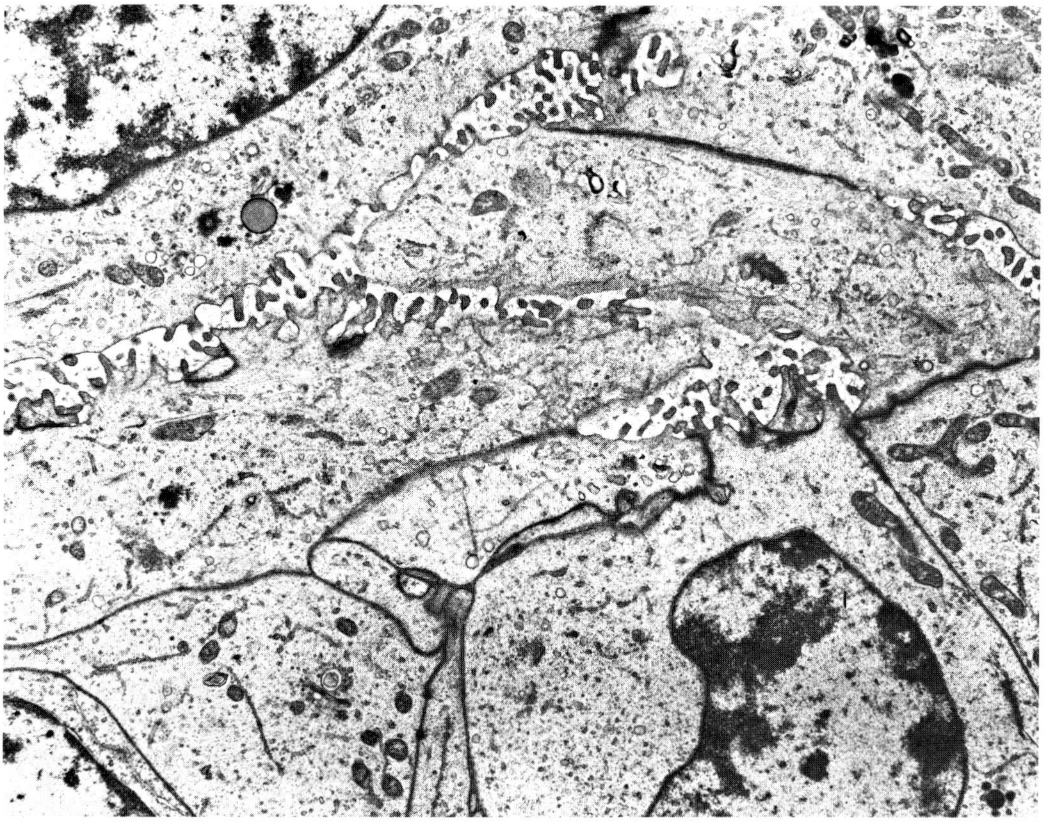

Figure 3-18. Ultrastructure of the epithelioid component of a biphasic tendosynovial sarcoma. Note the prominent microvilli-lined intercellular lumina and the tight junction between adjacent cells (×8,000).

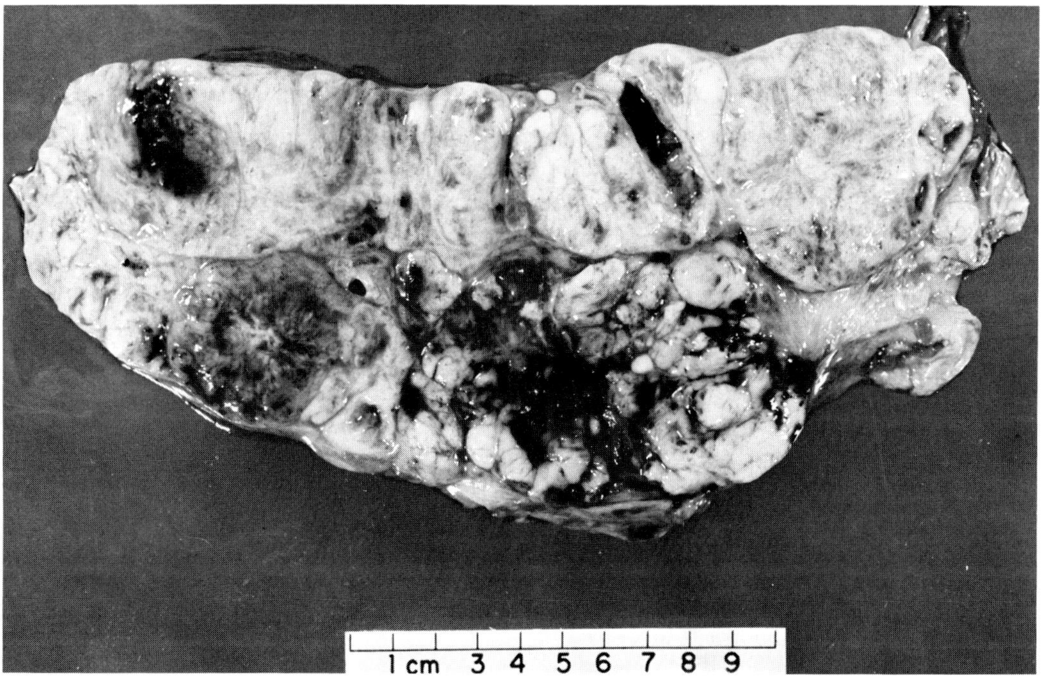

Figure 3-19. There is little variation in the consistency and color of various tendosynovial sarcomas. This figure shows a solid multilobular mass with hemorrhagic areas and numerous small papillary growths.

dle-shaped cells with elongated poorly preserved cytoplasms and prominent cigar-shaped nuclei. Stout (1953), Cadman et al (1965), and Moberger et al (1968) all came to the same conclusion that in all probability this pattern represents a monophasic type of tendosynovial sarcoma rather than fibrosarcoma. Even today there are pathologists who are unwilling to accept the existence of "monophasic" tumors. Lattes, for example, stated at the Soft Tissue Tumor Seminar of the American Society of Clinical Pathologists, in 1973, that "the diagnosis of monophasic synovial sarcoma is unwise because of all the many pitfalls associated with it." He did not state, however, his preference. My view is that, according to logic, if the term *biphasic* is used to describe a tumor with both spindle cell areas and pseudoglandular cleft-like spaces lined by "cuboidal" cells, then there is no doubt that *monophasic* tendosynovial sarcoma exists.

The tumor cells in monophasic spindle cell tumors are arranged in sheets and parallel cords. The stroma is minimal and finely reticular without collagen formation. Somewhat shorter tumor cells, with the same general morphology, are seen to be arranged as a cellular collar around capillary vessels. Mitotic figures are rare and the tumor is almost completely devoid of giant cells. The reader's attention is directed to a rare histopathologic form of monophasic tendosynovial sarcoma, the so-called *sclerosing form*. In this tumor cluster-forming tumor cells appear trapped in collagenous dense stroma; however, cytologically the tumor cells are similar to those in other forms of monophasic tendosynovial sarcomas. In conclusion, histologically, monophasic spindle cell types of tendosynovial sarcomas are similar to biphasic tendosynovial sarcomas, short of the pseudoglandular or epithelioid tubular structures (Figs. 3-20, 3-21, 3-22, 3-23).

It is my personal conviction that the term *monophasic spindle cell type of tendosynovial sarcoma* is worthy of attention if for no other reason than its high grade malignancy. Our experience with these tumors (Hajdu et al, 1977) shows that only 26% of the 59 patients who had this tumor survived for 5 years. Most of these tumors are bigger than 5 cm and usually are deeply seated tendosynovial lesions. They are found most commonly in the thigh, foot, and shoulder (Figs. 3-13, 3-24). (See also Fig. 1-59 and Table 1-15.)

Monophasic Pseudoglandular Tendosynovial Sarcomas. These tendosynovial sarcomas are far less common than the monophasic spindle cell forms. In these tumors the majority of the tumor cells are in gland-like or tubule-like structures. The pseudoglandular spaces are lined by mostly clear cells with prominent nuclei and nucleoli, the type described in biphasic forms. There is a minimal reticular stroma between the tightly arranged tubules and cords of clear cells. One rarely sees areas of calcification and chondroid or osteoid metaplasia. In our series, 34 tumors were classified as pseudoglandular. Size and anatomic site of the primary tumor seem to be important in prognosis (Figs. 3-13, 3-25).

Epithelioid Sarcoma. The origin of epithelioid sarcoma and clear cell sarcoma from tendosynovial or aponeurotic mesenchymal cells was implied from the time they were first described because of their topographic and microscopic appearance (Lejars and Rubens-Duval, 1910; Phemister, 1931; Sabrazes et al, 1934; Black, 1936; Berger, 1938; DeSanto et al, 1941; Laskowski, 1971). Enzinger introduced and popularized these terms in 1970 and 1965, respectively, in two concise studies. Since then, more of these neoplasms have been recognized.

Epithelioid sarcomas are composed, histologically, of short oval and round or polygonal cells similar to the epithelioid cells of biphasic and pseudoglandular tendosynovial sarcomas. However, the long cigar-shaped or oval cells that are dominant in the monophasic spindle cell tumors and also contribute to the stroma

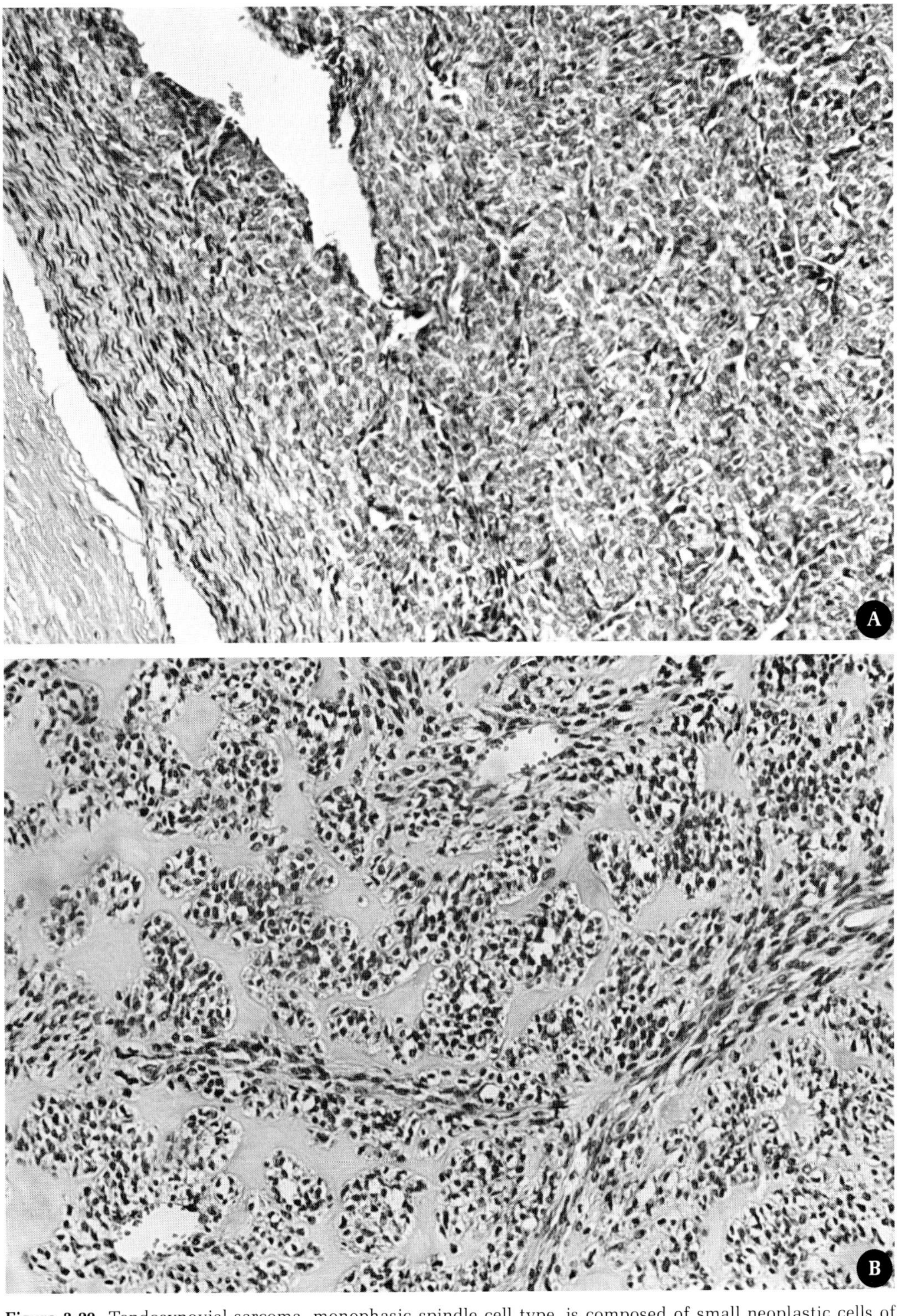

Figure 3-20. Tendosynovial sarcoma, monophasic spindle cell type, is composed of small neoplastic cells of uniform size. There is no particular arranged pattern in these tumors; however, the tumor cells have a tendency to line slits **(A)** and form clusters or cell cords **(B)**. Between cell clusters it is not uncommon to see geographically distributed acellular or sclerosing areas (**A,** H & E, ×140; **B,** H & E, ×140).

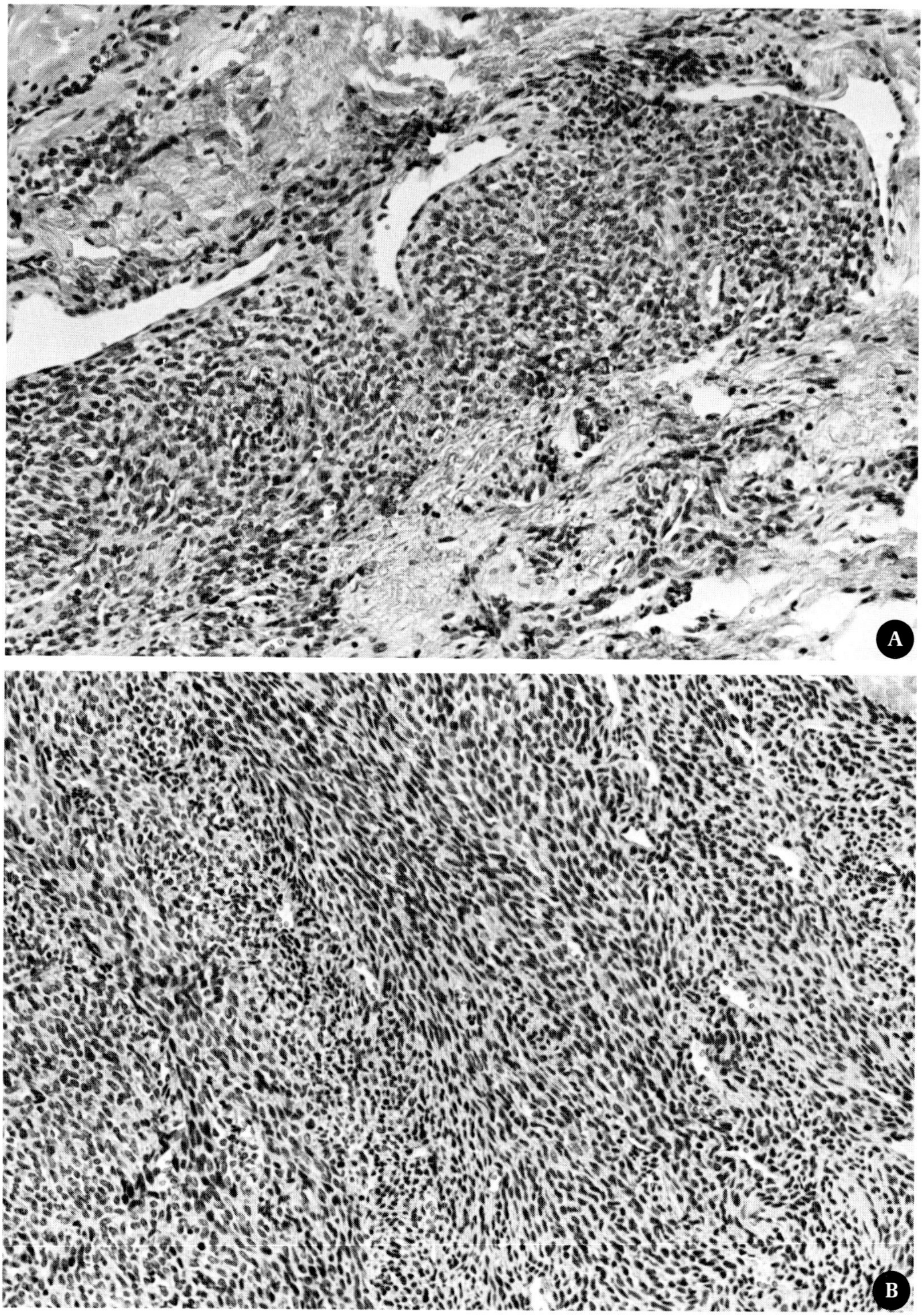

Figure 3-21. Tendosynovial sarcoma, monophasic spindle cell type.

A, The tumor infiltrates along adjacent tissue spaces and forms tumor nodules which blend into adjacent sclerosing fibrovascular tissues (H & E, ×140).

B, A highly cellular and richly vascular portion of a monophasic spindle cell type of tendosynovial sarcoma. The tumor cells are uniform, and the intercellular stroma is minimal (H & E, ×140).

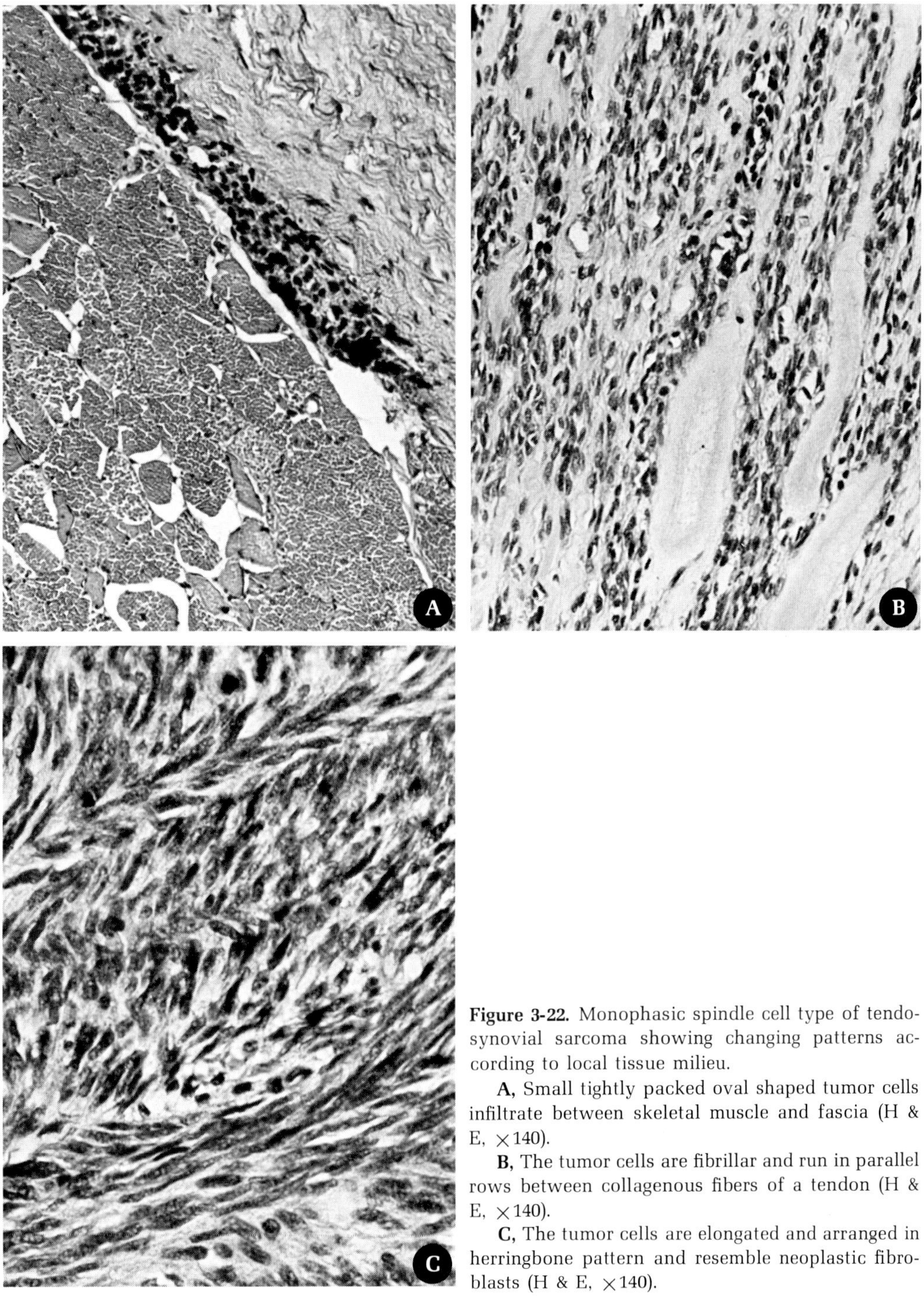

Figure 3-22. Monophasic spindle cell type of tendosynovial sarcoma showing changing patterns according to local tissue milieu.

A, Small tightly packed oval shaped tumor cells infiltrate between skeletal muscle and fascia (H & E, ×140).

B, The tumor cells are fibrillar and run in parallel rows between collagenous fibers of a tendon (H & E, ×140).

C, The tumor cells are elongated and arranged in herringbone pattern and resemble neoplastic fibroblasts (H & E, ×140).

of biphasic neoplasms are not seen. Also missing are the pseudoglandular or tubular structures which are so apparent in biphasic and pseudoglandular tumors. The tumor cells may have a multinodular arrangement along tendons, tendon sheaths, and blood vessels. It is not uncommon to see slightly acidophilic staining of the tumor cells. Around the tumor nodules commonly there is peripheral condensation of various reactive cells which may give the impression of an in-

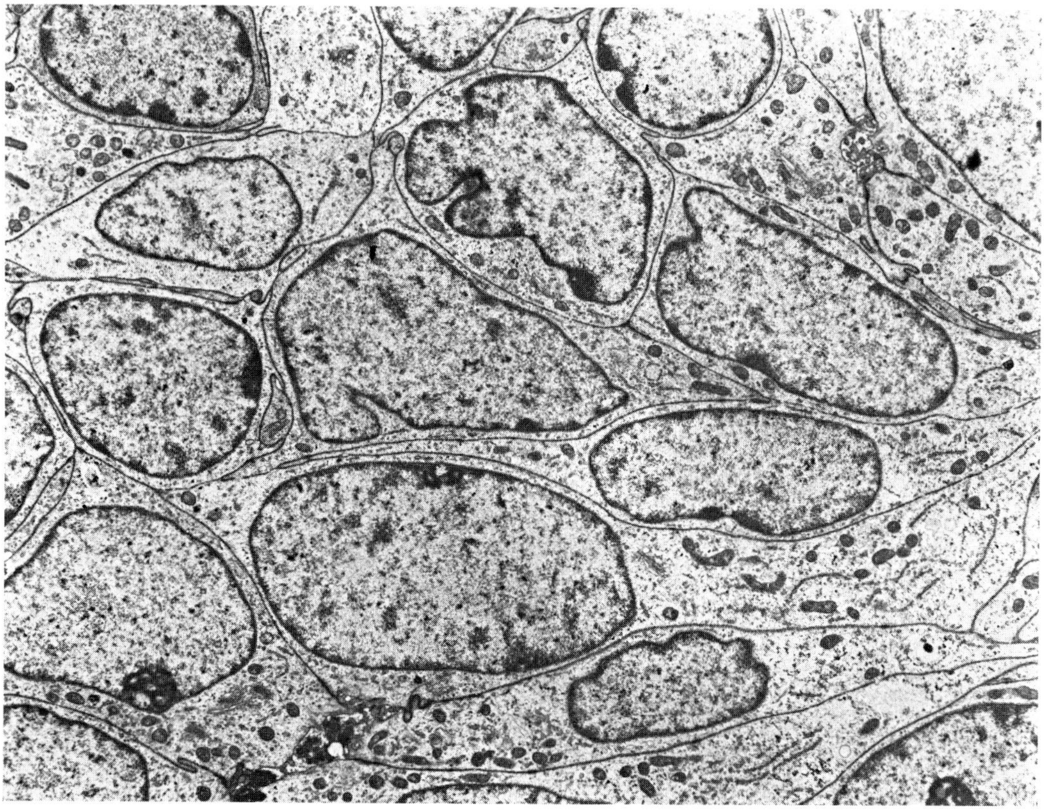

Figure 3-23. Ultrastructure of monophasic tendosynovial sarcoma, spindle cell type. The tumor consists of tightly packed undifferentiated mesenchymal cells without any particular distinguishing features (×4,800).

flammatory process. Granulomatous tissue reaction and necrosis can be considerable. In a few cases we were able to demonstrate that some of the necrotic or hyalinized areas were actually dilated blood vessels containing nests of neoplastic cells. Extensive deposits of collagenous material may divide cords and sheets of uniform tumor cells for innocuous-looking cell clusters and contribute to the sclerosing appearance of these neoplasms. (Figs. 3-26, 3-27).

Since Sabrazes et al, in 1934, first used the term *epitheliosarcoma* and Berger, in 1938, referred to the *epitheliosarcomatous* aspect of synovial sarcomas, numerous case reports and a number of review articles have been published. Enzinger's article, published in 1970, was followed by Dehner's report (1970) describing a penile primary tumor; Laskowski's 1961 article appearing in translation in 1971 described an "aponeurotic sarcoma" composed of multinodular dermal or subcutaneous firm masses fixed to fascia or tendon. Undeniably he described an epithelioid sarcoma. The article written by Santiago et al in 1972 is the first review of epithelioid sarcomas. They found 70 published cases and added their own 9 cases. In the same year, Seemayer et al found 92 reported cases in the literature and found that 49% of the patients were alive without evidence of the disease. Twenty-four percent died with metastatic tumor and the remaining 28% were alive with apparent evidence of the disease.

Gabbiani et al (1972), Frable et al (1973), and Patchefsky et al (1977) studied epithelioid sarcomas with the electron microscope and concluded that ultrastructural features (junctional complexes, scanty RER, few Golgi and mitochondria, the presence of clear and dark cells) *support*

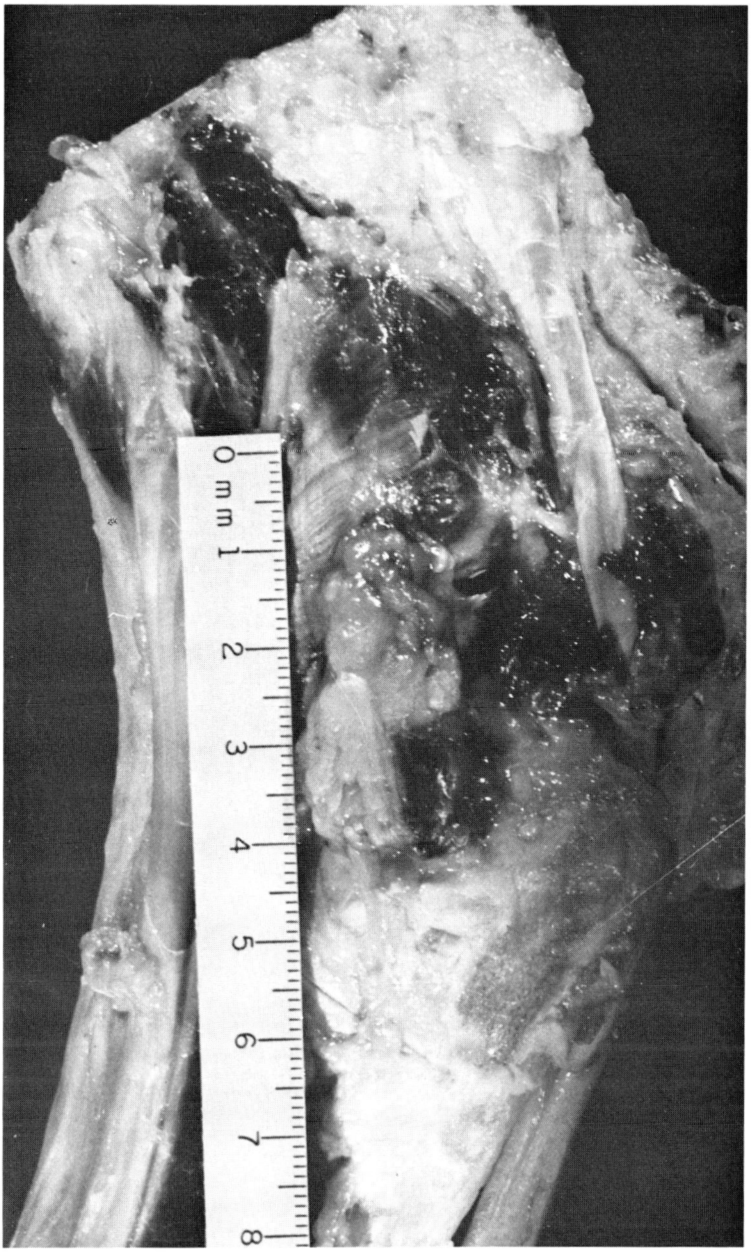

Figure 3-24. A deeply seated tendosynovial sarcoma infiltrating adjacent vessels and tendons.

the concept of synovial origin of these neoplasms. Since the concept that synovial tissue is modified connective tissue has been clearly established, the futility of discussions such as whether epithelioid sarcomas are fibroblastic or synovial in origin must be pointed out.

In our series of 12 cases (Hajdu et al, 1977), and also in the study reported by Prat et al, in 1978, in which they described 10 additional cases, the multifocal and superficial presentation of epithelioid sarcomas was demonstrated. Epithelioid sarcomas are located most commonly in exposed areas such as forearms, hand, leg, and foot (Figs. 3-28, 3-29). Seven of our 12 patients survived for 5 years. Epithelioid sarcomas have a tendency to metastasize to regional lymph nodes more frequently than any other tendosynovial sarcoma,

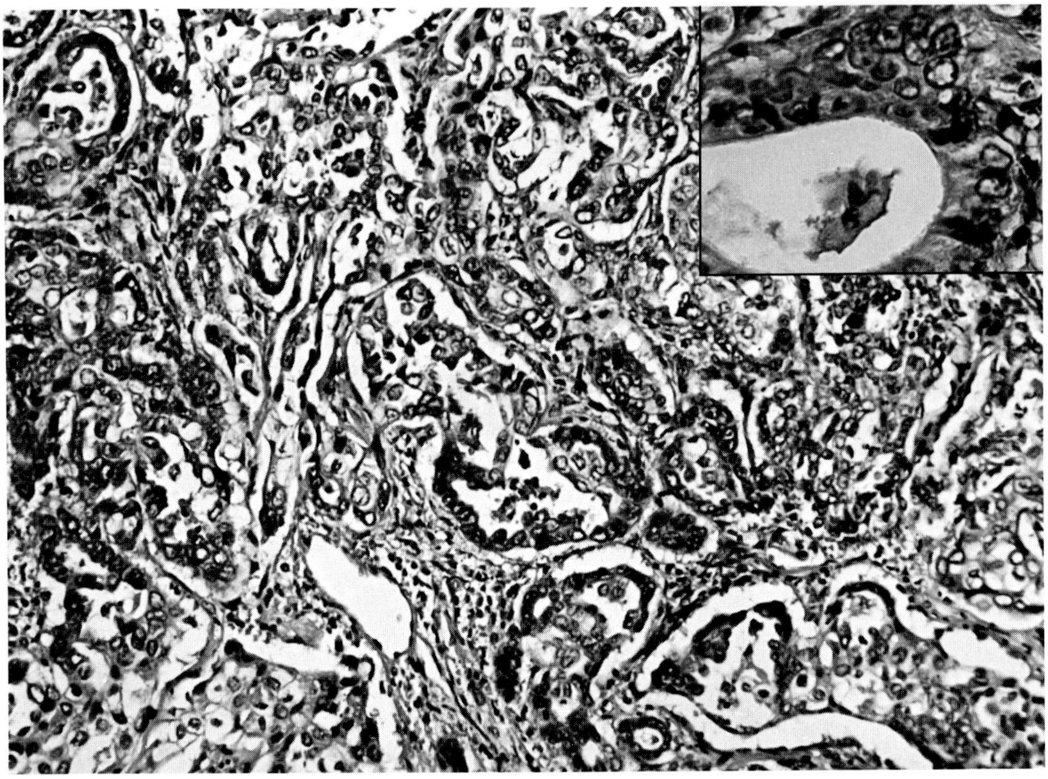

Figure 3-25. Tendosynovial sarcoma, monophasic pseudoglandular type. The tumor is predominantly composed of uniform round or cuboidal cells in clusters, cords, and alveolar nests. The pseudoglandular spaces are lined by tumor cells with distinct epithelioid features (see inset); however, they also show intimate relationship with surrounding stromal cells (H & E, ×140; inset, ×350).

and two of our patients died with disseminated intravascular coagulopathy (DIC).

Clear Cell Sarcoma. This is a rare and uncommon variety of tendosynovial sarcoma. The term *clear cell sarcoma* was introduced and popularized by Enzinger, in 1965, by reporting 21 cases. Undoubtedly the first description of these neoplasms was made by Phemister, in 1931, who called them "undifferentiated round-cell sarcoma." Bennett (1947) reported a series of 32 cases of synovial sarcomas among which he listed two tumors he considered a "more solid and simplified type of sarcoma derived from synovial tissues." Histologically these tumors are composed of pale staining clear round cells with prominent nuclei and nucleoli. The majority of the tumor cells contain moderate to large amounts of intracytoplasmic glycogen. Most of the tumor cells are arranged in clusters or in sheets with small amounts of intercellular stroma which is stainable with alcian blue and PAS (Figs. 3-30, 3-31).

The general histologic appearance of clear cell sarcomas is that of certain areas in the monophasic pseudoglandular tendosynovial sarcomas without gland-like or tubular structures. Kubo (1969), by studying the ultrastructure of a clear cell sarcoma of the patellar tendon, found that tendosynovial sarcoma may give the histologic pattern of clear cell sarcoma and added that *clear cell sarcoma should be considered a form of synovial sarcoma.* Kahn (1973) by studying malignant giant cell tumor of the tendon sheath with the electron microscope came to the conclusion also that *tendon sheath tumors may contain clear cell areas.*

Dutra (1970) reported 3 cases of clear cell sarcoma in which diastase-resistant, PAS-positive, intracytoplasmic granules

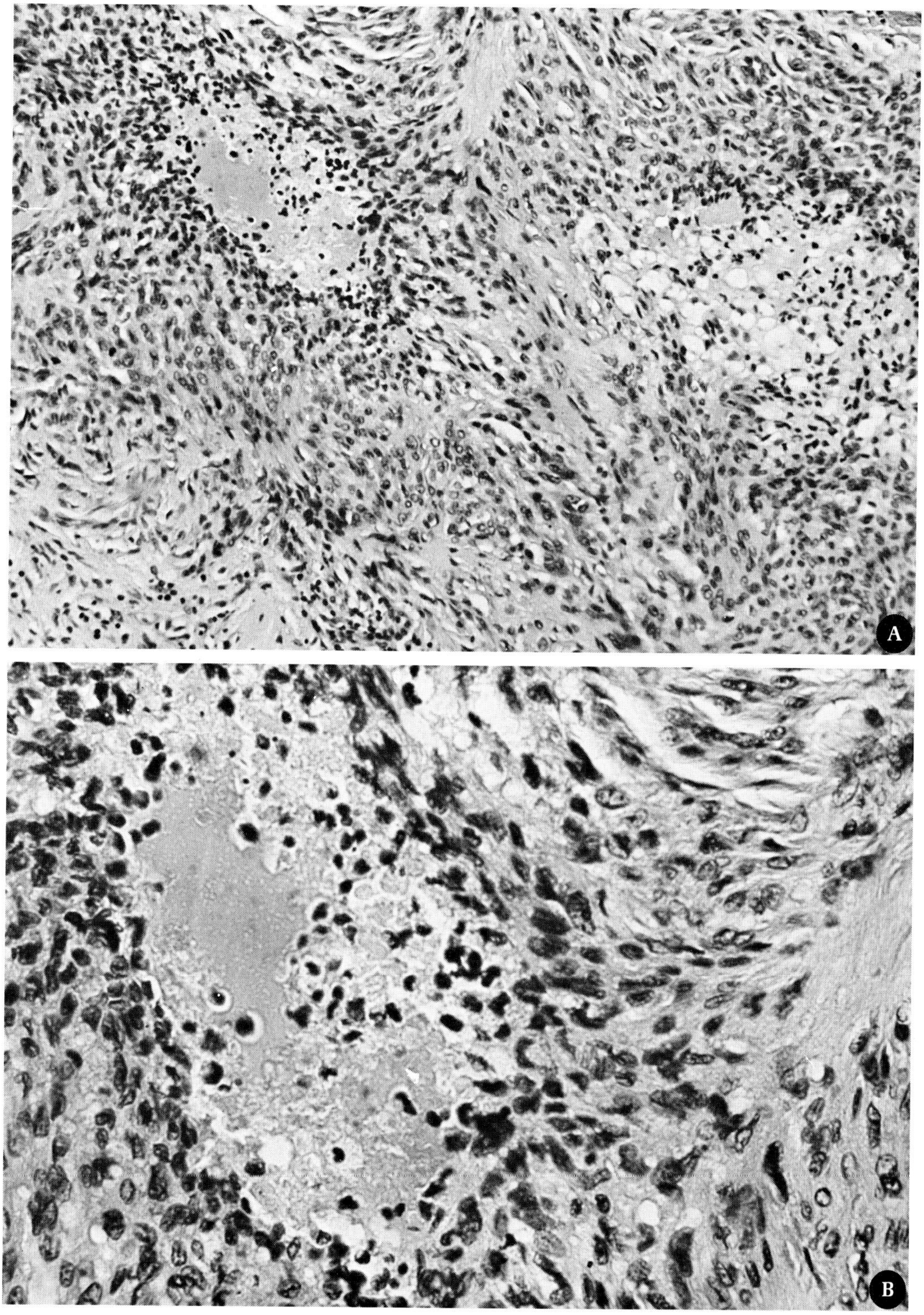

Figure 3-26. Tendosynovial sarcoma, so-called epithelioid sarcoma. The sarcoma is composed of fairly uniform oval or short spindle cells. The neoplastic cells cluster around necrotic centers and diffusely infiltrate the partly collagenous stroma. Note occasional lymphocytes and foam cells (**A,** H & E, ×140; **B,** H & E, ×350). (**A** from Hajdu, S. I., Shiu, M. H., and Fortner, J. G.: Tendosynovial sarcoma. A clinicopathologic study of 136 cases. Cancer 39:1201, 1977.)

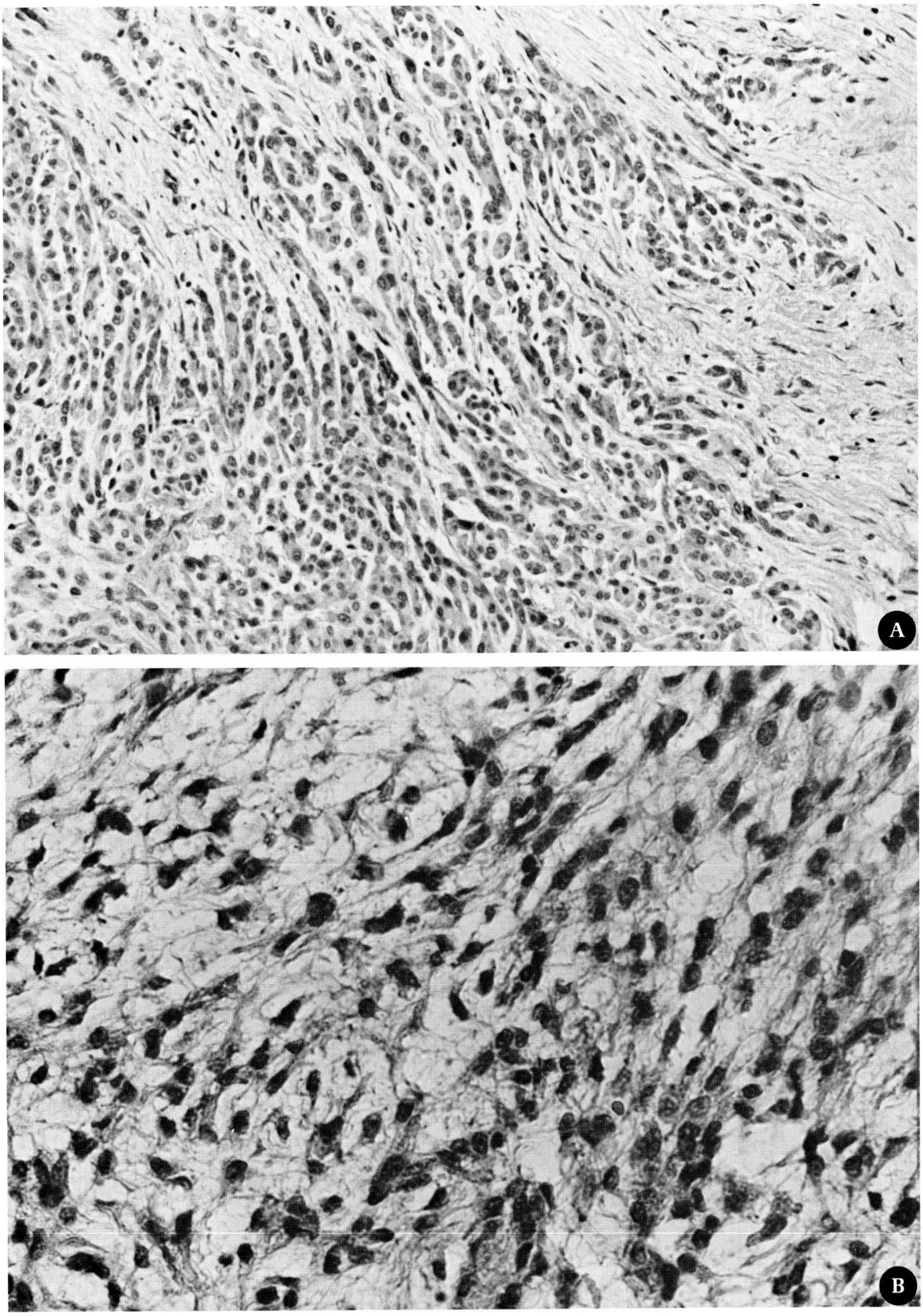

Figure 3-27. Tumor cells of epithelioid sarcoma form cell cords and infiltrates along collagenous cords of a tendon (H & E, ×140).

B, Epithelioid sarcoma of tendosynovial origin metastatic to intermuscular fascia proximal to the site of the primary tumor (H & E, ×350).

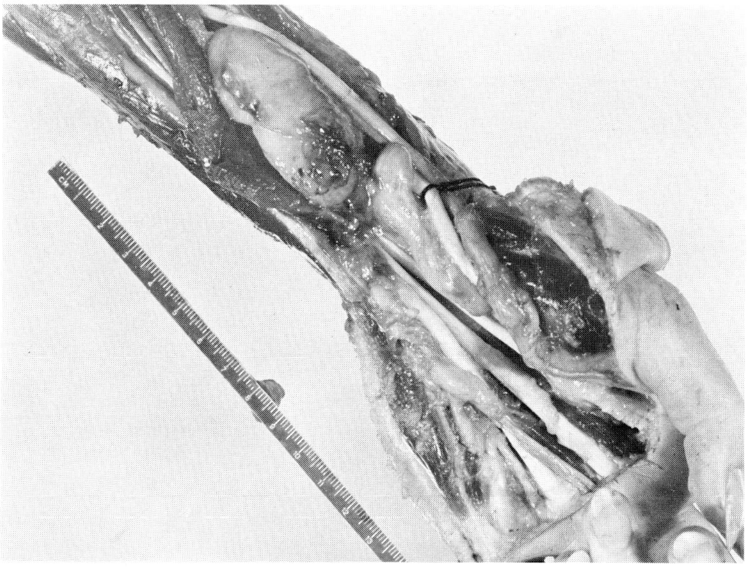

Figure 3-28. Multinodular subcutaneous presentation, limited to one anatomic region, along tendons, tendon sheaths, or fascia and from small to moderate size are characteristic features of tendosynovial epithelioid sarcoma (From Hajdu, S. I., Shiu, M. H., and Fortner, J. G.: Tendosynovial sarcoma. A clinicopathologic study of 136 cases. Cancer 39:1201, 1977).

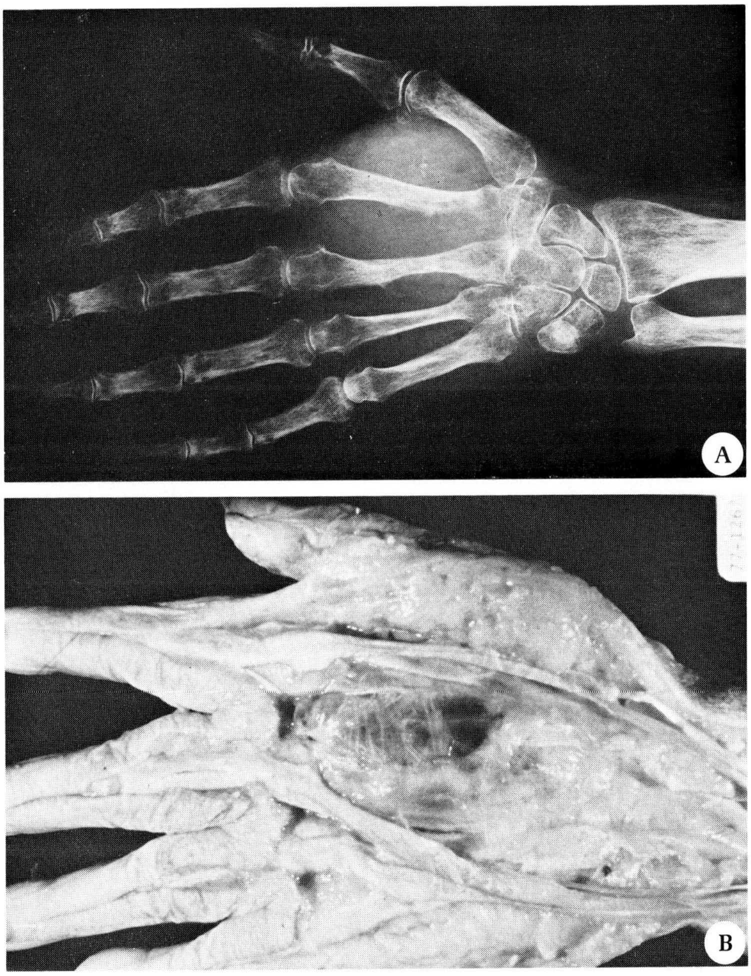

Figure 3-29. A, A poorly defined globoid mass, epithelioid sarcoma of the hand. **B,** Note the globoid brownish mass and its relation to adjacent tendons.

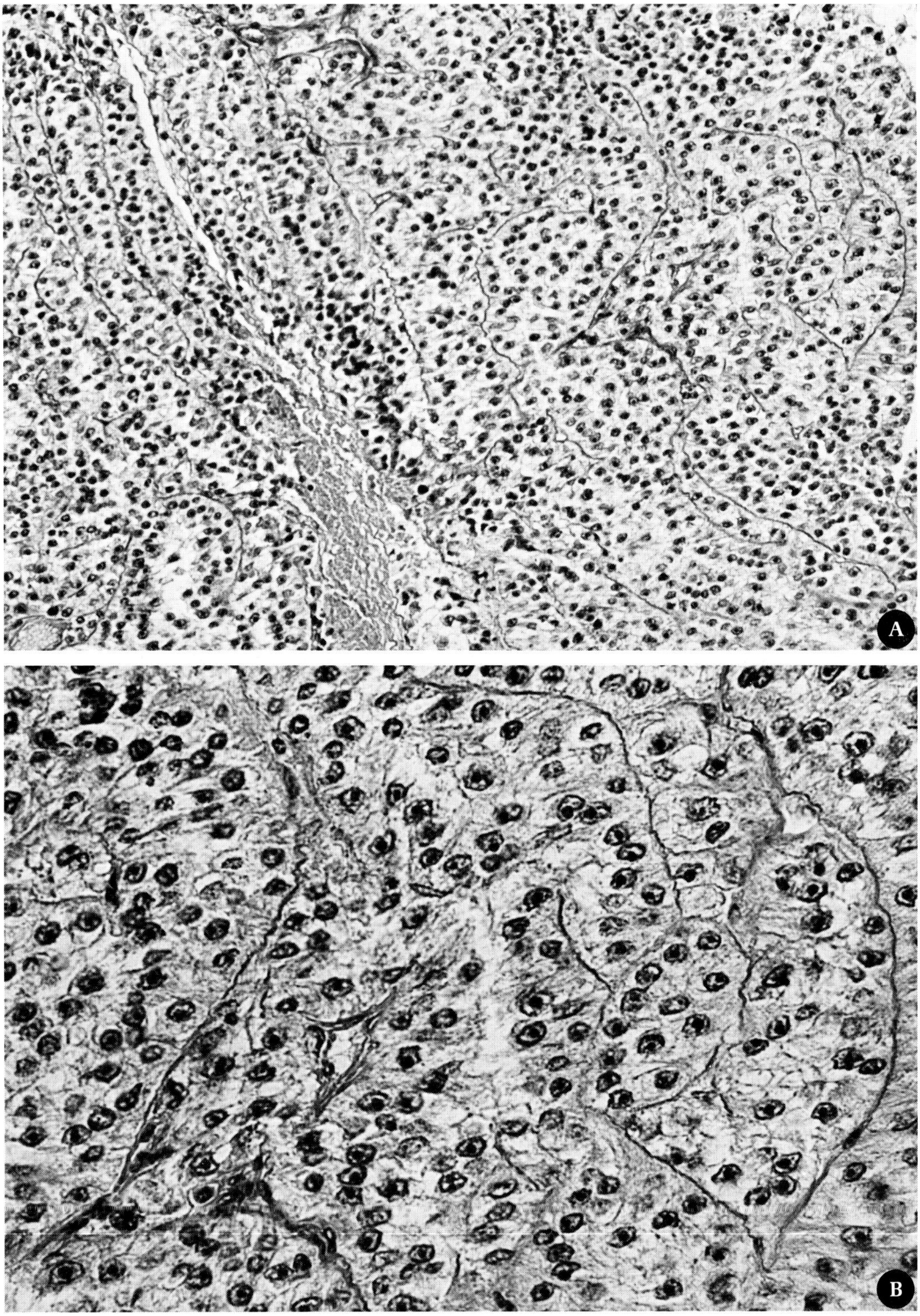

Figure 3-30. Tendosynovial sarcoma of the clear cell type, so-called clear cell sarcoma. This tumor is composed of uniform cuboidal, round, or short columnar cells arranged in clusters, cords, and lumenless tubular structures. The cytoplasm of the tumor cells is finely granular and sharply demarcated. The nuclei are round and uniform with prominent nucleoli. Note the absence of pleomorphic and giant cells which are so common in malignant melanoma. (**A,** H & E, ×140; **B,** H & E, ×350). (**B** from Hajdu, S. I., Shiu, M. H., and Fortner, J. G.: Tendosynovial sarcoma. A clinicopathologic study of 136 cases. Cancer 39:1201, 1977.)

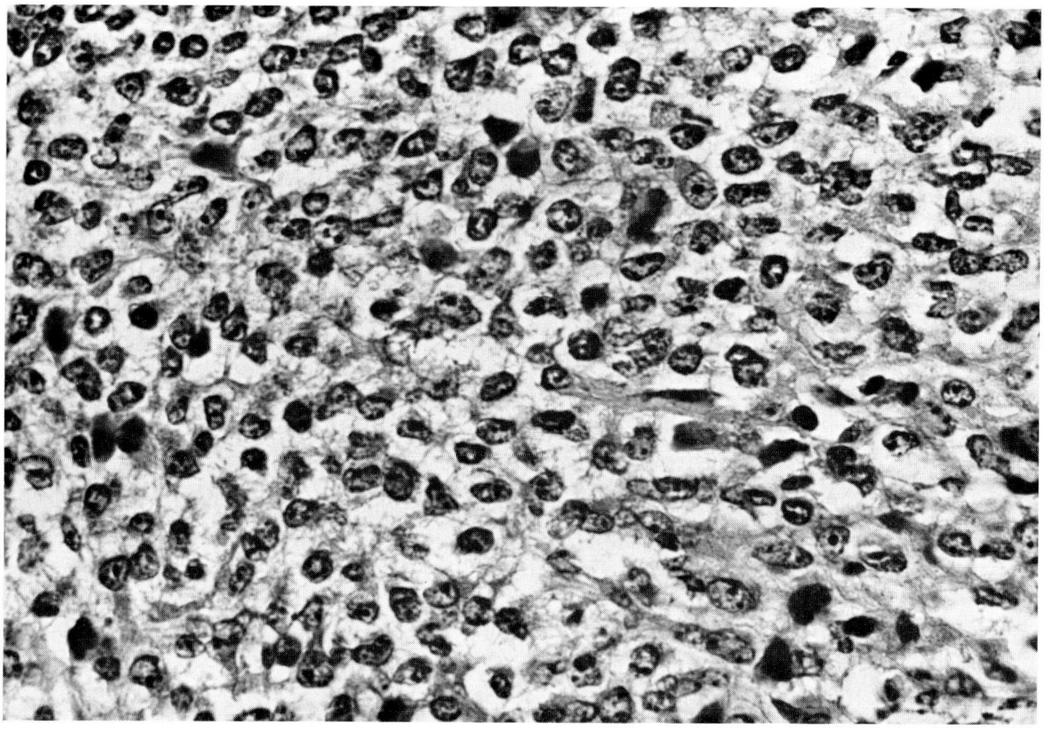

Figure 3-31. Tendosynovial clear cell sarcoma metastatic to the lung. The tumor cells are still well defined, uniform, round granular cells with prominent nuclei and clear cytoplasm; however, the arranged pattern illustrated in Figure 3-31 is not recognizable (H & E, ×350).

were evident. Hoffman and Carter reported a so-called clear cell sarcoma, which at the time of metastasis showed the presence of melanin pigment in the cytoplasm. Berman et al (1975) also reported a clear cell sarcoma which contained melanin. In light of these and other reports, a question should be raised about the true identity of some of the reported clear cell sarcomas.

Experienced surgical pathologists know that a number of neoplasms may have clear cell features. Among these are renal cell carcinoma, histiocytic lymphoma, alveolar cell carcinoma, mesonephric or mullerian carcinomas, certain skin adnexal neoplasms, malignant melanoma, paraganglioma, adrenal cortical carcinoma, hepatoma, schwannoma, leiomyoblastoma, histiocytic fibrous histiocytoma, hemangioendothelioma, and tendosynovial sarcoma.

Despite the heterogeneous and almost ubiquitous nature of the clear cells, it seems the term *clear cell sarcoma* should be retained and used with circumspection *after melanoma and other clear cell neoplasms have been ruled out* to identify this extremely rare form of tendosynovial neoplasm. Our experience with clear cell sarcomas (Hajdu et al, 1977), based on histochemical, ultrastructural, cytologic, and topographic studies, indicates not only that these neoplasms exist as tendosynovial neoplasms, but also that clear cell sarcomas are capable of showing features of other types of tendosynovial sarcomas when they recur or metastasize (Figs. 3-10, 3-11; Tables 3-9, 3-10). It is unfortunate that some authors consider all tendosynovial clear cell sarcomas as neuroectodermal tumors because in a number of the cases in their experience they were able to demonstrate intracytoplasmic melanin pigment and/or melanosomes. This oversimplification is misleading just as it would be wrong to consider all clear cell carcinomas as renal neoplasms. Clear

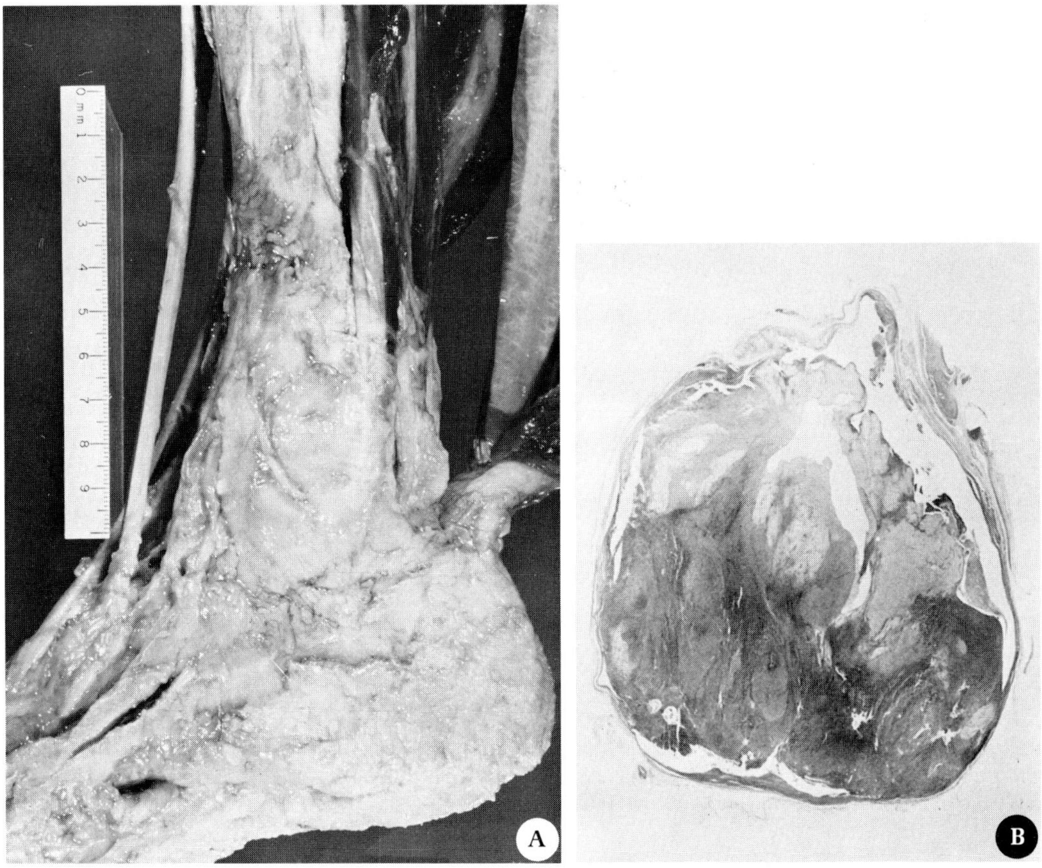

Figure 3-32. Tendosynovial sarcoma of the lower leg.

A, The tumor spread along the tendons and fibroconnective tissue compartments in the form of small discrete nodules.

B, Cross section of a tendon showing growth of the tumor within the tendon sheath with cystic degeneration and destruction of the tendon.

cell sarcoma of the tendosynovium is, without doubt, an entity. However, it must be remembered that a number of other tumors, including sarcomas, may have microscopic areas that resemble clear cell sarcoma, and one must study these tumors after adequate sampling by all available techniques and with full knowledge of the clinical presentation.

The fully malignant nature of clear cell sarcomas is apparent from published reports. They may occur at any site of the body, but they have particular predilection for the tendinous areas of the extremities (Fig. 3-32).

Chordoid Sarcoma. The term *chordoid tumor* or *chordoid sarcoma* was coined by Stewart, in 1948, but it was apparently Seidelin, in 1932, who reported the first authentic case under the title, "Liposarcoma with chordoma-like cells." If the case reports by Simard (1938), Laskowski (1955), Dutra (1960), Martin et al (1973), Weiss (1976), Hajdu et al (1977), and Dabska (1977) are considered acceptable, the total number of reported cases is less than two dozen. Our recent experience with 4 cases in addition to the two previously reported is summarized in Table 3-11.

Grossly chordoid tumors are fairly well-defined, grayish-looking lesions with a gelatinous consistency. They are extremely rare neoplasms found most commonly in the hand or wrist of middle-aged patients. The proximity, or direct relation, of the tumor to tendons, tendon sheaths, bursae, or chondrosynovial junctions can be established in almost every instance.

Histologically, chordoid tumors are composed of small oval or round cells with prominent nuclei and nucleoli. The cytoplasm is minute and dense and may appear polygonal. The tumor cells are loosely arranged in cords, clusters, or villous nodules. The stroma is almost completely devoid of cells but rich in mucopolysaccharides which stain faintly positive with PAS and alcian blue. Small ill-defined cartilaginous nodules scattered in the tumor give a distinct appearance to this otherwise harmless looking neoplasm (Figs. 3-33, 3-34). These neoplasms are apparently slowly growing, locally recurring malignant tumors with less than a 30% chance to metastasize and cause death (Table 3-13).

Prognosis

The rate of recurrence of tendosynovial sarcomas varies considerably from one reported series to another (Table 3-7). Nevertheless, there is general agreement that the majority of partially excised tumors will recur within a year and the rapidity of recurrence suggests a poor prognosis (Fig. 3-35).

Table 3-12 shows the rate of metastasis of tendosynovial sarcomas to regional lymph nodes, bone, and lung. We found (Hajdu et al, 1977) that biphasic, epithelioid, and clear cell sarcomas metastasize to lymph nodes more commonly than neoplasms without epithelioid or clear cell components (Fig. 3-36).

For the majority of the patients who die with tendosynovial sarcoma the direct cause of death is attributed to massive pleuropulmonary metastasis, but haphazard dissemination of the tumor to other organs can be expected terminally (Figs. 3-37, 3-38, 3-39). As would be expected, the survival of patients with tendosynovial sarcoma is influenced by a number of factors: duration of symptoms; size, anatomic site, and histologic type of the tumor; sex and age of the patient. In our series of 136 cases, we found that the overall 5-year survival rate of 40% was

TABLE 3-11. ***Series of Chordoid Tumors***

	AGE	SEX	SITE	THERAPY	RECURRENCE	THERAPY	FOLLOW-UP
Dabska (1977)	47	F	Ankle	Exc	7 yr.	Exc	NED, 7 yr.
	52	M	Knee	Exc	No	—	NED, 6 yr.
	18	M	Thigh	Exc	No	—	NED, 20 yr.
	12	M	Arm	Exc	No	—	NED, 10 yr.
	29	F	Back	Exc	19 yr.	Exc	NED, ?
	50	F	Groin	Exc	No	—	NED, 1 yr.
	22	F	Wrist	Exc	No	—	NED, 6 yr.
	25	F	Thigh	Exc	—	—	None
	28	F	Hand	Exc	2 yr.	—	NED, 5 yr.
	62	M	Buttock	Exc	No	—	NED, 5 yr.
Martin et al (1973)	32	F	Foot	Exc	No	—	NED, 10 yr.
	60	M	Foot	Exc	5 yr.	Amp	None
	52	M	Leg	Amp	—	—	NED, 12 yr.
	36	M	Foot	Exc	1 yr.	Exc	DcD, 7 yr.
Hajdu (unpublished)	40	M	Hand	Exc	2 yr.	Amp	NED, 6 yr.
	38	F	Thigh	Exc	1 yr.	Exc	DcD, 4 yr.
	62	F	Buttock	Exc	6 yr.	Exc	NED, 10 yr.
	42	M	Hand	Exc	—	—	None
	54	F	Knee	Exc	No	—	NED, 10 yr.
	59	M	Hand	Exc	2 yr.	Amp	NED, 3 yr.

Exc = excision; Amp = amputation; NED = no evidence of disease; DcD = died with disease.

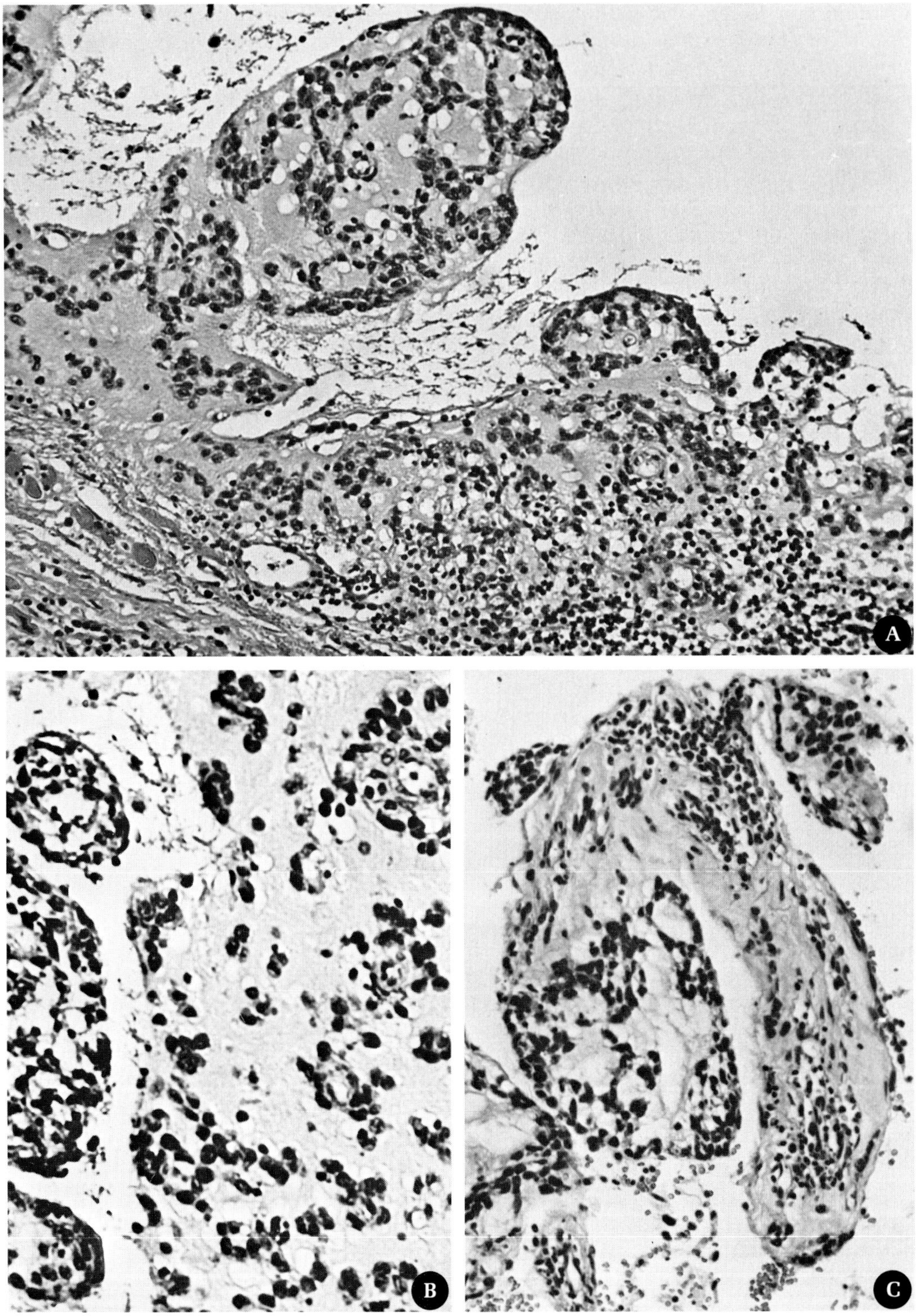

Figure 3-33. Chordoid sarcoma is composed of predominantly round or stellate cells in a myxoid stroma. The tumor cells are arranged in distinct villous papillae, clusters, or pseudoglands and the tumor cells near the surface of such structures have a tendency to form a delicate lining. (**A, C,** H & E, ×140; **B,** H & E, ×200). (**A** from Hajdu, S. I., Shiu, M. H., and Fortner, J. G.: Tendosynovial sarcoma. A clinicopathologic study of 136 cases. Cancer 39:1201, 1977.)

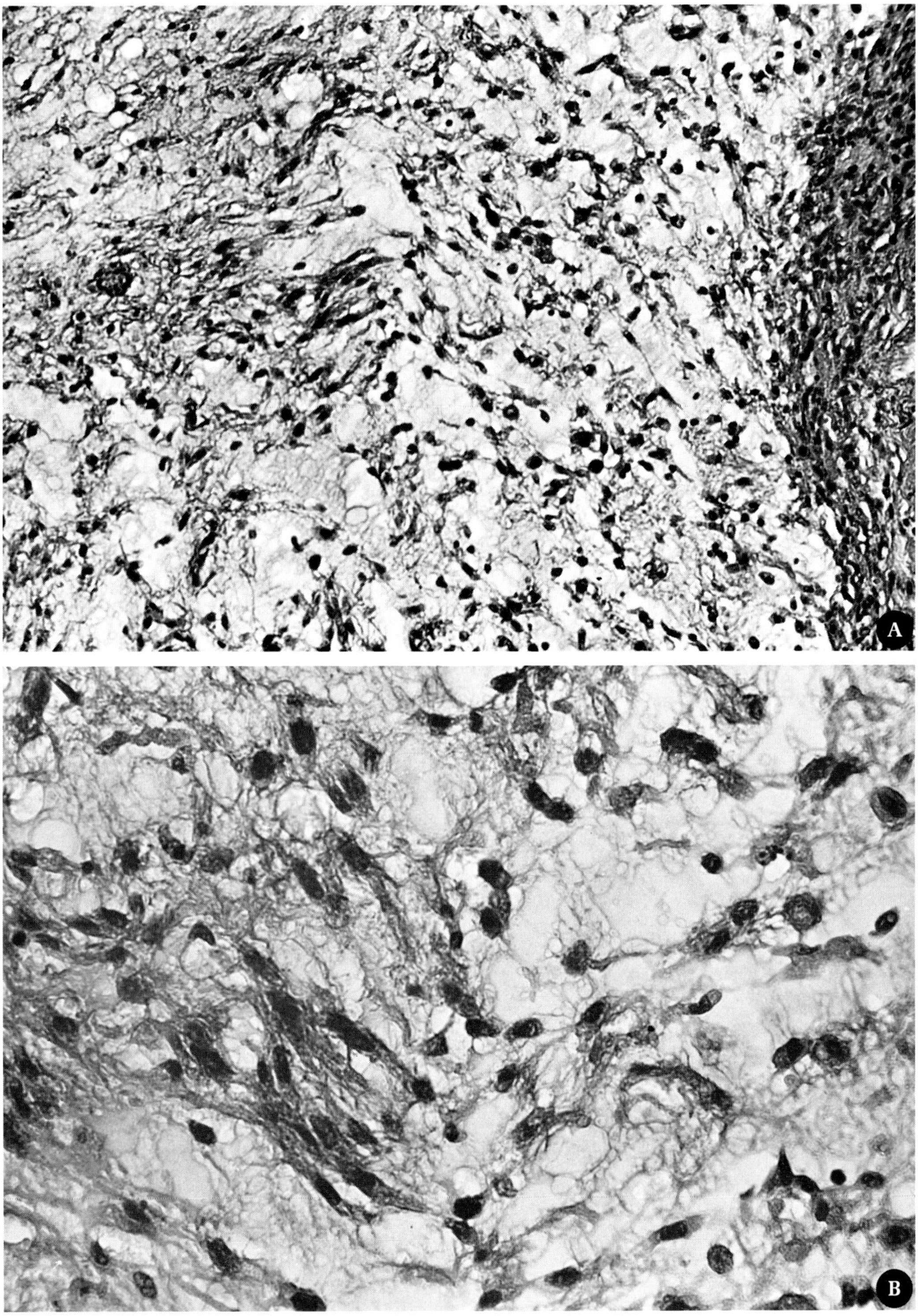

Figure 3-34. Stellate or polygonal tumor cells of chordoid sarcoma near the edge of the tumor. The tumor cells are joined together by fine cytoplasmic filaments. Note the mucopolysaccharide-rich granular and vacuolated stroma (**A,** H & E, ×140; **B,** H & E, ×350).

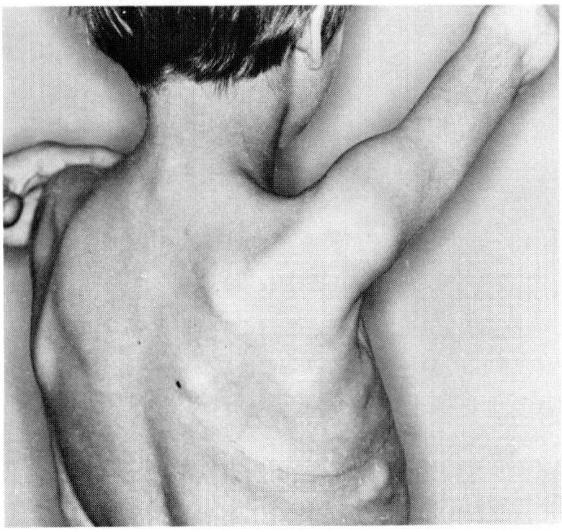

Figure 3-35. Subcutaneous nodules of metastatic tendosynovial sarcoma.

favorably influenced by the small size of the tumor (74%, 5-year survival), location at distal parts of the extremities (53%, 5-year survival), histologic type (biphasic, 55%, 5-year survival; epithelioid sarcoma, 58%, 5-year survival), and age of the patients (70%, 5-year survival during the first decade; 48%, 5-year survival after the sixth plus decades) (Figs. 3-9, 3-11, 3-13, 3-40; Table 3-6). (See also Fig. 1-59 and Table 1-15).

According to our findings (Hajdu et al, 1977; Shiu et al, 1979) the modality of surgical treatment is not a significant factor in 5-year survival of patients. The rates were 40% and 36%, respectively, when the tumor was removed by excision and am-

TABLE 3-12. ***Rate of Metastasis of Tendosynovial Sarcomas***

		METASTASES (%)		
AUTHORS	NUMBER REPORTED CASES	REGIONAL LYMPH NODE	BONE	LUNG
Pack and Ariel (1950)	60	19	8	65
Cadman et al (1965)	107	23	20	81
Hajdu et al (1977)	136	12	10	74

TABLE 3-13. ***Miscellaneous Findings in 136 Cases of Tendosynovial Sarcoma***

	TOTAL NO. OF PATIENTS	NO. OF PATIENTS ALIVE
Long duration of symptoms	15	3
Metastatic at diagnosis	5	0
Local recurrence	51	27
Local invasion of vessels	6	0
Local invasion of bone	12	1
Metastatic to bone	11	0
Metastatic to regional nodes	16	0
Metastatic to distant nodes	4	0
Metastatic to lung	99	8
Pulmonary resection	11	2
Malignant effusion	0	0

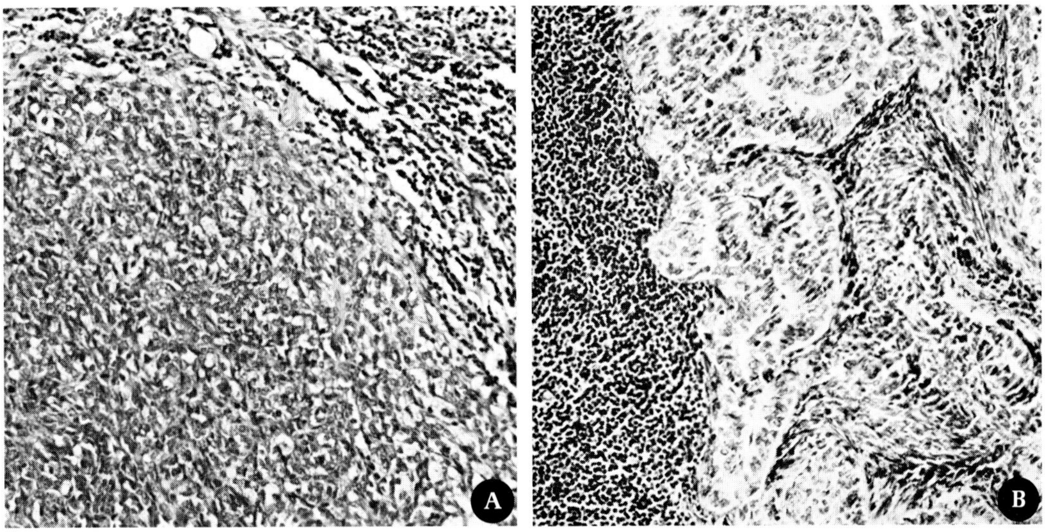

Figure 3-36. A, Epithelioid sarcoma metastatic to lymph node is composed of monophasic small stellate cells (H & E, $\times 140$).

B, Biphasic tendosynovial sarcoma metastatic to lymph node growing as monophasic pseudoglandular tendosynovial sarcoma (H & E, $\times 140$).

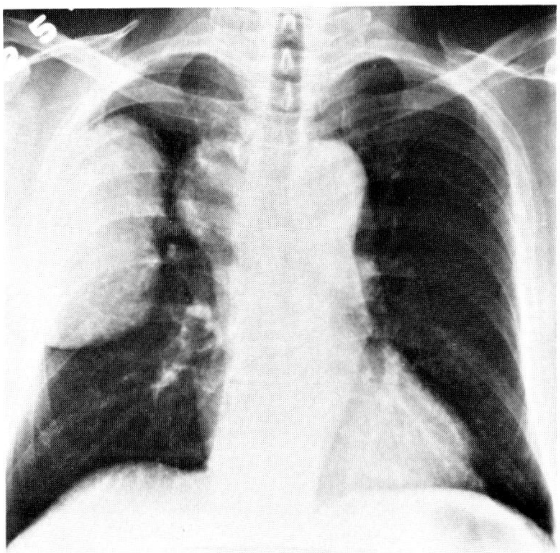

Figure 3-37. Massive and fatal pleuropulmonary metastasis of a tendosynovial sarcoma.

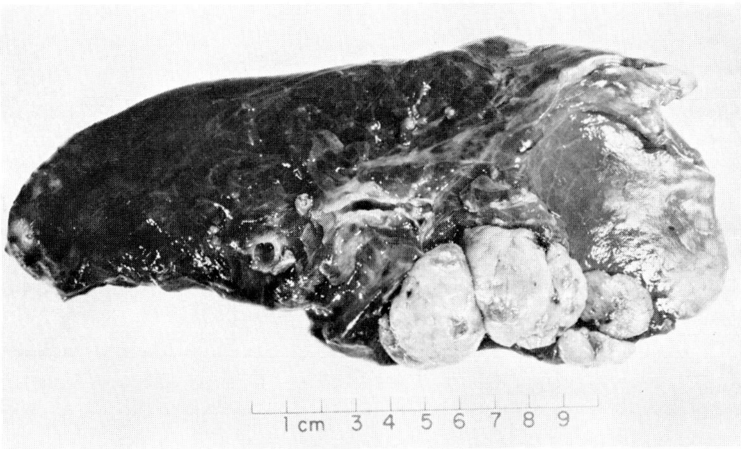

Figure 3-38. Resected lung with multiple solid pleuropulmonary nodules of metastatic tendosynovial sarcoma.

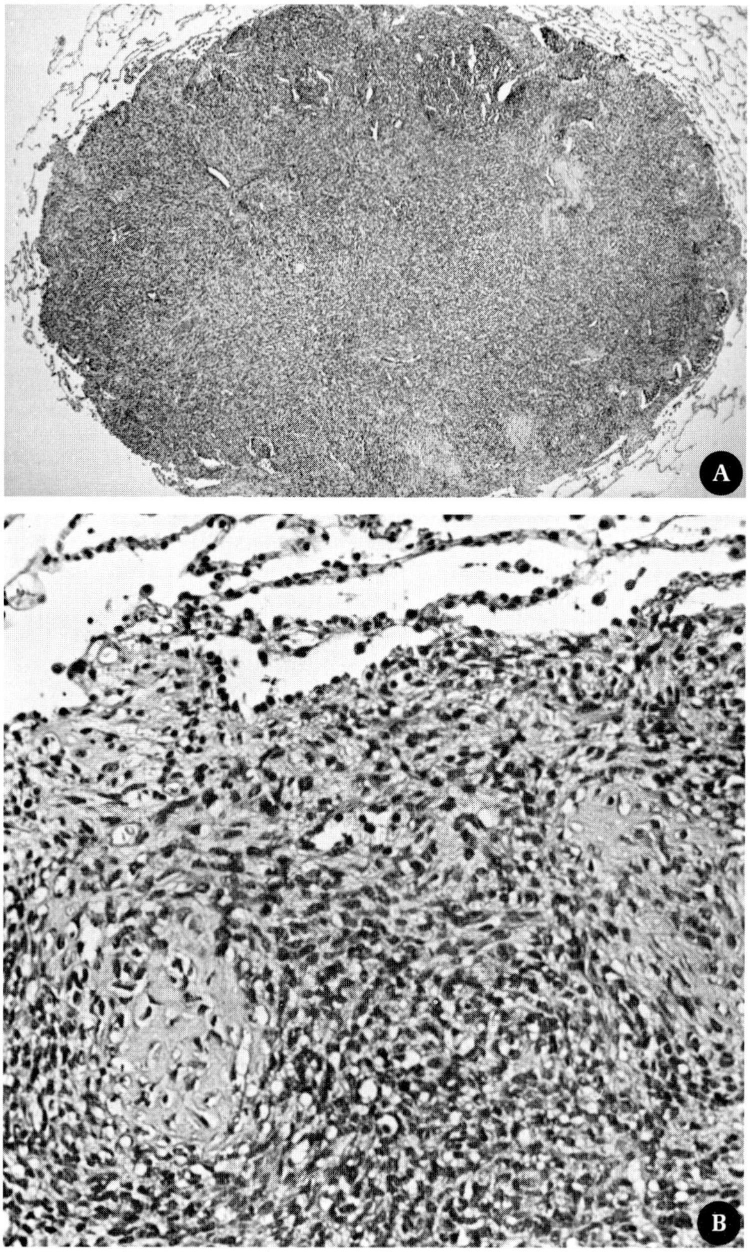

Figure 3-39. A circumscribed pulmonary nodule of a metastatic biphasic tendosynovial sarcoma.

A, The tumor is confined to one area and apparently grows by peripheral extension as a monophasic spindle cell type of tumor (H & E, ×35).

B, Note extension of tumor cells into the alveolar septa and absence of the biphasic pattern (H & E, ×140).

putation. However, with the inclusion of the size of the tumor it became apparent that 72% of the patients with small tumors and only 26% with large tumors (larger than 5 cm) survived for 5 years when the surgical treatment was short of amputation. Table 3-8 also shows that 76% of the patients with small tumor and only 25% of the patients with large tumor survived following amputation or more radical surgery. Therefore, it can be concluded that *the size of the primary tumor is per-*

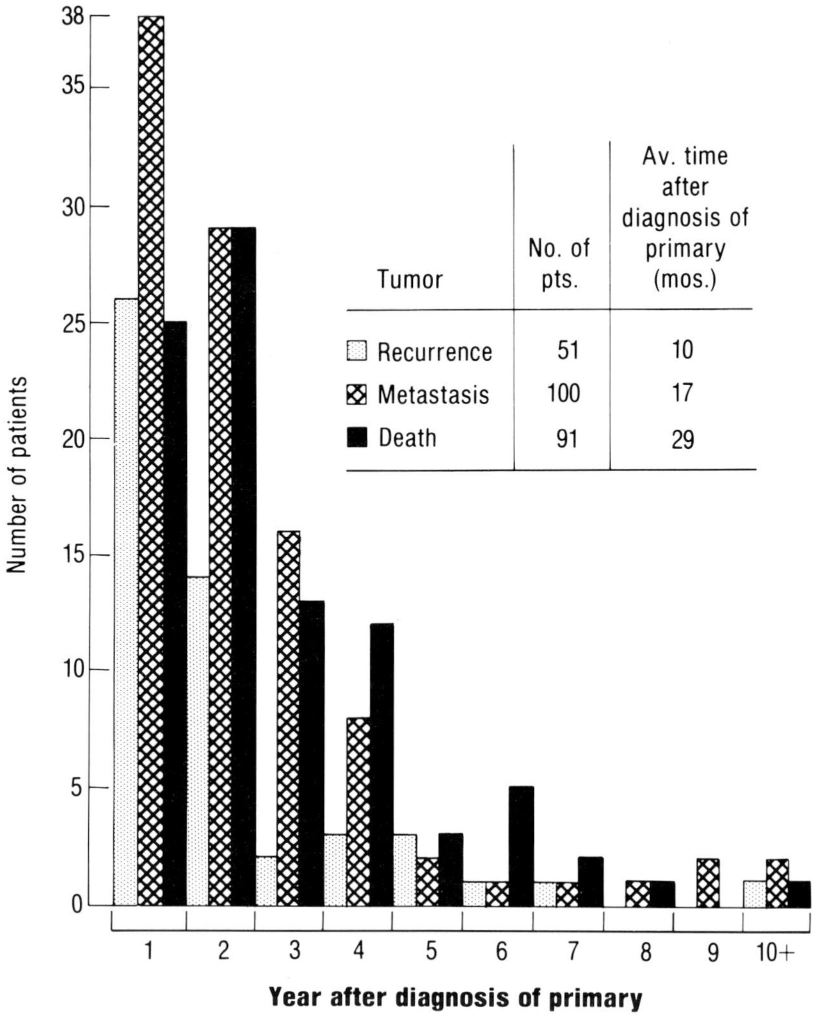

Figure 3-40. Most tendosynovial sarcomas recurred within a year after diagnosis of the primary lesion, metastasized within 2 years, and caused death less than 3 years after primary diagnosis. (From Hajdu, S. I., Shiu, M. H., and Fortner, J. G.: Tendosynovial sarcoma. A clinicopathologic study of 136 cases. Cancer 39:1201, 1977.)

haps more decisive in prognosis than anatomic site, histologic type, or modality of surgical treatment (Table 3-13; Fig. 3-41).

Differential Diagnosis

In the differential diagnosis of tendosynovial sarcomas a spectrum of neoplasms should be considered. *Malignant fibrous histiocytomas* can be easily distinguished from tendosynovial sarcomas; however, deeply seated fibroblastic fibrous histiocytomas may resemble monophasic spindle cell type sarcomas, but the cleft formations and villous projections of monophasic tumors are distinctly missing from fibrous histiocytomas. Similarly, schwannomas and leiomyosarcomas do not possess the same distinguishing features (see Chapter 2).

Biphasic tendosynovial sarcomas may resemble the pseudoglandular forms of *skin adnexal tumors* or other types of *adenocarcinomas*. However, the biphasic morphology, the non-cytoplasmic nature

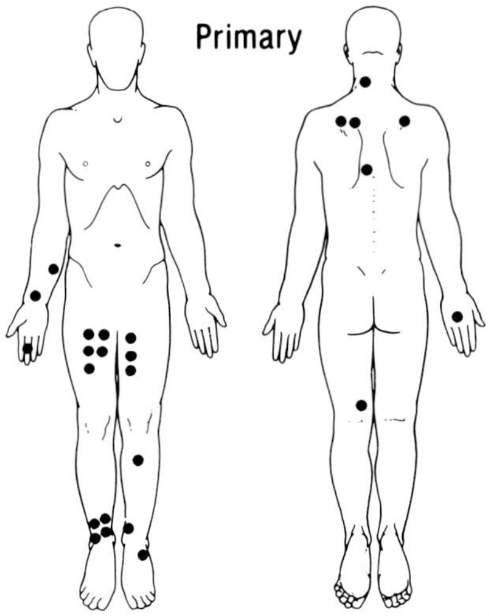

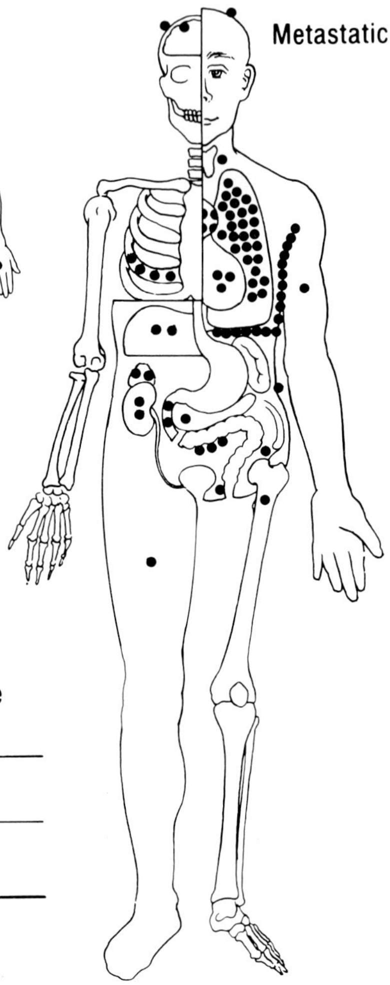

	No. of Patients	Average Age
Male	**18**	**30**
Female	**8**	**21**
	26	**26**

Figure 3-41. Postmortem findings show that tendosynovial sarcomas have a predilection to spread to pleuropulmonary and subcutaneous tissues (see Appendix).

of mucicarminophilic material, and the absence of pleomorphic cells are permanent findings in pseudoglandular tendosynovial sarcomas. In addition, *epithelioid mesothelioma* should be considered in the differential diagnosis but by virtue of its pleomorphism and collagenous and nonmucicarminophilic nature rarely if ever should cause diagnostic problems.

In limited biopsy material *epithelioid sarcoma* may contain areas that are indistinguishable from benign necrotizing or granulomatous processes. However, generous sampling almost invariably will disclose the non-inflammatory, multinodular, and infiltrative nature of epithelioid sarcoma.

Clear cell sarcoma is an extremely rare tendosynovial sarcoma that should be considered if the lesion is topographically tendosynovial in nature and melanin as well as mucicarmine stains are negative. The majority of neuroectodermal tumors such as *clear cell* or *nevoid schwannomas, blue nevi,* and *malignant melanomas* either stain positive with melanin stain or contain melanosomes or premelanosomes. Most of the *epithelial clear cell tumors,* on the other hand, contain in the cytoplasm either mucicarminophilic material or nondigestible PAS-positive granules.

Chordoid sarcoma is far less common than any of the other tendosynovial neoplasms. In differential diagnosis one should consider *mesenchymal chondrosarcoma* of soft parts. Mesenchymal chondrosarcoma is usually more compact, more cellular, more cartilaginous, more pleomorphic, and less mucinous or myxoid in appearance than chordoid sarcoma. (See Chapter 8.)

REFERENCES

References are listed in chronological order in each category.

INTRODUCTION

Bonn: De Continuationibus Membranarum. Amsterdam, 1763.

Winslow, J. B.: Exposition Anatomique de la Structure du Corps Humain. Paris, 1782.

Bichat, X.: Traite de Membranes. Paris, 1800.

Velpeau, A.: Traite complet d'anatomie chirurgical. Paris, 1837.

Von Kolliker, A.: Mikroskopische Anatomie. Leipzig, W. Engelmann, 1850.

Henle, F. G. J.: Handbuch der systematischen Anatomie des Menschen. Braunschweig, Vieweg & Sohn, 1855–71.

Hueter, C.: Zur Hist. d. Gelenkflaechen u. Gelenkkapsein. Virchows Arch. 66:1876.

Soubbotine, A.: Recherches histologiques sur la structure des membranes synoviales. Arch. physiol. norm. path. 2:532, 1880.

Masson, P., and Peyron, A.: A propos des tumeurs mixtes des glandes salivaires. Bull. Assoc. franc. Cancer 7:219, 1914.

Mayeda, T.: Experimentelle histologische Studie uber die Synovialmembrane. Mitt. med. Fakult. Tokyo 23:393, 1920.

Vaubel, E.: The form and function of synovial cells in tissue culture. J. Exp. Med. 58:63, 1932.

King, E. S. J.: The Golgi apparatus of synovial cells under normal and pathological conditions and with reference to the formation of synovial fluid. J. Pathol. 41:117, 1935.

Meyer, K., Smyth, E. M., and Dawson, M. H.: The isolation of a mucopolysaccharide from synovial fluid. J. Biol. Chem. 128:319, 1939.

Castor, C. W.: Production of mucopolysaccharides by synovial cells in simplified tissue culture medium. Proc. Soc. Exp. Biol. Med. 94:51, 1957.

Ropes, M. W.: Examination of synovial fluid. Bull. Rheum. Dis. 7:(Suppl. 5), 1957.

Lever, J. D., and Ford, E. H. R.: Histological, histochemical and electron microscopic observations on synovial membrane. Anat. Rec. 132:525, 1958.

Peach, R., Williams, G., and Chapman, J. A.: A light and electron optical study of regenerating tendon. Am. J. Pathol. 38:495, 1961.

Barland, P., Novikoff, A. B., and Hamerman, D.: Electron microscopy of the human synovial membrane. J. Cell Biol. 14:207, 1962.

Shaw, N. E., and Martin, B. F.: Histological and histochemical studies on mammalian knee joint tissues. J. Anat. 96:359, 1962.

Ball, J., Chapman, J. A., and Muirden, K. D.: The uptake of iron in rabbit synovial tissue following the intra-articular injection of iron dextran. A light and electron microscopic study. J. Cell Biol. 22:351, 1964.

Blau, S., Janis, R., Hamerman, D., and Sandson, J.: Cellular origin of hyaluronate proteins in the human synovial membrane. Science 150:353, 1965.

Good, A. E., and Frishette, W. A.: Crystals in dried smears of synovial fluid. JAMA 198:80, 1966.

Sutton, J. S., and Weiss, L.: Transformation of monocytes in tissue culture into macrophages, epithelioid cells, and multinucleated giant cells. An electron microscope study. J. Cell Biol. 28:303, 1966.

Evanson, J. M., Jeffrey, J. J., and Krane, S. M.: Human collagenase: identification and characterization of an enzyme from rheumatoid synovium in culture. Science 158:499, 1967.

Mitchell, N. S., and Cruess, R. L.: Synovial regeneration after synovectomy. Can. J. Surg. 10:234, 1967.

Palmar, D. G.: Synovial villi. Arthritis Rheum. 10:451, 1967.

Peacock, E. E.: Dynamic aspects of collagen biology. II. Degradation and metabolism. J. Surg. Res. 7:481, 1967.

Greenlee, T. K.: The fine structure changes in differentiation of tendon fibroblasts. South. Med. J. 61:711, 1968.

Ghadially, F. N., and Roy, S.: Ultrastructure of Synovial Joints in Health and Disease. London, Butterworths, 1969.

Hahn, K. J., and Hahn, M.: Hyaluronate synthesis by human synovial cells in monolayer culture under treatment with indomethacin and phenylbutazone. Pharmacology 5:97, 1971.

Kishner, I., and Somerville, J. A.: Permeability

of human synovial membrane to plasma proteins. Arthritis Rheum. 14:560, 1971.
Hirohata, K.: Electron microscopic observation of synovial tissue in health and disease. *In* Biochemistry and Pathology of Connective Tissue. Edited by Y. Otaka. Tokyo, Igaku Shoin, 1974.
Werb, Z., and Gordon, S.: Secretion of a specific collagenase by stimulated macrophages. J. Exp. Med. 142:346, 1975.
Bub, V., Lippert, H., Zech, M., and Arnold, G.: Zur Biomechanik menschlicher Sehnen: Zusammenhange von Relaxation und Spannungsruckgewinn. Arch. Orthop. Unfallchir. 80:169, 1976.

NON-NEOPLASTIC LESIONS

Cruveilhier, J.: Anatomie pathologique du corps humain. Paris, Bailliere, 1829–1835.
Wilks, S.: Lectures on Pathological Anatomy. London, Longman, 1859.
Clark, W. C.: The pathogenesis of ganglia. Surg. Gynecol. Obstet. 7:56, 1908.
Dowd, C. N.: Villous arthritis of the knee. Ann. Surg. 56:363, 1912.
Robineau, S.: Chondromatose articulaire. Bull. Mem. Soc. Chir. Paris 14:491, 1919.
Chauvin and Roux: Fibro-chondrome de la gaine tendineuse de l'extenseur du quatrième orteil. Bull. Mem. Soc. Anat. Paris 90:75, 1920.
Fisher, A. G. T.: A study of loose bodies composed of cartilage and bone occurring in joints. With special reference to their pathology and etiology. Br. J. Surg. 6:493, 1921.
Carp, L., and Stout, A. P.: A study of ganglia with special reference to treatment. Surg. Gynecol. Obstet. 47:460, 1928.
Reimann, H., and Kienbock, R.: Uber Gelenks-Osteochondromatose mit Sarkombildung. Roentgenpraxis 3:942, 1931.
Bearse, C.: Ganglions of tendon sheaths: Method of treatment. JAMA 109:1626, 1937.
Coggeshall, H. C., Warren, C. F., and Bauer, W.: The cytology of normal human synovial fluid. Anat. Rec. 77:129, 1940.
Kautz, F. G.: Capsular osteoma of the knee joint, report of four cases. Radiology 45:162, 1945.
Bennett, G. A.: Reactive and neoplastic changes in synovial tissue. Proc. Inst. Med. Chicago 18:26, 1950.
Sherman, M.: The non-specificity of synovial reactions. Bull. Hosp. Joint Dis. 12:110, 1951.
Brooks, D. N.: Nerve compression by simple ganglia: a review of 13 collected cases. J. Bone Joint Surg. 34B:391, 1952.
Trevor, D.: A case of synovial chondromatosis of the temporomandibular joint. Postgrad. Med. J. 28:408, 1952.
Becker W. F.: Hydrocortisone therapy in ganglia. Industr. Med. Surg. 22:555, 1953.
Fisk, G. R.: Bone concavity caused by a ganglia. J. Bone Joint Surg. 37B:663, 1955.
Hicks, J. D.: Synovial cysts in bone. Aust. N.Z. J. Surg. 26:138, 1956.
Jones, R. S., and Carter, Y.: Experimental arthritis. I. Morphologic alterations of the guinea pig after the parenteral injection of bacterial extracts. Arch. Pathol. 63:472, 1957.
Nixon, J. E., Frank, G. R., and Chambers, G.: Synovial osteochondromatosis. With report of four cases, one showing malignant change. U.S. Armed Forces Med. J. 11:1434, 1960.
Page-Thomas, D. P., Dingle, J. T., and Cook, E. R.: Synovial proliferation induced by polysaccharides. Nature 186:251, 1960.
McCarty, D. J., and Hollander, J. L.: Identification of urate crystals in gouty synovial fluid. Ann. Intern. Med. 54:452, 1961.
Murphy, F. P., Dahlin, D. C., and Sullivan, C. R.: Articular synovial chondromatosis. J. Bone Joint Surg. 44A:77, 1962.
Davis, J. M. G.: The ultrastructural changes that occur during the transformation of lung macrophages to giant cells and fibroblasts in experimental asbestosis. Br. J. Exp. Pathol. 44:568, 1963.
Hamerman, D., Sandson, J., and Schubert, M.: Biochemical events in joint disease. J. Chronic Dis. 16:835, 1963.
Barland, P., Novikoff, A. B., and Hamerman, D.: Structure and cytochemistry of the rheumatoid synovial membrane with special reference to lysosomes. Am. J. Pathol. 44:853, 1964.
Curtiss, P. H.: Changes produced in the synovial membrane and synovial fluid by disease. J. Bone Joint Surg. 46A:873, 1964.
Dao, L.: A new method of treatment of ganglia and synovial cysts. J. Occup. Med. 6:217, 1964.
Goldman, R. L., and Lichtenstein, L.: Synovial chondrosarcoma. Cancer 17:1238, 1964.
Gristma, A. G., and Wilson, P. D.: Popliteal cysts in adults and children. Arch. Surg. 88:357, 1964.
Hollander, J. L., McCarty, D. J., Astorga, G., and Castro-Murillo, E. I.: The "R.A. cell" and a working hypothesis. Ann. Intern. Med. 62:271, 1965.
Mullins, F., Berard, C. W., and Eisenberg, S. H.: Chondrosarcoma following synovial chondromatosis. Cancer 18:1180, 1965.
Schmid, F. R., and Ogata, R. I.: Synovial fluid evaluation in joint disease. Med. Clin. North Am. 49:165, 1965.
Derbyphiro, R. L.: Observation of the treatment in ganglia. Am. J. Surg. 112:636, 1966.

Grimley, P. M., and Sokoloff, L.: Synovial giant cells in rheumatoid arthritis. Am. J. Pathol. 49:931, 1966.

Malinin, T. I., Pekin, T. J., Bauer, H., and Zvaifler, N. J.: Vacuoles in synovial fluid leukocytes. Am. J. Clin. Pathol. 45:728, 1966.

Norton, W. L., and Ziff, M.: Electron microscopic observations on the rheumatoid synovial membrane. Arthritis Rheum. 9:589, 1966.

Soren, A.: Pathogenesis and treatment of ganglion. Clin. Orthop. 48:173, 1966.

Hageman, P. O.: Sporotrichosis tendovitis and tendosynovitis. Trans. Am. Clin. Climatol. Assoc. 79:193, 1967.

Jeffreys, T. E.: Synovial chondromatosis. J. Bone Joint Surg. 49B:530, 1967.

Bender, G., Aszodi, K., and Barsony, I.: Maligne Umbildung einer synovialen Osteochondromatosis. Z. Orthop. 105:208, 1968.

Gaucher, A., Faure, G., Netter, P., Pourel, J., and Duheiller, J.: Application de la microscopie electronique a balayage a l'evaluation de la teneur en fer de la membrane synoviale humaine. Sem. Hop. Paris 52:1543, 1968.

Muirden, K. D., and Senator, G. B.: Iron in the synovial membrane in rheumatoid arthritis and other joint diseases. Ann. Rheum. Dis. 27:38, 1968.

Schumacher, H. R.: The synovitis of pseudogout: Electron microscopic observations. Arthritis Rheum. 11:426, 1968.

Jayson, M. I. V., and Dixon, A. S. J.: Valvular mechanism in juxta articular cysts. Ann. Rheum. Dis. 29:415, 1970.

Ryan, G. B., and Spector, W. G.: Macrophage turnover in inflamed connective tissue. Proc. R. Soc. Lond. 175:269, 1970.

Andrew, L., and Elken, O.: Arthrographic studies on wrist ganglia. J. Bone Joint Surg. 53A:299, 1971.

Sim, F. H., and Dahlin, D. C.: Ganglion cysts of bone. Mayo Clin. Proc. 46:484, 1971.

Barthel, C. H., Huncan, J. R., and Ross, R. F.: Histologic and histochemical characterization of synovial membrane from normal and Mycoplasma hyorhinis-infected swine. Am. J. Vet. Res. 33:2501, 1972.

Dehaven, J. D.: Sporotrichosis arthritis and tenosynovitis. J. Bone Joint Surg. 54A:874, 1972.

Lussier, A., Medicis, R., Brochu, N. A., and Myhal, D.: Les microcristaux et leur implication cytopathogenique dans les arthrites. Union Med. Can. 101:2672, 1972.

Toyama, W. M.: Familial popliteal cysts in children. Am. J. Dis. Child. 124:586, 1972.

Bowerman, J. W., and Muhletaler, C.: Arthrography of rheumatoid synovial cysts of the knee and wrist. J. Can. Assoc. Radiol. 24:24, 1973.

Naib, Z. M.: Cytology of synovial fluids. Acta Cytol. 17:279, 1973.

Taylor, A. R., and Rana, N. A.: A valve, an explanation of the formation of popliteal cysts. Ann. Rheum. Dis. 32:419, 1973.

Marrocco, G. R., Tihen, W. S., Goodnough, C. P., and Johnson, R. J.: Granulomatous synovitis and osteitis caused by Sporothrix schenckii. Am. J. Clin. Pathol. 64:345, 1975.

Broderick, P. A., Corvese, N., Pierik, M. G., Pike, R. F., and Mariorenzi, A. L.: Exfoliative cytology interpretation of synovial fluid in joint disease. J. Bone Joint Surg. 58A:396, 1976.

Dayer, J. M., Krane, S. M., and Russell, R. G. G.: Production of isolated adherent rheumatoid synovial cells. Proc. Natl. Acad. Sci. USA 73:945, 1976.

Holm, C. L.: Primary synovial chondromatosis of the ankle. J. Bone Joint Surg. 58A:878, 1976.

Lenz, W., Klein, W., and Huth, F.: Punktatdiagnostik von Gicht und Pseudogicht. Beitr. Pathol. 157:161, 1976.

Trias, A., and Quintana, O.: Synovial chondrometaplasia: Review of world literature and a study of 18 Canadian cases. Can. J. Surg. 19:151, 1976.

Akhtar, M., Mahajan, S., and Kott, E.: Synovial chondromatosis of the temporomandibular joint. J. Bone Joint Surg. 59A:266, 1977.

Dayer, J. M., Russell, R. G. G., and Krane, S. M.: Collagenase production by rheumatoid synovial cells: stimulation by a human lymphocyte factor. Science 195:181, 1977.

Dryll, A., Lansaman, J., Peltier, A. P., Cazalis, P., de Seze, S., and Bariety, J.: Ultrastructural study of human synovial membrane with immunoperoxidase. Lab. Invest. 36:68, 1977.

Mainardi, C. L., Werb, Z., and Harris, E. D.: Proliferative synovitis in hemophilia: morphologic and biochemical observations. Arthritis Rheum. 20:127a, 1977.

Werb, Z., Mainardi, C. L., Vater, C. A., and Harris, E. D.: Endogenous activation of latent collagenase by rheumatoid synovial cells. N. Engl. J. Med. 296:1017, 1977.

Someren, A., and Merritt, W.H.: Tenosynovial chondroma of the hand: A case report with a brief review of the literature. Hum. Pathol. 9:476, 1978.

Villacin, A. B., Brigham, L. N., and Bullough, P. G.: Primary and secondary chondrometaplasia. Human Pathol. 10:439, 1979.

NEOPLASTIC LESIONS

Bichat, M. F. X.: Anatomie Generale Traite des Membranes. Paris, Brosson, 1806.

Lebert, H.: Physiologie Pathologique. Paris, Bailliere, 1845.
Robin, M. C.: Sur l'existence de deux especes nouvelles d'elements anatomique qui se trouvent dans le canal medullaire de os. C. R. Soc. Biol. 1:119, 1849.
Chassaignac, M.: Tumeur des gaines tendinéuses. Gaz. Hop. (Paris) 47:185, 1852.
Henle, F. G. J.: Handbuch der systematischen Anatomie des Menschen. Braunschweig, Vieweg & Sohn, 1855–71.
Wells, S.: Tumor from the flexor tendon of a forefinger. Trans. Pathol. Soc. London, pp. 379–380, 1857.
Wilks, S.: Lectures on Pathological Anatomy. London, Longman, 1859.
Broca, M.: Tumeur a myeloplaxes de la main. Bull. Soc. Chirurgie 1:342, 1860.
Simon, G.: Exstirpation einer sehr grossen, mit dicken Stiele angewachsenen Kneigelenkmaus mit gluklichem Erfolge. Arch. Klin. Chir. 6:573, 1865.
Czerny, V.: Fibrosarcome de la gaine tendineuse du quatrieme doigt. Arch. Klin. Chir. 10:904, 1869.
Rustizky, J.: Epithelialcarcinom der Dura mater mit hyaliner degeneration. Virchows Arch. (Pathol. Anat.) 59:191, 1874.
Gross: Tumeur sarcomateuse myeloide de la paume de la main gauche. Bull. Mem. Soc. Chir. Paris 4:281, 1878.
Hagen-Torn, O.: Entwickelung und Bau der Synovialmembranen. Arch. mikr. Anat. 21:591, 1882.
Heurtaux, A.: Myelome des gaines tendineuses. Arch. gén. Méd. 28:40; 160, 1891.
Stuer, J.: Eine ungewohnliche Geschwulst der Ellenbogenge lenksgegend. Mang. Diss. Wurzburg, 1893.
Bonjour, S.: Tumeurs fibro-tendineuses a myeloplaxes. These de Paris, 1897.
Targett, J. H.: Giant-celled tumours of the integuments. Trans. Pathol. Soc. London 48:230, 1897.
Dor, L.: Relation des tumeurs a myeloplaxes et des Xanthoms. Cong. franc. Chir. Paris, 1898.
Marsh, H.: Primary sarcoma of the synovial membrane of the kneejoint. Lancet 1330, 1898.
Venot, A.: Myelome des gaines tendineuses a point de part ossuex. Rev. Chir. 17:232, 1898.
Bellamy, H. F.: The myeloid tumor of tendon sheaths. J. Pathol. Bacteriol. 7:465, 1901.
Tomaselli, R.: Myeloma della guaine tendinee. La Reforma Medica, 1901, page 770.
Marsh, H.: Discussion of cases of sarcoma of synovial membrane of the knee joint. Lancet 1:1398, 1902.
Bloodgood, J. C.: Haemangiomatous elephantiasis. Prog. Med. 4:154, 1903.
Suter, F. A.: Zur Casuistik der Fingertumoren. Arch. Klin. Chir. 75:624, 1905.
Lejars, F., and Rubens-Duval, H.: Les sarcomes primitifs des synoviales articulaires. Rev. Chir. 41:751, 1910.
Dowd, C. N.: Villous arthritis of the knee (sarcoma). Ann. Surg. 56:363, 1912.
Smirnoff, A.: Sur les tumeurs de burses sereuses de l'articulation du genou. Chirour. Arch. Bel. 27:193, 1912.
Spiess, P.: Zur Lehre der von Schnenscheiden und Aponeurosen ausgehenden Riesenzellensarkome. Frankfurt. Z. Pathol. 13:1, 1913.
Tourneux, J. P.: Les sarcomes des gaines tendineuses. Rev. Chir. 47:817, 1913.
Beekman, F.: Giant-cell tumors of the tendon sheaths. Ann. Surg. 62:738, 1915.
Bolognesi, G.: Les tumeurs primitives des aponeuroses. Rev. Chir. 51:876, 1916.
Ely, L. W.: Giant cell growth of bone and tendon sheath. Ann. Surg. 68:426, 1918.
Broders, A. C.: Benign xanthic extraperiosteal tumor of the extremities containing foreign body giant cells. Ann. Surg. 70:574, 1919.
Ewing, J.: Neoplastic Diseases, 2nd edition. Philadelphia, W. B. Saunders Co., 1922.
Krogins, A.: So-called xanthosarcoma of tendon sheaths. Finska läk-Sällsk. Handl. 44:102, 1922.
Buxton, St. J. D.: Tumours of the tendon and tendon sheaths. Br. J. Surg. 10:469, 1923.
Faccini, U.: Un caso di peritelioma sarcomatoso della capsula articolare del ginocchio destro. Arch. ital. Chir. 7:481, 1923.
Brandro, F.: Lipoma arborescens of tendon sheaths. Chir. Organi Mov. 9:235, 1925.
Christopher, F.: Giant-cell sarcoma apparently arising from the aponeurosis of the forearm. JAMA 87:167, 1926.
Levy, G.: Xanthelasma et xanthome. Ann. Anat. Pathol. 2:247, 1925.
Vermooten, V.: Xanthosarcoma of thumb: A central benign giant cell tumor of the proximal phalanx of the thumb. Ann. Surg. 81:851, 1925.
Smith, L. W.: Synoviomata. Am. J. Pathol. 3:355, 1927.
Carp, L., and Stout, A. P.: A study of ganglia with special reference to treatment. Surg. Gynecol. Obstet. 47:460, 1928.
Geschickter, C. F., and Copeland, M.M.: Osteitis fibrosa and giant cell tumor. Arch. Surg. 19:169, 1929.
Dudley, H. D.: Giant cell tumors of tendon sheaths. Northwest Med. 29:217, 1930.
Pryn, P.: Synoviales Sarkoendotheliom des Kniegelenks. Virchows Arch. 279:71, 1930.
Wagner, L. C.: Intraarticular endothelial tumors arising from the synovial membrane. Ann. Surg. 92:421, 1930.

Diez, J.: El endotelioma sinovial articular. Prensa med argent. 18:487, 1931.

Hunter, W. C.: Benign polymorphocellular tumors of the knee region. Am. J. Pathol. 7:13, 1931.

Phemister, D. B.: Undifferentiated round-cell sarcomas. Ann. Surg. 93:125, 1931.

King, M. C. S.: The pathology of ganglion. Aust. N.Z. J. Surg. 1:367–381, 1932.

Seidelin, H.: Liposarcoma with chordoma-like cells. Acta Pathol. Microbiol. Scand. 9:289, 1932.

Geschickter, C. F., and Lewis, D.: Tumors of tendon sheaths, joints and bursae. Am. J. Cancer 22:96, 1934.

Lewis, D.: Tumors of the tendon sheaths. Surg. Gynecol. Obstet. 59:344, 1934.

Morton, J. J.: Tumors of the tendon sheaths, their close biological relationship to tumors of the joints and bursae. Surg. Gynecol. Obstet. 59:441, 1934.

Sabrazes, J., Loubat, E., De Grailly, R., and Magendie, J.: Synovial sarcomes. Gaz. hebd. Sci. méd. Bordeaux 55:754, 1934.

King, E. S. J.: The Golgi apparatus of synovial cells under normal and pathological conditions and with reference to the formation of synovial fluid. J. Pathol. Bacteriol. 41:117, 1935.

Black, W. C.: Synovioma of the hand. Report of a case. Am. J. Cancer 28:481, 1936.

Knox, L. C.: Synovial sarcoma. Am. J. Cancer 28:461, 1936.

Coley, B. L., and Pierson, J. C.: Synovioma: Report of fifteen cases with review of literature. Surgery 1:113, 1937.

Mason, M. L.: Tumors of the hand. Surg. Gynecol. Obstet. 64:129, 1937.

Berger, L.: Synovial sarcomas in serous bursae and tendon sheaths. Am. J. Cancer 34:501, 1938.

Simard, L. C.: Tumor of the palm having the structure of a mixed tumor of the salivary glands. Am. J. Cancer 33:182, 1938.

Thannhauser, S. J., and Magendantz, H.: Different clinical groups of xanthomatous diseases: Clinical physiological study of 22 cases. Ann. Intern. Med. 11:1652, 1938.

Brunschwig, A.: Tumors of the synovia, tendons and joint capsules of the hands and feet. Surgery 5:101, 1939.

Galloway, J. D. B., Broders, A. C., and Ghormley, R. K.: Xanthoma of the tendon sheaths and synovial membranes. A clinical and pathologic study. Arch. Surg. 40:485, 1940.

Lewis, R. W.: Roentgen recognition of synovioma. Am. J. Roentgenol. 44:170, 1940.

DeSanto, D. A., Tennant, R., and Rosahn, P. D.: Synovial sarcomas in joints, bursae and tendon sheaths. A clinical and pathological study of sixteen cases. Surg. Gynecol. Obstet. 72:951, 1941.

Jaffe, H. L., and Lichtenstein, L.: Sarcoma (synovioma). Bull. Hosp. Joint Dis. 2:3, 1941.

Jaffe, H. L., Lichtenstein, L., and Sutro, C. J.: Pigmented villonodular synovitis, bursitis and tenosynovitis. Arch. Pathol. 31:731, 1941.

Ewing, J.: Neoplastic Diseases, 4th edition. Philadelphia, W. B. Saunders Co., 1942.

Fisher, H. R.: Synovial sarcomesothelioma (sarcoendothelioma). Am. J. Pathol. 18:529, 1942.

Haagensen, C. D., and Stout, A. P.: Synovial sarcoma. Ann. Surg. 120:826, 1944.

Bennett, G. A.: Malignant neoplasms originating in synovial tissues (synoviomata): a study of thirty-two specimens registered at the Army Institute of Pathology during the war-time period, 1941–1945. J. Bone Joint Surg. 29:259, 1947.

Foster, L. N.: The benign giant cell tumor of tendon sheaths: An example of sclerosing hemangioma. Am. J. Pathol. 23:567, 1947.

Stewart, F. W.: Case 24, Division of Laboratories and Research, Albany, New York, 1948.

Stewart, M. J.: Benign giant-cell synovioma and its relation to "xanthoma." J. Bone Joint Surg. 30B:522, 1948.

Kobak, M. G., and Perlow, S.: Xanthomatous giant cell tumors arising in soft tissue. Report of an instance of malignant growth. Arch. Surg. 59:909, 1949.

Wright, C. J. E.: Rapid recurrence of a giant-cell synovioma of tendon sheath. J. Pathol. Bacteriol. 61:271, 1949.

Murray, M. R., Stout, A. P., and Pogogeff, I. A.: Synovial sarcoma and normal synovial tissue cultivated *in vitro*. Ann. Surg. 31A:619, 1949.

Eisenberg, R. B., and Horn, R. C.: Synovial sarcoma of chest wall: report of case. Ann. Surg. 131:281, 1950.

Pack, G. T., and Ariel, M.: Synovial sarcoma (malignant synovioma): a report of 60 cases. Surgery 28:1047, 1950.

Spencer, H., and Whimster, I. W.: The development of giant-celled tendon sheath tumors and related conditons (chronic villonodular synovitis and cutaneous histiocytoma). J. Pathol. Bacteriol. 62:411, 1950.

Fletcher, A. G., and Horn, R. C.: Giant cell tumors of tendon sheath origin; a consideration of bone involvement and report of two cases with extensive bone destruction. Ann. Surg. 133:374, 1951.

Tillotson, J. F., McDonald, J. R., and Janes, J. M.: Synovial sarcomata. J. Bone Joint Surg. 33A:459, 1951.

Wright, C. J. E.: Benign giant cell synovioma:

An investigation of 85 cases. Br. J. Surg. 38:257, 1951.

Berkheiser, S. W.: Synovioma-like tumor (synovial sarcoma) of abdominal wall: Report of a case. Ann. Surg. 135:114, 1952.

Harkness, G. G.: Malignant synovioma; with special reference to diversity of tissue differentiation. Aust. N.Z. J. Surg. 22:60, 1952.

King, E. S. J.: Tissue differentiation in malignant synovial tumors. J. Bone Joint Surg. 34B:97, 1952.

Wright, C. J. E.: Malignant synovioma. J. Pathol. Bacteriol. 64:585, 1952.

Stout, A. P.: Tumors of the Soft Tissues. Washington, D.C., Armed Forces Institute of Pathology, 1953.

Decker, J. P., and Owen, B. J.: An invasive giant cell tumor of tendon sheath in the foot. Bull. Ayer Clin. Lab. 4:43, 1954.

Jernstrom, P.: Synovial sarcoma of the pharynx. Report of a case. Am. J. Clin. Pathol. 24:957, 1954.

Lederer, H., and Sinclair, A. J.: Malignant synovioma simulating "adamantinoma of the tibia." J. Pathol. Bacteriol. 67:163, 1954.

Price, C. H. G., and Valentine, J. C.: Malignant giant-cell synovioma of phalanx. J. Clin. Pathol. 7:231, 1954.

Craig, R. M., Pugh, D. G., and Soule, E. H.: The roentgenologic manifestations of synovial sarcoma. Radiology 65:837, 1955.

Devas, M. B., and Thompson, A. D.: Malignant synovioma. Proc. R. Soc. Med. 48:168, 1955.

Laskowski, J.: Zarys onkologii. *In* Pathology of Tumors. Edited by H. Kolodziejska. Warszawa, PZWL, 1955.

Lichtenstein, L.: Tumors of synovial joints, bursae and tendon sheaths. Cancer 8:861, 1955.

Martens, V. E.: Unusual synovial tumors. JAMA 157:888, 1955.

Hicks, J. D.: Synovial cysts in bone. Aust. N.Z. J. Surg. 26:138, 1956.

Breiner, C. W., and Freiberger, R. H.: Bone lesions associated with villonodular synovitis. Am. J. Roentgenol. 79:618, 1958.

Crocker, D. W., and Stout, A. P.: Synovial sarcoma in children. Cancer 12:1123, 1959.

Phalen, G. S., McCormack, L. J., and Gazale, W. J.: Giant cell tumor of the tendon sheath (Benign synovioma) in the hand. Evaluation of 56 cases. Clin. Orthop. 15:140, 1959.

Stout, A. P., and Gorman, I. G.: Mixed tumors of skin of the salivary gland type. Cancer 12:537, 1959.

Dutra, R. R.: Mixed tumor, salivary gland type of deep fascial region of thigh. Arch. Pathol. 70:562, 1960.

Luse, S. A.: A synovial sarcoma studied by electron microscopy Cancer 13:312, 1960.

McMaster, P. E.: Pigmented villonodular synovitis with invasion of bone. J. Bone Joint Surg. 42A:1170, 1960.

Harrison, E. G., Black, B. M., and Devine, K. D.: Synovial sarcoma primary in the the neck. Arch. Pathol. 71:137, 1961.

Cade, S.: Synovial sarcoma. J. R. Coll. Surg. 8:1, 1962.

Smith, J. H., and Pugh, D. G.: Roentgenographic aspects of articular pigmented villonodular synovitis. Am. J. Roentgenol. 87:1146, 1962.

Marsh, H. O., Shellito, J. G., and Callahan, W. P.: Synovial sarcoma of the sternoclavicular region. J. Bone Joint Surg. 45A:151, 1963.

Snook, G. A.: Pigmented villonodular synovitis with bony invasion: Report of two cases. JAMA 189:424, 1963.

Cadman, N. L., Soule, E. H., and Kelly, P.: Synovial sarcoma: An analysis of 134 tumors. Cancer 18:613, 1965.

Enzinger, F. M.: Clear-cell sarcoma of tendons and aponeuroses. An analysis of 21 cases. Cancer 18:1163, 1965.

Johnson, E. W.: Adjacent and distant spread of giant cell tumors. Am. J. Surg. 109:163, 1965.

Raben, M., Calabrase, A., Higinbotham N. L., and Philips, R.: Malignant synovioma. Am. J. Roentgenol. 93:145, 1965.

Gravanis, M. B.: Malignant giant-cell tumors of tendon sheaths. Bull. Pathol. 9:130, 1966.

Hirohata, K., and Kumon, H.: Pigmented villonodular synovitis and bursitis. Clin. Orthop. Surg. 1:769, 1966.

Mackenzie, D. H.: Synovial sarcoma. A review of 58 cases. Cancer 19:169, 1966.

McCallum, D. E., Musser, A. W., and Rhangos, W. C.: Experimental villonodular synovitis. South. Med. J. 59:966, 1966.

Ross, R., and Greenlee, T. K.: Electron microscopy: Attachment sites between connective tissue cells. Science 153:997, 1966.

Stern, A. L.: Pigmented villonodular synovitis. J. Am. Podiatry Assoc. 56:26, 1966.

Batsakis, J. G., Nishiyama, R. H., and Sullinger, G. D.: Synovial sarcomas of the neck. Arch. Otolaryngol. 85:327, 1967.

Matthews, J. L., Martin, J. H., Race, G. J., and Collins, E. J.: Giant-cell centrioles. Science 155:1423, 1967.

Bliss, B. O., and Reed. R. J.: Large cell sarcoma of tendon sheath: malignant giant cell tumors of tendon sheath. Am. J. Clin. Pathol. 49:776, 1968.

Byers, P. D., Cotton, R. E., Deacon, O. W., Lowy, M., Newman, P. H., Sissons, H. A., and Thomson, A. D.: The diagnosis and treatment of pigmented villonodular synovitis of the temporomandibular joint. J Bone Joint Surg 50B:290, 1968

Eisenstein, R.: Giant-cell tumor of tendon

sheath. Its histogenesis as studied in the electron microscope. J. Bone Joint Surg. 50A:476, 1968.
Hampole, M. K., and Jackson, B. A.: Analysis of 25 cases of malignant synovioma. Can. Med. Assoc. J. 90:1025, 1968.
Holmes, K. V., and Choppin, P. W.: On the role of microtubules in movement and alignment of nuclei in virus-induced syncytia. J. Cell Biol. 39:526, 1968.
Moberger, G., Nilsonne, U., and Friberg, S.: Synovial sarcoma. Acta Orthop. Scand. (Suppl.) 11:3, 1968.
Murphy, E., and Margarit, E.: Synovial sarcoma of the anterior abdominal wall. Ann. Surg. 168:928, 1968.
Schajowicz, F., and Blumenfeld, I.: Pigmented villonodular synovitis of the wrist with penetration into bone. J. Bone Joint Surg. 50B:312, 1968.
Scott, P. M.: Bone lesions in pigmented villonodular synovitis. J. Bone Joint Surg. 50B:306, 1968.
Sirsat, M. V., and Doctor, V. M.: Synovial sarcoma in Indians: Observations on 22 cases with emphasis on morbid anatomy. Indian J. Cancer 5:160, 1968.
Gewheiler, J. A., and Wilson, V. W.: Diffuse biarticular pigmented villonodular synovitis. Radiology 93:137, 1969.
Jones, F. E., Soule, E. H., and Coventry, M. B.: Fibrous xanthoma of synovium (giant cell tumor of tendon sheath, pigmented nodular synovitis). J. Bone Joint Surg. 51A:76, 1969.
Kubo, T.: Clear-cell sarcoma of patellar tendon studied by electron microscopy. Cancer 24:948, 1969.
McClatchie, S.: An example of a clear cell sarcoma of tendon. E. Afr. Med. J. 46:524, 1969.
Zippel, H.: Zur Diagnose, Differentialdiagnose und Therapi der Synovialome. Abl. Chir. 94:958, 1969.
Attie, J. N., Steckler, R. M., and Platt, N.: Cervical synovial sarcoma. Cancer 25:759, 1970.
Campanacci, M., Cervellati, C., and Olmi, R.: Aspetti neoplastiformi della sinovite villonodulare pigmentosa. Chir. Organi Mov. 60:464, 1970.
Dehner, L. P., and Smith, B. H.: Soft tissue tumors of the penis. Cancer 25:1431, 1970.
Dutra, F. R.: Clear cell sarcoma of tendons and aponeuroses. Three additional cases. Cancer 25:942, 1970.
Enzinger, F. M.: Epithelioid sarcoma. A sarcoma simulating a granuloma or a carcinoma. Cancer 26:1029, 1970.
Hale, J. E., and Calder, I. M.: Synovial sarcoma of abdominal wall. Br. J. Cancer 24:471, 1970.
Pickren, J. W., Valenzula, L., and Elias, E. G.: Synovial sarcoma. Proc. Natl. Cancer Conf. 6:795, 1970.
Gabbiani, G., Kaye, G. I., Lattes, R., and Majoni, G.: Synovial sarcoma, electron microscopic study of a typical case. Cancer 28:1031, 1971.
Johnson, R. T., and Rao, P. N.: Nuclear-cytoplasmic interaction in the achievement of nuclear synchrony in DNA synthesis and mitosis in multinucleated cells. Biol. Rev. 46:97, 1971.
Laskowski, J.: Aponeurotic sarcoma. Pol. Med. J. 10:12, 1971.
Sim, F. H., and Dahlin, D. C.: Ganglion cysts of bone. Mayo Clin. Proc. 46:484, 1971.
Arthaud, J. B.: Pigmented nodular synovitis: Report of 11 lesions in non-articular location. Am. J. Clin. Pathol. 58:511, 1972.
Farmer, C. B., and Viamonte, M.: Angiography in synovial disease. Clin. Orthop. 85:101, 1972.
Fisher, E. R., and Horvat, B.: The fibrocytic derivation of the so-called epithelioid sarcoma. Cancer 30:1074, 1972.
Gabbiani, G., Fu, Y. S., Kaye, G. I., Lattes, R., and Majoni, G.: Epithelioid sarcoma. A light and electron microscopic study suggesting a synovial origin. Cancer 30:468, 1972.
Gambert, J.: Villonodular synovitis of the knee in children. Ann. Chir. 26:1011, 1972.
Kolar, J., and Thyssen, H.: The radiological findings in malignant synovialoma. Radiol. Diagn. 13:355, 1972.
Salm, R., and Sissons, H. A.: Giant-cell tumours of soft tissues. J. Pathol. 107:27, 1972.
Santiago, H., Feinerman, L. K., and Lattes, R.: Epithelioid sarcoma. A clinical and pathological study of nine cases. Hum. Pathol. 3:133, 1972.
Seemayer, T., Dionne, P. G., and Tabah, E. J.: Epithelioid sarcoma. Can. J. Surg. 17:1, 1972.
Soule, E. H., and Enriquez, P.: Atypical fibrous histiocytoma–malignant fibrous histiocytoma, malignant histiocytoma and epithelioid sarcoma: A comparative study of sixty-five tumors. Cancer 30:128, 1972.
Von Andel, J. G.: Synovial sarcoma—a review and analysis of treated cases. Radiol. Clin. Biol. 41:145, 1972.
Castro, E. B., Hajdu, S. I., and Fortner, J. G.: Surgical therapy of fibrosarcoma of extremities. Arch. Surg. 107:284, 1973.
Feinstein, M., and Rubin, L.: Pigmented villonodular synovitis. ACSF Journal 12:77, 1973.
Frable, W. J., Kay, S., Lawrence, W., and Schatzki, P. F.: Epithelioid sarcoma: An electron microscopic study. Arch. Pathol. 95:8, 1973.
Hoffman, G. J., and Carter, D.: Clear cell sarcoma of tendons and aponeuroses with melanin. Arch. Pathol. 95:22, 1973.

Kahn, L. B.: Malignant giant cell tumor of tendon sheath. Ultrastructural study and review of the literature. Arch. Pathol. 95:203, 1973.

Lapayowker, M. S., Miller, W. T., Levy, W. M., and Harwick, R. D.: Pigmented villonodular synovitis of the temporomandibular joint. Radiology 108:313, 1973.

Martin, R. F., Melnick, P. J., Warner, N. E., Terry, R., Bullock, W. K., and Schwinn, C. P.: Chordoid sarcoma. Am. J. Clin. Pathol. 59:623, 1973.

Papadimitriou, J. M., Sforsina, D., and Papaelias, L.: Kinetics of multinucleate giant cell formation and their modification by various agents in foreign body reactions. Am. J. Pathol. 73:394, 1973.

Rubin, L., and Feinstein, M. H.: Pigmented villonodular synovitis. J. Foot Surg. 12:77, 1973.

Black, M. M., and Epstein, W. L.: Formation of multinucleate giant cells in organized epithelioid cell granulomas. Am. J. Pathol. 74:263, 1974.

Bryan, R. S., Soule, E. H., Dobyns, J. H., Pritchard, D. J., and Linscheid, R. L.: Primary epithelioid sarcoma of the hand and forearm: A review of thirteen cases. J. Bone Joint Surg. 56A:458, 1974.

Lee, S. M., Hajdu, S. I., and Exelby, P. R.: Synovial sarcomas in children. Surg. Gynecol. Obstet. 138:701, 1974.

Mackenzie, D. H.: Clear cell sarcoma of tendon and aponeuroses with melanin production. J. Pathol. 114:231, 1974.

Mariano, M., and Spector, W. G.: The formation and properties of macrophage polykaryons (inflammatory giant cells). J. Pathol. 113:1, 1974.

Moussavi, H., and Ghodsi, S.: Synovial sarcoma of the tongue: report of a case. J. Laryngol. Otol. 88:795, 1974.

Berman, R. M., Noe, J., and Kempson, R. L.: Clear cell sarcoma with melanin pigment. Cancer 36:977, 1975.

Mathews, R. S., and Hart, J. A. L.: Benign synovioma (Pigmented villonodular synovitis). Surg. Forum 26:513, 1975.

Roth, J. A., Enzinger, F. M., and Tannenbaum, M.: Synovial sarcoma of the neck: a follow-up study of 24 cases. Cancer 35:1243, 1975.

Shiu, M. H., Castro, E. B., Hajdu, S. I., and Fortner, J. G.: Surgical treatment of 297 soft tissue sarcomas of the lower extremity. Ann. Surg. 182:597, 1975.

Hajdu, S. I., and Hajdu, E. O.: Cytopathology of Sarcomas and Other Nonepithelial Malignant Tumors. Philadelphia, W. B. Saunders Co., 1976.

Mitcherling, J. J., Collins, E. M., Tomich, C. E., Bianco, R. P., and Cooper, W. K.: Synovial sarcoma of the neck: Report of a case. J. Oral Surg. 34:64, 1976.

Sapp, J. P.: An ultrastructural study of nuclear and centriolar configurations in multinucleated giant cells. Lab. Invest. 34:109, 1976.

Weiss, S. W.: Ultrastructure of the so-called "chordoid sarcoma." Cancer 37:300, 1976.

Dabska, M.: Parachordoma. A new clinicopathologic entity. Cancer 40:1586, 1977.

Hajdu, S. I., Shiu, M. H., and Fortner, J. G.: Tendosynovial sarcoma. A clinicopathologic study of 136 cases. Cancer 39:1201, 1977.

Mackenzie, D. H.: Monophasic synovial sarcoma—a histological entity? Histopathology 1:151, 1977.

Miyamoto, Y., Tani, T., and Hamaya, K.: Pigmented villonodular synovitis of the temporomandibular joint. Plast. Reconstr. Surg. 59:283, 1977.

Patchefsky, A. S., Soriano, R., and Kostianovsky, M.: Epithelioid sarcoma. Ultrastructural similarity to nodular synovitis. Cancer 39:143, 1977.

Stern, R. E., and Gauger, D. W.: Pigmented villonodular tenosynovitis. J. Bone Joint Surg. 59A:560, 1977.

Boudreaux, D., and Waisman, J.: Clear cell sarcoma with melanogenesis. Cancer 41:1387, 1978.

Alguacil-Garcia, A. Unni, K. K., and Goellner, J. R.: Giant cell tumor of tendon sheath and pigmented villonodular synovitis. An ultrastructural study. Am. J. Clin. Pathol. 69:6, 1978.

Koivuniemi, A., and Nickels, J.: Synovial sarcoma diagnosed by fine-needle aspiration biopsy. Acta Cytol. 22:515, 1978.

Massarelli, G., Tanda, F., and Salis, B.: Synovial sarcoma of the soft palate: Report of a case. Hum. Pathol. 9:341, 1978.

Prat, J., Woodruff, J. M., and Marcove, R. C.: Epithelioid sarcoma. Cancer 41:1472, 1978.

Shiu, M. H., McCormack, P., Hajdu, S. I., and Fortner, J. G.: Surgical treatment of tendosynovial sarcoma. Cancer 43:889, 1979.

chapter 4

Tumors of Adipose Tissue

NON-NEOPLASTIC LESIONS

- *Fat Necrosis*
- *Lipogranuloma*
- *Lipodystrophia*
- *Piezogenic Papules*
- *Adiposis Dolorosa*
- *Steatopygia*

NEOPLASTIC LESIONS

- *Lipoma*
  - Well-Differentiated Lipoma
  - Myxoid Lipoma
  - Fibroblastic Lipoma
  - Pleomorphic Lipoma
  - Angiolipoma
  - Angiomyolipoma
  - Myelolipoma
  - Lipoblastoma
  - Hibernoma
- *Liposarcoma*
  - Well-Differentiated Liposarcoma
  - Myxoid Liposarcoma
  - Lipoblastic Liposarcoma
  - Fibroblastic Liposarcoma
  - Pleomorphic Liposarcoma

ALTHOUGH adipose tissue constitutes, in normal conditions, about from 15% to 25% of the human body, and in obese individuals fat may contribute more than 40% of body weight, it received little attention prior to the 1960's when a number of publications appeared on the morphology, physiology, and biochemistry of adipose tissue. Formation of adipose tissue begins during the fifth month of intrauterine life and reaches its peak of normal development soon after birth. Morphologically and functionally the adipose tissue is classified into two main types: *white* and *brown*.

It is believed that both white and brown *adipose cells may arise from undifferentiated fibroblasts and tissue histiocytes, as well as from primitive mesenchymal cells* which are abundant about blood vessels. The factors influencing the differentiation of these precursor cells into adipose cells are not well understood, but it is certain that the quantity and distribution of fat is influenced by hormonal, nutritional, and genetic factors. Unfortunately, confusion still exists as to the precise origin of fat cells, since even recent studies have not ruled out that fat cells may also arise from predetermined anlage. Bell (1909) reviewed and summarized all the early investigations on the nature of fat cells.

According to medical historians, Toldt, in 1870, first stated that the adipose tissue is a specialized tissue, an organ on its own, and entirely distinct from other tissues. He held that the appearance of vacuolated *adipocytes* (mature fat cells) is preceded by the formation of granular *lipoblasts* (embryonal fat cells).

That fat cells are highly specialized is shown by their inability to multiply under normal condition. However, even the most distended adipocytes are active functionally and capable of taking up granules of vital stains and diminishing the large cytoplasmic fat globules to small refractile granules (Clark and Clark, 1940). According to Margaillan (1929) the chemical composition and functional role of fat are different from one anatomic region of the body to another. This variation was described by Strandberg, in 1915. Skin lost from one hand of a young girl because of a burn was replaced by a skin graft, including subcutaneous tissue, from the abdominal wall. As the patient grew older and somewhat obese, the transplanted skin accumulated the same amount of fat as the abdominal wall so that the hand had the grotesque appearance of a boxing glove.

Morphologically, the white adipose tissue is composed of large spherical or globoid fat cells. Each cell contains one large globule of fat which is formed by the conglomerate of small fat droplets. The intracytoplasmic fat can be stained with such dyes as Oil red-O or Sudan black. The cytoplasm of mature fat cells is reduced to a thin rim that surrounds the fat globule and contains a flattened or crescent shape nucleus.

Depending on location and age, fat cells vary in size and shape from spindle- or spherical-shaped fibroblast-like cells (prolipoblasts), round cells (lipoblasts), containing little lipid, multivacuolated cells (preadipocytes) to mature fat cells with globoid fat vacuoles (adipocytes) (Fig. 4-1). The accumulation of lipid is an obvious criterion for distinguishing fat cells from other cells. Normally there is one large lipid droplet within the fat cell, but smaller lipid droplets can be seen in the outer cytoplasmic rim. Ultrastructurally, intracytoplasmic lipid droplets are often crenated and unrelated morphologically to any cell organelles. The ink-blot outline of lipid droplets may be caused by a combination of factors, e.g., fixation, polymerization, and sectioning.

According to Napolitano (1963), during differentiation adipose cells go through a sequence of modification of cell organelles. At the earliest stage in differentiation of adipose cells, numerous lipid inclusions appear toward one pole of the *pre-adipose fibroblast* (prolipoblast).

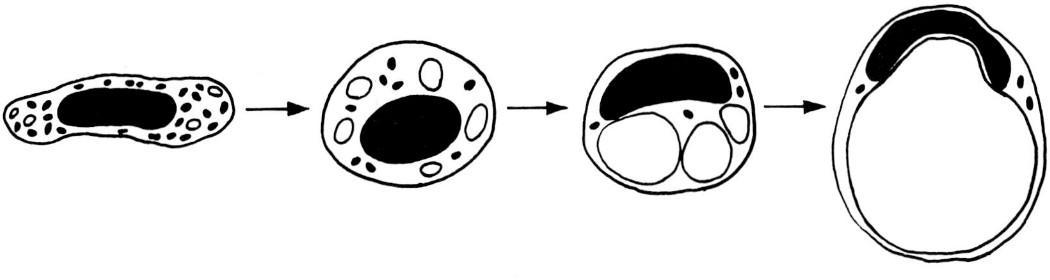

Figure 4-1. Schematic illustration of pathway of differentiation of fat cells. The prolipoblast is a short spindle or elongated oval cell which contains in the cytoplasm a few fat vacuoles and many glycogen granules. The lipoblast is a round or oval cell which contains in the cytoplasm fat vacuoles and some glycogen granules. The nucleus is round and prominent. The preadipocyte contains numerous fat vacuoles and minimal collagen. The nucleus is eccentrically placed in the cytoplasm. The adipocyte or mature fat cell contains a solitary large fat vacuole, compressed and minimal cytoplasmic organelles and an eccentrically placed nucleus.

These smooth-surfaced vesicles, containing material of low electron opacity (lipomicrons), continue to be present throughout the differentiation of fat cells.

Later in differentiation glycogen appears (lipoblast) in addition to lipid droplets, but it is transitory because glycogen is rarely observed in mature adipose cells. In mature fat cells (adipocytes) the cell organelles can be found throughout the peripheral rim of the cytoplasm. The cytoplasm of fat cells is bounded by a plasma membrane which is surrounded by an external lamina as well as a network of collagen fibers.

The adipose nature of the fat cell makes tissue processing for proper microscopic studies relatively difficult. According to Lever (1957) and Napolitano (1963) the ultrastructural characteristics of fat cells are essentially the same as those of other connective tissue cells. Ewing referred to the highly vascular nature of adipose tissue in a lecture at Memorial Hospital for Cancer in 1935 and said, "steatoblasts and lipoblasts are derived from the adventitial layers of the blood vessels." Capillary vessels are indeed close to the surface membrane of fat cells, but they are separated by their basement membranes and small bundles of collagen; however, it is possible that pericytes, being multipotential cells, may play a role in the histogenesis of fat cells.

A small amount of multiglobular adipose tissue, the brown fat, is present at birth throughout the body, but particularly in the subcutaneous tissues about the shoulders and neck, in the axillae, in the mediastinum, in the retroperitoneum, around the joints, and around the heart. This richly vascularized nodular reddish tissue is believed to arise from the so-called primitive fat organs during fetal life and gradually disappear postnatally. However, Melicow, in 1977, by examining adipose tissue removed with adrenal pheochromocytoma found histologic evidence of brown fat in 18 of 29 cases.

According to historians, brown fat was first described by Velsch, in 1670, in hibernating animals, and it has been the subject of a considerable number of investigations since the report of Hatai, in 1902, in which he compared the "interscapular gland" of human embryos to the hibernating gland of animals. Brown fat is different from white fat not only in color, which is mainly due to the high concentration of *cytochrome pigments* in the mitochondria, but also in cytomorphology as well as in function. It is composed of lobulated masses of multinucleated fat cells containing a number of small fat globules centrally placed around vesicular nuclei. The brown fat is richly innervated, and nerve fibers are frequently observed in the fibrous septae separating gland-like lobules. The fine structure of brown fat, according to Napolitano and Fawcett (1958), is characterized by granularity, size, and complex internal structure of its mitochondria. Picard et al, in 1966, demonstrated that the fat cells in brown adipose tissue are lined by a 70 to 80 angstrom membrane with close connection to endoplasmic reticulum.

The brown fat has a greater oxygen consumption, a lower respiratory quotient, and a greater anaerobic glycolysis than ordinary white fat. Selye and Timiras as early as 1949 emphasized that under certain conditions the brown fat can take up the function of the adrenal cortex and participate in the alarm reaction. Dawkins et al, in 1966, localized catecholamines in brown fat and postulated their role in the hydrolysis of triglycerides and oxidation of fatty acids. Smith, in 1969, reported that brown fat is primarily a heat-producing tissue and can be activated by norepinephrine. It is possible that repeated stimulation of brown fat may lead to its hypertrophy or hyperplasia (see Hibernoma).

The old belief that white adipose tissue is mainly a supportive tissue is not true. The literature on the physiology and biochemistry of adipose tissue is extensive, but it is beyond the scope of this work to review functional aspects of adipose tissue in detail. Among the multifaceted roles of adipose cells the most important are (1) *lipogenesis and lipid deposition,* (2) *the mobilization of lipid, and* (3) *the maintenance of the stored lipid.*

Williamson, in 1964, was the first to attempt to correlate structure with function by studying deposition and mobilization of lipid in mammalian adipose cells. He found that lipid droplets are free in the cytoplasm and morphologically unrelated to any of the organelles but suggested that the numerous micropinocytotic invaginations and vesicles in active fat cells reflect a two-way transport mechanism. He postulated that the first and perhaps the most important mechanism is the "direct-entry" or "direct-release" by dissolution of lipid by lipid-lipid interaction. The second transport mechanism involves liposomes which may transfer lipid aggregates into the storage droplet.

Slavin, in 1972, described a series of morphologic changes which took place in progressive loss of lipids. The reduction of intracytoplasmic lipid droplets was found to be associated with the appearance of membrane-bound dense bodies, irregularity of the cell surface, and rosette-like arrangement of the micropinocytotic vesicles. He believes that the *lipid-depleted fat cells resemble the brown fat cells and the electron dense granules are probably mucopolysaccharide material.*

Today two routes of fat synthesis are accepted: one is the *reversed beta-oxidation* in the mitochondria and the other is the so-called *extra-mitochondrial pathway.* Not every step of these processes is clearly understood, but it is certain that their reversal results in breakdown of fat with subsequent release of energy (Shapiro and Wertheimer, 1956).

Furthermore, Picard et al, in 1966, found an intimate morphologic relationship between the endoplasmic reticulum, mitochondria, and lipid granules of brown fat cells, suggesting possible structure-function relationship. Carpentier et al, in 1977, found that the morphologic changes of the plasma membrane of adipocytes in obese mice is not due to size increase only but may be a reflection of a more profound metabolic alteration. Available evidence suggests that changes in the metabolism and differentiation of adipose cells are associated with marked ultrastructural changes. These and other observations that have been published in an attempt to explain and correlate structural and functional changes in non-neoplastic fat cells may lay the groundwork for better understanding of the pathophysiology and morphology of neoplastic cells.

NON-NEOPLASTIC LESIONS

FAT NECROSIS

Fat necrosis was first described by Balser, in 1882, in association with acute hemorrhagic pancreatitis. Since then it has become well known that fat necrosis may develop at the site of trauma or contact with bile or pancreatic secretion. However, it is less well known that when adipose tissue is traumatized the breakdown products of fat may act as a foreign body and initiate local *inflammatory* and *proliferative changes*. Additional changes such as fibrosis and calcification may be produced by fatty acids alone or in combination with calcium. Fat necrosis of adipose tissue of the subcutis in infants and in children, as well as in adults, is relatively common. The female breast is especially prone to develop fat necrosis. According to Adair and Munzer (1947) the incidence of fat necrosis of the breast is nearly 3% in patients considered to have mammary carcinoma. Pancreatitis frequently causes fat necrosis in the omentum and retroperitoneum, but occasionally other areas such as the pericardium, bone marrow and subcutaneous tissues are also involved. Szymanski and Bluefarb (1961) and Schrier et al (1965) reported on subcutaneous nodular fat necrosis (panniculitis) in pancreatitis.

Grossly, subcutaneous fat necrosis appears as an indurated, fairly well-circumscribed semifirm nodule or mass. Following surgical excision the cross section of the lesion may show areas of hemorrhagic necrosis or cystic degeneration.

Microscopically, the dominant elements are large polyhedral and granular lipoblasts and various acute and chronic inflammatory cells. Occasionally one may find elongated or bizarre multinucleated fat cells and areas of vasculitis (Fig. 4-2). The treatment of choice is simple surgical excision with the exception of the infantile form which is usually self-limited and resolves in a couple of months.

LIPOGRANULOMA

Lipogranuloma is known under a dozen terms. The most commonly used ones are *nodular panniculitis* and *sclerosing panniculitis.* The term, *sclerosing lipogranuloma,* introduced by Smetana and Bernhard, in 1950, is one of the most commonly used designations. The designation often varies according to the anatomic site of the lesion (see review by Reske and Namiki, in 1975). Lipogranulomas occur as irregular and hard nodules. Most of these lesions probably represent a self-limited reparative process initiated by physical or chemical trauma or perhaps infectious organisms. Most of the reported lipogranulomas occur either in the *abdomen* or in the *retroperitoneum.* Microscopically these lesions are composed of aggregates of chronic inflammatory cells, sparsely vascular and focally necrotic adipose tissue, and partially hyalinized fibrous tissue. Cholesterol clefts and areas of calcification are not uncommon findings (Fig. 4-3). One cannot escape from the feeling that some of the lipogranulomas are perhaps nothing else than inflamed and proliferative fat necrosis. It may be difficult to distinguish lipogranuloma from sclerosing lipoma and pleomorphic lipoma.

There is general agreement in the literature that the treatment should be limited surgery, since there are numerous reported cases of spontaneous recovery (Smetana and Bernhard, 1948; Steinberg, 1953; and French et al, 1966).

Numerous lipogranulomatous lesions, so-called *paraffinomas,* were produced by injection of oils and paraffins for therapeutic and cosmetic purposes (Whitaker et al, 1948). Castillo-Oertel and Johnson, in 1977, reported their experience with lipogranuloma of male genitalia. It is of interest that they were able to identify, in most of the cases, exogenous paraffin hydro-

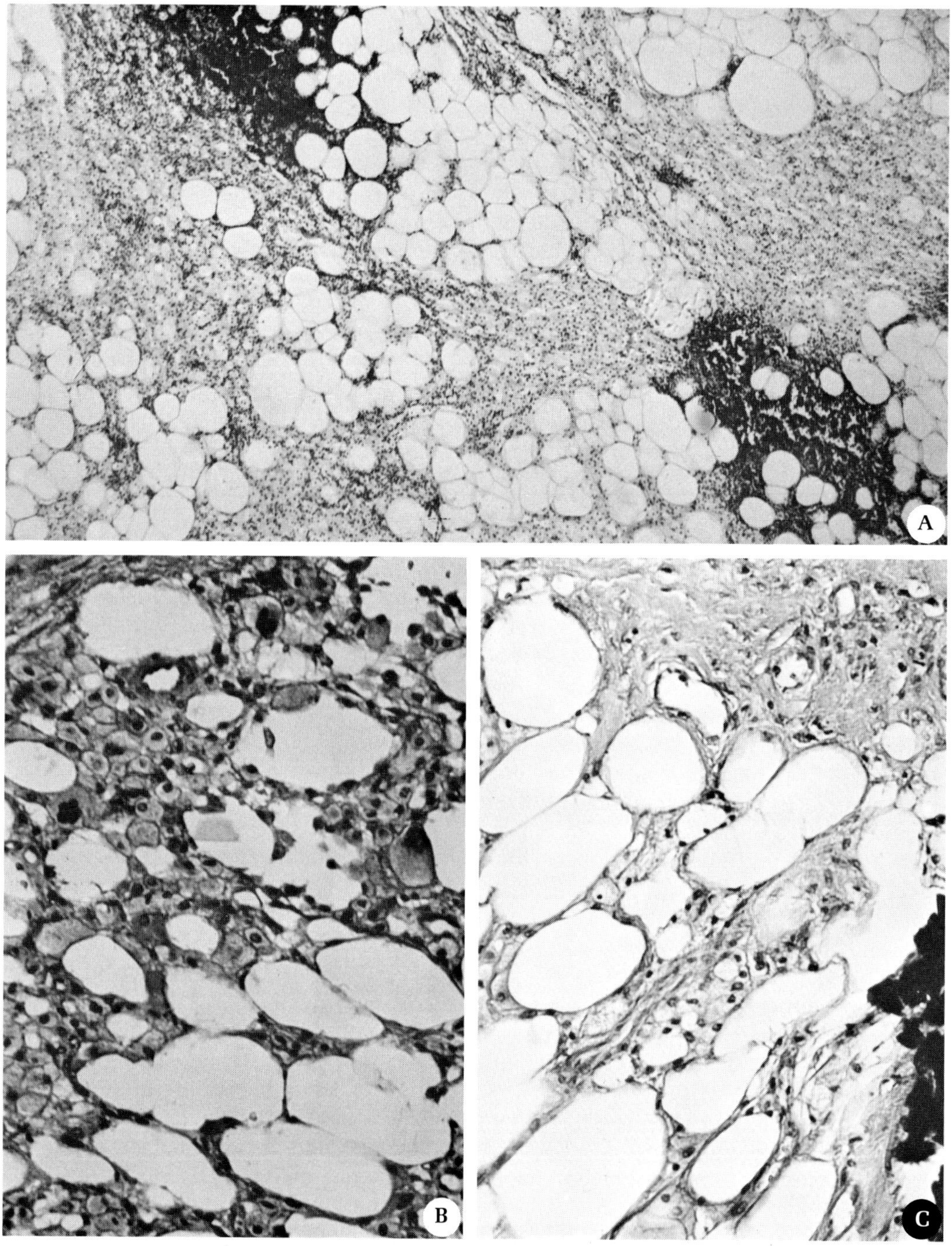

Figure 4-2. Fat necrosis. This lesion consists of a mixture of adipocytes, lipoblasts, and various inflammatory cells. The perivascular and intercellular stroma contain histiocytes **(B)** and appear fibrous **(C).** Note an area of calcification in **C** (**A,** H & E, ×35; **B,** & **C,** H & E, ×140).

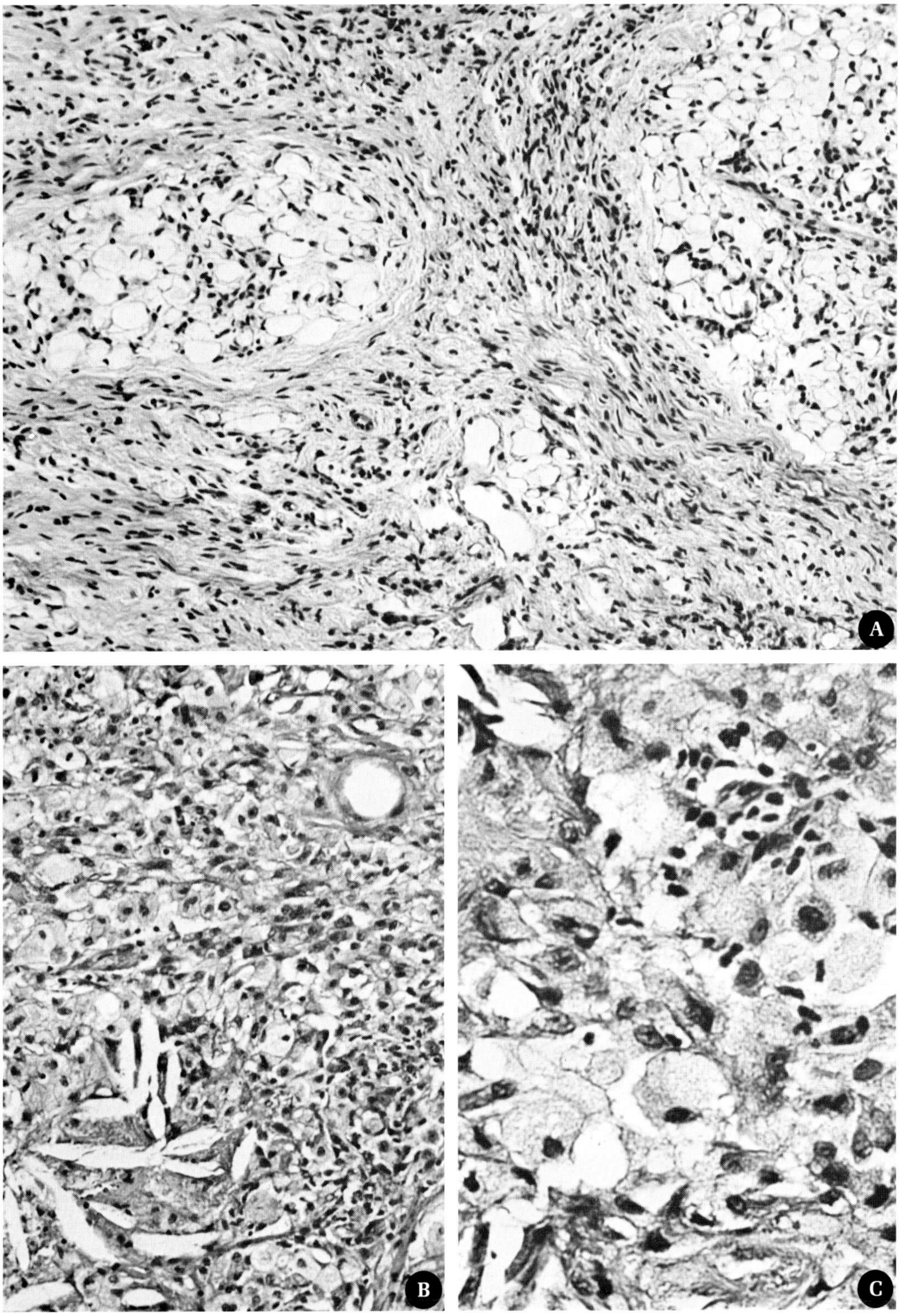

Figure 4-3. Lipogranuloma.

A, Adipocytes are encircled and compressed by laminated ring of slender fibroblasts (H & E, ×85).

B, A collection of chronic inflammatory cells forms a solid, cohesive, and tightly packed pattern. Note the cholesterol crystals (H & E, ×140).

C, Foam cells and other fibrous histiocytic elements (H & E, ×350).

carbons by infrared absorption spectrophotometry.

LIPODYSTROPHIA

There are several forms of lipodystrophia. Since all of these conditions are associated with specific endocrine abnormalities, they cannot be confused with tumors of the adipose tissue. Perhaps one of the most common forms is the so-called *dystrophia adiposogenitalis,* otherwise known as pituitary obesity with infantilism or Fröhlich's syndrome which was first described by Mohr in 1840, more than 60 years prior to the report by Fröhlich.

It is fairly well established that human obesity is in large measure determined by nutritional, hormonal, and hereditary factors. Less well known are the causative factors in *lipodystrophia progressiva,* which chiefly affects middle-aged females. It is characterized by irregular distribution of fat in subcutaneous tissue, e.g., there may be complete loss of fat in the upper part of the body while there is abundant or excessive adipose tissue below the waist line. Hormonal imbalance and the disturbance of autonomic trophic regulations are suspected as etiologic factors.

Congenital diffuse lipomatosis is a rare abnormality and usually is confined to one or two limbs. It is a progressive enlargement of the extremity during childhood associated with corresponding skeletal and vascular abnormalities.

PIEZOGENIC PAPULES

Piezogenic papules, first described by Shelly and Rawnsley in 1968, are cystic *herniations of subcutaneous fat* (dermatocele) into the dermal collagen. This term is derived from the Greek word *piezo* which means "pressure." These papules appear as cobblestone-like nodules on the medial and lateral aspects of the heels on weight-bearing (Fig. 4-4). It is a disease of obese patients, and according to Schlappner (1972) the papules can be painful or non-painful. There is no apparent sex, age, or family predominance. The lesion itself is composed of tiny herniated nodules of subcutaneous adipose tissue into the dermis, associated with focal fat necrosis and hyalinization of dermal collagen. Usually supportive orthotic treatment is sufficient, and surgical excision is rarely required.

ADIPOSIS DOLOROSA

Adiposis dolorosa or Dercum's disease is a syndrome rather than a disease. The cardinal signs are *adiposity, asthenia, pain, and psychic abnormality.* It is a rare systemic abnormality with localized overgrowth of subcutaneous fat by painful and tender tumor-like masses.

The name *adiposis dolorosa* was first proposed by Dercum at the meeting of the American Neurological Association, in 1888. He subsequently, in 1892, described three cases in detail (see Fig. 1-28). It is a disease of unknown etiology and affects predominantly middle-aged females. The fat deposit may be diffuse or nodular, symmetrical or irregular. Kling, in 1937, reviewed 112 cases and found that accumulation of fat most commonly appeared around joints of the knee, elbow, and ankle. It is of historical interest that one of the first *in vitro* cultures of fat cells, established by Marinesco and Minea, in 1916, derived from the adipose tissue of Dercum's disease. It is estimated that there are approximately 400 reported cases of Dercum's disease in the literature. At present there is no known definitive therapy for this abnormality.

STEATOPYGIA

Steatopygia is a symmetrical accumulation of adipose tissue in the buttocks. It is accepted as normal and a sign of distinction in the women of some African tribes.

There are somewhat similar symmetrical multinodular lipomatous deposits in the neck, first described by Brodie in 1846, but commonly known as *fat neck of Madelung,* because of his report in 1888. It is a rare disorder probably induced by hormonal imbalance and chiefly affects middle-aged Caucasian males (Fig. 4-5).

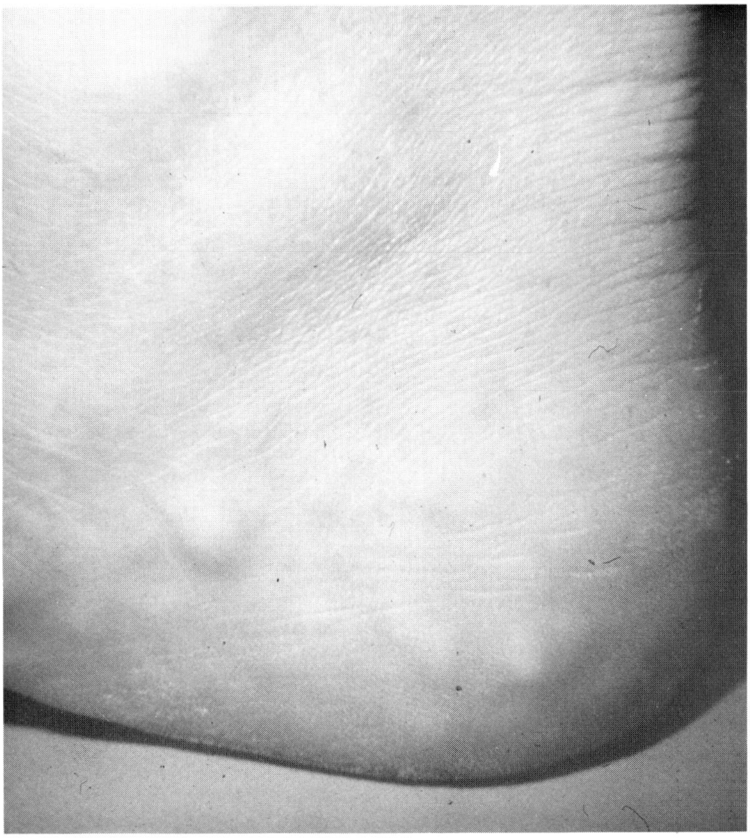

Figure 4-4. Piezogenic pedal papules are essentially fat herniations involving the heel pad on obese individuals. Similar fat herniations may also be seen in the metatarsal area. (Courtesy Berlin, S. J.; Soft Somatic Tissues of the Foot. Mount Kisco, N.Y., Futura Publishing Co., 1976.)

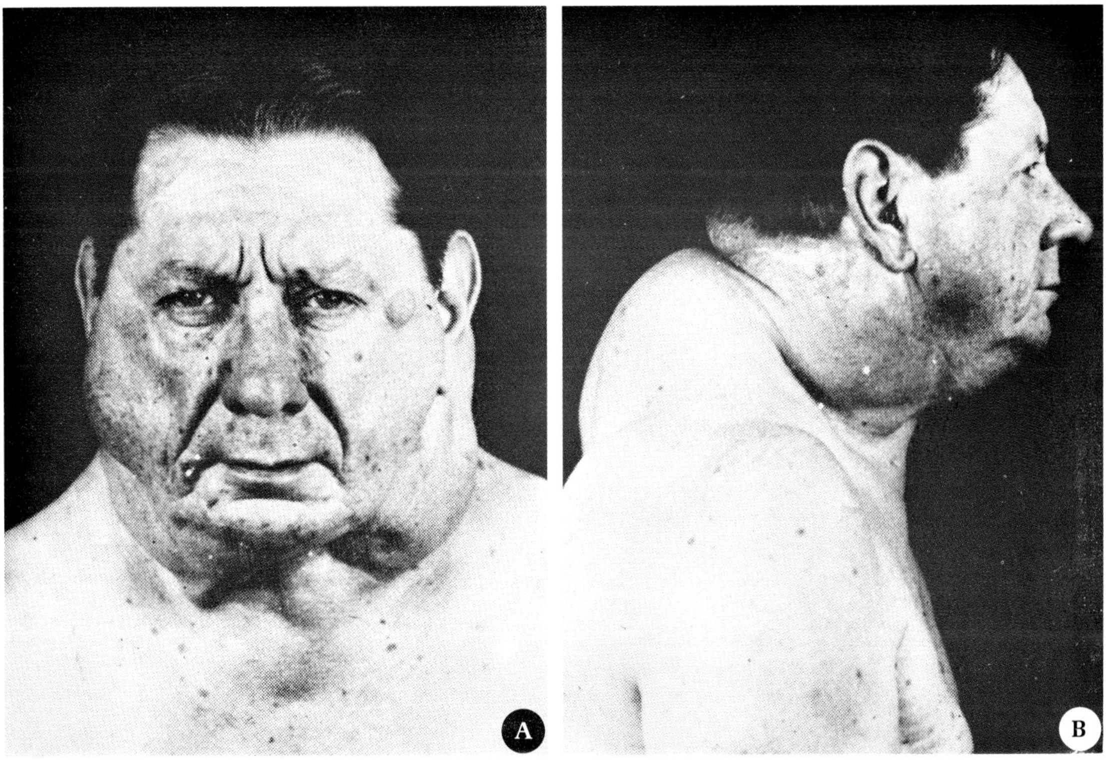

Figure 4-5. Fat neck of Madelung, (From Pack, G. M., and Ariel, I. M. (eds.): Tumors of the Soft Somatic Tissues and Bone. New York, Harper & Row, 1964, Figure 7-7, p. 117.)

NEOPLASTIC LESIONS

LIPOMAS*

Lipomas are the most common neoplasms of adipose tissue. The first reference to a tumor, probably a lipoma, arising from fat is in the *Papyrus Ebers*, written 1552 B.C.: "If the tumor goes and comes under your finger, trembling even when your hand is still, it is a fatty tumor, and treat it with the knife." There are innumerable references to lipomas in the literature. Among the most notable contributions are the large series reported by Adair et al, in 1932; Geschickter, in 1934; and Pack and Pierson, in 1954 (Fig. 4-6). Lipomas, to a certain extent, are analogous to steatopygous deposits in their growth pattern and familial tendency but dissimilar in regional distribution and have no racial predilection (see Steatopygia).

The etiology of lipomas is not known, but hereditary and hormonal factors may play a role in their development. Ewing (1928) classified lipomas into three groups: (1) replacement lipomatosis, (2) homologous lipomas, and (3) heterologous lipomas. Today, lipomas, like most other tumors, are classified on the basis of microscopic appearance (Table 4-1).

Well-differentiated Lipoma. These so-called simple lipomas occur mostly in persons after the age of 40 and are more common in females than males. Adair et al, in 1932, reported that in their series of 134 patients, 73% were women. *Congenital lipomas* and lipomas in children have been reported, but they are extremely rare. Lipomas may occur in any location, but they are most common in the subcutaneous tissue of the shoulder, back, chest, neck, and thigh; they are rare in the face, scalp, feet, and hands. They may vary in size from small nodules to huge masses and can be solitary or multiple, symmetrical or unilateral. According to the records, the largest lipoma was reported by Delamater, in 1859. The estimated weight of the tumor was more than 200 pounds, but the patient weighed only 90 pounds (see Chapter 1, Fig. 1-27). Martin, in 1928, reported a benign subcutaneous lipoma of the back which in 58 years grew to a weight of 59 pounds. Wells, in 1940, reported a huge lipoma weighing 69 pounds. Multiple lipomas may show a familial tendency or may be associated with neurofibromas (see Chapter 7).

The clinical diagnosis of even such common tumors as lipomas can sometimes be difficult. In most cases microscopic examination is required to ascertain their benign nature. Lipomas are usually slow growing, asymptomatic, and non-tender masses, but nerve compression with pain, hypoesthesia, and other funtional abnormalities are frequently associated with deep lipomas. Varga and Balazsy, in 1976, reported two cases in which lipoma compressed the radial nerve.

Well-differentiated lipomas are of a lighter color than the surrounding fat and as a rule are encapsulated and sharply demarcated from the surrounding tissues, except of the so-called infiltrating lipomas. The capsule is a thin, fibrous, membrane-like structure with broad fibrous trabeculae projecting inward between the fat lobules. The consistency of

TABLE 4-1. ***Classification of Lipomas***

Well-differentiated lipoma
Myxoid lipoma
Fibroblastic lipoma
Pleomorphic lipoma
Angiolipoma
Angiomyolipoma
Myelolipoma
Lipoblastoma
Hibernoma

**Synonyms and related terms:* simple lipoma, myxolipoma, lipomyxoma, myxofibrolipoma, lipoblastoma, hibernoma, myelolipoma, lipoma arborescens, lipoma dolorosa, angiolipoma, angiomyolipoma, pleomorphic lipoma, myolipoma, infiltrating lipoma, troublesome lipoma, lipoma telangiectodes, adenolipomatosis, Madelung's disease.

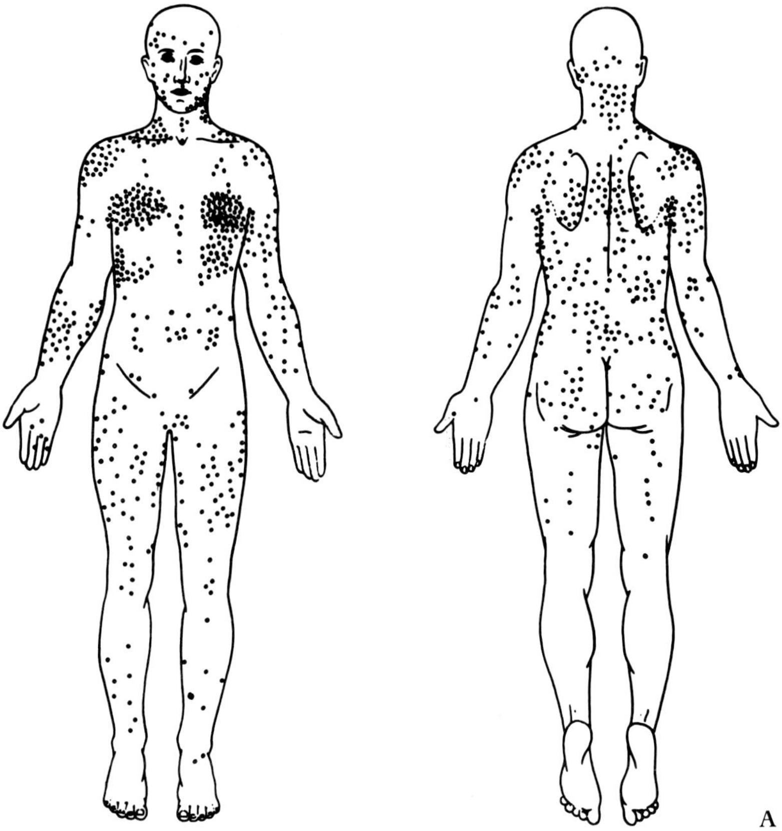

A

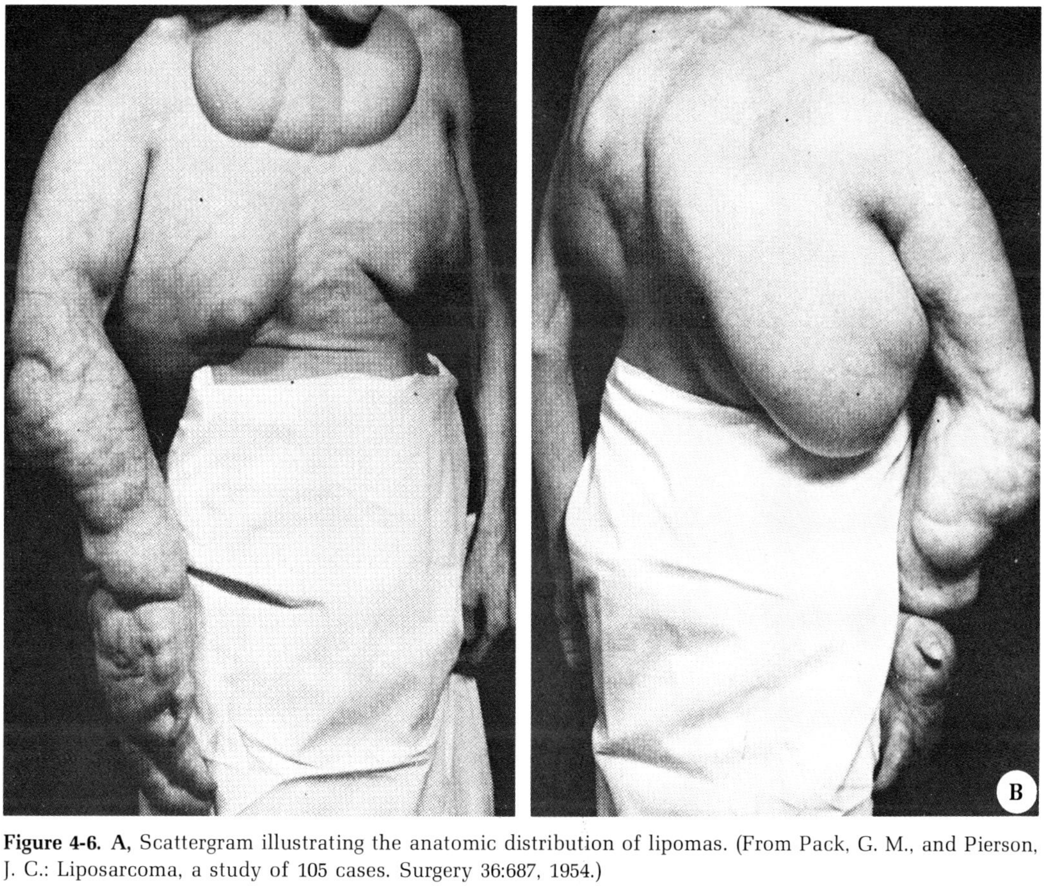

B

Figure 4-6. A, Scattergram illustrating the anatomic distribution of lipomas. (From Pack, G. M., and Pierson, J. C.: Liposarcoma, a study of 105 cases. Surgery 36:687, 1954.)

B, Diffuse lipomatosis involving chiefly the neck, shoulder and right arm. (From Pack, G. M., and Ariel, I. M.: Tumors of the Soft Somatic Tissues and Bone. New York, Harper & Row, 1964.)

the tumor depends upon the quantity of fibrous, vascular, and other connective tissue elements. Cystic areas, as the result of fat necrosis or liquefaction, are not uncommon findings in traumatized and large tumors.

Microscopically lipomas are composed of fat cells and other connective tissue elements. The fat cells may vary from large, spherical, and distended mature fat cells, with the typical "chicken wire" appearance, to small polyhedral embryonic or myxoid cells in disarranged pattern. The cytomorphology of most lipomas is fairly uniform and monotonous, but rarely there is an admixture of different microscopic patterns in the same tumor. The tumor cells are tightly adherent to each other and arranged in lobules bounded by collagenous fibroblasts and blood vessels (Fig. 4-7).

Lipomas exhibit a number of interesting features, e.g., the skin over a lipoma is cooler than in other areas because of the insulating quality of fat. Although lipomas histologically and chemically are similar to ordinary fat, the wasting body, in case of starvation, cannot utilize the fat of lipomas.

Lipomas should be excised, surgically, with clean surgical margin to ensure complete removal.

There are no organs in the human body in which lipomas have not been reported. Lipomas have occurred in unusual sites such as the *heart* (Brewis, 1905; Estevez et al, 1964), *eye* (Soebo, 1948), *the larynx* (Walford, 1930), *the mediastinum*

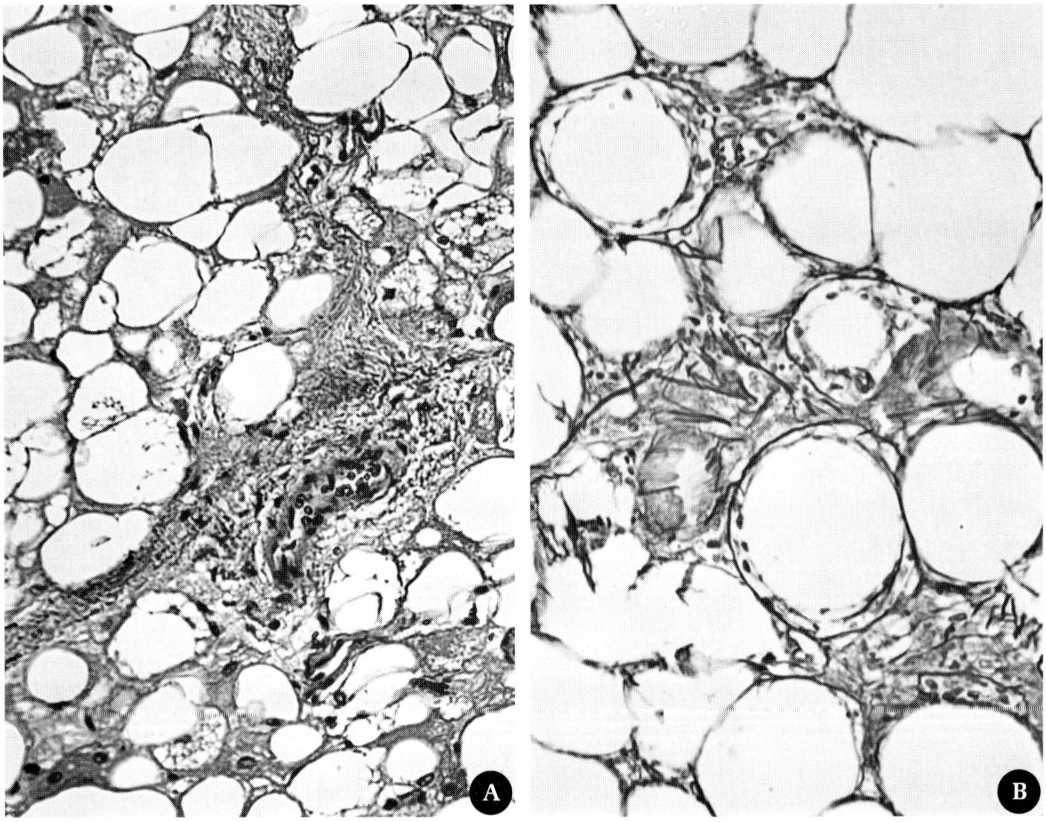

Figure 4-7. Well-differentiated lipoma.

A, An area with perivascular fibrosis. Note the branching extension of slim fibrous cords between mature adipocytes and a few foam cells (H & E, ×140).

B, Reticulum stain demonstrates fragmented collagen (type III) fibers. Also notice the way reticulum fibers encircle the fat cells (Retic. stain, ×140).

(Mackay-Dick et al, 1956), *bone* (Oosthuizen and Barletson, 1947; Child, 1955), *meniscus* (Stedfeld, 1955), *lung* (Watts et al, 1946; Krause and Ross, 1962; Politis et al, 1979), *the scrotum* (Hinman and Gibson, 1924; Cecil, 1927; Leyson et al, 1976), *the mesentery* (Bass, 1941), and *tendosynovium* (Strauss, 1922; Eibel, 1966).

The literature on lipomas is extensive, and it is beyond the scope of this volume to review all available publications and every organ site. It seems, however, that the intracranial, retroperitoneal, gastrointestinal, and intramuscular lipomas because of their unique clinicopathology deserve separate listing.

The most common site of *intracranial lipomas* is the corpus callosum. Lipomas of the central nervous system are usually associated with congenital anomalies such as spina bifida and meningomyelocele (Baker and Adams, 1938; Cant and Astley, 1952). Caram et al, in 1957, reported intradural lipomas of the spinal cord. Lipomas in children are rare but are found most commonly either intracranially or in the retroperitoneum.

Retroperitoneal lipomas may attain huge size. As a rule only less than one-third of the adipose tumors of the retroperitoneum, in adults, are benign. Symptoms usually are vague but an intravenous pyelogram frequently shows ureteral displacement. Surgical exploration and excision of the tumor is necessary in an attempt to prevent compression and obstruction of vital structures (Golding et al, 1972). Farbman, in 1950, reviewed all published reports of retroperitoneal lipoid tumors from 1937 to 1947. A review article published by Harvard, in 1953, lists all of the reported retroperitoneal lipomas in children.

Gastrointestinal lipomas are rare, but structurally they are similar to common subcutaneous lipoma. They can be single or multiple, sessile or pedunculated. They can arise anywhere in the gastric or intestinal wall, but the majority are *submucosal* in location. Comfort, in 1931, reviewed 181 cases of gastrointestinal lipomas, 92 of which were in the colon, 65 in the small intestine, and 24 in the stomach. Mayo et al, in 1963, reported that 110 of the 186 lipomas of the intestinal tract occurred in the large intestine. According to reports, the two most common sites of origin of lipomas in the gastrointestinal tract are the prepyloric region of the stomach and the ileocecal valve. Boquist et al, in 1972, reported 10 cases of lipomas arising from the ileocecal valve. They pointed out that the so-called lipohyperplasia and fatty degeneration of the ileocecal valve which are frequently associated with the "ileocecal valve syndrome" should be regarded as lipomas. The treatment of choice according to reports is enterotomy with local excision, although resection may be necessary in neglected cases.

Often it is difficult to establish the exact site of origin of a lipoma arising in deep soft tissues. One apparent site of origin, and perhaps the most common one, is *muscle*. According to historians, the first intramuscular lipoma within the trapezius muscle was described by Paget, in 1853, and Morestin, in 1898, reported the first congenital intramuscular lipoma. These neoplasms should not be confused with fatty replacement of skeletal muscle in obesity, muscular atrophy, and degeneration. In all of these conditions, the vascular component that is so prominent in lipomas is absent or minimal.

According to estimates more than 40% of intramuscular lipomas are in the arm and the shoulder region and there is a preponderance for males. Intramuscular lipomas are usually unencapsulated, and Regan et al, in 1946, coined the term of *infiltrating lipoma*. Indeed, in most cases there is extensive dissociation and infiltration of the surrounding muscle fibers giving the impression of other than a benign neoplastic process.

It is claimed (Kindblom et al, 1974) that intramuscular lipomas are more radiotranslucent than the surrounding soft tissues and appear radiologically as an ill-defined area. Grossly these tumors have an innocuous soft consistency and flat contour when the muscle is relaxed which change to a firm consistency and spherical contour when the muscle is contracted. The relatively common occurrence of these lesions is shown by the fact that Behrend, in 1929, was able to collect 190 reported cases from the literature. Dione and Seemayer, in 1974, reviewed 27 cases of deep-seated lipomas and emphasized the tendency of intramuscular lipomas to recur after local excision (Table 4-2).

Myxoid Lipoma. Most of the lipomas, regardless of the site of origin, are composed of spherical or globoid mature fat cells. A less common form, the so-called myxoid lipoma, a term first used by Salzer, in 1888, is also ubiquitous. This tumor is found most commonly in the retroperitoneum, around the genitourinary organs, and in the alimentary canal. It is a neoplastic growth composed of small and medium-sized adipocytes, moderate amounts of fibroblasts, and prominent capillary vessels (Fig. 4-8). The mucinous material surrounding many of the tumor cells gives a myxoid or myxomatous appearance to these tumors. Rarely, one may find in highly vascular areas a few hematopoietic elements, including megakaryocytes (see Chapter 2, Myxoma).

Fibroblastic Lipoma. Also called spindle cell lipoma, sclerosing lipoma, or fibrolipoma, fibroblastic lipoma is an admixture of fat cells and elongated slender fibroblasts in a myxomatous-like stroma. The branching cytoplasmic processes of fibroblasts between palisading capillary vessels give a semitransparent spiderweb-like appearance to these tumors. Not uncommonly the monotonous fibromyxoid appearance is interrupted by clusters of inflammatory cells, histiocytes, and granular lipoblasts. According to Enzinger and Harvey (1975) these tumors occur almost exclusively in middle-aged male patients and nearly all of the reported tumors were excised from the posterior neck and the shoulder region (Fig. 4-9). Evans et al, 1979, reviewed 30 cases of lipoid tumors that were formerly classified as well-differentiated liposarcomas and concluded that most of the tumors could be reclassified as "atypical" lipomas with myxoid, fibrous, or pleomorphic components.

Pleomorphic Lipoma. This rare bizarre neoplasm must be distinguished from fat necrosis, lipogranuloma, and pleomorphic liposarcoma. It has a quiescent myxoid or fibroblastic lipoma appearance, in most areas, but the nests of bizarre mononuclear or multinuclear histiocytic-looking giant cells make it distinct from all other lipomas (Fig. 4-10). Most of the 40 cases reported by Enzinger, in 1977, occurred in middle-aged males in the subcutaneous tissues of the shoulder and posterior neck.

Angiolipoma. Although Bowen, in 1912, was the first to describe a case of angiolipoma, it was Howard and Helwig, in 1960, who established angiolipoma as an entity. The distinctive features of this lesion are the striking predominance of blood vessels, their infiltrative nature, and the notorious tendency to recur after simple excision. Most of the cases in the series of Howard and Helwig were not infiltrating; however, in later publications the nonencapsulated and infiltrating nature of these lesions was emphasized (Gonzalez-

TABLE 4-2. ***Infiltrating Lipomas****

	NO. OF CASES	MEAN AGE, YR.	MOST COMMON SITE	RECURRENCE
Infiltrating lipoma	13	50	Lower extremity	62%
Infiltrating angiolipoma	14	35	—	50%

*Modified from Dione, G. P., and Seemayer, T. A.: Infiltrating lipomas and angiolipomas revisited. Cancer 33: 732, 1974.

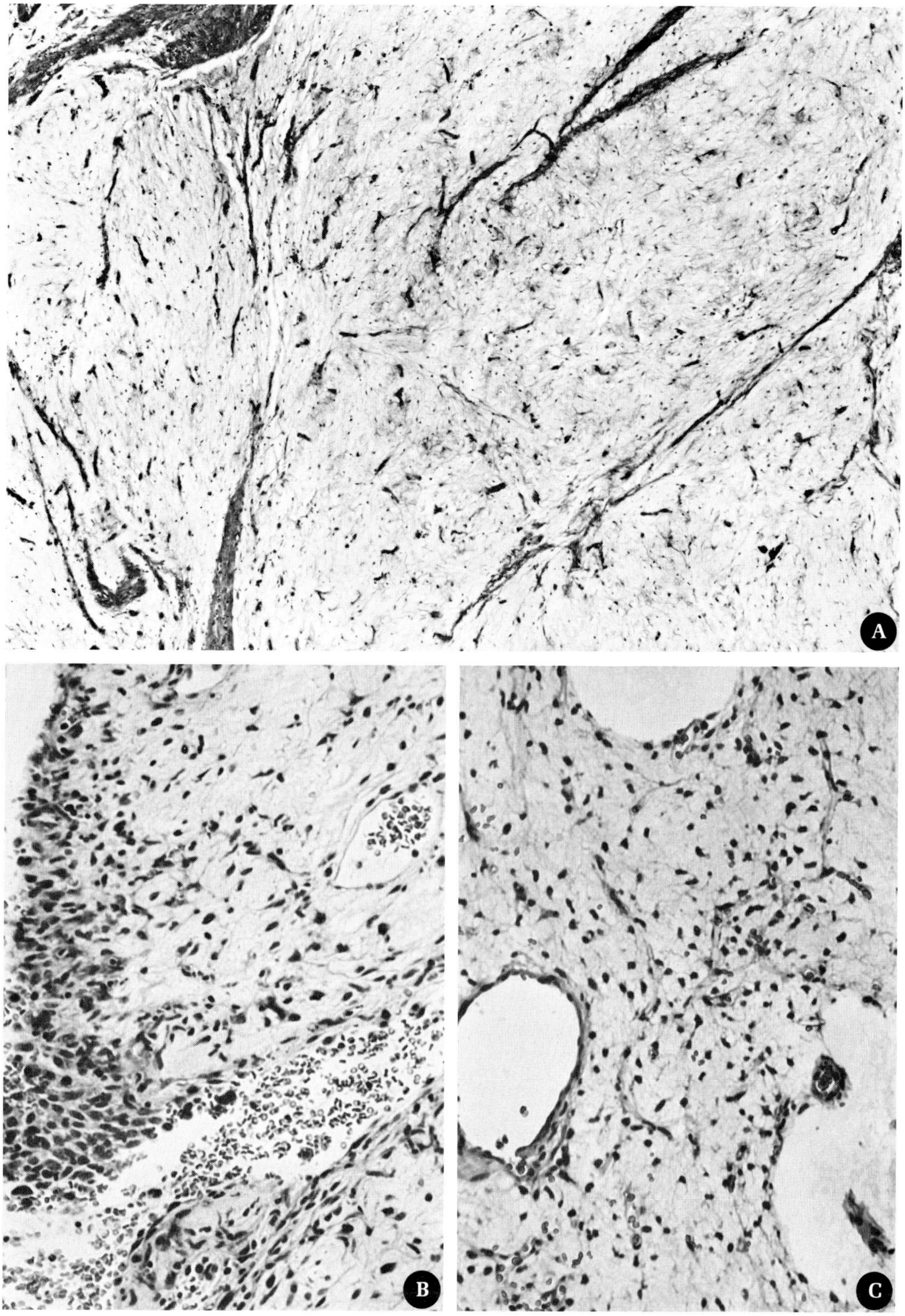

Figure 4-8. Myxoid lipoma. The fat cells are mostly immature short, spindle-shaped prolipoblasts and multivacuolated preadipocytes. The stroma is rich in mucopolysaccharides. Collection of lipoblasts around vascular spaces **(C)** and at the edge of the fat lobules **(B)** may give a solid consistency and solid appearance (**A,** H & E, ×35; **B** & **C,** H & E, ×85).

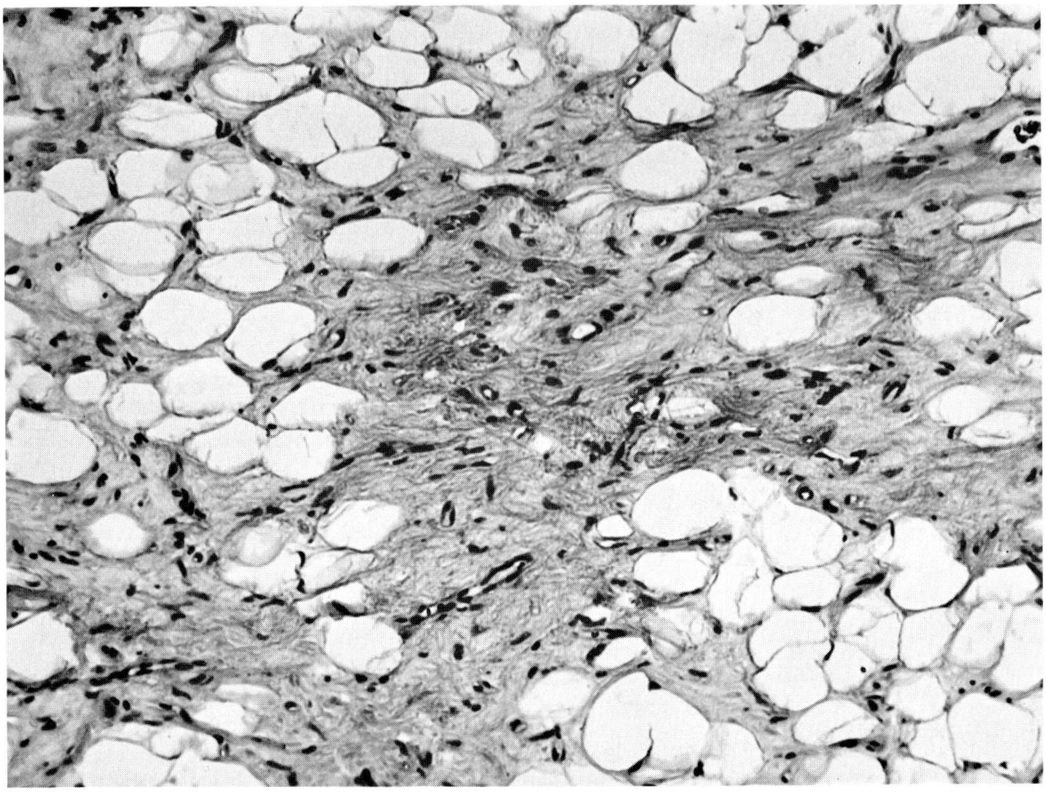

Figure 4-9. Fibroblastic or sclerotic lipoma. Sparsely branching cellular fibroconnective tissue is positioned between adipocytes. Immature fat cells are conspicuously absent (H & E, ×140).

Crussi et al, 1966; Dionne and Seemayer, 1974; Lin and Lin, 1974). They are usually subcutaneous in origin but many examples of infiltrating fascia, muscle, periosteum, and bone have been described. Lin and Lin, in 1974, reviewed the English literature on infiltrating angiolipomas and found 23 cases with documentation of infiltration into bone (Table 4-3).

Microscopically, they are composed of proliferating capillary blood vessels, mature and immature fat cells, and fibroconnective tissue arranged in a haphazard fashion (Fig. 4-11). The vessels are usually lined by plump endothelial cells and in the lumen there may be fibrous thrombi. The wall of the blood vessels may be thickened, but there is no sign of atypism. The postulate that angiolipomas may represent hamartomas is supported by the younger mean age of the patients (Table 4-4). Despite the infiltrating and often worrisome proliferative nature of angiolipomas, there is no one reported instance of malignant transformation. The management of these tumors is similar to that of other lipomas, but perhaps the excisional margin should be a little bit more generous.

Angiomyolipoma. The term *angiomyolipoma* was first used by Morgan et al, in 1951, but the first reference to a lesion that histologically corresponds to angiomyolipoma was first described by Fischer, in 1911. Since tuberous sclerosis was first described by Bourneville, in 1880, many authors pointed out the association of renal tumors and tuberous sclerosis. According to Critchley and Earl (1932) renal tumors occur in 80% of patients with tuberous sclerosis; however, we have been unable to substantiate this claim by reviewing our 27 cases and 130 reported cases in the literature. Table 4-5 is a summary and comparison of pertinent data from our article (Hajdu and Foote, 1969).

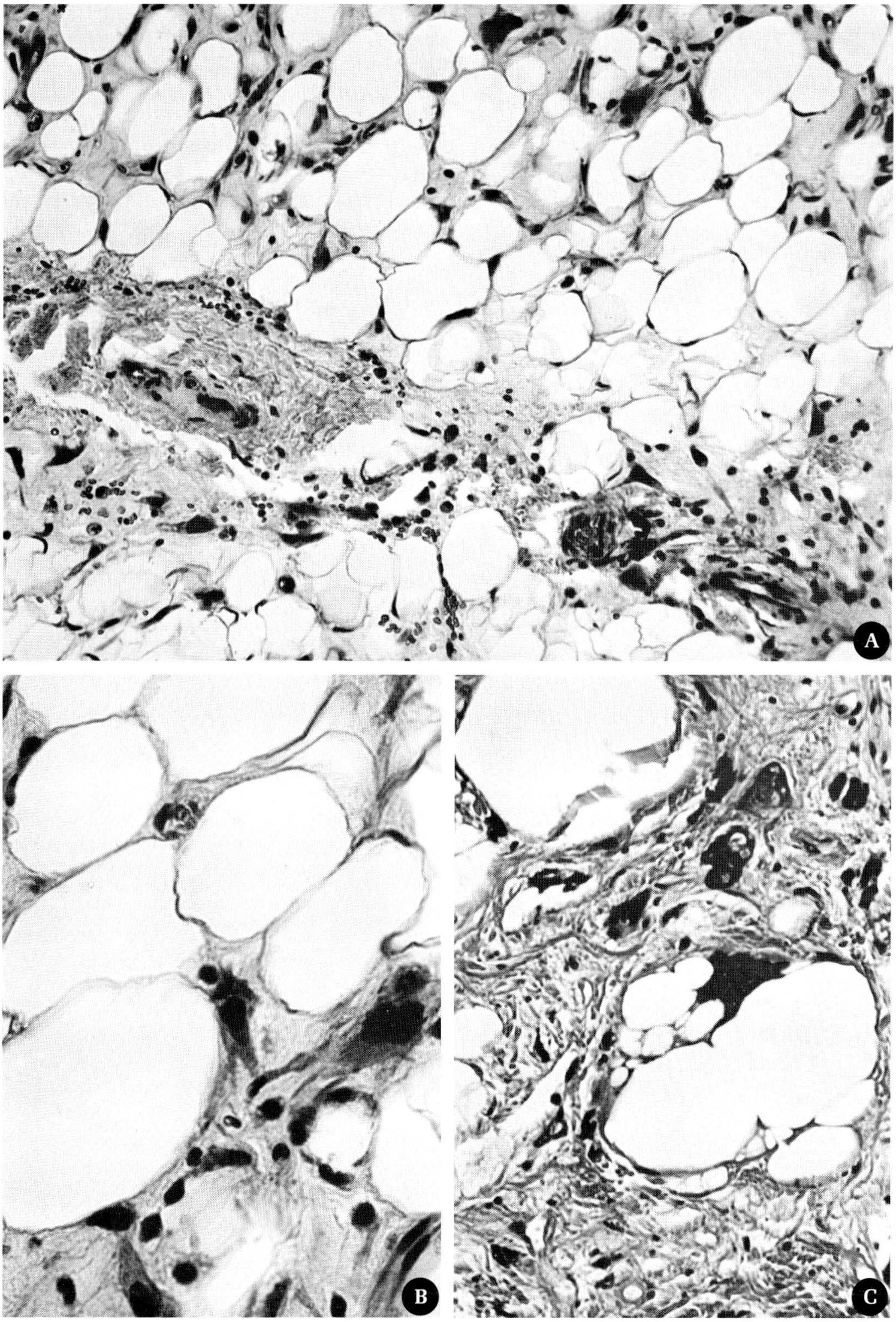

Figure 4-10. Pleomorphic lipoma. This tumor is predominantly composed of mature fat cells; however, there are occasional round lipoblasts and other immature forms interpositioned between adipocytes and stromal cells. The pleomorphic cells are found in the fibroreticular stroma, and they range in size and shape from enlarged fibroblasts **(B)** to bizarre "monster cells" with branching cytoplasmic filaments **(C).** The heaviest concentration of such cells is usually found about or near capillary vessels and interlobular spaces (**A,** H & E, ×140; **B,** H & E, ×350).

TABLE 4-3. ***The Relative Proportion of Various Histologic forms in a Series of 459 Cases of Lipomas****

HISTOLOGIC TYPE	NUMBER OF CASES
Well-differentiated lipoma	388
Fibroblastic lipoma	39
Angiolipoma	25
Hibernoma	4
Myxoid lipoma	3

*Modified from Lin, J. J., and Lin, F.: Two entities in angiolipoma: A study of 459 cases of lipoma with review of the literature on infiltrating angiolipoma. Cancer 34: 720, 1974.

In essence, we were able to accept only 9 of the 53 renal tumors which occurred in patients with tuberous sclerosis as angiomyolipomas. Most of the renal tumors were either hyernephromas or tubular adenomas. It seems that the number of reported cases of angiomyolipoma without tuberous sclerosis far outnumbers the ones with tuberous sclerosis. None of the 32 patients reported by Farrow et al, in 1968 and none of our cases had tuberous sclerosis. It seems the association of angiomyolipoma with tuberous sclerosis is unwarrantedly overestimated in the literature and it is not appreciated that *angiomyolipoma is more common without tuberous sclerosis than with it.*

Clinically and morphologically angiomyolipoma can masquerade as several other renal lesions: simple cyst, renal cell carcinoma, sarcoma, and polycystic kidney, just to mention the most common ones. Clark and Palubinskas, in 1972, reviewed 26 cases angiographically and concluded that in 68% of the cases the vascularity was indistinguishable from renal cell carcinoma, 28% from pseudo-

TABLE 4-4. ***Comparison of Certain Lipomas****

TUMOR TYPE	NO. OF PATIENTS WITH FOLLOW-UP	MEDIAN AGE	MALES (%)	RECURRENCE (%)	MOST COMMON SITES
Fibroblastic lipoma	63	55	91	0	Posterior neck Shoulder
Intramuscular lipoma	46	44	73	15	Thigh Shoulder
Pleomorphic lipoma	22	60	76	4	Posterior neck Shoulder

*Modified and reproduced with permission from Enzinger, F. M.: Benign lipomatous tumors simulating a sarcoma. *In* M. D. Anderson Hospital and Tumor Institute, Houston: Management of Primary Bone and Soft Tissue Tumors. © 1977 by Year Book Medical Publishers, Inc., Chicago.

TABLE 4-5. ***Comparison of Reported Cases of Renal Angiomyolipoma with or without Tuberous Sclerosis****

	NO. CASES	MALE	FEMALE	SEX UNKNOWN	AV. AGE YR.	SIZE OF TUMOR <1 cm	>1 cm
Renal tumors with tuberous sclerosis	53	17	24	12	17	22	31
Renal angiomyolipomas without tuberous sclerosis	104	14	87	3	50	26	78

*Modified from Hajdu, S. I., and Foote, F. W.: Angiomyolipoma of the kidney. Report of 27 cases and review of the literature. J. Urol. 102:396, 1969.

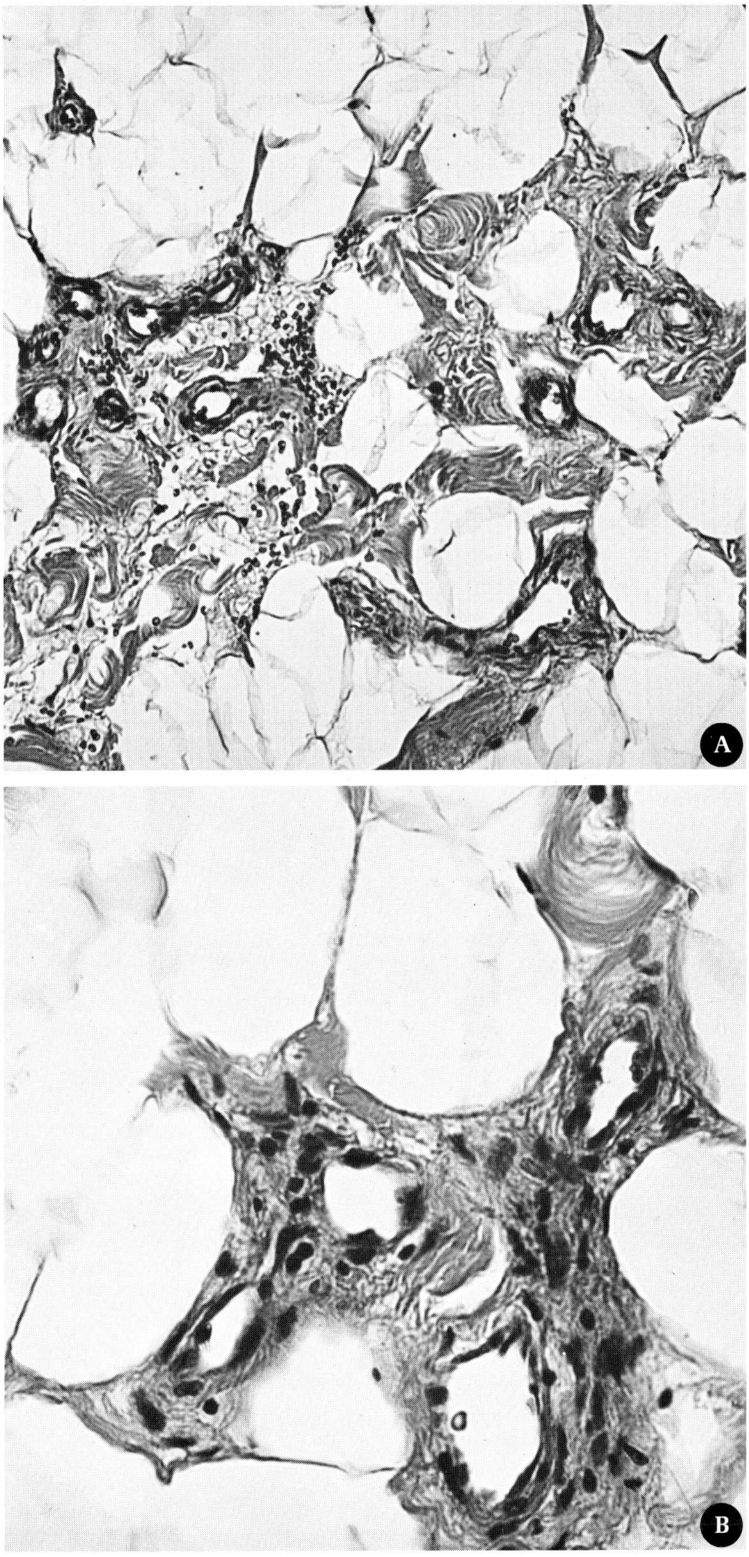

Figure 4-11. Angiolipoma. Hyperplastic capillary vessels with prominent endothelial and pericytic cells in the stromal partitions between adipocytes. There is also accumulation of wavy fibroreticular material about the vessels (**A,** H & E, ×140; **B,** H & E, ×350).

aneurysm, and 4% avascular. The gross appearance at operation is also an unreliable guide. These tumors may range in size from small intraparenchymal nodules to huge size with adherence to the renal capsule and direct extension into perirenal tissues such as fat and hilar lymph nodes. They are usually single and unilateral lesions. In 80% of the cases the location is the right side, and female patients outnumber male patients 4 to 1.

On cut surface these tumors may vary from yellow to gray according to the proportion of fat and other connective tissue elements.

Histologically, angiomyolipomas can be quite bizarre and pleomorphic. They are frequently misdiagnosed microscopically either as liposarcoma or leiomyosarcoma. The tumors are composed of fat, smooth muscle, and blood vessels. The proportion of these elements varies from case to case. Some angiomyolipomas are predominantly leiomyomatous, whereas others are predominantly composed of adipose tissue. The vascular component of these tumors consists of thick-walled, often tortuous blood vessels. They may display the characteristic sunburst or whorled appearance of hamartomatous blood vessels. The lumen of the blood vessels may vary widely in diameter and shape. Most of the blood vessels are surrounded by collars of smooth muscle cells extending as strands into the adjacent adipose tissue (Fig. 4-12).

As a rule, angiomyolipomas are sharply demarcated from the renal parenchyma, but they may extend into adjacent lymph nodes and soft tissues. There are at least three known cases with extension into the renal vein. Since the first report of a *malignant angiomyolipoma* by Ehrmann, in 1914, two additional cases of malignant angiomyolipoma have been reported (Berg, 1955 and Hartveit and Hallerbraker, 1960). Without questioning that a malignant form of this lesion may occur, one should be aware that pleomorphism of bizarre smooth muscle fibers, adipocytes, and blood vessels is one of the characteristics of benign angiomyolipomas. As far as I know there is not a single well-documented case of metastasizing or locally recurring angiomyolipoma in the literature, despite the fact that some of the tumors were twice the size of the kidney.

Myelolipoma. This tumor is composed of adipose tissue and hematopoietic elements. It is found most commonly in the adrenal gland but extra-adrenal cases have been reported. Parsons and Thompson, in 1959, reviewed the literature and reported a symptomatic myelolipoma of adrenal which weighed 1,250 grams. Adrenal myelolipomas are not known to be associated with blood dyscrasias; however, most of the reported lesions of extra-adrenal sites such as the omentum, mediastinum, and thyroid were found in association with various hematologic abnormalities. Occasionally myelolipomatous areas can be found in the form of solid nodules in any type of lipoma.

Lipoblastoma. This growth of embryonal lipoblasts can be localized (lipoblastoma) or diffuse (lipoblastomatosis). The term *lipoblastoma* was coined by Jaffe, in 1926. Lipoblastomatosis was first reported by Goormaghtigh et al, in 1936, but was not widely known prior to the report by Vellios et al in 1958. Many of these lesions were reported in the literature under names such as *lipoma foetocellular, congenital lipomatoid tumor,* and *embryonal lipoma.* It affects infants and young children. According to Chung and Enzinger, in 1973, the majority of these lesions occur during the first 3 years of life, and boys afflicted outnumber girls by a ratio of 2 to 1. The subcutis of the extremities is the most common site of these lesions. They are considered to be the childhood counterpart of lipoma simplex and diffuse lipomatosis. It is believed that they arise from persistent embryonic tissue, but the histogenesis is far from settled.

Histologically, lipoblastomas are composed of vacuolated adipocytes, granular lipoblasts, and elements of poorly differentiated mesenchymal cells. The tumor

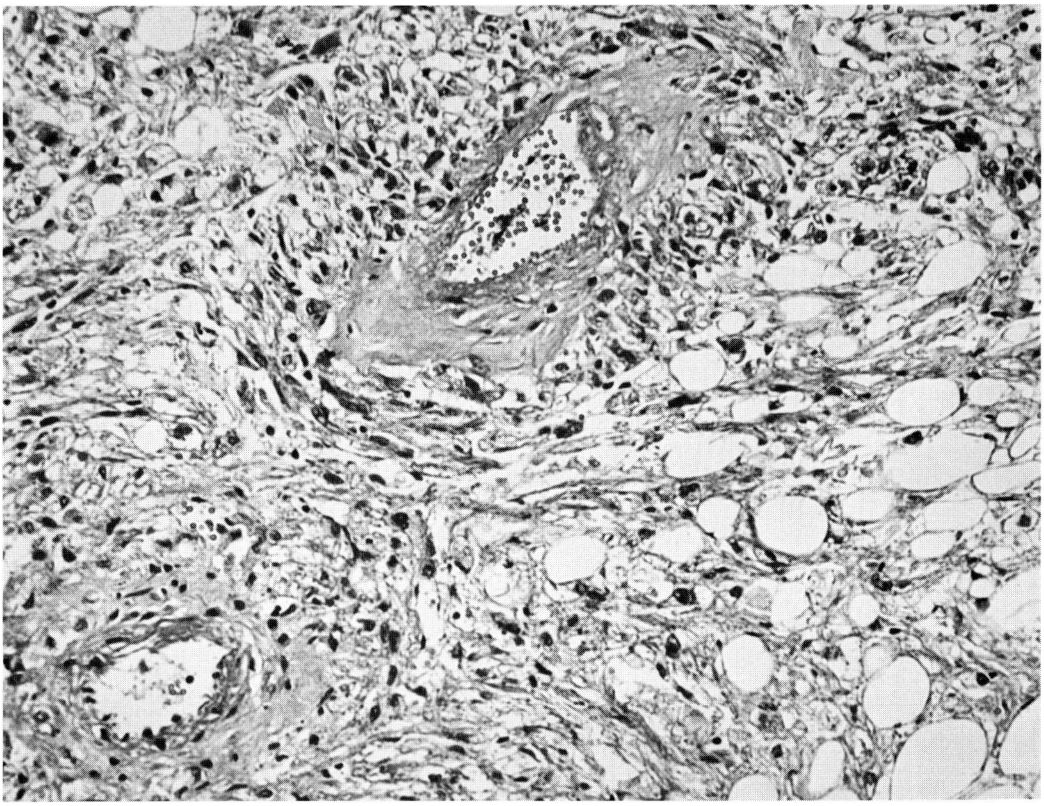

Figure 4-12. Angiomyolipoma. Note the delicate blending of hamartomatous blood vessels, long fibromuscular cells, and adipocytes into a conglomerate of cellular tumor (H & E, ×140).

cells are arranged in distinct lobular masses with arranged plexiform capillaries and myxoid stroma. It is almost certain that a number of hibernomas were included in some of the reports. Due to the resemblance of lipoblasts to the lipoblasts in lipoblastic liposarcoma attention should be paid to the *uniformity, lobular arrangement, sparse cellularity, and admixture of adipocytes and lipoblasts in lipoblastomas* (Figs. 4-1, 4-13).

The benign nature of these lesions is demonstrated by their limited tendency to recur, from 10 to 15%, and by their lack of metastasis.

Hibernoma. Hibernoma or lipoma of brown adipose tissue is also known as lipoma glandulare and atypical lipoma. Probably the first example of these rare lesions was described by Merkel, in 1906. The word *hibernoma* was introduced in a seminar by Gery while discussing the case reported by Bonnel, in 1914. Hibernomas are found most commonly in the subcutaneous tissue of the back, shoulder, neck, axilla, and occasionally in the mediastinum. It is generally believed that the tissue of origin is the brown fat, a special form of adipose tissue which corresponds to the hibernating glands in animals (Dardick, 1978).

The physiology and morphology of the hibernating gland, brown fat, and hibernoma have been reviewed by Brines and Johnson, in 1949, and by Sutherland et al, in 1952. Mesara and Batsakis, in 1967, reviewed 26 cases of hibernoma from the literature and added one additional case of their own (Table 4-6). Grossly these tumors have a lobular contour and distinct brownish color due to the high concentration of lipochrome pigments.

Hibernoma is a slowly growing benign neoplasm of adults. It is composed mainly

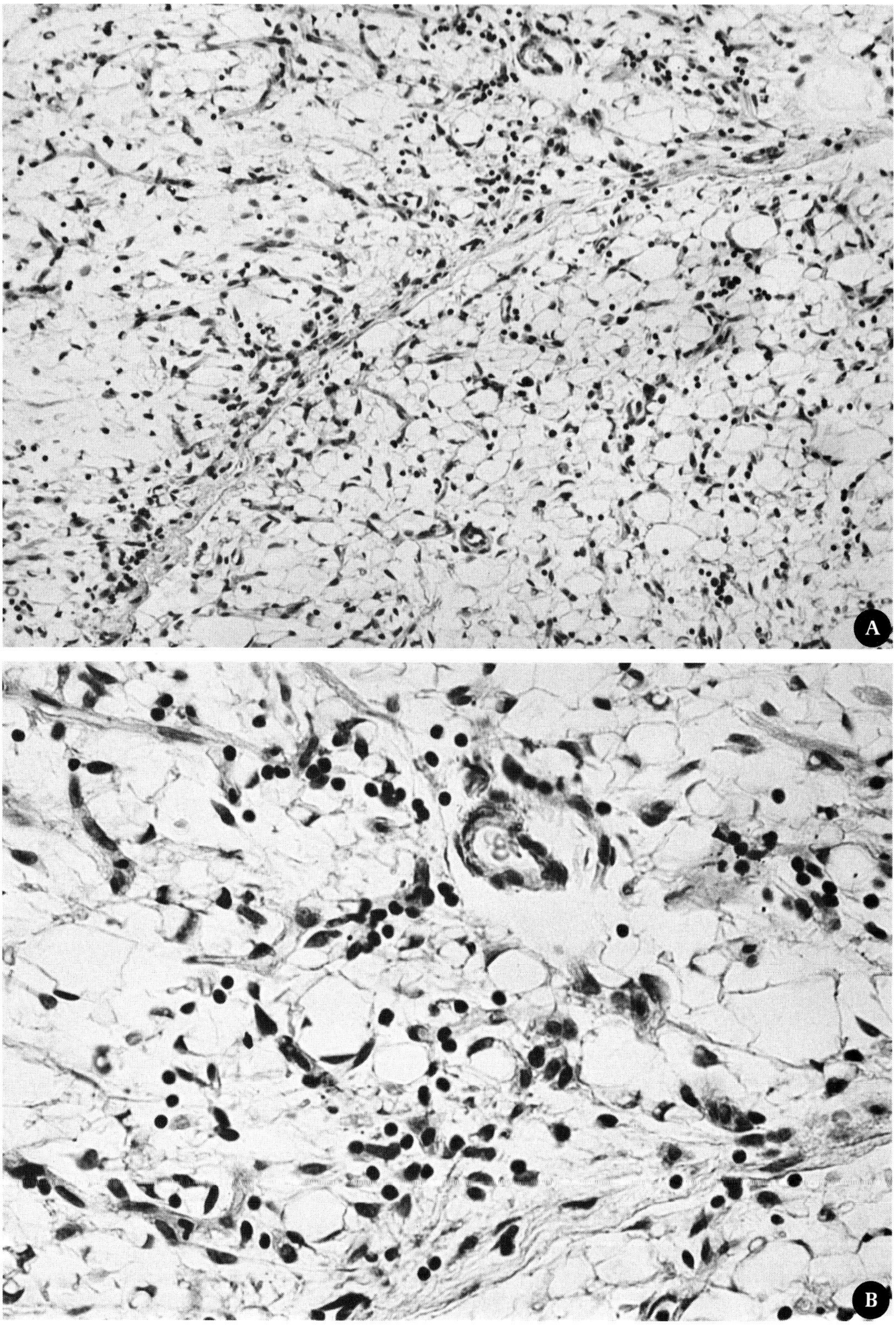

Figure 4-13. Lipoblastoma is composed of glycogen-rich round lipoblasts, mature adipocytes, and multivacuolated and stellate preadipocytes in well-defined lobular compartments (**A**). Note the sparsely vascular stroma and absence of pleomorphic elements (**A,** H & E, ×35; **B,** H & E, ×140).

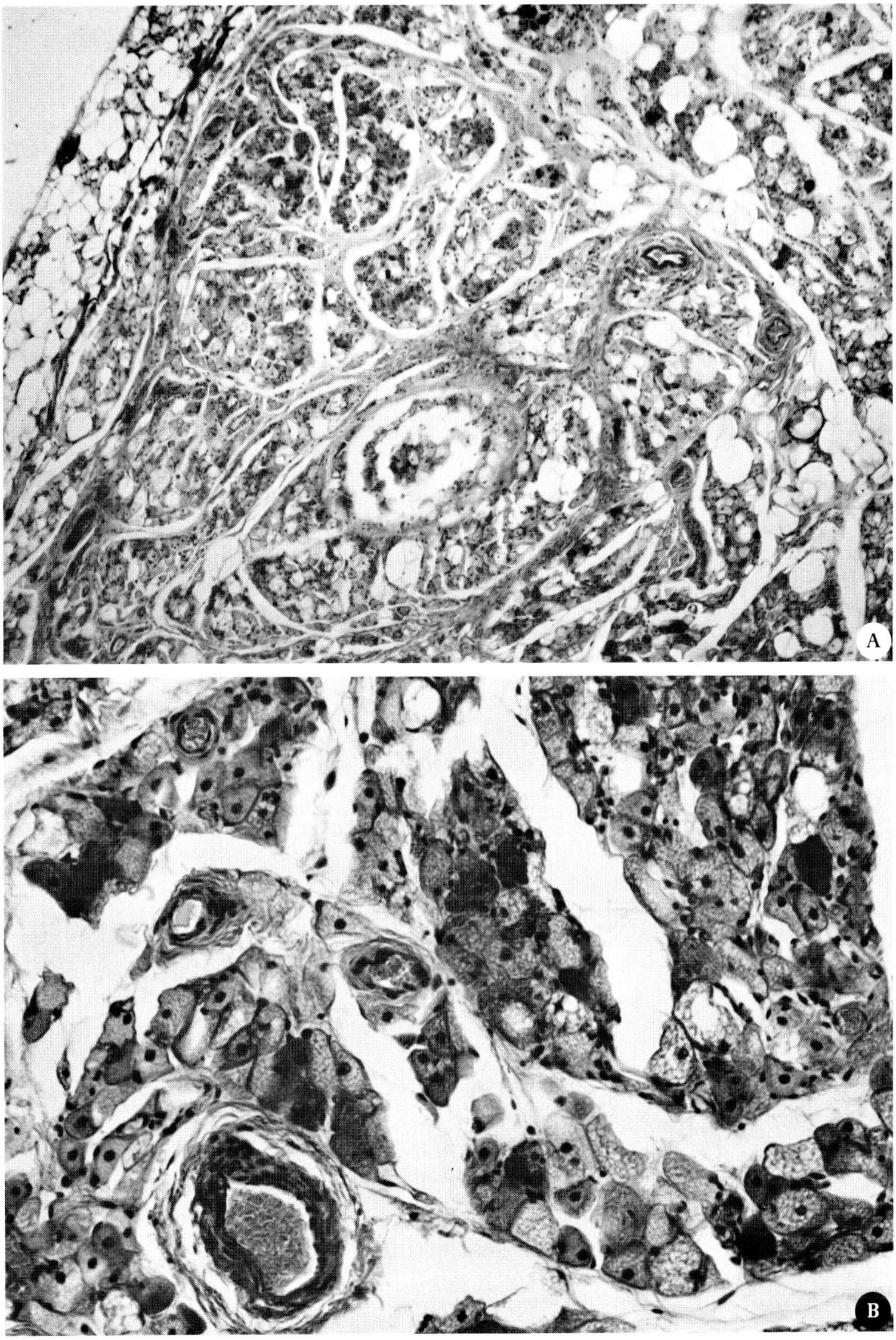

Figure 4-14. Hibernoma.

A, Granular cytoplasmic embryonal fat cells arranged in lobular nests (H & E, ×35).

B, The cytoplasm of the fat cells is granular with a round or polyhedral contour. The nuclei are punctate and centrally positioned in the cytoplasm (H & E, ×140).

TABLE 4-6. ***Hibernomas Reported in the Literature****

SITE	NO. OF CASES
Back	12
Mediastinum	4
Buttocks	4
Axilla	3
Neck	2
Abdomen	2

*Modified from Mesara, B. W., and Batsakis, J. G.: Hibernoma of the neck. Arch. Otolaryngol. 85:95, 1967.

of multinucleated globoid and lipid-rich adipocytes with central dark nuclei and granular cytoplasms. The tumor cells usually are arranged in tightly composed lobules. Because the interlobular septae are highly vascular, some of these tumors may be detected by angiography. According to Gross and Wood (1953), in unstained formalin-fixed frozen sections and sections stained with Sudan black, anisotropic crystals resembling cholesterol crystals can be seen in the cytoplasm of many tumor cells. No convincing example of malignant hibernoma or malignant transformation of hibernoma has been reported. However, Symmers, in 1944, reported a possible malignant form in a 3-month-old boy who died with brownish-red nodules throughout the abdominal cavity which on histologic examination resembled brown fat. The superficial resemblance of hibernomas, microscopically, to *granular cell myoblastoma* (see Chapter 9), *lipoblastoma,* and *histiocytic fibrous histiocytoma* (see Chapter 2) should be kept in mind at the time of diagnosis (Fig. 4-14).

The first case of *malignant transformation* in a lipoma was reported by Wohlgemuth, in 1910. Since this publication, 10 additional cases have been reported in the literature (Table 4-7). It is indeed surprising, considering the great frequency of lipomas, that liposarcomas do not develop more frequently in preexisting benign lipomas. In the light of these cases, careful gross and histopathologic examination of lipomas is indicated. Any unusually firm and grayish areas should be sampled for microscopic examination. My personal experience with benign lipomas that turned to malignant neoplasms amounts to 10 cases (Table 4-7). The common features of these neoplasms are their predominantly myxoid nature and the presence of a mass for several years at the site of the subsequent liposarcoma.

LIPOSARCOMA*

Although the first report of a tumor corresponding to liposarcoma was that of Zappoli in 1843, the first clear description of a malignant tumor of the adipose tissue was by Virchow in 1857. In the same year Foerster reported a tumor he described as "myxo-sarcoma" of the thigh, which recurred despite excisions. Following these reports, a number of case reports appeared in the literature. Notable descriptions are Senftleben's (1858) account of a liposarcoma in a child and Waldeyer's (1865) report of a liposarcoma which metastasized to the liver and the lungs. The first series of 6 cases of myxoliposarcoma of the groin were reported by Hellman in 1888, and Lenger, in 1899, described the first authentic example of retroperitoneal liposarcoma. As early as 1910 Beriel attempted to classify the so-called malignant lipomas and Wohlgemuth called attention to a myxosarcoma which arose from a lipoma (Table 4-7).

Robertson, in 1916, was able to collect from the literature 51 cases of liposarcoma and stressed the occurrence of a spectrum of morphologic patterns of the tumors he called "lipoma myxomatodes." Ewing, in 1928, published the first case of primary *intraosseous liposarcoma* to which Stewart added three cases in 1931, all with fatal courses, and Goldman described one additional case in 1964.

**Synonyms and related terms:* lipomyxosarcoma, myxoma lipomatodes, lipoblastic lipoma, myxoliposarcoma, fibroblastic liposarcoma, epithelioid liposarcoma, pleomorphic liposarcoma, round-cell liposarcoma. Also see Table 4-8.

TABLE 4-7. ***Liposarcoma Arising in Lipoma****

AUTHOR	YR. OF REPORT	NO. OF CASES	AGE	SEX	SITE	HISTOLOGIC TYPE	FOLLOW-UP
Wohlgemuth	1910	1	43	F	Arm	Myxoid	—
Schiller	1918	2	67	F	Thigh	Myxoid	—
			67	F	Trunk	—	—
Blavet di Briga	1923	1	Adult	M	—	—	—
Geschickter	1934	2	39	F	Retroperit.	Myxoid	Alive, 8 yr.
			Adult	F	Thigh	Myxoid	Died, 16 yr.
Wright	1948	1	60	F	Thigh	—	Alive, 9 mo.
Sternberg	1952	1	56	M	Back	Myxoid	Alive, 3 yr.
Pack and Pierson	1954	2	Adult	M	Chest	Myxoid	Alive, 8 yr.
			Adult	M	Thigh	—	—
Sampson et al	1960	1	79	F	Back	Myxoid	Alive, 9 mo.
Hajdu	(unpublished)	10	63	F	Retroperit.	Well-diff.	Died, 7 yr.
			67	M	Thigh	Well-diff.	Died, 30 yr.
			55	M	Thigh	Myxoid	Alive, 16 yr.
			40	F	Retroperit.	Myxoid	Died, 13 yr.
			53	F	Trunk	Myxoid	Died, 13 yr.
			38	M	Back	Myxoid	Died, 8 yr.
			54	F	Back	Myxoid	Died, 18 yr.
			44	M	Thigh	Myxoid	Died, 5 yr.
			55	F	Thigh	Myxoid	Died, 5 yr.
			52	F	Thigh	Lipoblastic	Died, 12 yr.

*Compiled from the literature and personal experience.

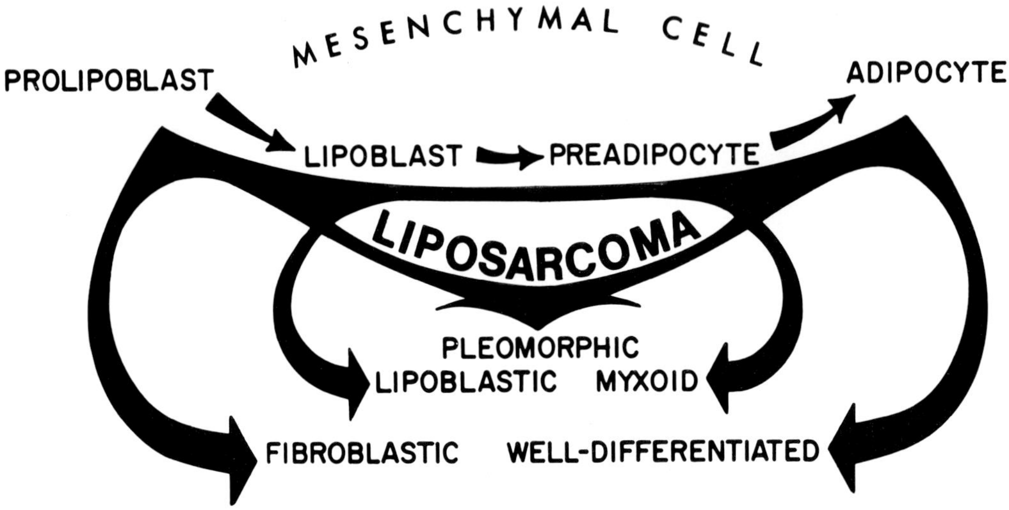

Figure 4-15. Schematic illustration of the pathway of maturation of fat cells and the relationship between various fat cells and malignant neoplasms. Fibroblastic liposarcoma is predominantly composed of prolipoblasts; lipoblastic or round cell liposarcoma is composed of lipoblasts. Preadipocyte will dominate in myxoid liposarcoma. Well-differentiated liposarcoma is composed of mature fat cells (adipocytes), and in pleomorphic liposarcoma one may find, in combination, neoplastic forms of all of the basic cells (see Figures 4-1 and 4-24).

Jaffe, in 1926, proposed classifying malignant lipomatous tumors into three groups: *lipoblastoma,* composed of immature fat cells, *lipoma pseudomyxomatodes,* composed of mature fat cells, and *liposarcoma,* which is characterized by anaplasia of fat cells. Ewing, in 1935, defined myxoid liposarcoma and called attention to its radiosensitivity. Ewing divided malignant lipomatous tumors into two groups: the *myxoliposarcoma* with vascular stroma and the *granular cell lipoblastoma* (Table 4-8). Pack and Anglem, in 1939, reported 6 cases of liposarcomas in children and reviewed 7 other cases from the literature.

Murray and Stout, in 1943, studied two metastatic liposarcomas in tissue culture and the following year Stout reported the first large series, 41 cases, of liposarcomas. Stout separated malignant tumors of the adipose tissue into three categories: well-differentiated myxoid liposarcoma, poorly differentiated myxoid liposarcoma, and so-called round cell or adenoid type of liposarcoma. Practically all the writers who reported on liposarcomas mentioned the wide and overlapping morphologic patterns in liposarcomas. Ackerman and Wheeler (1942) felt that it does not appear justified to divide liposarcomas into specific types. Their opinion was seconded by Evans (1968) who stated, "Despite the diversity and variation in degree of differentiation manifested by different tumors and by different regions of the same tumor, liposarcomas constitute a single group of neoplasms, the subdivisions of which, based on histological features are of limited value." From studies reported by others and from my personal experience has evolved the classification of liposarcomas listed in Tables 4-9 and 4-10 and Fig. 4-15.

While lipomas are more common in the subcutaneous tissue, liposarcomas have a predilection for the deeper soft tissues. Stout stated (1953): "If a tumor is deep, bulky and nodular, often it proves to be a liposarcoma." Fortunately, the majority of tumors arising from the adipose tissues are benign. Geschickter (1934) reported 12 liposarcomas among 490 tumors of fat, and Pack and Pierson (1954) stated that one of every 120 adipose tumors is sarcoma.

Liposarcomas may occur wherever adipose tissue is present. In order of fre-

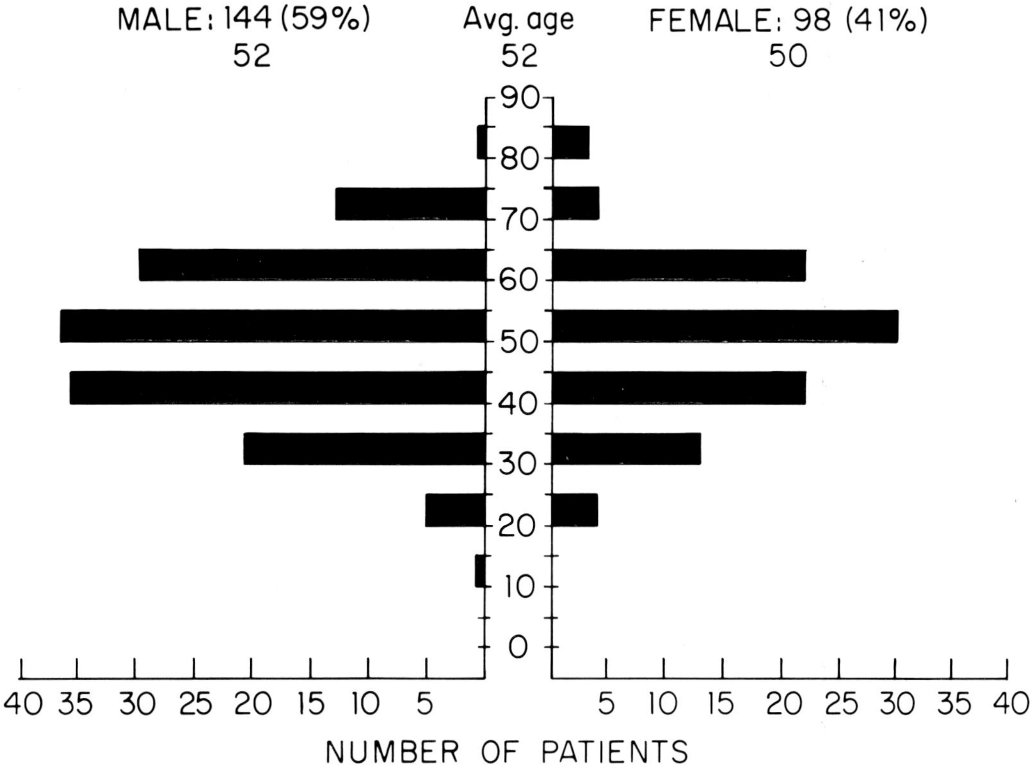

Figure 4-16. Age and sex distribution of 242 patients treated at Memorial Sloan-Kettering Cancer Center for liposarcoma of soft tissues.

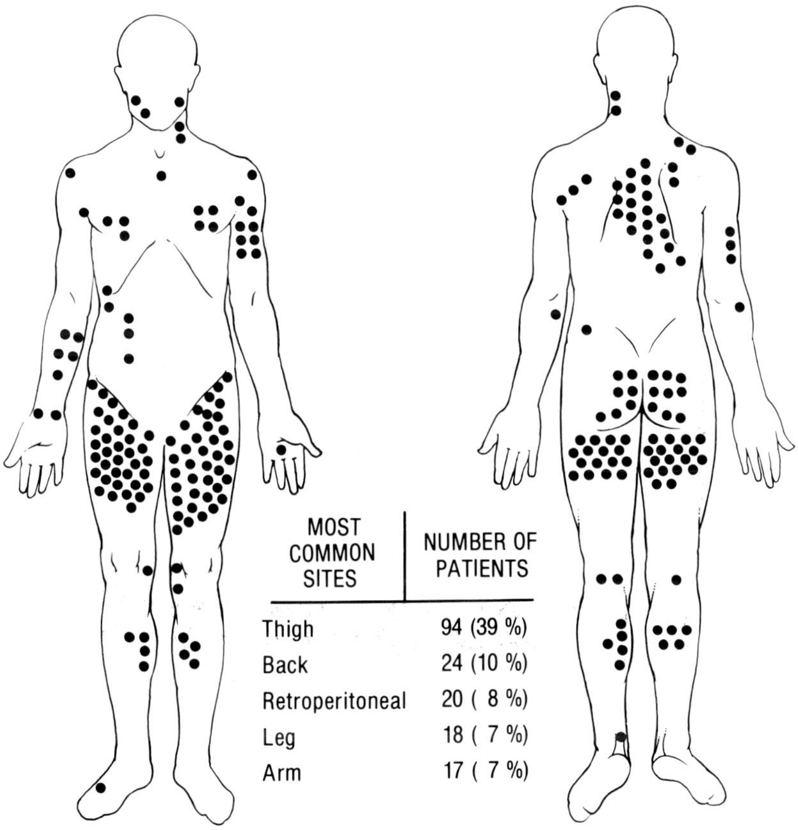

Figure 4-17. Scattergram illustrates the anatomic distribution of liposarcomas. (Retroperitoneal tumors are not included).

TABLE 4-8. *Classification and Terminology of Liposarcomas*

Robertson (1916)	1. Liposarcoma, adult type 2. Liposarcoma, embryonic type
Jaffe (1926)	1. Lipoma pseudomyxomatodes 2. Lipoblastoma 3. Liposarcoma
Ewing (1935)	1. Embryonal lipomyxosarcoma 2. Granular cell liposarcoma
Stout (1944)	1. Well-differentiated myxoid liposarcoma 2. Poorly differentiated myxoid liposarcoma 3. Round cell or adenoid liposarcoma
Enterline et al (1960)	1. Lipoma-like liposarcoma 2. Well-differentiated myxoid liposarcoma 3. Poorly differentiated myxoid liposarcoma 4. Myxoid mixed liposarcoma 5. Nonmyxoid liposarcoma
Enzinger and Winslow (1962)	1. Myxoid liposarcoma 2. Round cell liposarcoma 3. Well-differentiated liposarcoma 4. Pleomorphic liposarcoma
Reszel et al (1966)	1. Myxoid liposarcoma 2. Lipogenic liposarcoma 3. Pleomorphic liposarcoma
Kindblom et al (1975)	1. Well-differentiated liposarcoma 2. Myxoid liposarcoma 3. Well-differentiated liposarcoma with pleomorphic or round cell areas 4. Myxoid liposarcoma with round cell or pleomorphic areas 5. Round cell liposarcoma 6. Pleomorphic liposarcoma

quency the lower extremity, the upper extremity, and the retroperitoneum are the most common primary sites. Stout, in 1953, in his review of soft tissue sarcomas found that 41% of the liposarcomas occurred in the lower extremities. We also found (see Shiu et al, 1975) in our review of soft tissue sarcomas of the lower extremity that liposarcoma is the commonest (28%) malignant soft tissue tumor of the lower extremity and *has particular predilection to the inner thigh and the popliteal space.* It has been also reported that retroperitoneal liposarcomas are somewhat more common on the left than on the right.

The etiology of liposarcomas, as with all other soft tissue sarcomas, is not clear. The possibility that trauma serves occasionally as a trigger mechanism deserves attention. Ewing (1942) stated that "Since transition to fat tissue is often followed by marked proliferation of fat cells and progressive productive inflammation, it is not unreasonable to assume that under special circumstances the proliferation may take on a malignant character." Although a number of investigators—Eilber and

TABLE 4-9. ***Histologic Classification of Liposarcomas****

1. Well-differentiated liposarcoma
2. Myxoid liposarcoma
3. Lipoblastic liposarcoma
4. Fibroblastic liposarcoma
5. Pleomorphic liposarcoma

*This classification and subdivision was developed by reviewing 368 liposarcomas treated at Memorial Sloan-Kettering Cancer Center during a period of 25 years (1950–1975).

Morton (1970); Gyorkey et al (1971)—suggested that a viral agent is associated with liposarcomas there is no convincing evidence that viruses can be implicated in the etiology.

In general, liposarcomas develop in the late years of life but may appear at any time. They occur almost twice as commonly in males than in females. Enzinger and Winslow (1962) noted that patients with liposarcoma in the lower limb were significantly younger than those with retroperitoneal primary lesions. Age and sex of 242 patients treated for liposarcoma at Memorial Sloan-Kettering Cancer Center are illustrated in Fig. 4-16. The anatomic distribution of the tumors is given in Figure 4-17 and Table 4-11. Notice that our findings closely correspond to data reported in various series (Table 4-12).

Grossly, liposarcomas are firmer, less easily compressed, and more fixed to adjacent tissues than lipomas. Most of the liposarcomas are oval with the major axis of the tumor parallel to the longitudinal axis of the nearby muscle. They may appear encapsulated and may attain huge sizes, especially in the retroperitoneum, the largest being that of Hirsch and Wells (1920) which weighed 169 pounds.

Liposarcomas usually begin as a painless mass or swelling of the deep soft tissues. They grow steadily but not rapidly (Figs. 4-18, 4-19). Most of the tumors are unifocal and grossly well-defined lesions; however, multicentric and irregular tumors, especially in the retroperitoneum, have been reported. The surfaces of liposarcomas do not present definite encapsulation although they are fairly sharply demarcated. They appear distinctly different in appearance from the adipose tissue which is almost invariably brighter yellow, less lobular, and softer in consistency.

On cut section the tumor has the appearance of solid, glistening, friable, or gelatinous pale white, lobulated adipose tissue in which there are focal gray and brownish areas. The bulky part of the tumor appears partially compartmentalized by fibrous strands which appear to grow into the surrounding fibromuscular tissues. The muscle fibers often blend imperceptibly with the edge of the tumor (Fig. 4-20). In larger tumors it is not uncommon to see areas of hemorrhage and cystic degeneration (Fig. 4-21).

Grossly, liposarcomas may resemble lipomas, especially the lipoblastic types. Occasionally it is difficult to distinguish, even with the microscope, cellular lipomas and well-differentiated liposarcomas. Differentiation is further complicated by the fact that a liposarcoma may arise from a preexisting lipoma, but in general liposarcomas are considered to

TABLE 4-10. ***Terminology of Lipomas and Liposarcomas According to Cell of Origin***

LIPOMA	DOMINANT CELL	LIPOSARCOMA
Well-differentiated	Adipocyte	Well-differentiated
Myxoid	Preadipocyte	Myxoid
Lipoblastoma	Lipoblast	Lipoblastic
Fibroblastic	Prolipoblast	Fibroblastic
Pleomorphic	—	Pleomorphic

TABLE 4-11. ***The Most Common Anatomic Sites of Liposarcoma According to Sex***

NUMBER OF PATIENTS			
MALE: 144		FEMALES: 98	
Thigh	57 (40%)	Thigh	37 (38%)
Back	18 (12%)	Retroperitoneum	12 (12%)
Groin	10 (7%)	Leg	10 (10%)
Arm	9 (6%)	Arm	8 (8%)
Buttock	9 (6%)	Buttock	7 (7%)

arise de novo, not as a consequence of malignant transformation of benign lipomas (Table 4-7). It is of interest that in almost all of the 20 cases of liposarcoma arising in lipoma there is a long history of a lipoma-like lesion which suddenly, prior to the biopsy, started to increase in size.

The first authentic case of *multicentric liposarcoma* was reported by Siegmund, in 1934, in which one tumor was intermuscular in the thigh and several others were in the subcutaneous tissues throughout the body. Siegmund considered his case to be an example of systemic malignant disease of adipose tissue. Ackerman (1944) reported a case with 5 primary tumors, and Georgiades et al (1969) described a patient who developed, in sequence, 12 histologically similar liposarcomas in a period of 9 years without apparent evidence of metastasis. Enzinger and Winslow (1962) referred to 20 liposarcomas with possible multiple sites and Reszel et al (1966) included 5 proven cases in their report (Table 4-12).

It is difficult to decide clinicopathologically in any specific case whether a tumor arising in a site unusual for metastasis but common for a primary tumor is actually a metastasis or another primary tumor of the same type. As a general rule, multicentric tumors must develop in ana-

TABLE 4-12. ***Reported Series of Liposarcomas***

AUTHOR(S)	NO. OF CASES	PRIMARY SITE	MEDIAN AGE (YR.)	SEX: MALE (%)	SEX: FEMALE (%)	RECURRENCE (%)
Stout (1944)	41	Extremities, 56% Trunk, 17% Retroperitoneum, 10%	53	59	41	—
Pack and Pierson (1954)	105	Extremities, 74% Others, 13%	52	57	43	33
Enterline et al (1960)	53	Lower extremity, 36% Others, 74%	53	55	45	48
Enzinger and Winslow (1962)	103	Lower extremity, 57% Retroperitoneum, 43%	51	57	43	54
Reszel et al (1966)	222	Lower extremity, 76% Upper extremity, 24%	50	62	38	70
Spittle et al (1970)	60	Lower extremity, 68% Others, 32%	53	57	43	73
Hajdu, Erlandson, and Fortner (in press)	242	Lower extremity, 61% Upper extremity, 10% Trunk, 17% Retroperitoneum, 8% Others, 4%	52	59	41	55

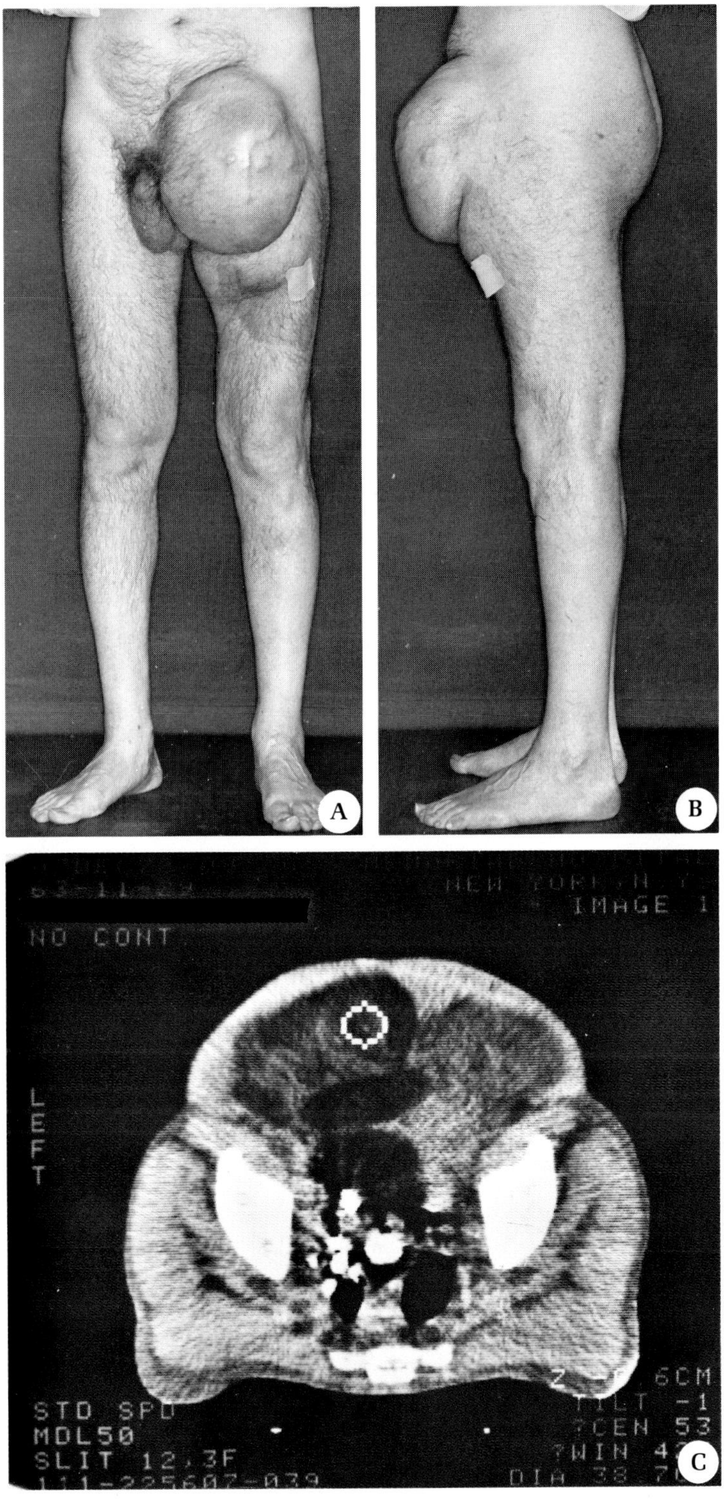

Figure 4-18. Recurrent and neglected myxoid liposarcoma of 43-year-old male. Following hemipelvectomy, the patient died with metastatic tumor.

C, The average density of a large myxoid liposarcoma is measured by computerized transaxial tomography (CT) (For comparison see Figure 2-71B. (Courtesy Dr. R. Watson, Memorial Sloan-Kettering Cancer Center).

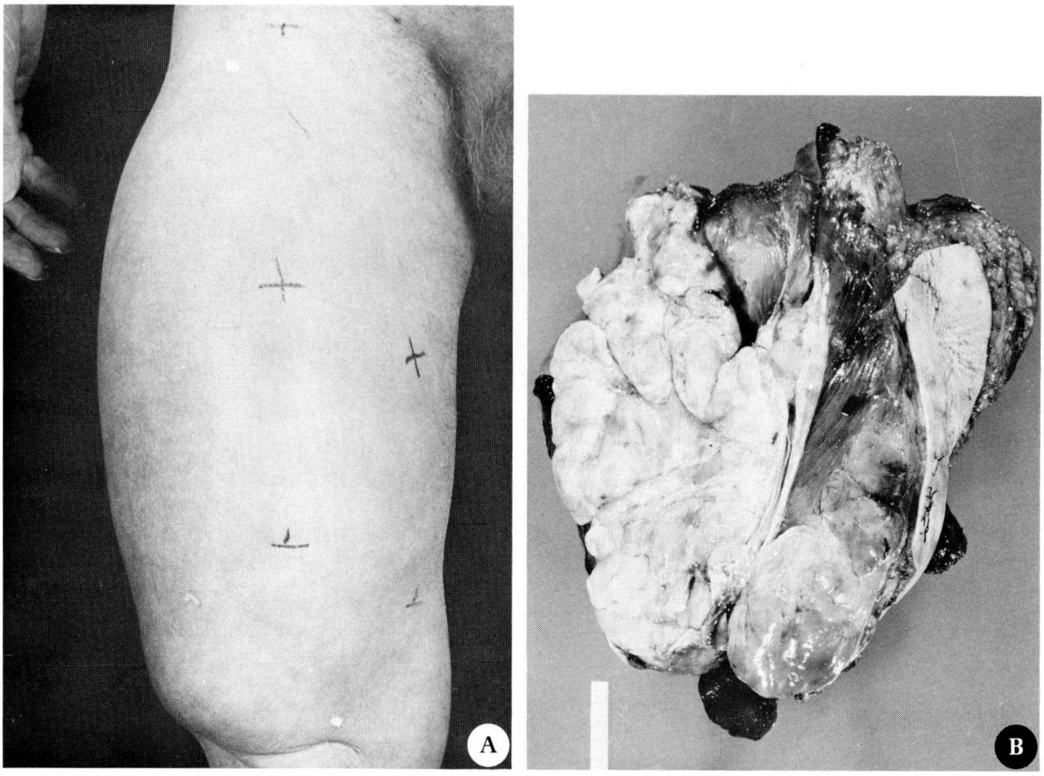

Figure 4-19. Well-differentiated liposarcoma of the thigh removed by muscle group resection. The tumor measured 30 × 15 cm. The patient died without any evidence of tumor 2 years after surgery.

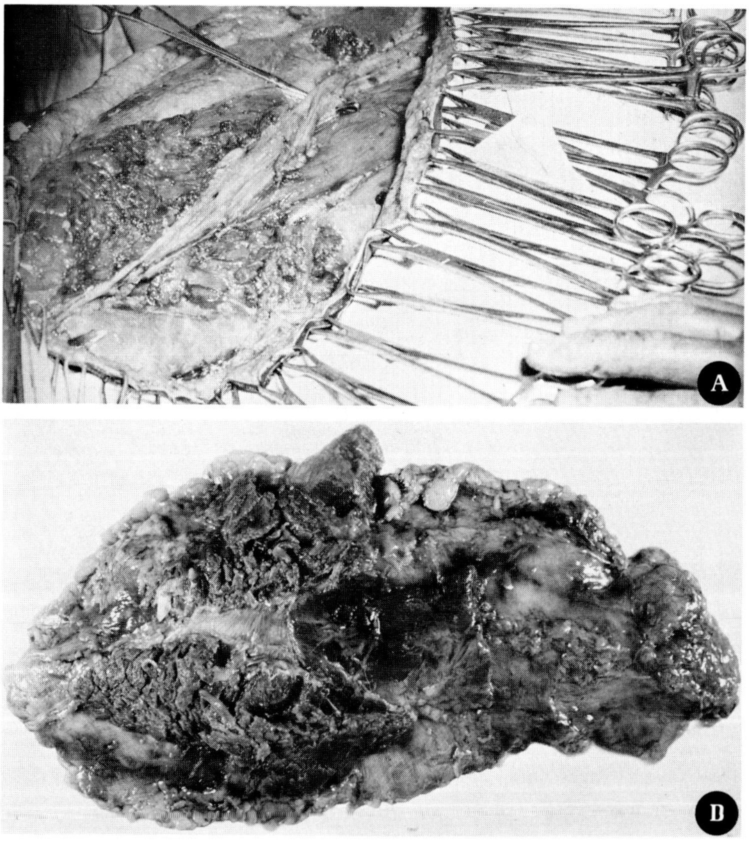

Figure 4-20. A, Surgical dissection of the back for myxoid liposarcoma.

B, Surgical specimen of fibroblastic liposarcoma after excision with clean margin. Note the intimate blending of the tumor in consistency and color with adjacent fibromuscular tissues.

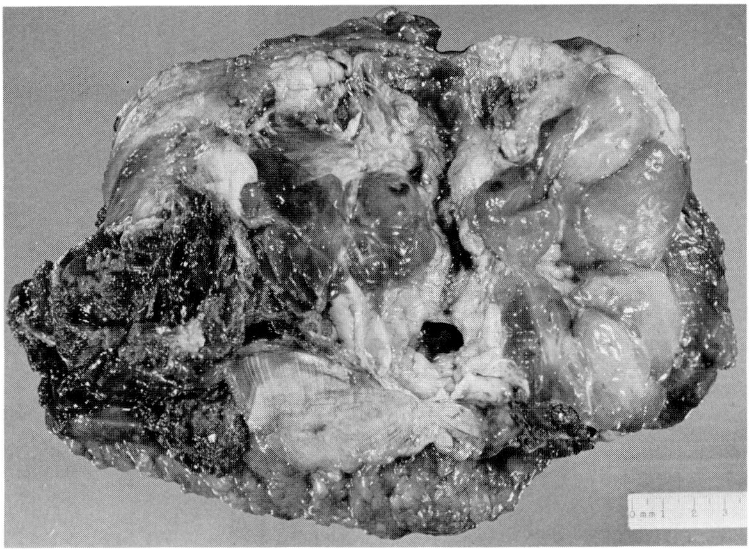

Figure 4-21. Myxoid liposarcoma consists of multiple yellowish-white tumor nodules. At the left and lower part of the specimen there are a portion of skeletal muscle, fascial aponeurotic tissue, and benign fat.

tomic sites where liposarcomas usually develop and there must be no tumors in sites where liposarcomas usually metastasize and a reasonably long follow-up without evidence of disseminated metastatic spread of the tumor. In the series of liposarcomas I studied only 2 cases could be accepted as multicentric primary tumors.

Liposarcomas in unusual sites such as the *breast* have been reported (McGregor, 1960). Only one of the 242 liposarcomas I studied arose in the breast.

Primary *intraosseous liposarcomas* are scarce. The only recorded cases are the ones reported by Stewart (1931) and Goldman (1964).

The *gastrointestinal tract* is rarely the site of liposarcoma. However, well-documented cases have been reported by Menne and Birge (1936), Abrams and Turberville (1941), and Hawkins and Terrell (1965).

Froug (1941) reported a case of liposarcoma arising in the *kidney* and reviewed the literature. One of the liposarcomas reviewed at Memorial Sloan-Kettering Cancer Center was a primary tumor of the *spermatic cord*.

Liposarcomas of the *head and neck* regions were reviewed by Saunders et al (1979). They added 4 cases of the 25 previously reported cases and concluded that less than 50% of patients were alive without evidence of disease and that the prognosis corresponds to the cell type of the tumor.

Radiologic diagnosis of liposarcomas may be feasible, since liposarcomas may contain sufficient amounts of fat to be radiotranslucent. Due to the high vascularity of liposarcomas, especially the myxoid variants, angiographic studies may help to establish the diagnosis (Lester et al, 1971).

Liposarcomas are notorious for their great variety of microscopic features and lack of homogeneity. Traditionally liposarcomas have been classified as predominantly well-differentiated, predominantly myxoid, predominantly round-cell, and predominantly pleomorphic types. Since liposarcomas seldom appear in pure forms, some writers (Akerman, 1944; Evans, 1968; Das Gupta, 1970) questioned the value of subclassification. Others, on the other hand, found the histologic differences between subtypes so considerable that they questioned whether liposarcoma should be considered as a single entity (Enzinger and Winslow, 1962) (Fig. 4-22).

The general rule of thumb in histologic

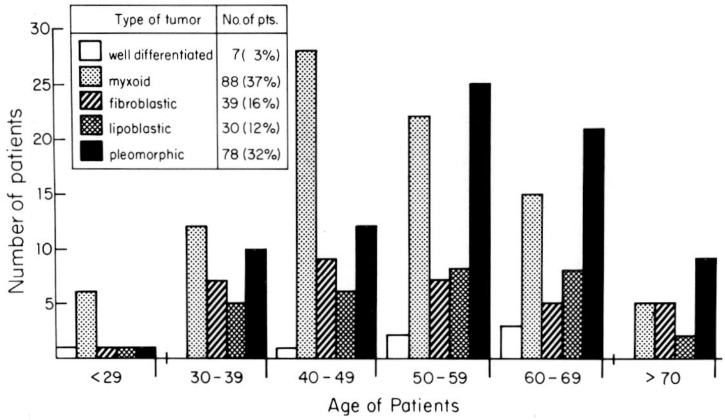

Figure 4-22. Histologic types of liposarcomas encountered in a series of 242 cases, according to age of the patients. Note that the majority of pleomorphic liposarcomas occur about two decades later than myxoid liposarcomas.

classification of liposarcomas is that *the proportion of intracytoplasmic fat globules diminishes and the pleomorphism of the tumor cells, as well as the number of abnormal mitoses, increases with the grade of malignancy.* The scheme of classification presented here (Fig. 4-15; Table 4-9) follows, in general, the classification employed by others; however, there are some differences (Table 4-8). The major differences are (1) introduction of a subtype called fibroblastic liposarcoma, (2) classification of the so-called round cell tumor as a lipoblastic liposarcoma, and (3) the emphasis that transitional forms between any two or more tumors of each of the five forms can exist (Figs. 4-23 color, 4-24, 4-25; Tables 4-13, 4-14).

According to our experience, the tumor cells derived from liposarcomas in tissue

TABLE 4-13. ***Subclassification of Liposarcomas***

	WELL-DIFFERENTIATED	MYXOID	FIBROBLASTIC	LIPOBLASTIC	PLEOMORPHIC
Mature fat cells (adipocytes)	+++	+	+−	−	+
Vacuolated fat cells (pre-adipocytes)	++	+++	+	+−	+
Lipoblasts	+−	+	++	+++	+−
Fibroblast-like cells (prolipoblasts)	+−	+−	+++	+	+
Foam cells	+	+	+	+	+−
Tumor giant cells	+−	+−	+	+	+++
Multinucleated tumor cells	+−	−	+−	+−	+++
Myxoid stroma	+	+++	+−	+−	+−
Fibrous stroma	+	+−	+++	+	+−
Vascular stroma	+−	+++	++	+++	+
Mitotic activity	−	+	++	+++	+++
Fat stain	++	++	+	+	++
PAS stain	+−	+−	++	+++	++

+++ = most common; ++ = common; + = uncommon; +− = may be present; − = absent.

TABLE 4-14. *Histologic Type and Anatomic Site of Liposarcomas*

HISTOLOGIC TYPE	TOTAL NO. OF PATIENTS	NO. OF PATIENTS			
		HEAD AND NECK	TRUNK	RETROPERITONEUM	EXTREMITIES
Well-differentiated	7	1	—	1	5
Myxoid	86*	3	12	8	63
Fibroblastic	39	1	8	2	28
Lipoblastic	29†	2	5	3	19
Pleomorphic	78	—	15	6	57
	239	7	40	20	172

*2 pelvic primary tumors are not included.
†1 primary tumor of the spermatic cord is omitted.

culture (Fig. 4-26) in cytologic preparations (Fig. 4-25), and nude mice (Figs. 4-27, 4-30) are different from those of fibrosarcoma or fibrous histiocytoma (Hajdu and Hajdu, 1976; Sethi et al, 1977; Hajdu, Lemos, et al, 1979). Most investigators who studied liposarcomas with the electron microscope distinguished three cell types which correspond to light microscopic observations: stellate cells, fibroblast-like spindle cells, and round cells (Scarpelli and Greider, 1962; Morton et al, 1969; Kalderon and Fethiere, 1973; Kindblom and Save-Soderbergh, 1979; Reddick et al, 1979).

Well-differentiated Liposarcoma. Although believed to be a nonmetastasizing type of tumor, a well-differentiated liposarcoma may infiltrate locally and recur if not adequately removed. The difficulty in distinguishing microscopically between lipomas and well-differentiated liposarcomas has been pointed out by numerous authors. Enzinger and Winslow (1962) proposed the subclassification of well-differentiated liposarcomas for the "lipoma-like" and the "sclerosing" forms of liposarcomas. These forms basically correspond to the well-differentiated adipocytic and well-differentiated lipoblastic liposarcomas according to the scheme presented in Figure 4-15 and Table 4-9. If a sufficient number of sections are available for microscopic examination, the diagnosis presents no difficulty; however, in a limited biopsy the diagnosis of well-differentiated liposarcoma is difficult.

The well-differentiated adipocytic liposarcomas are composed of globoid mature adipocytes not too different from those commonly seen in simple lipomas and myxoid liposarcomas (see Tables 4-10 and 4-13). However, the tumor cells show from slight to moderate pleomorphism which is most pronounced in the nuclei. The peculiar notched nucleus, a common finding in most of the other forms of liposarcomas, as well as in the well-differentiated ones, was first described by Unna in 1895 and referred to as Unna's Lochkern. According to Plaut (1957), this nuclear characteristic may be used for differentiating malignant neoplastic fat cells from the non-malignant forms. Clusters of multivacuolated preadipocytes and granular or stellate lipoblasts are interspaced between well-differentiated globoid adipocytes. The number of elongated fibroblast-like prolipoblasts is limited, but in the fibrous forms they may be numerous (Fig. 4-28).

The heaviest concentration of non-vacuolated cells is usually seen around capillary vessels, nerves, and the edge of the tumor. The fibrillar cytoplasmic processes of the spindle cells may form irregular reticular bundles running multidirectionally like an ink patch. The fibrillar processes, which stain positive with retic-

Figure 4-23. A, Well-differentiated liposarcoma is a low-grade malignant neoplasm characterized by the mixture of monovesicular benign adipocytes and immature multivesicular preadipocytes and granular lipoblasts. The presence of the latter two cell types warrants its classification as a malignant neoplasm.

In the background of these mixed elements which supply the link between the distinctly lobular arrangement there is a rich capillary network. Note the absence of inflammatory cells and histiocytic foam cells (H & E, ×140).

B, Myxoid liposarcoma is a low-grade malignant neoplasm. This neoplasm is composed of small stellate and multivesicular preadipocytes with pyknotic nuclei and irregular cytoplasm ending in fine reticular filaments. The tumor cells nest in a richly myxoid stroma which stains positive with alcian blue and are arranged about branching capillary vessels.

The rich chain-link or chicken-wire-like network of capillary vessels and the intimate relation between tumor cells and capillary vessels suggest perhaps more than an interesting morphologic pattern. For example, on the basis of microscopic pattern, it would not be wrong to call these myxoid neoplasms "myxoid pericytomas"; however, the stellate cells are also rich in intracytoplasmic lipids which warrants classification of the neoplasms as myxoid liposarcoma (H & E, ×140).

C, Lipoblastic liposarcoma (round cell liposarcoma) is a high-grade and fully malignant neoplasm. It is composed of fairly uniform round or slightly oval mononuclear lipoblasts. The tumor cells are rich in intracytoplasmic glycogen and contain fat vacuoles. The cytoplasmic membrane is well outlined and follows the contour of the nuclei.

The tumor cells are adherent and packed between a network of capillary vessels (H & E, ×350).

D, Fibroblastic liposarcoma is a high-grade, malignant neoplasm. It is composed of uniform, slender spindle cells containing pyknotic solitary nuclei and fibrillar or granular cytoplasms. The cytoplasm, which is long and extends into branching, often tangled processes, stains positive with reticulum stain.

The tumor cells are about branching capillary vessels and follow in their position the arranged chicken-wire pattern of the capillary vessels. The capillary network of fibroblastic liposarcomas is identical with that of myxoid liposarcomas. The tumor cells, prolipoblasts, in individual cell morphology and arrangement show striking resemblance to the storiform pattern often seen in fibroblastic fibrous histiocytomas (see Chapter 2) and schwannomas (see Chapter 8) (H & E, ×140).

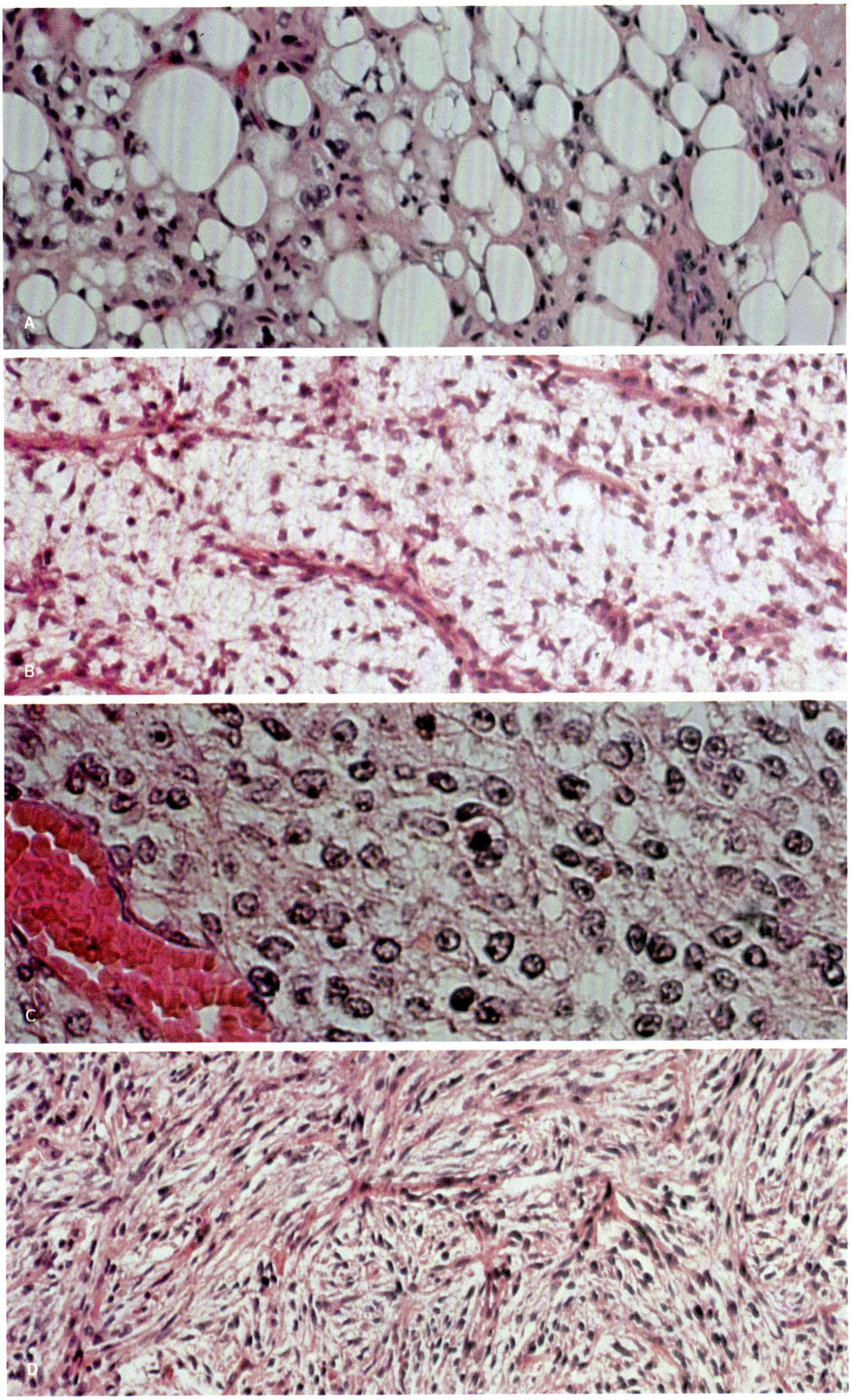

Figure 4-23.

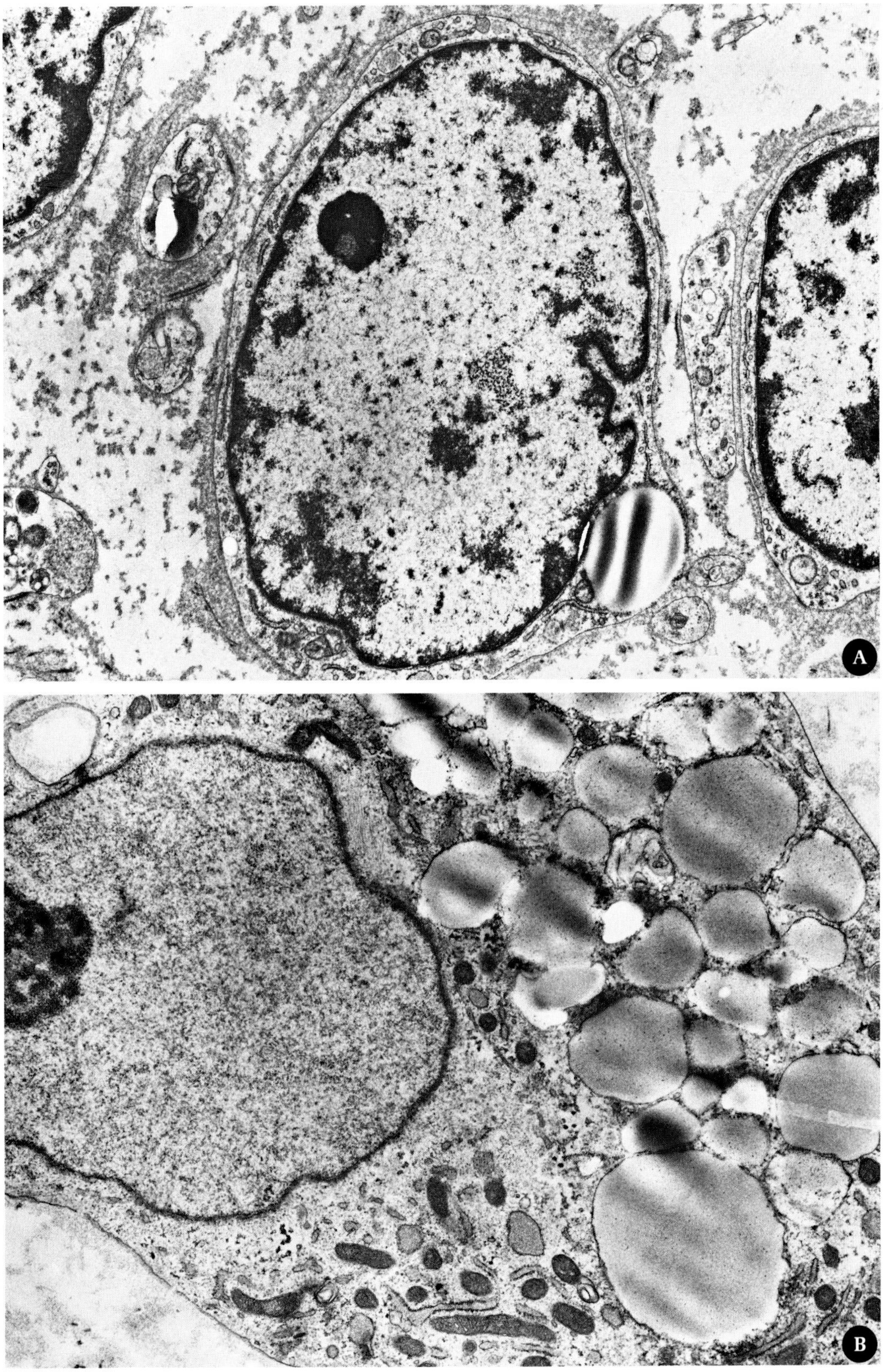

Figure 4-24. A, Ultrastructure of lipoblastic liposarcoma. A neoplastic lipoblast contains one lipid droplet in a narrow cytoplasm. Note the large oval nucleus and the myxoid stroma (×9,200) (also see Figures 4-1 and 4-24).

B, Myxoid liposarcoma. Portion of a neoplastic preadipocyte. There are numerous lipid droplets in the cytoplasm (×12,000).

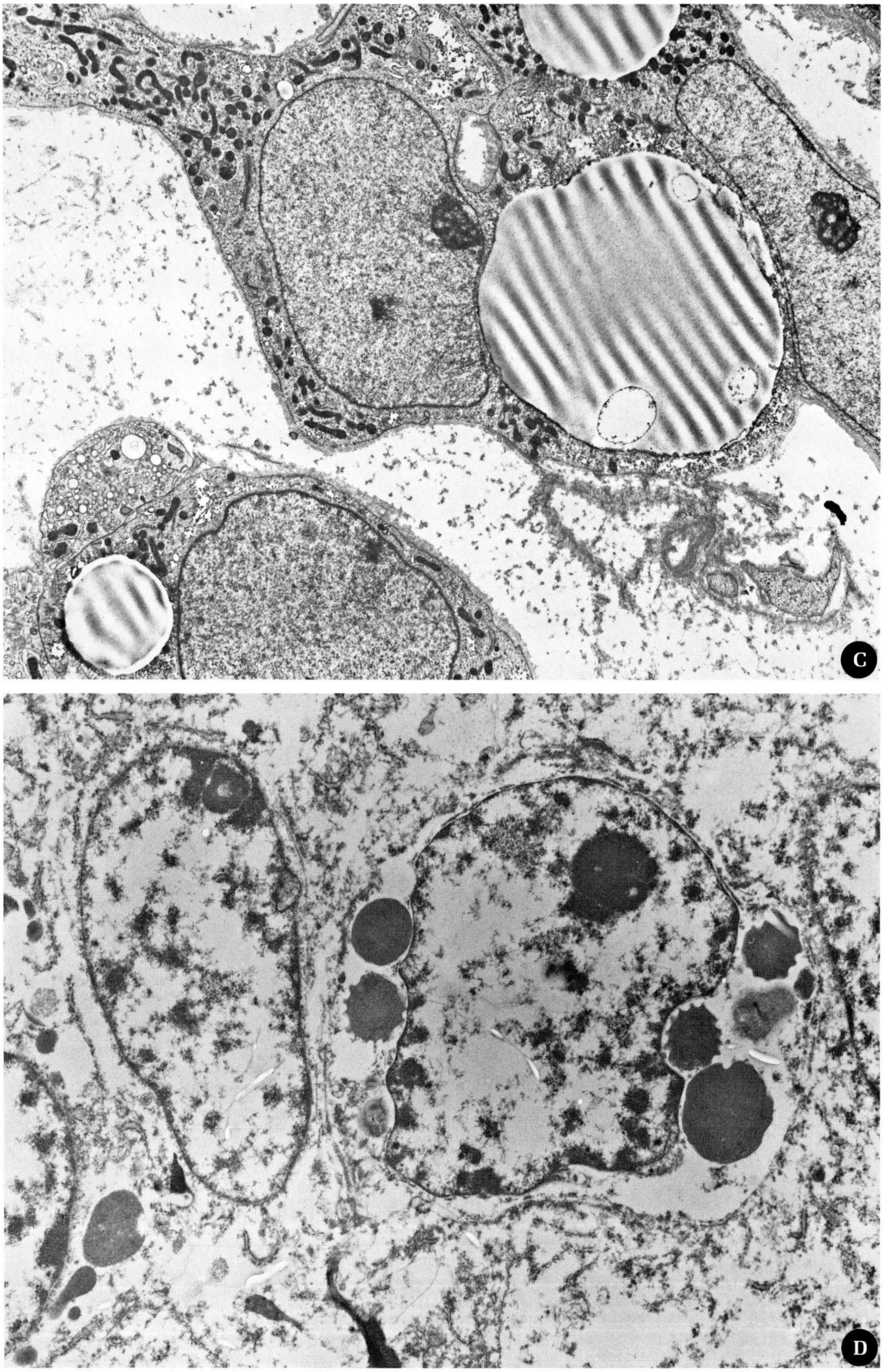

Figure 4-24 (cont.). C, Adipocytes of a well-differentiated liposarcoma. Note the large lipid droplets, glycogen granules, and electron-dense mitochondria (×4,800).

D, Pleomorphic liposarcoma. This material was processed for electron microscopy from paraffin-embedded tissue. Note the electron-dense lipid-like inclusions, some of which look crenated, in the cytoplasm of neoplastic cells (×8,000). (See also Appendix.)

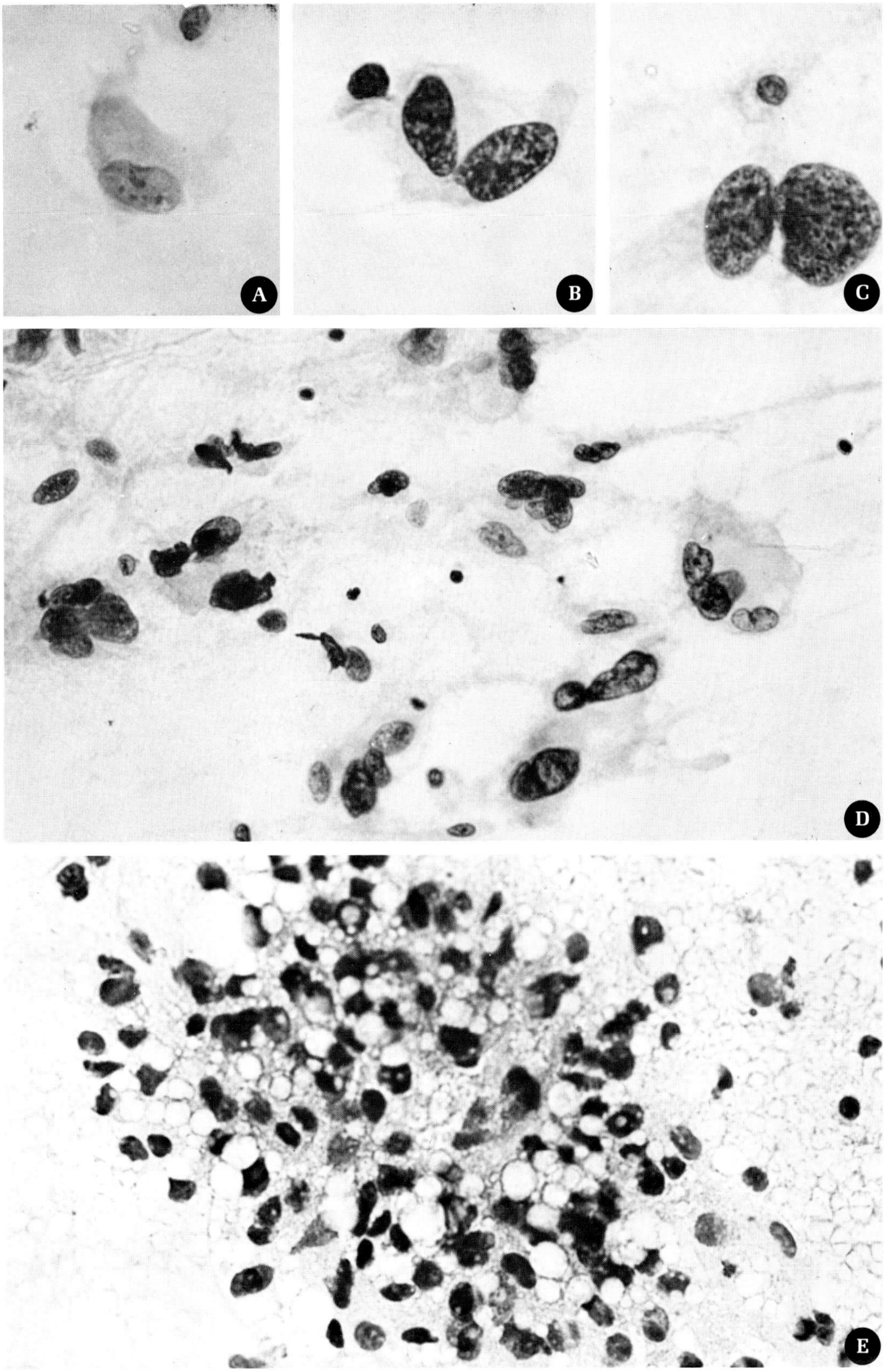

Figure 4-25. Exfoliated cells of liposarcoma in sputum **(A)** and pleural effusion **(B, C).** The oval-shaped prominent nuclei are adherent to each other and surrounded by transparent cytoplasm (Pap stain, ×570).

D, Imprint smear of pleomorphic liposarcoma. Note the variation of size and shape of nuclei as well as cytoplasm. (H & E, ×450).

E, Lipoblastic liposarcoma. Section of cell block prepared from aspiration specimen. Granular cytoplasmic and vacuolated neoplastic fat cells in a cohesive cluster (H & E, ×350). (From Hajdu, S. I., and Hajdu, E. O.: Cytopathology of Sarcomas. Philadelphia, W. B. Saunders Co., 1976).

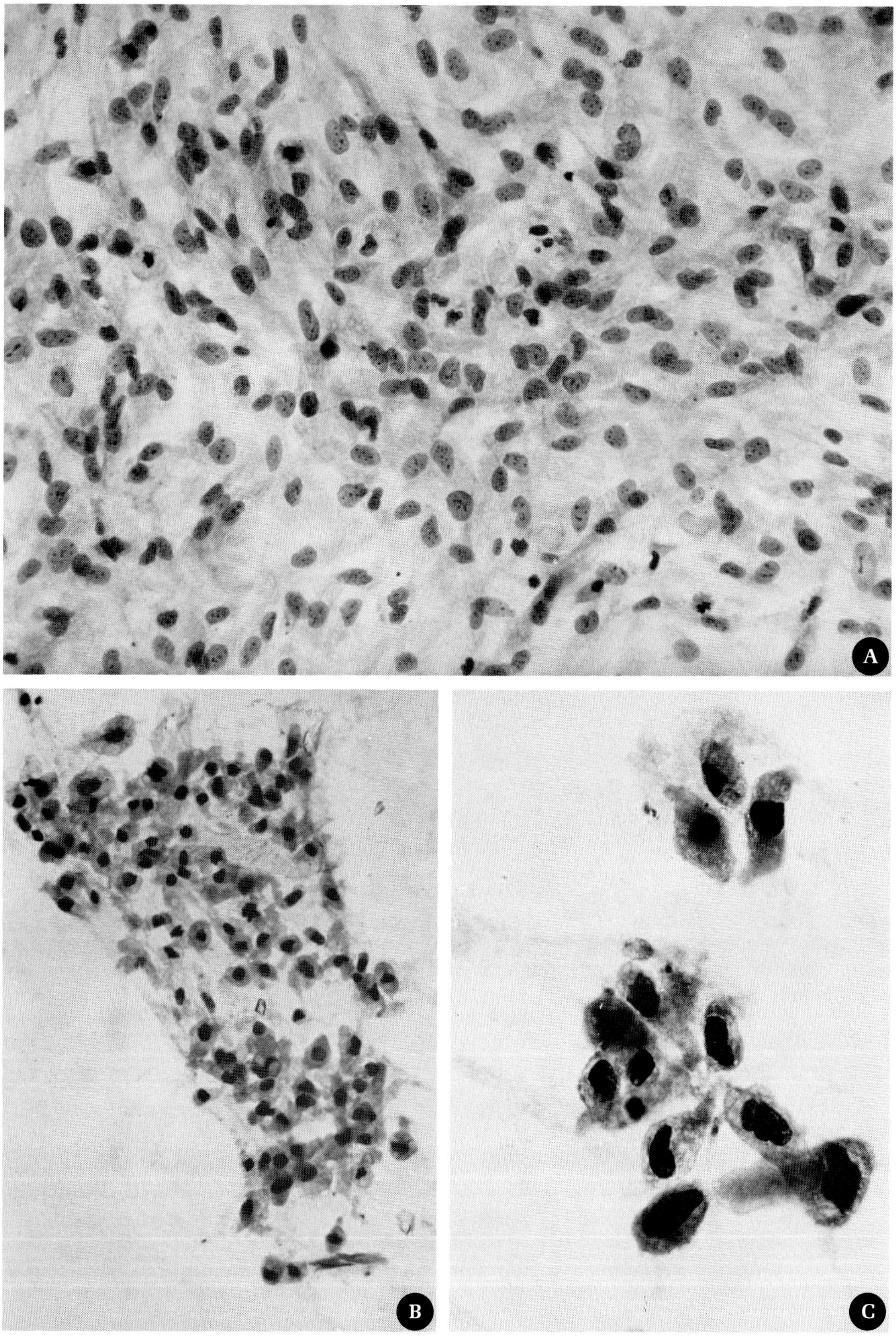

Figure 4-26. Liposarcoma in tissue culture. Monolayer tissue culture of a fibroblastic and lipoblastic liposarcoma (**A,** Pap stain, ×140).

B, C, Smear of trypsinized monolayer culture of the tumor illustrated in **A.** The tumor cells are clusters forming mostly granular cytoplasmic oval or round cells (**B,** Pap stain, ×140; **C,** Pap stain, ×570).

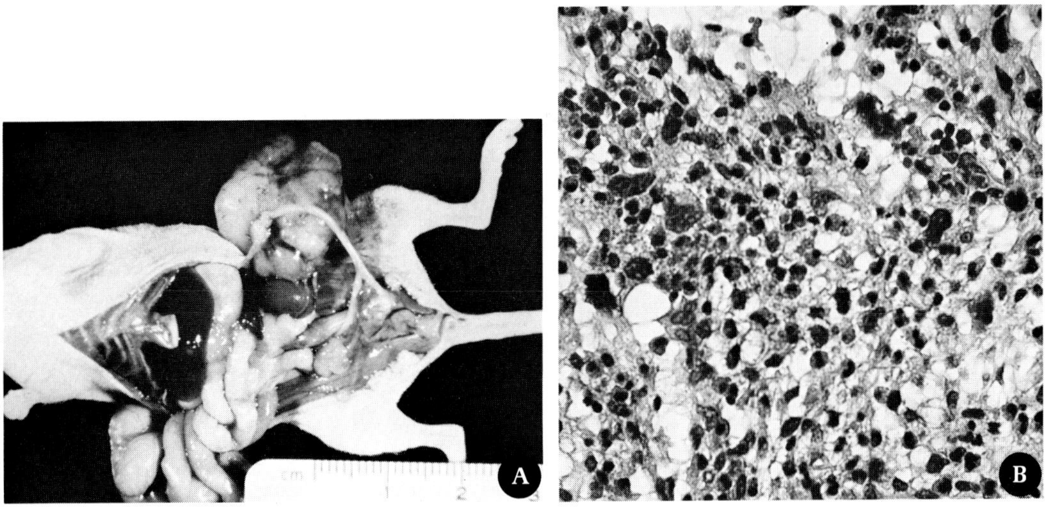

Figure 4-27. Cell suspension of lipoblastic liposarcoma of Figure 4-39, injected into the peritoneal cavity of nude mouse. Multiple tumor nodules appeared and reached the size seen in **A** in 3 weeks.

B, Microscopic appearance of one of the tumor nodules excised from the nude mouse (H & E, ×350). (See and compare with Figure 4-39.)

ulum stain (collagen type III), are often difficult to discern, or they are completely absent, around large uniglobular adipocytes. It seems as the fat cell expands the extracellular fibrillar processes undergo attenuation. Mitotic figures are exceedingly rare and the vascularity is moderate (Fig. 4-29).

The proportion of comingling of vacuolated neoplastic fat cells, preadipocytes and adipocytes, and fibrillar prolipoblasts and roundish lipoblasts will decide whether the tumor is predominantly adipocytic or myxoid, lipoblastic, or fibroblastic (Table 4-10).

In a series of 242 liposarcomas studied by us (Hajdu, Erlandson, and Fortner, 1979) there were 7 well-differentiated liposarcomas. Two of these were fibrous histologically, and both patients died with metastatic tumors 7 and 13 years, respectively, after initial diagnosis. The other 5 patients are alive without apparent evidence of the disease 3, 4, 7, 20, and 30 years, respectively, following initial diagnosis (see Table 4-14). The two tumors which caused the death of the patients were primary lesions in the retroperitoneum and the thigh. The primary sites of the others were the groin, leg, thigh, face, and buttock.

Myxoid Liposarcomas. Like the well-differentiated forms, myxoid liposarcomas can be subdivided on the basis of the proportion of lipoblastic and adipocytic elements (Figs. 4-1, 4-15). The vascularity of myxoid liposarcomas is pronounced. The capillary vessels may run in an irregular fashion, so-called chicken track form. An irregular network of fine reticular fibers may run along the vessels. Almost invariably a number of pyknotic tumor cells are trapped among the fibrillar processes. Occasionally round or stellate granular or finely vacuolated cells may dominate certain areas. Areas where these cells are found may be completely devoid of mucoid stroma.

Ewing (1935) believed that the so-called myxosarcomas arise from fat cells and there are transitional forms between myxosarcomas and bona fide liposarcomas. He said that "the process of the embryonal growth of fat tissue begins with the proliferation of capillaries and arterioles, the adventitial or endothelial cells of which, instead of going on to produce fat, yield chiefly mucus and occasionally embryonal fat tissue." He noted that "the structure of myxoliposarcoma, with its fine capillary blood vessels suggests the source of the high radiosensi-

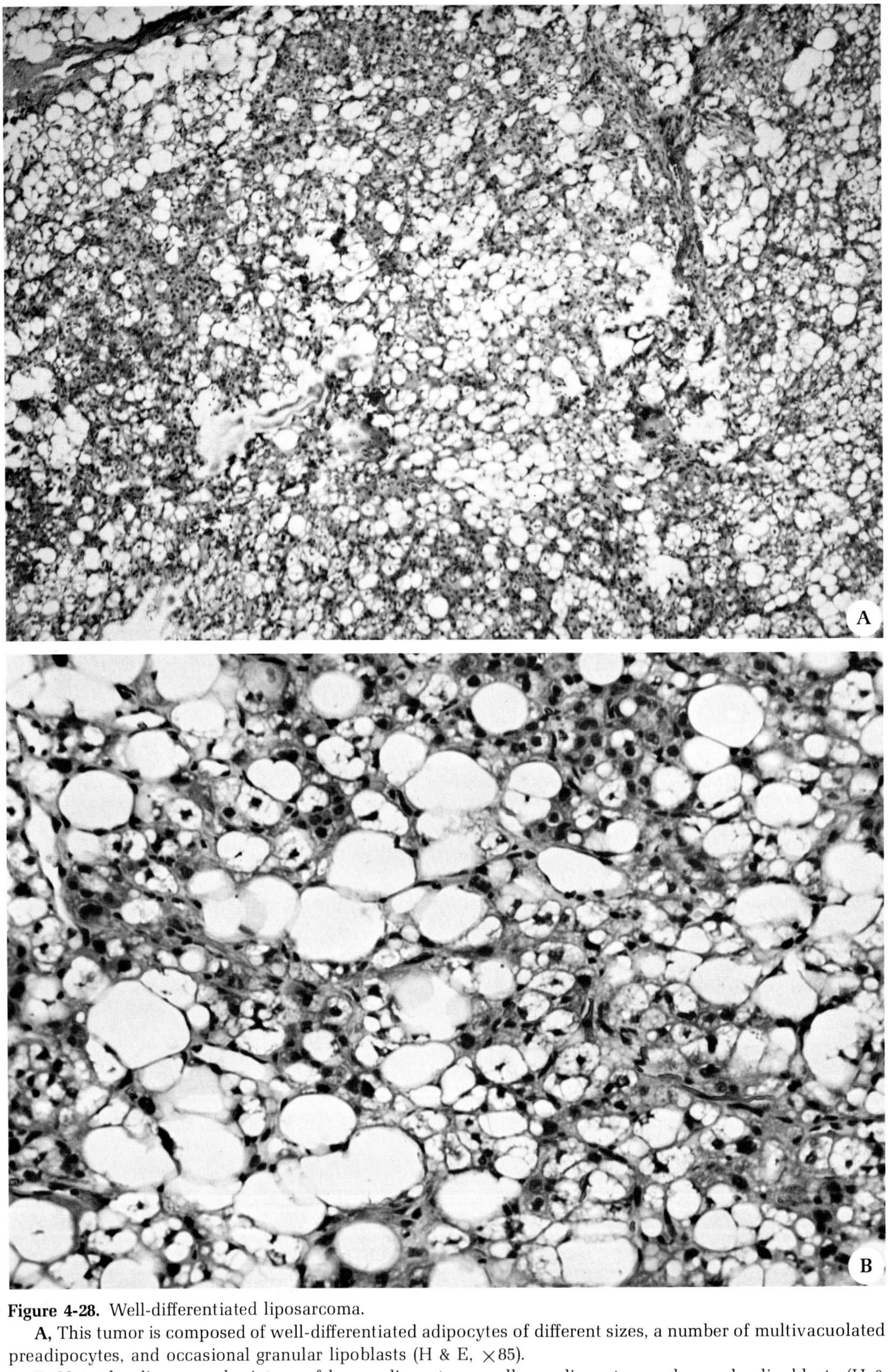

Figure 4-28. Well-differentiated liposarcoma.

A, This tumor is composed of well-differentiated adipocytes of different sizes, a number of multivacuolated preadipocytes, and occasional granular lipoblasts (H & E, ×85).

B, Note the disarranged mixture of large adipocytes, small preadipocytes, and granular lipoblasts (H & E, ×140).

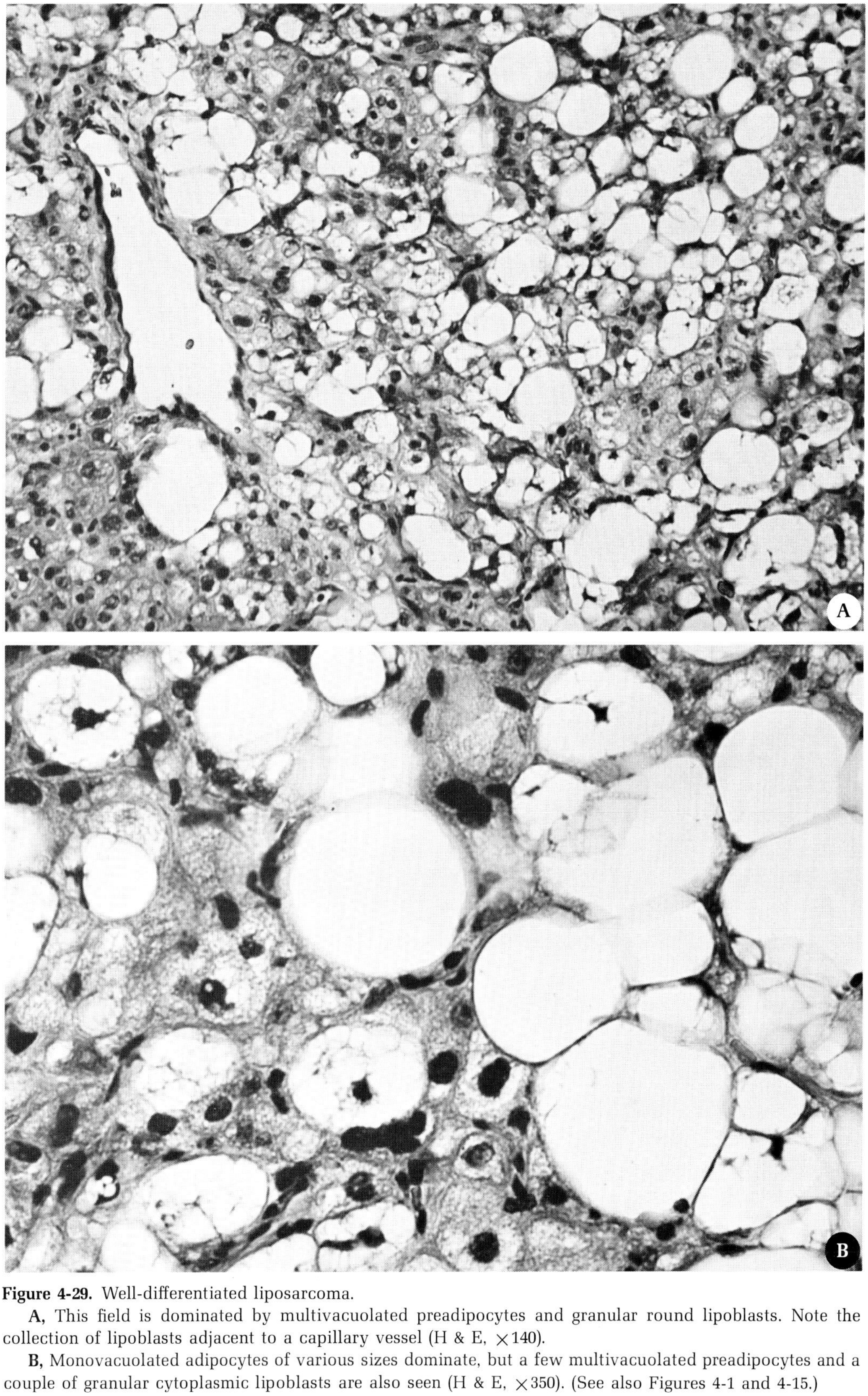

Figure 4-29. Well-differentiated liposarcoma.

A, This field is dominated by multivacuolated preadipocytes and granular round lipoblasts. Note the collection of lipoblasts adjacent to a capillary vessel (H & E, ×140).

B, Monovacuolated adipocytes of various sizes dominate, but a few multivacuolated preadipocytes and a couple of granular cytoplasmic lipoblasts are also seen (H & E, ×350). (See also Figures 4-1 and 4-15.)

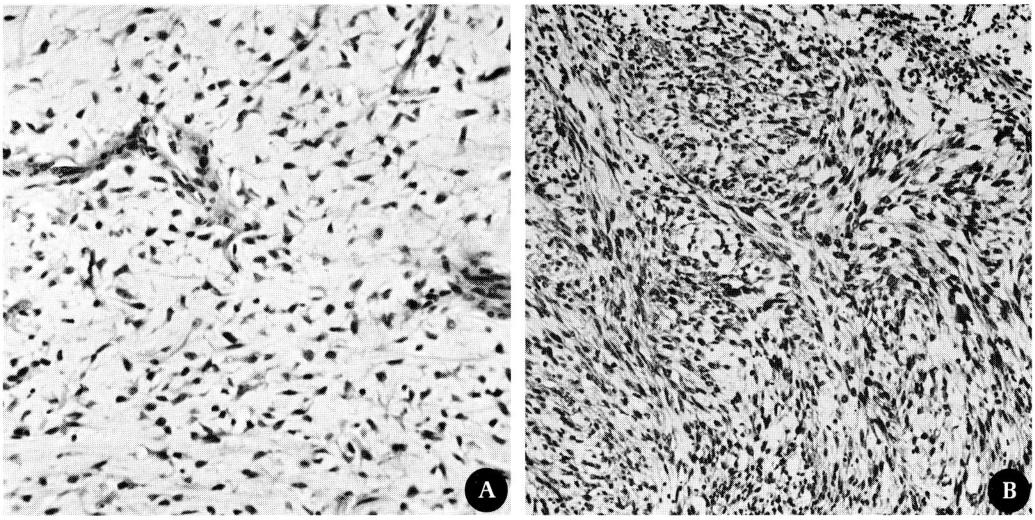

Figure 4-30. **A,** Myxoid liposarcoma from the patient's biopsy specimen injected into nude mouse (H & E, ×140). **B,** Malignant tumor excised from the nude mouse 5 weeks after the injection looks more fibroblastic than myxoid. (See Hajdu and Fogh, 1978.)

tivity which has sometimes been exhibited by this tumor."

Myxosarcomas were the subject of several reports, the first being by Virchow, in 1863. He did not know the exact origin of these tumors but noted the frequent presence of fat cells in the tumor which he regarded as a form of fatty degeneration. He also noticed that these so-called myxosarcomas were found most commonly in regions where fat tissue is abundant. Some of the later authors confused myxosarcomas with fibrosarcoma (Hellmann, 1888) due to the presence of fibroblast-like cells, fibrillar collagen-like material, and scarcity of vacuolated fat cells.

Without doubt, *most of the reported so-called myxosarcomas are actually myxoid liposarcomas,* and certain numbers perhaps are myxoid variants of fibrous histiocytomas or benign myxomas (see Chapter 2 and Table 4-15). The dominant cells in myxoid liposarcoma are stellate or oval mononuclear fat cells. In the cytoplasm there is a single eccentric nucleus and small vacuoles surrounded by scanty eosinophilic cytoplasm. Some of

TABLE 4-15. ***Special Stains in Differential Diagnosis***

	MYXOMA	LIPOID TUMORS	TENDOSYNOVIAL TUMORS	CHONDROID TUMORS	EPITHELIAL TUMORS
Intracytoplasmic PAS-positive granules	+	+	+	+	+
Intracytoplasmic PAS-positive granules after diastase digestion	−	−	−	−	+
Stroma with Alcian blue	+	+	+	+	−+
Stroma with Alcian blue after hyalurinodase digestion	−	−	−+	+	−

these cells may assume a typical signet-ring form (adipocyte) because of the intracytoplasmic vacuole. There are no appreciable numbers of mitotic figures, and the number of pleomorphic tumor cells is limited. However, small nests of lipoblasts are not uncommon, especially near blood vessels and interlobular fibrous septae (Figs. 4-31, 4-32). If the proportion of stellate or oval cells decreases in favor of fusiform fibrillar cells (prolipoblasts), the tumor should be classified as fibroblastic liposarcoma.

The myxoid stroma of myxoid liposarcoma is rich in acid mucopolysaccharides. This substance is stainable with Alcian blue and PAS and is digested by hyaluronidase and diastase (Table 4-15).

The two types of cells characteristic of myxoid liposarcoma were seen by Kalderon and Fethiere (1973) with the electron microscope. The *fibroblast-like cells,* (prolipoblasts) contain bundles of intracytoplasmic fibrils and clusters of mitochondria and numerous pinocytic vesicles; the other cells *preadipocytes* and *adipocytes,* contain ribosome-studded vacuoles, fat droplets, and eosinophilic lipoprotein granules (Figs. 4-1, 4-15, 4-24).

Myxoid liposarcomas are the most common type of liposarcomas occurring in the thigh, groin, trunk, and popliteal areas (Table 4-14). Enterline (1960) found that more myxoid than non-myxoid liposarcomas were encountered in young people. Our experience with these lesions shows it is important to distinguish myxoid liposarcomas from the *fibroblastic* and *lipoblastic* forms. Myxoid liposarcomas are far more common and less malignant neoplasms than these other forms (Figs. 4-33, 4-34, 4-35; and see Figs. 4-40, 4-42, 4-45).

On the average, myxoid liposarcomas appear in patients 15 or 20 years younger than the patients with lipoblastic and pleomorphic liposarcomas (Fig. 4-22). Eight of the 88 myxoid liposarcomas occurred in the retroperitoneum and 4 of the 8 patients are alive without evidence of the disease. Although all forms have a tendency to recur after excision, the rate of recurrence of the myxoid liposarcoma is 50%, lower than that of the more aggressive forms (Table 4-16). Almost all liposarcomas that originated in pre-existing lipomas were histologically the myxoid type (Table 4-7).

Fibroblastic Liposarcoma. This form of liposarcoma is predominantly composed of slender, fibroblast-like cells, prolipoblasts (see Figs. 4-1 and 4-15). The tumor cells follow the paths of the ubiquitous and branching capillary vessels. The vascular pattern of fibroblastic liposarcomas is strikingly similar to the cross-link or chicken wire-like arrangement of capillary vessels in myxoid liposarcomas. In many of the fibroblastic liposarcomas signet-ring type or stellate preadipocytes and granular cytoplasmic lipoblasts are admixed with elongated glycogen and fat-containing prolipoblasts (Fig. 4-36). Occasionally, avascular areas may show storiform arrangement of prolipoblasts and may resemble fibroblastic fibrous histiocytoma and non-collagenous schwannoma (Table 4-13). The term *fibroblastic liposarcoma* should be used only when the fibroblast-like prolipoblasts are the dominant elements of the tumor (Fig. 4-37).

Age, sex, and site of fibroblastic liposarcomas correspond to those of myxoid liposarcomas. However, the tendency of these neoplasms to recur is higher (62%), and they also carry a much higher mortality (60%) than myxoid liposarcomas (Table 4-18 and see Figs. 4-34, 4-44, and 4-45).

The intimate relationship between the tumor cells and the rich capillary network in these tumors, as in the myxoid and

TABLE 4-16. ***Retroperitoneal Liposarcoma***

Well-differentiated liposarcoma	1/1
Myxoid liposarcoma	4/8
Fibroblastic liposarcoma	2/2
Lipoblastic liposarcoma	3/3
Pleomorphic liposarcoma	5/6
	15/20

Numerator = number of patients dead.
Denominator = total number of patients.

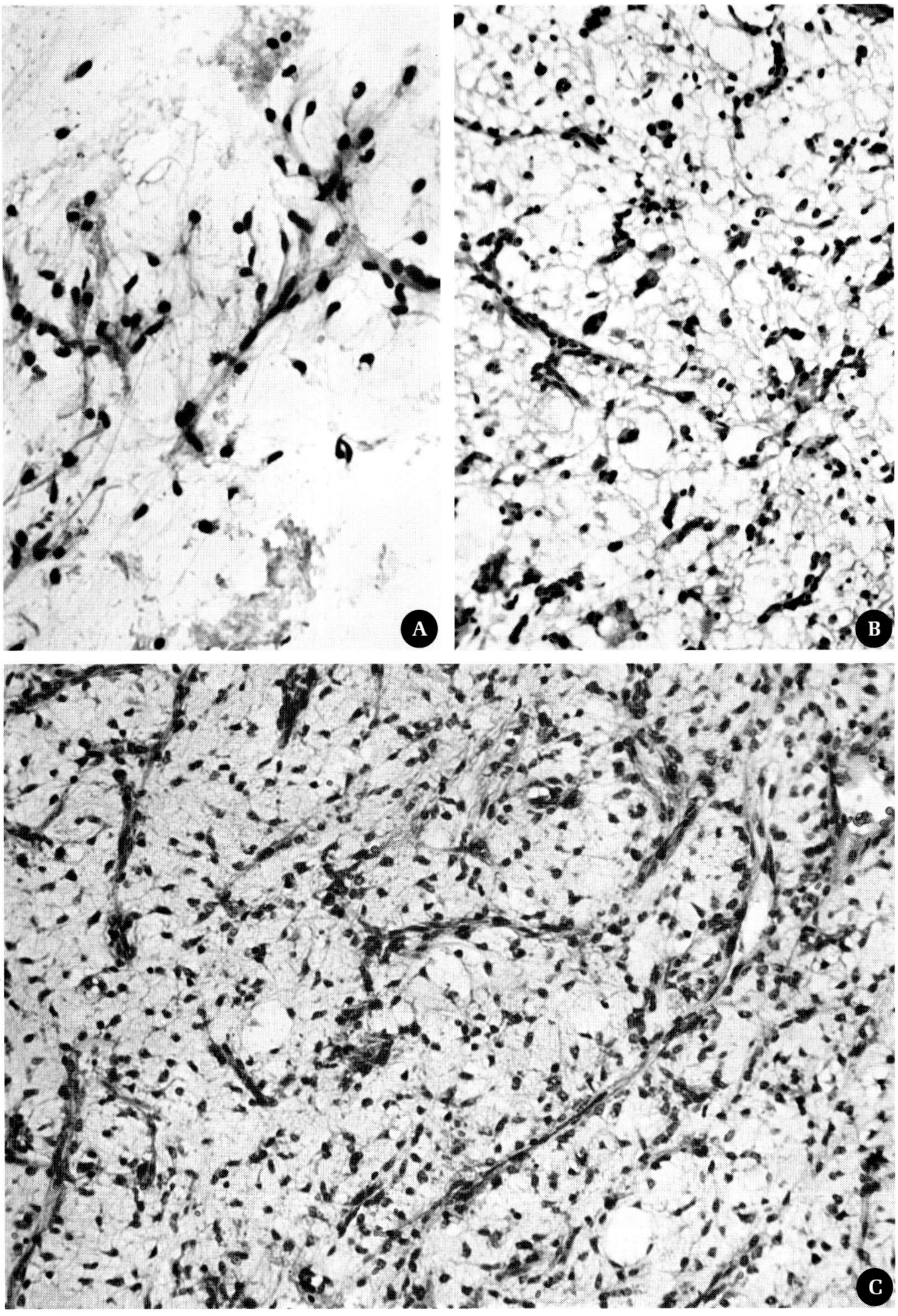

Figure 4-31. Myxoid liposarcoma.

A, Percutaneous aspiration smear prepared from an inguinal myxoid liposarcoma. The slender reticular and myxoid cells are arranged about capillary vessels (H & E, ×140).

B, C, Tissue sections of myxoid liposarcoma showing a monomorphic pattern of finely vacuolated preadipocytes. Watch the linear or crosslink-arranged capillary network (H & E, ×140).

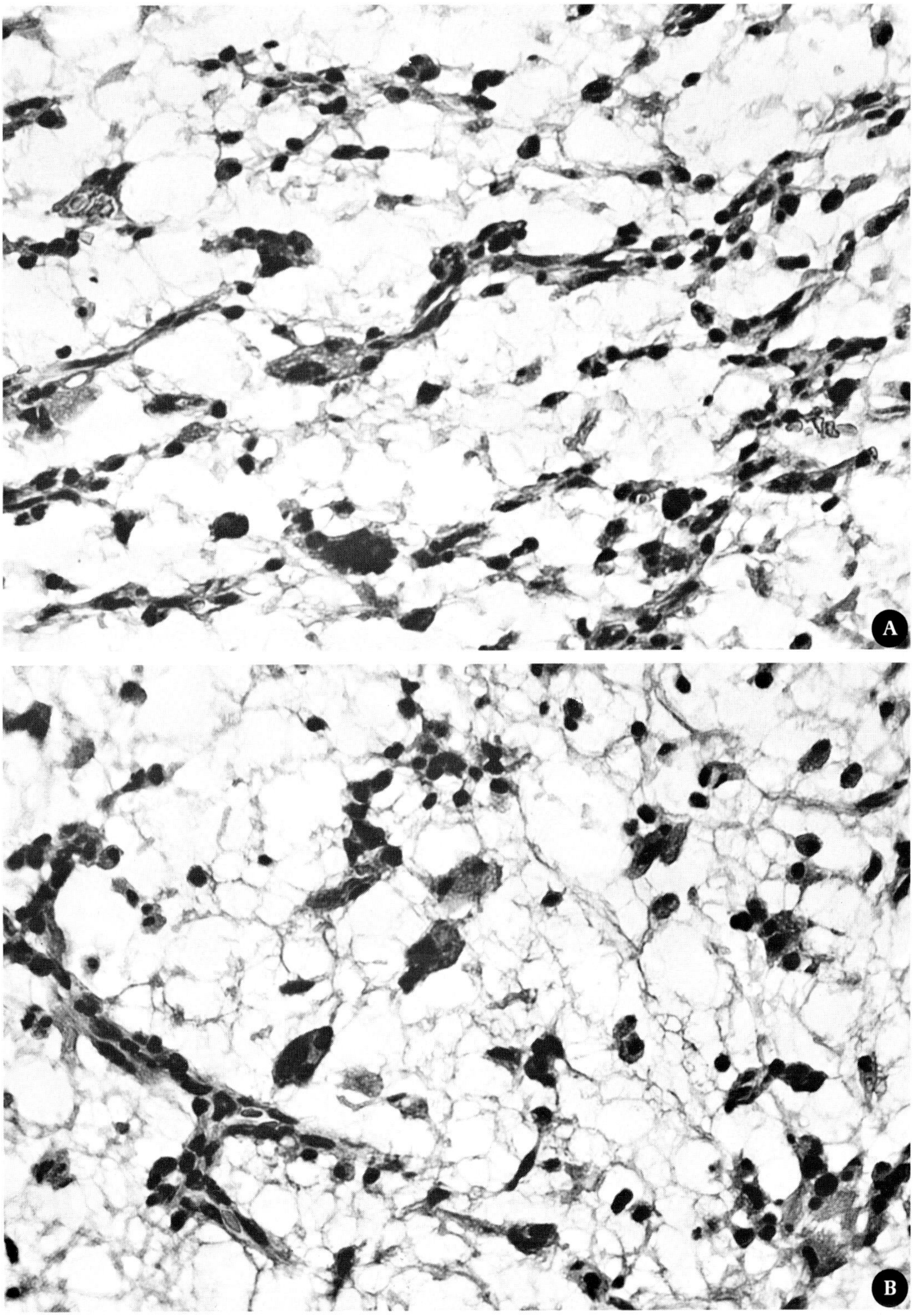

Figure 4-32. Myxoid liposarcoma. At this magnification the multivacuolation of preadipocytes and their adherent relation to the capillary wall or capillary pericytes are well seen. Also note a few granular cytoplasmic lipoblasts (H & E, ×350). (See Figures 4-1 and 4-15.)

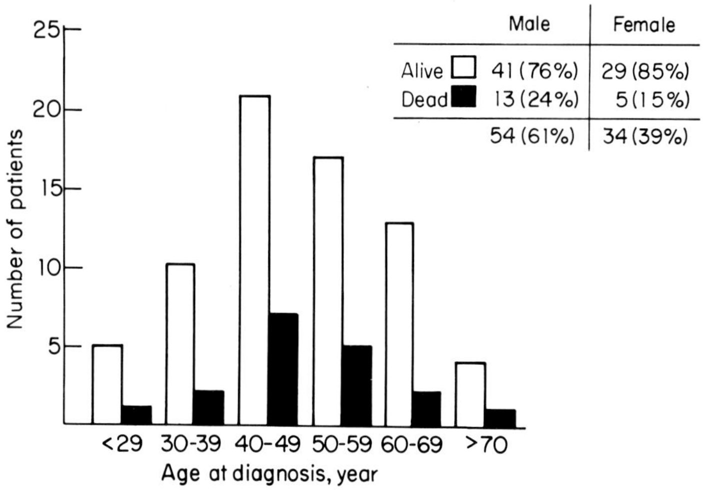

Figure 4-33. Age distribution and mortality of 88 patients treated at Memorial Sloan-Kettering Cancer Center for myxoid liposarcoma (see also Figure 4-44).

lipoblastic forms, suggests perhaps more than plain morphologic peculiarity. Although it is generally accepted (Reszel et al, 1966; Spittle et al, 1970; Kalderon and Fethiere, 1973; Hajdu and Hajdu, 1976; Gould et al, 1976; Desai et al, 1978; and Kindblom, 1979) that the different subtypes of liposarcoma reflect the wide cellular spectrum of differentiation of adipose tissue and that all liposarcomas are histogenetically related, the histogenesis of liposarcomas is far from settled. It is quite possible, as Ewing suggested in 1935, that the tumor cells in myxoid tumors arise from aberrant capillary vessels.

Lipoblastic Liposarcoma. This so-called round cell or epithelioid type of liposarcoma is predominantly composed of oval or round cells, lipoblasts and preadipocytes, in a myxomucinous or fibrillar background (Figs. 4-1, 4-15). Most commonly the stroma is myxoid rather than fibrillar; hence, the lipoblastic liposarcoma *may show resemblance to myxoid liposarcoma.* The individual cells are most commonly uniform round cells with granular pinkish and finely vacuolated, ill-defined cytoplasm. The nuclei may vary slightly in size and shape, the majority being round or oval with prominent

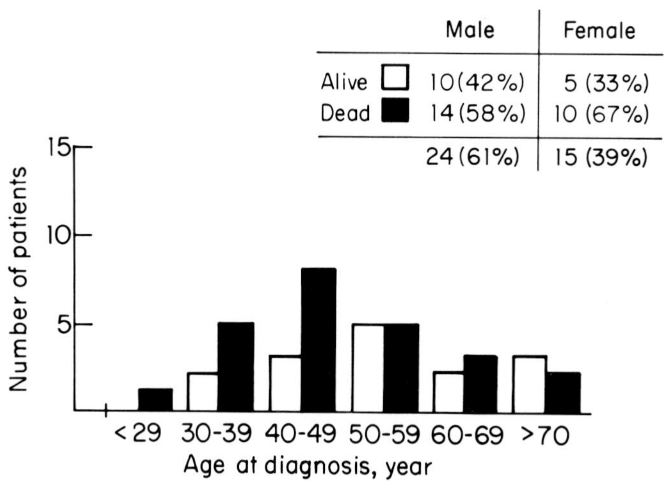

Figure 4-34. Mortality and age distribution of 39 patients treated at Memorial Sloan-Kettering Cancer Center for fibroblastic liposarcoma (see also Figures 4-15 and 4-44).

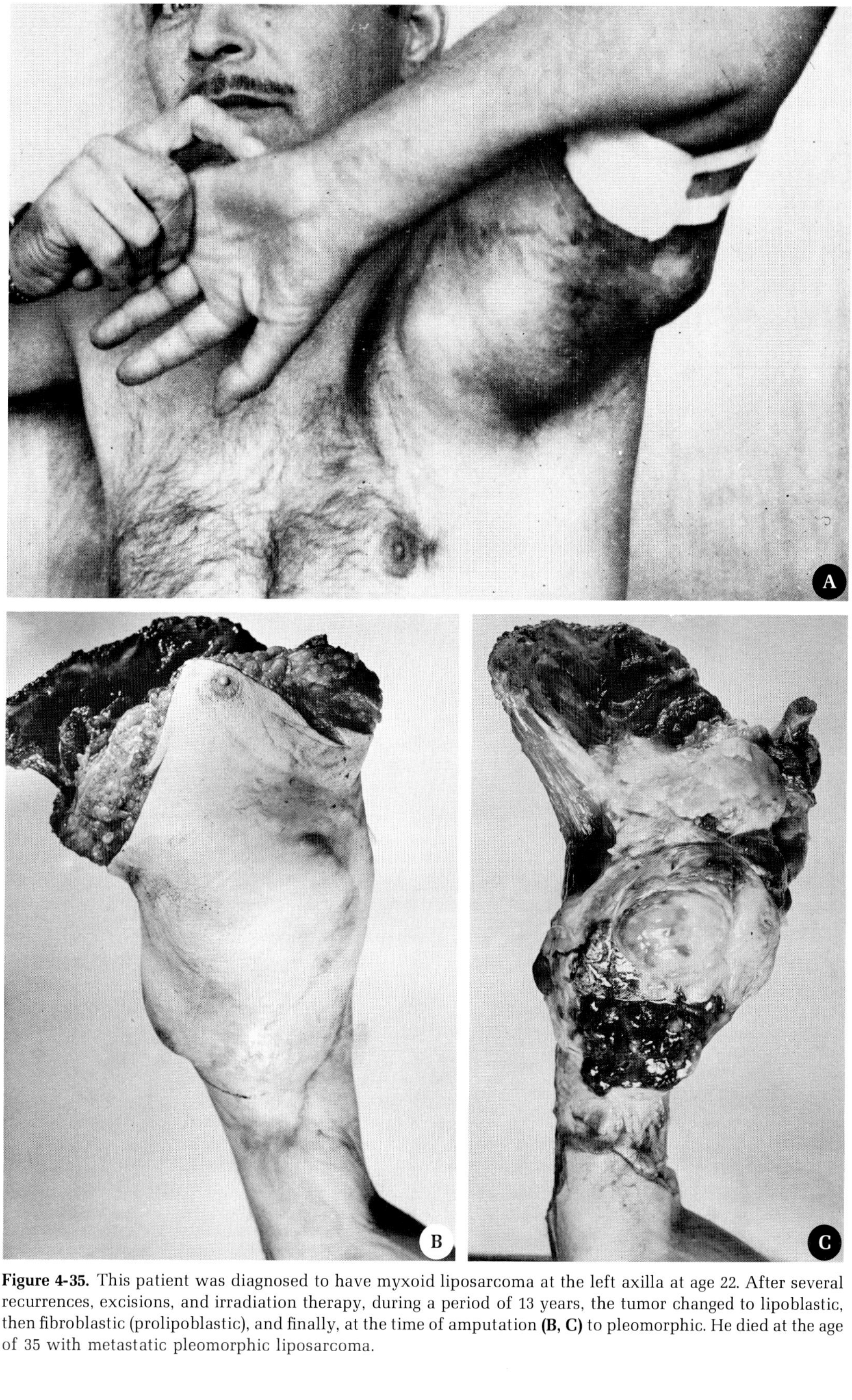

Figure 4-35. This patient was diagnosed to have myxoid liposarcoma at the left axilla at age 22. After several recurrences, excisions, and irradiation therapy, during a period of 13 years, the tumor changed to lipoblastic, then fibroblastic (prolipoblastic), and finally, at the time of amputation **(B, C)** to pleomorphic. He died at the age of 35 with metastatic pleomorphic liposarcoma.

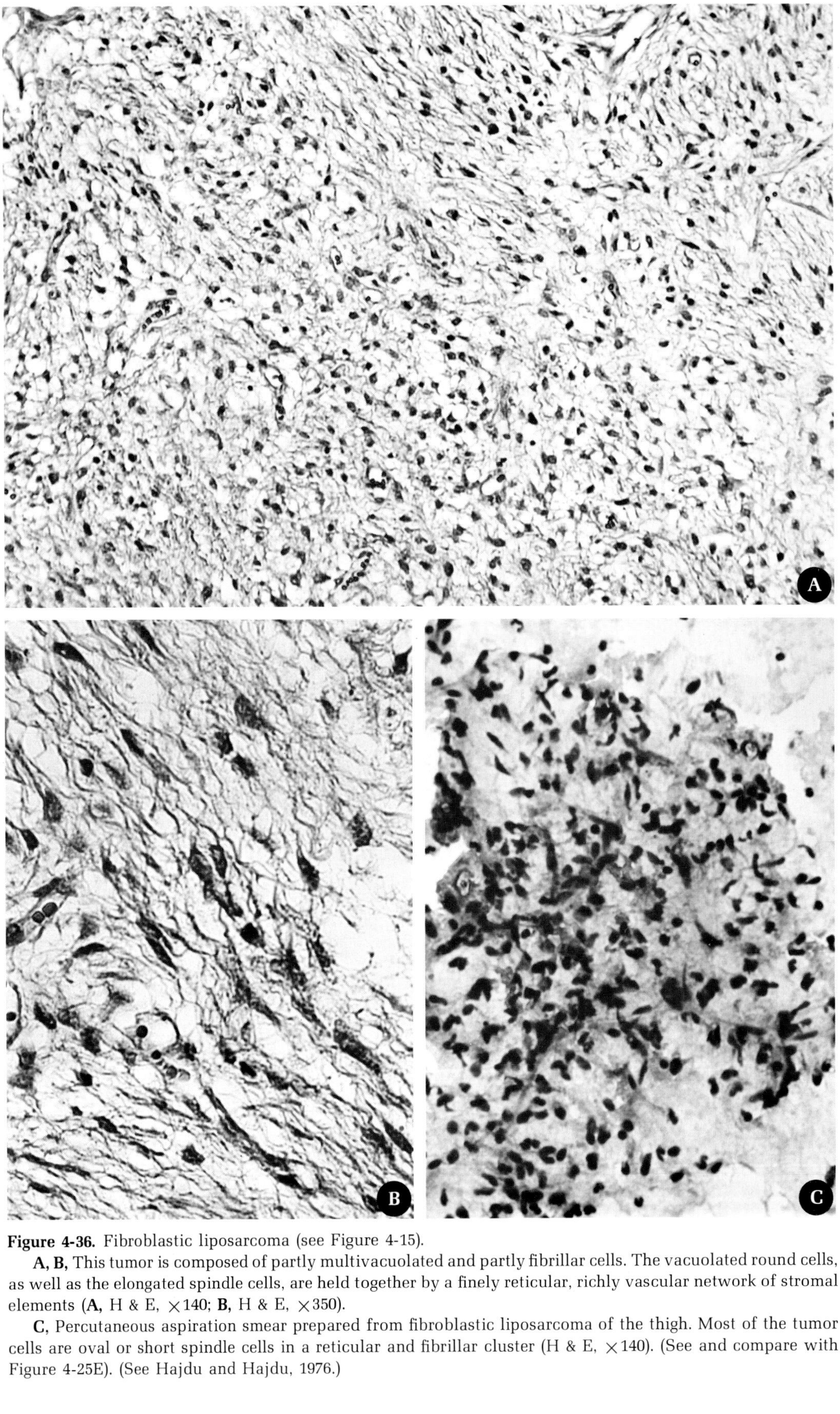

Figure 4-36. Fibroblastic liposarcoma (see Figure 4-15).

A, B, This tumor is composed of partly multivacuolated and partly fibrillar cells. The vacuolated round cells, as well as the elongated spindle cells, are held together by a finely reticular, richly vascular network of stromal elements (**A,** H & E, ×140; **B,** H & E, ×350).

C, Percutaneous aspiration smear prepared from fibroblastic liposarcoma of the thigh. Most of the tumor cells are oval or short spindle cells in a reticular and fibrillar cluster (H & E, ×140). (See and compare with Figure 4-25E). (See Hajdu and Hajdu, 1976.)

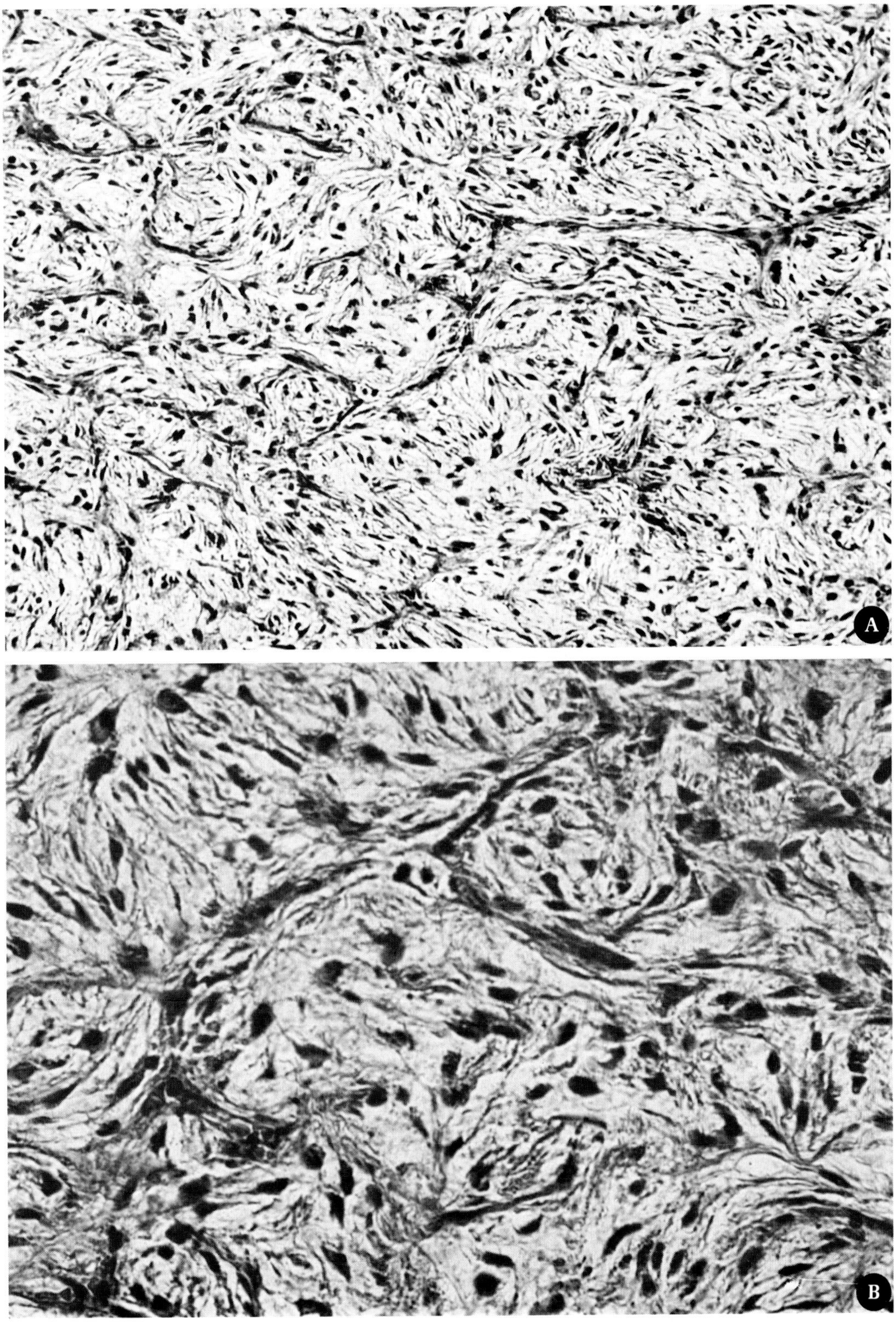

Figure 4-37. Fibroblastic liposarcoma. Note the complete obstruction of the space between capillary vessels by slender fibroblastic cells (prolipoblasts). The arranged pattern of these cells resembles the storiform pattern commonly seen in fibroblastic fibrous histiocytomas (see Figure 2-24) and certain neurogenic tumors (see Figure 7-24). However, the linear or cross-link type of capillary network is distinctly that associated with liposarcomas, e.g., myxoid liposarcoma (see Figures 4-28 and 4-29).

B, The intimate relationship between capillary vessels and individual tumor cells is so unique that one cannot rule out possible histogenetic connection between capillaries and tumor cells (**A,** H & E, ×140; **B,** H & E, ×350).

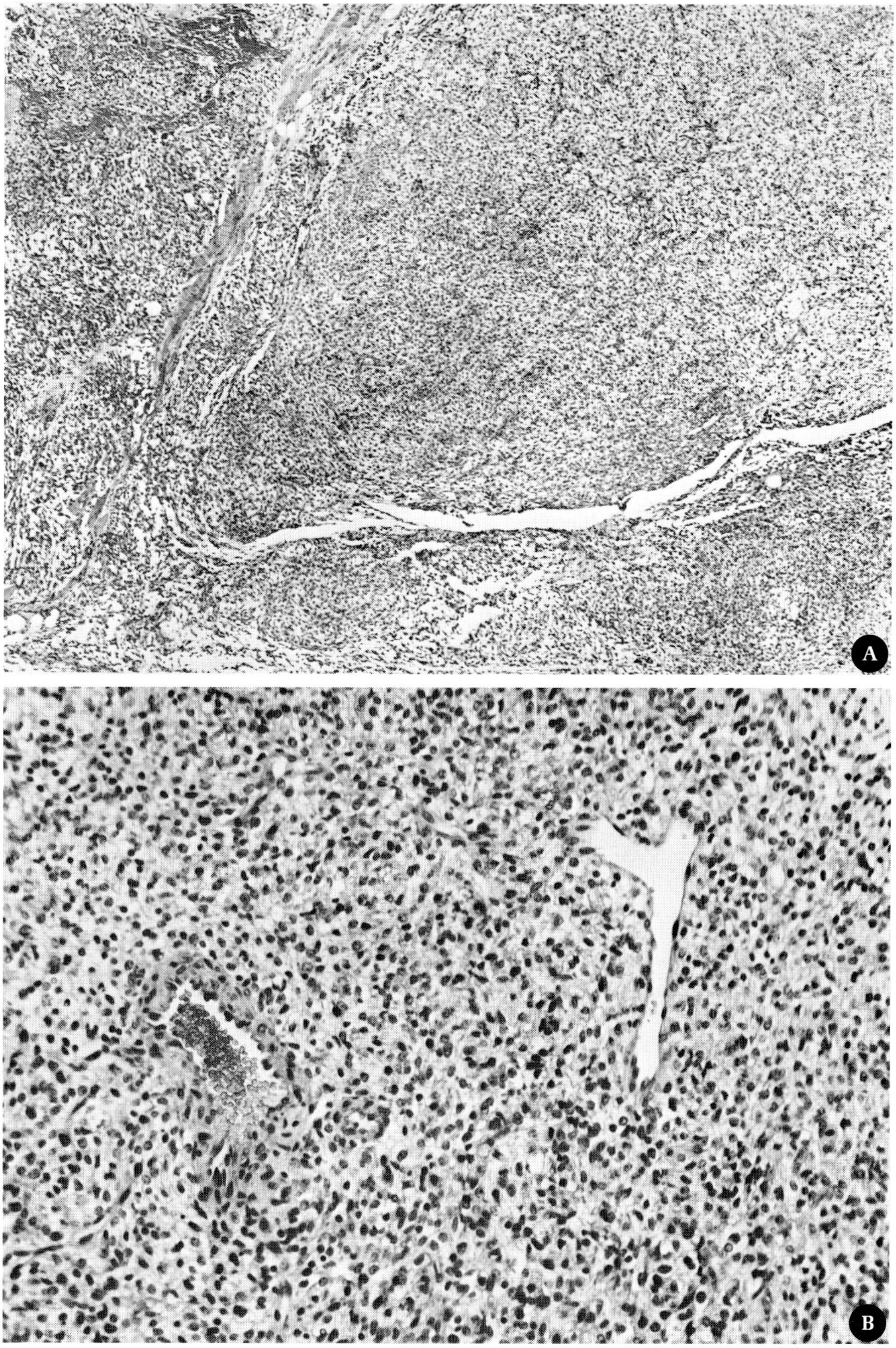

Figure 4-38. Lipoblastic (or so-called round cell) liposarcoma consists of uniform round lipoblasts. Note the homogeneous spread of the tumor cells between capillary vessels (**A,** H & E, ×35; **B,** H & E, ×140).

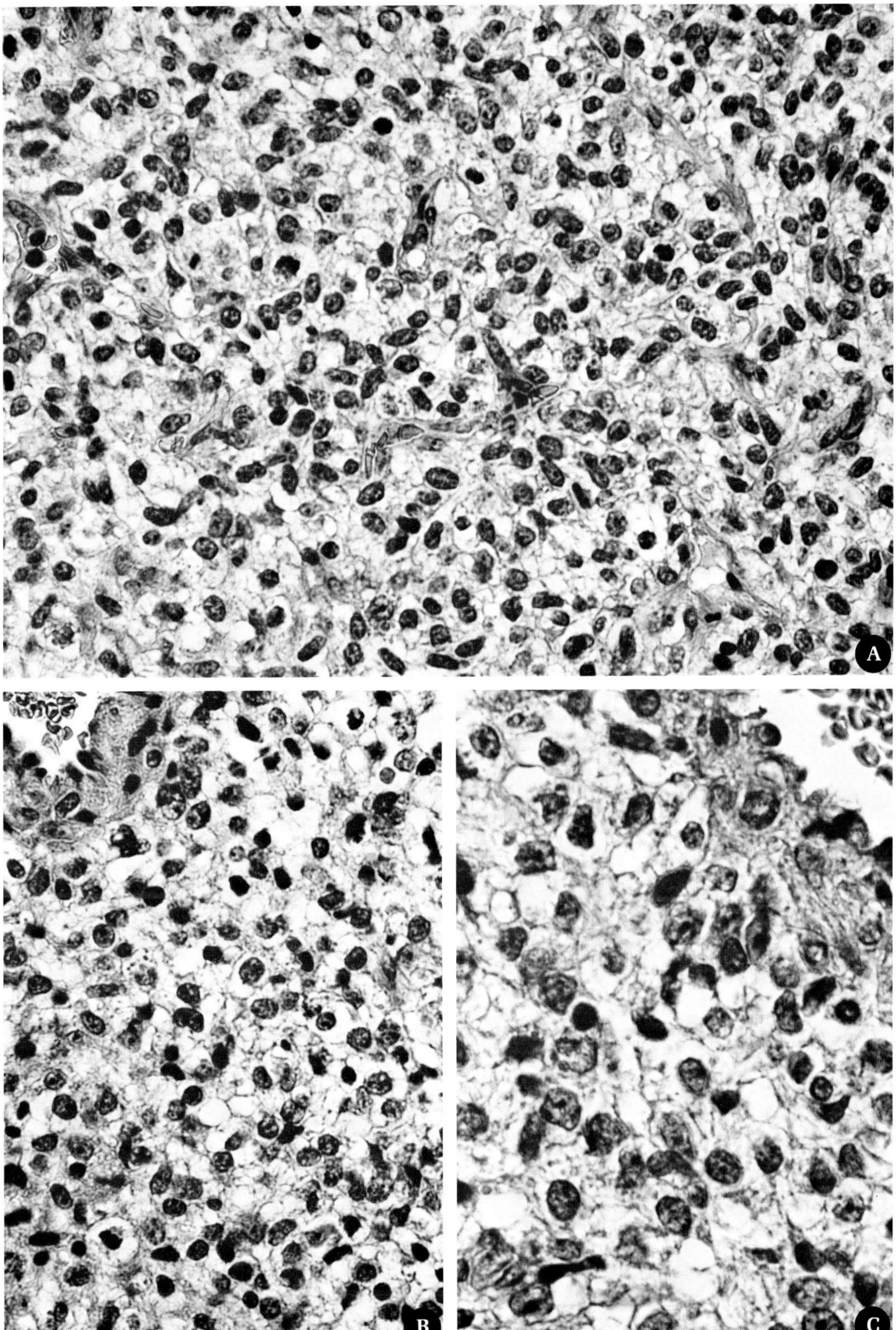

Figure 4-39. Lipoblastic liposarcoma (see Figure 4-15).

This tumor is characterized by mononuclear granular cytoplasmic lipoblasts arranged in a lacy or mosaic pattern. Note the glycogen granules as well as occasional lipoid vacuoles in the cytoplasm. **B, C,** The tumor cells seem to have direct contact with pericytes of the capillary vessels (**A, B,** ×350; **C,** H & E, ×470).

nucleoli. The nuclei may be scalloped and pushed peripherally by lipid droplets. Occasionally one may see a few rounded vacuolated lipoblasts with pyknotic nuclei resembling cells in the hibernoma (Figs. 4-38, 4-39). Rarely one may find a few hematopoietic elements in highly vascular myxoid areas.

Lipoblastic liposarcomas can be exceedingly cellular, and the cellularity may obscure the intricate meshwork of capillaries. The quantity of mucinous material may vary from case to case. The mucoid lakes so common in myxoid liposarcomas are rare findings in these lesions. However, whatever quantity is present, it is stainable with Alcian blue and completely removable from the sections by prior treatment with hyaluronidase. Because of the microscopic similarity of some of these tumors to chordoid tumors or mesenchymal cartilaginous tumors, the hyaluronidase treatment of sections has differential diagnostic significance, since the sulfated mucopolysaccharides of these latter lesions are not depolymerized by hyaluronidase (Table 4-15).

Our review of lipoblastic liposarcomas (Hajdu, Erlandson, and Fortner, 1979) at Memorial Sloan-Kettering Cancer Center is summarized in Table 4-12 and Figure 4-40. Although this neoplasm, the lipoblastic liposarcoma (or the so-called round cell liposarcoma) can be further subdivided histologically for adipocytic and spindle cell forms, the 30 cases studied did not show significant differences in relation to site, size, rate of recurrence, and prognosis. Twenty of the 30 tumors were primary neoplasms in the extremities, recurred in 67% of the cases, and caused death in 20 of the 30 patients (Table 4-18; Fig. 4-44).

Pleomorphic Liposarcomas. The pleomorphic types are so strikingly different from liposarcomas of other microscopic forms that it is often difficult to prove lipoid origin of these tumors. Especially the pleomorphic liposarcoma which contains prolipoblasts can look similar to fibroblastic fibrosarcoma or malignant fibrous histiocytoma. Liposarcomas containing a great number of cells with eosinophilic granular cytoplasm may be difficult to distinguish not only from pleomorphic fibrous histiocytomas but also from rhabdomyosarcoma (see Differential Diagnosis).

Several sections and diligent search for myxoid preadipocytes, granular lipoblasts, or tumor cells containing intracytoplasmic hyalin globules may be required before a diagnosis can be made. Frozen sections stained with fat stain help to disclose the true identity of most of these tumors. The large quantities of intracytoplasmic lipid material are easily demonstrable in the majority of the tumor cells. The highly malignant nature of these tumors is demonstrated by the numerous mitotic figures. The size of the tumor cells may range from slender spindle cells in a compact arrangement to immense tumor giant cells with giant nuclei and granular or foamy cytoplasms. The PAS-positive, non-diastase digestible hyalin globules, the so-called pink globules, are found most often in the cytoplasm of bizarre giant cells, but occasionally they may be seen in the form of piles of globules between loosely arranged cells in the richly vascular stroma (Fig. 4-23; Tables 4-13, 4-15).

The *presence of lipid droplets, however, is not necessarily diagnostic for liposarcoma.* Many other types of tumors, especially tumors of the fibrous histiocytic type, may contain tumor cells with lipid droplets due to degenerative changes or phagocytic activity. The hyalin globules, on the other hand, are mostly observed in tumors of fat origin. The first description of these pink globules was given by Wright, in 1948, in a case report of a liposarcoma arising in a pre-existing lipoma: "A striking feature of the tumor is the presence of deeply eosinophilic intra-cytoplasmic globoid bodies ranging in size up to 10 or 12 microns." Similar globoid hyalin bodies were described and illustrated by Kindblom et al, in 1975. The resemblance of these bodies to hyalin

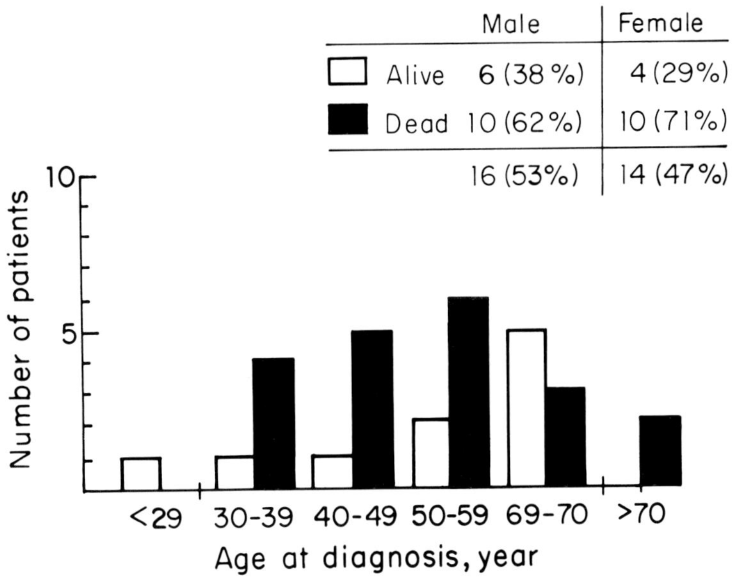

Figure 4-40. Age distribution and mortality of 30 patients with lipoblastic liposarcoma.

droplet degeneration is remarkable. Although it is possible that they result from degenerative changes and their pathophysiology is uncertain, they should be considered as aids in diagnosis of many of the otherwise unrecognizable lipoid neoplasms (Fig. 4-24D).

Pleomorphic liposarcomas of the adipocytic or vacuolated type are more easily identifiable with the microscope than with the pleomorphic lipoblastic types, but they are both bizarre neoplasms in their cytologic composition. The tumor cells may range in size from small vacuolated preadipocytes to gigantic multinucleated cells. Most of the tumors are loosely arranged in a sparsely cellular but highly vascular stroma. It is of interest that despite the multiplicity of bizarre cells, epulis-type giant cells or Touton giant cells are rarely seen in untreated or untraumatized liposarcomas (Fig. 4-41).

The cytoplasm of the tumor cells is ill-defined and may contain a number of small round vacuoles. Many cells contain only a few small discrete vacuoles in the foamy, finely granular, spidery cytoplasms, but other cells may contain as many as three dozen or more fat vacuoles in their distended cytoplasms. Fat stain is usually not required for proper diagnosis of these neoplasms, but in case of doubt it is rewarding to submit an unfixed section for fat stain or for electron microscopic examination (Fig. 4-24).

Enzinger and Winslow (1962) found that pleomorphic liposarcomas occur more frequently in older patients than the myxoid or lipoblastic types. This fact was confirmed by our review of 78 pleomorphic liposarcomas (Fig. 4-42). Evaluation of clinicopathologic findings disclosed that pleomorphic liposarcomas are highly malignant neoplasms with a rate of recurrence of 56% and an overall mortality rate of 77% (Table 4-18; Fig. 4-44). In anatomic distribution and age and sex of patients, pleomorphic liposarcomas did not show any particular predilection. Approximately 20% of the neoplasms which were ultimately classified as pleomorphic liposarcomas showed at an earlier stage of the disease either myxoid or lipoblastic growth patterns.

Incidence and Prognosis

Although liposarcoma is a disease of the adult, rare instances have been reported in children. Kauffman and Stout in

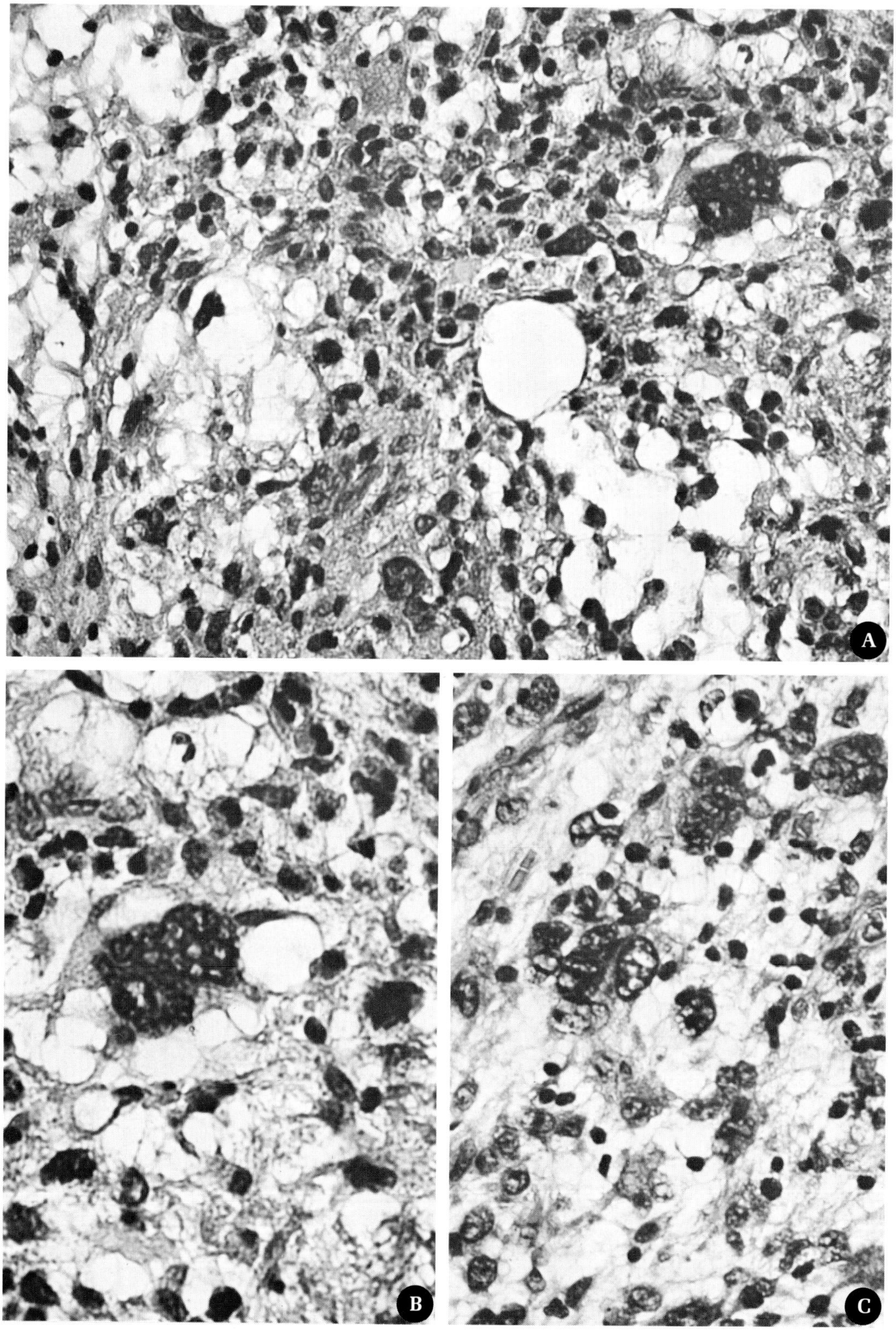

Figure 4-41. Pleomorphic liposarcoma.

Haphazard mixture of neoplastic fat cells at various stages of differentiation (see Figures 4-1 and 4-15). Note the many mono- and multinucleated forms and the granular cytoplasmic lipoblasts (H & E, ×350).

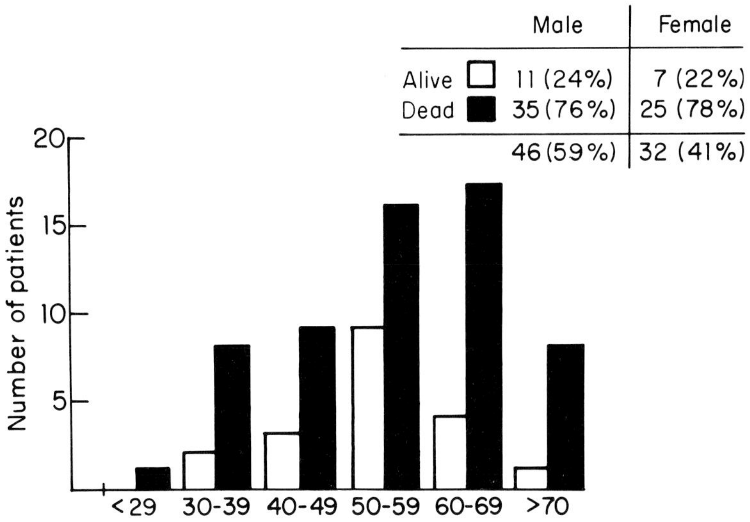

Figure 4-42. Age distribution and mortality of 78 patients treated at Memorial Sloan-Kettering Cancer Center for pleomorphic liposarcoma.

1959 found 15 reported cases in the literature and added 13 cases of their own. Of the 28 cases, only one metastasized, but the duration of the follow-up was too short in many cases to draw a conclusion. My personal experience with liposarcoma in children is limited to a half dozen cases. Most of the lipoid tumors in children are lipoblastomas rather than liposarcomas (see Fig. 4-16).

Kinne et al (1973) analyzed 34 cases of primary *retroperitoneal liposarcomas* representing 14% of the liposarcomas treated during the same period of time. Twenty-three of 34 tumors were myxoid liposarcomas. The overall 5-year survival rate was 4%; however, only 4 of the 34 patients were completely free of disease (Tables 4-16, 4-17). Farbman (1950) by reviewing the literature on retroperitoneal tumors found that the average size of retroperitoneal liposarcoma was 7.4 kg. *Hypoglycemia* may be found in association with many bulky, benign or malignant, retroperitoneal or intraperitoneal neoplasms because the tumor secretes a polypeptide with a molecular weight similar to that of insulin (Fig. 4-43).

Almost all of the investigators agree that there is a definite correlation between histologic type, size, and histologic grade of the tumors and survival. According to Reszel et al (1966) the 5-year survival varies from 75% (low-grade tumors) to 32% (high-grade tumors). Enzinger and Winslow (1962) gave a range of survival from 85% (well-differentiated liposarcoma) to 21% (pleomorphic liposarcoma) in a series of 103 patients (Table 4-12).

Investigators who consider desmoid tumors as non-malignant neoplasms because desmoids, according to them, do not metastasize, accept well-differentiated liposarcomas as malignant neoplasms. For example, Kauffman and Stout (1959) wrote, "Although well-differentiated liposarcoma is not known to metastasize, we have chosen to retain it in the liposarcoma group because of its local invasiveness and its inexorable tendency to recur."

Liposarcomas are known for their *tendency to recur* (Table 4-18). Rates of local recurrence have been reported by Pack and Pierson (1954) as 33%, by Enterline et al (1960) as 48%, by Kimbrough and Soule (1971) as 61%, and by Enzinger and Winslow (1962) as between 53 and 85%, depending on histologic types. Reszel et al (1966) stated that histologic grade and type of malignancy remained constant with each recurrence except in 1 of 22 cases. In an earlier report Van Meurs

TABLE 4-17. ***Primary Retroperitoneal Sarcomas of Soft Parts****

			NO. OF PATIENTS											
	NO. PATIENTS	AVG. AGE	MALE	FEMALE	PARTIAL SURG. RESEC.	TOTAL SURG. RESEC.	OP. MORTA-LITY	POST OP. RAD.	CHEMO-THERAPY	5-YR SURV.	OVERALL SURV.	CAUSE OF DEATH LOC.	MET.	BOTH
Liposarcoma	27	53	10	17	5	14	2	8	6	13	3	16	–	2
Leiomyo-sarcoma	17	45	9	8	7	2	3	5	5	2	1	11	2	2
Rhabdomyo-sarcoma	17	29	12	5	6	1	1	?	?	3	?	6	6	3
Fibrosarcoma	15	41	8	7	?	?	2	6	?	6	?	9	–	1
Malignant schwannoma	10	50	6	4	?	6	3	3	?	1	0	9	–	1
Undiff. sarcoma	7	50	4	3	2	2	0	3	?	1	?	3	–	3
Alveolar soft part sarcoma	1	49	–	1	?	?	?	?	?	0	–	?	?	?
Hemangio-pericytoma	1	40	–	1	?	?	–	?	?	0	–	?	?	?

Turnbull, A., and Hajdu, S. I.: Unpublished data.

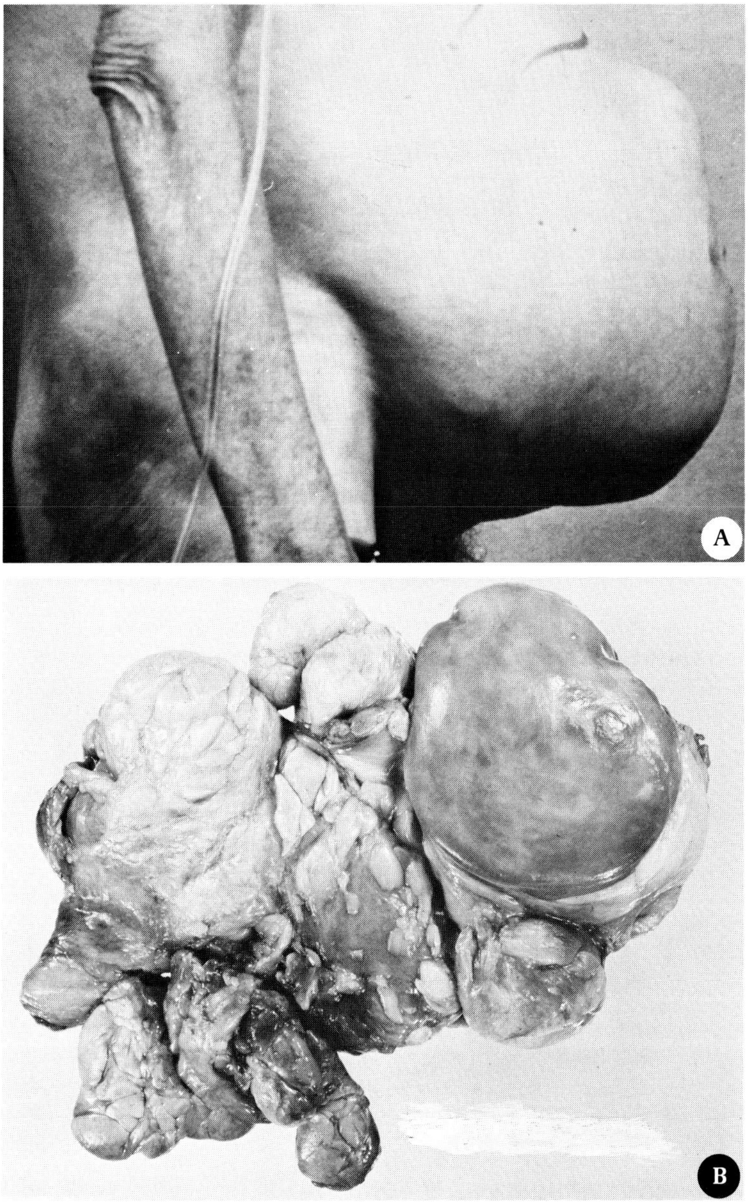

Figure 4-43. Retroperitoneal liposarcoma. A huge multilobular tumor mass was removed from the retroperitoneum. Of interest in this case, besides the enormous size of the tumor, is that some of the tumor nodules were microscopically benign while others showed a spectrum of differentiation from well-differentiated to pleomorphic liposarcoma.

(1946) presented a case of liposarcoma which had a tendency toward a better maturation with each recurrence until it finally resembled lipoma. In the series of 242 liposarcomas studied at Memorial Sloan-Kettering Cancer Center, about 25% *of the tumors changed toward higher grade and less differentiated forms with each recurrence,* e.g., from myxoid to fibroblastic or from myxoid to lipoblastic or pleomorphic forms. The clinical implication of this is apparent, since we found that the fibroblastic tumors had less favorable prognosis than the myxoid ones and pleomorphic forms are more malignant in their behavior than any other form (Figs. 4-44, 4-45; Table 4-19).

It seems that the anatomic distribution

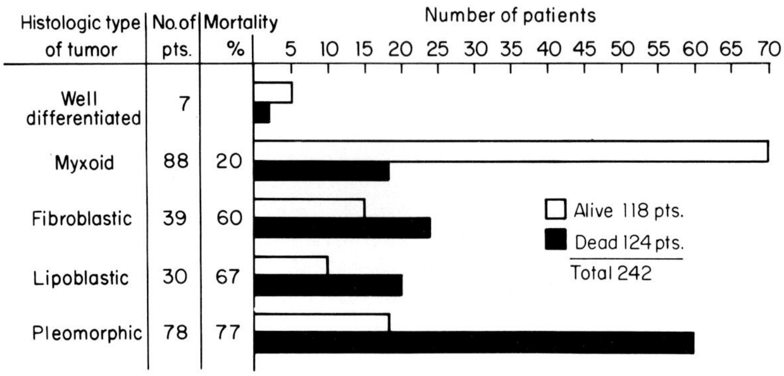

Figure 4-44. Correlation of histologic type and mortality in a series of 242 liposarcomas.

of any particular type of tumor is not influenced by the sex or age of the patient, but it is worth noticing that only three tumors occurred in the distal part of the extremities—one in the hand, one in the foot, and one behind the ankle. It is of interest that tumors of "exposed" regions did not differ significantly in prognosis from those which were in "unexposed" areas. (In reference to grade and stage see Chapter 1, Fig. 1-59 and Table 1-15.)

Despite the bulky and infiltrating nature of many of these tumors invasion of the *skin* (2 cases), major *blood vessels* (5 cases), major *nerves* (12 cases), and *bone* (5 cases) were not common findings. Only three of the tumors metastasized to regional lymph nodes and 14 spread to bones (Fig. 4-46).

Twenty-nine of the 242 patients (12%) had a second primary malignant neoplasm among which primary tumors of

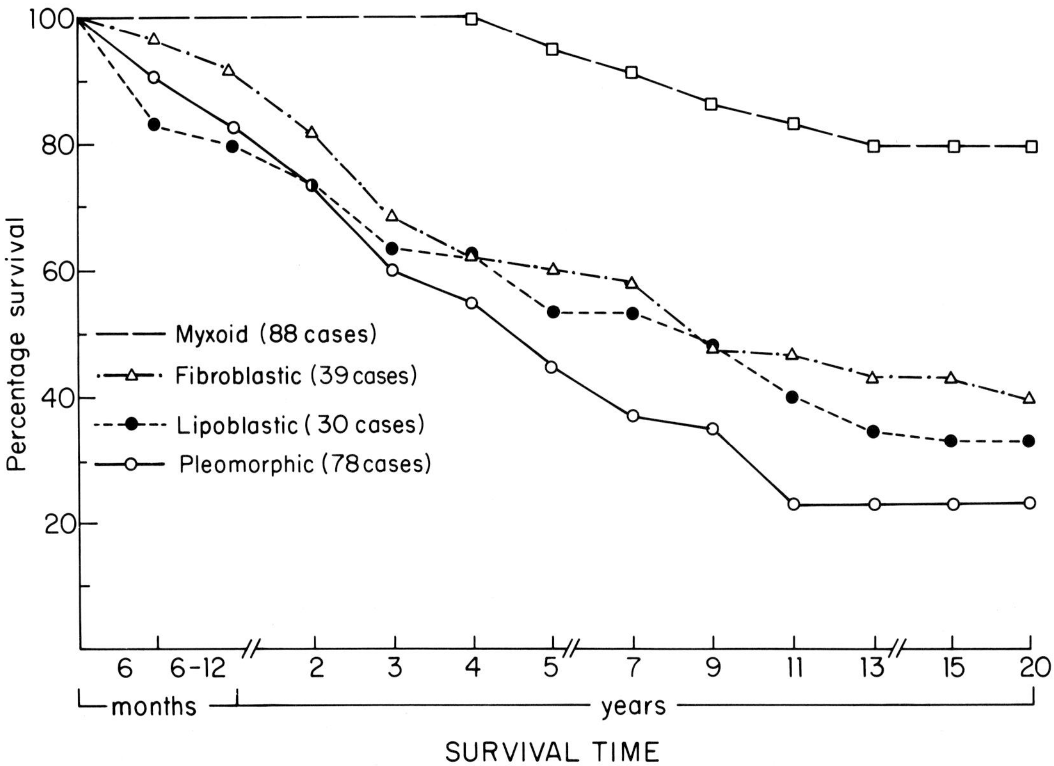

Figure 4-45. Percentage of survival of patients with various liposarcomas. (See Hajdu et al, 1979.)

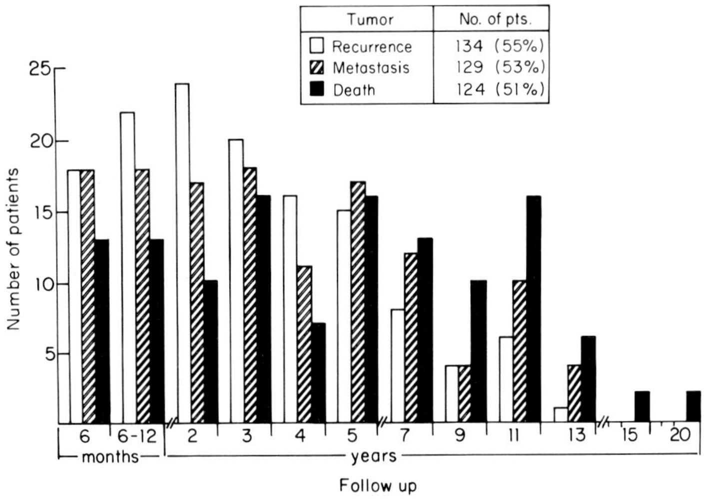

Figure 4-46. Rate and time of recurrence and metastasis of 242 liposarcoma. (See Hajdu et al., 1979.)

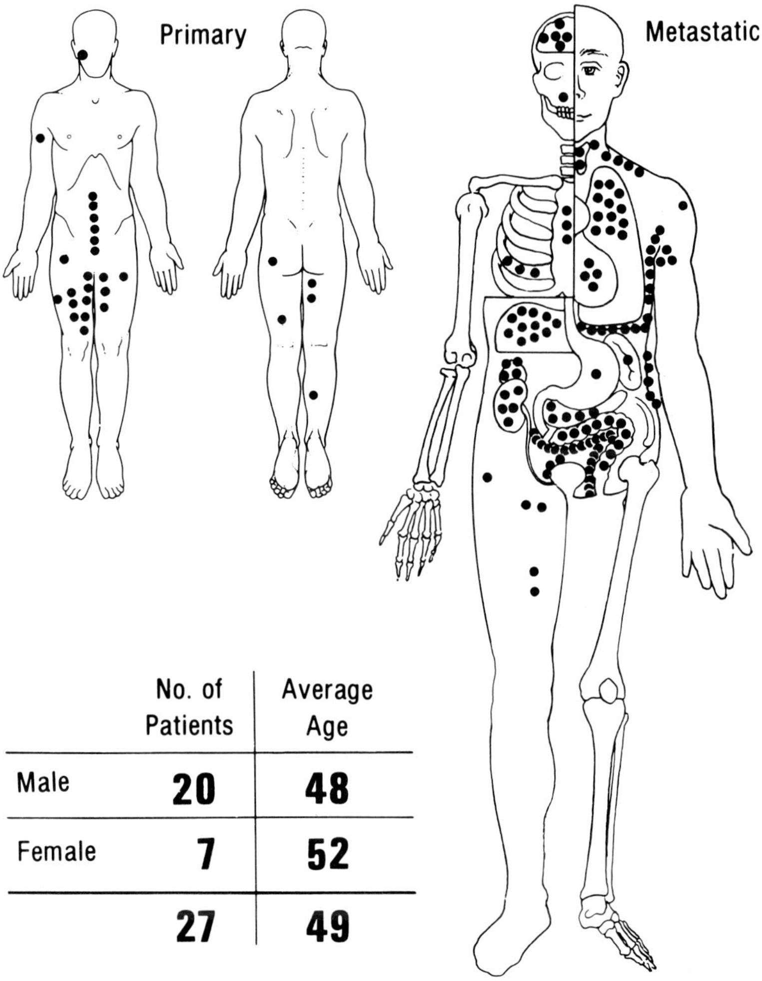

	No. of Patients	Average Age
Male	**20**	**48**
Female	**7**	**52**
	27	**49**

Figure 4-47. Distribution of metastatic sites of liposarcomas of 27 autopsied patients. Note the relatively high rate of spread to the liver and gastrointestinal tract, including the pancreas, and sparse involvement of the lung.

TABLE 4-18. *Rate of Recurrence of Liposarcomas*

HISTOLOGIC TYPE	NO. OF PATIENTS
Well-differentiated	2/7 (29%)
Myxoid	44/88 (50%)
Fibroblastic	24/39 (62%)
Lipoblastic	20/30 (67%)
Pleomorphic	44/78 (56%)
	134/242(55%)

the colon (8 cases), breast (7 cases), lung (2 cases), and ovary (2 cases) were the most common. Eighteen patients had histologically benign neoplasms. It is of interest that 12 patients had histologically benign lipoma in areas anatomically unrelated to the liposarcoma and in five of these cases the lipomas were multiple.

Many of these findings are somewhat in variance with those reported by others. For example, in the series of liposarcomas studied by Reszel et al (1966), 48% of the sarcomas were the myxoid type, and only two of these tumors metastasized. In the series of 242 liposarcomas studied by us (Hajdu, Erlandson, and Fortner, 1979) 37% were the myxoid type and 20% of the patients died with metastatic tumor. The most common sites of metastasis, according to our postmortem findings, are the lungs, liver, peritoneal surface, and brain (Fig. 4-47).

Among the various types of soft tissue sarcomas, liposarcoma is known to be one of the most *radiosensitive* (Shiu et al, 1975). As early as the late 1920's, Ewing and Stewart called attention to the radiosensitivity of these tumors.

Spittle et al (1970) observed local recurrence in 20% of the liposarcomas which were irradiated after surgery, whereas a recurrence rate of 74% was observed in tumors that were not irradiated. According to reports, local surgery combined with radiotherapy appears to be promising and may obviate the need for amputation in many cases. Many of the 242 tumors studied were treated by a combination of surgery and irradiation. No long-lasting beneficial effect was achieved by radiation therapy without surgery.

Little has been written about the beneficial effect of chemotherapy. Gottlieb et al (1972) reported complete remission in 3 out of 7 cases of liposarcomas treated with a combination of adriamycin and dimethyl triazenoimidazole carboxamide.

In most cases, wide excision or en bloc resection with postoperative irradiation is recommended. In case of well-differentiated liposarcomas and some of the better differentiated myxoid liposarcomas, if surgical removal, with clean margin, can be carried out, the patient should not be subjected to irradiation (Table 4-19).

Differential Diagnosis

The matter of differential diagnosis of liposarcomas is relatively simple, except

TABLE 4-19. *Surgical Treatment of Liposarcomas*

	NUMBER OF PATIENTS				
		PRIMARY TUMOR		RECURRENT TUMOR	
HISTOLOGIC TYPE	TOTAL	EXCISION	AMPUTATION	EXCISION	AMPUTATION
Myxoid	88	5/36(14%)	1/8	7/32(21%)	5/12
Fibroblastic	39	8/14(67%)	0/1	15/20(75%)	1/4
Lipoblastic	30	3/4 (75%)	4/6	11/18(61%)	2/2
Pleomorphic	78	15/22(68%)	11/11	20/29(68%)	14/15
	235	31/76(51%)	16/26(62%)	53/99(54%)	22/33(67%)

Numerator = number of patients dead.
Denominator = total number of patients.

for tumors that are at the two ends of the spectrum: well-differentiated liposarcomas and pleomorphic liposarcomas.

Certain *lipomas* with areas of fat necrosis may resemble well-differentiated liposarcoma because of foam cells, increased cellularity, and vacuolated adipocytes. However, most of the lipomas are small, subcutaneous lesions far less vascular than liposarcomas.

Myxoma may resemble myxoid liposarcoma but is much less innocuous and vascular in appearance and also does not contain multivacuolated lipoblasts. The arranged, mostly acellular, reticular or collagenous tissue is rarely a feature in liposarcomas (see Chapter 2).

Fibrous histiocytoma, especially the ones with prominent myxoid areas, may resemble myxoid liposarcoma, but the lack of lipoblasts, arranged blood vessels, and the absence of the pooling phenomenon helps to differentiate fibrous histiocytoma from liposarcoma (See Chapter 2).

In *pleomorphic fibrous histiocytoma* stainable lipid may be present in the polymorphic cells; however, the absence of adipocytes, lipoblasts, and bizarre giant cells with hyalin globules and the presence of mononuclear or multinucleated histiocytic forms, especially Touton giant cells, help to rule out liposarcoma (see Chapter 2).

The *pleomorphic rhabdomyosarcoma* should contain either cross-striated rhabdomyoblasts or embryonal rhabdomyoblasts to ascertain the diagnosis of the tumor. The presence of myoblasts with longitudinal myofilaments in combination with embryonal rhabdomyoblasts should also be accepted as diagnostic for rhabdomyosarcoma (see Chapter 5).

Chordoma, extraskeletal chondrosarcoma, and mesenchymal chondrosarcoma are characteristically arranged in lobules and contain numerous binucleated tumor cells. Histochemical demonstration of mucopolysaccharides is helpful in the differential diagnosis. Intracellular, diastase-digestible, PAS-positive polysaccharide granules of chondrocytes are not present in well-differentiated and myxoid liposarcomas; on the other hand, stromal and mucopolysaccharide substances in liposarcomas are digestible with testicular hyaluronidase but are unaffected by hyaluronidase in the sulfated form in chondroid tumors and chordoma. Of course, the characteristic multivacuolated and multinucleated bizarre adipocytes are absent in chondroid tumors as well as in chordoma (Table 4-15).

REFERENCES

References are listed in chronological order in each category.

INTRODUCTION

Toldt, C.: Lehrbuch der Gewebelehre mit vorzugsweiser Berucksichtingung des menschlichen Korpers. Stuttgart, Euke, 1870.

Hatai, S.: On the presence in human embryos of an interscapular gland corresponding to the so-called hibernating gland of lower mammals. Anat. Anz. 21:369, 1902.

Klotz, O.: Studies upon calcareous degeneration. The process of pathological calcification. J. Exp. Med. 7:633, 1905.

Bell, E. T.: On the occurrence of fat in the epithelium, cartilage and muscle fibres of the ox. Am. J. Anat. 9:412, 1909.

Bonnot, E.: The interscapular gland. J. Anat. 43:47, 1908–1909.

Strandberg, J.: A case of skin transplantation with unique results. Hygiea 77:373, 1915.

Lewis, M. R.: The formation of the fat droplets in the cells of tissue culture. Science 48:398, 1918.

Cramer, W.: On glandular adipose tissue, and its relation to other endocrine organs and to the vitamine problem. Br. J. Exp. Pathol. 1:184, 1920.

Rasmussen, A. T.: The so-called hibernating gland. J. Morphol. 38:147, 1923.

Margaillan, L.: Sur la regularite des variations des caracteres des huiles extraites d'un meme animal en fonction du point de prelevement. C. R. Acad. Sci. 188:1630, 1929.

Clark, E. R., and Clark, E. L.: Microscopic studies of new formation of fat in living adult rabbits. Am. J. Anat. 67:255, 1940.

Wells, H. G.: Adipose tissue, a neglected subject. JAMA 114:2177, 1940.

Wertheimer, E., and Shapiro, B.: The physiology of adipose tissue. Physiol. Rev. 28:451, 1948.

Fawcett, D. W., and Jones, I. C.: The effects of hypophysectomy, adrenalectomy and of

thiouracil feeding on the cytology of brown adipose tissue. Endocrinology 45:609, 1949.
Selye, H., and Timiras, P. S.: Participation of "brown fat" tissue in the alarm reaction. Nature 164:745, 1949.
Shapiro, B., and Wertheimer, E.: The metabolic activity of adipose tissue. Metabolism 5:79, 1956.
Lever, J. D.: The fine structure of adipose tissue in the rat with observations on the cytologic changes following starvation and adrenalectomy. Anat. Rec. 128:361, 1957.
Napolitano, L., and Fawcett, D. W.: The fine structure of brown adipose tissue in the newborn mouse and rat. J. Biophys. Biochem. Cytol. 4:685, 1958.
Napolitano, L.: The differentiation of white adipose cells. An electron microscopic study. J. Cell Biol. 18:663, 1963.
Williamson, J. R.: Adipose tissue. Morphological changes associated with lipid mobilization. J. Cell Biol. 20:57, 1964.
Irving, J. T.: Lipids and calciphylaxis. Arch. Oral Biol. 10:189, 1965.
Williamson, J. R., and Lacy, P. E.: Adipose Tissue. *In* Handbook of Physiology. Edited by A. E. Renold and G. F. Cahill, Jr. Washington, D. C., American Physiology Society, 1965.
Dawkins, M. J. R., Duckett, S., and Pearse, R. G. E.: Localization of catecholamines in brown fat. Nature 209:1144, 1966.
Picard, D., Tasso, F., and Cotte, G.: Aspect ultrastructural de la lipogenese dans le tissu adipeux brun. Z. Zellforsch. 69:260, 1966.
Smith, R. E.: Brown fat regulatory function and control. Bull. N.J. Acad. Sci., 93, 1969.
Berczi, I.: Fatty acids and soft tissue calcification. Exp. Med. Surg. 28:245, 1970.
Slavin, B. C.: The cytophysiology of mammalian adipose cell. Int. Rev. Cytol. 33:297, 1972.
Carpentier, J. L., Perrelet, A., and Orci, L.: Perturbation of the adipose cell plasma membrane in obese (ob/ob) mice. Lab. Invest. 37:260, 1977.
Melicow, M. M.: One hundred cases of pheochromocytoma at the Columbia-Presbyterian Medical Center, 1926–1976. Cancer 40: 1987, 1977.

NON-NEOPLASTIC LESIONS

Mohr, B.: Hypertophie der Hypophysis cerebri und dadurch bedingter Druck auf die Hirngrundflache, insbesondere auf die Sehnerven, das Chiasma derselben und den linkseitigen Hirnschenkel. Wochenschr. ges. Heilk. 6:565, 1840.
Brodie, B. C.: Clinical Lectures on Surgery. Delivered at St. George's Hospital. Philadelphia, Lea & Blanchard, 1846.
Balser, W.: Ueber Fettnekrose, eine zuweilen tödliche Krankheit des Menschen. Virchows Arch. Pathol. Anat. 90:520, 1882.
Madelung, O. W.: Ueber den Fatthals (diffuses Lipom des Halses). Arch. Klin. Chir., 37:106, 1888.
Dercum, F. X.: Three cases of hitherto unclassified affection resembling in its grosser aspects obesity, but associated with special nervous symptoms; adiposis dolorosa. Am. J. Med. Sci. 104:521, 1892.
Frölich, A.: Ein Fall von Tumor der Hypophysis cerebri ohne Akromegalie. Wien. Klin. Rdsch. 15:883; 906, 1901.
Marinesco, G., and Minea, J.: Deux cas de maladie de Dercum avec culture des tumeurs "in vitro". C.R. Soc. Biol. 79:866, 1916.
Miller, G. S.: Steatopygy and acromegaly. Am. J. Phys. Anthropol. 14:79, 1930.
Kling, D. H.: Juxta-articular adipose dolorosa. Arch. Surg. 34:599, 1937.
Wohl, M. G., and Pastor, N.: Adiposis dolorosa (Dercum's disease). JAMA 110:1261, 1938.
Adair, F. E., and Munzer, J. T.: Fat necrosis of the female breast. Am. J. Surg. 74:117, 1947.
Whitaker, W. G., Walker, E. T., and Canipelli, J.: Lipogranuloma of the peritoneum: Report of three cases following the intra-abdominal use of liquid petrolatum. JAMA 138:363, 1948.
Smetana, H. F., and Bernhard, W.: Sclerosing lipogranuloma. Arch. Pathol. 50:296, 1950.
Steinberg, B.: Systemic nodular panniculitis. Am. J. Pathol. 29:1059, 1953.
Cameron, A. H., and McMillan, D. H.: Lipomatosis of skeletal muscle in Maffucci's syndrome. J. Bone Joint Surg. 38B:692, 1956.
Szymanski, F. J., and Bluefarb, S. M.: Nodular fat necrosis and pancreatic disease. Arch. Dermatol. 83:224, 1961.
Schrier, R. W., Melmon, K. L., and Fenster, L. F.: Subcutaneous nodular fat necrosis in pancreatitis. Arch. Intern. Med. 116:832, 1965.
El-Kateb, H.: Experimental fat necrosis. Egypt. M.A.J. 48:382, 1965.
French, W. E., Bale, G. F., and Winborn, W. B.: Lipodystrophy of mesenteric fat. Surg. Gynec. Obstet. 122:1046, 1966.
Shelly, W. B., and Rawnsley, H. M.: Painful feet due to herniations of fat. JAMA 205:308, 1968.
Grant, J.: Piezogenic pedal papules. Arch. Dermatol. 101:619, 1970.
Urback, F., Johnson, W. C., and Davies, R. E.: Generalized paraffinoma (sclerosing lipogranuloma). Arch. Dermatol. 103:277, 1971.
Schlappner, O. L.: Painful and non-painful piezogenic pedal papules. Arch. Dermatol. 106:729, 1972.

Kipfer, R. E., Moertel, C. G., and Dahlin, D. C.: Mesenteric lipodystrophy. Ann. Intern. Med. 80:582, 1974.
Reske, M., and Namiki, H.: Sclerosing mesenteritis. Am. J. Clin. Pathol. 64:661, 1975.
Castillo-Oertel, Y., and Johnson, F. B.: Sclerosing lipogranuloma of male genitalia. Arch. Pathol. 101:321, 1977.

NEOPLASTIC LESIONS

Zappoli, A.: Liposarcoma. Bull d. Sc. med. Bologna 3:5, 1843.
Foerster, J.: Ueber die Bildung von Pigment und Fett in den Bindegewebszellen. Virchows Arch. [Pathol. Anat.] 12:197, 1857.
Virchow, R.: Ein Fall von Bosartigen, zun Theil in der Form des Neuromas auftretenden Fellgeschwulsten. Virchows Arch. [Pathol. Anat.] 11:281, 1857.
Senftleben, H.: Zur casuistik seltener Geschwulste. Virchows Arch. [Pathol. Anat.] 15:356, 1858.
Delamater, J.: Mammoth tumor. Cleve. M. Gaz. 1:31–40, 1859.
Virchow, R.: Die krankhaften Geschwulste. Berlin, A. Hirschwald, 1863.
Waldeyer, W.: Grosses Lipo-myxom des Mesenteriums mit secondaren sarcomatosen Heerden in der Leber und Lunge. Virchows Arch. [Pathol. Anat.] 32:543, 1865.
Arnold, J.: Ein Fall von angebornem lipomatosem Teratom der Stirngegend. Virchows Arch. [Pathol. Anat.] 43:181, 1868.
Bourneville, D. M.: Contribution a l'etude de l'idiotie. Sclerose tubereuse des circonvolutions cerebrales; idiotie et epilepsie hemiplegique. Arch. Neurol. 1:81, 1880.
Watson, E.: Non-malignant tumors of the spermatic cord, and their diagnosis from hernia. Lancet 1:792, 1885.
Hellman, L.: Ueber den Ursprungsort der Weichteilsarcome der Regio inguinalis. Wurzburg, H. Sturtz, 1888.
Salzer, F.: Myxoma lipomatodes capsulae adiposae renis. Wien. Klin. Wochenschr. 1:199, 1888.
Unna, P. G.: Zur Kenntnis den Kerne. Monatsschr. Prakt. Dermat. 20:597, 1895.
Adami, J. G.: On retroperitoneal and perirenal lipomata. Montreal Med. J. 25:529, 1897.
Morestin, M.: Lipome intra-musculaire congenital. Bull. Soc. Anat. 72:939, 1897.
Lenger, L.: Liposarcome de la capsule surrenale droite. Ann. Soc. Chir. 7:128, 1899.
Brewis, A. R.: Case of lipoma in right ventricle of heart. Lancet 2:829, 1905.
Merkel, H.: Uber ein Pseudolipom der Mamma (eigenartiger Fettzelltumor). Beitr. Pathol. Anat. 39:152, 1906.
Beriel, L.: A propos de la classification de certain tumeurs malignes: les lipomes malins. Lyon chir. 4:537, 1910.
Wohlgemuth, H.: Demonstration eines Myxosarkome aus einem Lipom enstanden. Verh. Berl. med. Gesellsch. 40:22, 1910.
Fischer, W.: Die Nierentumoren bei der Tuberosen Hirsklerose. Zeigler Beitr. path. anat. U.Z. allg. Path. 50:235, 1911.
Bowen, J. T.: Multiple subcutaneous hemangiomas, together with multiple lipomas, occurring in enormous numbers in an otherwise healthy, muscular subject. Am. J. Med. Sci. 114:189, 1912.
Kuttner, H., and Landois, F.: Die chirurgie der Quergestreiften Muskulatur. Dtsch. Chir. 25:228, 1913.
Bonnel, F.: Tumeur du creux de l'aisselle. Bull. Mem. Soc. Anat. Paris 89:110, 1914–1919.
Ehrmann, W. B.: Ein eigenartiges Angioliposarkom der Niere. Frankfurt. Z. Pathol. 15:51, 1914.
Robertson, H. E.: Lipoma myxomatodes. J. Med. Res. 35:131, 1916.
Schiller, H.: Lipoma of the funiculus spermaticus. Ann. Surg. 68:269, 1918.
Hirsch, E. F., and Wells, H. G.: Retroperitoneal liposarcoma. Report of an unusually large specimen with chemical analysis. Am. J. Med. Sci. 159:356, 1920.
Strauss, A.: Lipoma of tendon sheaths; with report of case and review of literature. Surg. Gynec. Obstet. 35:161, 1922.
Beyers, C. F.: A case of "subpleural" lipoma in a child. Lancet 1:283, 1923.
Blavet di Briga, C.: Transformazione sarcomatosa di un lipoma mixomatoso. Arch. Sci. Med. 46:204, 1923.
Hinman, F., and Gibson, T. E.: Tumors of the epididymis, spermatic cord and testicular tunics. A review of the literature and report of three new cases. Arch. Surg. 8:100, 1924.
Jaffe, R. H.: Recurrent lipomatous tumors of the groin. Liposarcoma and lipoma pseudomyxomatodes. Arch. Pathol. 1:381, 1926.
Moriconi, L. M.: Lipoma intramuscular del muscolo gran dorsale de destra nella sua porizone ascellare. Policlinico 33:366, 1926.
Cecil, A. B.: Intrascrotal lipomata. J. Urol. 17:557, 1927.
Inglis, K.: So-called interscapular gland and tumors arising therein. J. Anat. 61:452, 1927.
Ewing, J.: Neoplastic Diseases, 3rd edition. Philadelphia, W. B. Saunders Co., 1928.
Martin, H. S.: Massive lipoma of the subcutaneous tissue of the back. JAMA 90:2013, 1928.
Babes, A.: Sur l'histopathologie du lipome recidivant du type du lipome glandulaire proliferant. Bull. Cancer (Paris) 18:334, 1929.
Behrend, M.: Intermuscular lipomas. Report of three cases. Am. J. Surg. 7:857–860, 1929.

Walford, A.: Lipoma of larynx. J. Laryngol. Otol. 45:548, 1930.
Comfort, M. W.: Submucous lipomata of the gastrointestinal tract. Report of 28 cases. Surg. Gynec. Obstet. 52:101, 1931.
Stewart, F. W.: Primary liposarcoma of the bone. Am. J. Pathol. 7:87, 1931.
Adair, F. E., Pack, G. T., and Farrior, J. H.: Lipomas. Am. J. Cancer 16:1104, 1932.
Critchley, M., and Earl, C. J. C.: Tuberosa sclerosis and allied conditions. Brain 55:311, 1932.
Jones, T. E., and McClintock, J. C.: Liposarcoma. Ann. Surg. 98: 470, 1933.
Geschickter, C. F.: Lipoid tumor. Am. J. Cancer 21:617, 1934.
Siegmund, H.: Lipoblastic sarcomatose. Virchows Arch. [Pathol. Anat.] 293:458, 1934.
Ewing, J.: Fascial sarcoma and intermuscular myxoliposarcoma. Arch. Surg. 31:507, 1935.
Geormatigh, N., Venderlinden, P., and dePuysselier, R.: Lipocytomes et lipocyteses (lipoblastomes et lipoblastoses). Cancer (Bruxelles) 13:3, 1936–1937.
Haagensen, C. D., and Krehbiel, O. F.: Liposarcoma produced by 1:2-benzpyrene. Am. J. Cancer 27:474, 1936.
Menne, F. R., and Birge, R. F.: Primary liposarcoma of great omentum. Arch. Pathol. 22:823, 1936.
Shaw, A. F. B.: Embryonal cell liposarcoma. J. Pathol. Bacteriol. 43:277, 1936.
Baker, A. B., and Adams, J. M.: Lipomatosis of central nervous system. Am. J. Cancer 34:214, 1938.
Pack, G. T., and Anglem, T. J.: Tumors of soft somatic tissue in infancy and childhood. J. Pediat. 15:373, 1939.
Wells, H. G.: Adipose tissue, a neglected subject. JAMA 114:2177, 1940.
Abrams, H. J., and Turberville, J. S.: Liposarcoma of stomach. South. Surg. 10:891, 1941.
Bass, M. H.: Lipoma of mesentery in child aged 2 years. J. Mt. Sinai Hosp. 7:289, 1941.
Froug, C.: Liposarcoma of kidney; review of literature and case report. J. Urol. 45:290, 1941.
Ackerman, L. V., and Wheeler, P.: Liposarcoma. South. Med. J. 35:156, 1942.
Ewing, J.: Neoplastic Diseases, 4th edition. Philadelphia, W. B. Saunders Co., 1942.
Murray, M. R., and Stout, A. P.: Characteristics of liposarcoma grown "in vitro." Am. J. Pathol. 19:751, 1943.
Ackerman, L. V.: Multiple primary liposarcomas. Am. J. Pathol. 20:789, 1944.
Stout, A. P.: Liposarcoma—malignant tumor of lipoblasts. Ann. Surg. 119:86, 1944.
Symmers, D.: Spindle and giant cell sarcoma arising from unidentified precordial bodies. Arch. Pathol. 37:180, 1944.
Regan, J. M., Bickel, W. H., and Broders, A. C.: Infiltrating benign lipomas of the extremities. W.J. Surg. Obstet. Gynecol. 54:87, 1946.
Van Meurs, D. P.: Transformation of embryonic lipoma to common lipoma. Br. J. Surg. 34:282, 1946–1947.
Watts, C. F., Clagett, O. T., and McDonald, J. R.: Lipoma of the bronchus. J. Thorac. Surg. 15:132, 1946.
Oosthuizen, S. F., and Barletson, J.: Two cases of lipomatosis involving bone. Br. J. Radiol. 20:426, 1947.
Soebo, J.: Lipoma conjuctivae in 3 generations. Acta Ophthalmol. 26:447, 1948.
Wright, C. J. E.: Liposarcoma arising in a simple lipoma. J. Pathol. Bacteriol. 60:484, 1948.
Brines, O. A., and Johnson, M. H.: Hibernoma a special fatty tumor. Am. J. Pathol. 25:467, 1949.
Farbman, A. A.: Retroperitoneal fatty tumors: Report of case and collective review of literature from 1937 to 1947. Arch. Surg. 60:343, 1950.
Kittle, C. F., Boley, J. O., and Schafer, P.W.: Resection of an intrathoracic "Hibernoma." J. Thorac. Surg. 19:830, 1950.
Ayres, W. W., Firminger, H. I., and Hamilton, P. K.: Birefringent and sudanophilic lipoids in the adrenal cortex in disease and sudden death. Milit. Surg. 109:503, 1951.
Morgan, G. S., Straumfjord, J. V., and Hall, E. J.: Angiomyolipoma of the kidney. J. Urol. 65:525, 1951.
Cant, W. H. P., and Astley, R.: Lipoma of corpus callosum. Arch. Dis. Child. 27:478, 1952.
Sternberg, S. S.: Liposarcoma arising within a subcutaneous lipoma. Cancer 5:975, 1952.
Sutherland, J. C., Callahan, W. P., and Campbell, G. L.: Hibernoma. Cancer 5:364, 1952.
Gross, S., and Wood, C.: Hibernoma. Cancer 6:159, 1953.
Stout, A. P.: Tumors of the Soft Tissue. Washington, D.C., Armed Forces Institute of Pathology, 1953.
Caputo, N. T., and Spaulding, E. D.: Mediastinal liposarcoma. Harper Hosp. Bull. 11:122, 1953.
Harvard, M. B.: Retroperitoneal lipoma in children; report of a case and review of literature. J. Urol. 70:159, 1953.
Knowles, C. H., and Huggill, P. H.: Liposarcoma: with report of a case in a child. J. Pathol. Bacteriol. 68:235, 1954.
Pack, J. T., and Pierson, J. C.: Liposarcoma, a study of 105 cases. Surgery 36:687, 1954.
Yui, S.: Retroperitoneal liposarcoma in adult: a case report and review of literature. Gann, Tokyo 45:269, 1954.
Berg, J. W.: Angiolipomyosarcoma of kidney (malignant hamartomatous angiolipo-

myomata) in a case with solitary metastasis from a bronchogenic carcinoma. Cancer 8:764, 1955.

Brandenburg, W.: Beitrag zur Kenntnis der Riesenzellgeschwulste (Myxo-lipo-fibrosarcoma). Zentralbl. Allg. Pathol. 93:400, 1955.

Child, P. L.: Lipoma of the os calcis: report of a case. Am. J. Clin. Pathol. 25:1050, 1955.

Stedfeld, G.: Echte Lipome des Meniskus. Arch. Orthop. Unfallchir. 47:399, 1955.

Kanter, A. E., and Zummo, B. P.: Lipomas of gynecologic interest. Am. J. Obstet. Gynecol. 71:376, 1956.

Mackay-Dick, J., Harrison, G. K., and Rothnil, N. G.: Lipothymoma: report of a case and review of the literature. J. R. Army Med. Corps 102:39, 1956.

Caram, P. C., Scarcella, G., and Carton, C. A.: Intradural lipomas of spinal cord; with particular emphasis on "intermedullary" lipomas. J. Neurosurg. 14:28, 1957.

Plaut, A.: The notched nucleus of the fat cell (Unna's Lochkern). J. Mt. Sinai Hosp. 24:1112, 1957.

Vellios, F., Baez, J., and Shumacker, H. B.: Lipoblastomatosis: A tumor of fetal fat different from hibernoma. Am. J. Pathol. 34:1149, 1958.

Kauffman, S. L., and Stout, A. P.: Lipoblastic tumors of children. Cancer 12:912, 1959.

Parsons, L., and Thompson, J. E.: Symptomatic myelolipoma of the adrenal gland. Report of a case and review of the literature. N. Engl. J. Med. 260:12, 1959.

Enterline, H. T., Culbertson, J. D., Rochlin, D. B., and Brady, L. W.: Liposarcoma. A clinical and pathological study of 53 cases. Cancer 13:932, 1960.

Hartveit, F. and Hallerbraker, B.: Report of three angiolipomyomata and one angiolipomyosarcoma. Acta Pathol. Microbiol. Scand. 49:329, 1960.

Howard, W. R., and Helwig, E. B.: Angiolipoma. Arch. Dermatol. 82:924, 1960.

McGregor, J. D.: Liposarcoma of the breast. Case report and review of the literature. Can. Med. Assoc. J. 82:781, 1960.

Sampson, C. C., Saunders, E. H., Green, W. E., and Laurey, J. R.: Liposarcoma developing in a lipoma. Arch. Pathol. 69:506, 1960.

Winslow, D. J., and Enzinger, F. M.: Hyaluronidase-sensitive acid mucopolysaccharides in liposarcomas. Am. J. Pathol. 37:497, 1960.

Enzinger, F. M., and Winslow, D. J.: Liposarcoma: A study of 103 cases. Virchows Arch.[Pathol. Anat.] 335:367, 1962.

Krause, L. B., and Ross, C.: Intrathoracic lipomas. Arch. Surg. 84:444, 1962.

Phelan, J. T., and Perez-Mesa, C.: Liposarcoma of the superficial tissues. Surg. Gynecol. Obstet. 115:609, 1962.

Scarpelli, D. G., and Greider, M. H.: A correlative cytochemical and electron microscopic study of a liposarcoma. Cancer 15:776, 1962.

White, W. L., and Hanna, D. C.: Troublesome lipomata of the upper extremity. J. Bone Joint Surg. 44A:1353, 1962.

Catto, M., and Stevens, J.: Liposarcoma of bone. J. Pathol. Bacteriol. 86:248, 1963.

Mayo, C. W., Pagtalunan, R. J. G., and Brown, D. J.: Lipoma of the alimentary tract. Surgery 53:598, 1963.

Cox, R. W.: Hibernoma—the lipoma of immature adipose tissue. J. Pathol. Bacteriol. 68:511, 1964.

Estevez, J. M., Thompson, D. S., and Levinson, J. P.: Lipoma of the heart. Review of the literature and report of two autopsied cases. Arch. Pathol. 77:638, 1964.

Goldman, R. L.: Primary liposarcoma of the bone. Am. J. Clin. Pathol. 42:503, 1964.

Booher, R. J.: Lipoblastic tumors of the hands and feet. Review of the literature and report of 33 cases. J. Bone Joint Surg. 47A:727, 1965.

Hawkins, P. E., and Terrell, G. K.: Liposarcoma of the stomach. JAMA 191:154, 1965.

Ashby, B. S., and MacGillivray, J. B.: Paratesticular lipoma. Br. J. Surg. 53:828, 1966.

Eibel, P.: Juxtamalleolar lipomata. Clin. Orthop. 49:191, 1966.

Gonzalez-Crussi, F., Enneking, W. F., and Arean, V. M.: Infiltrating angiolipoma. J. Bone Joint Surg. 48A:1111, 1966.

James, D. H., Johnson, W. W., and Wrenn, E. L.: Effective chemotherapy of an abnormal liposarcoma. J. Pediatr. 68:311, 1966.

Reszel, P. A., Soule, E. H., and Conventry, M. B.: Liposarcoma of the extremities and limb girdles. A study of 222 cases. J. Bone Joint Surg. 48A:229, 1966.

Tanquada, R. E.: Subcutaneous lipomas of sites of insulin injection. Diabetes 15:807, 1966.

Mesara, B. W., and Batsakis, J. G.: Hibernoma of the neck. Arch. Otolaryngol. 85:95, 1967.

Panders, A. K., and Scherpenisse, L. A.: Oral lipoma. Br. J. Oral Surg. 5:33, 1967.

Shear, M.: Lipoblastomatosis of the cheek. Br. J. Oral Surg. 5:173, 1967.

Evans, W. R.: Tumors of adipose tissue. *In* Histological Appearances of Tumors. Baltimore, Williams & Wilkins, 1968.

Farrow, G. M., Harrison, E. G., Utz, D. C., and Jones, D. R.: Renal angiomyolipoma. A clinicopathologic study of 32 cases. Cancer 22:564, 1968.

Newman, P. H., and Silen, W.: Myelolipoma of the adrenal gland. Arch. Surg. 97:637, 1968.

Georgiades, D. E., Alcalais, C. B., and Karabela, V. G.: Multicentric well-differentiated liposarcomas. Cancer 24:1091, 1969.

Hajdu, S. I., and Foote, F. W.: Angiomyolipoma

of the kidney. Report of 27 cases and review of the literature. J. Urol. 102:396, 1969.

Morton, D. L., Hall, W. T., and Malmgren, R. A.: Human liposarcoma: tissue cultures containing foci of transformed cells with viral particles. Science 165:813, 1969.

Das Gupta, T. K.: Tumors and tumor-like conditions of the adipose tissue. Curr. Probl. Surg., April, 1, 1970.

Eilber, F. R., and Morton, D. L.: Immunologic studies of human sarcomas. Cancer 26:588, 1970.

Haasan, M. A.: Subcutaneous liposarcoma of forearm followed by liposarcoma of omentum. Br. J. Surg. 57:393, 1970.

Spittle, M. F., Newton, K. A., and Mackenzie, D. H.: Liposarcoma: A review of 60 cases. Br. J. Cancer 24:696, 1970.

Gyorkey, F., Sinkovics, J. G., and Gyorkey, P.: Electron microscopic observations on structures, resembling myxovirus in human sarcomas. Cancer 27:1449, 1971.

Kimbrough, R. F., and Soule, E. B.: Liposarcoma of the extremities. Clin. Orthop. 19:140, 1971.

Lester J., Rosenklint, A., Rovsing, T., Stephenson, N., and Struve-Christenson, E.: Angiography in tumors of the extremities. Acta Orthop. Scand. 42:152, 1971.

McCullough, D. L., Scott, R., and Seybolt, H. M.: Renal angiomyolipoma (hamartoma): Review of the literature and report of 7 cases. J. Urol. 105:32, 1971.

Zapata, J. E.: El liposarcoma a la luz del cultivo de tejidos. Rev. Clin. Esp. 122:191, 1971.

Boquist, L., Bergdahl, L., and Andersson, A.: Lipomatosis of the ileocecal valve. Cancer 29:136, 1972.

Clark, R. E., and Palubinskas, A. J.: The angiographic spectrum of renal hamartoma. Am. J. Roentgenol. 114:715, 1972.

Golding, P. L., Singh, M., and Worthington, B.: Bilateral ureteric obstruction caused by benign lipomatosis. Br. J. Surg. 59:69, 1972.

Gottlieb, J. A., Baker, L. H., Quagliana, J. M., Luce, J. K., Whitecar, J. P., Sinkovics, J. G., Rivkin, S. E., Brownlee, R., and Frei, E.: Chemotherapy of sarcomas with a combination of adriamycin and dimethyl triazenoimidazole carboxamide. Cancer 30:1632, 1972.

Chung, E. B., and Enzinger, F. M.: Benign lipoblastomatosis: An analysis of 35 cases. Cancer 32:482, 1973.

Kalderon, A. E., and Fethiere, W.: Fine structure of two liposarcomas. Lab. Invest. 28:60, 1973.

Kinne, D. W., Chu, F. C. H., Huvos, A. G., Yagoda, A., and Fortner, J. G.: Treatment of primary and recurrent retroperitoneal liposarcoma. Cancer 31:53, 1973.

Wanebo, H. J., Shah, J., Knapper, W., Hajdu, S. I., and Booher, R.: Reappraisal of surgical management of sarcoma of the buttock. Cancer 31:97, 1973.

Dione, G. P., and Seemayer, T. A.: Infiltrating lipomas and angiolipomas revisited. Cancer 33:732, 1974.

Kindblom, L. G., Angervall, L., Stener, B., and Wickbom, I.: Intermuscular and intramuscular lipomas and hibernomas: A clinical, roentgenologic, histologic and prognostic study of 46 cases. Cancer 33:754, 1974.

Lin, J. J., and Lin, F.: Two entities in angiolipoma: A study of 459 cases of lipoma with review of the literature on infiltrating angiolipoma. Cancer 34:720, 1974.

Enzinger, F. M., and Harvey, D. A.: Spindle cell lipoma. Cancer 36:1852, 1975.

Kindblom, L. G., Angervall, L., and Svendsen, P.: Liposarcoma. A clinicopathologic, radiographic and prognostic study. Acta Pathol. Microbiol. Scand. Suppl. 253:1, 1975.

Shiu, M. H., Castro, E. B., Hajdu, S. I., and Fortner, J. G.: Surgical treatment of 297 soft tissue sarcomas of the lower extremity. Ann. Surg. 182:597, 1975.

Shiu, M. H., Chu, F., Castro, E. B., Hajdu, S. I., and Fortner, J. G.: Results of surgical and radiation therapy in the treatment of liposarcoma arising in an extremity. Am. J. Roentgenol. 123:577, 1975.

Flenker, H.: Myxoid liposarcoma. Light and electron microscopic investigation. Virchows Arch. [Pathol. Anat.] 371:171, 1976.

Gould, V. E., Jao, W., Gould, N. S., and Soto, J. M.: Comparative ultrastructure of hibernomas and myxoid and pleomorphic liposarcomas. Lab. Invest. 34:316 (abstract), 1976.

Hajdu, S. I., and Hajdu, E. O.: Cytopathology of Sarcomas and Other Nonepithelial Malignant Tumors. Philadelphia, W. B. Saunders Co., 1976.

Leyson, J. F. J., Doroshow, L. W., and Robbins, M. A.: Extratesticular lipoma. Report of 2 cases and a new classification. J. Urol. 116:324, 1976.

Varga, A., and Balazsy, S.: A supinator csatornaban elhelyezkedo lipoma okozta nervus radialis laesio. Magy. Traumatol. Orthop. 19:269, 1976.

Walker, D. E., Barry, J. M., and Hodges, C. V.: Angiomyolipoma: Diagnosis and treatment. J. Urol. 116:712, 1976.

Enzinger, F. M.: Benign lipomatous tumors simulating a sarcoma. *In* Management of Primary Bone and Soft Tissue Tumors. Chicago, Year Book Medical Publishers, 1977.

Sethi, J., Hirshaut, Y., Hajdu, S. I., and Clements, L. G.: Growing human sarcomas in culture. Cancer 40:744, 1977.

Baden, E., and Newman, R.: Liposarcoma of the oropharyngeal region. Review of the literature and report of two cases. Oral Surg. 44:889, 1977.

Dardick, I.: Hiberoma: A possible model of brown fat histogenesis. Hum. Pathol. 9:321, 1978.

Desai, U., Ramos, C. V., and Taylor, H. B.: Ultrastructural observations in pleomorphic liposarcoma. Cancer 42:1284, 1978.

Hajdu, S. I., and Fogh, J.: The nude mouse as a diagnostic tool in human tumor cell research. *In* The Nude Mouse in Experimental and Clinical Research. Edited by J. Fogh and B. C. Giovanella. New York, Academic Press, 1978.

Evans, H. L., Soule, E. H., and Winkelmann, R. K.: Atypical lipoma, atypical intramuscular lipoma and well-differentiated retroperitoneal liposarcoma. A reappraisal of 30 cases formerly classified as well-differentiated liposarcoma. Cancer 43:574, 1979.

Kindblom, L. G., and Save-Soderbergh, J.: The ultrastructure of liposarcoma. A study of 10 cases. Acta Pathol. Microbiol. Scand. Sect. A 87:109, 1979.

Politis, J., Funahashi, A., Gehlsen, J. A., DeCock, D., Stengel, B. F., and Choi, H.: Intrathoracic lipomas. J. Thorac. Cardiovasc. Surg. 77:550, 1979.

Reddick, R. L., Michelitch, H., and Triche, T. J.: Malignant soft tissue tumors (malignant fibrous histiocytoma, pleomorphic liposarcoma, and pleomorphic rhabdomyosarcoma): An electron microscopic study. Hum. Pathol. 10:327, 1979.

Saunders, J. R., Jaques, D. A., Casterline, P. F., Percarpio, B., and Goodloe, S., Jr.: Liposarcomas of the head and neck. A review of the literature and addition of four cases. Cancer 43:162, 1979.

Hajdu, S. I., Lemos, L. B., Kozakewich, H., Helson, L., and Beattie, E. J. Jr.: Growth pattern and differentiation of human soft tissue sarcomas in nude mice. Cancer 47:90, 1981.

Hajdu, S. I., Erlandson, R., and Fortner, J. G.: Classification and histologic grading of liposarcomas. Cancer (in press).

Fortner, J.G., Martin, S., Hajdu, S.I., and Turnbull, A.: Primary sarcoma of the retroperitoneum. Semin. Oncol. (In press).

chapter 5

Tumors of Muscle

NON-NEOPLASTIC LESIONS

- ***Atrophy***
- ***Dystrophy***
- ***Myositis***
  - Polymyositis
  - Rhabdomyolysis
  - Myositis Ossificans
  - Proliferative Myositis
- ***Fibromatosis***
- ***Fasciitis***

NEOPLASTIC LESIONS

Tumors of Smooth Muscle

- ***Leiomyoma***
- ***Angiomyolipoma***
- ***Leiomyosarcoma***
- ***Leiomyoblastoma***

Tumors of Striated Muscle

- ***Rhabdomyoma***
- ***Embryonal Rhabdomyosarcoma***
  - Alveolar Rhabdomyosarcoma
  - Botryoid Sarcoma
- ***Pleomorphic Rhabdomyosarcoma***
- ***Rhabdomyoblastoma***

THE normal development of muscle progresses from small round cells (*myoblasts*) through a spindle cell form (*myocyte*) to multinucleate the muscle fiber. Longitudinal striation and, in the case of skeletal muscle, transverse striation appear at the most advanced stage of differentiation. Histologically, it was Leeuwenhoek, in 1721, who first distinguished smooth and striated muscle fibers (see Chapter 1, Fig. 1-9B).

The myoblast of the 7- to 9-week-old fetus is a small cell with little cytoplasm and a deeply stained homogeneous ovoid or spherical nucleus. As the myoblast acquires more cytoplasm, bipolar myocytes develop and longitudinal myofibrils appear. Myofibrils gradually increase in number, filling the cytoplasm and finally pushing the nucleus to its adult peripheral position. Muscle fibers fuse and multinucleated fibers appear at about 12 weeks during embryonic life.

In normal muscle, the muscle fibers lie in apposition to one another and present a polygonal appearance. Sarcolemmal nuclei are small and peripherally positioned. The diameter of muscle fibers varies with age and sex. At one year of age the average diameter of fibers is 15 μ, and there is a steady yearly increase of 2 to 4 microns until adult size is reached at 12 to 15 years of age.

Muscle has been studied intensively with both the light and the electron microscope. Details of structure and function of muscle are considered in a number of review articles (Pepe, 1967; Zachs, 1970).

Skeletal muscle is composed of multinucleated *muscle fibers* of various lengths. Each muscle fiber is surrounded by an electrically polarized membrane, the *sarcolemma*. In the cytoplasm or sarcoplasm of each muscle cell are the *myofibrils*, the contractile apparatus, and the *sarcoplasmic reticulum*, a complex tubular system which plays an important role in the activation and relaxation of the contractile system. In addition to these elaborate and highly differentiated components, the cytoplasm also contains lipid droplets, glycogen granules, and other elements such as mitochondria and RNA particles (Fig. 5-1).

Ultrastructurally the sarcolemma has two components, the *plasma membrane* and the *basement membrane*. The basement membrane stains positive with PAS stain and is believed to play an important role in maintaining the shape of individual cells.

The model for striated muscle with the double array of filaments, originally proposed by Hanson and Huxley in 1953, has remained essentially unchanged. According to this model each *myofibril* contains a number of *myofilaments* of various lengths and thicknesses. The characteristic dark and light banding of each myofibril, which gives the typical striated pattern of the whole muscle fiber, is due to the highly ordered and repetitious arrangements of the myofilaments. The dark

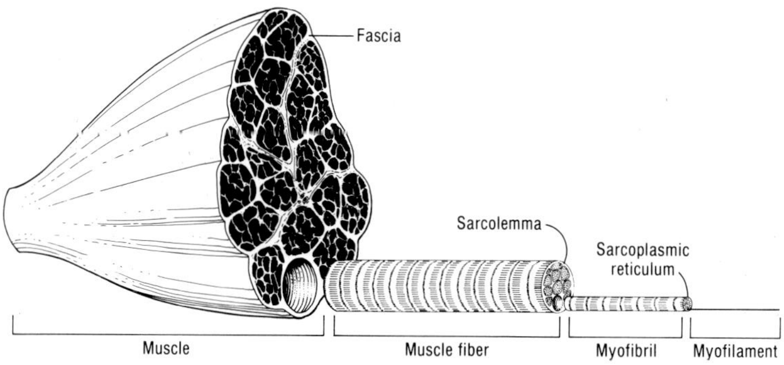

Figure 5-1. Schematic illustration of skeletal muscle and the relationship between various basic components.

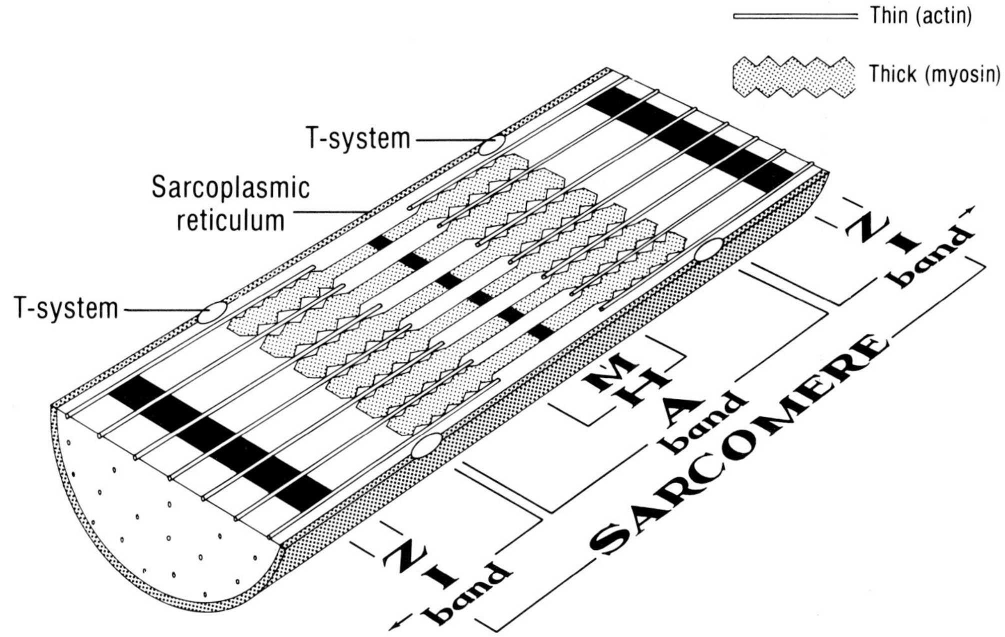

Figure 5-2. Schematic illustration of the structural unit, the sarcomere, of a myofibril. The band pattern of the myofibrils is caused by the highly ordered arrangement of the myofilaments (see also Figure 5-44).

band is anisotropic and is called the A band. The light band is isotropic and is called the I band. At the center of each A band is a pale H zone which is bisected by an M line; each I band is bisected by a dense Z line. The structural unit delineated by two successive Z lines is called a *sarcomere.* The average length of a sarcomere varies from 2 to 3 μ (Fig. 5-2).

The myofilaments are designated as *thick,* 100 Å in diameter (myosin), and *thin* (actin and tropomyosin) filaments. The A band is composed of interdigitating thick and thin filaments. The thick filaments are found only in the A band. The thin filaments, on the other hand, form the I band and extend into the A band as far as the H zone.

The thick filaments appear rough under the electron microscope, owing to the presence of lateral projections at regular intervals which seem to touch the adjacent segments of the thin filaments. Histochemical studies indicate that ATPase activity is confined to the site of projections between the thick and thin filaments. The ultrastructure of the Z line and its relationship to the thin filaments forming the I band is not well understood, but according to Price (1963) the ends of opposing I band filaments are interconnected with each other by finer filaments within the Z line. In muscle contraction the thick and thin filaments are driven past each other by a stereospecific interaction between the actin and myosin molecules, and the chemical bonds between these filaments are strongest during contraction.

The precise chemical composition of Z bands is far from ascertained, but Henson-Stiennon's (1965) description of "Z-bodies" as precursors of Z band material is generally accepted. This concept was furthered by Kelly (1969) who advanced the theory that in the genesis of Z bands from Z bodies the formation of a skein-like network of fine strands (myofilaments) is essential. *The skein-like network is an important component of many mesenchymal cells,* e.g., fibroblasts and chondroblasts, and usually is located at the cell periphery. According to Becher and Nachman (1973) platelets and megakaryocytes also contain a contractile protein, thrombosthenin, which biochemically resembles the actomyosin of smooth muscle (Rikihisa and Mizuno, 1977; Yablonka and Yaffe, 1977).

In the muscle cell each filament of skein appears to serve as the initial focus for attachment of the 1 μ long actin filaments. The synthesis of the actin filaments remains to be determined, but it is known that actin filaments are present near the skeins. Therefore, it is not unreasonable to believe that when muscle cells differentiate, the process begins with the elaboration of skeins (myofilaments composed of tropomyosin). This is followed by the appearance of Z-bodies prior to assembly of myosin filaments in the ribosome-rich interior of the cell. The formation of these components into A and I bands takes place in a gradual fashion. The earliest phase of this elaborate sequence probably corresponds to the *non-striated fibril stage* described by Holtzer, in 1961. The Z bands are merely formed as a consequence of the tension during registration throughout a myofibril, and they serve as filament-to-filament attachment sites between sarcomeres (Alexander and Bossen, 1978).

According to Zacchei and Caravita (1972) trypsin-dissociated muscle cells in tissue culture re-establish a structure similar to muscle tissue, but a disorder of the contractile units within the sarcoplasm indicates that the factors responsible for the orientated disposition of myofibrils is ineffective in tissue culture.

Veratti, in 1902, while working in Golgi's laboratory, demonstrated a fibrillar network, the *sarcomplasmic reticulum,* which surrounds the myofibrils and is composed of a complex network of *tubules* arranged in a coordinated pattern and having the striations of the myofibrils. This individual reticular sheath with its transverse tubular structure was ignored until it was rediscovered in 1953, by Bennett and Porter. The exact role of the sarcoplasmic reticulum is debated, but it is known to play a role in the return of the contracted fiber to a relaxed position. It apparently represents a communication network capable of storing and transferring intra- and extracellular information from the neuromuscular junction to mechanical action.

The *Golgi apparatus* is a rather inconspicuous structure in normal skeletal muscle and the *mitochondria* appear no different from those of other cells. The mitochondrion lies beneath the sarcolemma adjacent to the nucleus and is present in the A band region.

The nuclei of mature skeletal muscle are located in the periphery of the muscle fiber adjacent to the sarcolemma. Multinucleated skeletal muscle fibers form by the fusion of cells. Fusion is initiated by the recognition of homotypic cells and is mediated by specific molecular markers on the cell surface (Cooper and Konigsberg, 1961; Okazaki and Holtzer, 1966). With various histochemical stains, including adenosine triphosphatase (ATPase), two major types of fibers (Type I and Type II) can be distinguished in the human skeletal muscle (Table 5-1).

TABLE 5-1. ***Characteristics of Human Skeletal Muscle Fibers***

TYPE I	TYPE II
Stain dark with H & E	Stain light with H & E
Stain light with PAS	Stain dark with PAS
Stain light with ATPase	Stain dark with ATPase
Red *in vivo*	White *in vivo*
Slow contractile	Fast contractile
1/3 of muscle	2/3 of muscle
Male: 62 μ	Male: 69 μ
Female: 58 μ	Female: 50 μ

NON-NEOPLASTIC LESIONS

The basic non-neoplastic histopathologic diseases of muscle are atrophy, dystrophy, and myositis. Today, histochemical typing of muscle fibers using the myosin ATPase reaction is considered essential for complete histopathologic interpretation of muscle (Table 5-1). The information available from formalin-fixed, paraffin-embedded, longitudinal sections of muscle frequently complements that obtained from frozen transverse sections. Gross examination of the muscle tissue in non-neoplastic lesions is only rarely of diagnostic value.

ATROPHY

In general, atrophy of muscle means abnormally small myofibers. Atrophy may result from denervation disuse, metabolic changes, and a number of other causes. The earliest sign of *denervation atrophy* is the "rounding up" and central migration of the nuclei and increased nucleolar size. Occasional myofibers may be fragmented and vacuolated. In long-standing cases the myofibers disappear, hyaline bodies appear within myofibers, and the interstitial spaces are filled with fibroadipose tissue (Fig. 5-3). The amount of glycogen stainable with PAS is decreased, whereas the myosin ATPase activity is only slightly affected. If only a portion of the nerve is affected, there is a scattering of atrophic myofibers among normal appearing myofibers. This form of atrophy may be seen in many forms of neuropathy induced by *metabolic, toxic,* or *infectious agents.* While the division of muscle lesions into neurogenic atrophy and primary myopathy has proved useful, recent evidence suggests the distinction may be less valid than previously thought,

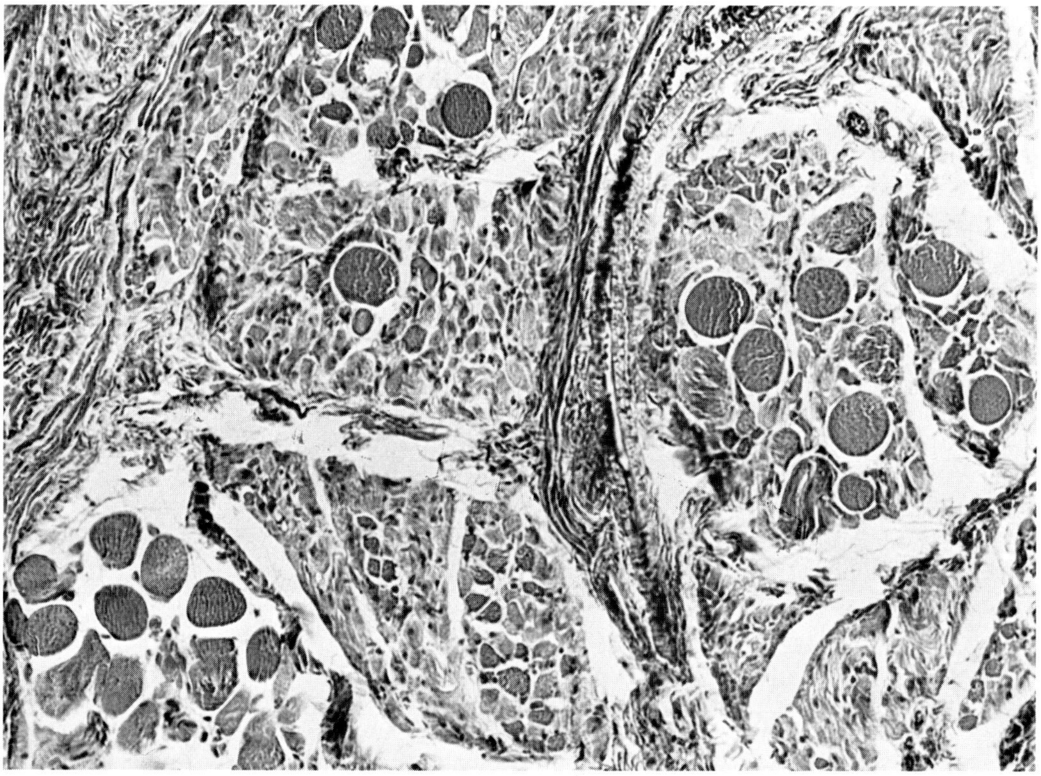

Figure 5-3. Denervation atrophy of skeletal muscle. Many myofibers are collapsed and replaced by fibroadipose tissue (H & E, ×35).

TABLE 5-2. *Comparison of Microscopic Features*

DENERVATION ATROPHY	MUSCULAR DYSTROPHY
Affects Type I and Type II fibers	Atrophy of myofibers Type I
Loss of myofibers	Patchy hypertrophy of fibers
Necrosis of fibers	Variation of myofiber size
Target fibers	Focal necrosis of fibers
Decrease in size of myofibrils	Myofibrillar eosinophilia
Loss of myofilaments	Rounded myofibers
Disorganized Z bands	Longitudinal splitting of fibers
Increased number of nuclei	Ring fibers
Clumping of sarcolemmal nuclei	Fatty and fibrous replacement
Basophilia	Basophilia
Fibers replaced by fat and fibrous tissue	Sarcoplasmic swelling
Loss of mitochondria	Sarcoplasmic histiocytic infiltrate
	Absence of myosin ATPase activity

since similar muscular changes are observed not infrequently in myasthenia gravis, muscular dystrophy, disuse atrophy, malnutrition, and carcinomatous myopathy.

In denervation atrophy the normal mosaic pattern of type I and type II fibers is missing. Both types of fibers are affected; however, in chronic denervation atrophy there are large groups of either type I or type II myofibers. Other suggestive or specific changes are summarized in Table 5-2. Exclusive atrophy of type II fibers has been described in disuse and steroid-induced myopathies.

Partial or complete muscle necrosis or localized unilateral or bilateral muscle hypertrophy of unknown etiology (e.g., in the masseter) may simulate a malignant tumor clinically. In most of these conditions biopsy is essential to establish the nature of the lesion.

DYSTROPHY

The classification and subclassification of clinical varieties of muscular dystrophy have been the subject of numerous articles (Pearse and Walton, 1962; Oteruelo et al, 1972; Oxenhandler et al, 1977). With the exception of *myotonic dystrophy,* a disease of type I fibers, the clinical varieties of muscular dystrophy cannot be distinguished one from another on the basis of muscle biopsy. In myotonic dystrophy, as well as in muscular dystrophy, Huvos and Pruzinski (1967) found that all types of muscle—skeletal, smooth, and cardiac—are involved. The distinguishing features of myotonic dystrophy are myofiber hypertrophy, long chains of central nuclei, and no sign of regeneration.

All observers agree that the histologic morphology of the muscle in *nonmyotonic muscular dystrophy* depends more upon the stage of the disease than upon clinical presentation. The most commonly seen changes in dystrophic muscles are summarized in Table 5-2.

In addition to myopathies such as those induced by toxic substances and infectious agents, Zacks (1970) listed a number of newer forms of myopathies (nemaline myopathy, central core disease, centronuclear myopathy, vacuolar myopathy, mitochondrial myopathy) all of which are without known etiology. *Carcinomatous neuromyopathy* is found not uncommonly in patients with advanced neoplasms. According to Croft and Wilkinson (1963), 6% of the men with carcinoma of the lung and 4% of the women with mammary carcinoma have carcinomatous neuromyopathy. Landing et al (1974) reported that in addition to muscular dystrophy the number of nuclei of the myofiber per millimeter, the surface area of fiber per nucleus, and the cytoplasmic volume per nucleus increase with fiber diameter in *Pompe's disease* and *Down's syndrome*. It has been suggested that an increase in the number of nuclei per millimeter of fiber in these and other myopathies is a response to fiber weakness (Fig. 5-4).

Subsarcolemmal *tubular aggregates* represent a relatively nonspecific response of striated muscle fibers to a variety of injuries. Schiaggino et al (1977) proposed that this material derives from the Z bands and is formed by the rearrangement of the sarcoplasmic reticulum.

More and more investigators think that many forms of muscular dystrophy are not purely muscular disorders but also include some fundamental neuronal defect. Hence, it is certain that better understanding and treatment of muscular dystrophies will emerge from better delineation of electrochemical processes in skeletal muscle.

MYOSITIS

While a mass appearing in the muscle must be regarded as a neoplasm from the clinical point of view, microscopic examination of such a lesion often reveals some type of benign non-neoplastic lesion. Localized myositis may mimic a neoplasm and may result from *ischemia, thromboembolic* or *granulomatous diseases, bacterial* and *viral infections,* as well as from *parasitic* or *protozoal infestation.*

Polymyositis. The least understood form of myositis is polymyositis. On the basis of vascular deposits of IgG in polymyositis, it has been proposed that one possible mechanism leading to muscle injury is through immune complexes (Whitaker and Engel, 1972; Oxenhandler et al, 1977). It is a nonhereditary disease which affects predominantly the girdle muscles. Two thirds of the patients have cutaneous (*dermatomyositis*) as well as muscular

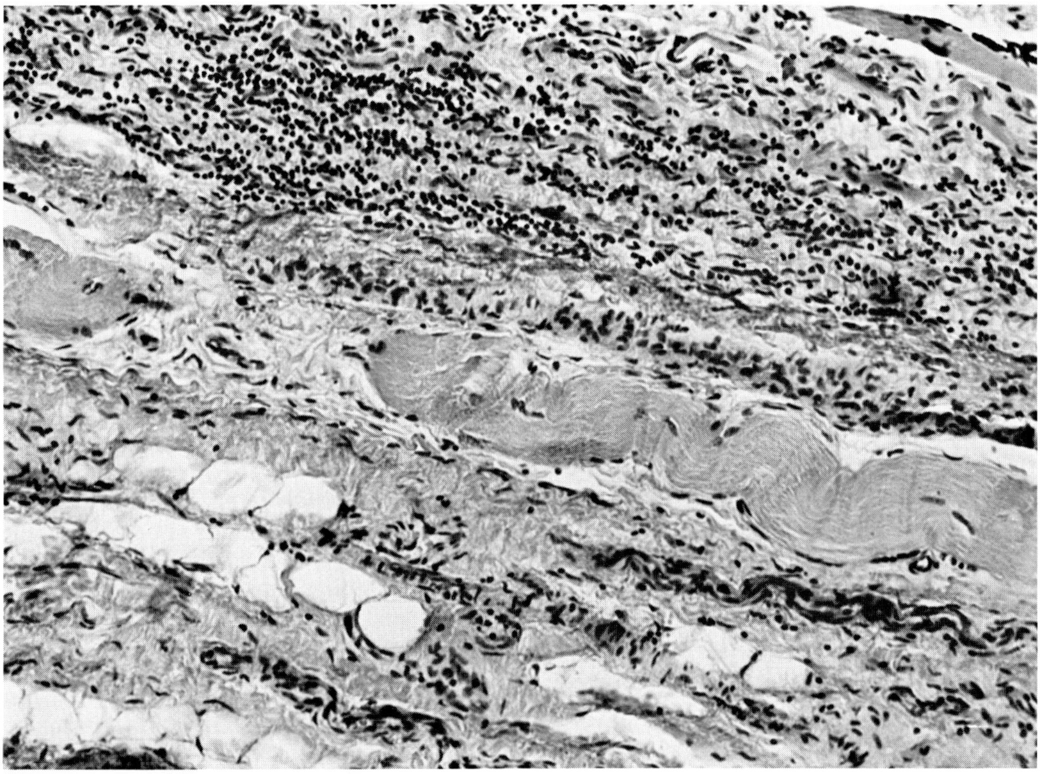

Figure 5-4. In muscular dystrophy there is evidence of myofiber hypertrophy with many centrally placed nuclei, longitudinal breakdown of muscle fibers, and replacement by fibroadipose tissue. Notice the florid inflammatory infiltrate (H & E, ×85).

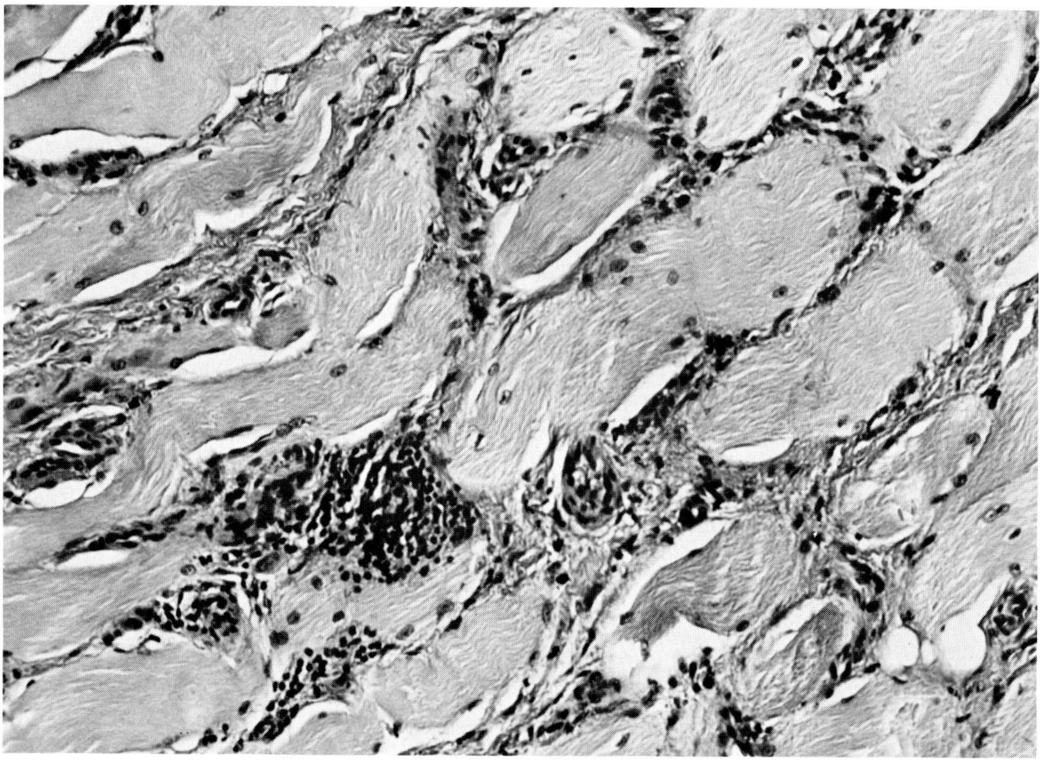

Figure 5-5. The perimysium is infiltrated by inflammatory cells in myositis. There is also evidence of focal necrosis and degeneration of muscle fibers (H & E, ×85).

changes and the incidence of malignant neoplasms is estimated to be 20%. Polymyositis can be clinically acute or chronic. *Histologically the end stage of the disease cannot be distinguished from muscular changes in denervation atrophy and muscular dystrophy.* At the early stage of the disease, one may find segmental degeneration, necrosis, and regeneration of muscle fibers with areas of inflammatory infiltrate of the endomysium and perimysium and sarcoplasmic degeneration (Fig. 5-5). Loss of myosin and ATPase activity are other nonspecific findings.

Rhabdomyolysis. A form of myositis that may be paroxysmal, gives rise to *myoglobinuria,* and is related to strenuous physical exercise is known as rhabdomyolysis. It is not uncommonly complicated by *oliguria* and elevated *creatine phosphokinase* as well as *lactic dehydrogenase* activity in the serum. In the muscle there is generalized necrosis of muscle fibers with concomitant attempts of regeneration. The destruction of muscle fibers is more severe than in polymyositis, but despite severe inflammatory infiltrate the endomysium and sarcolemma remain intact.

Focal collection of inflammatory cells associated with various degrees of muscle necrosis can be seen in a number of diseases, e.g., *rheumatoid arthritis, scleroderma, lupus erythematosus* and *dermatomyositis.* It is doubtful, however, whether muscle biopsy adds anything to the clinical and laboratory findings.

Myositis Ossificans.* This disease is characterized by deposits of ectopic bone in muscle as the result of trauma. The first case of myositis ossificans was reported in 1740 by Freke. However, according to historians the first example of myositis ossificans is the much discussed "femoral exostosis" of the Pithecanthropus erectus.

* *Synonyms and related terms:* myositis ossificans progressiva, localized myositis ossificans, myositis ossificans conscripta, Münchmeyer's disease.

Munchmeyer, in 1869, gave to the disease the name, earlier suggested by Dusch, and reported a series of 12 cases. It is usually a self-limited oval or round lesion with well-delineated, often partly calcified bony trabeculae in sparsely cellular fibroconnective tissue (Fig. 5-6). Rarely is it more than a localized lesion. Helferisch noted *microdactylia* in connection with the so-called systemic or progressive form which is believed to be a hereditary bone disorder. In most instances myositis ossificans is a benign non-neoplastic condition as a sequela to trauma and nothing more than local surgical excision is indicated. In a handful of cases myositis ossificans turned to a malignant neoplasm. Pack and Braund, in 1942, reported three fatal malignant tumors which arose from myositis ossificans.

Proliferative Myositis. Also known as myositis proliferans, proliferative myositis is an inflammatory pseudotumor of skeletal muscle. Kern, in 1960, reported a series of 7 cases of rapidly growing muscular lesions consisting of an ill-defined proliferation of fibroblasts and bizarre ganglion-like giant cells. He named the condition proliferative myositis. A possible relationship of proliferative myositis to myositis ossificans was suggested, and there are a few known cases of proliferative myositis with osteoid formation (Enzinger and Dulcey, 1967). Unlike nodular fasciitis, proliferative myositis does not primarily involve the subcutaneous tissues or fascia of the upper extremity, nor does it contain hypercellular pseudosarcomatous areas. Heffner et al, in 1977, reported 16 cases of so-called focal myositis that presented as rapidly enlarging and painful soft tissue tumors, and affected both children and adults.

Grossly, the nodule of proliferative myositis may range from a few to several centimeters. It is usually a deeply seated, rapidly growing lesion of the muscles of the shoulder, upper arm, thigh, or buttock. It is predominantly a disease of middle-aged males and is virtually nonexistent in children.

Microscopically, the lesion is poorly defined and affects mainly the perimysium, epimysium, and fascia. The two chief microscopic components of proliferative myositis are proliferating fibroblasts and loosely arranged nests of polygonal, ganglion-like, basophilic giant cells of the pleomorphic histiocytic type (Fig. 5-7). The treatment by local excision almost always assures no recurrence.

FIBROMATOSIS

(See Chapter 2.)

FASCIITIS

(See Chapter 2.)

NEOPLASTIC LESIONS

Tumors of Smooth Muscles

The first illustration of a tumor of apparently smooth muscle origin, a submucosal uterine leiomyoma, was published by Hody in 1747. Virchow (1854) is credited with the first use of the word *myoma.* The first two reported cases of malignant smooth muscle tumors were primary tumors of the saphenous vein and the inferior vena cava (Aufrecht, in 1868; and Perl, in 1871). The first report of a leiomyosarcoma in the United States was published by Mason, in 1883. A vascular myoma of the uterus with intravascular extension was reported by Sitzenfrey, in 1911, and the first account of multiple primary leiomyomas of the lung was made by Deussing, in 1912.

Bartkowiak, in 1936, first used the term *leiomyoblastoma* in reporting a case. In 1939, Nelson demonstrated that prolonged administration of estrogen may produce a smooth muscle tumor in the uterus, and Steiner reported on matastasizing leiomyoma of the uterus. Ackerman and Stout, in 1947, reported a case of leiomyosarcoma of the arm and Stout and Hill, in 1958, summarized their experience with leiomyosarcomas of soft tissues.

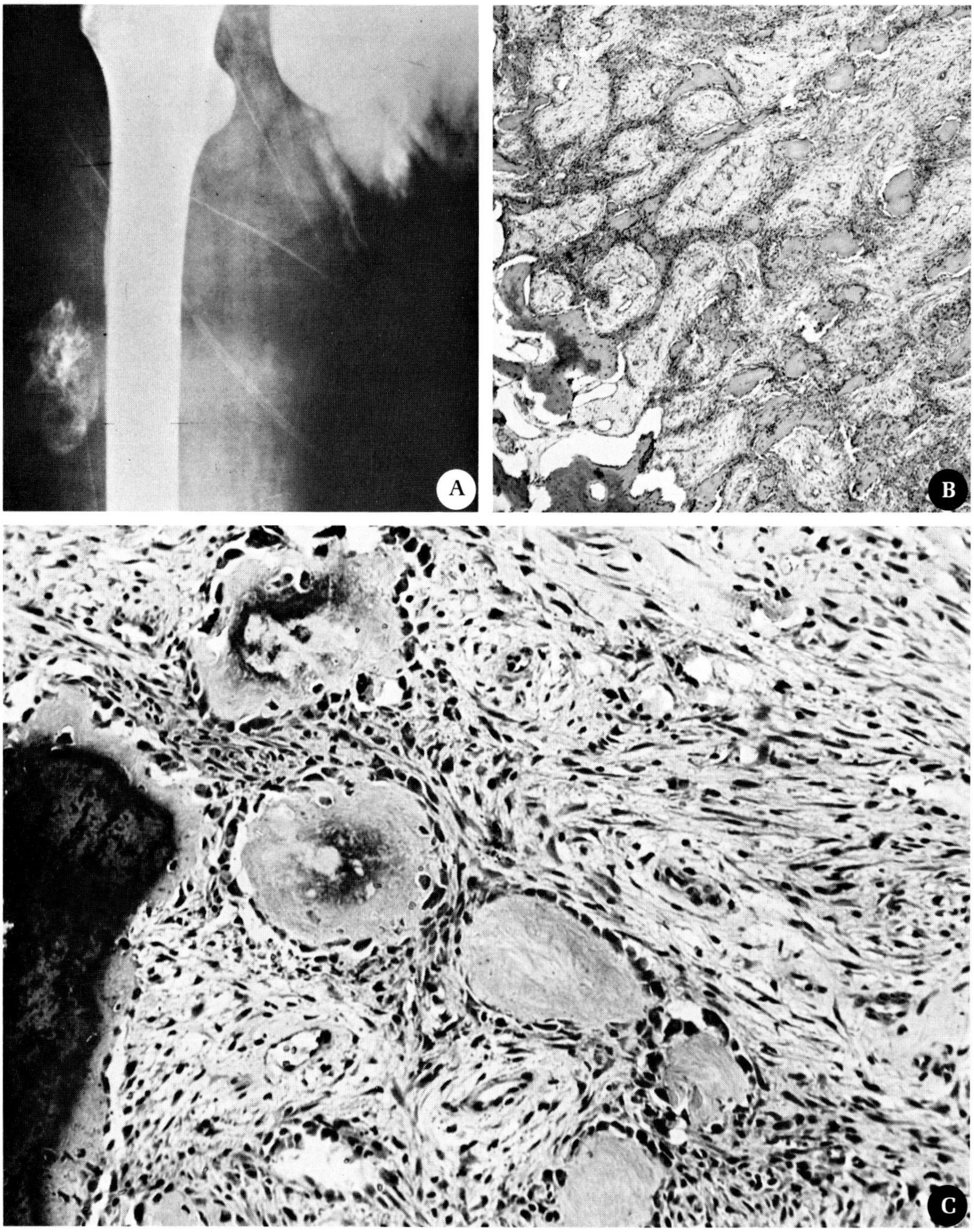

Figure 5-6. Myositis ossificans.

A, Irregular partially calcified lesion lateral to the midshaft of the femur.

B, Trabecular new bone formation in inflamed and fibrous skeletal muscle (right half of picture). There is evidence of sclerosis and calcification of newly formed bone (left lower corner) (H & E, ×35).

C, Islands and fragmented trabeculae of newly formed bone surrounded by highly vascular mesenchymal tissue predominantly composed of slender spindle cells. Note an almost completely calcified bone spicule at the left corner (H & E, ×85).

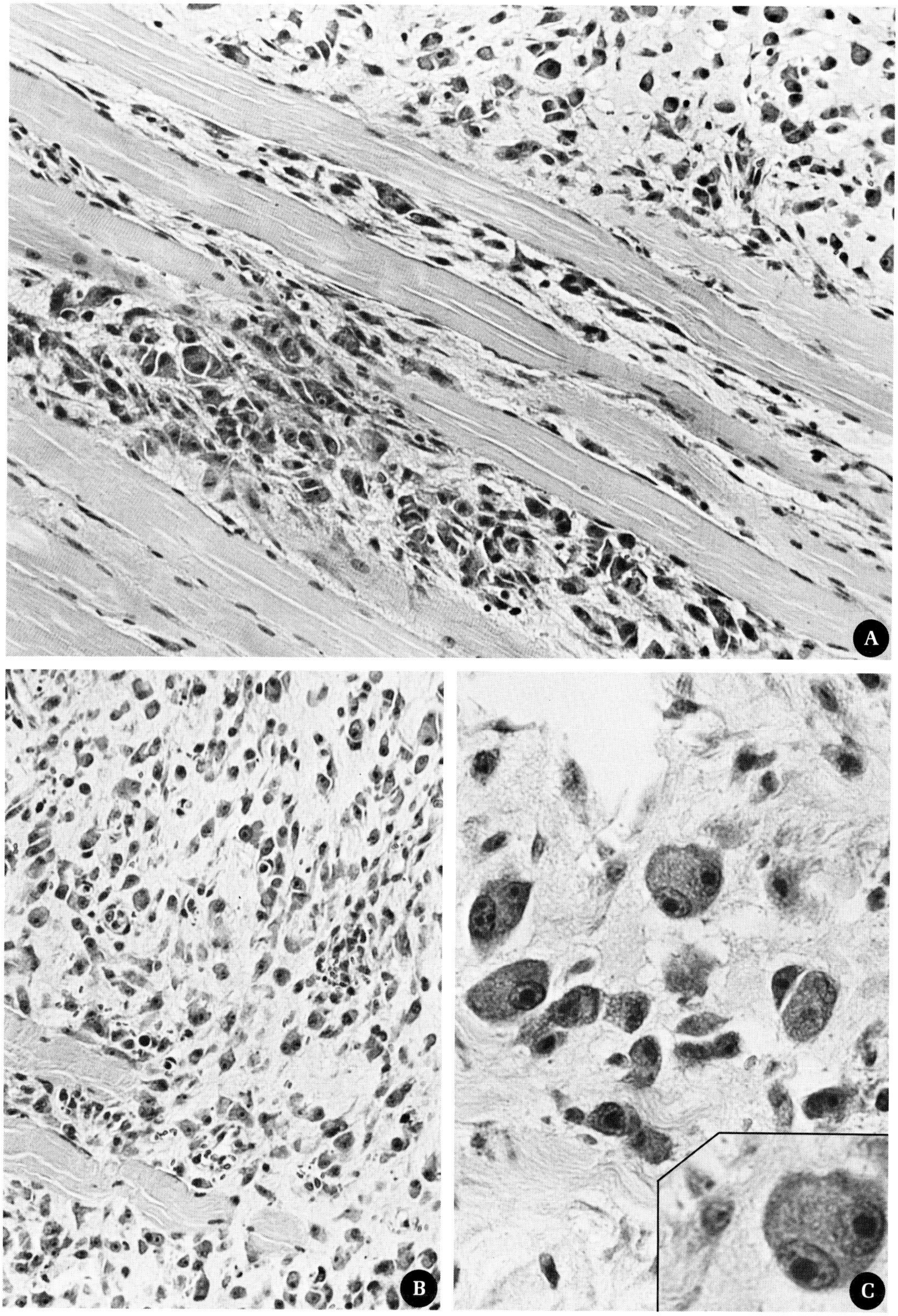

Figure 5-7. Proliferative myositis. The muscle fibers are separated and partially destroyed by polygonal and round histiocytic looking cells. Many of the cells are binucleated and have sharply demarcated granular cytoplasm (**A,** H & E, ×140; **B,** H & E, ×85; **C,** H & E, ×350; inset, H & E, ×570).

Martin et al, in 1960, reported a series of 6 cases of bizarre smooth muscle tumors of the stomach, apparently the first account of gastric leiomyoblastomas. Spiro and McPeak, in 1966, summarized their experience with so-called metastasizing leiomyomas. In 1969, Cornog studied the ultrastructure of leiomyoblastoma and Hajdu and Koss described the cytomorphology of exfoliated cells of metastatic leiomyosarcomas.

Smooth muscle and myoblasts are ubiquitous in the human body. They are present in every organ from the arrectores pilorum of the dermis to the smooth muscle fibers of the blood vessels. Considering the abundance of smooth muscle, it is surprising that benign as well as malignant smooth muscle tumors are not more common (Fig. 5-8).

LEIOMYOMA *

Leiomyoma is the most common benign tumor of smooth muscle. It can grow in any place where smooth muscle is found, for example, the skin, lung, kidney, and retroperitoneum.

Grossly leiomyoma may vary in size from a nodule less than a centimeter to a bulky mass. It is usually well demarcated from surrounding tissues and its consistency is usually firm or semisolid.

* *Synonyms and related terms:* leiomyomatosis, hereditary leiomyoma, vascular leiomyoma, fibroleiomyomatous hamartoma, metastasizing leiomyoma, leiomyomatosis peritonealis disseminata, angioleiomyoma, leiomyoma cutis.

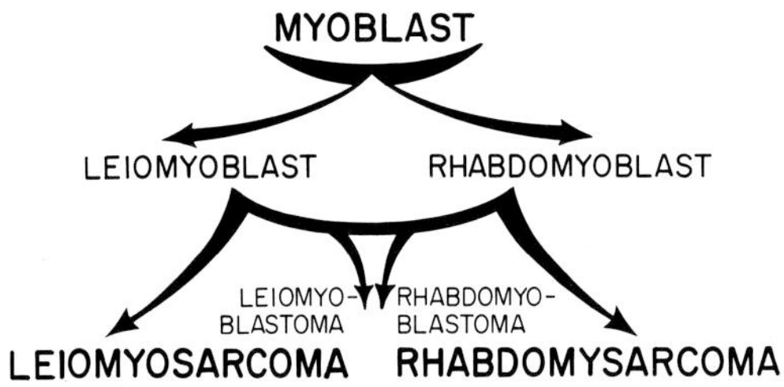

Figure 5-8. Myoblast is the earliest recognizable cell which is committed to becoming either a leiomyoblast or rhabdomyoblast. These forms play an important role in the genesis as well as histologic classification of muscle tumors.

Leiomyoma is composed of interlacing branches of smooth muscle associated with varying amounts of fibrous tissue between bundles. The smooth muscle cells are slender forms with nuclei showing blunt ends. The overall picture is that of monotony and cellular uniformity except for occasional polymorphic giant cells in myxomatous or necrotic areas. In the leiomyoma it is not uncommon to find blood vessels with thickened walls and areas of hyalin degeneration.

Cutaneous Leiomyomas. These tumors are either solitary or multiple (Stout, 1937; Kloepfer et al, 1958; Duhig and Ayer, 1959). The solitary tumors are thought to originate from blood vessel walls, and the multiple forms are considered to be derived from the arrectores pilorum (Fig. 5-9).

Leiomyoma cutis is predominantly a disease of middle-aged females. The etiology is unknown, but there are a few known familial cases (Kloepfer et al, 1958). The first well-documented case is that of Virchow (1854), who reported a 32-year-old male with multiple perimamillary tumors. Stout, in 1937, reviewed 80 cases from the literature and added 15 cases of his own. The largest single series of 83 cases was reported by Duhig and Ayer, in 1959. These authors noted that the majority of the lesions were in the lower legs and some of the leiomyomas had close relationship to dermal hemangiomas. The most satisfactory treatment of cutaneous leiomyomas is complete excision. Recurrence is rare but appearance of a second or additional leiomyoma is not uncommon following the excision of the first one.

In the literature there are a number of case reports of leiomyomas of unusual sites, e.g., *liver* (Demel, 1926), *nasopharynx* (Maesaka et al, 1968), *colon* (Freni and Keeman, 1977).

Vascular or Intravascular Myomas. The so-called vascular or intravascular myomas or angiomyomas are a group of neoplasms which are usually multiple and painful subcutaneous lesions and pre-

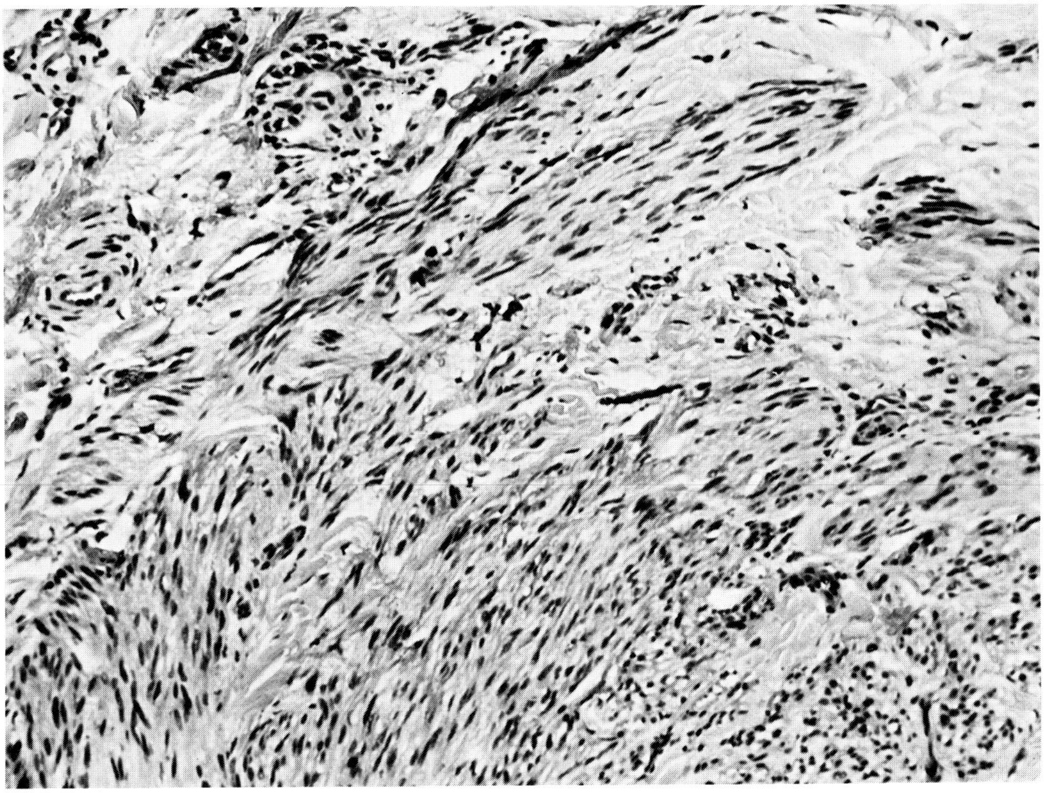

Figure 5-9. Cutaneous leiomyoma is composed of long and slender smooth muscle cells arranged in bundles and fascicles. There is usually no sharp demarcation between proliferating muscle fibers and surrounding tissues; it is not uncommon to see a few bizarre giant cells (H & E, ×85).

dominantly affect females during childbearing age. Sitzenfrey, in 1911, reported the first case in the uterus to which Harper and Scully (1961) and Scharfenberg and Geary (1974) added additional cases. Duhig and Ayer, in 1959, reported 61 cases. Lin and Svoboda (1971) reported a case of multiple vascular leiomyomas in a newborn baby (Fig. 5-10).

Pulmonary Leiomyomas. These so-called pulmonary fibroleiomyomatous hamartomas, solitary or multiple, are exceedingly rare benign lung lesions seen most commonly in middle-aged females. Since the first case report of this entity was published by Deussing, in 1912, approximately 16 additional cases have been reported in the literature (Franco, 1929; Aaxhus and Mylins, 1962; Silverman and Kay, 1976). Horstmann et al, in 1977, reported a case of multiple pulmonary leiomyoma with spontaneous regression during pregnancy. They stated that since these lesions cannot be distinguished from so-called benign metastasizing leiomyoma on the basis of clinical, roentgenographic, and histopathologic features all should be regarded as pulmonary metastases from a low-grade primary uterine neoplasm. However, this view is not shared by most observers. Most authors who reported on the subject feel that the benign course and the presence of epithelial components, in the majority of the cases, support the view that *pulmonary leiomyomas are benign hamartomatous rather than metastatic lesions.*

Metastasizing Leiomyomas. The exact nature of leiomyomatosis and so-called metastasizing leiomyomas is debated in the literature, since the first case of a metastasizing leiomyoma of the uterus was reported by Steiner, in 1939. He defined this entity as ". . . . a tumor com-

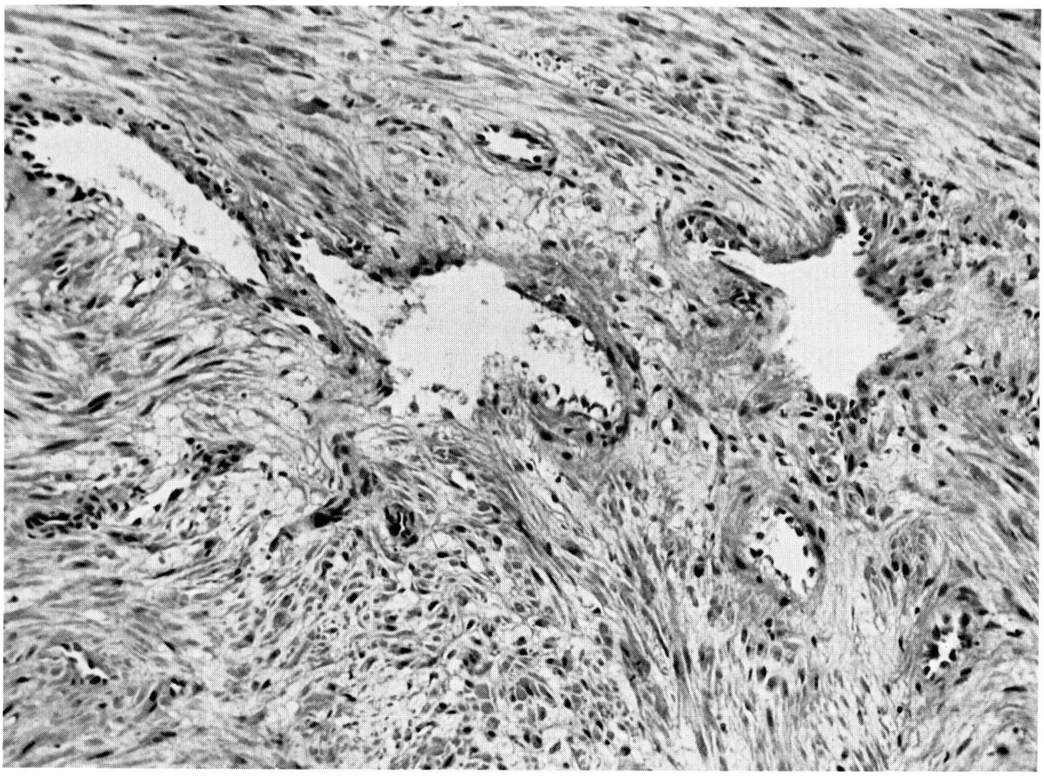

Figure 5-10. Vascular leiomyoma excised from subcutaneous tissue over the Achilles tendon. Either the smooth muscle cells arise from the wall of vessels or there is an intimate association between blood vessels and surrounding muscle cells (H & E, ×85).

posed histologically, in both the primary growth and its metastases, of benign appearing, fully differentiated smooth muscle cells and dense connective tissue." The difficulty in understanding the nature of these lesions is partly due to the lack of precise histologic criteria in assessing the degree of malignancy of smooth muscle tumors, especially that of cellular leiomyomas or so-called borderline tumors. The experience with metastasizing leiomyoma has been limited to fewer than 2 dozen cases in the literature. Short of a better explanation it is felt by most observers that metastases from adequately sampled benign appearing smooth muscle tumors represent an advanced stage of intravenous leiomyomatosis (Harper and Scully, 1961; Spiro and Koss, 1965).

Disseminated Peritoneal Leiomyomatosis. The so-called disseminated peritoneal leiomyomatosis is another unusual smooth muscle lesion which is characterized by the development of multiple peritoneal nodules. The nodules may involve both the parietal and visceral peritoneum of abdominal organs such as the bowel, urinary bladder, uterus, adnexa, and liver. It should be pointed out that disseminated peritoneal leiomyomatosis is a benign condition. In none of the 10 well-documented cases has there been metastasis to extra-abdominal organs or lymph nodes. The fact that almost all cases have been associated with pregnancy or functioning ovarian tumors implicates hormonal stimulus as an etiologic factor (Aterman et al, 1977). It has been suggested, on the basis of ultrastructural observations, that the cell of origin is the multipotent subcelomic mesenchymal cell, which retains the capacity to differentiate into several tissues, including smooth muscle (Goldberg et al, 1977; Nogales et al, 1978).

ANGIOMYOLIPOMA

(See Chapter 4).

TABLE 5-3. *Estimated Incidence of Leiomyosarcoma According to Primary Site of Origin*

SITE OF ORIGIN	% MALIGNANT NEOPLASMS
Uterus	2
Small intestine	50
Stomach	2
Colon	0.2
Lung	0.2
Soft tissues	2

LEIOMYOSARCOMA

Leiomyosarcomas are malignant neoplasms that arise from smooth muscle. The majority of these tumors are primary neoplasms of the uterus and gastrointestinal tract because of the predominance of smooth muscle in these organs (Table 5-3). The origin of leiomyosarcomas in soft tissues is rare. It is believed that most of these tumors arise primarily from veins.

Stout and Hill, in 1958, reported a series of 36 superficial leiomyosarcomas out of which 19 metastasized to the lungs and 4 of the tumors also spread to lymph nodes. One third of the primary tumors were in the thigh and one fourth in the head and neck areas. An earlier case report was written by Ackerman and Stout in 1947 and a case report was published by White in 1971. Since Aufrecht reported the first case of leiomyosarcoma of the saphenous vein in 1868 and Perl reported the first sarcoma of the vena cava in 1871, at least 38 primary leiomyosarcomas of the inferior vena cava and 16 cases arising in the saphenous vein or other veins have been reported (Table 5-4) (Harland and Clamen, 1960; Szasz et al, 1969; Jurayj et al, 1970; Kevorkian and Cento, 1973; Jernstrom and Gowdy, 1975; Bailey et al, 1976; and Brewster et al, 1976). Apparently primary sarcoma of the superior vena cava is even less common. Since the report of Ehrenberg in 1911 only one additional case has been reported (Davis et al, 1976) (Fig. 5-8).

Leiomyosarcoma of major veins is a disease primarily of middle-aged women. The most common vessel which gives rise to these tumors is the inferior vena cava. The middle third of the vena cava is given as the site of origin in more than 50% of the cases. Symptoms depend on the location of the tumor, its rate of growth, and the presence of any associated complication, e.g., thrombosis (Table 5-4).

Grossly, *leiomyosarcomas of soft parts* appear as fairly well-circumscribed or pseudoencapsulated lesions that are not usually firmly fixed to surrounding soft tissues (Fig. 5-11). Histologically, most of these lesions show a degree of malignancy ranging from low to moderate. Our experience with soft tissue leiomyosarcomas is summarized in Table 5-5. Most of the tumors are composed of fairly uniform elongated cells with blunt-end nuclei. The

TABLE 5-4. *Leiomyosarcoma of Major Veins**

	INFERIOR AND SUPERIOR VENA CAVA†	SAPHENOUS AND FEMORAL VEINS	OTHER VEINS
Number of cases	48	18	10
Male	13	10	4
Female	35	8	6
Average age	54	44	43
Symptoms	Pain Edema	Mass Edema	Mass Pain
Dead	28	10	4
No follow-up	7	4	3

*Compiled from the literature and personal experience.
†With 3 exceptions all inferior vena cava lesions.

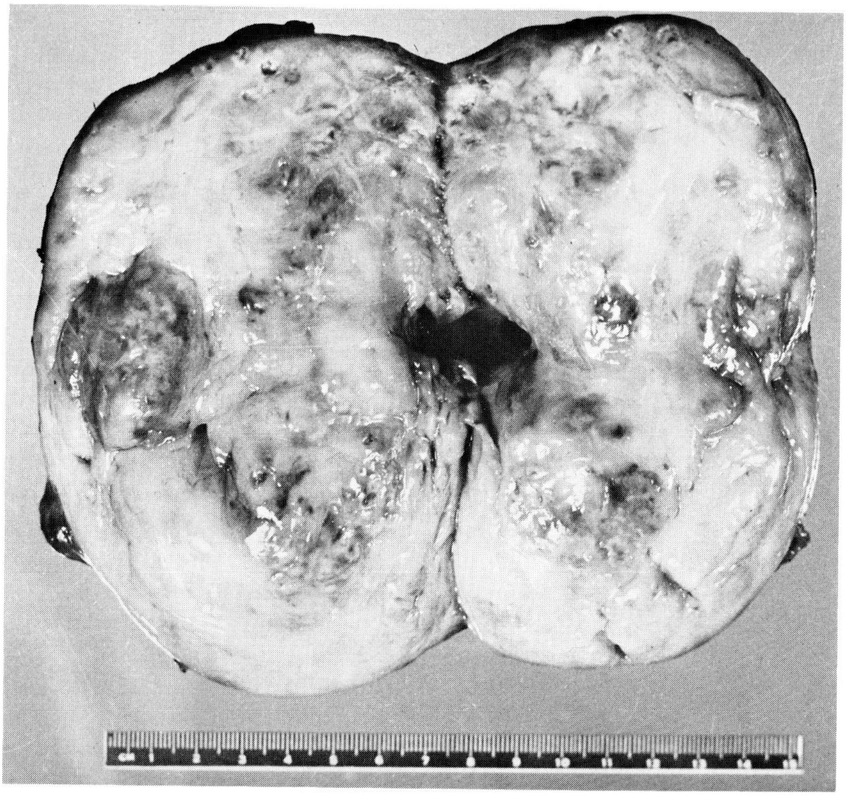

Figure 5-11. Leiomyosarcoma of the buttock showing solid and cystic areas on the cut surface. The tumor is surrounded by a well-defined pseudocapsule.

tumor cells show little tendency of pleomorphism, except in areas of degeneration and necrosis, and are organized in interlacing cords. Our findings confirm the statement by Stout and Hill (1958) that ". . . if a smooth muscle tumor is 2.5 cm or more in diameter and shows any evidence of mitotic figures, then the tumor should be considered malignant" (Fig. 5-12).

Although tumors of *major vessels* are grossly alarming lesions, it is because of their slow growth and relatively low potential to metastasize that cure or long-term surgical palliation is feasible. According to reports, surgical resection of the tumor is possible in more than 50% of the cases and local recurrences (36%) should not discourage re-excision.

Yannopoulos and Stout (1962) and Bothing and Soule (1965) reported the two largest series of *smooth muscle tumors in children,* and found an approximately equal incidence of leiomyoma and leiomyosarcoma. Estimation of the biologic potential of smooth muscle tumors can be especially difficult in children, since even benign cellular lesions may contain occasional bizarre forms and mitotic figures.

Leiomyosarcoma of the oral or nasal cavity is an unusually rare finding. Dropkin et al (1976) found 14 reported cases of leiomyosarcoma of the nasal cavity and paranasal sinuses in the literature to which they added a case of their own. This is a disease of females as well as males. The majority of tumors (72%) recurred after surgical resection and about 50% of the patients died with the disease, most of them in less than 3 years following initial diagnosis.

Brandjord et al (1977) summarized their experience with leiomyosarcoma of the oral cavity and reviewed the literature. Eight of the 18 tumors recurred locally. Despite various therapeutic attempts all 8 patients with recurrence and 2 additional

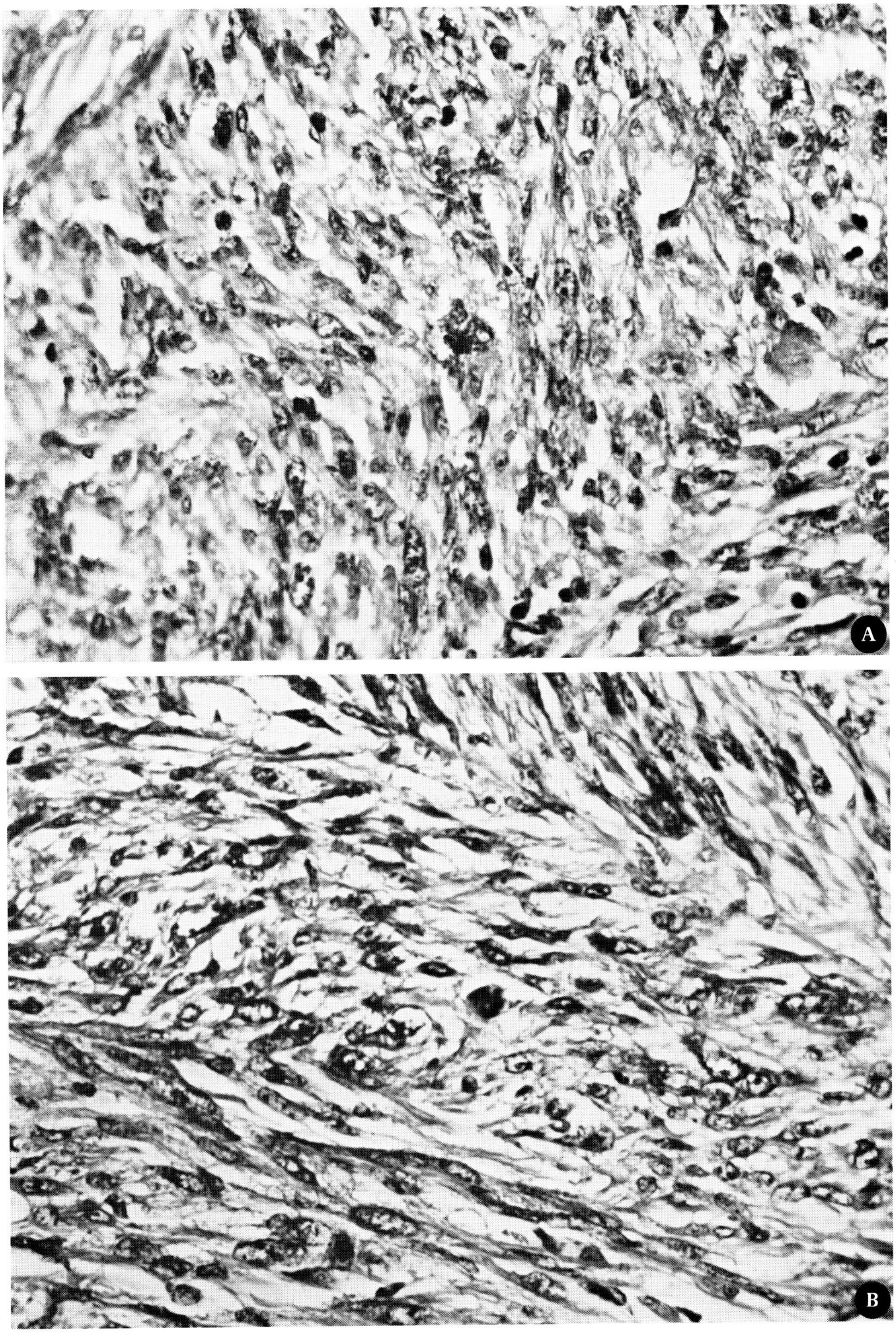

Figure 5-12. Histologically high grade leiomyosarcoma excised from the thigh of an adult male. The tumor cells are tightly packed, fairly uniform spindle cells.

The tumor cells run mostly in one direction in **A.** However, in **B** the tumor cells attempt to form a poorly designed herringbone pattern. There are numerous cells in mitosis, and the stroma is illusory (H & E, ×350).

TABLE 5-5. ***Leiomyosarcomas of Soft Tissues****

	NO. OF PATIENTS†
Total	22
Male	11
Female	11
Site of Primary Tumor	
Buttock	9‡
Thigh	7§
Shoulder	4
Other	2
Follow-up	
Died with metastatic disease—5 yr	16
Alive with no evidence of disease—2 to 21 yr	6

*Primary retroperitoneal leiomyosarcomas are not included (see Chapter 4).

†The average age was 54 years.

‡Seven of the 9 patients were female.

§Six of the 7 patients were male.

patients died with the diseases, less than 2 years after initial biopsy. Additional cases of leiomyosarcoma of the head and neck region were reported by Dobben, 1958; Mindell et al, 1975; Jakobiec et al, 1977.

Leiomyosarcoma of the genitourinary system with the exception of primary lesions of the prostate and urinary bladder is rare (Mackenzie et al, 1971; Tolia et al, 1973). When Greenwood et al, in 1972, reviewed the literature on leiomyosarcoma of the *penis*, they found 13 reported instances to which they added a case of their own. Three of the 9 patients with adequate follow-up information died with the disease.

Since the first case of a *sarcoma of the spermatic cord* was reported by Mason in 1883, a number of case reports and review articles have appeared in the literature (Arlen et al, 1969; Malek et al, 1972). The grave prognosis (the range of mortality is from 65 to 78%) is emphasized by all reviewers. It is of interest that in 8 cases the sarcoma developed in a pre-existing leiomyoma.

Yasuma and Yanaka, in 1971, reviewed 93 cases of *sarcoma of the gall bladder* from the literature. They found that it is a disease of elderly females and carries a grave prognosis. Masur et al, in 1975, reported 2 cases of primary *hepatic leiomyosarcoma* and reviewed 7 published case reports. Evaluation of these 9 cases disclosed that 6 of 7 patients, with follow-up information, died with metastatic disease (Fig. 5-13).

Primary *pulmonary leiomyosarcomas* are exceedingly uncommon. Approximately 32 cases of primary pulmonary leiomyosarcoma are recorded in the English language literature. The majority appear to arise from smooth muscle fibers in the bronchial wall and the prognosis is guarded (Martini et al, 1971). The role of cytologic examination of tracheobronchial secretion in early detection of such lesions is emphasized by recent reports (Hajdu and Koss, 1969; Takeda and Burechailo, 1969; Hajdu and Hajdu, 1976, Krumerman, 1977)(Fig. 5-14).

In the *retroperitoneum,* leiomyosarcomas according to our experience are one of the most common primary soft tissue neoplasms. Our findings (see Chapter 4, Table 4-17) concur with the findings of others (Ranchod and Kempson, 1977) that retroperitoneal leiomyosarcomas are almost invariably fatal neoplasms.

Leiomyosarcomas of the gastrointestinal tract are rare. It is estimated that fewer than 4% of the malignant tumors are leiomyosarcoma. Similarly, with the exception of the rectum, leiomyosarcomas of the large intestine are extremely uncommon lesions. On the other hand, leiomyosarcomas of the small intestine are second only to carcinoid tumors (Ranchod and Kempson, 1977; Akwari et al, 1978).

It is generally accepted that the criteria for the diagnosis of uterine leiomyosarcoma cannot be applied to smooth muscle tumors of soft parts. However, despite the fact that absence of mitoses does not preclude malignancy, the frequency of mitotic figures is the most useful single criterion for the diagnosis of leiomyosarcoma of soft parts.

The significance of *eosinophilic infiltrates* in smooth muscle and other tumors and of the occasional accompanying eo-

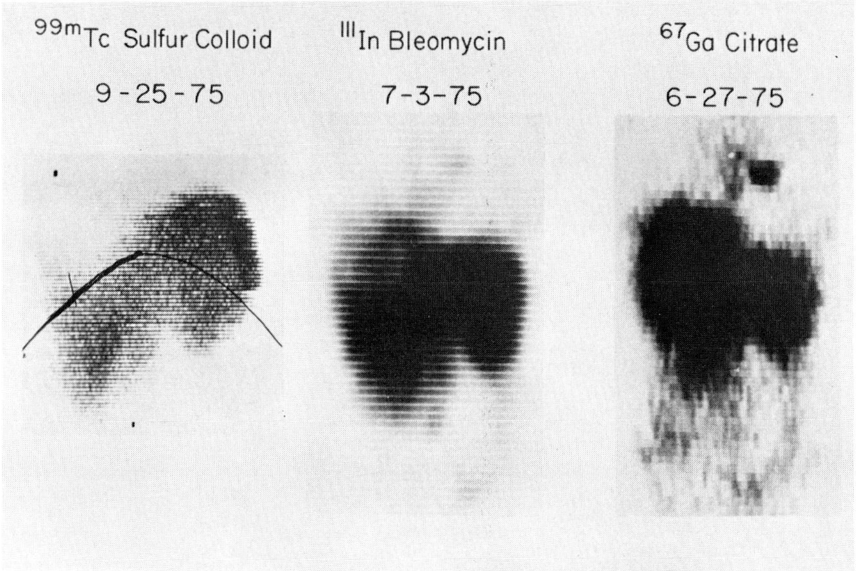

Figure 5-13. Gallium and bleomycin scans of the liver of a 37-year-old female with uterine leiomyosarcoma. At the time of follow-up examination, metastatic tumor was found as indicated here by increased uptake of gallium and bleomycin in the liver and left pulmonary hilum (Courtesy Dr. S. Yeh, Memorial Sloan-Kettering Cancer Center).

sinophilia is obscure. Some writers have suggested that eosinophilic response indicates good prognosis and favorable response to irradiation therapy.

Ultrastructurally leiomyosarcomas of soft tissues and malignant leiomyoblastomas are not different from malignant smooth muscle tumors of organs such as the uterus or urinary bladder. Malignant smooth muscle cells, in general, have more variable and less well-developed organelles than their benign or non-neoplastic counterparts. Of the five organelles commonly present in benign smooth muscle cells—arranged cytoplasmic actin filaments, pinocytotic vesicles, basement membranes, dense plaques, and electron-dense cytoplasmic bodies—only the latter two appear to be limited to smooth muscle cells. The fact that occasionally typical smooth muscle tumors are completely devoid of dense plaques or dense bodies indicates that smooth muscle tumors may show characteristic microscopic pattern prior to the development of any of the specific fine organelles (Fig. 5-15).

Although at present electron microscopic observation offers little aid in predicting the nature, whether it is benign or malignant, of any smooth muscle tumor, it helps to establish the myogenic origin of many neoplasms which cannot be classified by any other technique (Cornog, 1969; Ferenczy et al, 1971; Hajdu et al, 1972; Morales et al, 1975; Chang et al, 1977).

It has been shown that various soft tissue sarcomas share a common antigen; however, they are unable to react with specific antibodies when tissue sections are examined in an immunofluorescence system. Pertschuk (1975) studied a number of benign and malignant smooth muscle tumors and came to the conclusion that *immunofluorescence using anti-smooth-muscle antibodies is of no value in the diagnosis of leiomyosarcoma.* It is apparent that neoplastic cells of other than smooth muscle origin may show reaction with smooth muscle antibody, since actin-like contractile microfilaments may assemble in fibroblasts, fibroblast-like cells, and other mesenchymal cells when the cells are stimulated by cell-to-cell contact (Toh et al, 1976).

Leiomyosarcomas grow readily under in vitro conditions and are transplantable into animals (Hajdu and Fogh, 1978; Hajdu et al, 1979) (Fig. 5-16). If leiomyo-

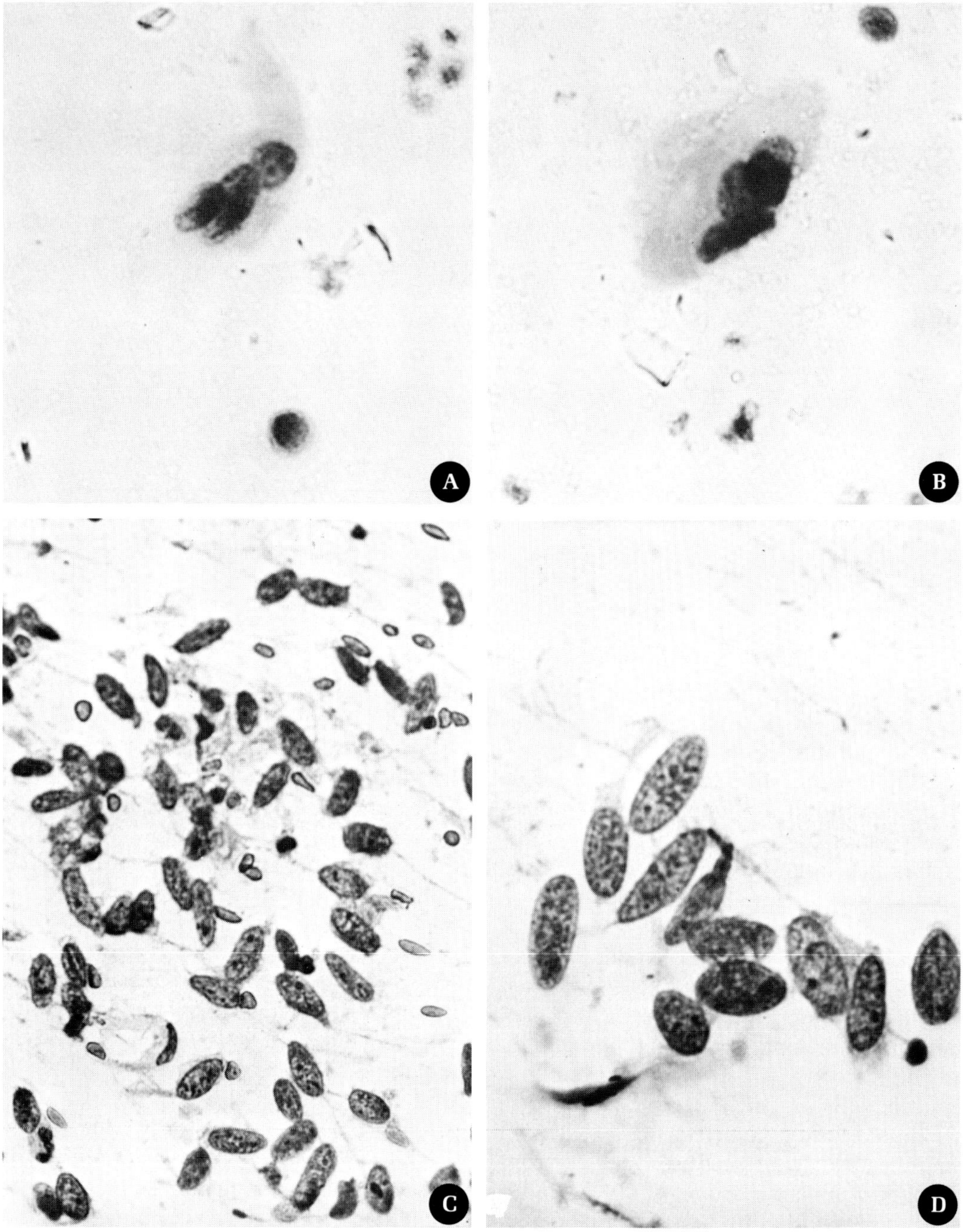

Figure 5-14. **A** and **B**, Exfoliated tumor cells of metastatic leiomyosarcoma. The tumor cells are bizarre multinucleated forms with ill-defined cytoplasmic borders (Pap stain, ×570).

C and **D**, Imprint smear of a well-differentiated leiomyosarcoma. Note the uniform cigar-shaped nuclei and the "fish-bone" arrangement of nuclear chromatin (**C**, Pap stain, ×450; **D**, Pap stain, ×570).

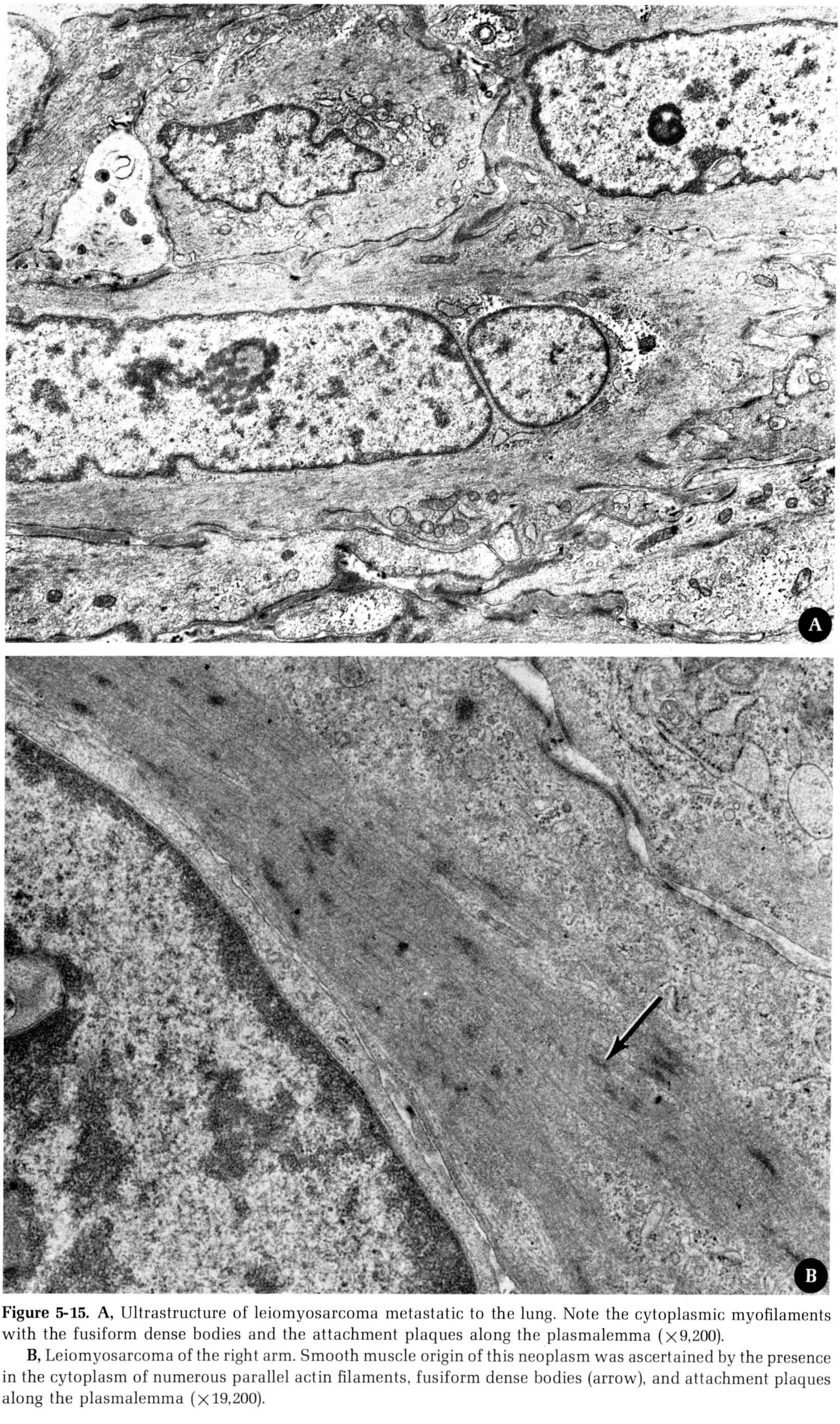

Figure 5-15. A, Ultrastructure of leiomyosarcoma metastatic to the lung. Note the cytoplasmic myofilaments with the fusiform dense bodies and the attachment plaques along the plasmalemma (×9,200).

B, Leiomyosarcoma of the right arm. Smooth muscle origin of this neoplasm was ascertained by the presence in the cytoplasm of numerous parallel actin filaments, fusiform dense bodies (arrow), and attachment plaques along the plasmalemma (×19,200).

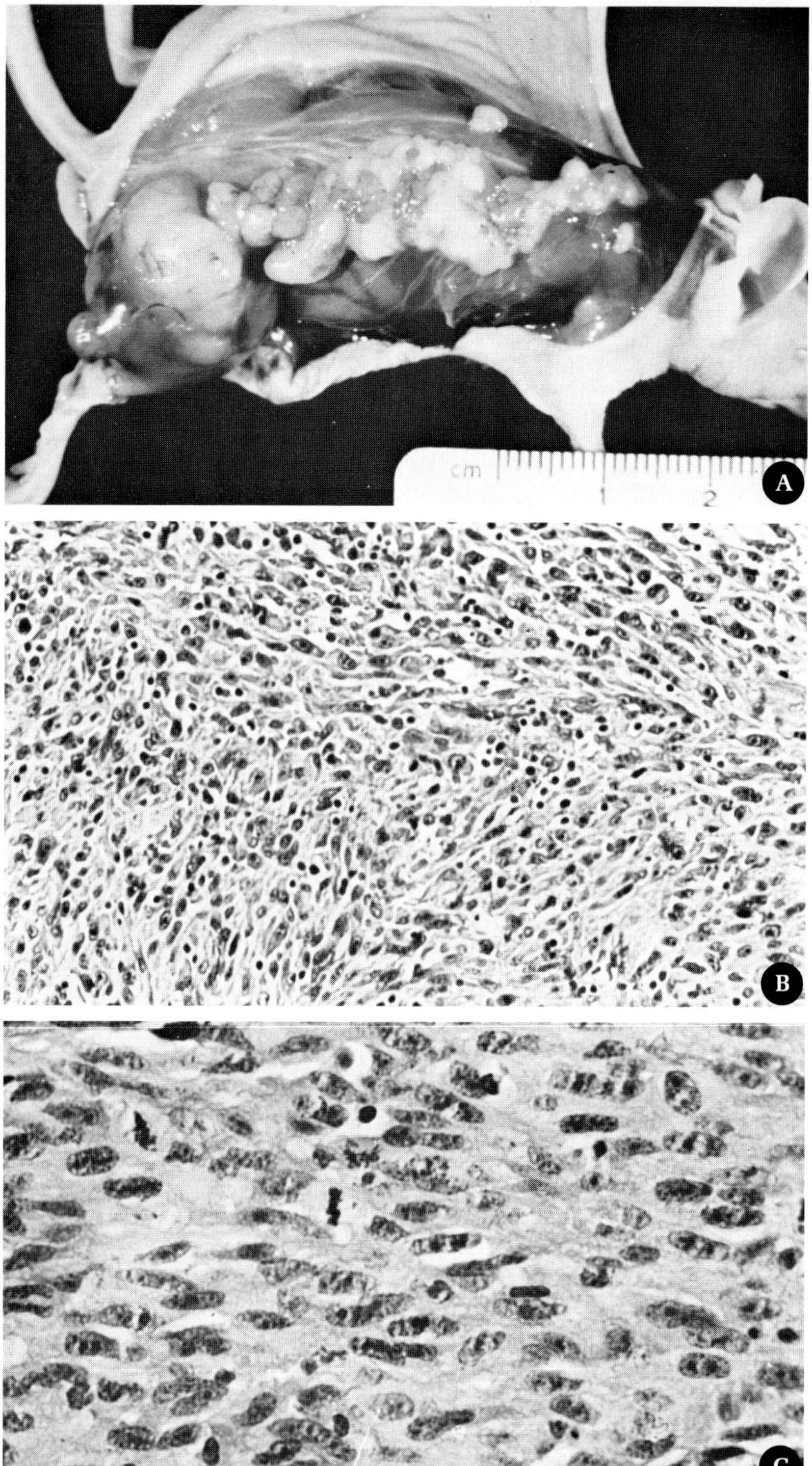

Figure 5-16. A, This nude mouse was sacrificed 5 weeks after subcutaneous injection of a cell suspension of human leiomyosarcoma.

B, Poorly differentiated metastatic leiomyosarcoma from which the inoculum was prepared (H & E, ×140).

C, Leiomyosarcoma, moderately well differentiated, excised from the nude mouse 5 weeks after injection of cell suspension of human leiomyosarcoma (H & E, ×250). (See Hajdu and Fogh, 1978.)

sarcomas of soft tissues are larger than 5 cm and deeply situated and contain more than 5 mitotic figures per 10 high-power fields, they should be considered fully malignant neoplasms (Fig. 5-17). (See Fig. 1-59 and Table 1-15.)

LEIOMYOBLASTOMA *

Since Bartkowiak first used the term *leiomyoblastoma,* in 1936, and Martin et al, in 1960, reported 6 cases of bizarre intramural gastric neoplasms, a number of case reports and review articles have accumulated on the clinicopathology and ultrastructure of leiomyoblastomas or so-called epithelioid leiomyomas (Stout, 1953; Cornog, 1969; Hajdu et al, 1972; Lavin et al, 1972; Appelman and Helwig, 1976; Chang et al, 1977). It is apparent from all available information that leiomyoblastomas are bizarre round cell smooth muscle tumors which can be just like the spindle cell variants, either benign or malignant (Fig. 5-8).

The clarity of the cytoplasm, which is one of the characteristics of the leiomyoblast, is due to intracytoplasmic vacuolization. The precise histogenesis, the histopathology, and the line of demarcation between benign and malignant lesions are widely debated in the literature. By reviewing the literature one gets the impression that leiomyoblastomas are almost always primary gastric neoplasms. In 1972, we reviewed our experience with 44 cases of gastric and extragastric leiomyoblastomas (Lavin et al, 1972). Although many of the cases were primary neoplasms, 18 of the 44 cases were extragastric in origin. However, only 2 of the 18 tumors arose from soft tissues, one of the neck and the other one of the retroperitoneum (Tables 5-6, 5-7; Fig. 5-18).

Leiomyoblastoma is a disease of males as well as females. The gross size of the tumor may range from less than 1 cm to several inches. Microscopically, these tumors are composed predominantly of round and vacuolated myoblasts in various stages of differentiation. When a sufficient number of sections are available for microscopic examination, in malignant tumors it is almost always possible to demonstrate in every other high-power field one or two of the structural qualities commonly seen in leiomyosarcomas, i.e., pleomorphism of the tumor cells, pyknotic bizarre nuclei, tumor giant cells, and occasional mitotic cells. In the evaluation of malignancy of any smooth muscle tumor it is apparent that in leiomyoblastomas, as well as in atypical smooth muscle tumors, consideration must be given to factors such as nuclear *hyperchromatism, pleomorphism, mitotic activity, necrosis, size* and *anatomic site* (Figs. 5-19, 5-20).

It is apparent from Table 5-7 that leiomyoblastomas larger than 10 cm, especially the ones that are extragastric in location, should be considered fully malignant neoplasms. Smaller tumors composed of well-differentiated round vacuolated uniform leiomyoblasts should be considered either as low-grade malignant

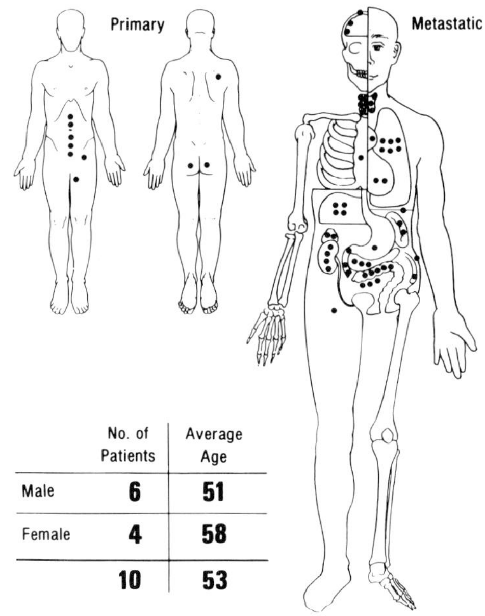

	No. of Patients	Average Age
Male	6	51
Female	4	58
	10	53

Figure 5-17. Postmortem findings of patients who died with metastatic leiomyosarcoma of soft tissues show that the intestines, lungs, vertebrae, kidneys, and liver are the most commonly involved organs.

* *Synonyms and related terms:* epithelioid leiomyoma, epithelioid leiomyosarcoma, clear cell leiomyosarcoma, bizarre leiomyosarcoma.

TABLE 5-6. *Anatomic Location of Leiomyoblastomas and Survival of Patients**

PRIMARY SITE	TOTAL	NO. OF PATIENTS: ALIVE OR DEAD WITHOUT NEOPLASM	NO. OF PATIENTS: DIED WITH NEOPLASM
Stomach	26	16	10
Neck	1	1	0
Esophagus	1	0	1
Duodenum	1	0	1
Jejunum	2	0	2
Ileum	2	1	1
Colon	2	1	1
Rectum	1	1	0
Retroperitoneum	1	0	1
Uterus	6	3	3
Vulva	1	1	0
Total	44	24	20

*Modified from Lavin, P., Hajdu, S. I., and Foote, F. W.: Gastric and extragastric leiomyoblastomas. Cancer 29:305, 1972.

neoplasms or as neoplasms with malignant potential.

Tumors of Striated Muscle

Malignant tumors of skeletal muscle, which were occasionally called *malignant rhabdomyomas,* were recognized almost a century prior to the first description of a truly *benign rhabdomyoma* by Schmincke, in 1922. The first authentic sarcomas of the striated muscle were reported by Stafford in 1839 and Guersant in 1854. Weber and Wilks are credited with the first use of the term *rhabdomyosarcoma* in 1854 and 1859, respectively. There can be little doubt that Weber described a rhabdomyosarcoma. The patient was a 21-year-old man with a tumor of the tongue made up of "muscle cells in all stages of differentiation from adult to embryonal forms." Wilks pointed out that "cancer is not unfrequently met within the muscle surrounding cancerous tumors of epithelial variety but I think it is rare as primary disease." Although *embryonal rhabdomyosarcoma* was described in a number of early case reports (Stafford, 1839; Guersant, 1854; Targett, 1892), it was Berard, in 1894, who coined the term by describing a tumor he called "Tumeur embryonnaire du muscle strié." A few

TABLE 5-7. *Factors Influencing Survival of Patients with Gastric and Extragastric Leiomyoblastomas**

	NO. OF PATIENTS DIED WITH DISEASE
Gastric leiomyoblastoma	10/26 (38%)
Extragastric leiomyoblastoma	10/18 (55%)
Symptomatic > 6 months	16/23 (69%)
Size > 10 cm	17/20 (80%)
Metastatic	20/21 (95%)

Numerator: Died.
Denominator: Number of patients.
*Modified from Lavin, P., Hajdu, S. I., and Foote, F. W.: Gastric and extragastric leiomyoblastoma. Cancer 29:305, 1972.

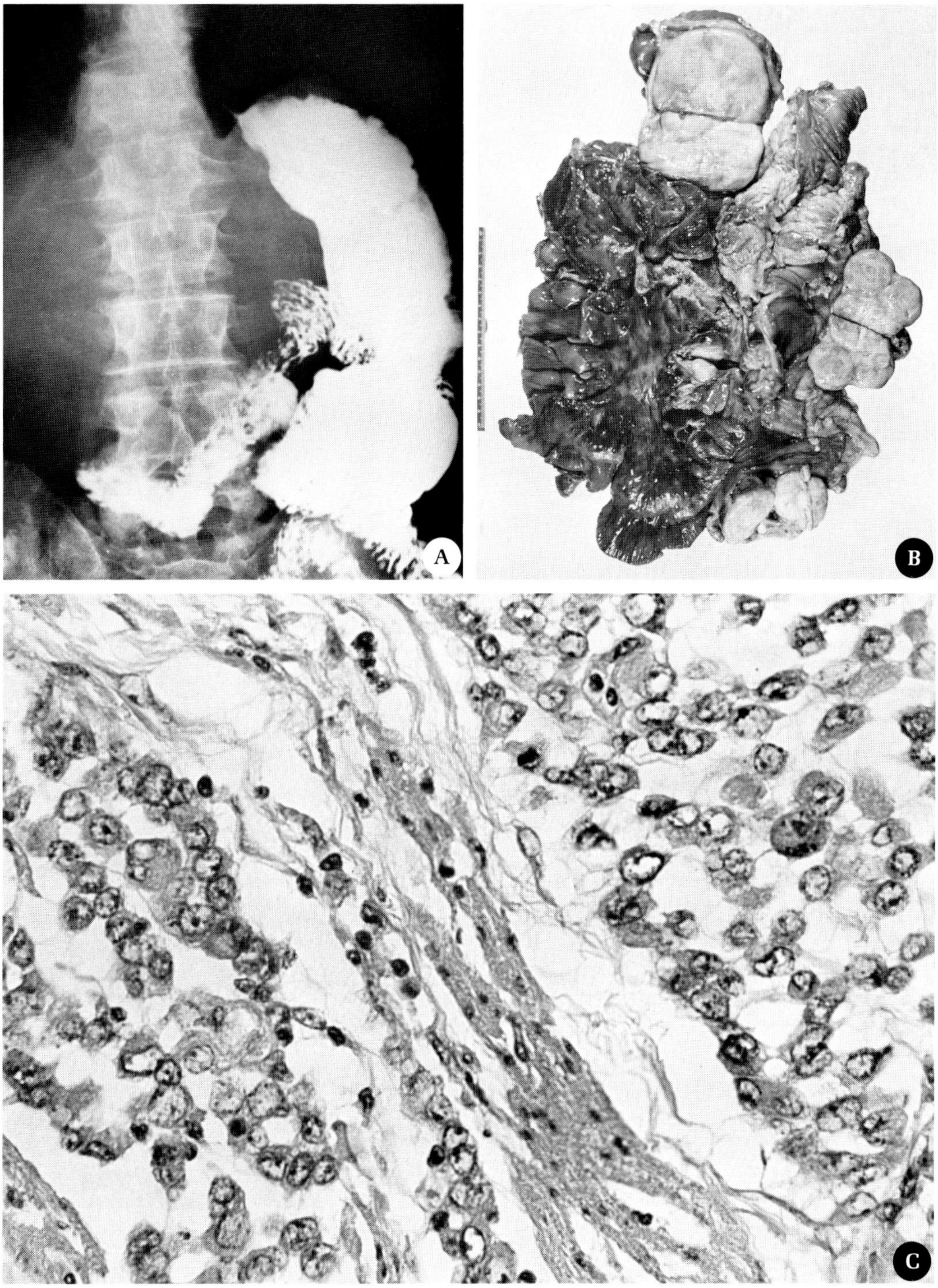

Figure 5-18. **A** and **B,** Extragastric leiomyoblastoma composed of a conglomerate of several tumor masses involving loops of intestines, mesentery, and retroperitoneum. Some of the smaller tumor nodules appear pedunculated and polypoid.

C, An innocuous-looking area from one of the smaller tumor nodules shows predominantly uniform round cells in a fibromyxoid stroma (H & E, ×140).

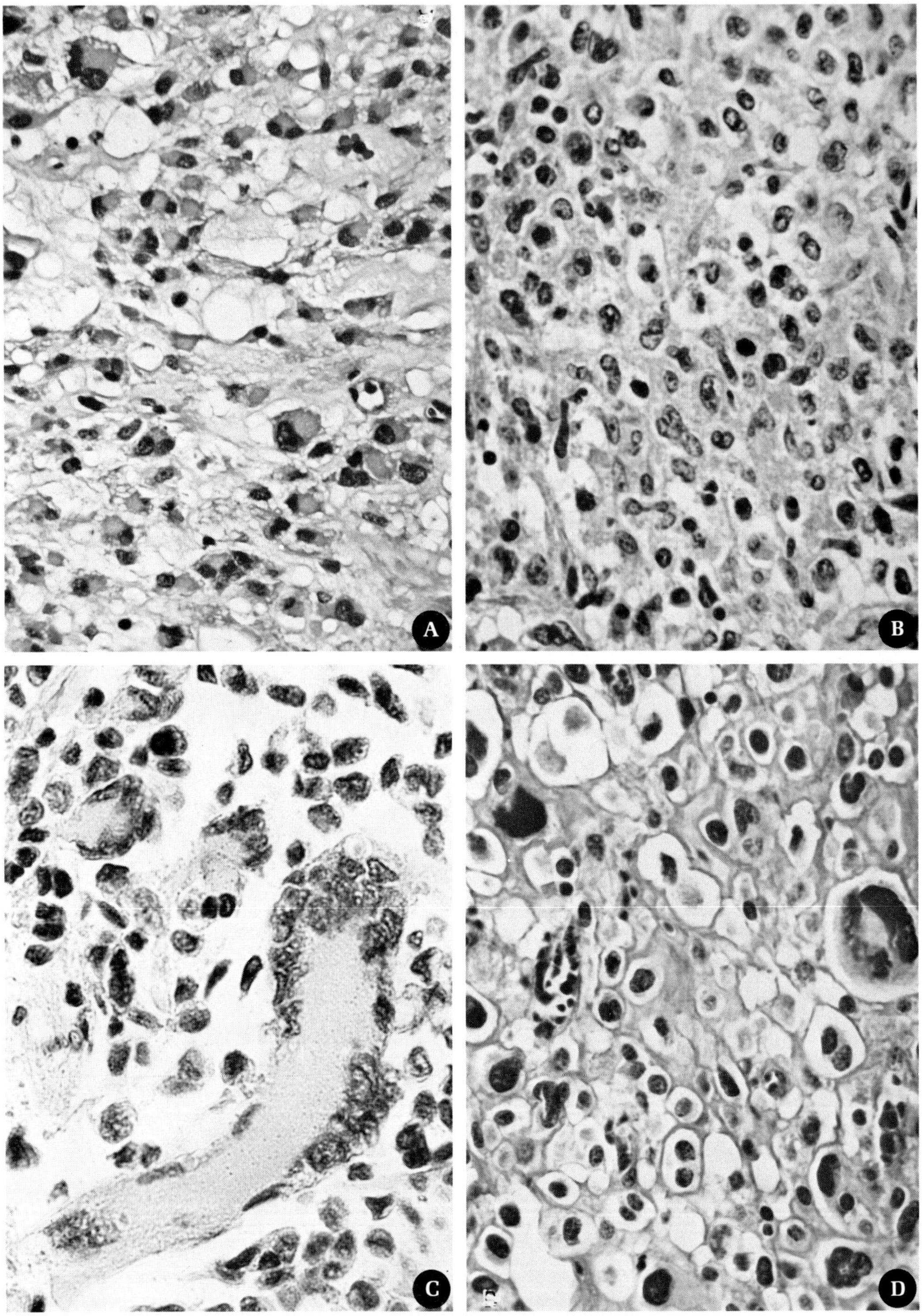

Figure 5-19. Microscopic appearance of leiomyoblastoma or so-called epithelioid leiomyosarcoma. The size of the tumor cells may range from small granular round cells to large vacuolated and bizarre forms. There is a cohesive tendency between tumor cells, and fused or cluster-forming cells are not uncommon. Notice an abortive muscle fiber or "myotube" with several adherent cells in **C** (H & E, ×140). (See also Figure 5-49.)

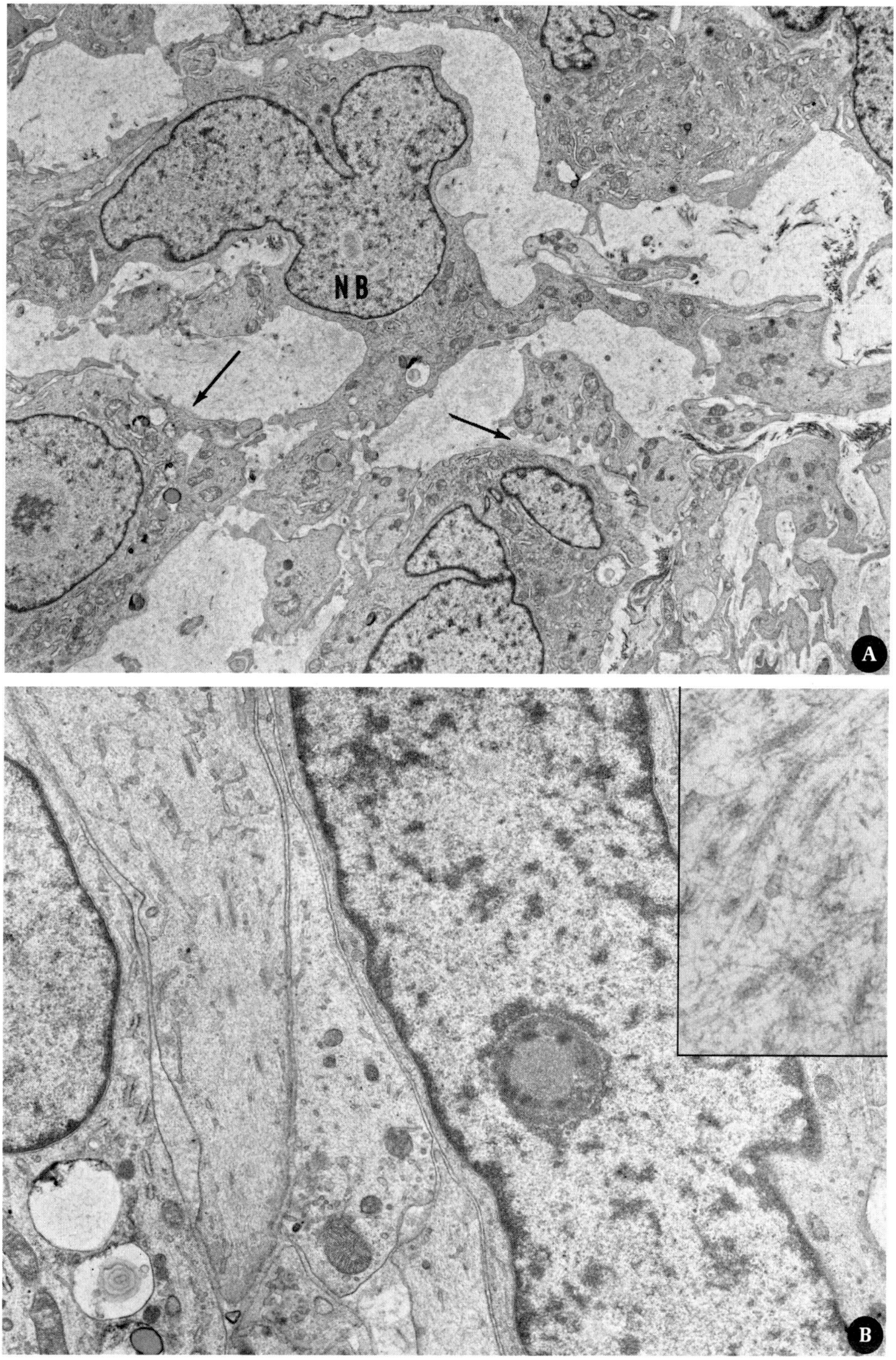

Figure 5-20. Ultrastructural features of a gastric leiomyoblastoma.

A, Tumor cells are surrounded by a granular matrix containing dispersed collagenous fibrils. Note the nuclei (NB) and discontinuous basement membrane at the cell surface (arrows) (×5,280).

B, Neoplastic smooth muscle cell with ring nucleus and cytoplasmic myofilaments (×13,200). Inset shows cytoplasmic myofilaments at higher magnification (×50,400). (From Hajdu, S. I., Erlandson, R. A., and Paglia, M. A.: Light and electron microscopic studies of a gastric leiomyoblastoma. Arch. Pathol. 93:36, 1972. Copyright 1972, American Medical Association.)

years later, Montpellier (1929), reporting on "rhabdomyomas," introduced the term *sarcome alveolaire* meaning *alveolar rhabdomyosarcoma*. He summarized all reported cases of rhabdomyomas and discussed the histogenesis and morphology in tissue culture. The term *rhabdomyoma* for sarcomas was first proposed by Zenker in 1864, and Borst introduced the term *myoblastic sarcoma* (Fig. 5-8).

Two excellent monographs on tumors of the striated muscle were written by Despres (1866) and Peyron (1929). The first significant review article on skeletal muscle tissue tumors was written by Wolfensberger, in 1894. This was followed by the concise review of rhabdomyosarcomas by Stout in 1946 and Stobbe and Dargeon's much quoted article on embryonal rhabdomyosarcoma in 1950. The first ultrastructural study of rhabdomyosarcoma was reported by Chaoman et al in 1963, and Cornog and Gonatas, in 1967, published the first article dealing with the ultrastructure of rhabdomyoma. The first successful use of combination chemotherapy and irradiation in the treatment of embryonal rhabdomyosarcomas is claimed by many people, but it should be credited to Edland who reported his 5-year survival results in 1967.

It has been estimated that about 0.5% of tumors and from 10% to 25% of all sarcomas of the soft tissues are rhabdomyosarcomas. The comparative rarity of rhabdomyosarcomas is partly explained by the fact that striated muscle cells are differentiated, out-of-cycle cells and do not undergo mitoses in postnatal life. Nevertheless, it is astonishing, considering the weight and extent of skeletal muscle in the body, that it has fewer tumors than any other tissues.

The etiology of rhabdomyosarcomas is not known. Congenital factors warrant consideration because of the frequency with which rhabdomyosarcomas occur in the newborn.

RHABDOMYOMA

Rhabdomyoma is a benign tumor of the striated muscle. It is exceedingly rare, but examples have been reported in the heart and skeletal muscles. According to Walter and Guerbaoui (1976) 44 cases of extracardiac rhabdomyoma have been reported.

It is doubtful that mature striated muscle can ever give rise to a tumor and it is generally accepted that rhabdomyomas arise de novo from fetal rests. However, there is no general agreement whether they should be considered hamartomas or true neoplasms.

Rhabdomyoma is predominantly a disease of adult males between the ages of 25 and 40 years and almost all tumors occur *in the head and neck regions*. However, rare examples in the *stomach* (Tuazon, 1969) and *vagina* (Gad and Eusebi, 1975; Gold and Bossen, 1976) have been reported (Table 5-8).

Wolfensberger, in 1894, is credited with the first description of a case of rhabdomyoblastoma, but the term *myoblastoma* appeared earlier, in the mid-1800's, in the literature. Cappell and Montgomery, in 1937, wrote the first comparative report on rhabdomyomas and myoblastomas; Cornog, in 1967, reported the first ultrastructural study of rhabdomyoblastoma. *Grossly,* rhabdomyoblastomas usually appear as multinodular yellowish gray fairly well-demarcated, glistening nodules ranging in size from 0.5 to 3 cm.

Histologically, they are customarily subdivided for the so-called *adult type* and *fetal type* (Table 5-8). However, most observers agree that these two types merely represent two different stages of the same tumor. The fetal form consists of haphazardly oriented bundles of undifferentiated mesenchymal cells and fairly typical strap cells, some with cross striation in a loosely arranged and sparsely cellular stroma. Fetal rhabdomyoma must be distinguished from sarcoma botryoides. Rhabdomyoma contains numerous well-differentiated rhabdomyoblasts, is rarely ulcerated, lacks the characteristic cambium layer of sarcoma botryoides, and seldom contains pleomorphic and mitotic cells. Most of the patients with rhabdomyoma are adults or children of older

TABLE 5-8. *Soft Tissue Rhabdomyoma**

ANATOMIC SITES	MALE	FEMALE	MEDIAN AGE
Oral or nasal cavities	10	2	54
Neck	8	2	49
Head	5	1	1
Larynx	6	1	52
Vagina or vulva	—	8	47
Other	2	2	38
	31	16	

*Compiled from the literature and personal experience.

age groups than those with botryoid sarcoma.

The so-called adult types of rhabdomyomas are predominantly composed of fairly uniform, closely packed polygonal rhabdomyoblasts with eosinophilic, granular, and vacuolated cytoplasms. Occasionally irregularly arranged, basophilic, crystal-like inclusions or filaments, first described by Moran ad Enterline, in 1964, which stain with PTAH stain and ultrastructurally have been shown to be condensed myofilaments and hypertrophic Z-band material (Chernobilsky et al, 1968; Gold and Bossen, 1976) are seen (Fig. 5-21). The superficial resemblance of rhabdomyoma to so-called granular cell myoblastoma can be striking. However, arranged myofilaments or crystalline-like material has not been demonstrated in granular cell lesions. Local excision, it seems, is the treatment of choice. Only two of the reported cases recurred after excision.

The resemblance of rhabdomyoma of striated muscle and that of the heart is more than a superficial one. In both lesions, partially polygonal and vacuolated myoblasts are present. Although ultrastructural studies failed to resolve the exact histogenesis of rhabdomyoma of the heart, which is the most common primary tumor of infancy and frequently is associated with the tuberous scelerosis complex, they clearly attest to its myogenic nature (Silverman et al, 1976). Since von Recklinghausen, in 1862, first described *cardiac rhabdomyoma*, numerous review articles have appeared. Fenoglio et al, in 1976, reported in a series of 36 patients that 78% were under one year of age and 90% had multiple cardiac lesions. They postulated that cardiac rhabdomyoblastomas are congenital hamartomas rather than true neoplasms but admitted that the individual cells closely resemble embryonic cardiac muscle cells.

EMBRYONAL RHABDOMYOSARCOMA

The term *embryonal* in connection with rhabdomyosarcoma was first used by Berard (1894) in describing a case in a 2-year-old child. However, a number of tumors apparently of the same nature were reported much earlier (Stafford, 1839; Guersant, 1854; Pfannenstiel, 1892; Targett, 1892). The first series of 63 cases of rhabdomyosarcoma was reported by Wolfensberger in 1894. Thirty-eight of the tumors he reported were primary neoplasms of the urogenital system, and there were 4 orbital, 7 cervical, and 14 miscellaneous rhabdomyosarcomas.

Burgess, in 1914, reported a metastatic rhabdomyosarcoma of the thigh. The patient was a 19-year-old female who died with metastatic tumor involving lung, bones, breast, and lymph nodes. He pointed out that he had seen several of these "malignant rhabdomyomas" in young people and "to such tumors, the terms—sarcoma and alveolar sarcoma—or other indefinite names would probably be applied in the ordinary course of routine pathological examination." He also emphasized that "only after a very ex-

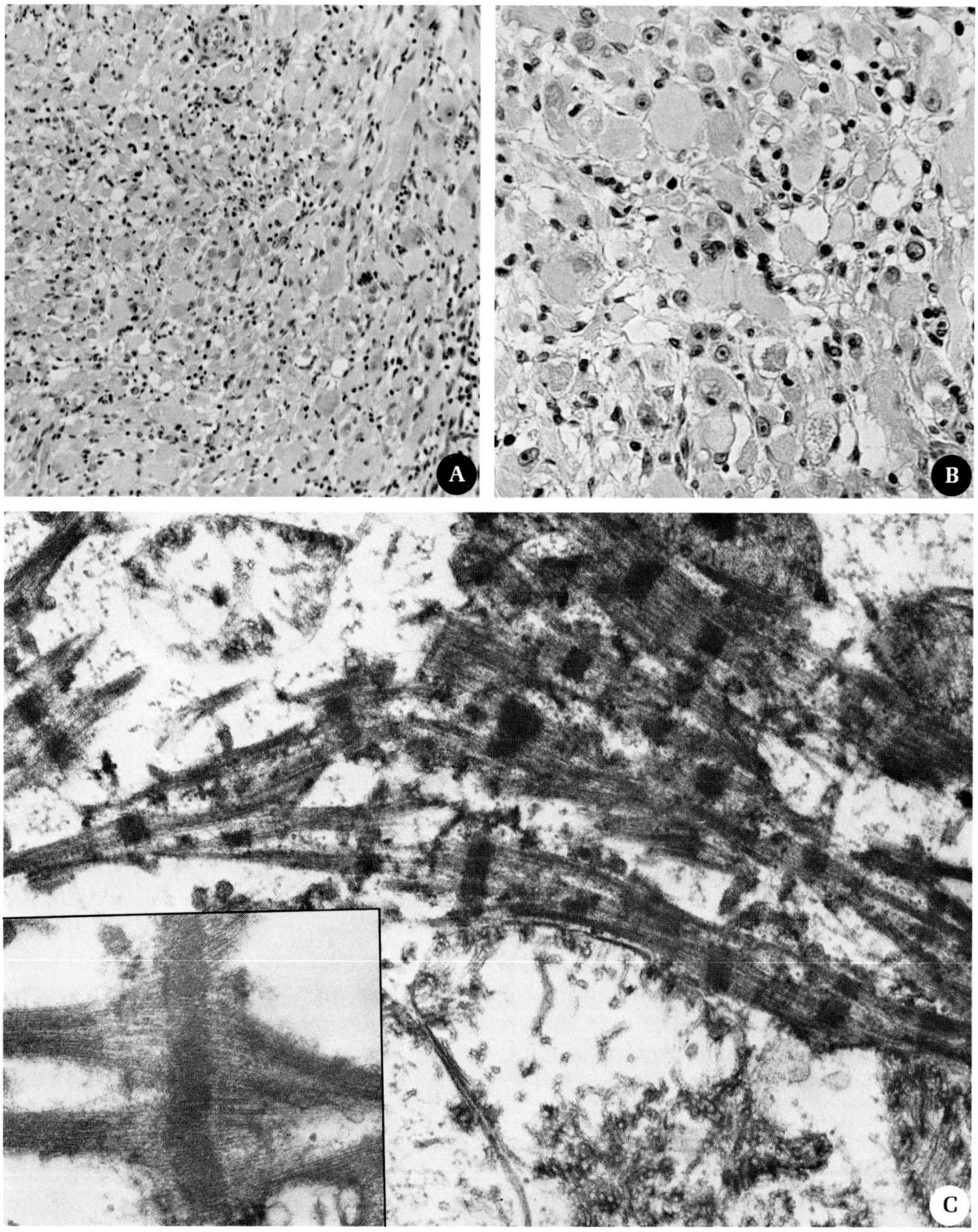

Figure 5-21. Rhabdomyoma is composed of well-defined mature rhabdomyocytes in a piled-up and haphazardly arranged form. There is no recognizable pattern or organization and the stroma is minimal. There are, however, a number of clearly visible inflammatory and fat cells throughout the tumor. The granular and arranged cytoplasmic material is also visible (**A,** H & E, ×85; **B,** H & E, ×140). (See also Chapter 9.)

C, Electron micrograph of a mediastinal rhabdomyoma showing abundant bundles of myofilaments with prominent Z bands (×27,000). Inset, Hypertrophied Z band and lighter I band (×32,000). (Courtesy Miller, R., Kurtz, S. M., and Powers, J. M.: Mediastinal rhabdomyoma. Cancer 42:1983, 1978.)

TABLE 5-9. ***Reported Series of Rhabdomyosarcomas***

AUTHORS	NO. OF CASES	TYPE STUDIED	SURVIVAL (%)
Stout (1946)	121	Embryonal and pleomorphic	3
Stobbe and Dargeon (1950)	15	Embryonal	13
Linscheid et al (1965)	82	Pleomorphic	36*
Soule et al (1969)	75	Embryonal	21*
Enzinger and Shiraki (1969)	102	Embryonal	8*
Ghavimi et al (1975)	27	Embryonal	Stage I 92 Stage II 50 Stage III 40
Ariel and Briceno (1975)	110	Embryonal and pleomorphic	32*
Maurer et al (1977)	423	Embryonal	Stage I 92 Stage II 90 Stage III 79 Stage IV 50
Hajdu et al† (unpublished)	121	Pleomorphic	21*

*5-year survival.
†In reference to Grade and Stage see Fig. 1-59 and Table 1-15.

tended search was it possible to find tumor cells which had reached a sufficient degree of differentiation to enable them to be recognized as striated muscle cells" (Fig. 5-8).

The review articles prior to 1950, including the article written by Stout in 1946, did not distinguish between pleomorphic and embryonal rhabdomyosarcomas (Table 5-9). Stobbe and Dargeon, of Memorial Sloan-Kettering Cancer Center, drew attention to the embryonal type of rhabdomyosarcoma in 1950. Horn and Enterline, in 1958, contributed to the better understanding of rhabdomyosarcomas by subclassifying them into four categories: *pleomorphic, alveolar, embryonal, and botryoid.* Stout and Lattes (1967), who suggested that there is little prognostic value in differentiating the histologic types of embryonal rhabdomyosarcoma, grouped alveolar, botryoid, and embryonal types together as juvenile rhabdomyosarcoma. Our experience with embryonal rhabdomyosarcoma at Memorial Sloan-Kettering Cancer Center supports their view. However, we are not in favor of introducing the term *juvenile,* since we have seen more than a few embryonal rhabdomyosarcomas in adult and elderly patients (Table 5-10). If it were understood

TABLE 5-10. ***Embryonal Rhabdomyosarcomas in Adults***

	NO. OF PATIENTS*
Total	42
Male	27
Female	15
Most Common Sites	
Extremities	18
Trunk	12
Head and neck	6
Other	6
Follow-up	
Alive	8

*The average age was 31 years.

that *alveolar* is a descriptive term indicating the presence of tubular or alveolar microscopic arrangement of some of the tumor cells and *botryoid* indicates nothing else than polypoid or grape-like gross appearance of some of the embryonal rhabdomyosarcomas and that these terms should be used for the purpose of subclassification rather than classification of rhabdomyosarcomas, we would all be better off.

Apparently most of the rhabdomyosarcomas arise from undifferentiated mesoderm rather than from myotome-derived skeletal muscle. In general, the gross appearance of embryonal rhabdomyosarcomas, with the exception of botryoid sarcoma, is not different from that of pleomorphic rhabdomyosarcoma or most of the other types of soft tissue sarcomas. They are fairly well-circumscribed, nonbulky neoplasms with moderately soft or gelatinous consistency.

Sarcoma botryoides, first described by Guersant, in 1854, is an inappropriate term, as I indicated before, unless it is used parenthetically to denote only gross appearance. It was actually Pfannenstiel, in 1892, who pointed out the botryoid or grape-like appearance. Since then it is known that embryonal rhabdomyosarcomas with gross botryoid features are the most common tumors found in the urogenital tract of infants and children. In girls, they occur chiefly in the vagina and less often in the bladder. In boys, they occur more often in the bladder and less often in the urethra, prostate, and spermatic cord. Tumors with similar (botryoid) gross appearance have also been noted in the oropharynx and nasopharynx and the common bile duct (Daniel et al, 1959).

Microscopically, in most embryonal rhabdomyosarcomas several different patterns are found: solid, myxoid, trabecular, and alveolar or tubular. Most of the tumors are highly vascular, and the tumor cells may have a prominent pericytic arrangement. In such areas it is not uncommon to see heavy mostly acellular fibrous bands separating the blood vessels and the tumor cells. The basic cell type most commonly seen is a thin tapering embryonal rhabdomyoblast with bipolar cytoplasmic processes and a small usually eccentrically placed nucleus. The cytoplasm is eosinophilic and relatively small. Pinkish, PAS-positive, diastase-soluble, finely granular material is often visible in the cytoplasm adjacent to the nucleus (Figs. 5-22, 5-37).

These cells may appear as small, oval, undifferentiated mesenchymal cells without any distinctive features or as round cells, myoblasts, with prominent vesicular nuclei. More differentiated forms are the spindle-shaped or strap-shaped monocytes. In these forms, longitudinal and occasionally cross striation can be identified. Myxomatous areas usually contain large numbers of differentiated myocytes. Binucleation is not uncommon, but multinucleated forms are an exceedingly rare finding (Figs. 5-23, 5-24).

Experience shows that in most tumors adequately sampled one finds an admixture of the various types of tumor cells. If the undifferentiated small oval and round cells (embryonal myoblasts) are predominant, the tumor may show striking resemblance to Ewing's sarcoma (see Chapter 8). Maurer et al (1977) in their review subclassified embryonal rhabdomyosarcomas according to these features and found no apparent correlation between histologic subtypes of the tumor and prognosis.

Alveolar or tubular arrangement of some of the tumor cells in embryonal rhabdomyosarcoma, an apparent imitation of an embryonal myotubular pattern of growth, has been described by Burgess (1914) and Peyron (1929) and rediscovered by Riopelle and Theriault in 1956. Montpellier, as early as 1929, stated that "les sarcomes alveolaires" are composed of small neoplastic myocytes in arranged pattern. The alveolar pattern of presentation as a pure form, without other components, is rare. A number of publications compared the clinicopathologic features of alveolar and nonalveolar types of

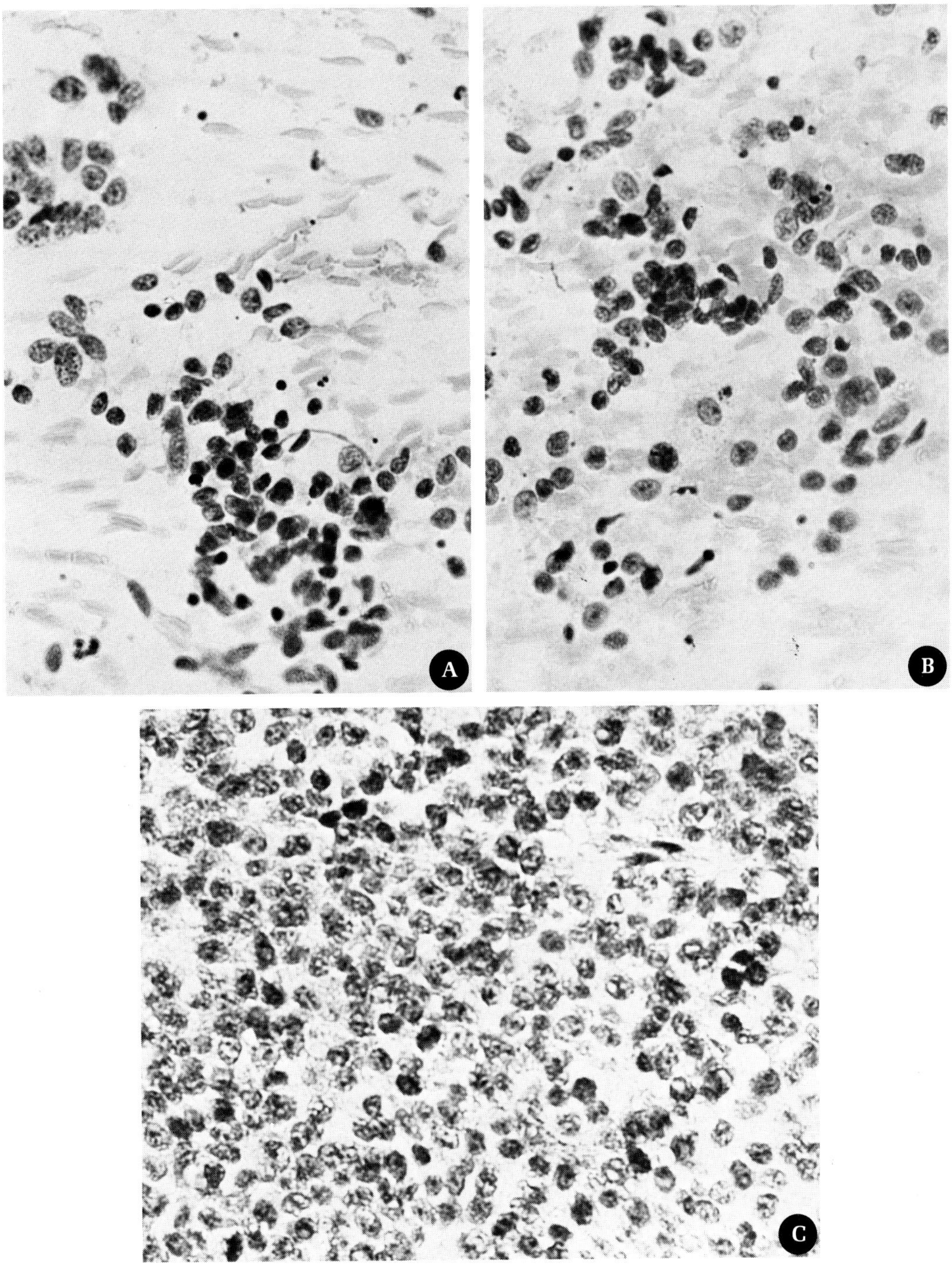

Figure 5-22. **A** and **B**, Smears prepared from percutaneous aspirate of an embryonal rhabdomyosarcoma. The tumor cells are small and uniform and form clusters and pseudorosettes **(A)**. The cytoplasm is small and poorly defined (**A** and **B**, H & E, ×350).

C, Tissue section of embryonal rhabdomyosarcoma cut from cell block of aspirate. Notice poorly preserved and uniform neoplastic cells with "washed-out" cytoplasm and nuclei, and adherence between tumor cells (H & E, ×350).

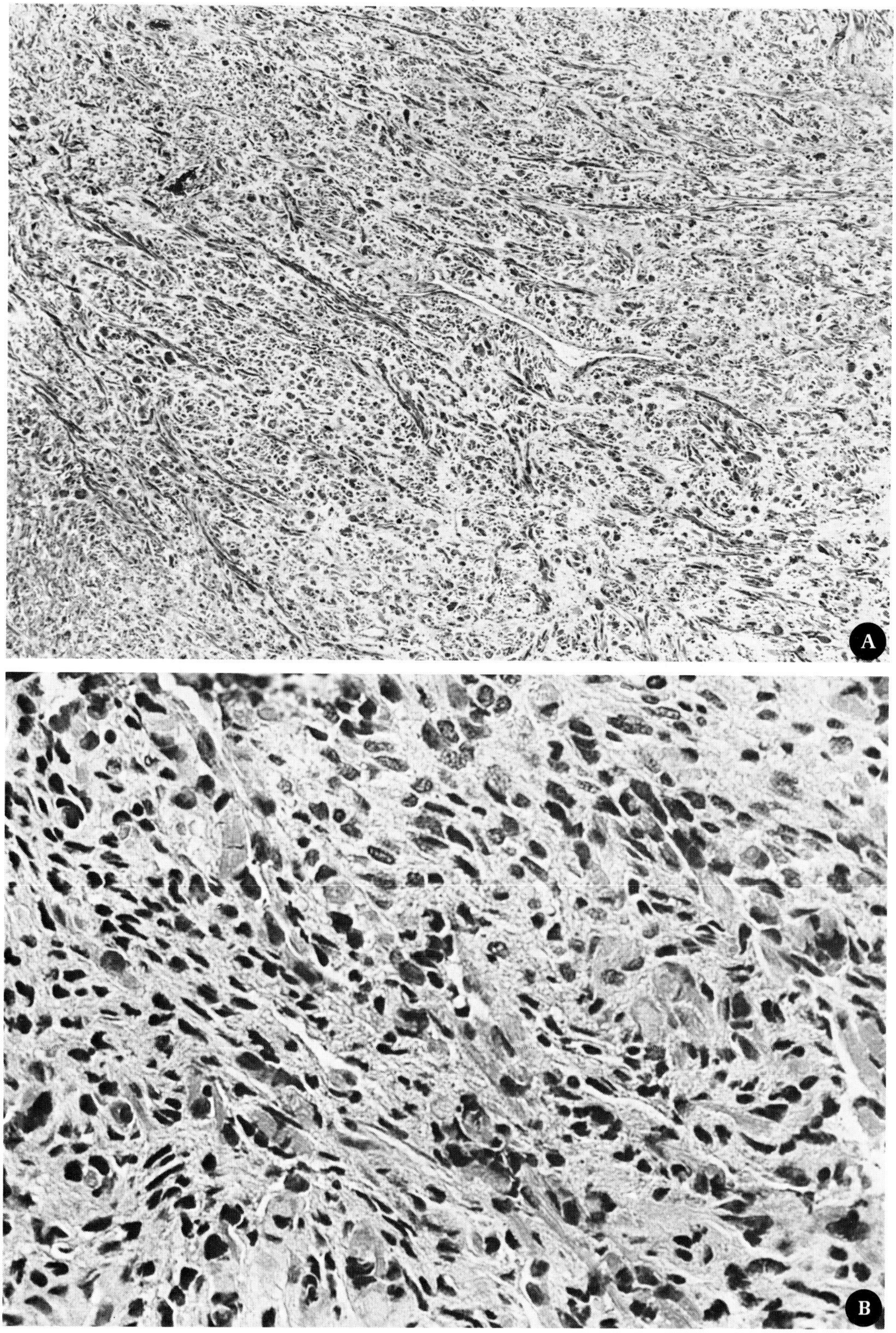

Figure 5-23. Embryonal rhabdomyosarcoma of the prostate of a young child. There is perhaps more pleomorphism than usually seen in most embryonal rhabdomyosarcomas, but the dominant cells are small pyknotic oval cells or short spindle cells. Numerous capillary vessels and tissue slits are visible in the tumor (**A,** H & E, ×35; **B,** H & E, ×350).

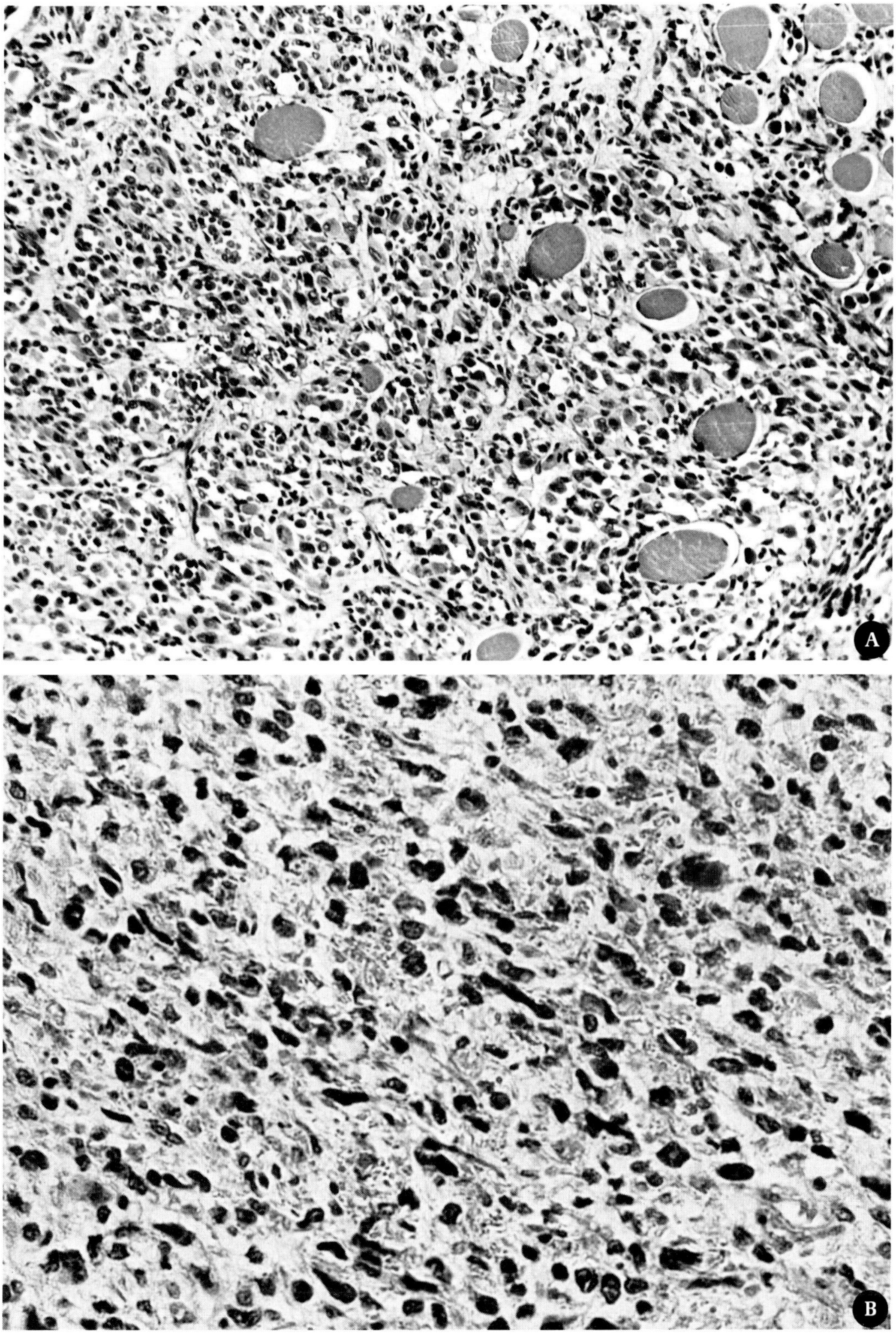

Figure 5-24. Embryonal rhabdomyosarcoma of the thigh.

A, Tumor cells either infiltrate the muscle or indicate the site of neoplastic transformation. Tumor cells form numerous pseudorosettes or alveoli either by cohesion or by taking over the fibroreticular frame of destroyed muscle fibers (H & E, ×140).

B, The nuclei of the tumor cells are pyknotic, the cytoplasm is granular, and the stroma is myxoid. Note a number of binucleated forms. (H & E, ×350).

rhabdomyosarcomas without making consistent conclusions (Enterline and Horn, 1958; Enzinger and Shiraki, 1969; Schuster et al, 1972) (Figs. 5-25, 5-26).

Our experience with these tumors shows that most of the embryonal rhabdomyosarcomas contain more than one of the described patterns and are composed of a spectrum of tumor cells (Table 5-11).

Embryonal rhabdomyosarcoma is the most common soft tissue sarcoma in children, and the number of case reports and review articles on this topic attest to that (Stobbe and Dargeon, 1950; Dito and Batsakis, 1962; Lawrence et al, 1964; Masson and Soule, 1965; Nelson, 1968; Soule et al, 1969; Exelby, 1974). It is estimated that from 4 to 8% of all malignant tumors in children under 15 years of age are embryonal rhabdomyosarcoma. Histologically identical tumors may also occur in other than children in the pediatric ages, but they are uncommon (Table 5-10; Figs. 5-27, 5-28).

The age incidence of children with embryonal rhabdomyosarcoma varies according to the primary site of the tumor, but the median age in most studies is listed as 5 years. Tumors of the *head and neck, extremities,* and *trunk* may be seen at any age in childhood. *Paratesticular lesions* are primarily seen in children after the age of 9 years, with the peak incidence being in adolescents between 14 and 17 years of age. Embryonal rhabdomyosarcomas of the *bladder, prostate,* and *vagina* are usually seen in infants.

TABLE 5-11. ***Embryonal Rhabdomyosarcomas of Soft Tissues***

PRIMARY SITE	NO. OF PATIENTS
Head and neck	133
Upper extremity	20
Trunk	39
Lower extremity	67
Other	9
Total	268

Miller and Dalager, in 1974, found by studying the death certificates of 1,170 children who died of rhabdomyosarcoma that there are two peaks in age distribution. One occurs soon after birth and is mainly due to head and neck and genitourinary lesions and the other peak during late adolescence is mainly due to tumors of the paratesticular structures (Fig. 5-29).

Our experience and the experience of others shows that one third to 50% of the embryonal rhabdomyosarcomas are primary neoplasms of the head and neck region, 20% arise in the extremities, and the remaining are either visceral or trunk lesions.

The rate of *metastasis to lymph nodes,* in various studies, ranges from 15 to 25%. It is felt that the rate and modality of metastasis is influenced by anatomic site, size, and clinical stage of the tumor.

Familial distribution of embryonal rhabdomyosarcoma was suggested by Li and Fraumeni, in 1969. They found that in families of 5 of 418 children studied, all of whom died with embryonal rhabdomyosarcoma, a second child also had a soft tissue sarcoma and a high frequency of other cancers; e.g., mammary carcinoma occurred among female relatives of the children.

Embryonal rhabdomyosarcoma is prone to occur where striated muscle is not usually found, e.g., bile duct, urinary bladder, vagina, spermatic cord, and prostate. It is the most common malignant neoplasm involving the pelvis of children. Sporadic examples have been found in the *lungs, heart, larynx, esophagus, brain,* and *gastrointestinal tract.* The origin of striated muscle tumors in organs in which normally no striated muscle is found has not been explained satisfactorily; however, if one considers the ubiquitous presence of mesectodermal remnants, it is easy to understand the origin of rhabdomyosarcomas at unusual sites (Zimmerman et al, 1972). Sandborn et al (1967) found two layers of atypical striated muscle in the intestine of the larvae of Drosophila. They also mentioned Auber's work which described striated muscle fibers in the intestine of the scorpion.

Davis et al, in 1969, reviewed 18 reported cases of *embryonal rhabdomyosarcoma of bile ducts* and added 5 of their own cases. Primary tumors of the biliary tree occur more frequently in females than in males, and most of the tumors appear prior to 4 years of age and resemble botryoid sarcoma grossly and microscopically. On the average, patients in all known cases died because of local complications in less than 6 months after initial diagnosis.

Embryonal rhabdomyosarcoma of the urinary bladder almost always presents in the form of botryoid sarcoma. Metastases to regional lymph nodes and distant sites are a relatively late occurrence.

Medical historians believe that it was Rokitansky, who first described a *paratesticular embryonal rhabdomyosarcoma,* but it was without question Neuman, in 1866, who first reported the results of a histologic examination of a rhabdomyosarcoma in a 3-year-old child. Paratesticular embryonal rhabdomyosarcoma is extremely rare. It is estimated that less than 1% of intrascrotal neoplasms are rhabdomyosarcomas. According to Littmann et al (1972) and Beccia et al (1976) only a third of all reported cases of paratesticular rhabdomyosarcomas occurred in patients older than 16 years (Fig. 5-30). According to Exelby (1979), the combination of chemotherapy, irradiation, and surgical treatment (orchiectomy; groin, pelvic, and retroperitoneal node dissection) of patients with paratesticular embryonal rhabdomyosarcoma assures 2-year survival for 80% and a 5-year disease-free period for 50% of patients. This result is achieved despite the fact that approximately 10% of the deep groin nodes and 60% of the retroperitoneal lymph nodes above the bifurcation are found to contain metastatic tumor.

Head and neck regions, including the orbit and middle ear, are the most common sites of embryonal rhabdomyosarcoma (Table 5-12). *Intracranial* (Deutsch et al, 1972) and *intraocular* sites (Zimmerman et al, 1972) are exceedingly rare sources of origin (Fig. 5-31).

The intrinsic *larynx* is an equally rare site of origin of embryonal rhabdomyosarcoma (Kernan and Cracovaner, 1935; Kratz and Ritterhoff, 1961; Canalis et al, 1976). Of the approximately two dozen reported cases less than half occurred in children, and most of the patients were males.

Recent years have witnessed major advances in the management of embryonal rhabdomyosarcoma. Combined treatment with surgery, irradiation therapy, and multiagent chemotherapy is the standard current management of patients with embryonal rhabdomyosarcoma. As a result of diligent use of various combination therapy protocols, today more than 50%

TABLE 5-12. ***Embryonal Rhabdomyosarcoma of the Orbit***

AUTHORS	NO. OF CASES	SITE OF ORIGIN			
		ORBIT	EYELID	CONJUNCTIVA	OTHER
Calhoun and Reese, 1942	19	10	4	4	1
Frayer and Enterline, 1959	12	10	1	0	1
Ashton and Morgan, 1965	33	19	11	3	0
Jones et al, 1965	62	47	12	2	1

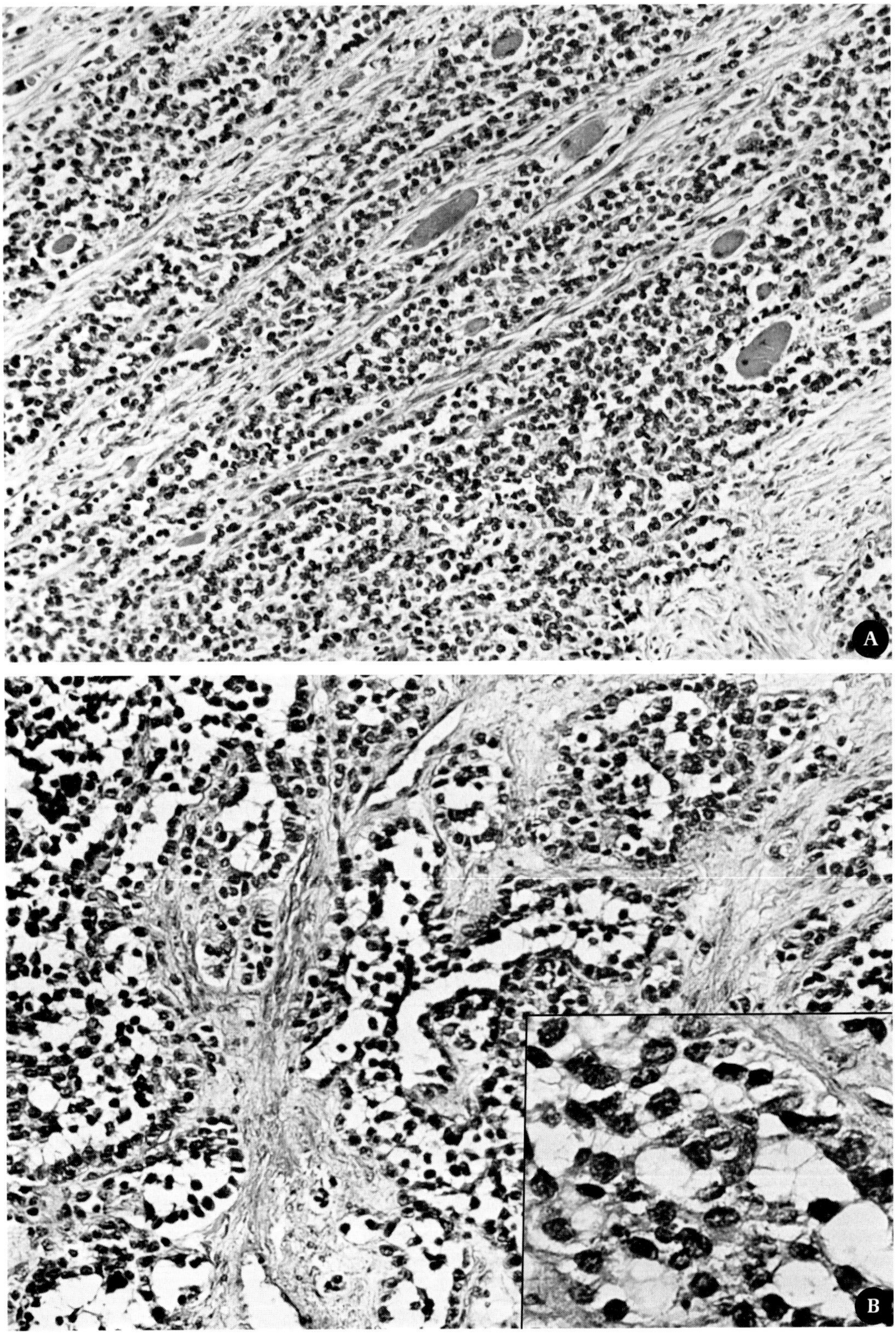

Figure 5-25. Embryonal rhabdomyosarcoma of the so-called alveolar type. The fairly typical neoplastic embryonal rhabdomyoblasts use the existing reticular network of the striated muscle to infiltrate and form the characteristic alveoli. The partition between alveolar nests is formed by sparsely cellular fibrovascular connective tissue elements (**A,** H & E, ×140; **B,** H & E, ×350; inset ×570).

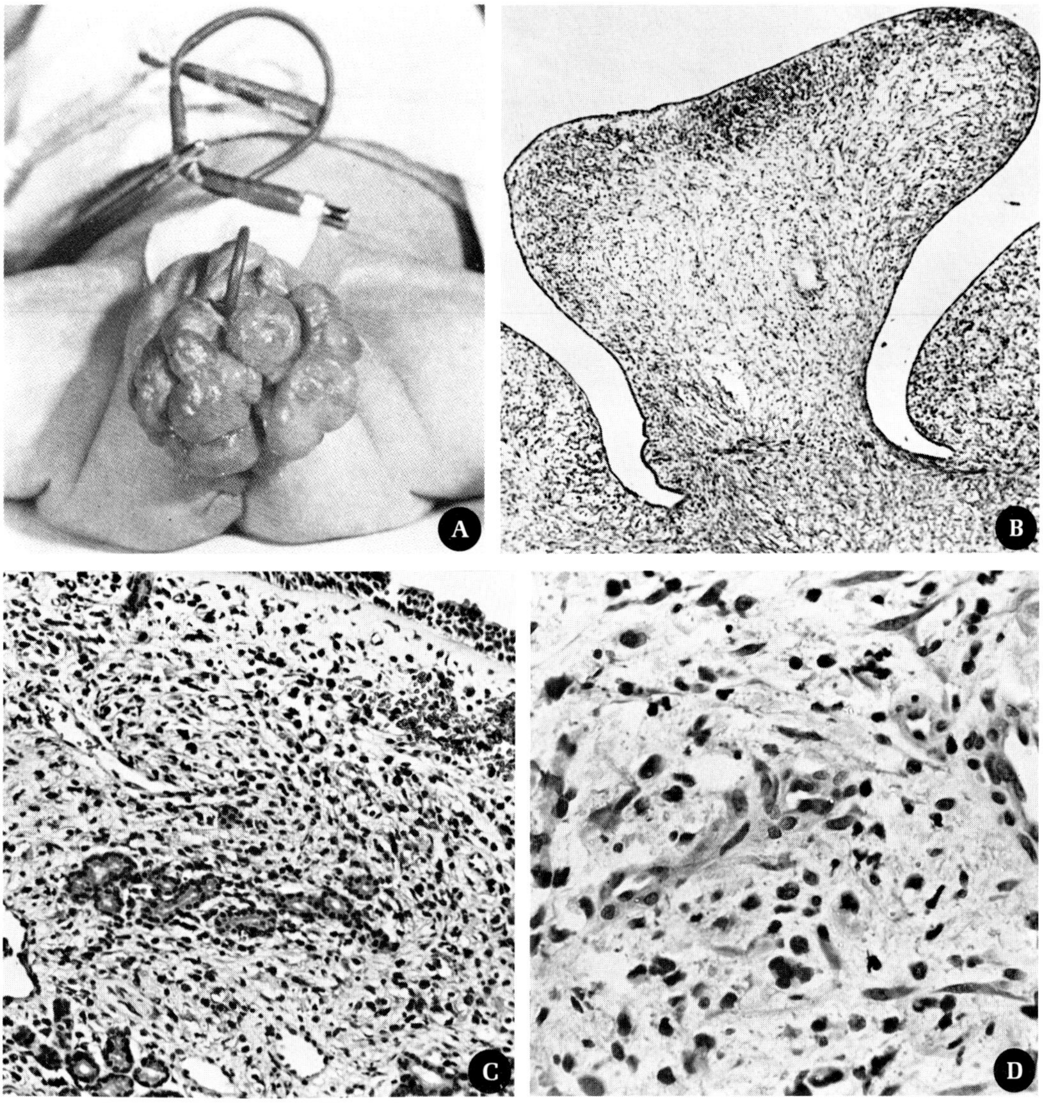

Figure 5-26. A, Botryoid sarcoma of the vagina of a 2-month-old infant presenting as a polypoid perineal mass. (From Pack, G. M., and Ariel, I. M.: Tumors of Somatic Tissues and Bone. New York, Harper and Row, 1964.)

B, Typical polypoid appearance with dense clusters of neoplastic cells near the mucosal lining (H & E, ×35).

C and **D,** Botryoid sarcoma of the nasopharynx. Pyknotic neoplastic embryonal rhabdomyoblasts in a loosely arranged fibrovascular submucosal stroma. There are numerous binucleated and elongated spindly forms between the network of hypertrophic capillary vessels in **D** (**C,** H & E, ×85; **D,** H & E, ×350).

of the patients survive beyond 5 years. It seems that anatomic site and stage of the diseases greatly influence survival (Table 5-13). For example, in most reports it is shown that orbital and genitourinary lesions have a more favorable prognosis than tumors of the extremities. It is certain that recent survival figures will be further improved by more proper clinical staging and by more appropriate selection of chemotherapeutic drugs as well as the sequence of their administration and dosage (Fig. 5-32 and see Fig. 1-59 and Table 1-15).

Embryonal rhabdomyosarcoma must be distinguished from other small cell malignant neoplasms, e.g., *neuroblastoma, Ewing's sarcoma, primitive neuroectodermal tumor,* and *lymphoreticular neoplasms.* In this respect it is mandatory that

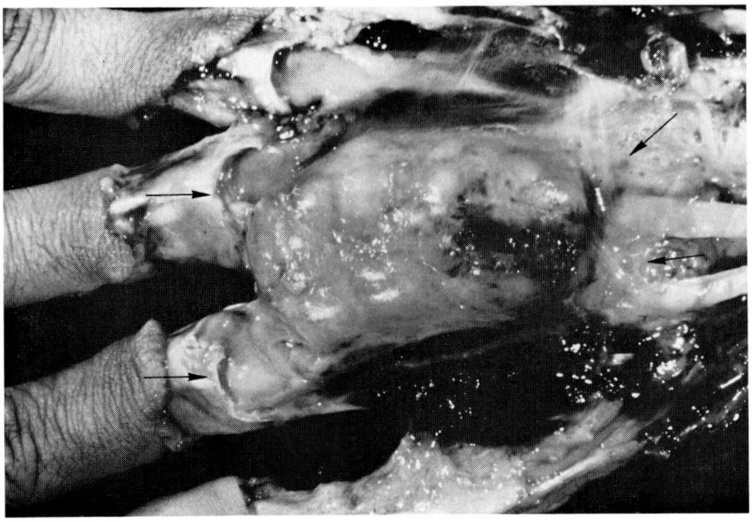

Figure 5-27. Amputated hand of a child after dissection shows embryonal rhabdomyosarcoma invading tendons (arrows) and other soft tissues (From Hajdu, S. I., and Hajdu, E. O.: Cytopathology of Sarcomas. Philadelphia, W. B. Saunders Co., 1976).

the pathologist study the microscopic slides with full knowledge of pertinent clinical information and laboratory findings. Almost invariably, if a sufficient number of sections are prepared, one will find at least traces of embryonal rhabdomyoblasts and areas suggestive of either alveolar or botyroid patterns in embryonal rhabdomyosarcomas (see Chapters 7 and 8). According to Sarnat et al (1979) myofibrils are clearly identifiable with ATPase and nicotinamide adenine dinucleotide tetrazolium reductase (NADH-TR) may show longitudinal and cross striations that are not demonstrable with hematoxylin and eosin and PTAH stains.

PLEOMORPHIC RHABDOMYOSARCOMA

The literature on pleomorphic rhabdomyosarcoma is scarce. In most studies on rhabdomyosarcomas the pleomorphic forms are admixed with the embryonal forms (Table 5-9; Fig. 5-8) (Linscheid, 1965; Keyhani and Booher, 1968; Kaloyannides, 1969). Pleomorphic rhabdomyosarcomas

TABLE 5-13. ***Outline of Study Design Used in the American Intergroup Rhabdomyosarcoma Study***

GROUP	STUDY DESIGN
I	Localized disease, completely resected (regional nodes not involved)
	(a) Confined to muscle or organ of origin
	(b) Contiguous involvement—infiltration outside the muscle or organ of origin, as through fascial planes
II	(a) Grossly resected tumor with microscopic residual disease (nodes negative)
	(b) Regional disease, completely resected (nodes positive or negative)
	(c) Regional disease with involved nodes, grossly resected, but with evidence of microscopic residual disease
III	Incomplete resection or biopsy with gross residual disease
IV	Metastatic disease present at onset

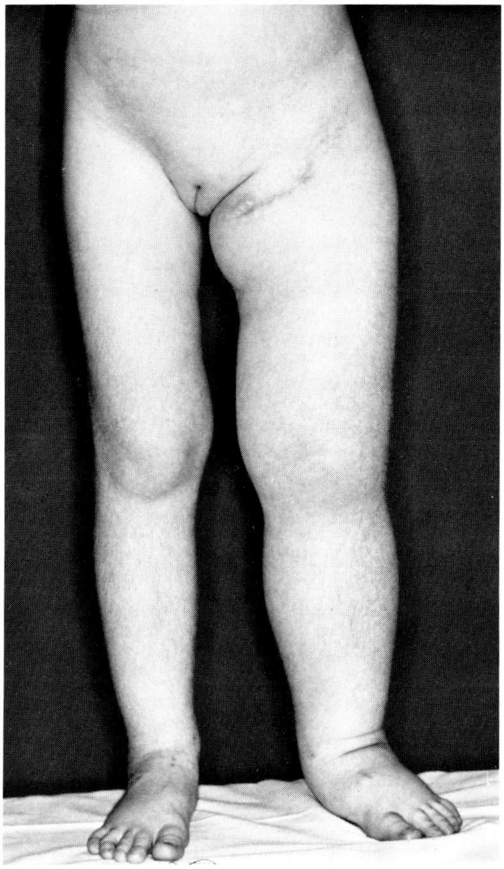

Figure 5-28. Embryonal rhabdomyosarcoma of the left groin of a 3-year-old girl. There is marked swelling and lymphedema of the whole extremity.

have always been a source of fascination and frustration because of their diverse morphology.

Pleomorphic rhabdomyosarcoma is predominantly a disease of adults, in contrast to embryonal rhabdomyosarcoma which predominantly affects males under the age of 16 years. Pleomorphic rhabdomyosarcoma has the highest incidence during the fifth decade, and males and females are affected in almost equal proportion. Although this trend in age distribution holds up in most cases, age should not be considered as a barrier to the occurrence of pleomorphic or embryonal forms of rhabdomyosarcoma. Our experience with pleomorphic rhabdomyosarcoma is summarized in Figures 5-33 and 5-34 and Table 5-9.

Pleomorphic rhabdomyosarcomas are usually silent in growth. Although most of the tumors reach a considerable size prior to diagnosis, they are usually less bulky than liposarcomas (see Chapter 4). They are moderately firm and freely movable deep-seated lesions. Changes in shape and consistency with relaxation or contraction of the muscle are important features that point to a muscular location of the tumor. The consistency of the tumor, however, may vary from case to case according to the amount of collagen and other stromal components.

Stout (1946) stated that if a soft tissue

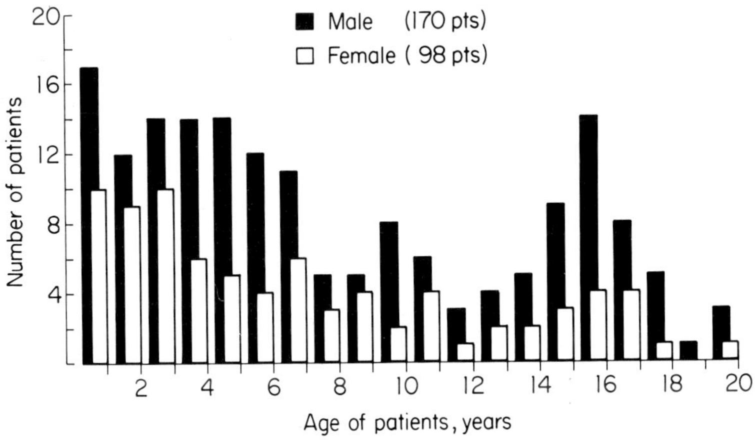

Figure 5-29. Age and sex distribution of 268 patients treated for embryonal rhabdomyosarcoma at Memorial Sloan-Kettering Cancer Center.

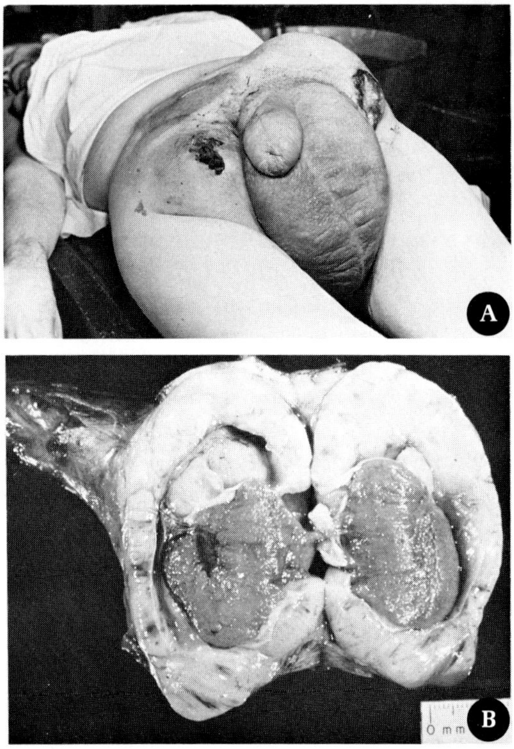

Figure 5-30. **A**, Paratesticular embryonal rhabdomyosarcoma with bilateral inguinal and pelvic metastases.

B, Paratesticular embryonal rhabdomyosarcoma removed by orchiectomy. The sarcoma encircles and invades the cross-sectioned testis. (From Hajdu, S. I., and Hajdu, E. O.: Cytopathology of Sarcomas and Other Nonepithelial Malignant Tumors. Philadelphia, W. B. Saunders Co., 1976.)

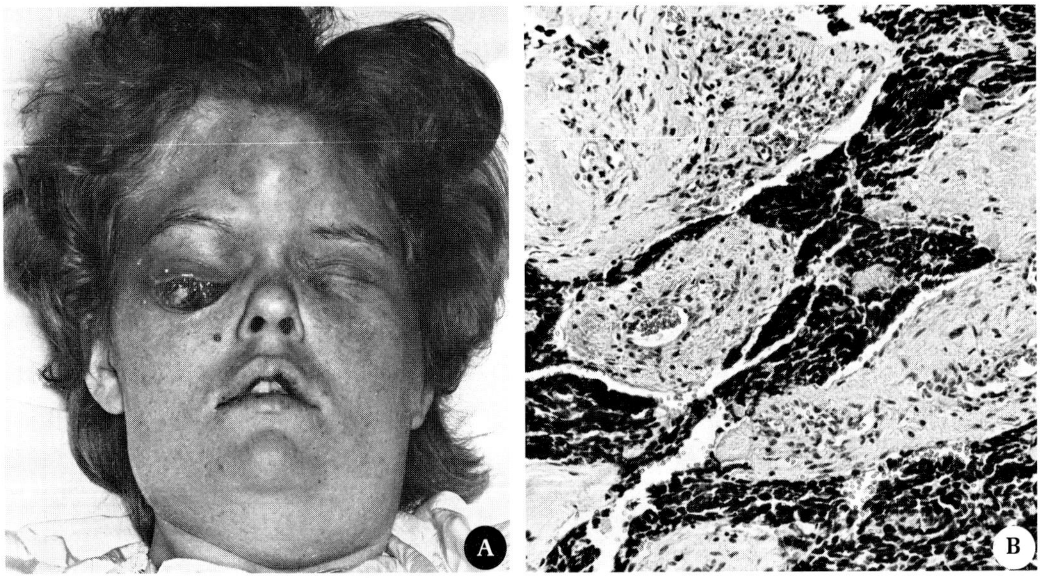

Figure 5-31. Fatal embryonal rhabdomyosarcoma of the orbit in a teenager. Microscopically, embryonal rhabdomyosarcoma in head and neck areas may show pile-up of the tumor cells between dense fibrovascular clefts. Note the perivascular fibrous tissue and the pyknotic and compressed, oat cell-looking, tumor cells (H & E, ×85).

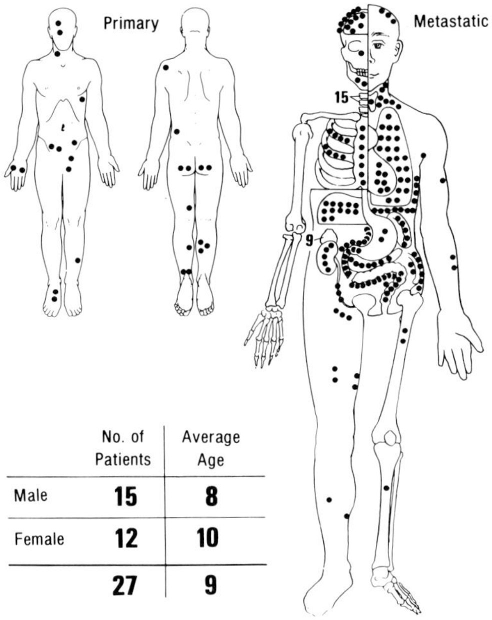

Figure 5-32. At autopsy it is shown that no organ or organ system is spared by metastatic embryonal rhabdomyosarcoma. Vertebrae, ribs, sternum, iliac bones, as well as long bones, lungs, liver, skull, mesentery, heart, pancreas, kidneys, and skin, are all targets of metastatic spread (see Appendix).

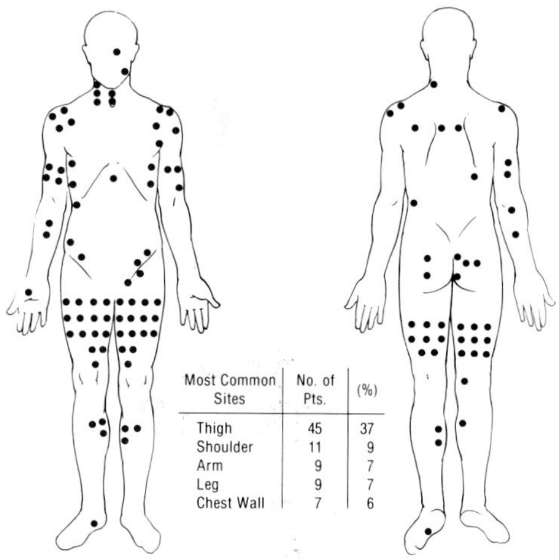

Figure 5-34. Scattergram illustrating regional distribution of 121 pleomorphic rhabdomyosarcomas.

tumor "starts deeply and grows into the skin producing a projecting, dark red, fungating mass, it may be a rhabdomyosarcoma." The gross appearance of the excised tumor is reddish brown and is influenced by the vascularity and amount of necrosis. On gross examination many of the tumors appear circumscribed and encapsulated. These features are almost always illusory, since the tumors usually extend far beyond the circumscribed growth.

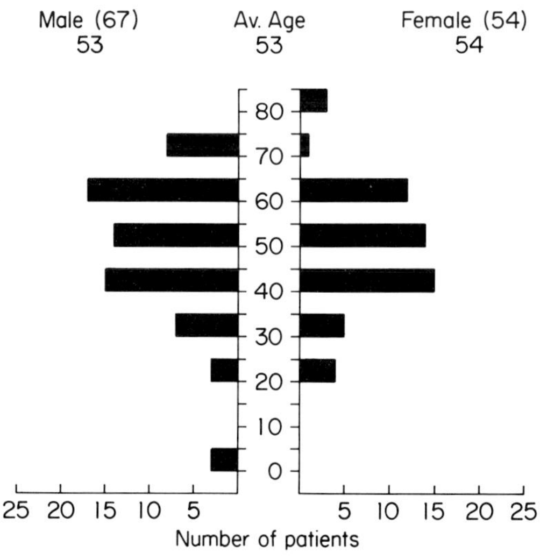

Figure 5-33. Age and sex distribution of 121 patients treated at Memorial Sloan-Kettering Cancer Center for pleomorphic rhabdomyosarcoma.

Anatomically, most of the pleomorphic rhabdomyosarcomas can be traced to inter- or intramuscular fascial tissues as the most probable source of origin. They appear most commonly in the thigh, shoulder, and upper arm (Fig. 5-34). The etiology is unknown and it is debated whether trauma or pre-existing intramuscular benign lesions (e.g., proliferative myositis, rhabdomyoma, or myositis ossificans) play a role in the appearance of certain rhabdomyosarcomas. I have seen two cases in which histologically proven myositis ossificans was present in the same muscle compartment for 7 and 9 years, respectively, where rhabdomyosarcoma appeared subsequently, but I have yet to see transformation of myositis proliferans or rhabdomyoma to rhabdomyosarcoma (Figs. 5-35, 5-36).

Microscopically, pleomorphic rhabdomyosarcomas are composed of *rounded* (rhabdomyoblasts), *strap-shaped* (rhabdomyocytes), or *racquet-shaped* (dediffer-

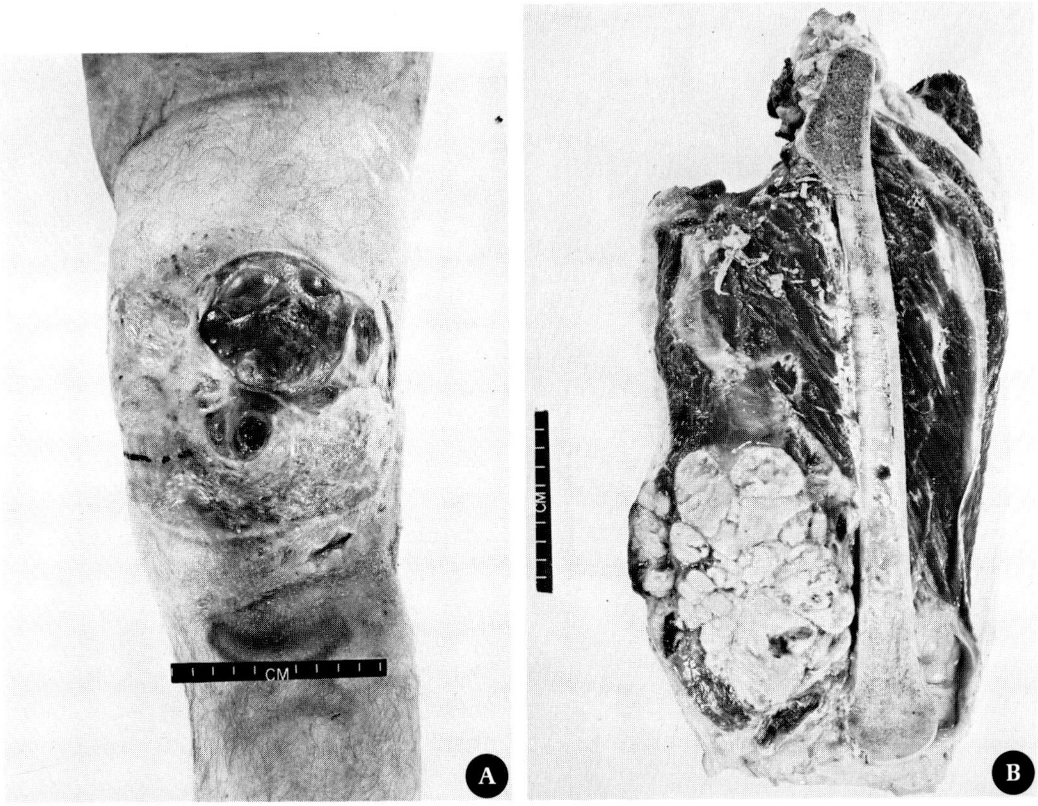

Figure 5-35. Pleomorphic rhabdomyosarcoma of the thigh before and after amputation. The sarcoma is fairly well defined and multilobular. Notice the satellite tumor nodules under the skin and adhesion of the tumor to the periosteum at one point.

entiated myocytes) cells (Figs. 5-37 color, 5-38, 5-39). The rounded malignant rhabdomyoblasts are polygonal or truly round, pink cells with large solitary nuclei and concentrically fibrillar, granular, and compact cytoplasms. There is considerable variation in the size of these cells, and it is not uncommon to see them in ill-defined areas in tumors predominantly composed of the other forms. However, malignant rhabdomyoblasts are rarely the sole components, and it seems appropriate to designate such neoplasms malignant rhabdomyoblastoma. Malignant rhabdomyoblasts are common findings in *paratesticular embryonal rhabdomyosarcoma, immature teratomas,* and *metastatic Wilms' tumors,* as well as in rhabdomyosarcomas following irradiation therapy. The resemblance of these cells to ganglion cells or cells of so-called granular cell myoblastoma can be so striking that pleomorphic rhabdomyosarcoma in which malignant rhabdomyoblasts predominate occasionally is classified as ganglioneuroblastoma or malignant granular cell myoblastoma.

Strap-shaped cells with two or more nuclei arranged in tandem may give the appearance of a spindle-cell tumor to rhabdomyosarcomas. However, the herringbone appearance of fibroblastic tumors (see Chapter 2) is rarely seen in these neoplasms. Multinucleation and longitudinal or cross striation of spindle cells are features of strap-shaped myocytes. Cross striation (Fig. 5-2) is a highly desirable finding for proper classification, but often even diligent search fails to produce arranged myofilaments. In the presence of characteristic microscopic features, such as malignant myoblasts, rhabdomyoblasts, racquet-shaped cells, and elements of embryonal rhabdomyoblasts cross striation is not mandatory for the diagnosis of rhabdomyosarcoma. As early as 1928 Wolbach said that the "myoblastic origin may be identified in the absence of definitely cross-striated cells by the presence of centriole clusters and abortive fibril formation" (Figs. 5-40, 5-41).

It is known from our own experience (Sethi et al, 1977; Hajdu and Fogh, 1978) and reports of others (White and Cox, 1967; McAllister et al, 1969; Nameroff et al, 1970; McAllister et al, 1971) that in tissue culture of muscle cells cross striation and longitudinal myofibrils are variable and may appear, disappear, and reappear within a cell.

The racquet-shaped dedifferentiated myocyte usually contains a single round nucleus at the expanded end of the tapering cytoplasm. The cytoplasm generally stains acidophilic with hematoxylin and eosin (H & E) and contains uniform granules, many of which stain positive with PAS and are digestible with diastase. It is not uncommon to find parallel longitudinal intracytoplasmic filaments extending outward with the cytoplasm for a variable distance. The longitudinal myofibrils, as well as the occasional cross-striated fibrils, stain positive with PTAH stain and scarlet with Masson trichrome. The myofibrils are often curved with twisted ends and bulb-shaped swellings. Longitudinal as well as cross-striated fibers were illustrated by Burgess, in 1913, in his article describing the first case of metastatic rhabdomyosarcoma (see Chapter 1). Rakov, as early as 1937, called attention to the presence of *tonofibrils* in malignant rhabdomyoblasts.

Neoplastic cells of the so-called *spider-web cells* are rare findings but an important morphologic form of malignant elements in pleomorphic rhabdomyosarcoma (Fig. 5-39). Despite the various characteristic cells (Figs. 5-42, 5-43), it should be noted that pleomorphic rhabdomyosarcomas may not show these cells in all parts of the tumor. *Fibroblastic, collagenous, lipoblastic, myxoid,* or *fi-*

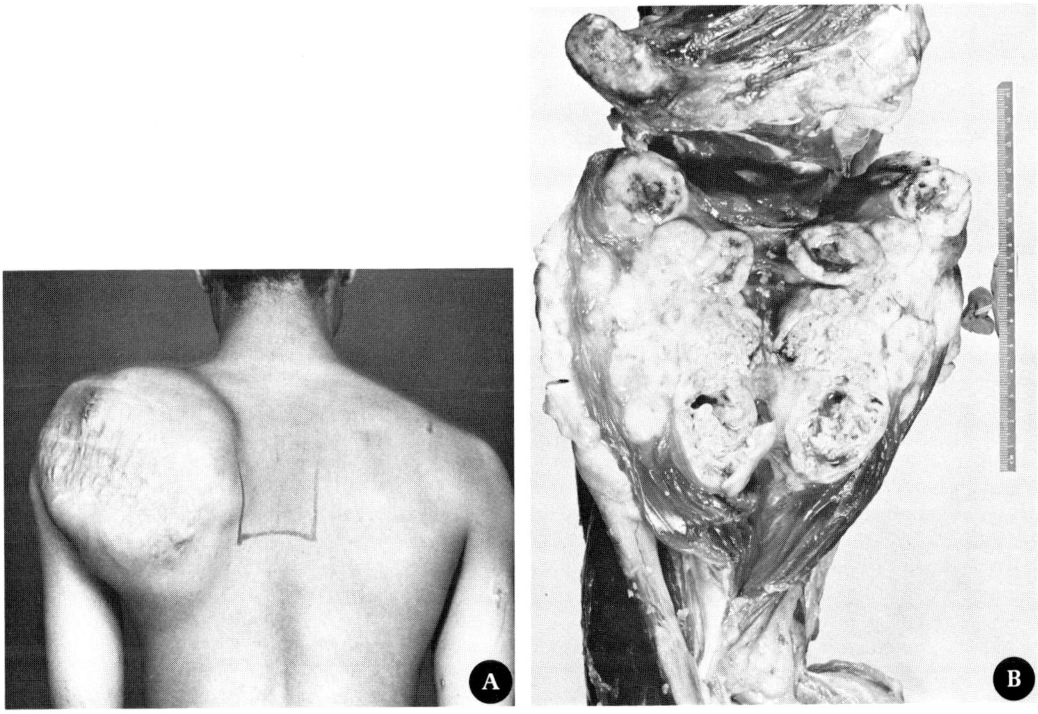

Figure 5-36. A, Massive recurrence of pleomorphic rhabdomyosarcoma. **B,** Multinodular spread of pleomorphic rhabdomyosarcoma with solid and cystic areas.

Figure 5-37. **A,** Leiomyosarcoma of the saphenous vein. This is a low-grade malignant neoplasm histologically; however, the location makes it a potentially dangerous tumor.

It is composed of spindle cells with cigar-shaped nuclei. The cytoplasm is long and fibrillar. The nuclei are moderately pleomorphic, centrally positioned, and darkly stained. The tumor cells have a wide one-directional position, and the intercellular stroma is loosely arranged and sparsely cellular (H & E, ×350).

B, Embryonal rhabdomyosarcoma should be considered as a fully malignant and high-grade neoplasm. It is composed of small cells with pyknotic nuclei and minute pinkish red cytoplasm. The nuclei are usually eccentrically positioned in the cytoplasm and not uncommonly binucleated forms.

Although the tumor cells are small, there is considerable variation in size; however, no multinucleated or giant cells are seen. The stroma is vascular and in areas where the tumor cells are in myxoid or fibrous surrounding the neoplastic rhabdomyoblast may assume a spindle shape (H & E, ×140).

C, Alveolar rhabdomyosarcoma is composed of neoplastic embryonal rhabdomyoblasts, the same type as the ones described in **B.** The distinguishing features of this neoplasm are the uniformity of the tumor cells and their characteristic alveolar arrangement. The alveolar pattern resembles the embryonal myotubules. The tumor cells, as illustrated, are in a loose myxofibrillar and richly vascular stroma (H & E, ×350).

D, Pleomorphic rhabdomyosarcoma is a high-grade malignant tumor. It is composed of a spectrum of pleomorphic neoplastic cells ranging in size and shape from small, round, histiocytic-like cells to polygonal, round, or strap cells. Although the pleomorphism of the tumor cells is a typical feature, it does not permit specific identification without demonstration of longitudinal or cross-striated myofilaments and the presence of embryonal rhabdomyoblasts. Perhaps the most important is to consider the uniform acidophilic staining of the cytoplasm, and several sections must be searched carefully for cross-striated tumor cells. The earliest form of cross striation can be seen best in longitudinal strap cells, as in this case, either by trichrome stain or PTAH stain (Trichrome, ×350).

E, Rhabdomyoblastoma. This term is introduced to call attention to this unique neoplasm. It is a high-grade neoplasm composed predominantly of acidophilic round or oval cells in a semicohesive or non-cohesive pattern. The tumor cells range in size from small embryonal rhabdomyoblasts to large ganglion cell-like globoid rhabdomyoblasts. Most of the tumor cells are mononuclear, but binucleated or multinucleated with piled-up nuclei are also seen. Most of the nuclei are pyknotic and eccentrically positioned in the granular, homogeneous, and pink cytoplasm (H & E, ×350).

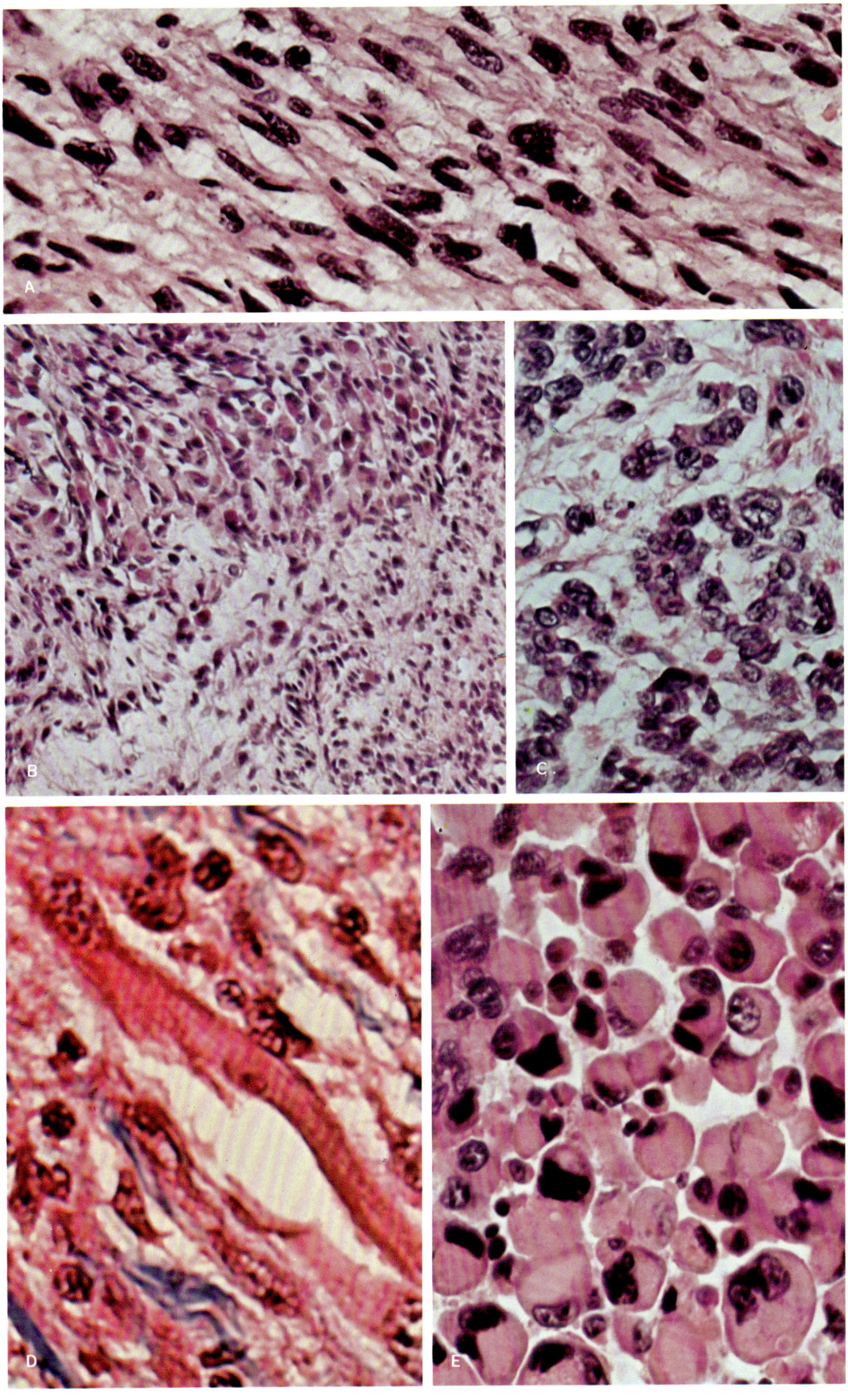

Figure 5-37.

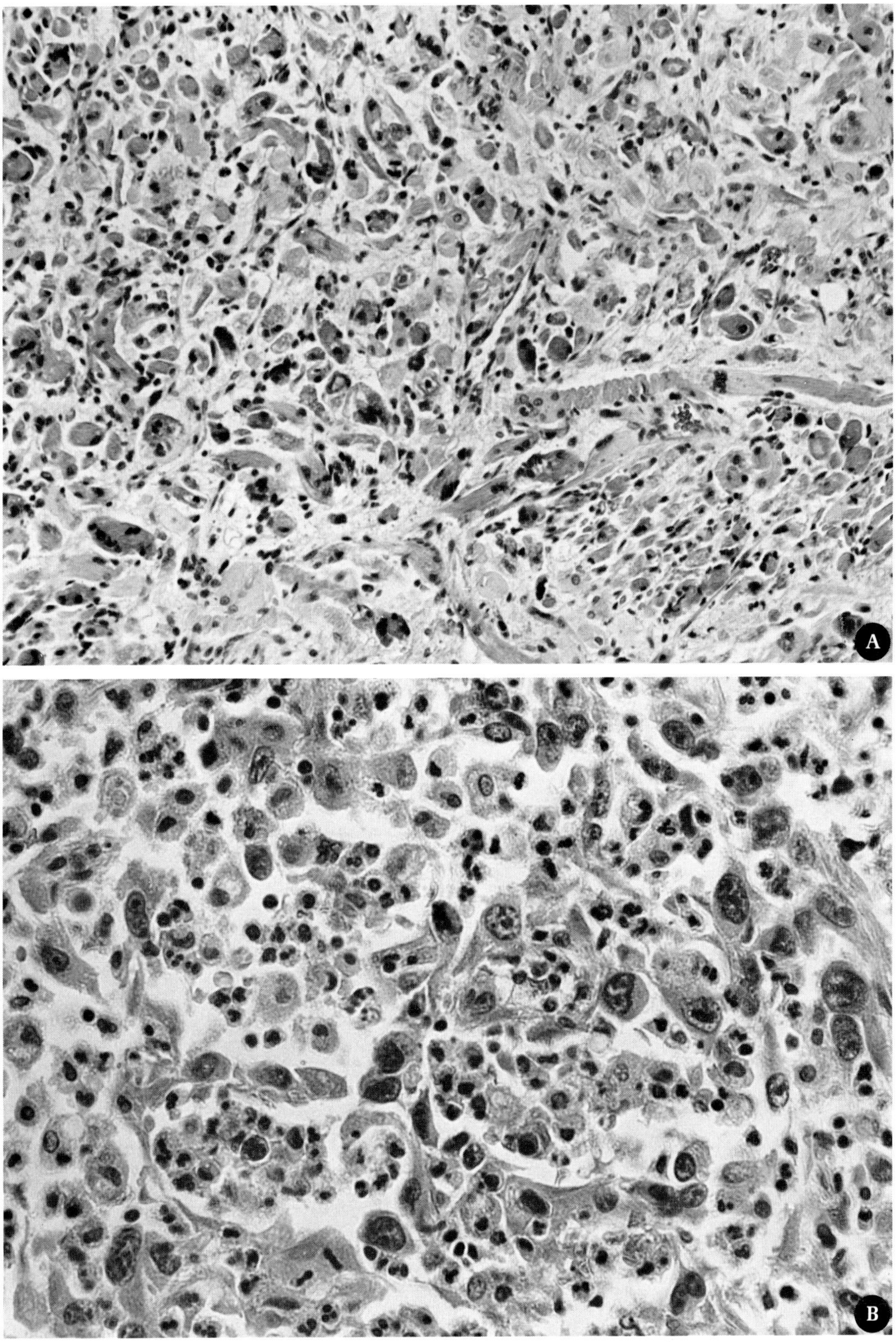

Figure 5-38. Pleomorphic rhabdomyosarcoma composed of polymorphic neoplastic rhabdomyoblasts ranging in size from small embryonal forms to multinucleated giant cells. The nuclei, as well as the cytoplasm, are well defined and both nuclei and nucleoli are prominent. There are numerous unpredictable contacts between neighboring cells (**A,** H & E, ×140; **B,** H & E, ×350).

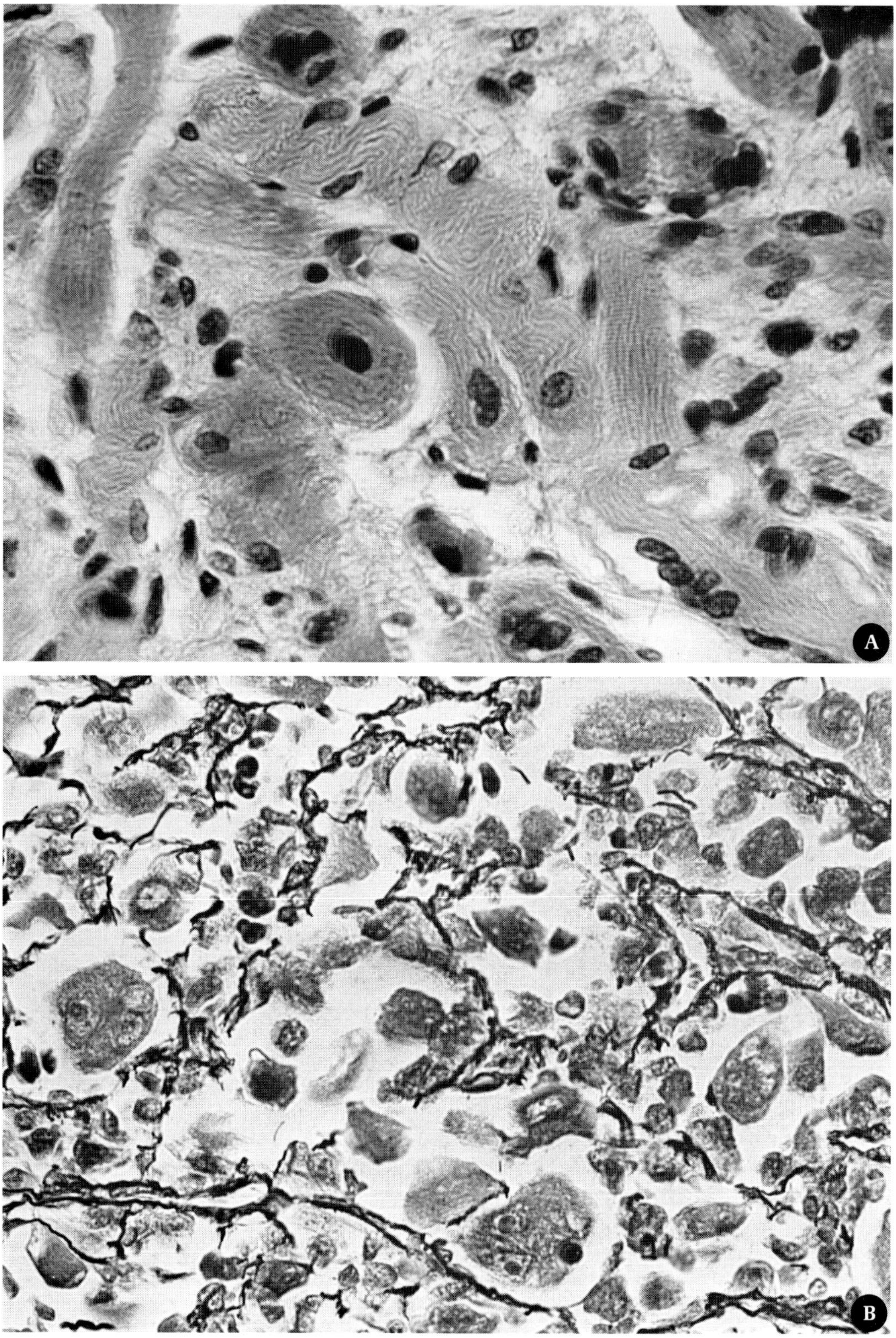

Figure 5-39. A, Pleomorphic rhabdomyosarcoma showing longitudinal and cross-striated cytoplasmic filaments. There are two well-defined round target cells and numerous distorted, multinucleated, and hyperplastic strap cells. In the background, note the embryonal rhabdomyoblasts (H & E, ×570).

B, Reticulin stain of pleomorphic rhabdomyosarcoma demonstrates the indifferent relationship between neoplastic cells and stromal fibers (×570). (Please notice that reticulin fibers in fibrous histiocytomas and fibrosarcomas are closely related to cytoplasmic processes. See Chapter 2.)

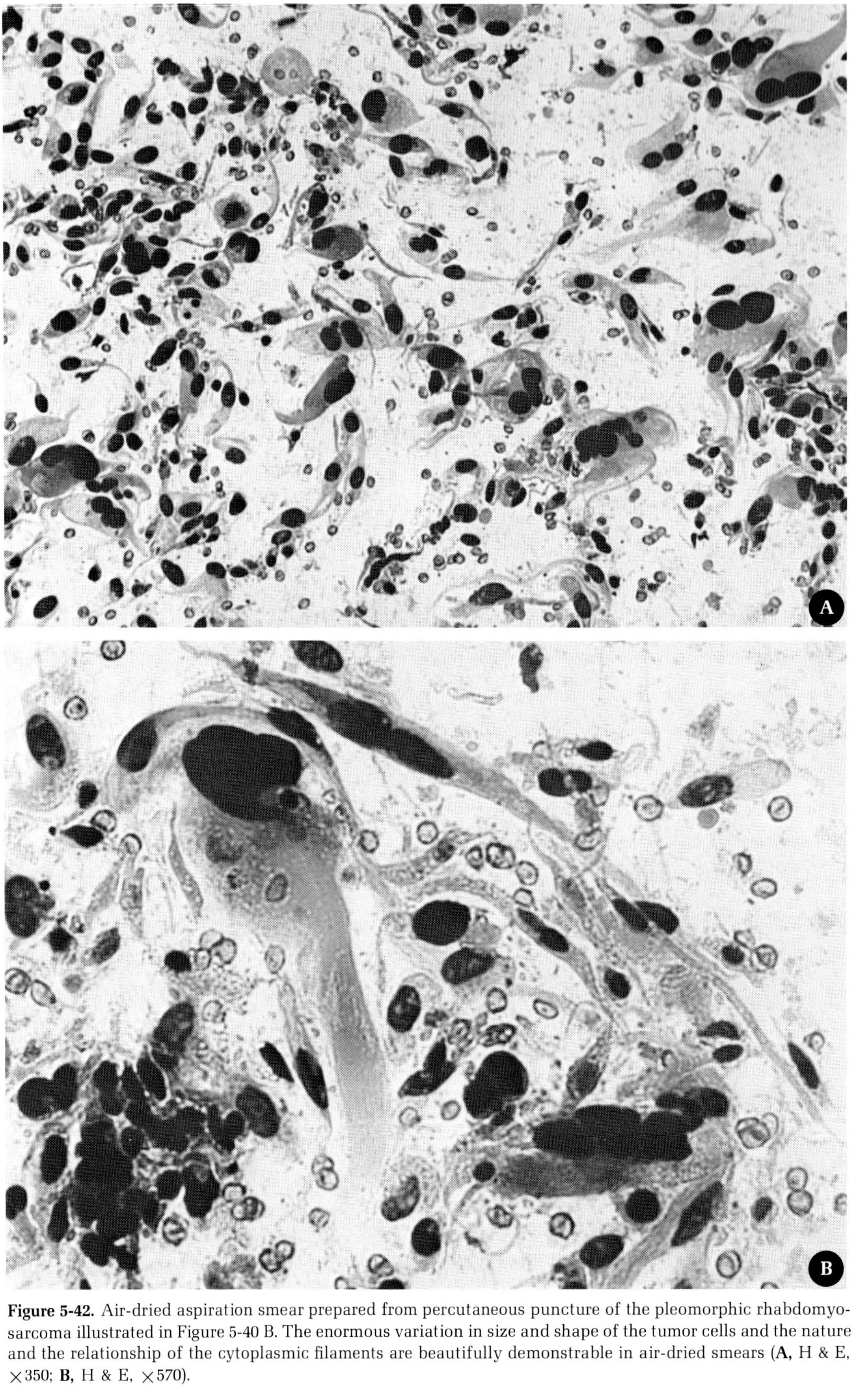

Figure 5-42. Air-dried aspiration smear prepared from percutaneous puncture of the pleomorphic rhabdomyosarcoma illustrated in Figure 5-40 B. The enormous variation in size and shape of the tumor cells and the nature and the relationship of the cytoplasmic filaments are beautifully demonstrable in air-dried smears (**A,** H & E, ×350; **B,** H & E, ×570).

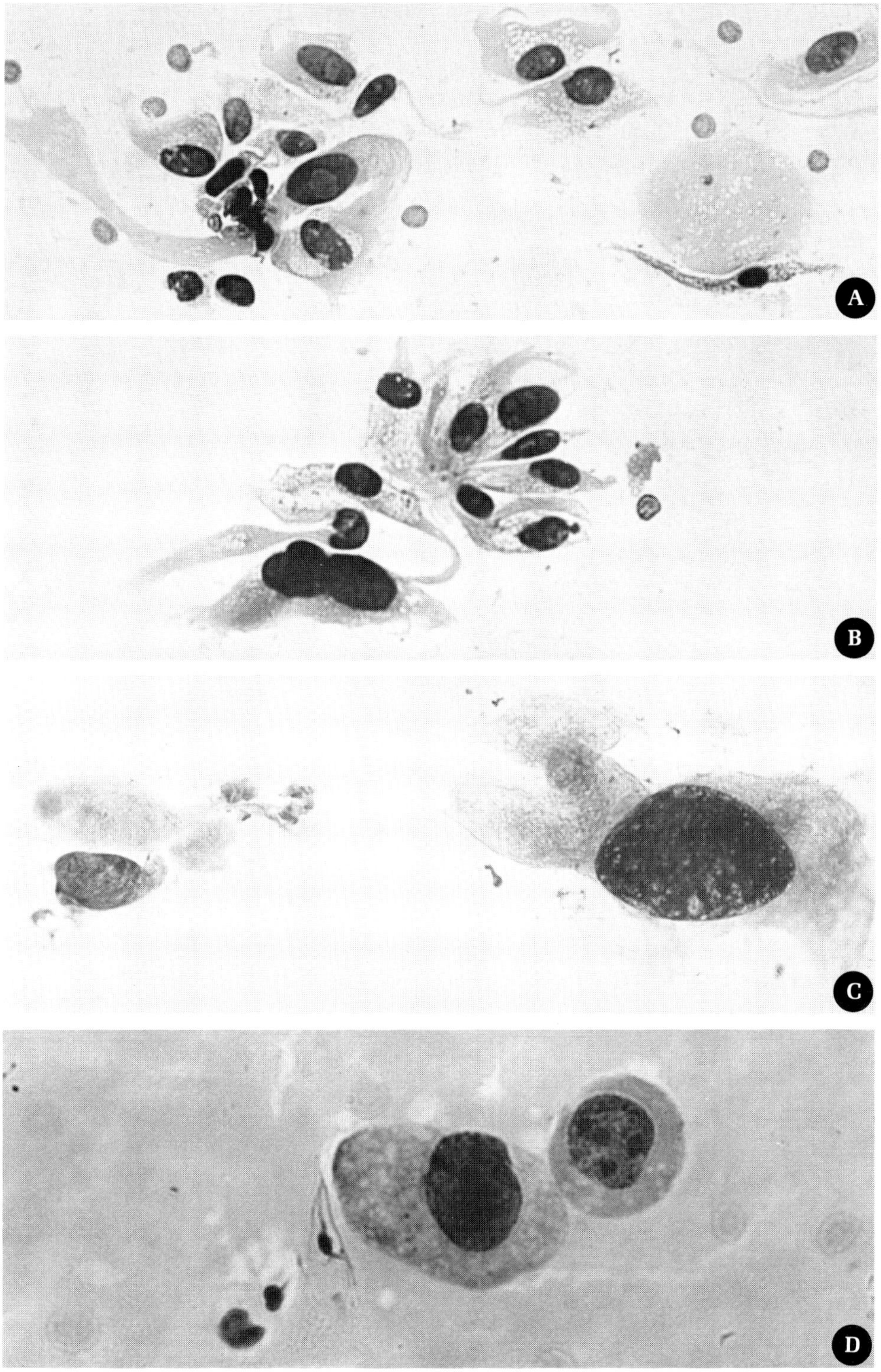

Figure 5-43. **A** and **B,** The tangled and intimate relationship of neoplastic cells of pleomorphic rhabdomysarcoma as seen in air-dried aspiration smear (H & E, ×350).

C and **D,** Exfoliated neoplastic cells of pleomorphic rhabdomyosarcoma in smears stained by the Papanicolaou technique (×570).

brous histiocytic areas indicate the multipotential ability of mesenchymal cells. Such findings do not indicate that pleomorphic rhabdomyosarcoma does not exist, and all such tumors should be called fibrous histiocytoma as proposed by certain writers. Ignoring characteristic, differentiated and dedifferentiated, cells would be wrong, just as it would be wrong to assume that osteogenic sarcoma does not exist because occasionally the bulky part of the tumor shows nothing else than fibroblastic and other undifferentiated mesenchymal cells and only traces of the malignant osteoids. On the other hand, it is true that every pleomorphic sarcoma having acidophilic cells is not necessarily a pleomorphic rhabdomyosarcoma (Table 5-14).

Apparently immunofluorescence techniques employing antiskeletal-muscle antibodies are of little value in the differentiation of rhabdomyosarcoma from other soft tissue sarcomas. Rhabdomyosarcomas either contain so little antigen that present methods lack sufficient sensitivity for its detection or are antigenically different from skeletal muscle and incapable of binding with antiskeletal muscle antibodies (Pertschuk, 1975).

Most of the tumor cells in pleomorphic rhabdomyosarcoma have sharply outlined cytoplasms. The tumor cells may lie adjacent to each other parallel and in arranged pattern, or they may be haphazardly grouped together without any apparent pattern. The stroma most often is finely reticular or collagenous with an irregular network of large capillary vessels.

TABLE 5-14. ***Diagnoses on Review of 214 Sarcomas Originally Diagnosed as Pleomorphic Rhabdomyosarcoma***

DIAGNOSIS ON REVIEW	NO. OF CASES
Pleomorphic rhabdomyosarcoma	121
Malignant fibrous histiocytoma	64
Liposarcoma	6
Fibrosarcoma	3
Leiomyosarcoma	9
Tendosynovial sarcoma	4
Embryonal rhabdomyosarcoma	3
Other	4

As a rule, mitoses in pleomorphic rhabdomyosarcoma are present but sparse. Other features such as *cannibalism, bizarre multinucleation, nuclear vacuolization, giant nucleolus* are rare findings and can be seen in many other pleomorphic sarcomas than rhabdomyosarcomas.

Ultrastructural examination of rhabdomyosarcoma reveals features characteristic of developing myoblasts and myocytes and often permits more exact subclassification than the classification feasible by light microscopy. Although a number of articles appeared on the subject (Toker, 1968; Horvat et al, 1970; Boram et al, 1972; Morales, 1972), no specific organelles have been found which would help to distinguish between benign and malignant rhabdomyoblasts (Figs. 5-44, 5-45).

The first electron microscopic study of rhabdomyosarcoma was that of Kroll et al in 1963. It has been stated by every observer in reference to the ultrastructure of rhabdomyosarcomas that tumor cells of rhabdomyosarcomas prior to the development of thick and thin filaments cannot be distinguished from other types of mesenchymal tumor cells.

Pleomorphic rhabdomyosarcoma is usually considered to be one of the most malignant forms of soft tissue sarcomas. Our experience shows that despite radical surgical ablation most patients died with metastatic disease less than 3 years after initial diagnosis (Fig. 5-46). It seems that irradiation and chemotherapy have no long-lasting beneficial effects (Fig. 5-47).

Considering the embryonal origin of myoblasts from undifferentiated mesenchymal cells, it is not surprising that pleomorphic mesenchymal tumors such as *pleomorphic fibrous histiocytoma* (see Chapter 2), *pleomorphic fibrosarcoma* (see Chapter 2) and *leiomyosarcoma* may cause differential diagnostic difficulties. However, the arranged stromal pattern, foam cells, giant cells of the Touton or

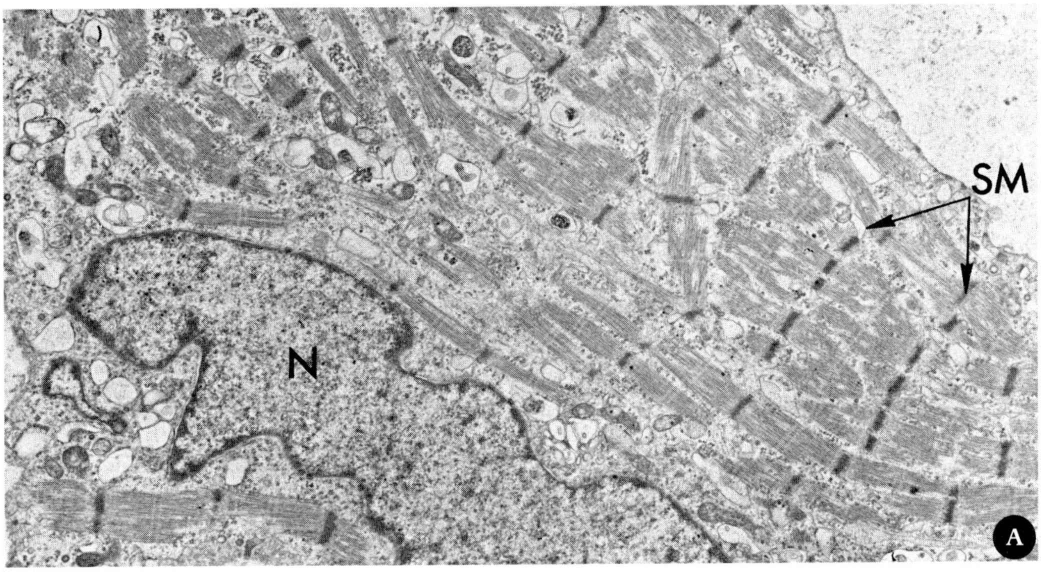

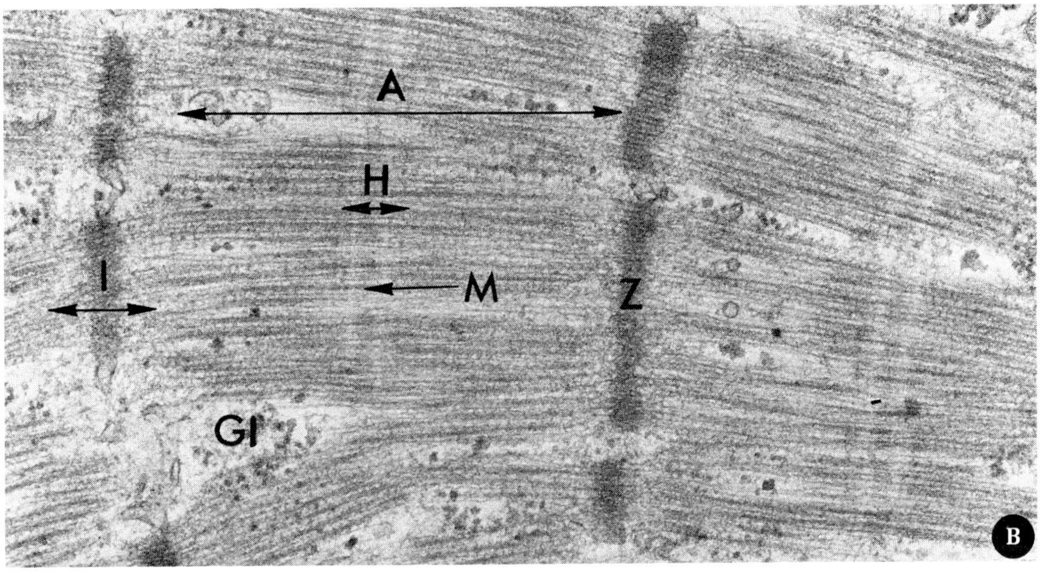

Figure 5-44. Ultrastructure of a neoplastic rhabdomyoblast.

A, Well-defined alignment of mature and banded sarcomeres (SM). This alignment is responsible for the "cross striations" in rhabdomyoblasts. N indicates the nucleus (×11,200).

B, Higher magnification of a well-developed sarcomere in a neoplastic rhabdomyblast, composed of I, A, H, M, and Z bands. Note scattered glycogen (Gl) particles between myofilaments and myofibrils (×40,000). (From Boram, L. H., Erlandson, R. A., and Hajdu, S. I.: Mesodermal mixed tumor of the uterus. A cytologic, histologic and electron microscopic correlation. Cancer 30:1295, 1972.) (See also Figures 5-1 and 5-2.)

foreign body type, and histiocytic forms commonly seen in fibrous histiocytomas are rare findings in rhabdomyosarcomas. Despite the occasional pleomorphism of fibrosarcomas, only traces of the herringbone pattern and trichrome-positive collagenous fibers that are highly specific features of fibrosarcomas are seen in rhabdomyosarcomas. The distinction between pleomorphic leiomyosarcoma and pleomorphic rhabdomyosarcoma depends on the presence of embryonal or mature

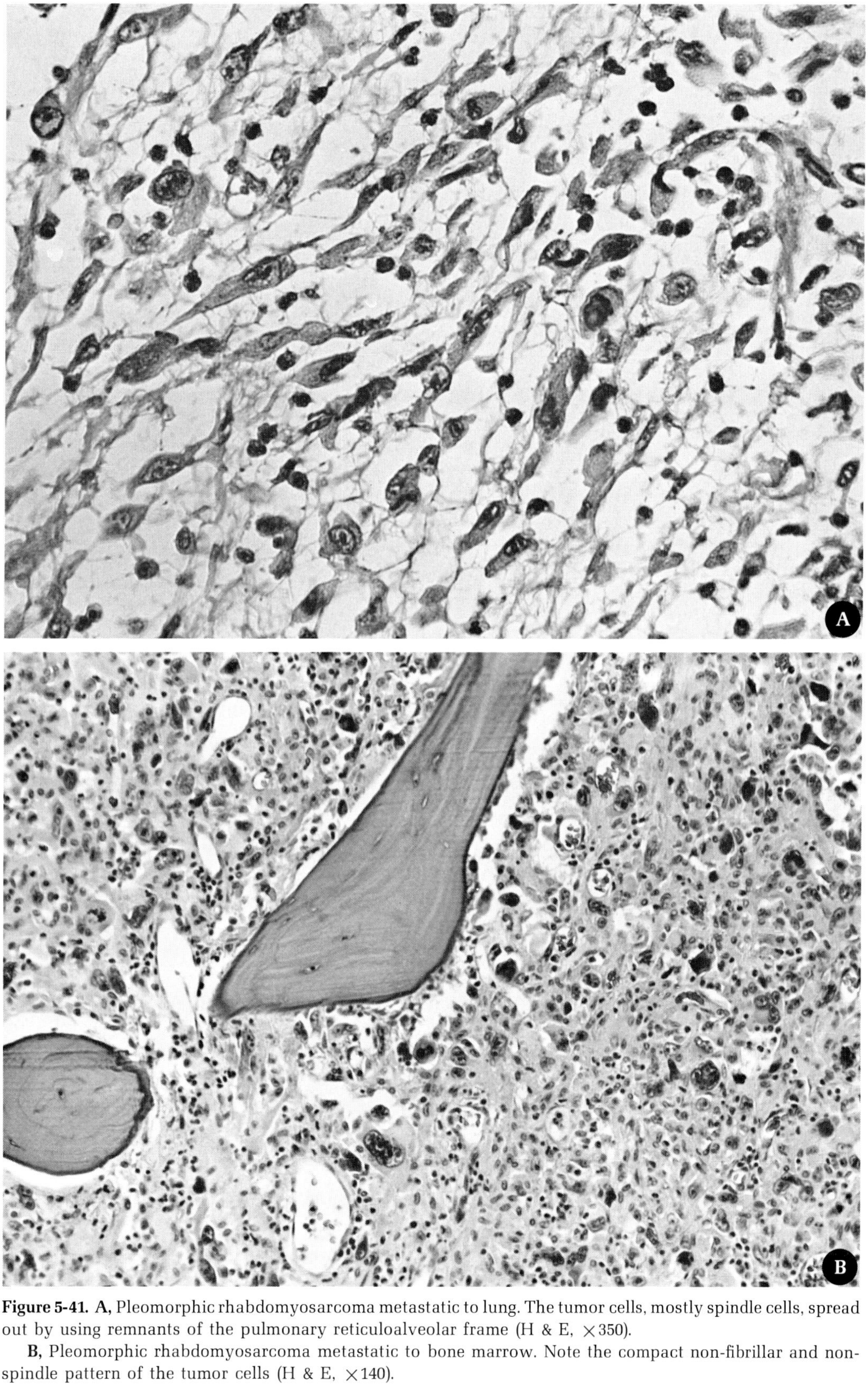

Figure 5-41. A, Pleomorphic rhabdomyosarcoma metastatic to lung. The tumor cells, mostly spindle cells, spread out by using remnants of the pulmonary reticuloalveolar frame (H & E, ×350).

B, Pleomorphic rhabdomyosarcoma metastatic to bone marrow. Note the compact non-fibrillar and non-spindle pattern of the tumor cells (H & E, ×140).

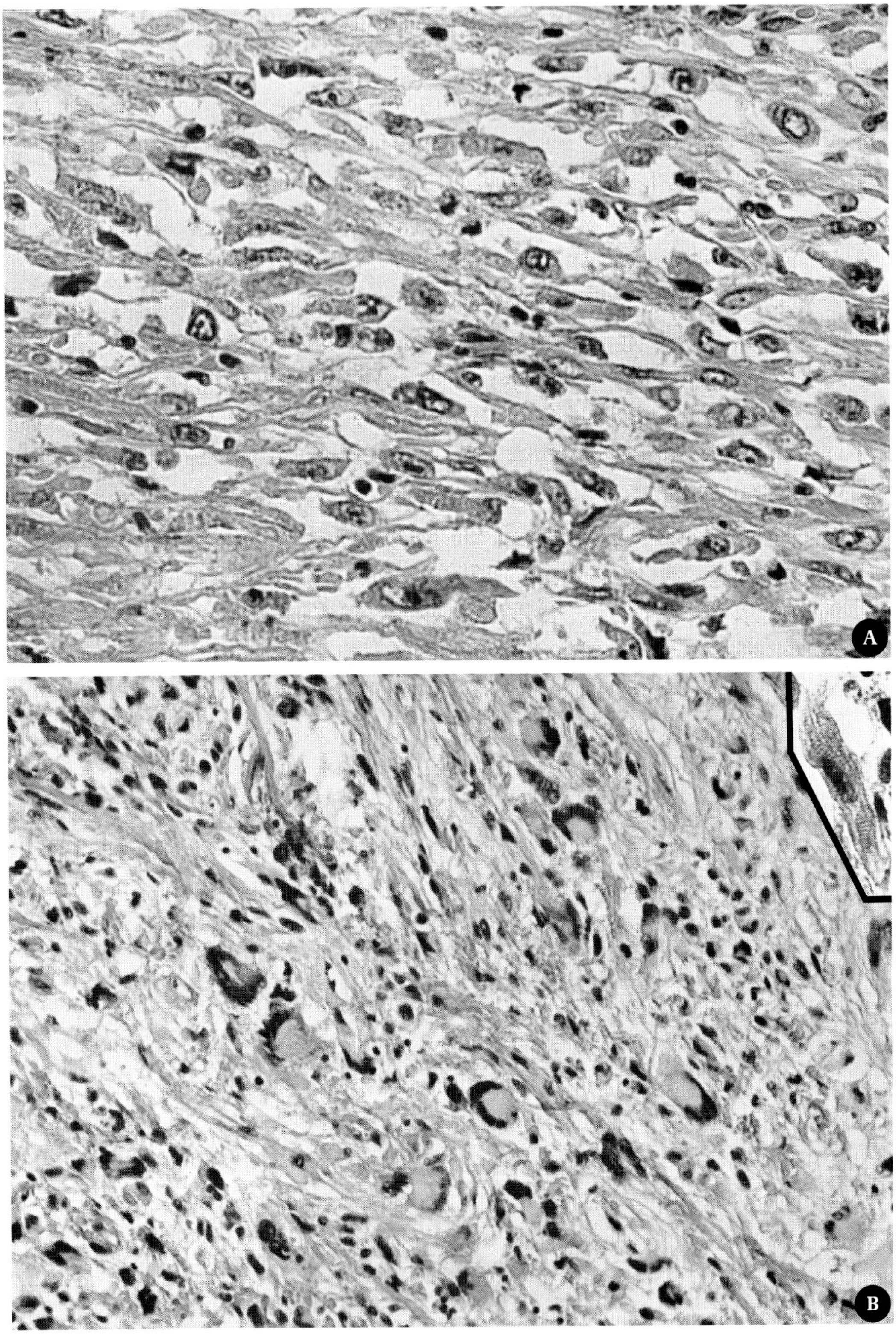

Figure 5-40. A, Arranged strap cells of pleomorphic rhabdomyosarcoma. Longitudinal as well as cross striation is seen in abundance (H & E, ×350).

B, Pleomorphic rhabdomyosarcoma with numerous undifferentiated and poorly differentiated mono- and multinucleated neoplastic cells. The multinucleated giant cells are strictly neoplastic and not the reactive type. Attempt to demonstrate cross striation in such tumors is difficult, if not impossible (see inset) (H & E, ×140; inset, ×570).

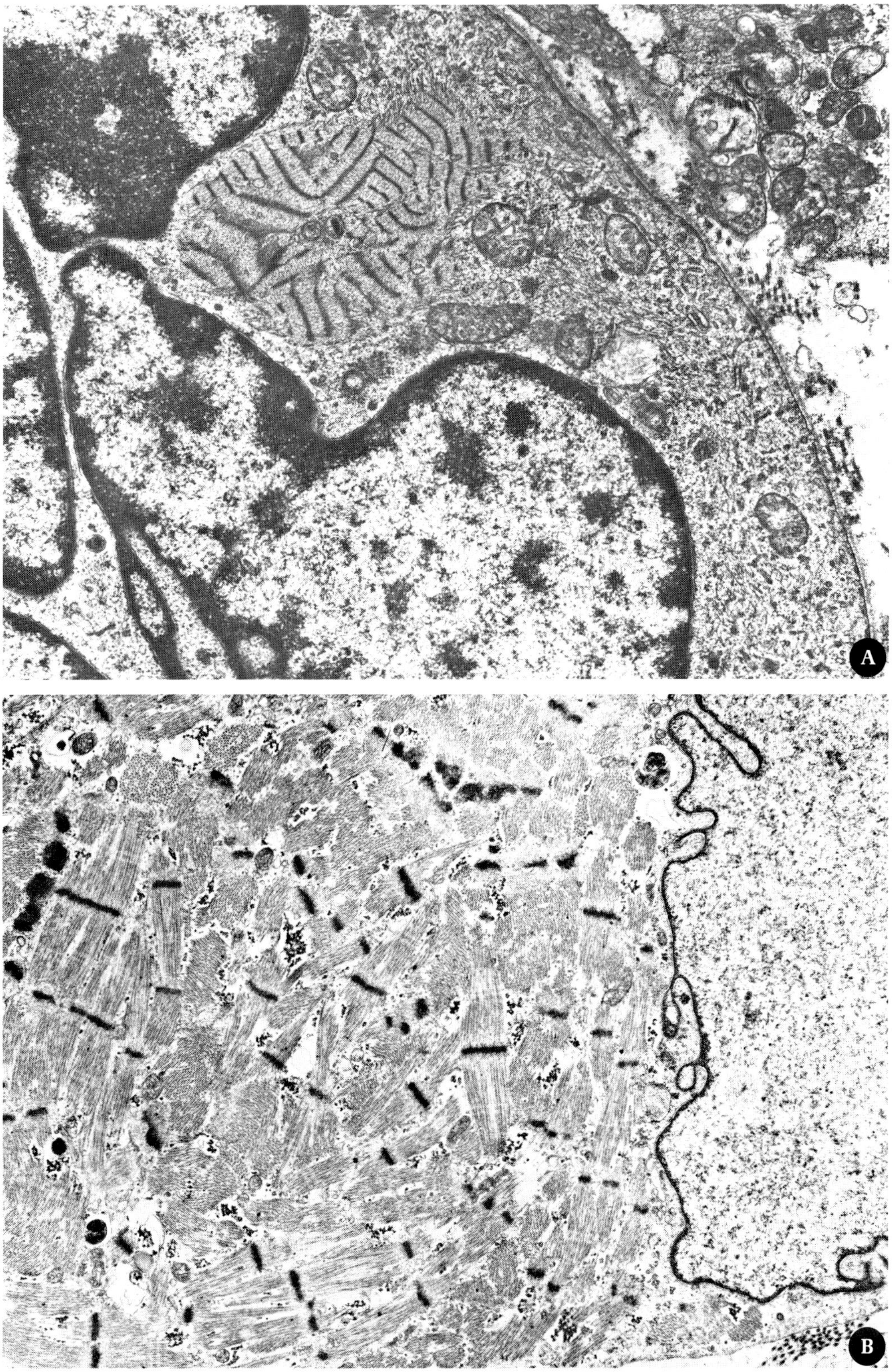

Figure 5-45. **A,** Ultrastructure of a portion of a poorly differentiated rhabdomyoblast. Note the geometrically arranged circular configuration of primitive sarcomeres, prominent basal lamina, and the multilobulated nucleus (×15,000).

B, Portion of a well-differentiated neoplastic rhabdomyoblast containing numerous disoriented sarcomeres in the cytoplasm. Note the prominent Z bands (×10,000).

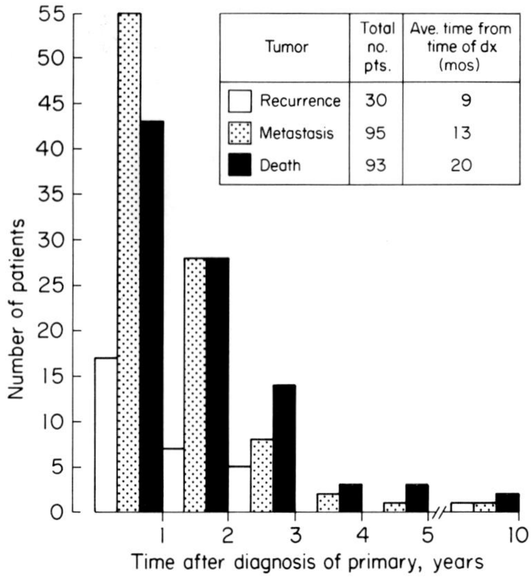

Figure 5-46. Summary of rate of recurrence and metastasis of 121 pleomorphic rhabdomyosarcomas treated at Memorial Sloan-Kettering Cancer Center during the period of 20 years. Note the high mortality rate (77%).

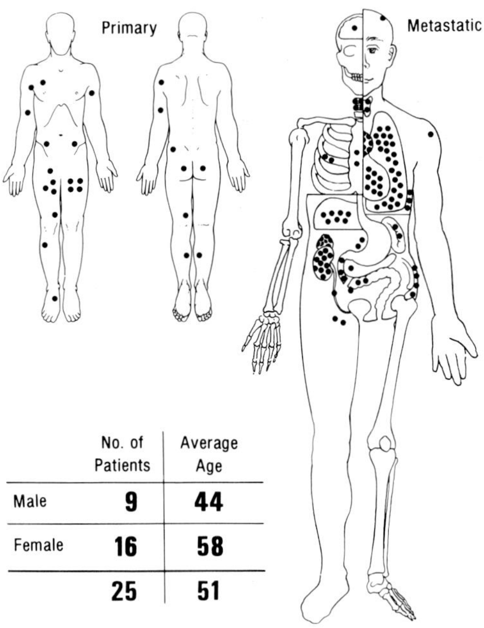

Figure 5-47. Scattergram illustrating the primary and metastatic sites of 25 pleomorphic rhabdomyosarcomas. Metastases are indicated according to autopsy findings. Lungs, kidneys, heart, adrenals, and mediastinum are the most common sites of secondary deposits (see Appendix).

rhabdomyoblasts, target cells, and cross-striated myofibrils in the latter and absence in the former.

RHABDOMYOBLASTOMA

At early stages of embryonic life rhabdomyoblasts of developing muscle are small round cells with little cytoplasm and dark round nuclei. As these early forms acquire more cytoplasm the cells become larger and rounder with an eccentrically displaced round nucleus in the cytoplasm (Fig. 5-8). The cytoplasm stains pinkish-red with H & E stain and contains coarse granules and fibrils arranged in a laminated pattern. These mature rhabdomyoblasts may be found in clusters or in isolated islands in embryonal as well as in pleomorphic rhabdomyosarcomas but occasionally are the sole or predominant components of a neoplasm. I feel that despite the rarity of such neoplasms, neoplasms predominantly composed of malignant rhabdomyoblasts should be distinguished from rhabdomyosarcoma because of their unique histologic morphology and the potential danger of confusing them with benign *rhabdomyoma. Pleomorphism of the cytoplasm, prominence of the nuclei, multinucleation, and the presence of intracytoplasmic longitudinal, cross-striated, or circular fibers are features characteristic of malignant rhabdomyoblasts.* These features are so apparent that malignant rhabdomyoblastomas can be easily distinguished from benign *rhabdomyoma* and *ganglioneuroblastoma* in the majority of the cases (Figs. 5-48, 5-49, 5-50, 5-51).

Histologically, benign myoblasts as well as malignant-looking rhabdomyoblasts are seen, in addition to rhabdomyosarcomas, not uncommonly in primary as well as in metastatic *germ cell tumors, Wilms' tumors, pulmonary blastomas,* and a number of *other tumors.* In a recent review of the records of 214 patients treated for pleomorphic rhabdomyosarcoma at Memorial Sloan-Kettering Cancer Center during a period of 25 years 11 pa-

TABLE 5-15. ***Rhabdomyoblastomas***

PATIENT	AGE	SEX	SITE OF PRIMARY TUMOR	SIZE OF TUMOR, cm	TREATMENT	RECURRENCE	METASTASIS	FOLLOW-UP
1	71	M	L. shoulder	15	Excision	—	3 mo.	DcD, 8 mo.
2	54	F	R. back	10	Excision	2 mo.	10 mo.	DcD, 13 mo.
3	45	F	L. thigh	20	Hemipel-vectomy	—	17 yr.	NED, 8 yr.
4	15	M	Paratestis	35	Excision	—	at admission	DcD, 9 mo.
5	58	F	R. thigh	25	Amputation	—	5 mo.	DcD, 10 mo.
6	3	M	L. buttock	3	Excision	—	—	NED, 8 mo.
7	21	M	Testis*	—	Orchi-ectomy	—	6 mo.	DcD, 14 mo.
8	7	M	Pelvis	12	Excision	—	4 mo.	DcD, 11 mo.
9	44	F	R. neck	20	Excision	4 mo.	4 mo.	DcD, 2 mo.
10	20	M	L. thigh	8	Excision	1 mo.	—	NED, 18 yr.
11	18	M	Retroperi-toneum	large	Excision	—	—	DcD, 14 mo.

*The primary tumor was embryonal carcinoma with teratoma elements which metastasized to the retroperitoneum in the form of pure rhabdomyoblastoma.

DcD = died with disease; NED = no evidence of disease.

tients actually had rhabdomyoblastoma (Table 5-15).

Although one may question the value of introducing a new term such as *rhabdomyoblastoma,* I feel there is merit to it, since it is a far more distinct tumor morphologically than leiomyoblastoma, alveolar rhabdomyosarcoma, or some other less distinct entities. Further studies are needed for precise definition and distinction of these neoplasms. The term of *rhabdomyoblastoma* should be used only when the neoplasm appears microscopically malignant. On the other hand, lesions predominantly composed of well-differentiated myocytes and exhibiting only foci of atypical rhabdomyoblastic elements should be considered atypical or borderline rhabdomyoblastomas. Admittedly, as in certain leiomyoblastomas, there will always be a case in which the level of differentiation is such that no statement can be issued without reservation as to the exact nature of the lesion.

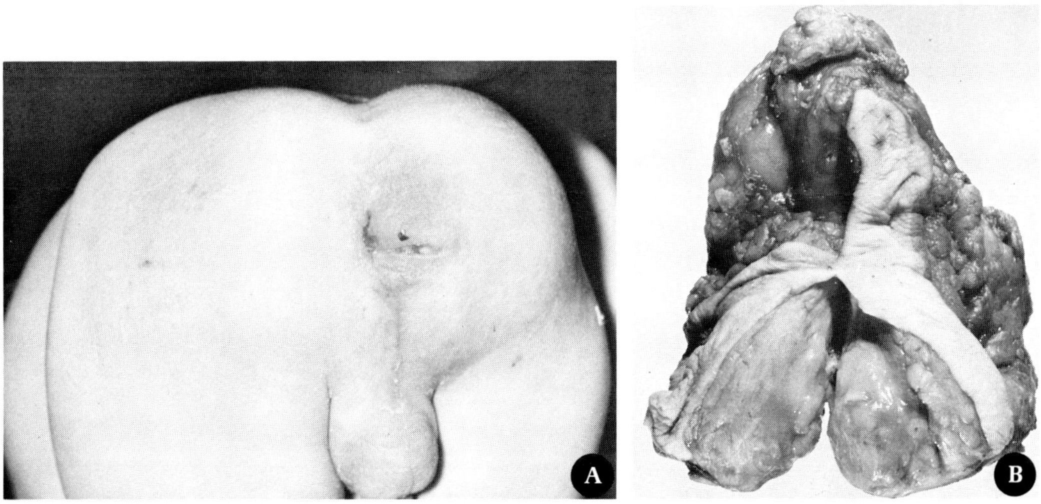

Figure 5-48. A, Rhabdomyoblastoma involving the perineum and buttock of a young child.

B, Rhabdomyoblastoma after resection showing well-defined, lobular contour and solid, non-cystic consistency of the tumor.

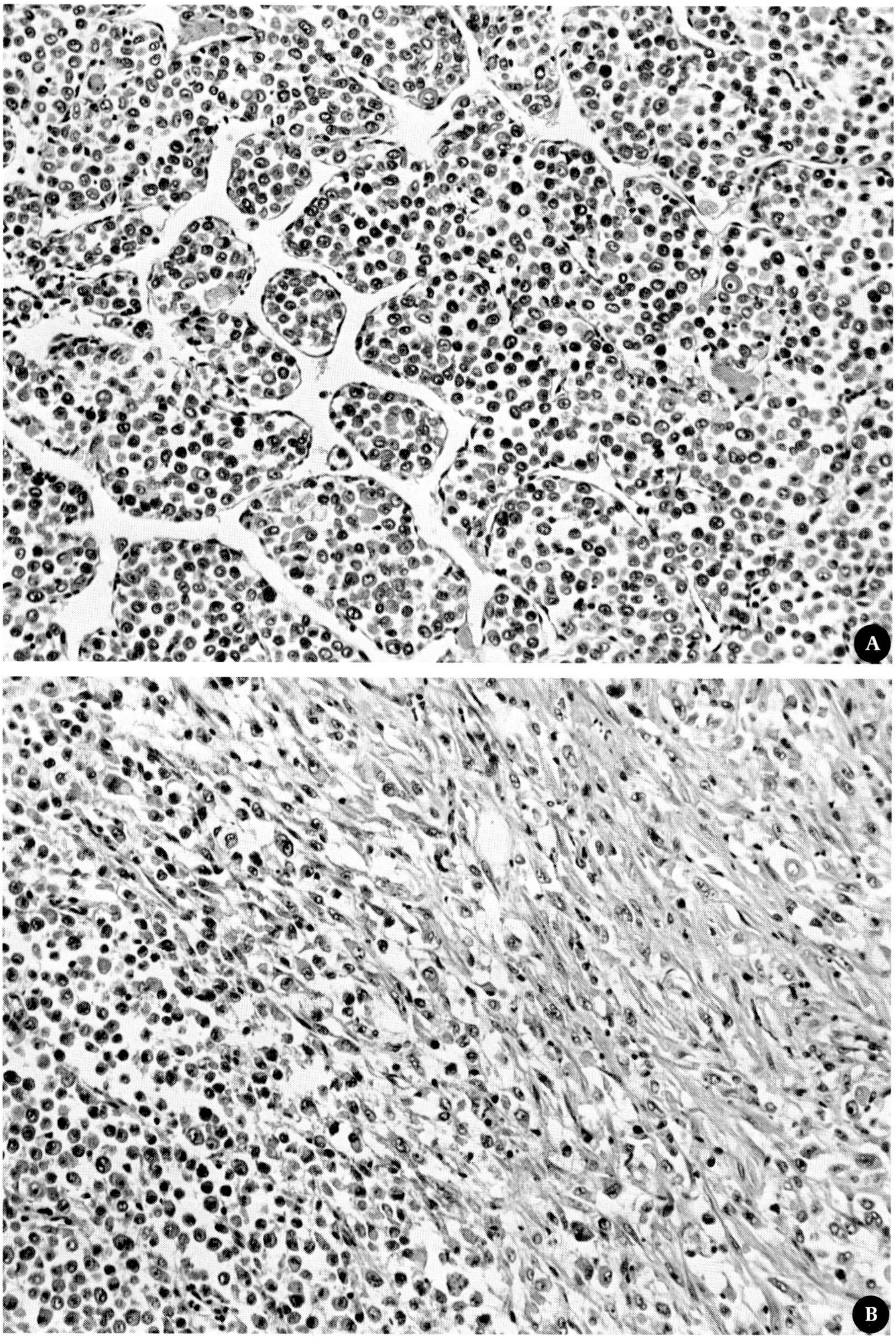

Figure 5-49. Rhabdomyoblastoma.

A, The tumor is composed of uniform small target or pebble-shaped neoplastic rhabdomyoblasts. The tumor cells are arranged in loosely formed bunches edged by a finely reticular frame (H & E, ×140). (Compare with Figure 5-19.)

B, In an area of the tumor illustrated in **A,** the round myoblasts are intermingled with elongated strap cells (H & E, ×140).

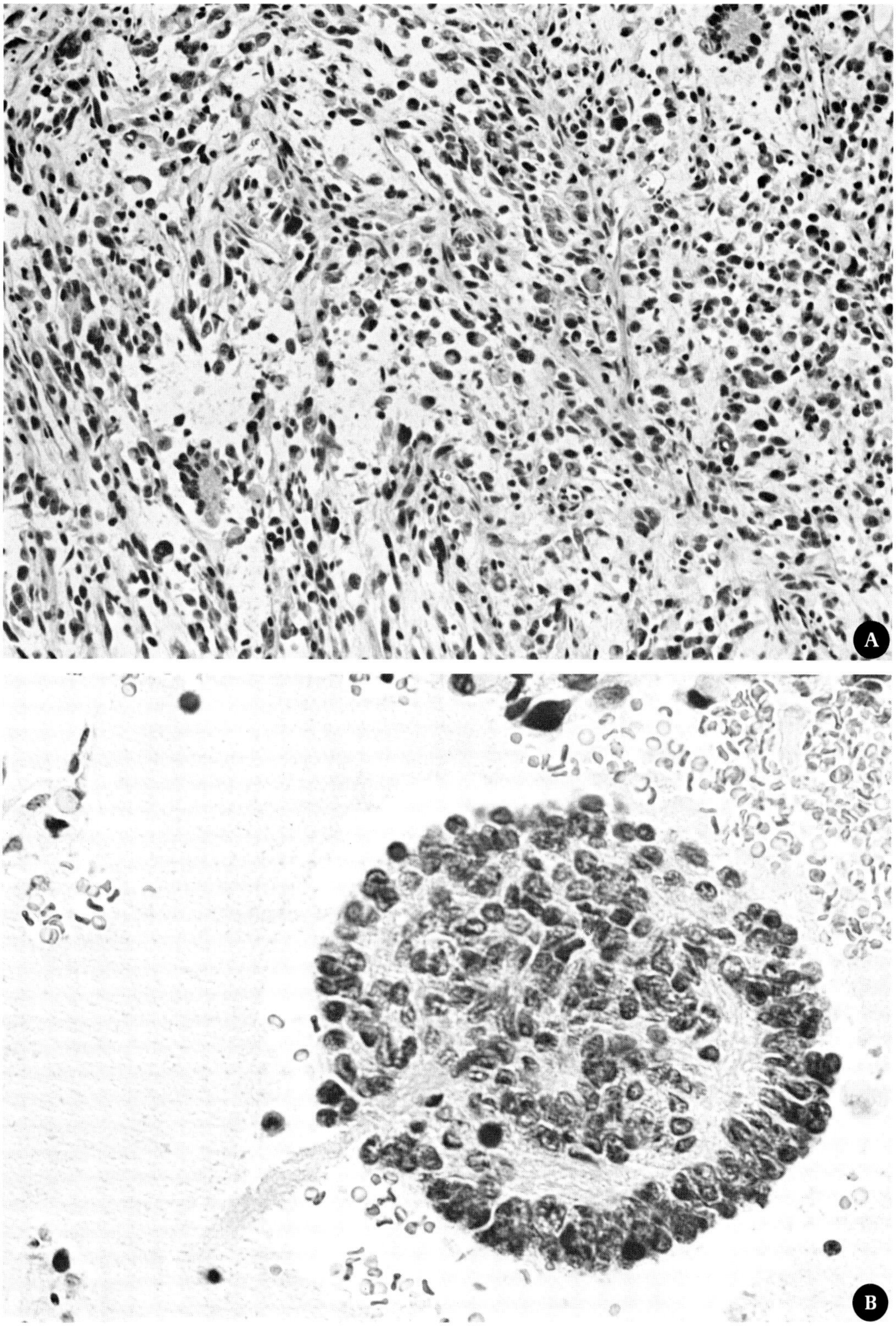

Figure 5-50. Rhabdomyoblastoma.

A, There is a mixture of well-defined round and pyknotic oval rhabdomyoblasts in a myxovascular stroma. Note the cohesive dandelion units of clustering neoplastic myoblasts (H & E, ×140).

B, The close-up view of one of these units shows a richly fibrillar network of longitudinal filaments between the minute nuclei. See one bundle of filaments extending out from the cluster like a stalk (H & E, ×350).

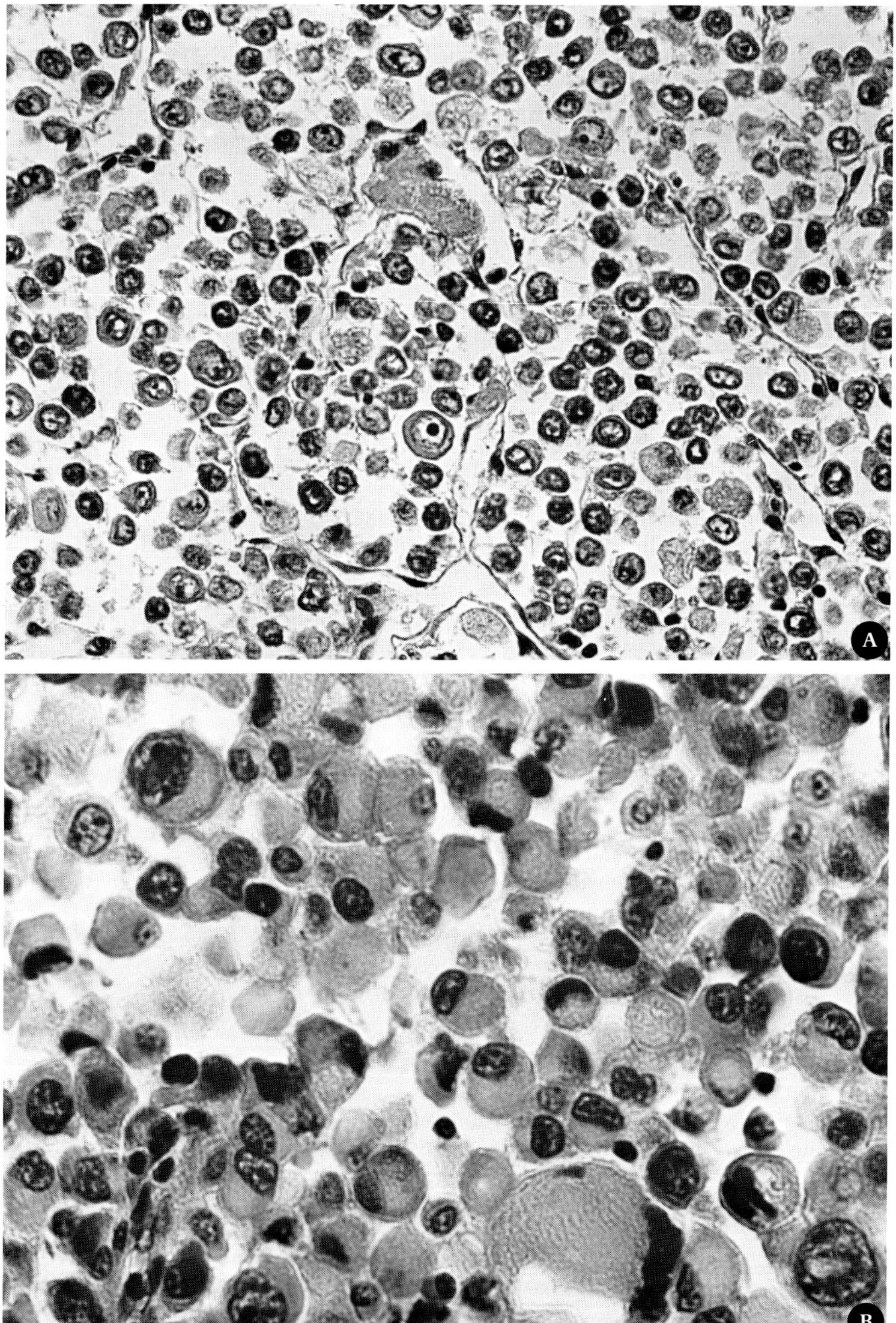

Figure 5-51. Rhabdomyoblastoma. At higher magnification the pebble- or target-shaped neoplastic rhabdomyoblasts show a rich fibrillar cytoplasmic network. Numerous ill-designed or abortive cross-striated fibers can be detected in the acidophilic cytoplasm of a number of tumor cells (**A,** H & E, ×350; **B,** H & E, ×570).

REFERENCES

References are listed in chronological order in each category.

INTRODUCTION

Leeuwenhoek, A.: Observations on the fibers of the muscles. Philos. Trans. 5:390, 1721.

Veratti, E.: Richerche sulla fine struttura della fibra muscolare striata. Mem. Ist. Lomb., Classe Sc. Mat. Nat. 19:87, 1902.

Wolback, S. B.: Centrioles and histogenesis of the myofibril in tumors of striated muscle origin. Anat. Rec. 37:255, 1928.

Nageotte, J., and Gayon, L.: Reticulin. Am. J. Pathol. 6:631, 1930.

Roskin, G.: La cellule myomateuse et quelques problemes relatifs a'la cellule musculaire. Bull. Assoc. franc. Cancer 23:172, 1934.

Pogogeff, I. A., and Murray, M. R.: Regeneration of adult mammalian skeletal muscle in vitro. Science 101:174, 1945.

Marsh, B. B.: Effects of adenosine triphosphate on fibre volume of muscle homogenate. Biochim. biophys. Acta 9:247, 1952.

Adams, R. D., Denny-Brown, D., and Person, C. M.: Diseases of Muscle. New York, P. B. Hoebner, 1953.

Bennett, H. S., and Porter, K. R.: An electron microscope study of sectioned breast muscle of the domestic fowl. Am. J. Anat. 93:61, 1953.

Hanson, J., and Huxley, H. E.: Structural basis of cross-striation in muscle. Nature 172:530, 1953.

Szent-Gyorgyi, A.: Chemistry of Muscular Contraction. New York, Academic Press, 1953.

Hibbs, R. G.: Electron microscopy of developing cardiac muscle in chick embryos. Am. J. Anat. 99:17, 1956.

Porter, K. R., and Palade, G. E.: Studies on the endoplasmic reticulum. Its form and distribution in striated muscle cells. J. Biophys. Biochem. Cytol. 3:269, 1957.

Holtzer, H.: Aspects of chondrogenesis and myogenesis. In Synthesis of Molecular and Cellular Structure. Edited by D. Rudnick. New York, Ronald Press, 1961.

Montgomery, R. D.: Growth of human striated muscle. Nature 195:194, 1962.

Huxley, H. E.: Electron microscopic studies in the structure of natural and synthetic protein filaments from striated muscle. J. Mol. Biol. 7:281, 1963.

Price, H. M.: The skeletal muscle fibre in the light of electron microscopic studies. Am. J. Med. 35:589, 1963.

Huxley, H. E.: Structural arrangements and the contraction mechanism in striated muscle. Proc. R. Soc. Lond. [Biol.] 160:442, 1964.

Allen, E. R., and Pepe, R. A.: Ultrastructure of developing muscle cells in the chick embryo. Am. J. Anat. 116:115, 1965.

Betz, E. H., Firket, H., and Reznik, M.: Some aspects of muscle regeneration. Int. Rev. Cytol. 19:203, 1965.

Dunn, A. W.: Anomalous muscle simulating soft tissue tumors in the lower extremities. J. Bone Joint Surg. 47A:1397, 1965.

Henson-Steinnon, J. A.: Morphogenese de la cellule musculaire striee etudiee au microscope electronique. J. Microscopie 4:657, 1965.

Okazaki, K., and Holter, H.: Myogenesis: fusion, myosin synthesis and mitotic cycle. Proc. Natl. Acad. Sci. USA 56:1484, 1966.

Firkey, H.: Ultrastructural aspects of myofibril formation in cultured skeletal muscle. Z. Zellforsch. 78:313, 1967.

Fischman, D. A.: An electron microscope study of myofibril formation in embryonic chick skeletal muscle. J. Cell Biol. 32:557, 1967.

Mintz, B., and Baker, W. W.: Normal mammalian muscle differentiation and gene control of isocitrate dehydrogenase synthesis. Proc. Natl. Acad. Sci. USA 58:592, 1967.

Pepe, F. A.: The myosin filament. J. Mol. Biol. 27:203, 1967.

Sandborn, E. B., Duclos, S., Messier, P. E., and Roberger, J. J.: Atypical intestinal striated muscle in Drosophila melanogaster. J. Ultrastruct. Res. 18:695, 1967.

Kelly, D. E.: Myofibrillogenesis and Z-band differentiation. Anat. Rec. 163:403, 1969.

Schotland, D. L.: An electron microscopic study of target fibers, target-like fibers and related abnormalities in human muscle. J. Neuropathol. Exp. Neurol. 28:214, 1969.

Edge, M. B., and Walker, S. M.: Evidence for a structural relationship between sarcoplasmic reticulum and Z lines in dog papillary muscle. Anat. Rec. 166:51, 1970.

Engel, W. K., Bishop, D. W., and Cunningham, G. G.: Tubular aggregates in type II muscle fibers: Ultrastructual and histochemical correlation. J. Ultrastruct. Res. 31:507, 1970.

Schiaffino, S., Hanzlikova, V., and Pierobon, S.: Relations between structure and function in rat skeletal muscle fibers. J. Cell Biol. 47:107, 1970.

Van de Velde, R. L., and Brown, B. A.: A modifed Bodian Protargol stain for identification of striated muscle elements. Am. J. Clin. Pathol. 54:768, 1970.

Zacks, S. I.: Recent contributions to the diagnosis of muscle disease. Hum. Pathol. 1:465, 1970.

Lewis, P. D., Pallis, C., and Pearse, A. G. E.: "Myopathy" with tubular aggregates. J. Neurol. Sci. 13:381, 1971.

Walker, S. M., and Edge, M. B.: The sacroplasmic reticulum and development of Z-lines in skeletal muscle fibers of fetal and postnatal rats. Anat. Rec. 169:661, 1971.

Zacchei, A. M., and Caravita, S.: Observations on the ultrastructure of chick-embryo cardiac myoblasts re-aggregated in long-term cultures. J. Embryol. Exp. Morphol. 28:571, 1972.

Becker, C. G., and Nachman, R. L.: Contractile proteins of endothelial cells, platelets and smooth muscle. Am. J. Pathol. 71:1, 1973.

Warren, R. H.: Interaction of the sacroplasmic reticulum with Z-lines during myogenesis in amphibian skeletal muscle. Anat. Rec. 177:225, 1973.

Becker, C. G., Hardy, A. M., and Dubin, T.: Contractile and relaxin proteins of smooth muscle, endothelial cells, and platelets. Thrombos. Diathes. Haemorrh. Suppl. 60:25, 1974.

Engel, W. K.: Fiber-type nomenclature of human skeletal muscle for histochemical purposes. Neurology 24:344, 1974.

Lazarides, E., and Weber, K.: Actin antibody: The specific visualization of actin filaments in non-muscle cells. Proc. Natl. Acad. Sci. USA 71:2268, 1974.

Ferrans, V. J., Maron, B. J., Buja, L. M., Ali, N., and Roberts, W. C.: Intranuclear glycogen deposits in human cardiac muscle cells: ultrastructure and cytochemistry. J. Mol. Cell. Cardiol. 7:373, 1975.

Goldman, R. D., Lazarides, E., Pollack, R., and Weber, K.: The distribution of actin in non-muscle cells. Exp. Cell Res. 90:333, 1975.

Slatkin, D. N., and Pearson, J.: Intramyofiber metastases in skeletal muscle. Hum. Pathol. 7:347, 1976.

Toth, B. H., Hard, G. C., Cauchi, M. N., and Muller, M. K.: Smooth-muscle-associated contractile proteins in renal mesenchymal tumor cells and in transformed cells from DMN-injected rats. Br. J. Cancer 34:533, 1976.

Oberc, M. A., and Engel, W. K.: Ultrastructural localization of calcium in normal and abnormal skeletal muscle. Lab. Invest. 36:566, 1977.

Rikhisa, Y., and Mizuno, D.: Demonstration of myosin on the cytoplasmic side of plasma membranes of guinea pig polymorphonuclear leukocytes with immunoferritin. Exp. Cell Res. 110:87, 1977.

Yablonka, Z., and Yaffe, D.: Synthesis of myosin light chains and accumulation of translatable mRNA coding for light chain-like polypeptides in differentiating muscle cultures. Differentiation 8:133, 1977.

Alexander, C. B., and Bossen, E.: Peripheral couplings in human skeletal muscle. Lab. Invest. 39:17, 1978.

NON-NEOPLASTIC LESIONS

Freke, J.: A case of extraordinary exostosis. Philos. Trans. No. 456, London, 1740.

Munchmeyer: Ueber myositis ossificans progressiva. Z. rat. Med. 34:9, 1869.

Helferisch, H.: Ein Fall v. sogen. Myositis ossificans progessiva. Aerztl. Intelligenzbl. 26: 1879.

Janicke, O.: Einen Fall von Myositis interstitialis. Dtsch. Med. Wochenschr. 21:117, 1895.

DeWitt, L. M.: Myositis ossificans with a report of two cases. Am. J. Med. Sci. 120:295, 1900.

Rosenstirn, J.: A contribution to the study of myositis ossificans progressiva. Ann. Surg. 68:485, 1918.

Dubois, E.: Uber die Haupt-merkmale des Femur von Pithecanthropus erectus. Anthropol. Anz. 4:131, 1927.

Mair, W. F.: Myositis ossificans progressiva. Edinburgh Med. J. 39:69, 1932.

Pack, G. T., and Braund, R. R.: The development of sarcoma in myositis ossificans. Report of three cases. JAMA 119:776, 1942.

Vero, F., Machacek, G. F., and Bartlett, F. H.: Disseminated congenital osteomas of skin, with subsequent development of myositis ossificans. JAMA 129:728, 1945.

Riley, H. D., and Christie, A.: Myositis ossificans progressiva. Pediatrics 8:753, 1951.

Ackerman, L. V.: Extraosseous localized nonneoplastic bone and cartilage formation (so-called myositis ossificans); clinical and pathologic confusion with malignant neoplasms. J. Bone Joint Surg. 40A:279, 1958.

Kern, W. H.: Proliferative myositis: a pseudosarcomatous reaction to injury. Arch. Pathol. 69:209, 1960.

Adams, R. D., Denny-Brown, D., and Pearson, C. M.: Diseases of Muscle. New York, P. B. Hoebner, 1962.

Engel, W. K.: The essentiality of histo- and cytochemical studies of skeletal muscle in the investigation of neuromuscular disease. Neurology 12:778, 1962.

Pearse, G. W., and Walton, J. N.: Progressive muscular dystrophy; the histopathological changes in skeletal muscle obtained by biopsy. J. Pathol. Bacteriol. 83:535, 1962.

Croft, P. B., and Wilkinson, M.: Carcinomatous neuromyopathy. Lancet 1:184, 1963.

Flynn, J. E., and Graham, J. H.: Myositis ossificans. Surg. Gynec. Obstet. 118:100, 1964.

Enzinger, F. M., and Dulcey, F.: Proliferative myositis. Report of thirty-three cases. Cancer 20:2213, 1967.

Huvos, A. G., and Pruzanski, W.: Smooth mus-

cle involvement in primary muscle disease. Arch. Pathol. 83:234, 1967.
Reid, J. D., Hajdu, S. I., and Attah, E.: Infantile cardiomyopathy: A previously unrecognized type with histiocytoid reaction. J. Pediatr. 73:335, 1968.
Porro, R. S., Webster, H., and Tobin, W.: Needle biopsy of skeletal muscle. J. Neuropathol. Exp. Neurol. 28:299, 1969.
Nakashima, N., Tamura, Z., Okamoto, S., and Gato, R.: Inclusion bodies in human neuromuscular disorder. Arch. Neurol. 22:270, 1970.
Zacks, S. I.: Recent contributions to the diagnosis of muscle disease. Hum. Pathol. 1:465, 1970.
Waldhart, E., and Lynch, J. B.: Benign hypertrophy of the masseter muscles and mandibular angles. Arch. Surg. 102:115, 1971.
Fisher, E. R., Gonzalez, A. R., Khurana, R. C., and Danowski, T. S.: Unique, concentrically laminated membranous inclusions in myofibers. Am. J. Clin. Pathol. 58:239, 1972.
Oteruelo, F. T., Hudson, A. J., and Haust, M. D.: Comparative ultrastructural studies of muscle in para-Duchenne and Duchenne types of muscular dystrophy. Am. J. Pathol. 66:39, 1972.
Whitaker, J. N., and Engel, W. K.: Vascular deposits of immunoglobulin and complement in idiopathic inflammatory myopathy. N. Engl. J. Med. 286:333, 1972.
Climie, A. R. W.: Muscle biopsy: Technic and interpretation. Am. J. Clin. Pathol. 60:753, 1973.
Landing, B. H., Dixon, L. G., and Wells, T. R.: Studies on isolated human skeletal muscle fibers. Hum. Pathol. 5:441, 1974.
Bohan, A., and Peter, J. B.: Polymyositis and dermatomyositis. N. Engl. J. Med. 292:344, 403, 1975.
Lagier, R., and Cox, J. N.: Pseudomalignant myositis ossificans. A pathological study of eight cases. Hum. Pathol. 6:653, 1975.
Heffner, R. R., Armbrustmacher, V. W., and Earle, K. M.: Focal myositis. Cancer 40:301, 1977.
Oxenhandler, R., Adelstein, E. H., and Hart, M. N.: Immunopathology of skeletal muscle. Hum. Pathol. 8:321, 1977.
Schiaggino, S., Severin, E., Cantini, M., and Sartore, S.: Tubular aggregates induced by anoxia in isolated rat skeletal muscle. Lab. Invest. 37:223, 1977.

TUMORS OF SMOOTH MUSCLES

Hody, E.: An account of a large boney-structure found in the womb. Philos. Trans. IX:191, 1747.
Virchow, R.: Ueber cavernose (erectile) Geschwulste und Telangiectasien. Arch. Path. Anat. Physiol. 6:553, 1854.
Aufrecht, E.: Ein myom der vena saphena. Virchows Arch. [Pathol. Anat.] 44:133, 1868.
Perl, L.: Ein fall von sarkom der vena cava inferior. Virchows Arch. [Pathol. Anat.] 53:378, 1871.
Mason, G. W.: Sarcoma of the spermatic cord with hernia of the vermiform appendix. Med. News 42:554, 1883.
Griffon and Segall: Sarcome de la vesicule propage au foie. Bull. Soc. Anat. 72:586, 1897.
Knauer, R.: Beitrag zur Anatomie der Uterusmyoma. Beitr. Geburtsch. Gynäk. 1:695, 1903.
Albrecht, D.: Uber Hamartome. Verhd. Dtsch. Ges. Pathol. 7:153, 1904.
Ehrenberg, L.: Zwei Falle von Tumor im Herzen. Dtsch. Arch. Klin. Med. 103:293, 1911.
Sitzenfrey, A.: Ueber Venenmyome des Uterus mit intravask-ularem Wachstum. Z. Geburtsch. Gynaek. 68:1, 1911.
Deussing, R.: Multiple primare Myome der Lunge. Thesis, Univ. of Munich, 1912.
Proper, M. S., and Simpson, B. T.: Malignant leiomyomata. Surg. Gynecol. Obstet. 29:39, 1919.
Evans, N.: Malignant myomata and related tumors of uterus. Surg. Gynecol. Obstet. 30:225, 1920.
Demel, P.: Ein operierter Fall von Leber myom. Virchows Arch. 281:881, 1926.
Franco, E. E.: Sopra un rarissimo voluminosa leiomyoma del pulmone. Tumori 15:27, 1929.
Bartkowiak, Z.: Ein Fall von Sarcoma leiomyoblasticum der Haut. Zentralbl. Allg. Pathol. 65:179, 1936.
Stout, A. P.: Solitary cutaneous and subcutaneous leiomyoma. Am. J. Cancer 29:435, 1937.
Nelson, W. O.: Atypical uterine growths produced by prolonged administration of estrogenic hormones. Endocrinology 24:50, 1939.
Steiner, P.: Metastasizing fibroleiomyoma of the uterus. Am. J. Pathol. 15:89, 1939.
Ackerman, L. V., and Stout, A. P.: Leiomyosarcoma of arm. J. Missouri Med. Assoc. 44:592, 1947.
Stout, A. P.: Tumors of the Soft Tissues. Washington, D.C., Armed Forces Institute of Pathology, 1953.
Ober, W. B., and Black, M. B.: Neoplasms of the subcelomic mesenchyme. Arch. Pathol. 59:698, 1955.
Borghard-Erdle, A. M. and Hirsch, E. F.: Glomus tumor of the uterus. Arch. Pathol. 65:244, 1958.

Dobben, G. D.: Leiomyosarcoma of the nasopharynx. Arch. Otolaryngol. 68:211, 1958.
Kloepfer, H. W., Krafchuk, J., Derbes, V., and Burks, J.: Hereditary multiple leiomyoma of the skin. Am. J. Hum. Genet. 10:48, 1958.
Stout, A. P., and Hill, W. T.: Leiomyosarcoma of superficial soft tissues. Cancer 11:844, 1958.
Duhig, J. T., and Ayer, J. P.: Vascular leiomyoma: a study of 61 cases. Arch. Pathol. 68:424, 1959.
Harland, W. A., and Clamen, M.: Leiomyosarcoma of the inferior vena cave with clinical features of Chiari syndrome. Can. Med. Assoc. J. 83:1064, 1960.
Martin, J. F., Baxin, P., Feroldi, J., and Cabanne, F.: Tumeurs myoides intramurales de l'estomac. Considerations microscopiques a propos de 6 cas. Ann. Anat. Pathol. 5:484, 1960.
Harper, R. S., and Scully, R. E.: Intravenous leiomyomatosis of the uterus. Obstet. Gynecol. 18:519, 1961.
Aaxhus, T., and Mylins, E.: Leiomyoma of the lung. Acta Chir. Scand. 124:373, 1962.
Stout, A. P.: Bizarre smooth muscle tumors of the stomach. Cancer 15:400, 1962.
Yannopoulos, K., and Stout, A. P.: Smooth muscle tumors in children. Cancer 15:958, 1962.
Bird, C. C., and Willis, R. A.: The production of smooth muscle by the endometrial stroma of the adult human uterus. J. Pathol. Bacteriol. 90:75, 1965.
Bothing, A. J., and Soule, E. H.: Smooth muscle tumors in children. Cancer 18:711, 1965.
Spiro, R. H., and Koss, L. G.: Myosarcoma of the uterus. Cancer 18:571, 1965.
Maesaka, A., Keyaki, Y., and Nakahashi, T.: Nasal angioleiomyoma and leiomyosarcoma. Otologia 12:42, 1966.
Spiro, R. H., and McPeak, C. J.: On the so-called metastasizing leiomyoma. Cancer 19:544, 1966.
Bulmer, J. H.: Smooth muscle tumors of the limbs. J. Bone Joint Surg. 49B:52, 1967.
Arlen, M., Grabstald, H., and Whitmore, W. F.: Malignant tumors of the spermatic cord. Cancer 23:525, 1969.
Cohen, M. L.: Intracardial leiomyosarcoma. N.Y. State J. Med. 69:1767, 1969.
Cornog, J. L.: The ultrastructure of leiomyoblastoma. Arch. Pathol. 87:404, 1969.
Hajdu, S. I., and Foote, F. W.: Angiomyolipoma of the kidney. Report of 27 cases and review of the literature. J. Urol. 102:396, 1969.
Hajdu, S. I., and Koss, L. G.: Diagnosis of metastatic myosarcomas. Acta Cytol. 13:545, 1969.
Szasz, I. J., Barr, R., and Scobic, T. K.: Leiomyosarcoma arising from veins: two cases and review of the literature of venous neoplasms. Can. J. Surg. 12:415, 1969.
Takeda, M., and Burechailo, F. A.: Smooth muscle cells in sputum. Acta Cytol. 13:696, 1969.
Jurayj, M. N., Midell, A. I., Bederman, S., Gruen, J., and O'Brien, P. H.: Primary leiomyosarcomas of the inferior vena cava—report of a case and review of the literature. Cancer 26:1349, 1970.
Ferenczy, A., Richart, R. M., and Okagaki, T.: A comparative ultrastructural study of leiomyosarcoma, cellular myoma and leiomyoma of the uterus. Cancer 28:1004, 1971.
Lin, J. L., and Svoboda, D. J.: Multiple congenital mesenchymal tumors. Multiple vascular leiomyomas in several organs of a newborn. Cancer 28:1046, 1971.
Mackenzie, A. R., Sharma, T. C., Whitmore, W. F., and Melamed, M. R.: Non-extirpative treatment of myosarcoma of the bladder and prostate. Cancer 28:329, 1971.
Martini, N., Hajdu, S. I., and Beattie, E. J.: Primary sarcoma of the lung. J. Thorac. Cardiovasc. Surg. 61:33, 1971.
White, A. G.: Leiomyosarcoma of the foot. Proc. R. Soc. Med. 64:56, 1971.
Yasuma, T. and Yanaka, M.: Primary sarcoma of the gallbladder. Acta Pathol. Jap. 21:285, 1971.
Boram, L. H., Erlandson, R. A., and Hajdu, S. I.: Mesodermal mixed tumor of the uterus. Cancer 30:1295, 1972.
Greenwood, N., Fox, H., and Edwards, E. C.: Leiomyosarcoma of the penis. Cancer 29:481, 1972.
Hajdu, S. I., Erlandson, R. A., and Paglia, M. A.: Light and electron microscopic studies of a gastric leiomyoblastoma. Arch. Pathol. 93:36, 1972.
Lavin, P., Hajdu, S. I., and Foote, F. W.: Gastric and extragastric leiomyoblastomas. Cancer 29:305, 1972.
Malek, R. S., Utz, D. C., and Farrow, G. M.: Malignant tumors of the spermatic cord. Cancer 29:1108, 1972.
Kevorkian, J., and Cento, D. P.: Leiomyosarcoma of large arteries and veins. Surgery 73:390, 1973.
Tolia, B. M., Hajdu, S. I., and Whitmore, W. F.: Leiomyosarcoma of the renal pelvis. J. Urol. 109:974, 1973.
Bolande, R. P.: The neurochristopathies: A unifying concept of disease arising in neural crest maldevelopment. Hum. Pathol. 5:409, 1974.
Scharfenberg, J. C., and Geary, W. L.: Intravenous leiomyomatosis. Obstet. Gynecol. 43:909, 1974.
Cabre-Fiol, V., Vilardell, F., Sala-Cladera, E., and Perez Mota, A.: Preoperative cytologic

diagnosis of gastric leiomyosarcoma. Gastroenterology 68:563, 1975.

Fleming, W. H., and Jove, D. F.: Primary leiomyosarcoma of the lung with positive sputum cytology. Acta Cytol. 19:14, 1975.

Jernstrom, P. and Gowdy, R. A.: Leiomyosarcoma of the long saphenous vein. Am. J. Clin. Pathol. 63:25, 1975.

Masur, H., Sussman, E. B., and Molander, D. W.: Primary hepatic leiomyosarcoma. A report of two cases. Gastroenterology 69:994, 1975.

Mindell, R. S., Calcaterra, T. C., and Ward, P. H.: Leiomyosarcoma of the head and neck. Laryngoscope 85:904, 1975.

Morales, A. R., Fine, G., Pardo, V., and Horn, R. C.: Ultra-structure of smooth muscle tumors with a consideration of the possible relationship of glomangiomas, hemangiopericytomas and cardiac myxomas. *In* Pathology Annual. Edited by S. C. Sommers. New York, Appleton-Century-Crofts, 1975.

Pertschuk, L. P.: Immunofluorescence of soft tissue tumors with anti-smooth-muscle and anti-skeletal muscle antibodies. Am. J. Clin. Pathol. 63:332, 1975.

Appelman, H. D., and Helwig, E. B.: Gastric epithelioid leiomyoma and leiomyosarcoma (leiomyoblastoma). Cancer 38:708, 1976.

Bailey, R. V., Stribling, J., Weitzner, S., and Hardy, J. D.: Leiomyosarcoma of the inferior vena cava. Report of a case and review of the literature. Ann. Surg. 184:169, 1976.

Brewster, D. C., Athanasoulis, C. A., and Darling, C.: Leiomyosarcoma of the inferior vena cava. Arch. Surg. 111:1081, 1976.

Davis, G. L., Bergmann, M., and O'Kane, H.: Leiomyosarcoma of the superior vena cava. J. Thorac. Cardiovasc. Surg. 72:408, 1976.

Dropkin, L. R., Tang, K. C., and Williams, J. R.: Leiomyosarcoma of the nasal cavity and paranasal sinuses. Ann. Otol. Rhinol. Laryngol. 85:399, 1976.

Hajdu, S. I., and Hajdu, E. O.: Cytopathology of Sarcomas and Other Nonepithelial Malignant Tumors. Philadelphia, W. B. Saunders Co., 1976.

Shen, S. C., and Yunis, E. J.: Leiomyosarcoma developing in a child during remission of leukemia. J. Pediatr. 89:780, 1976.

Silverman, J. F., and Kay, S.: Multiple primary leiomyomatous hamartomas. Cancer 38: 1199, 1976.

Toh, B. H., Muller, H. K., and Elrick, W. L.: Smooth muscle associated antigen in astrocytes and astrocytomata. Br. J. Cancer 33:105, 1976.

Aterman, K., Fraser, G. M., and Lea, R. H.: Disseminated peritoneal leiomyomatosis. Virchows Arch. Pathol. 374:13, 1977.

Brandjord, R. C., Reaume, C. E., and Wesley, R. K.: Leiomyosarcoma of the floor of the mouth: Review of the literature and report of case. J. Oral Surg. 35:590, 1977.

Chang, V., Aikawa, M., and Druet, R.: Uterine leiomyoblastoma. Ultrastructural and cytologic studies. Cancer 39:1563, 1977.

Freni, S. C., and Keeman, J. N.: Leiomyomatosis of the colon. Cancer 39:263, 1977.

Goldberg, M. S., Hurt, W. G., and Frable, W. J.: Leiomyomatosis peritonealis disseminata: Report of a case, review of the literature. Obstet. Gynecol. 49:46, 1977.

Horstmann, J. P., Pietra, G. G., Harman, J. A., Cole, N. G., and Grinspan, S.: Spontaneous regression of pulmonary leiomyomas during pregnancy. Cancer 39:314, 1977.

Jakobiec, F. A., Font, R. L., Tso, M. O. M., and Zimmerman, L. E.: Mesoectodermal leiomyoma of the ciliary body. Cancer 39:2102, 1977.

Krumerman, M. S.: Leiomyosarcoma of the lung. Primary cytodiagnosis in two consecutive cases. Acta Cytol. 21:103, 1977.

Overgaard, J., Frederiksen, P., Helmig, O., and Jensen, O. M.: Primary leiomyosarcoma of bone. Cancer 39:1664, 1977.

Ranchod, M., and Kempson, R. L.: Smooth muscle tumors of the gastrointestinal tract and retroperitoneum. Cancer 39:255, 1977.

Akwasi, O. E., Dozois, R. R., Weiland, L. H., and Beahrs, O. H.: Leiomyosarcoma of the small and large bowel. Cancer. 42:1375, 1978.

Nogales, F. F., Matilla, A., and Carrascal, E.: Leiomyomatosis peritonealis disseminata. An ultrastructure study. Am. J. Clin. Pathol. 69:452, 1978.

Hajdu, S. I., and Fogh, J.: The nude mouse as a diagnostic tool in human tumor cell research. *In* The Nude Mouse in Experimental and Clinical Research. Edited by J. Fogh and B. C. Giovanella. New York, Academic Press, 1978.

TUMORS OF STRIATED MUSCLE

Stafford, R. A.: A case of enlargement from melanoid tumor of the prostate gland in a child five years of age. Med. Chir. Trans. 22:218, 1839.

Guersant, M. P.: Polypes du vagin chez une petite fille de treize mois. Moniteur hopitaux 2:187, 1854.

Weber, C. O.: Anatomische Untersuchung einer hypertrophische Zunge nebst Bemerkungen uber die Neubildung quergestreifter Muskelfasern. Virchows Arch. [Pathol. Anat.] 7:115, 1854.

Wilks, S.: Lectures on Pathological Anatomy. London, Longman, 1859.

von Recklinghausen, F.: Verhandlungen der

Gesellschaft für Geburstshülfe, Herr v. Recklinghausen legt der Gesellschaft ein Herz von einem Neugeborenen. Monatsschr. Geburtsk. 20:1, 1862.

Despres, A.: Les Tumeurs des Muscles. Paris, 1866.

Neumann, E.: Ein Fall von Myoma striocellular am Hoden. Virchows Arch. 30:497, 1866.

Anderson, A., and Odmasnsson, E.: Rhabdomyosarcoma und mehrere andere Geschwulste in einem uterus. Nord. Med. Ark. 1:1, 1869.

Pfannenstiel, J.: Das traubige Sarcom de cervix uteri. Virchows Arch. [Pathol. Anat.] 127:305, 1892.

Targett, J. H.: Congenital myxosarcoma of the neck containing striped muscle cells. Trans. Pathol. Soc. London 43:157, 1892.

Berard, M.: Tumeur embryonnaire du muscle strie. Lyon Med. 77:52, 1894.

Wolfensberger, R.: Uber ein Rhabdomyom der Speiserohre. Beitr. Pathol. Anat. Allg. Pathol. 15:491, 1894.

Fujinami, A.: Ein Rhabdomyosarkom mit hyaliner Degeneration (cylindrom) im willkurlischen Muskel. Virchows Arch. [Pathol. Anat.] 160:203, 1900.

Miller, C. J., and Gurd, F. B.: Malignant rhabdomyoma of the vagina in children. Surg. Obstet. Gynecol. 11:391–397, 1910.

Burgess, A. M.: Malignant rhabdomyoma with multiple metastases. J. Med. Res. 29:447, 1914.

Schmincke, A.: Kongenitale Herzhypertrophie, bedingt durch diffuse Rhabdomyombildung. Beitr. Pathol. 70:513, 1922.

Abrikossoff, A. L.: Uber Myome, ausgehend von der quergestreiften willkurlichen Muskulatur. Virchows Arch. [Pathol. Anat.] 260:215, 1926.

Slobodnik, M.: Zur Grage der Kehlkopfsarcome. Z. Hals. Nas. Ohrenheilkd. 19:505, 1928.

Wolbach, S. B.: A malignant rhabdomyoma of skeletal muscle. Arch. Pathol. 5:775, 1928.

Houette, Ch.: Rhabdomyome diverticulaire congenital de la vessie. Ann. Anat. Pathol. 6:267, 1929.

Montpellier, J.: Les rhabdomyomes. Caracteres generaux et varietes anatomo-clinique. Bull. Assoc. franc. Cancer 18:538, 1929.

Peyron, A.: Les tumeurs des muscles. Atlas du Cancer Fasc. 7, Paris, Felix Alcan, 1929.

Lochrane, C. D.: Rhabdomyosarcoma of corpus uteri. Proc. R. Soc. Med. 26:1429, 1933.

Klemperer, P.: Myoblastoma of the striated muscle. Am. J. Cancer 20:324, 1934.

Kernan, J. D., and Cracovaner, A. J.: Rhabdomyosarcoma of the vocal cord—report of a case. Laryngoscope 45:891, 1935.

Cappell, D. F., and Montgomery, G. L.: On rhabdomyoma and myoblastoma. J. Pathol. Bacteriol. 44:517, 1937.

Rakov, A. I.: Malignant rhabdomyoblastoma of the skeletal musculature. Am. J. Cancer 30:445, 1937.

Moulonguet, P., and Pollosson, E.: Sarcomes des muscles et des coulees conjoctives des membres. J. Chir. 52:501, 1938.

De, M. N., and Tribendi, B. P.: Skeletal muscle tissue tumor. Br. J. Surg. 28:17, 1940.

Arkles, H. A.: Coincidence of rhabdomyosarcoma of the diaphragm, idiopathic hypoglycemia and retroperitoneal sarcoma. Med. Bull. Vet. Adm. 19:225, 1942.

Calhoun, S. P., and Reese, J. B.: Rhabdomyosarcoma of the orbit. Arch. Ophthalmol. 27:558, 1942.

Hill, R. P., and Stout, A. P.: Sarcoma of the breast. Arch. Surg. 44:734, 1942.

Howe, C. W., and Warren, S.: Myoblastoma. Surgery 16:319, 1944.

Stout, A. P.: Rhabdomyosarcoma of the skeletal muscles. Ann. Surg. 123:447, 1946.

Stobbe, G. D., and Dargeon, H. W.: Embryonal rhabdomyosarcoma of the head and neck in children and adolescents. Cancer 3:826, 1950.

Pack, G. T., and Eberhart, W. F.: Rhabdomyosarcoma of skeletal muscle. Report of 100 cases. Surgery 32:1023, 1952.

Riopelle, J. I., and Theriault, J. P.: Sur une forme meconnue de sarcome des parties molles: le rhabdomyosarcoma alveolaire. Ann. Anat. Pathol. 1:88, 1956.

Enterline, H. T., and Horn, R. C.: Alveolar rhabdomyosarcoma. Distinctive tumor type. Am. J. Clin. Pathol. 29:356, 1958.

Horn, R. C., and Enterline, H. T.: Rhabdomyosarcoma: a clinicopathological study and classification of 39 cases. Cancer 11:181, 1958.

Daniel, W. W., Koss, L. G., and Brunschwig, A.: Sarcoma botryoides of the vagina. Cancer 12:74, 1959.

Frayer, W. C., and Enterline, H. T.: Embryonal rhabdomyosarcoma of the orbit in children and young adults. Arch. Ophthalmol. 62:203, 1959.

Willis, R. A.: Pathology of Tumors, 3rd edition. London, Butterworths, 1960.

Kratz, R. C., and Ritterhoff, R.: Sarcoma of the larynx. Ann. Otol. Rhinol. Laryngol. 70:239, 1961.

Morales, J. B.: Congenital rhabdomyoma, tuberous sclerosis and splenic histiocytosis. A histochemical study. Arch. Pathol. 71:485, 1961.

Potenza, A. D., and Winslow, D. J.: Rhabdomyosarcoma of the hand. J. Bone Joint Surg. 43A:700, 1961.

Dito, W. R., and Batsakis, J. G.: Rhabdomyosarcoma of the head and neck: an appraisal of the biological behavior in 170 cases. Arch. Surg. 84:582, 1962.

Patton, R. B., and Horn, R. C.: Rhabdomyosarcoma: clinical and pathological features and comparison with human fetal and embryonal skeletal muscle. Surgery 52:572, 1962.

Portenfield, J. F., and Zimmerman, L. E.: Rhabdomyosarcoma of the orbit. Virchows Arch. [Pathol. Anat.] 335:329, 1962.

Albores-Saavedra, J., Martin, R. C., and Smith, J. L.: Rhabdomyosarcomata. Ann. Surg. 157:186, 1963.

Chaoman, G. B., Jones, K. S., and Spelsberg, W. W.: An electron microscopic study of rhabdomyosarcoma. Invest. Ophthalmol. 2:538, 1963.

Goldman, R. L.: Multicentric benign rhabdomyoma of skeletal muscle. Cancer 16:1609, 1963.

Kroll, A. J., Kowabara, T., and Howard, G. M.: Electron microscopy of rhabdomyosarcoma of the orbit: a study of two cases. Invest. Ophthalmol. 2:523, 1963.

Lawrence, W., Jegge, G., and Foote, F. W.: Embryonal rhabdomyosarcoma, a clinicopathologic study. Cancer 17:361, 1964.

Moran, J. J., and Enterline, H. T.: Benign rhabdomyoma of the pharynx. A case report, review of the literature and comparison with cardiac rhabdomyoma. Am. J. Clin. Pathol. 42:174, 1964.

Steinbridge, V. A., Luibel, F. J., and Askworth, C. T.: Soft tissue sarcomas: electron microscopic approach to histogenetic classification. South. Med. J. 51:772, 1964.

Ashton, N., and Morgan, G.: Embryonal sarcoma and embryonal rhabdomyosarcoma of the orbit. J. Clin. Pathol. 18:669, 1965.

Jones, I. S., Reese, A. R., and Krout, J.: Orbital rhabdomyosarcoma. Trans. Am. Ophthalmol. Soc. 63:224, 1965.

Linscheid, R. L., Soule, E. H., and Henderson, E. D.: Pleomorphic rhabdomyosarcoma of the extremities and limb girdles. J. Bone Joint Surg. 47A:715, 1965.

Masson, J. K., and Soule, E. H.: Embryonal rhabdomyosarcoma of the head and neck. Am. J. Surg. 110:585, 1965.

Papaioannou, A. N., and McPeak, C. J.: Rhabdomyosarcoma of the buttock producing hypoglycemia. Ann. Surg. 161:553, 1965.

Grice, H. C., and Mannell, W. A.: Rhabdomyosarcoma induced in rats by intramuscular injection of blue VRS. J. Natl. Cancer Inst. 37:845, 1966.

Cornog, J. L., and Gonatas, N. K.: Ultrastructure of rhabdomyoma. J. Ultrastruct. Res. 20:433, 1967.

Edland, R. W.: Embryonal rhabdomyosarcoma. Five-year survival of a patient treated by radiation and chemotherapy. Am. J. Roentgenol. 99:400, 1967.

Kroll, A. J.: Fine structural classification of orbital rhabdomyosarcoma. Invest. Ophthalmol. 6:531, 1967.

Lattes, R.: Sarcomas of the breast. JAMA 201:531, 1967.

Sanborn, E. B., Duclos, S., Messier, P. E., and Roberge, J. J.: Atypical intestinal striated muscle in Drosophilia melanogaster. J. Ultrast. Res. 18:695, 1967.

Stout, A. P., and Lattes, R.: Tumors of the soft tissue. *In* Atlas of Tumor Pathology, 2nd series. Washington, D.C., Armed Forces Institute of Pathology, 1967.

Legier, J. F., and Willis, H. A.: Primary cerebellar rhabdomyosarcoma. J. Neurosurg. 26:436, 1967.

Mahour, G. H., Soule, E. H., Mills, S. D., and Lynn, H. B.: Rhabdomyosarcoma in infants and children. J. Pediatr. Surg. 2:402, 1967.

White, L., and Cox, D.: Chromosome changes in a rhabdomyosarcoma during recurrence and in cell culture. Br. J. Cancer 21:684, 1967.

Chernobilsky, B., Cornog, J. L., and Enterline, H. T.: Rhabdomyoma. Am. J. Clin. Pathol. 49:782, 1968.

Keyhani, A. and Booher, R. J.: Pleomorphic rhabdomyosarcoma. Cancer 22:956, 1968.

Nelson, A. J.: Embryonal rhabdomyosarcoma. Cancer 22:64, 1968.

Ross, C. F.: Rhabdomyoma of sternomastoid. J. Pathol. Bacteriol. 95:556–558, 1968.

Toker, C.: Embryonal rhabdomyosarcoma; an ultrastructural study. Cancer 21:1164, 1968.

Battifora, H. A., Eisenstein, R., and Schild, J. A.: Rhabdomyoma of larynx. Ultrastructural study and comparison with granular cell tumors (myoblastomas). Cancer 23:183, 1969.

Burrington, J. D.: Rhabdomyosarcoma of the paratesticular tissues in children. Report of 8 cases. J. Pediatr. Surg. 4:503, 1969.

Davis, G. L., Kissane, J. M., and Ishak, K. G.: Embryonal rhabdomyosarcoma (sarcoma botryoides) of the biliary tree. Report of 5 cases and review of the literature. Cancer 24:333, 1969.

Enzinger, F. M., and Shiraki, M.: Alveolar rhabdomyosarcoma. An analysis of 110 cases. Cancer 24:18, 1969.

Hajdu, S. I., and Koss, L. G.: Diagnosis of metastatic myosarcomas. Acta Cytol. 13:545, 1969.

Kaloyannides, T. M.: Pleomorphic rhabdomyosarcoma of the gingiva. Oral Surg. 27:150, 1969.

Kay, D., Gerszten, E., and Denninson, S. M.:

Light and electron microscopic study of a rhabdomyoma arising in the floor of the mouth. Cancer 23:708, 1969.

Li, F. P., and Fraumeni, J. F.: Rhabdomyosarcoma in children: Epidemiologic study and identification of a familial cancer syndrome. J. Natl. Cancer Inst. 43:1365, 1969.

McAllister, R. M., Melnyk, J., Finklestein, J. Z., Adams, Jr., E. C., and Gardner, M. B.: Cultivation in vitro of cells derived from a human rhabdomyosarcoma. Cancer 24:520, 1969.

Soule, E. H., Geitz, M., and Henderson, E. D.: Embryonal rhabdomyosarcoma of the limbs and limb girdles. Cancer 23:1336, 1969.

Tuazon, R.: Rhabdomyoma of the stomach. Am. J. Clin. Pathol. 52:37, 1969.

Brasfield, R. D.: Granular cell myoblastoma. Cancer 25:415, 1970.

Garancis, J. C., Komorowski, R. A., and Kuzma, J. F.: Granular cell myoblastoma. Cancer 25:542, 1970.

Horvat, B. L., Caines, M., and Fisher, E. R.: The ultrastructure of rhabdomyosarcoma. Am. J. Clin. Pathol. 53:555, 1970.

Nameroff, M. A., Reznik, M., Anderson, P., and Hansen, J. L.: Differentiation and control of mitosis in a skeletal muscle tumor. Cancer Res. 30:595, 1970.

Sutow, W. W., Sullivan, M. P., Ried, H. L., Taylor, H. G., and Griffith, K. M.: Prognosis in childhood rhabdomyosarcoma. Cancer 25:1348, 1970.

Wyatt, R. B., Schochet, S. S., and McCormick, W. F.: Rhabdomyoma: light and electron microscopic study of a case with intranuclear inclusions. Arch. Otolaryngol. 92:2, 1970.

Adam, Y. G., and Farr, H. W.: Primary orbital tumors. Am. J. Surg. 122:726, 1971.

Fallon, G., Schiller, M., and Kilman, J. W.: Primary rhabdomyosarcoma of the bronchus. Ann. Thorac. Surg. 12:650, 1971.

Hesoda, S., Suzki, H., Kawabe, H., Watanabe, Y., and Isojima, G.: Embryonal rhabdomyosarcoma of the middle ear. Cancer 27:943, 1971.

McAllister, R. M., Nelson-Rees, W. A., Johnson, E. Y., Rangey, R. W., and Gardner, M. B.: Disseminated rhabdomyosarcoma formed in kittens by cultured human rhabdomyosarcoma cells. J. Natl. Cancer Inst. 47:603, 1971.

Boram, L. H., Erlandson, R. A., and Hajdu, S. I.: Mesodermal mixed tumor of the uterus. A cytologic, histologic and electron microscopic correlation. Cancer 30:1295, 1972.

Dehner, L. P., Enzinger, F. M., and Font, R. L.: Fetal rhabdomyoma. Cancer 30:160, 1972.

Deutsch, M., Leen, R., and Mercado, R.: Rhabdomyosarcoma of the middle cranial fossa. Cancer 31:1193, 1972.

Grosfeld, J. L., Smith, J. P., and Clatworthy, H. W.: Pelvic rhabdomyosarcoma in infants and children. J. Urol. 107:673, 1972.

Littmann, R., Tessler, A. N., and Velensi, Q.: Paratesticular rhabdomyosarcoma: A case presentation and review of the literature. J. Urol. 108:290, 1972.

Morales, A., Fine, G., and Horn, R. C.: Rhabdomyosarcoma: An ultrastructural appraisal. *In* Pathology Annual (Edited by S. C. Sommers), New York, Appleton-Century-Crofts, 1972.

Roszel, J. F.: Cytology of urine from dogs with botryoid sarcoma of the bladder. Acta Cytol. 16:443, 1972.

Schuster, S. A. D., Ferguson, E. C., and Marshall, R. B.: Alveolar rhabdomyosarcoma of the eyelid. Arch. Ophthalmol. 87:646, 1972.

Smith, B. H., and Dehner, L. P.: Sarcoma of the prostate gland. Am. J. Clin. Pathol. 58:43, 1972.

Tank, E. S., Fellmann, S. L., and Wheeler, E. S.: Treatment of urogenital tract rhabdomyosarcoma in infants and children. J. Urol. 107:324, 1972.

Zimmerman, L. E., Fort, R. L., and Anderson, S. B.: Rhabdomyosarcomatous differentiation in malignant intraocular medulloepitheliomas. Cancer 30:817, 1972.

Donaldson, S. S., Castro, J. R., Wilburn, J. R., and Jesse, R. H.: Rhabdomyosarcoma of head and neck in children. Combination treatment by surgery, irradiation and chemotherapy. Cancer 31:26, 1973.

Jaffee, N., Filler, R. M., Farber, S., Traggis, D. G., Vawter, G. F., Tefft, M., and Murray, J. E.: Rhabdomyosarcoma in children. Improved outlook with a multidisciplinary approach. Am. J. Surg. 125:482, 1973.

Kilman, J. W., Clatworthy, H. W., Newton, W. A., and Grosfeld, J. L.: Reasonable surgery for rhabdomyosarcoma. A study of 67 cases. Ann. Surg. 178:346, 1973.

Woodruff, J. M., Chernik, N. L., Smith, M. C., Millett, W. B., and Foote, F. W.: Peripheral nerve tumors with rhabdomyosarcomatous differentiation (malignant "Triton" tumors). Cancer 32:426, 1973.

Exelby, P. R.: Management of embryonal rhabdomyosarcoma in children. Surg. Clin. North Am. 53:849, 1974.

Heyn, R. M., Holland, R., Newton, W. A., Tefft, M., Breslow, N., and Hartmann, J. R.: The role of combined chemotherapy in the treatment of rhabdomyosarcoma in children. Cancer 34:2128, 1974.

Miller, R. W., and Dalager, N. A.: Fatal rhabdomyosarcoma among children in the

United States, 1960–69. Cancer 34:1897, 1974.

Ariel, I. M., and Briceno, M.: Rhabdomyosarcoma of the extremities and trunk. J. Surg. Oncol. 7:269, 1975.

Bale, P. M., and Reye, R. D. K.: Rhabdomyosarcoma in childhood. Pathology 7:101, 1975.

Gad, A., Eusebi, V.: Rhabdomyosarcoma of the vagina. J. Pathol. 115:179, 1975.

Ghavimi, F., Exelby, P. R., D'Amgio, G. J., Cham, W., Lieberman, P. H., Tan, C., and Murphy, L.: Multidisciplinary treatment of embryonal rhabdomyosarcoma in children. Cancer 35:677, 1975.

Helson, L., Krochmal, P., and Hajdu, S. I.: Diagnostic value of cytologic specimens obtained from children with cancer. Ann. Clin. Lab. Sci. 5:294, 1975.

Beccia, D. J., Krane, R. J., and Olsson, C. A.: Clinical management of non-testicular intrascrotal tumors. J. Urol. 116:476, 1976.

Canalis, R. F., Platz, C. E., and Cohn, A. M.: Laryngeal rhabdomyosarcoma. Arch. Otolaryngol. 102:104, 1976.

Fenoglio, J. J., McAllister, H. A., and Ferrans, V. J.: Cardiac rhabdomyoma: a clinicopathologic and electron microscopic study. Am. J. Cardiol. 38:241, 1976.

Gold, J. H., and Bossen, E. H.: Benign vaginal rhabdomyoma. A light and electron microscopic study. Cancer 37:2283, 1976.

Hajdu, S. I., and Hajdu, E. O.: Cytopathology of Sarcomas and Other Nonepithelial Malignant Tumors. Philadelphia, W. B. Saunders Co., 1976.

Liebner, E. J.: Embryonal rhabdomyosarcoma of head and neck in children. Cancer 37:2777, 1976.

Silverman, J. F., Kay, S., McCue, C. M., Lower, R. R., Brough, A. J., and Chang, C. H.: Rhabdomyoma of the breast. Ultrastructural study of three cases. Lab. Invest. 35:596, 1976.

Srouji, M. N., Donaldson, M. H., Chatten, J., and Koblenzer, C. S.: Perianal rhabdomyosarcoma in childhood. Cancer 38:1008, 1976.

Walter, P., and Guerbaoui, M.: Rhabdomyome foetal. Virchows Arch. [Pathol. Anat.] 371:59, 1976.

Weichert, K. A., Bove, K. C., Aron, B. S., and Lampkin, B.: Rhabdomyosarcoma in children. Am. J. Clin. Pathol. 66:692, 1976.

Fenoglio, J. J., Diana, D. J., Bowen, T. E., McAllister, H. A., and Ferrans, V. J.: Ultrastructure of a cardiac rhabdomyoma. Hum. Pathol. 8:700, 1977.

Lawrence, W., Hays, D. M., and Moon, T. E.: Lymphatic metastasis with childhood rhabdomyosarcoma. Cancer 39:556, 1977.

Maurer, H. M., Moon, T., Donaldson, M., Fernandez, C., Gehan, E. A., Hammond, D., Hays, D. M., Lawrence, W., Newton, W., Razab, A., Ramey, B., and Soule, E. H.: The intergroup rhabdomyosarcoma study. Cancer 40:2015, 1977.

Sethi, J., Hirshaut, Y., Hajdu, S. I., and Clements, L. G.: Growing human sarcoma in culture. Cancer 40:744, 1977.

Shrivastava, S., Jacks, J. J., White, R. S., and Edwards, J. E.: Diffuse rhabdomyomatosis of the heart. Arch. Pathol. 101:78, 1977.

Ueda, K., Guppo, R., Unger, R., Martin, L., and Bove, K.: Rhabdomyosarcoma of lung arising in congenital cystic adenomatoid malformation. Cancer 40:383, 1977.

Hajdu, S. I., and Fogh, J.: The nude mouse as a diagnostic tool in human tumor cell research. *In* The Nude Mouse in Experimental and Clinical Research. Edited by J. Fogh and B. C. Giovanella. New York, Academic Press, 1978.

Hildebrand, H., and Biserte, G.: Ultrastructural investigation of NI_3S_2-induced rhabdomyosarcoma in Wistar rat. Cancer 42:528, 1978.

Miller, R., Kurtz, S. M., and Powers, J. M.: Mediastinal rhabdomyoma. Cancer 42:1983, 1978.

Ramey, R. B., Hays, D. M., Lawrence, W., Soule, E. H., Tefft, M., and Donaldson, M. H.: Paratesticular rhabdomyosarcoma in childhood. Cancer 42:729, 1978.

Exelby, Ph. R.: Personal communication, 1979.

Sarnat, H., deMello, D. E., and Siddiqui, S. Y.: Diagnostic value of histochemistry in embryonal rhabdomyosarcoma. Am. J. Surg. Pathol. 3:177, 1979.

Hajdu, S. I., Lemos, L. B., Kozakewich, H., Hetson, L., and Beattie, E. J., Jr.: Growth pattern and differentiation of human soft tissue sarcomas in nude mice. Cancer 47:90, 1981.

chapter 6

Tumors of Vessels

NON-NEOPLASTIC LESIONS

Pyogenic Granuloma
Angioblastic Lymphoid Hyperplasia
Hereditary Hemorrhagic Telangiectasia
Arteriovenous Fistula

NEOPLASTIC LESIONS

Tumors of Blood Vessels

Hemangioma
Capillary Hemangioma
Cavernous Hemangioma
Venous Hemangioma
Papillary Endothelial Hyperplasia
Hypertrophic Hemangioma
Angiomatosis
Angiofibroma
Angiolipoma
Angiomyolipoma
Angiomyoma
Leiomyosarcoma
Glomus Tumor
Hemangiopericytoma
Hemangiosarcoma
Kaposi's Sarcoma
Hemangioblastoma

Tumors of Lymphatic Vessels

Lymphangioma
Cystic Hygroma
Lymphatic Cyst
Papillary Endothelial Hyperplasia
Lymphangiectasia
Lymphangiomyoma
Lymphangiosarcoma

BLOOD vessels consist of smooth muscle cells, endothelial cells, and pericytes. The endothelial cells are elongated and flattened and blend into the contour of the vessel.

The earliest network of endothelial cells in the human embryo develops in the third week from the mesoderm adjacent to the yolk sac. From this conglomerate of cells, the heart and the aorta are the first to appear, and then by progressive branching the capillary network develops (Sabin, 1917; Kramer, 1960).

Adjacent *endothelial cells* are interdigitated and form tight junctions. Endothelial cells contain numerous pinocytotic vesicles and Weibel-Palade bodies, rod-shaped intracytoplasmic structures measuring 0.1 μ to 3 μ (Weibel-Palade, 1964; Sengel and Stoebuer, 1970). The endothelial cells resemble each other, regardless of the size of the vessels, except for the abundance of lysosomes in the endothelial cells of venules (Movat and Fernando, 1964) (Fig. 6-1).

The *pericytes,* or perivascular cells also known as adventitial cells, are external to the endothelial cells and appear similar throughout the vascular system. Pericytes are surrounded by basal lamina which separates them from adjoining perivascular fibroblasts or "veil" cells. Pericytes do not form a continuous sheath around vessels. The spaces or gaps between pericytes vary according to type and size of vessels and anatomic site.

Pericytes possess a unique quality. They may become histiocytic, ameboid, or fibroblastic. Such cells no longer contain basement membrane and may act as phagocytic or fibrohistiocytic cells (see Chapter 2). Crocker et al (1970) demonstrated that during wound healing fibroblast-like primitive mesenchymal cells resembling pericytes are incorporated into the vessel wall and are surrounded by basal laminae.

The endothelial cells of lymphatic vessels contain intracytoplasmic organelles similar to those of the blood vessels, but their basal lamina is interrupted or completely absent. Pericytes do not surround lymphatic vessels, but lymphatic vessels have anchoring filaments which extend from the endothelial cells to the adjacent stroma (Rouvier, 1938; Weber, 1973).

Endothelial cells have been the subject of investigation by histologists, electron microscopists, physiologists, and recently immunologists. It has been proposed that endothelial cells may play an important role in such diverse processes as vascular permeability, hemostasis, and deposition of immune complexes along the basement membranes.

Contractile proteins, which have been found in many nonmyogenic cells, including endothelial cells, and platelets are apparently required for specialized functions of the cells such as mobility, secretion, and phagocytic activity. Endothelial cells, both in vivo and in vitro, have been shown by using immunofluorescence techniques to contain smooth muscle *actomyosin* (Becker and Nachman, 1973; Gabbiani et al, 1975; Moore et al, 1977).

Majno et al (1969) demonstrated that gaps between endothelial cells are widened because of contraction in response to histamine, serotonin, and bradykinin. Such widening of intercellular junctions permits contact between platelets and collagen-like tissue proteins which is known to lead to platelet adhesion, clot formation, and subsequently hemostasis. Furthermore, the discovery of antigenic similarity between the contractile apparatus of platelets and endothelial cells supports the theory that despite morphologic dissimilarity of the endothelial cell and the platelet there is an intimate functional relationship between these cells. This is supported by the findings of Lewis et al (1973) and Macarak et al (1977) that endothelial cells stained brilliantly with antibody against human thrombosthenin possess ABO blood group antigens and factor VIII antigen.

It has been shown by histologic and enzyme-histochemical techniques that

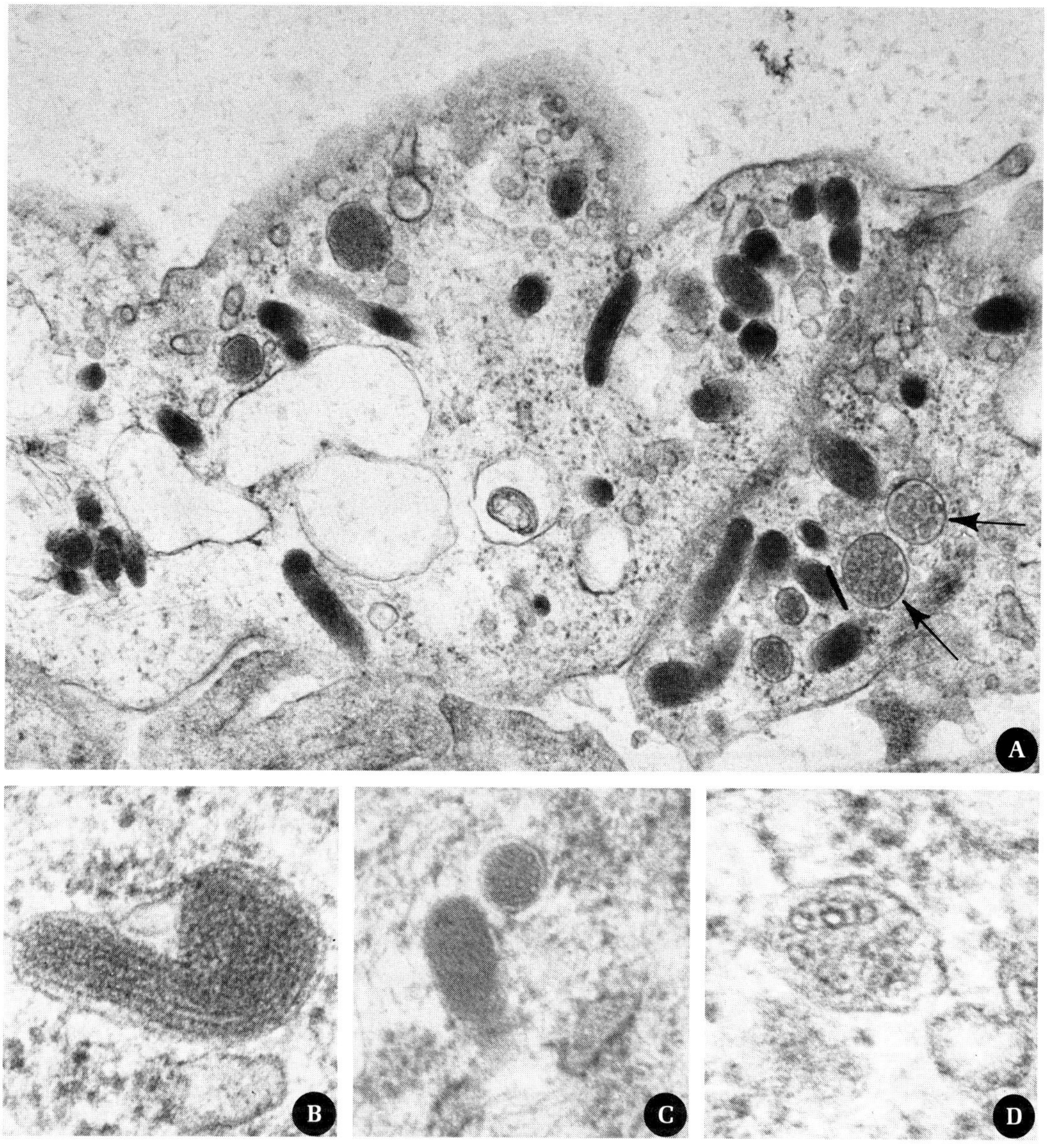

Figure 6-1. **A,** Endothelial cells containing numerous Weibel-Palade bodies. Arrows indicate multivesicular bodies, not to be mistaken for cross section of Weibel-Palade bodies (×22,000).

B, Club-formed Weibel-Palade body (×85,000).

C, Longitudinal and cross section of Weibel-Palade bodies (×45,000).

D, Multivesicular body (×85,000). (Courtesy Carstens, H. B., and Schrodt, G. R.: Ultrastructure of sclerosing hemangioma. Am. J. Pathol. 77:377, 1974.)

there is a marked difference between normal and proliferating endothelial cells. For example, the alkaline phosphatase activity is decreased (and is probably related to enlargement of endothelial cells), the ATP-ase activity is increased (and may be related to the increase in basement membrane material produced by the endothelial cell), and the 5-nucleotidase activity disappears completely in proliferating endothelial cells.

Two unique properties of endothelial cells, according to Handenschild et al (1976), are that in tissue culture they *do not respond to serum growth factors* and are able to synthesize DNA only when subconfluent; thus they differ from fibroblasts and muscle cells. It is speculated that this unique property of endothelial cells is required for the maintenance and integrity of blood vessel walls in vivo, since the blood is rich in growth-stimulating factors. It is possible that interruption of the continuity of the endothelium is a prerequisite to proliferation of endothelial cells as well as underlying smooth muscle cells, pericytes, and fibroblasts. Kelly et al (1976), found that while endothelial cells proliferate in tissue cultures of central nervous system tumors, fibroblasts do not grow in such cultures. On the other hand, Folkman (1972) observed that a diffusible *anti-angiogenetic* factor in neonatal cartilage is capable of inhibiting capillary proliferation induced by tumor *angiogenetic* factor. When angiogenetic and anti-angiogenetic factors are purified and properly characterized, the implications may be far reaching because it is known that when a neoplasm is deprived of its blood supply it is unable to grow.

NON-NEOPLASTIC LESIONS

PYOGENIC GRANULOMA*

Pyogenic granuloma is composed of small vessels arranged in lobules in an inflammatory and granulomatous background. The term *pyogenic granuloma* was introduced by Hartzell in 1904. This granuloma may occur anywhere under squamous mucosa and the skin. It may appear as a sessile or pedunculated growth with a minute stalk; however, most commonly, it is a slightly elevated plaque covered by intact mucosa or skin. The capillaries may appear extremely exuberant and *hypertrophic hemangioma, well-differentiated hemangiosarcoma, Kaposi's sarcoma,* and *glomus tumor* should be considered in the differential diagnosis (Fig. 6-2).

Pyogenic granuloma affects males as well as females. Angelopoulos (1971) stated that 60% of the reported cases occurred in patients between 10 and 40 years of age. The etiology is unknown, but most authors suggest that it is most likely due to trauma. Although pyogenic granuloma is not a neoplasm, it must be removed, preferably by excision, to prevent secondary infection or hemorrhage (Pinkus and Rudner, 1969).

**Synonyms and related terms:* granuloma pyogenicum, granulation hemangioma, granuloma gravidarum, granuloma telangiecticum, granuloma pediculatum.

ANGIOBLASTIC LYMPHOID HYPERPLASIA*

Angioblastic lymphoid hyperplasia or pseudopyogenic granuloma is a proliferative vascular lesion associated with hyperplastic changes of lymphoid tissue and containing infiltrates of eosinophils. According to Kawada et al (1965) it was Kimura et al, in 1948, who first called attention to this peculiar disease. Wilson-Jones and Bleehen, in 1969, reported a series of 14 cases and Wells and Whimster reported 9 cases in the same year. Six additional cases were described by Reed and Terazakis, in 1972, and Eady and Wilson-Jones (1977) added 6 new cases to the literature in which they performed histochemical and electron microscopic studies and concluded that the dermal lesions arise predominantly from venous capillaries.

These lesions occur almost exclusively on the face, neck, and scalp and around the ears (Fig. 6-3). Clinically it is characterized by flat or slightly elevated solitary or multiple dermal and/or subcutaneous nodules. The nodules may persist for years and affect predominantly middle-aged females.

Histologically, the angioblastic nodules are composed of proliferating blood ves-

**Synonyms and related terms:* pseudopyogenic granuloma, Kimura's disease, angiolymphoid hyperplasia with eosinophilia, eosinophilic lymphoid granuloma, eosinophilic granuloma of soft tissue, subcutaneous angiolymphoid hyperplasia, atypical pyogenic granuloma, papular angioplasia.

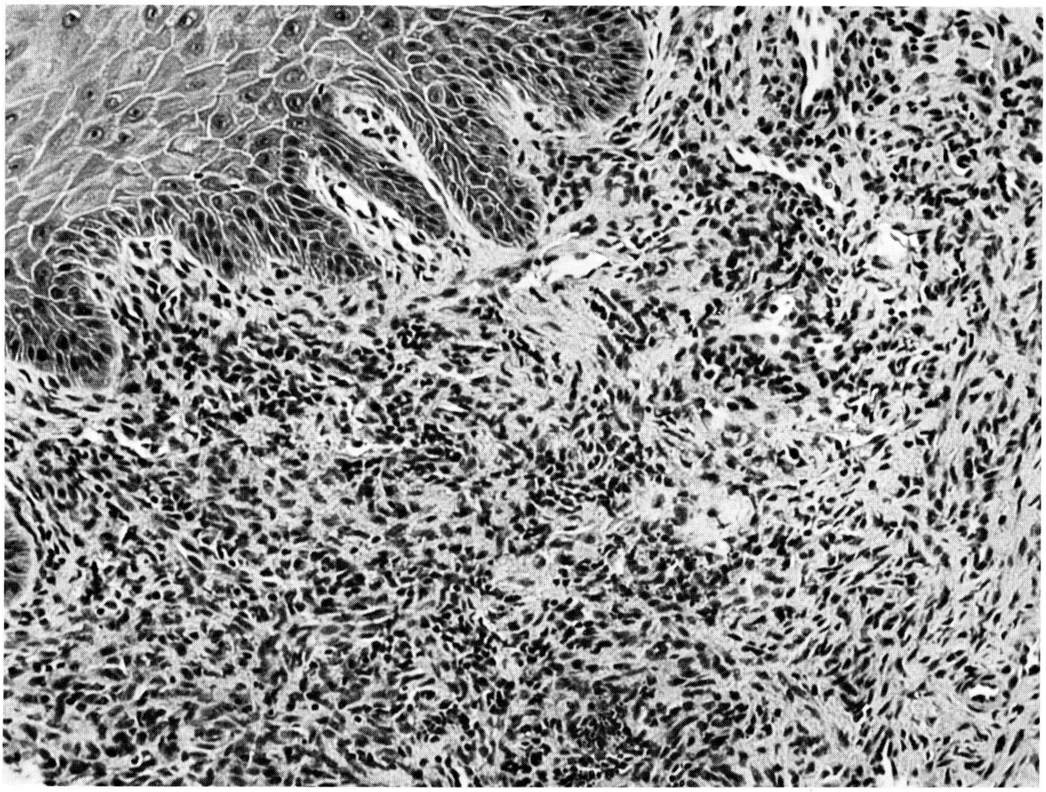

Figure 6-2. Pyogenic granuloma. Extensive but localized subepithelial infiltrate of various inflammatory cells. Note numerous short spindle cells and minuscule capillary vessels buried in the infiltrate (H & E, ×140).

sels and lymphatic vessels, with hypertrophic endothelial cells. The often tortuous vessels are surrounded by hyperplastic lymphoid tissue with well-preserved lymphoid follicles and infiltrates of eosinophils as well as mast cells. Although there is evidence of proliferation of dermal and subcutaneous fibroblasts and other stromal elements, there is only a remote possibility of confusing these lesions with *pyogenic granuloma, angiosarcoma, Kaposi's sarcoma, mycosis fungoides, lymphocytoma cutis, allergic vasculitis,* or *angiomatous lymphoid hamartoma.* Angiomatous lymphoid hamartomas are predominantly well-defined, deep-seated lymphoreticular lesions (Castleman, 1954; Harrison and Bernatz, 1963; Tung and McCormack, 1967; Boxer et al, 1972). The prominent histiocytic deposit around thick-walled blood vessels is a characteristic feature of *angiomatous lymphoid hamartomas. Lymphocytoma cutis* is a benign nonspecific inflammatory and granulomatous lesion, with no prominent vascular component. *Mycosis fungoides* exhibits a monomorphic diffuse lymphoreticular infiltrate in the dermis with the typical Pautrier's abscesses. *Allergic vasculitis* is panarteritis microscopically and is often drug-induced. The inflammatory cells, mononuclear cells, and eosinophils are deposited in nodular patterns in and around small arteries, arterioles, and venules (Mullich et al, 1979).

The etiology and the histogenesis of this vascular abnormality are unknown, but most observers agree that the initial process is active angiogenesis which is followed, at a later stage of the disease, by proliferation of lymphoid tissue. In about one third of the reported cases the skin lesions were found in association with *blood eosinophilia.* The significance of this association is obscure.

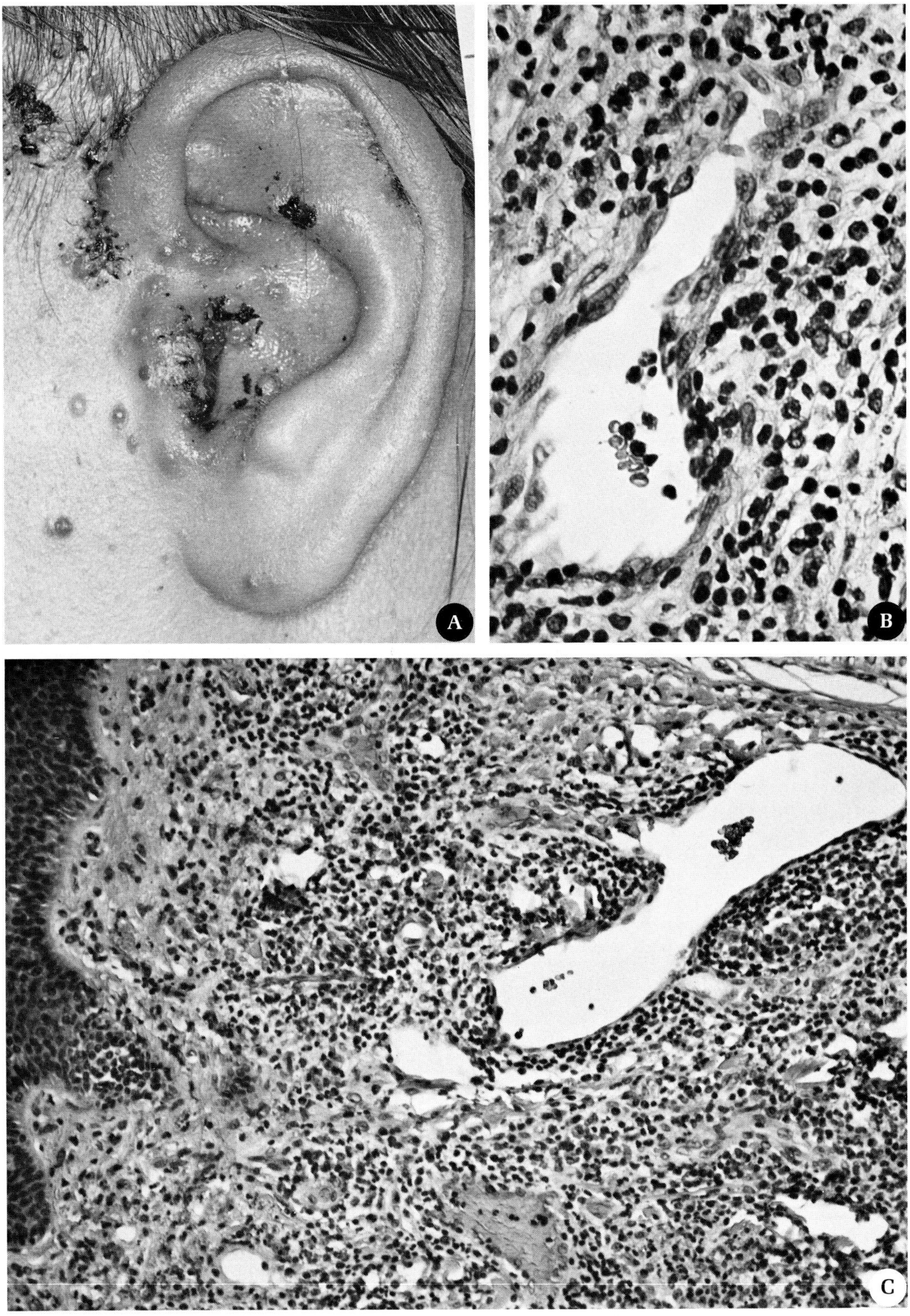

Figure 6-3. Angiofollicular lymphoid hyperplasia.

A, Fairly typical clinical presentation of the disease in the form of multiple papulomacular lesions.

B and **C,** Microscopically, angiofollicular lymphoid hyperplasia consists of diffuse and nodular lymphocytic and eosinophilic infiltrate in dermis and subcutis and hypertrophy and focal hyperplasia of capillary vessels. Lymphocytes may also appear in aggregates or may form lymphoid nodules with follicles (**B,** H & E, ×350; **C,** H & E, ×140).

There is no general agreement on the best modality of treatment, but observers have reported good results after local excision.

HEREDITARY HEMORRHAGIC TELANGECTASIA*

Hereditary hemorrhagic telangiectasia, or Osler-Weber-Rendu disease, is an autosomal dominant inherited vasculopathy characterized by telangiectasia of the skin, mucous membrane, and internal organs. The disease primarily involves capillaries, venules, and small muscular arteries, but aneurysms and arteriovenous fistulas also have been recorded (Fig. 6-4).

The pathogenesis of this disorder is not known, but it has been advanced that the telangiectasia is the result of defective development of vascular and perivascular fibroelastic tissues and capillary endothelial cells (Goldstein, 1931; Hashimoto and Pritzker, 1972; Sussman and Sternberg, 1975).

Repeated epistaxis, hemoptysis, hematuria, melena, and chronic anemia are the result of profuse bleeding from the widespread telangiectatic lesions. There are several references in the literature, dating back to Hippocrates, to "generalized telangiectasis" and hereditary epistaxis (Lotzbeck, 1859; Babbington, 1865), but the first cases of heredofamilial angiomatosis, in two families, was reported by Chiari, in 1887. Rendu, in 1896, reported a man with telangiectasis whose father had repeated attacks of melena. The patients of Osler (1901) and Weber (1907) had multiple cutaneous and mucosal telangiectasia and recurring hemorrhages. Ullman (1896) is credited with the first illustration of a case of multiple telangiectasia.

The onset of the disease may be during childhood, but the telangiectases become evident usually in the fourth and fifth decades of life. Approximately 20% of the patients will develop arteriovenous pulmonary malformations which may lead to arterial hypoxemia and secondary polycythemia and neurologic symptoms (Adams et al, 1977).

Goldstein (1931) found about 90 families and about 500 people affected with this disease and described splenomegaly in advanced cases. Muller et al (1978) studied a family in which 87 members, in six generations, possessed traits of hemorrhagic telangiectasia.

**Synonyms and related terms:* Osler-Weber-Rendu disease, hereditary hemorrhagic thromboasthenia, heredofamilial angiomatosis, multiple hereditary telangiectases.

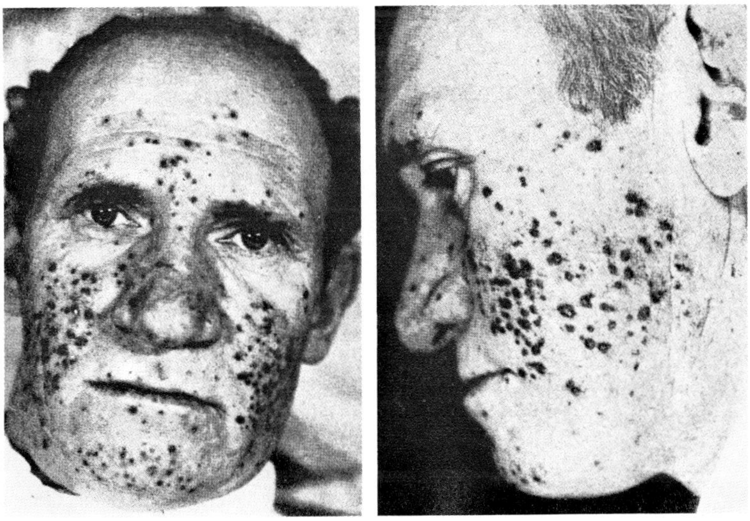

Figure 6-4. Hereditary hemorrhagic telangiectasis. Osler-Weber-Rendu disease. (From Pack, G., and Ariel, I. M.: Tumors of the Soft Somatic Tissues—A Clinical Treatise. New York, Harper and Bros., 1958.)

The multifocal nature of the lesions precludes effective therapy by surgery or cauterization. The therapeutic value of irradiation and steroids is also limited.

ARTERIOVENOUS FISTULA

Arteriovenous fistula is also known as arteriovenous malformation, vascular hamartoma, or cirsoid and racemose aneurysm. Hunter (1752) first described the thrill and bruit commonly found in association with arteriovenous fistulas. These lesions are characterized by dilated and predominantly thick-walled vascular channels lined by focally prominent endothelial cells. It is believed that most of these lesions are the result of congenital malformation or are traumatic in origin and there is a shunt between arteries and veins without a connecting capillary bed. Due to long-standing and constant irritation and pressure the vessel walls are hyalinized and thickened. The stroma between blood vessels may show fibrosis and calcification. If the lesion is localized, it may give the appearance of a tumor (Fig. 6-5). It is felt that angiography is valuable in preoperative assessment of the exact nature and boundaries of such lesions (Lawton et al, 1957).

NEOPLASTIC LESIONS

Tumors of Blood Vessels

Neoplasms of blood vessels are not uncommon. Fortunately the majority of tumors of blood vessels are benign hemangiomas.

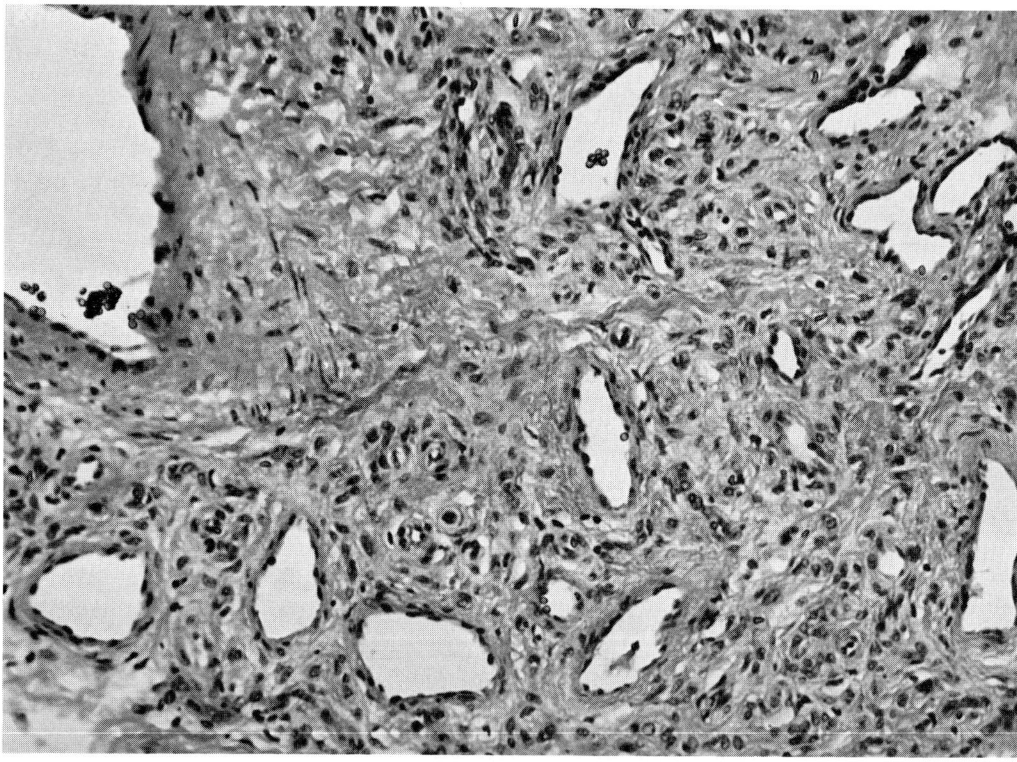

Figure 6-5. Arteriovenous fistula or so-called vascular hamartoma. The vessels are larger than capillary vessels and possess thick partially hyalinized walls. The stroma between the vessels is partly fibrous and contains a number of small and hypertrophic vessels, but the larger vessels' endothelial lining is not hyperplastic (H & E, ×140).

HEMANGIOMA*

Typically, hemangiomas are of capillary origin, but they may also arise from venules and arterioles. Angiomas at an early stage are composed of irregular, lumenless vascular channels and clusters of endothelial cells.

Reported studies of hemangiomas are numerous. Among the most important contributions are the articles written by Maffucci (1881) describing the first case of *Maffucci syndrome;* Shennan (1914) recording the first case of a so-called histologically nonmalignant angioma which metastasized; Masson (1923) calling attention to an entity known today as *papillary endothelial hyerplasia;* Burman and Milgram (1930) reviewing the subject of hemangioma of tendon and tendon sheath; Herrington (1953) reporting a case of congenital malformation involving the entire lower extremities; and Bendeck and Lichtenberg (1957) discussing cavernous hemangiomas of striated muscle.

Hemangiomas may remain unchanged in size or may enlarge with the growth of the child. In adults, hemangiomas usually do not increase in size, except during pregnancy and in case of arteriovenous malformations. Watson and McCarthy (1940) reviewed 1,056 hemangiomas and found a female preponderance (65%) and considered the majority congenital.

According to Geschickter and Keasbey (1935) more than 30% of the hemangiomas are discovered in children under 10 years of age and in about 5% of the cases multiple lesions are present. Lampe and Latourette (1959) studied 471 hemangiomas, of which about 50% occurred on the trunk, one third on the extremities and one sixth in the head and neck region. There are many theories as to the pathomechanism of hemangiomas, none of which is satisfactory.

Although subclassification of hemangiomas is arbitrary and the various forms often merge into each other, it is customary to distinguish capillary and cavernous forms (Table 6-1).

Capillary Hemangiomas. These are the most common of all hemangiomas and may occur in the skin or mucous membranes. Two thirds of the superficial angiomas are the capillary type, and congenital origin can be established in most cases (Johnson et al, 1956; Bean and Rather, 1963; Meitner and Pavur, 1965). They may be minute lesions, like the so-called De Morgan's spots and spider nevus or large like the port-wine stain. Histologically, capillary hemangiomas are composed of capillary vessels lined by a single layer of flattened or plump endothelial cells surrounded most commonly by a discontinuous layer of pericytes and reticulum fibers. The intervascular stroma is almost always sparsely cellular and myxomatous (Fig. 6-6).

Cavernous and Venous Angiomas. Cavernous angiomas are composed of dilated blood vessels and spaces lined by thin walls. Both arterial and venous vessels may form cavernous angiomas. Due to their connection with the general circulation cavernous hemangiomas may reach enormous size. Blood filled cul-de-sacs or sinuses are common findings especially in venous hemangiomas. According to Waisman (1968), cavernous hemangiomas occur in less than 5% of the newborn, and they tend to occur after infancy (Fig. 6-7).

TABLE 6-1. ***Most Common Sites of Hemangiomas***

	%
Head and neck	30
Liver	20
Extremities	19
Trunk	11
CNS	8
Other	12

* *Synonyms and related terms:* capillary hemangioma, cavernous hemangioma, venous hemangioma, intravascular papillary endothelial hyperplasia, hypertrophic hemangioma, juvenile hemangioma, De Morgan's spots, port-wine stain, fibrocavernous hemangioma, lipo-cavernous hemangioma, racemose or cirsoid aneurysmal hemangioma.

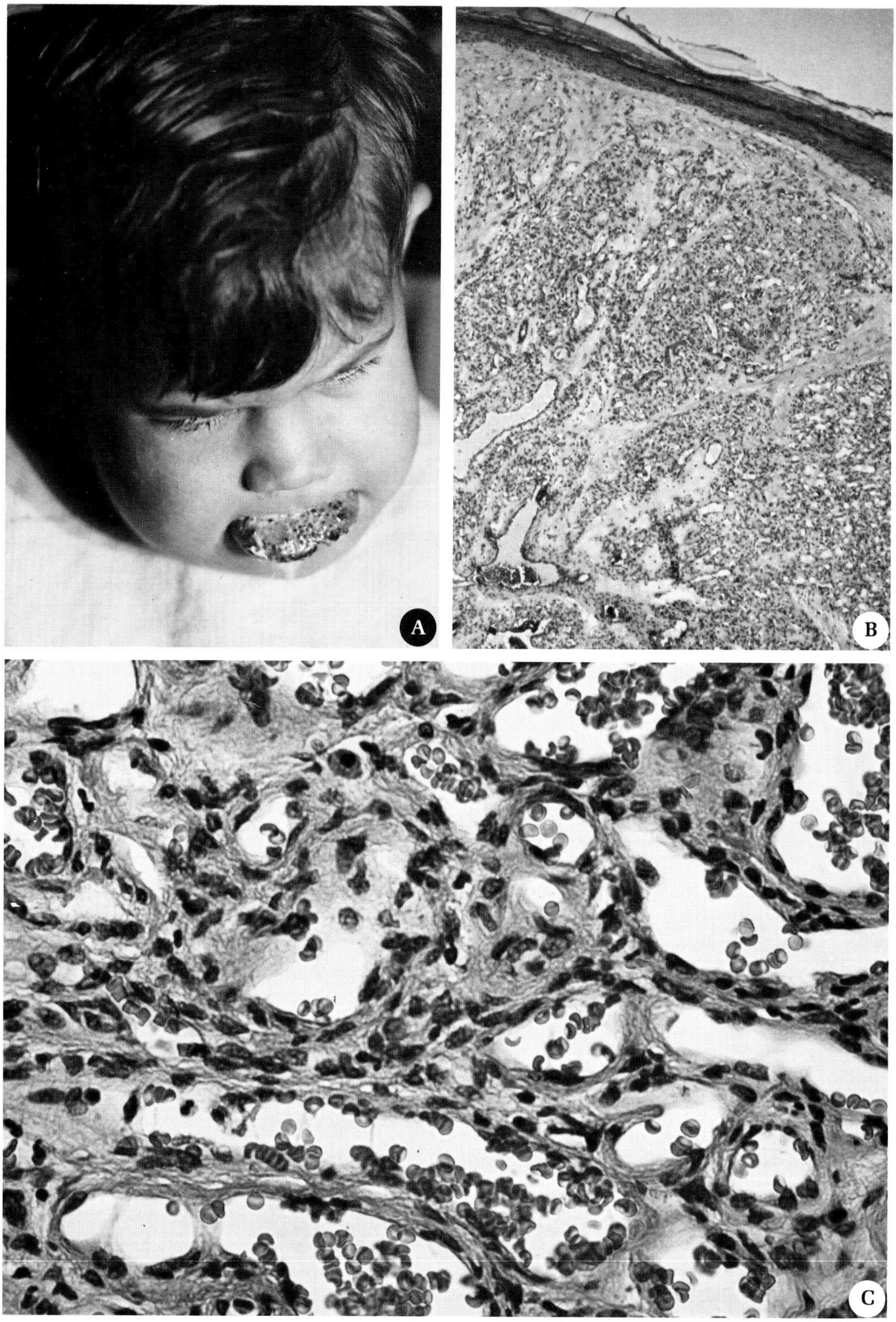

Figure 6-6. Capillary hemangioma.

A, Young child with congenital capillary hemangioma of the tip of the tongue.

B and **C,** Microscopically, capillary hemangioma is composed of interrelated, moderately dilated, and hypertrophic capillary vessels. There is no evidence of hyperplasia or atypia of endothelial cells and the stroma looks sparsely cellular (**A,** H & E, ×35; **B,** H & E, ×350).

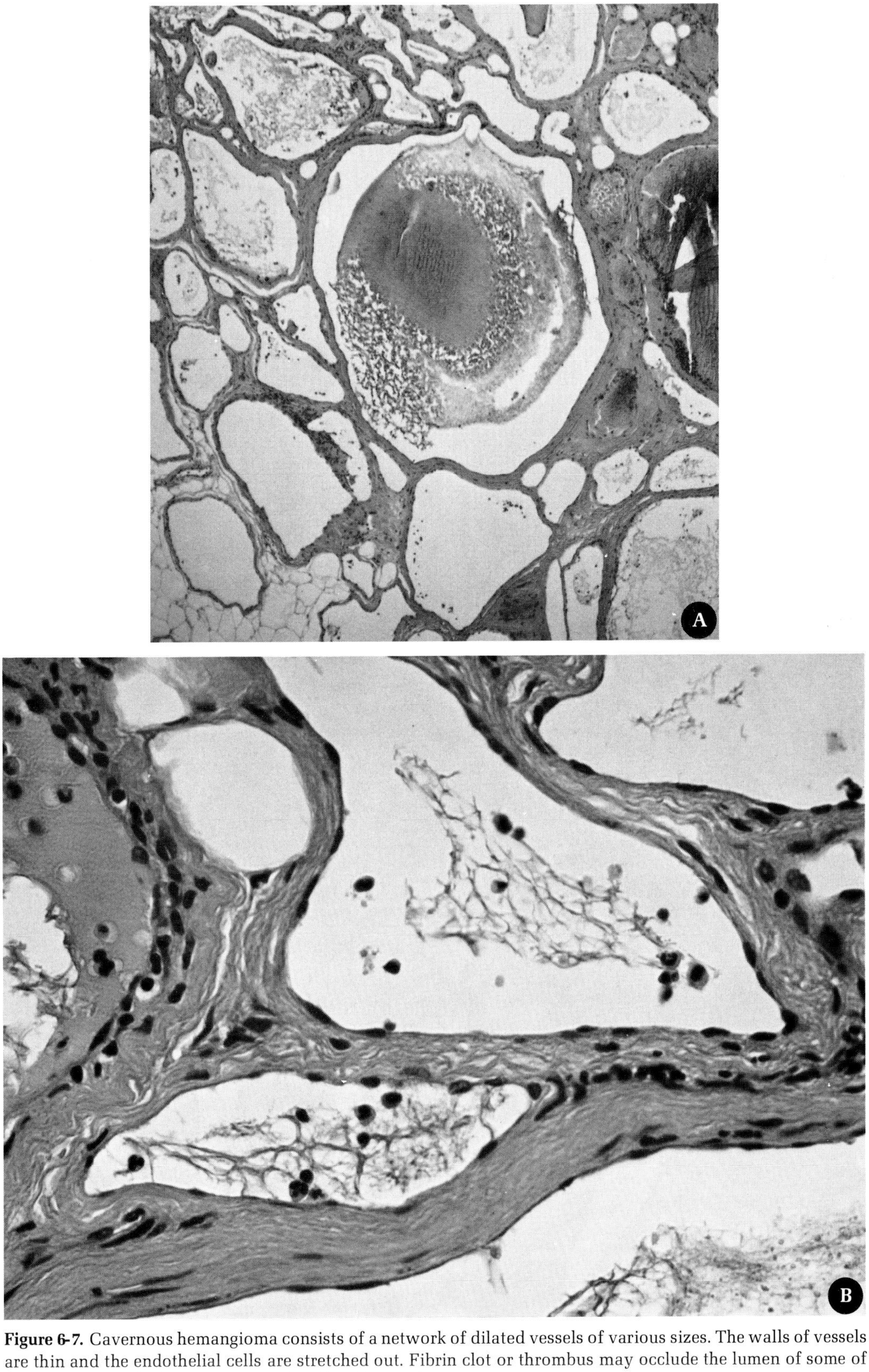

Figure 6-7. Cavernous hemangioma consists of a network of dilated vessels of various sizes. The walls of vessels are thin and the endothelial cells are stretched out. Fibrin clot or thrombus may occlude the lumen of some of the dilated vessels (**A,** H & E, ×35; **B,** H & E, ×570).

Hemangiomas, especially the ones which are *intramuscular* (Bendeck and Lichtenberg, 1957; Allan and Enzinger, 1972) or are located in deep soft tissues (Stone and Vincente, 1951; Waddel, 1967), often have prominent endothelial cells and intraluminal vascular projections. Jenkins and Delaney (1932), in a series of 256 cases of intramuscular hemangiomas, observed that 47% of the cases were congenital, and trauma played a role in the etiology of 17% of the cases. Intramuscular hemangiomas may grow and expand between muscle fibers, resulting in deposit of fibrous and adipose tissues, and may appear fibro- or lipocavernous (Fig. 6-8).

Papillary Endothelial Hyperplasia. A variant of benign vascular neoplasms is the so-called papillary endothelial hyperplasia.* The first reference to a case of such a lesion is in Ewing's book, *Neoplastic Diseases,* second edition, page 307, 1922. Ewing wrote that it is "a rare and somewhat obscure intravascular endothelioma. . . . The endothelium grows first in broad papillary masses which later become fused and enlarged, distending the vessel wall." He added that he has seen this neoplasm in dilated varicose veins and lymphatic vessels as well as in lymph nodes in chronic lymph stasis and referred to Schlagenhaufer who described such lesions in hemorrhoidal veins. Salyer and Salyer (1975) called attention to similar papillary lesions in organizing thrombi.

Despite Masson's (1923) reference to Ewing's original description in his case report "Hemangioendotheliome vegetant intravasculaire," which is based on a case of inflamed and ulcerated hemorrhoid of a 68-year-old man, some writers credit Masson with the first description of papillary endothelial hyperplasia.

**Synonyms and related terms:* intravascular papillary endothelial hyperplasia, intravascular angiomatosis, intravascular atypical vascular proliferation, pseudoangiosarcoma, vegetant intravascular hemangioendothelioma, intravascular hemangioendothelioma, endovascular papillary angioendothelioma.

Most of the time, these lesions are a peculiar benign, intravascular papillary endothelial growth. They have a predilection for the subcutis of the head and neck regions and distal parts of the extremities. Females are affected more commonly than males and it is more commonly seen in adults than in children (Table 6-2). The size of the lesion may range from less than a centimeter to several centimeters and the duration is several months.

Microscopically, the most striking feature is the *endothelial cell-lined papillary tufts which are projecting into the lumen of a dilated blood vessel or cavernous vascular space.* The endothelial cells are prominent and may form detached clusters or cell cords. One may find microscopic areas with solid growths of polygonal endothelial cells that resemble *hemangiosarcoma* (Fig. 6-9). However, careful consideration of certain characteristic microscopic features (Table 6-3) and the gross presentation of papillary endothelial hyperplasia and hemangiosarcoma will help to reach the right diagnosis in most instances without difficulty.

The histogenesis and the precise classification of papillary endothelial hyperplasia is far from settled and it may be a reactive rather than a neoplastic process. Whether the endothelial proliferation is a sequel to thrombosis or the thrombosis is secondary to the endothelial hyperplasia and papillary growths is debated in the literature. I personally believe that when the local circulation is compromised, both of these modalities may result in the formation of papillary endothelial tufts. The exact histogenesis often cannot be established purely on the basis of microscopic examination.

Hypertrophic Hemangioma.* This tumor of the blood vessels occurs almost exclusively in children and infants. It is characterized by proliferation of blood vessels, hyperplasia, and atypia of endo-

**Synonyms and related terms:* juvenile hemangioma, benign juvenile endothelioma, juvenile hemangioendothelioma.

TABLE 6-2. ***Papillary Endothelial Hyperplasia***

	NO. CASES WITH FOLLOW-UP	FEMALE-TO-MALE RATIO	AVG. AGE YR.	MOST COMMON SITES	RECURRENCE	FOLLOW-UP
Dabska (1969)	6	2:1	7	Head and neck	2	No evidence of disease*
Clearkin and Enzinger (1976)	31	6:5	39	Fingers Head and Neck Trunk	0	No evidence of disease
Kuo et al (1976)	14	2:1	40	Head and Neck Extremities	1	No evidence of disease
Personal observation	8	2:1	30	Head and Neck	2	No evidence of disease

*2 patients presented with metastasis to nodes; however, both patients were alive without evidence of disease 6 and 4 years later, respectively.

thelial cells. All observers agree that the occasional mitotic figures and exuberant growth of endothelial cells make these lesions more ominous looking than actually they are (Mallory, 1908; Stout, 1943; Schow et al, 1975). Microscopically, one should consider the fibromyxoid stromal partitions between branching blood vessels, lack of solid areas, and absence of invasion of the vessel walls and adjacent stroma, as well as the age of the patient in order to distinguish hypertrophic hemangioma from well-differentiated hemangiosarcoma. Taxy and Gray (1979) reported that electron microscopy is useful in the diagnosis of these often histologically worrisome lesions (Fig. 6-10). Due to their branching nature hypertrophic hemangiomas tend to be locally aggressive and will recur unless excised with clean margin.

Angiomatosis. The term *angiomatosis* usually means the presence of multiple and diffuse hemangiomas in infants. It is a congenital and systemic disease and usually occupies a portion of the trunk, extremity, or head and neck area. It usually follows the regional distribution of a major nerve or blood vessel. Due to the increased arteriovenous circulation there

TABLE 6-3. ***Distinguishing Microscopic Features of Papillary Endothelial Hyperplasia and Hemangiosarcoma***

	PAPILLARY ENDOTHELIAL HYPERPLASIA	HEMANGIOSARCOMA
Papillary pattern	Common	Rare
Solid pattern	Rare	Common
Thrombus	Common	Rare
Intravascular distribution	Common	Rare
Endothelial pleomorphism	Uncommon	Common
Nuclear atypia	Rare	Common
Mitotic endothelial cells	Rare	Common
Endothelial cells in sheets	Rare	Common
Necrosis	Rare	Common
Hemosiderin deposits	Common	Uncommon
Inflammatory cells	Common	Uncommon
Calcification	Occasional	Rare
Vasculitis	Common	Rare

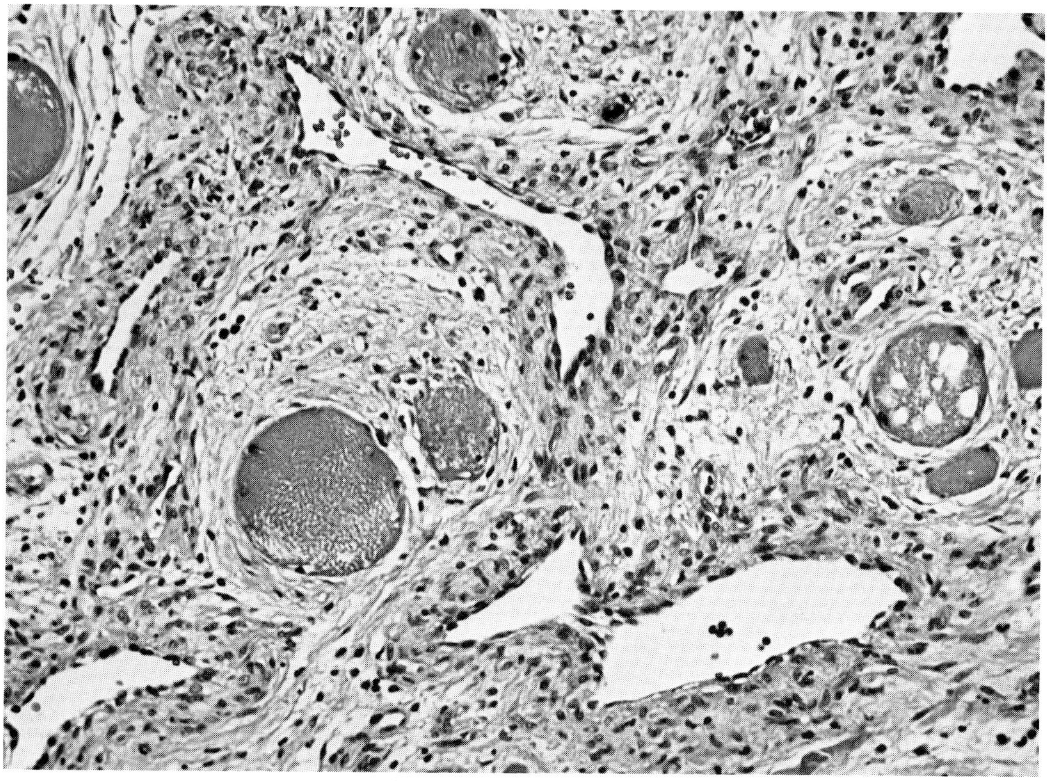

Figure 6-8. Intramuscular hemangioma. Note the striking resemblance of this lesion to the one illustrated in Figure 6-5. The vessels are tortuous, hypertrophic, and larger than capillary vessels and seem to carry with them a generous complement of fibrous tissue which is able to destroy muscle fibers. Note the proliferating pericytes (H & E, ×140).

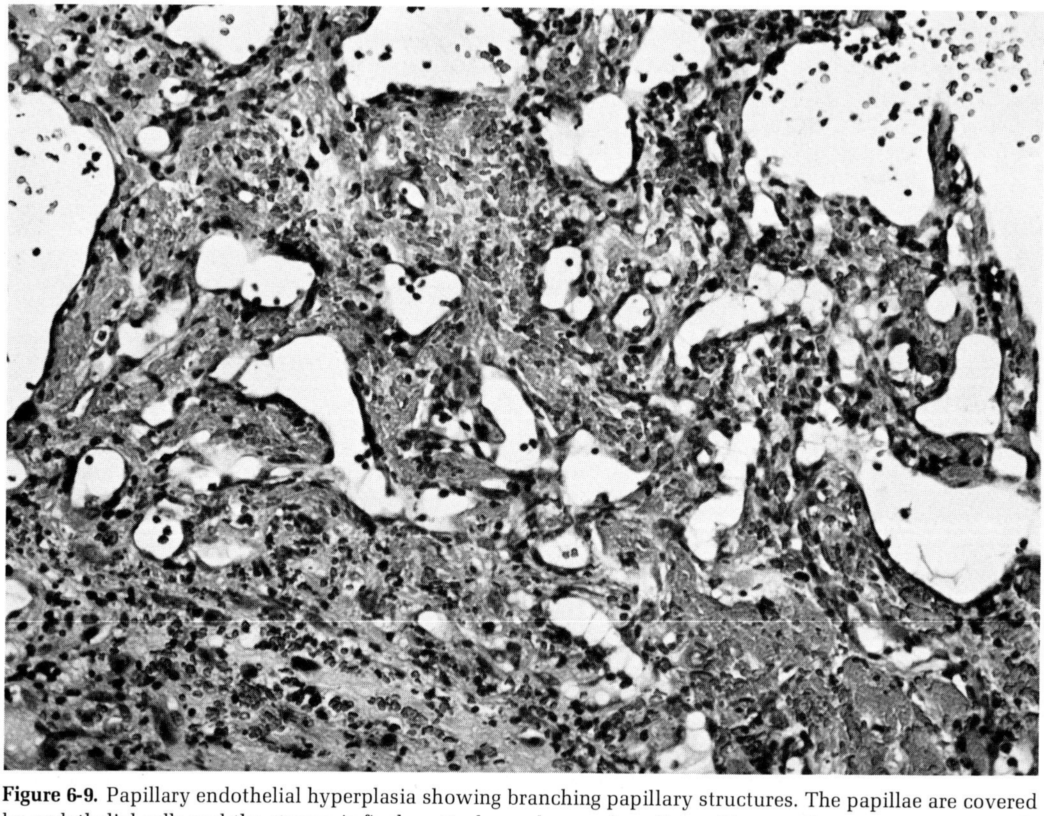

Figure 6-9. Papillary endothelial hyperplasia showing branching papillary structures. The papillae are covered by endothelial cells and the stroma is finely reticular and sparsely cellular. The papillary structures protrude into a cysticly dilated vascular lumen and fuse with each other (H & E, ×140).

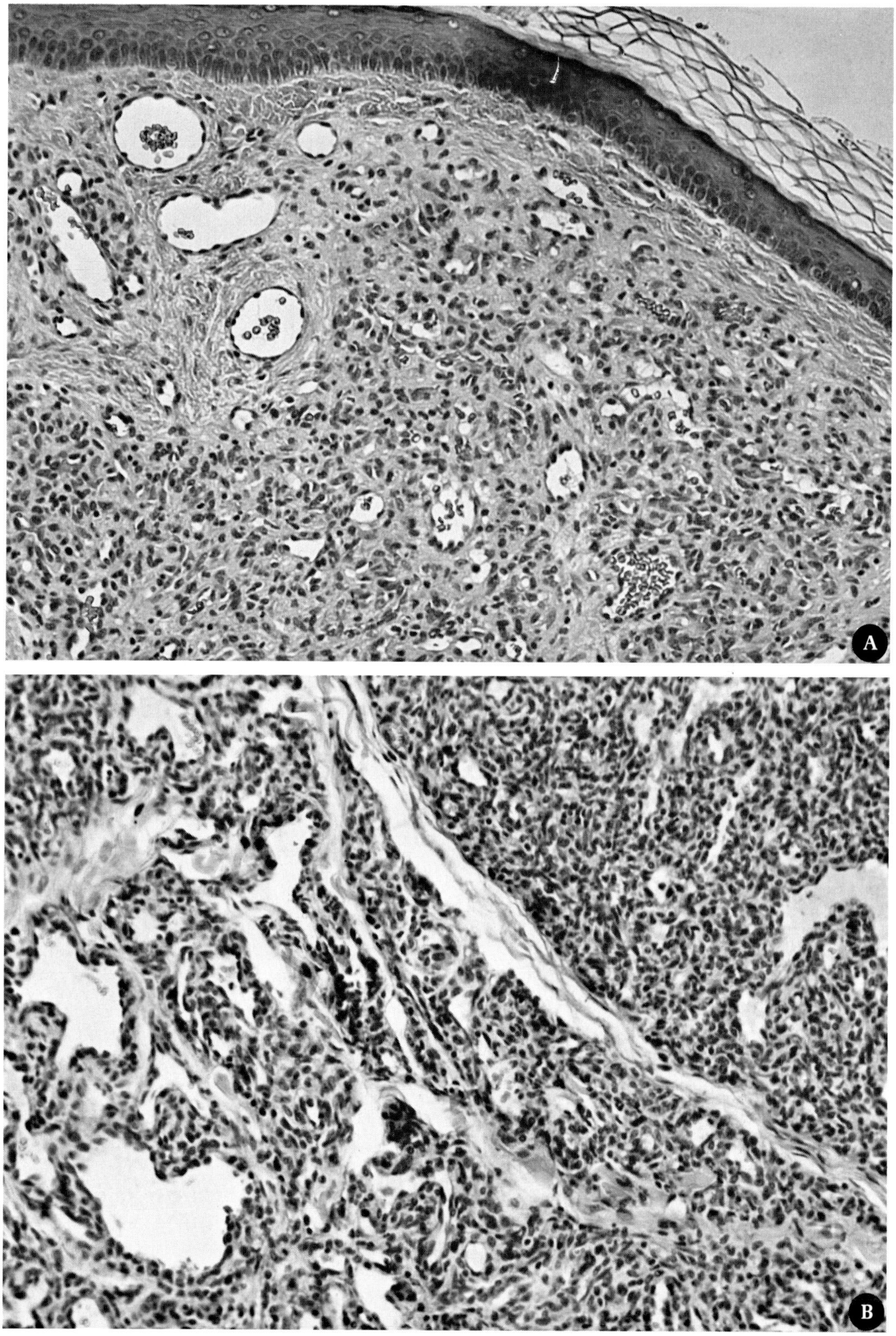

Figure 6-10. Hypertrophic hemangioma.

A, Innumerable hypertrophic capillary vessels are seen to form an anastomosing network in the dermis (H & E, ×140).

B, Focally this lesion is so cellular that the capillary lumen can be recognized only with great difficulty (right upper corner) (H & E, ×140).

may be pronounced hypertrophy of soft parts, bones, and parenchymal organs in the regions affected. A form of angiomatosis is frequently referred to as "blue-rubber-bleb nevus syndrome," a term introduced by Bean in 1955 and used by Rice and Fischer in 1962.

In some cases systemic angiomatosis is part of a basic embryonal maldevelopment which involves several organ systems, e.g., the *central nervous system* (ataxia-telangiectasia, Sturge-Weber or encephalotrigeminal angiomatosis and Lindau-von Hippel's disease or hemangiomatosis of the retina and cerebellum) and the *skeletal system* in the form of dyschondroplasia (Maffucci's syndrome) (Maffucci, 1881; Kuzman and King, 1948; Bean, 1955; Kings, 1975). Some of these lesions, analogous to the hypertrophic hemangiomas, undergo regression when the patients are getting older.

The treatment of hemangiomas ranges from ligation and occlusion to cryosurgery according to the nature and location of the lesion. Surgeons report that most hemangiomas bleed when incised or traumatized, but surgical removal with clean margins is almost a bloodless operation.

ANGIOFIBROMA*

Angiofibroma rarely occurs in any other site than the nasopharynx. It is a *benign neoplasm composed of angiomatous vessels in a fibromyxoid stroma.* It occurs almost exclusively in boys and may regress spontaneously after puberty.

According to medical historians, Hippocrates first described the "hard nasal polyp" and the name *juvenile nasopharyngeal fibroma* was coined by Chaveau in 1906. Jaques (1911), Denker (1912), and Delevan (1915) reported on the site of origin and the best modality of treatment including irradiation therapy. The first large series of 29 cases was reported by Martin et al in 1948. Sternberg, in 1954, summarized the experience with these lesions at Memorial Sloan-Kettering Cancer Center.

Nasopharyngeal angiofibroma has been the subject of numerous reports, among which the most notable ones are the summary of the invasive angiofibromas by English et al (1972); the review article, based on 120 cases, by Neel et al (1973); and the ultrastructural studies by Svoboda and Kirchner (1966) and Taxy (1977).

The signs and symptoms of nasopharyngeal angiofibroma are nasal obstruction, recurrent epistaxis, and deformity of the face. Grossly, most of the tumors appear encapsulated and covered by the nasal mucosa. On close examination, however, the majority of tumors are seen to invade adjacent structures, most commonly the maxillary sinus. The precise site of origin cannot be determined in the majority of cases, but Neel et al (1973) felt that "the specific point of origin is on the posterior lateral wall of the roof of the nose, where the sphenoidal process of the palatine bone meets the horizontal ala of the vomer bone and the root of the pterygoid process of the sphenoid bone." Although some tumors undergo spontaneous regression, others are aggressive, have a tendency to recur, and not uncommonly invade the middle cranial fossa.

Microscopically, angiofibroma is composed of a rich angiomatous network of blood vessels of varying sizes. The vascular channels are lined by a single layer of endothelial cells, slender smooth muscle cells, and scattering pericytes. The stroma is mostly composed of collagen fibrils, fibroblasts, and inflammatory cells such as histiocytes, plasma cells, and mast cells. Although most of the tumors are collagenous, it is not uncommon to find loosely arranged myxoid areas (Fig. 6-11).

English et al, in 1972, summarized various modalities of treatment and stated that cryosurgery combined with surgical excision proved to be the most satisfactory method of therapy. Biller (1978) reported that irradiation as the primary

* *Synonyms and related terms:* fibroma, hemangiofibroma, juvenile nasopharyngeal angiofibroma, juvenile angiofibroma.

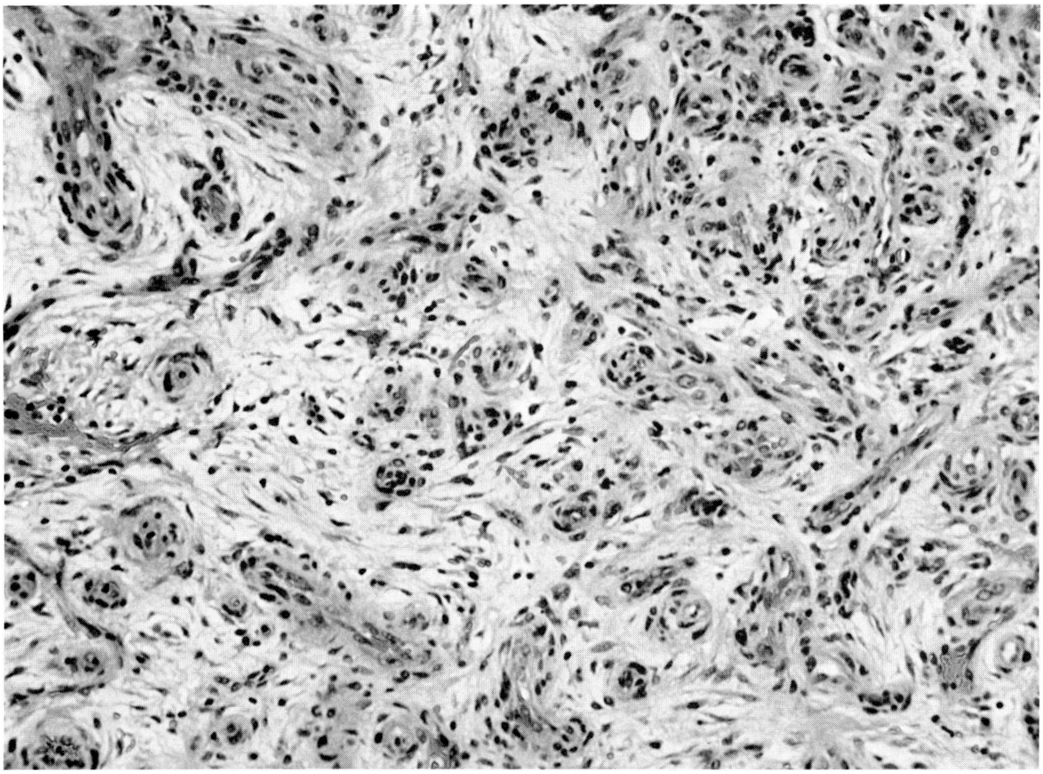

Figure 6-11. Angiofibroma.

Tightly packed conglomerate of small and medium-sized blood vessels in partly myxoid and partly collagenous fibrous stroma. The endothelial cells are flattened and somewhat compressed by the proliferating smooth muscle cells and pericytes (H & E, ×140).

treatment modality is contraindicated except in selected cases.

ANGIOLIPOMA

(See Chapter 4.)

ANGIOMYOLIPOMA

(See Chapter 4.)

LEIOMYOSARCOMA

(See Chapter 5.)

GLOMUS TUMOR*

Glomus tumor is closely related to hemangiopericytoma, angiomyoma and leiomyosarcoma of blood vessels. *It is a benign uncommon neoplasm of the skin and submucosal tissues arising from the so-called glomic end-organs or anastomosing arteriovenous capillaries.* Kolaczek, in 1878, is credited with the first description of such a tumor occurring subungually in the great toe. He erroneously called the tumor "Angio-Sarkom." Chandelux, in 1882, reported two cases of painful subcutaneous tumors he believed to be adnexal skin lesions. Masson, in 1919, conceived the idea that these lesions are bizarre arteriovenous anastomosis. The two articles by Barre and Masson and by Masson in 1924 are the first ones in which the name *glomus tumor* (tumeur du glomus neuromyoarteriel) appeared.

Glomus tumors are usually solitary, but according to reports they are multiple in 5 to 10% of the cases (Tannovski and Hashimoto, 1969; Goodman and Abele, 1971). There is no sex predilection, and they occur most commonly in persons between

* *Synonyms and related terms:* glomangioma, benign hemangiopericytoma, angioneuroma, benign pericytic tumor, angioneuromyoma, neuromyoarterial tumor.

20 and 40 years of age (Kobut and Stout, 1961). Glomus tumors may appear anywhere in the body, but the majority of the lesions are limited to the extremities, particularly to the nail bed and fingertips (Gupta et al, 1965; Goodman and Abele, 1971).

The size of glomus tumors usually ranges from a few millimeters to a couple of centimeters. Surgical excision is considered curative. Glomus tumors have no tendency to recur and no malignant transformation has been recorded.

Histologically, glomus tumor is an exuberant form of the normal glomus body (Fig. 6-12) with hyperplasia of thick-walled capillary vessels, glomus cells, and nonmyelinated nerve fibers. The glomus cells are usually arranged in cell cords or sheets about vascular spaces and blood vessels (Fine and Morales, 1973). Cytologically, they are uniform round or oval cells with well-formed granular cytoplasms and finely granular nuclear chromatin and rarely do they assume spindle shapes. In tissue culture Murray and Stout (1942) have identified the glomus cells as pericytes (Fig. 6-13).

Recent ultrastructural studies indicate that glomus cells resemble modified smooth muscle cells in that they possess intracytoplasmic myofilaments, pinocytotic vesicles, fusiform condensation, and attachment bodies (Toker, 1969; Tannovski and Hashimoto, 1969; Venkatachalam and Greally, 1969). Like smooth muscle cells, they are enveloped by basement membrane. Myofibrils within glomus cells were first suggested by Masson in 1924.

Although the ultrastructural resemblance of glomus cells to smooth muscle cells of muscular arteries is striking, one cannot overlook the fact that pericytes are multipotential cells and also have features of smooth muscle cells. It seems that the resemblance or phenotypic similarity of glomus cells to abortive smooth muscle cells does not exclude their origin from pericytes and as a fact it is quite possible that the histogenesis of both cells, glomus cells and pericytes, is the same.

HEMANGIOPERICYTOMA*

Rouget, in 1874, was the first to notice pericytes while studying the histology of the cat's eye, and for a while these cells were referred to as Rouget cells. The term *pericyte* was coined by Zimmerman in 1923. After studying pericytes in various animals and describing their histologic appearance, he proposed that pericytes are of smooth muscle origin. He said pericytes are small oval cells with branching cytoplasmic processes which encircle the capillaries "like a hand with slightly spread fingers which is gripping the other arm." Thus, it is not surprising that ultrastructural studies, 50 years later, disclosed the presence of myofilaments in certain pericytes. Schmidt (1937), using the term *gemmangioma* introduced by Orsos in 1934, reported a series of peculiar vascular tumors which should be distinguished from angiosarcoma and gave the first good description of hemangiopericytoma.

Although Stout and Murray first used the term and reported 9 cases in 1942, hemangiopericytoma was accepted as an entity only after Stout's second article in 1949. According to Stout and Murray (1942), "Hemangiopericytomas are composed of capillary blood vessels with one or more layers of rounded cells arranged about them, which cannot be called glomus tumors because they lack the organoid features of these encapsulated complex neoplasms, yet differ from simple capillary hemangiomata because of the presence of their perivascular cells." They added, ". . . the relationship between pericyte and smooth muscle cell is strongly suggested because the cells arranged about the tumor vessels vary all the way from the usual rounded pericyte through an intermediate phase of spindle shapes to a fully differentiated cell with myofibrils."

Aschoff was among the first to propose that pericytes should be considered multi-

* *Synonyms and related terms:* hemangioendothelioma, gemmangioma, perithelioma, juvenile hemangiopericytoma.

potential cells rather than smooth muscle cells. Today, all available evidence, especially that deduced from electron microscopic studies (Murad et al, 1968; Kuhn and Rosai, 1969; Bommer et al, 1976; Eiomoto, 1977; Waldo et al, 1977; Angervall et al, 1978) supports the theory, directly or indirectly, that *hemangiopericytes, like Schwann cells and primitive fibrous histiocytic cells, are multipotential cells and can be precursors of other cells such as smooth muscle cells, endothelial cells, rhabdomyoblasts, and fibroblasts.* It also supplies definite proof that the cell of origin of hemangiopericytomas is the pericyte. Murad et al (1968) should be credited with the first concise ultrastructural study of hemangiopericytomas, but they were also the first to point out that while glomus tumor cells resemble vascular smooth muscle cells, hemangiopericytomas are clearly composed of pericytes. The functional role of pericytes is not clear, but it has been postulated that because of their contractile powers they control the caliber of the vessels. The theory that pericytes are the constituents of two tumors, hemangiopericytoma and glomus tumor, is not held anymore.

Hemangiopericytoma is a rare tumor and is likely to exhibit a malignant clinical course. It may occur at any age but most commonly is found during the fourth and fifth decades. It may arise in almost any part of the body, but the most common sites are the lower extremities, the retroperitoneum, and the trunk. There is no apparent sex predilection, but it is felt that female patients tend to be somewhat older than the male patients. Hemangiopericytomas possess no particular gross appearance, except for their vascular appearance. Although they are usually small, they may attain considerable size, up to a dozen or more centimeters.

The *histologic appearance* of hemangiopericytomas is summarized by Stout and Murray (1942): "The tumor must be composed of groups of endothelial-lined tubes or impervious endothelial sprouts surrounded by round cells with a supporting network of reticulin fibers. The rounded cells may show a tendency to become elongated and in this form poorly defined myofibrils may be found. Usually, the vessels with their pericytes are distinct one from the other, separated by a fibrous stroma, but they may become so closely packed that the pericytes of one vessel may be in continuity with those of its neighbors." They gave a warning by saying: "One should be very certain, however, that the growth is basically vascular and not a tumor whose cells are nourished by a rich vascular network such as one sees in many tumors of endocrine organs, in some Ewing tumors of bone marrow, and elsewhere."

The fine structure of tumor cells of hemangiopericytoma is similar to that of fibroblasts. Unlike fibroblasts, neoplastic hemangiopericytes possess a basement membrane, occasional pinocytotic vesicles, and fine cytoplasmic filaments (Figs. 6-14, 6-15).

The ways and means of distinguishing so-called benign and malignant hemangiopericytomas are debated in the literature. According to Enzinger and Smith (1976) benign and malignant forms can be distinguished microscopically and "benign hemangiopericytomas outnumber malignant hemangiopericytomas by a sizeable margin and can be recognized by their lack of cellularity, their low mitotic rate and the absence of necrosis and hemorrhage." They also concluded that the so-called congenital or infantile hemangiopericytoma is a definite entity invariably having a benign prognosis.

My personal experience and the experience of others are in variance with the preceding view. Although microscopic appearance is important and without doubt borderline tumors exist, size, location, and resectability of hemangiopericytoma are factors that should be considered with more weight than the histologic appearance. This perhaps explains why most malignant forms occur in locations

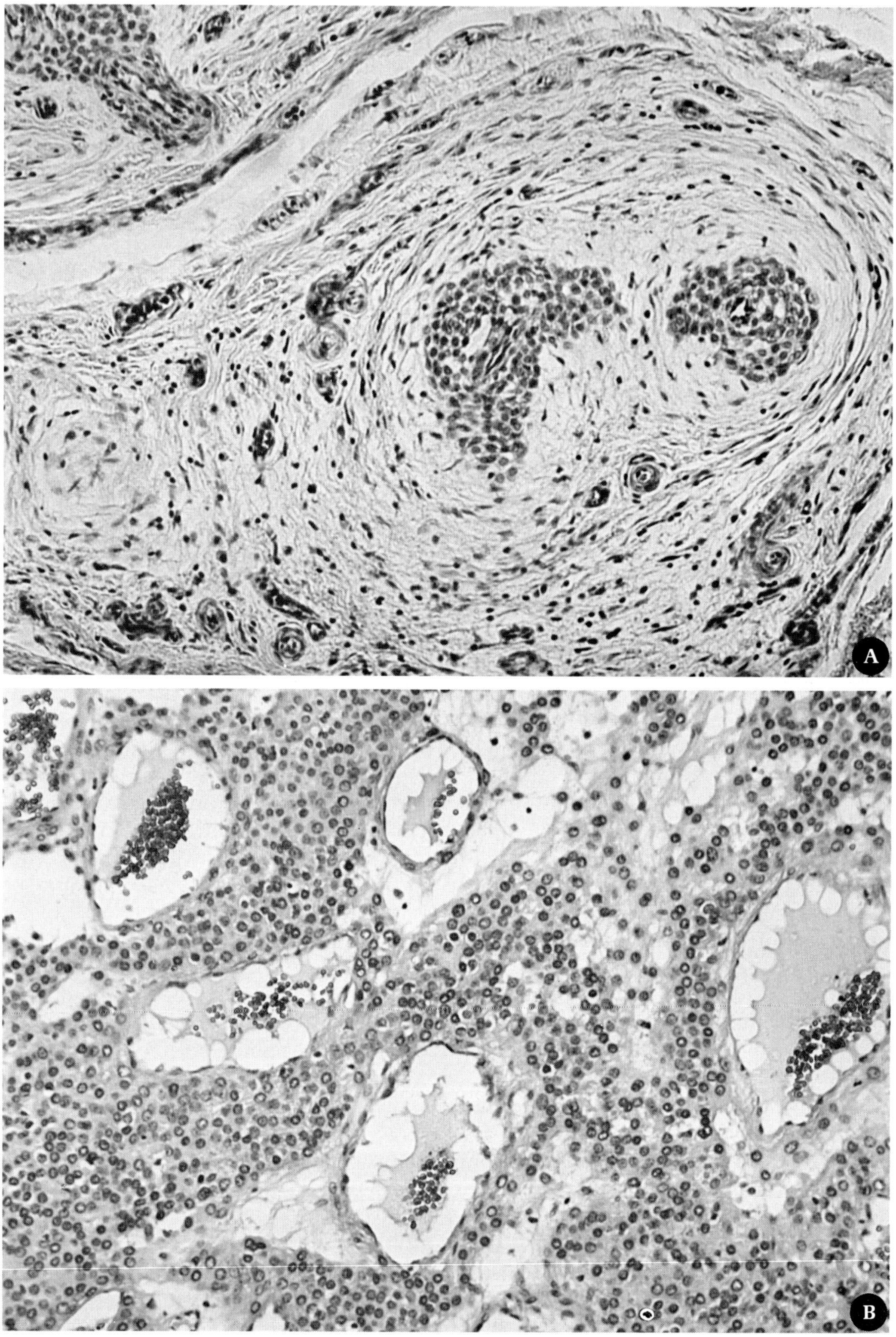

Figure 6-12. A, So-called sacrococcygeal glomus or Luschka's gland (H & E, ×85).

B, Glomus tumor of the tip of a finger. The tumor is composed of dilated capillary vessels which are lined by flat, stretched-out endothelial cells and have thin muscular coats and numerous piled-up glomus cells. Glomus cells have uniform round nuclei and branching ill-defined cytoplasms. They are arranged in cords which follow the contour of the blood vessels or aggregate in patterned sheets (H & E, ×140).

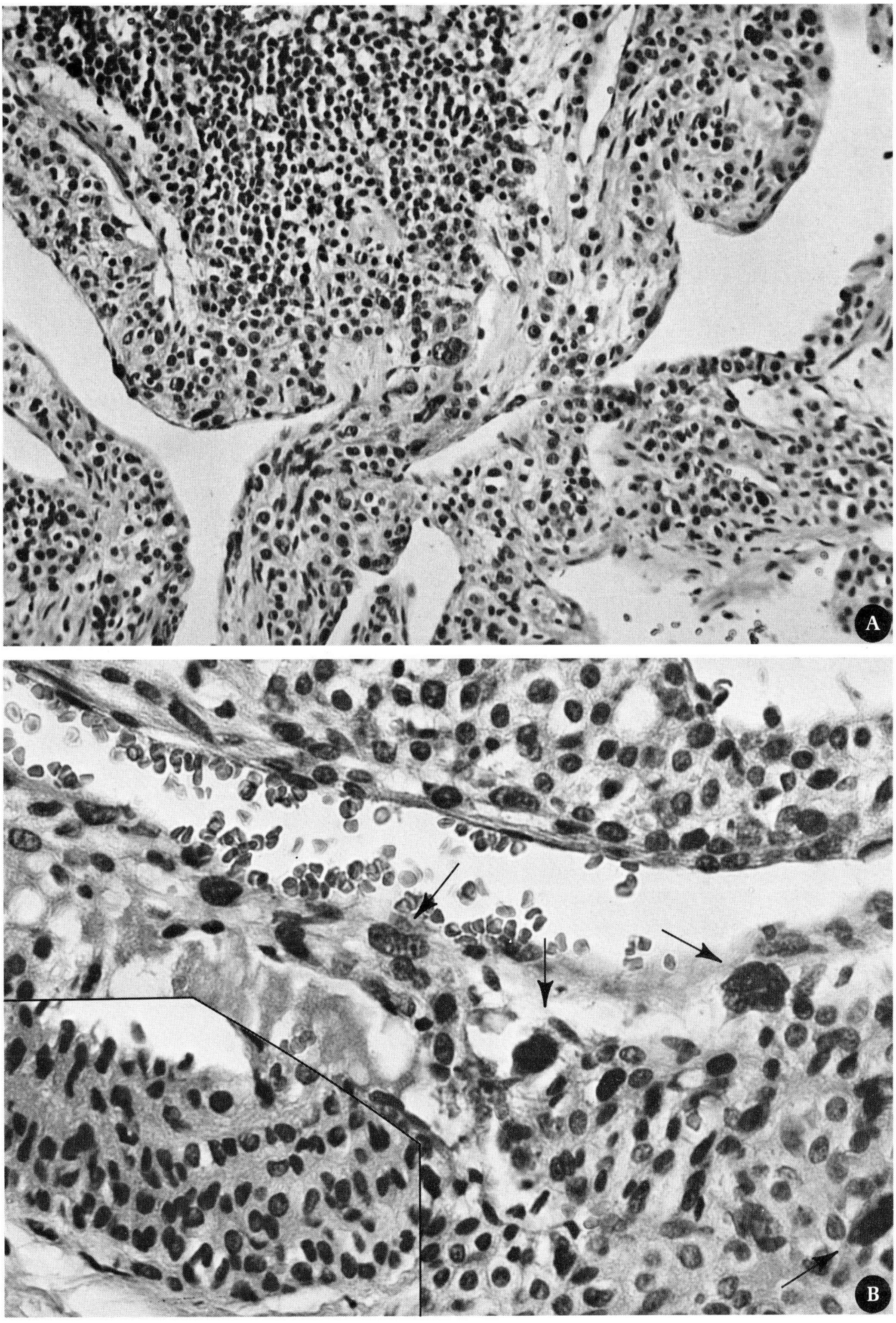

Figure 6-13. Atypical glomus tumor of the foot.

There is a distinct perivascular linear arrangement of mostly round and uniform glomus cells, but a few cells are displaced a certain distance from the vessel wall and others assume bizarre pleomorphic or fused nuclear forms (see arrows).

The basic units of glomus tumor, however, even in atypical tumors, is the multilayered uniform glomus cells (**A,** H & E, ×140; **B,** H & E, ×350; inset, ×350).

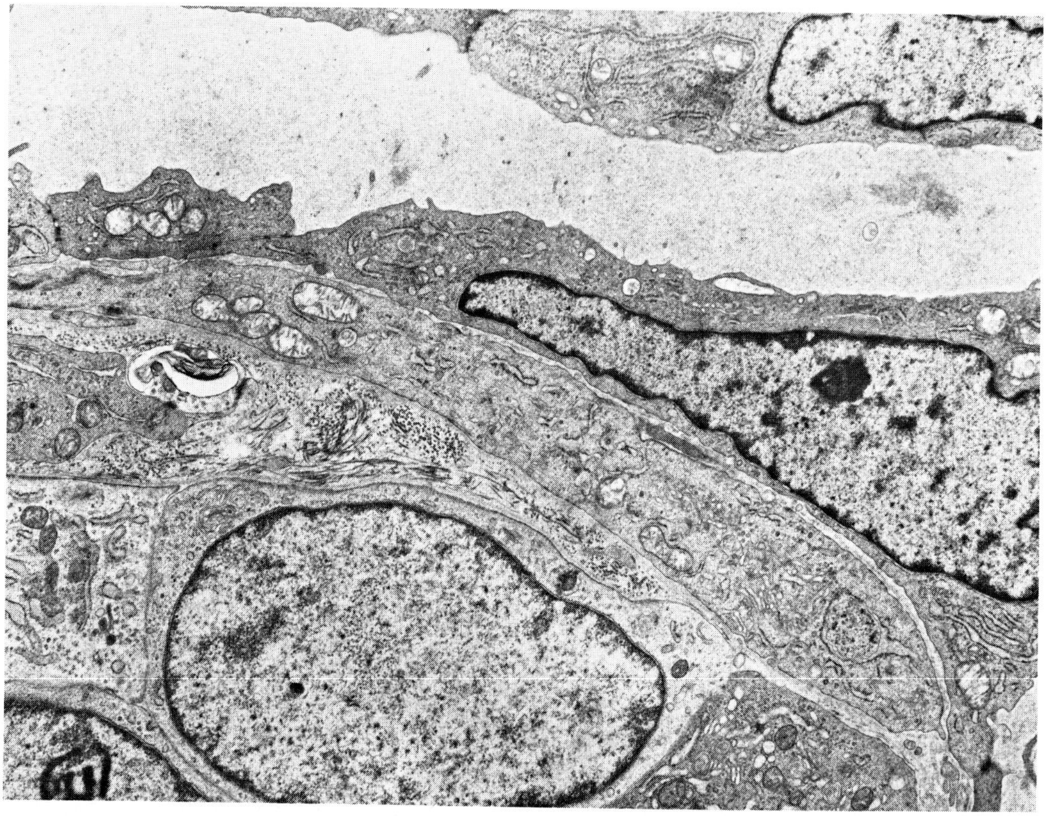

Figure 6-14. Hemangiopericytoma.
A capillary vessel is surrounded by neoplastic pericytes. Note the thin, discontinuous basal lamina surrounding the neoplastic pericytes (×8,000).

where complete extirpation cannot be accomplished. Stout reported his observations in 1942, 1949, and 1953 and repeatedly stated the difficulty in developing histologic criteria for malignancy of hemangiopericytomas. He added that the presence or absence of mitotic figures and of anything short of complete cellular anaplasia was not helpful in arriving at a diagnosis of malignancy. Purely on the basis of histomorphology, all hemangiopericytomas should be considered potentially malignant, analogous to carcinoid tumors or granulosa cell tumors, and the prognosis for each tumor should be based on size, location, and histologic grade of the tumor and age of the patient (Figs. 6-16, 6-17). (See also Figure 1-59 and Table 1-15.)

At least 400 examples of hemangiopericytoma have been reported in the literature (Table 6-4). Most hemangiopericytomas occurring in children are included in reports discussing tumors of adults. However, Kauffman and Stout, in two separate reports in 1960 and 1961, reviewed their experience with these tumors in pediatric patients and concluded that the presence of numerous mitotic figures and a high degree of anaplasia usually indicate a malignant course. The absence of these histologic features did not necessarily indicate a benign clinical course. Hollmann et al (1971) reviewed 276 cases of hemangiopericytomas from the literature, which included 65 tumors in children, and stated that the rate of malignancy for children (50%) was higher than that for adults.

No organ or region of the body is exempt from hemangiopericytoma. Primary *pulmonary hemangiopericytomas* were reported by Oshner and DeCamp (1958); Davis et al (1972); Meade et al (1974) and

Krishan et al (1975). Meade in 1974 reported 28 cases and stated that the mortality of female patients was 25%, whereas 66% of the males succumbed to the disease. Grode, in 1972, reported that only 2 of his 6 patients with hemangiopericytoma involving the *central nervous system* were alive without evidence of the tumor. Goellner et al (1978) reported their experience with 26 cases of hemangiopericytoma of the *meninges* and stated that 80% of the tumors recurred and 23% metastasized; only 3 patients were alive without evidence of the disease. Silverberg et al (1971) studied a *uterine primary hemangiopericytoma* with the electron microscope. Wilbanks et al described four *pelvic hemangiopericytomas* in a literature review in 1975.

There is general agreement in the literature that partial excision of hemangiopericytoma almost invariably results in recurrence. In reference to rate of metastasis, again there is general agreement, and the rate is given as 50% (Table 6-4).

All authors agree that the primary treatment of hemangiopericytoma should be surgical resection with a clean margin. Mira et al (1977) reported long-term (on the average 27 months) local control of the disease by radiation therapy in 11 patients and proposed that surgical excision should be combined with wide-field, high dose radiation therapy. Even in advanced cases, palliative irradiation is worthwhile. Bredt and Serpick (1969) reported a temporary response with actinomycin D and vincristine; however, most authors agree that, despite the diversity of chemotherapeutic agents used, no sustained objective

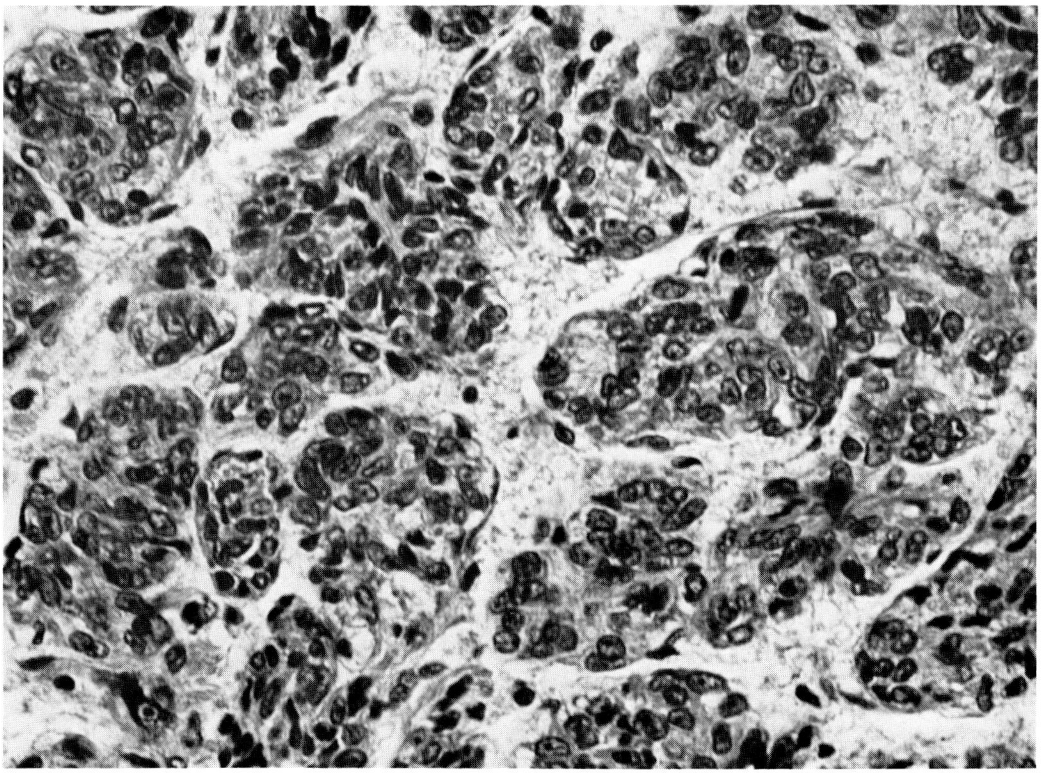

Figure 6-15. Hemangiopericytoma.

This is the type of hemangiopericytoma commonly referred to as benign, atypical, or borderline hemangiopericytoma. There is a distinct clustering of capillary vessels and neoplastic pericytes. These discrete units, vessels, and their hyperplastic coats are segregated by myxofibrillary stroma which gives a pseudoglandular appearance to the tumor (H & E, ×350).

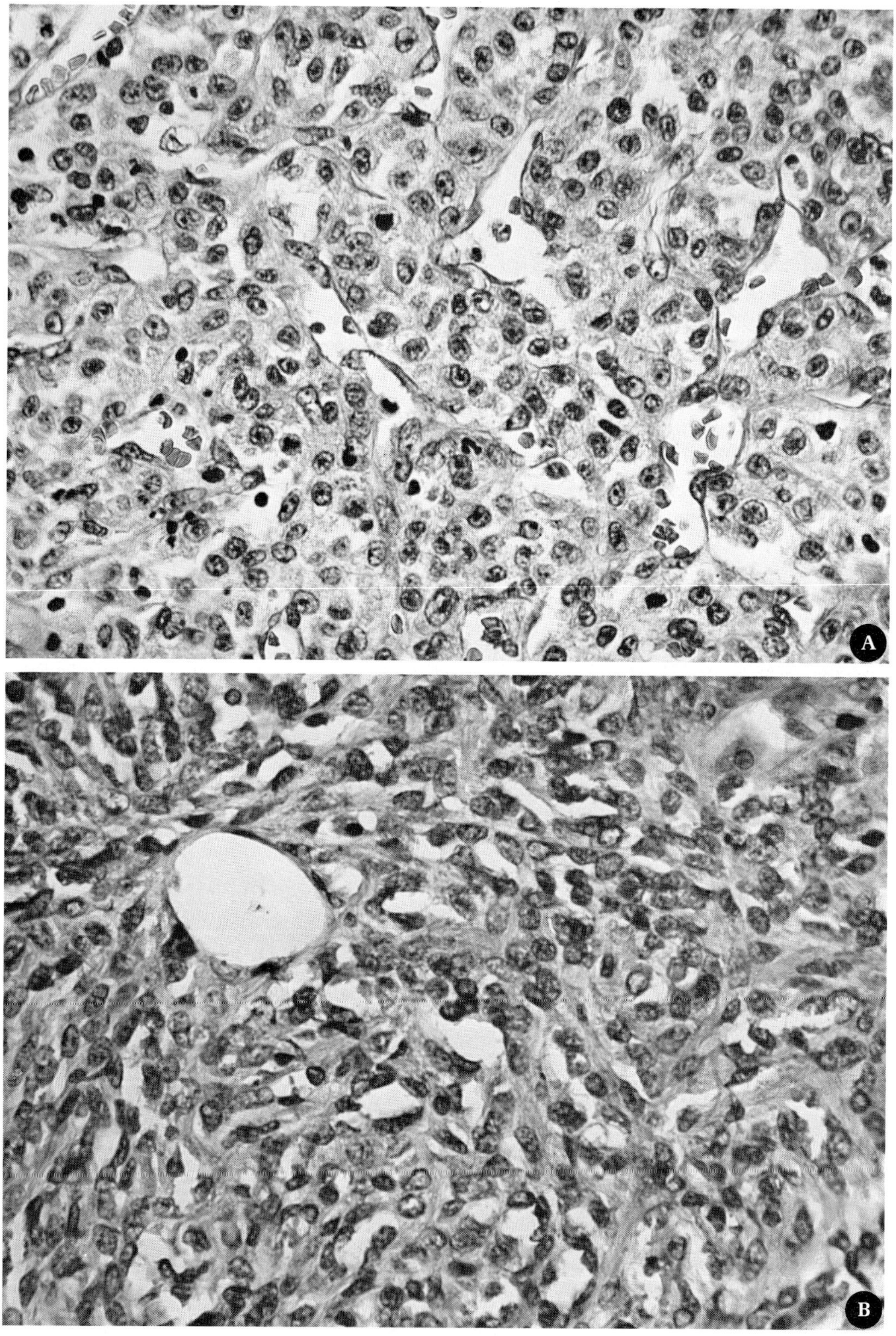

Figure 6-16. A, Hemangiopericytoma. Empty capillary lumen in a compact sea of uniform neoplastic pericytes. Note the direct contact between endothelial cells and pericytes. Monotonous perivascular arrangements and sparsity of mitotic figures are characteristics of this tumor (H & E, ×350).

B, This hemangiopericytoma consists of round as well as oval-shaped pericytes. Note the numerous small capillary lumens and somewhat disarranged distribution of the neoplastic pericytes (H & E, ×350).

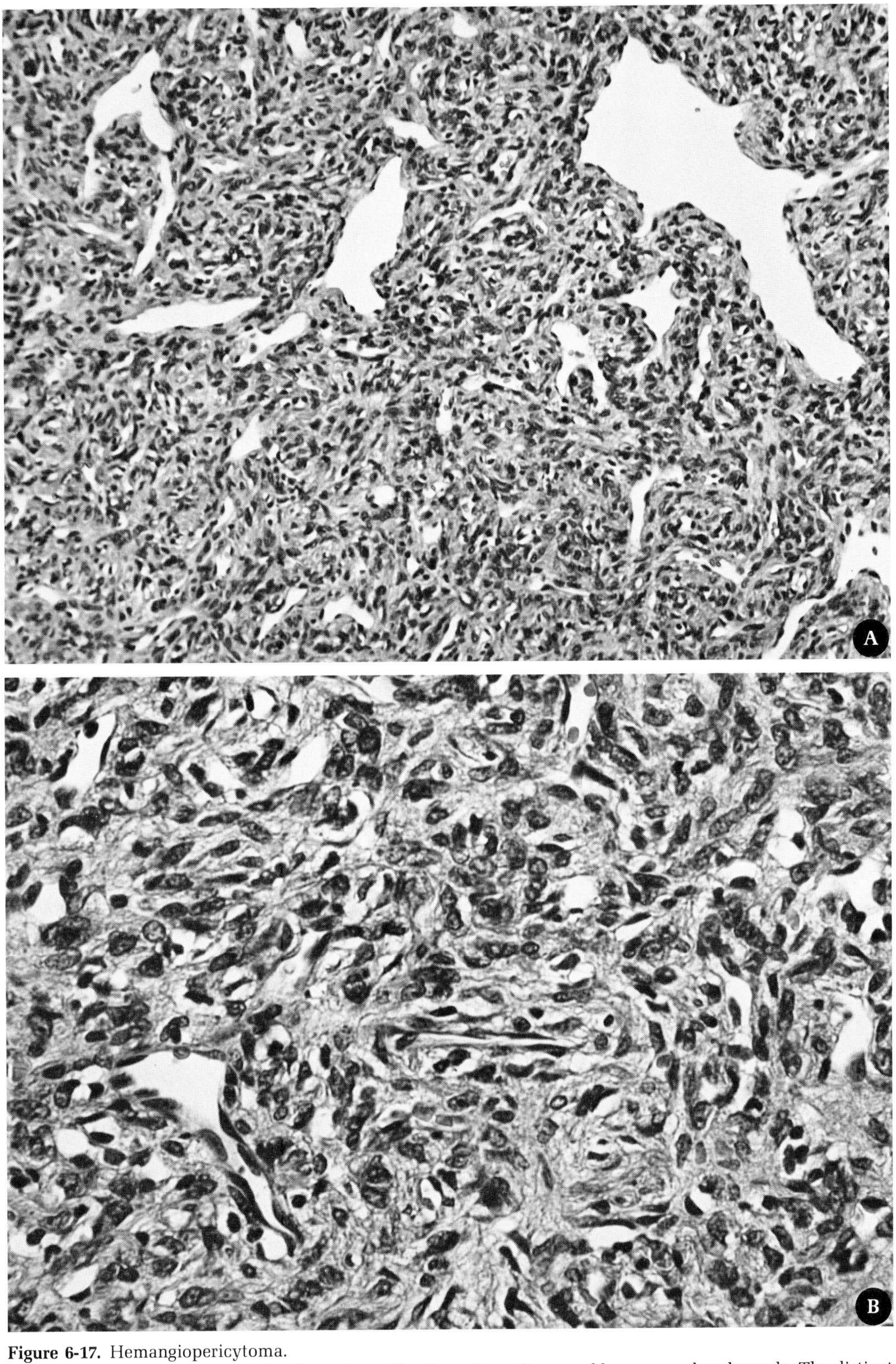

Figure 6-17. Hemangiopericytoma.

A, Hemangiopericytoma arising from the walls of small, medium, and large vascular channels. The distinct vascular lumina are not obstructed, and the crowding of neoplastic cells is strictly outside of the vessels' walls (H & E, ×140).

B, Hemangiopericytoma, predominantly composed of spindle and oval cells. Crowding of neoplastic pericytes and occasional bizarre and distorted pericytes characterizes this tumor (H & E, ×350).

TABLE 6-4. *Series of Hemangiopericytoma*

	NO. OF CASES WITH FOLLOW-UP	MOST COMMON SITES	RECURRENCE %	METASTASIS %	MORTALITY %
Stout and Murray (1942)	4	—	50	25	25
Stout (1949)	14	Retroperitoneum Trunk	28	35	43
O'Brien and Brasfield (1965)	23	Trunk Extremities	—	48	48
Gerner et al (1974)	13	Thigh Retroperitoneum	4	50	46
McMaster et al (1975)	60	Thigh Retroperitoneum	22	50	60
Enzinger and Smith (1976)	93	Lower extremities Retroperitoneum	—	—	30
Hajdu (personal experience)	64	Lower extremities	29	47	52

response was observed in any of the studies.

Without doubt, many soft tissue sarcomas which are rich in blood vessels are mistakenly classified as hemangiopericytoma. However, if one adheres to the histologic criteria described by Stout in 1942 and again in 1949, the diagnostic problems should be minimal. Among the tumors that may resemble hemangiopericytoma are tendosynovial sarcomas, fibrous histiocytomas, leiomyoblastoma, primitive neuroectodermal tumor, and mesenchymal chondrosarcoma.

Tendosynovial sarcomas, especially the monophasic type, can be extremely vascular. However, the slender and monomorphic spindle cells and the synovial clefts are characteristic features of tendosynovial sarcomas that distinguish them from hemangiopericytomas (see Chapter 3).

Fibrous histiocytomas, especially the fibroblastic types, may show prominent vascular patterns. However, the typical storiform or cartwheel patterns with occluded small capillary vessels rarely resemble the open and branching capillary spaces of hemangiopericytoma (see Chapter 2).

Leiomyoblastoma may show striking similarity to hemangiopericytoma microscopically, but the tumor cells in leiomyoblastoma are usually plump oval or round cells with well-defined nuclear and cytoplasmic membranes (see Chapter 5).

Primitive neuroectodermal tumor due to its primitive nature and mixed neuroectodermal and mesenchymal elements may mimic hemangiopericytoma. However, it is less vascular, less arranged, and more cellular than hemangiopericytoma (see Chapter 7).

Mesenchymal chondrosarcoma should not cause differential diagnostic problems if the tumor is adequately sampled, since the admixture of cellular myxoid, chondroid, and round cell elements in alveolar or lobular patterns is not a feature of hemangiopericytoma (see Chapter 8).

HEMANGIOSARCOMA*

In spite of the fact that blood vessels are ubiquitous, and benign vascular tumors are common, malignant tumors of blood vessels are exceedingly rare. One of the most fulminating malignant vascular tumors is the so-called angiosarcoma, properly called hemangiosarcoma. It is a disease of adults and affects males as well as females. Most of the hemangiosarcomas are deeply seated and bulky lesions, but it is not uncommon to see subcutaneous or submucosal distribution, especially in the head and neck regions (Figs. 6-18, 6-19, 6-20, color).

Kolaczek, in 1878, is credited with first using the term *Angio-Sarkom*. However, it is open to question whether the lesion he described was truly an angiosarcoma or a glomus tumor. Undoubtedly, the term *fungus haematodes* in Hey's book, *Practical Observation in Surgery,* published in 1803, meant, among other things, hemangiosarcoma. The first recorded instance of a metastatic angiomatous growth was that of Langhans in 1879. He reported a man 30 years old with multiple vascular tumors of the spleen and liver and regarded the hepatic lesions as metastases from the spleen.

The literature on the subject of hemangiosarcoma is confusing because hypertrophic hemangiomas, hemangioblastoma, arteriovenous malformations, multiple angiomatoid malformations, and so-called metastatic hemangioma have been included erroneously in this category (Shennan, 1914; Sherill and Graves, 1915; Wright, 1928; Robinson and Castleman, 1936). In a 1943 summary of his experience with 18 cases, Stout adopted the term *hemangioendothelioma,* devised by Mallory in 1908, and pointed out that he had "not been able to find any case which offers incontrovertible proof of the existence of such an anomaly as a benign metastasizing hemangioma." After reviewing the case reported by Robinson and Castleman, in 1936, as benign

**Synonyms and related terms:* angiosarcoma, malignant angioendothelioma, angiomyosarcoma, malignant metastasizing angioma, capillary angiosarcoma, hemangioendothelioma, hemangioendothelioblastoma, hemangioendotheliosarcoma, Kupffer cell sarcoma, angioplastic sarcoma, hemangioblastoma, malignant angioendotheliomatosis proliferans, malignant endovascular papillary angioendothelioma.

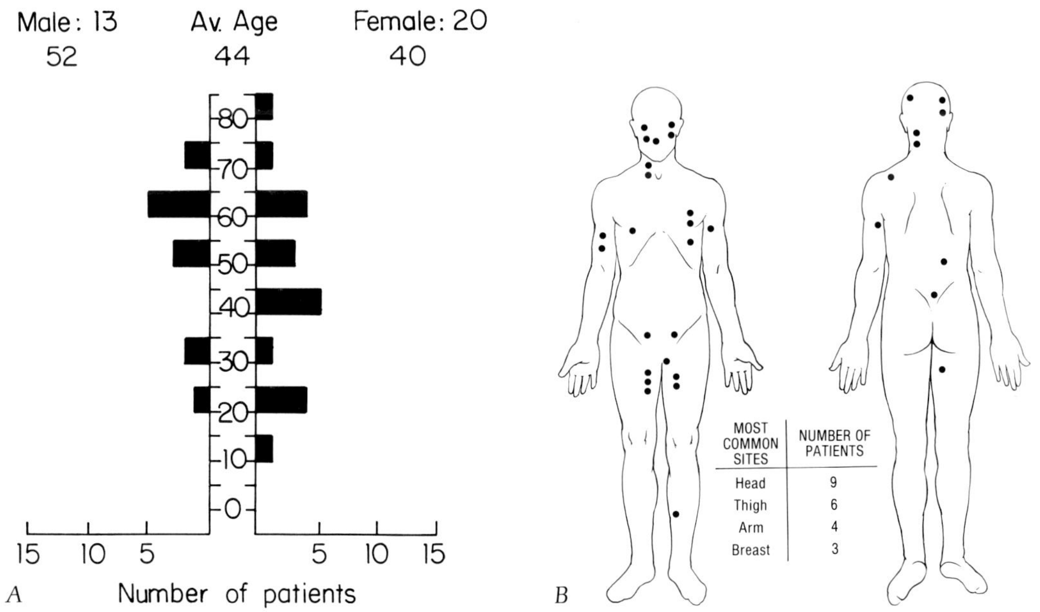

Figure 6-18. A, Age and sex distribution of 33 patients treated at Memorial Sloan-Kettering Cancer Center for hemangiosarcoma.

B, Anatomic sites of 33 hemangiosarcomas.

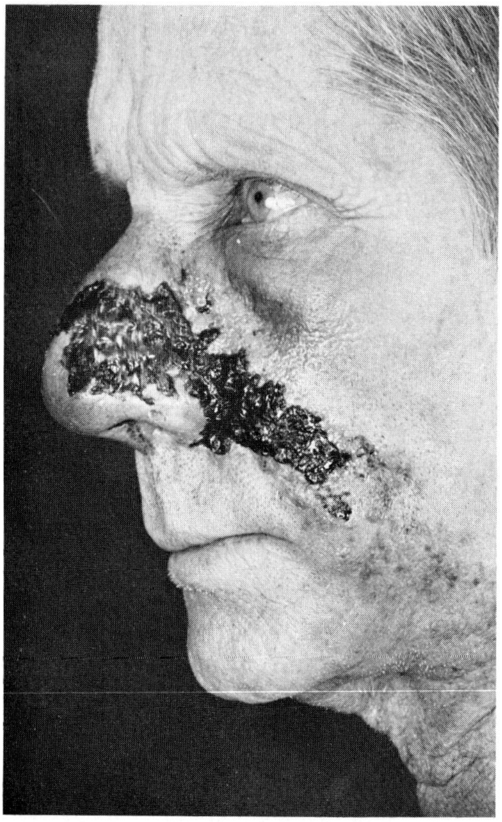

Figure 6-19. This 64-year-old male died, with disseminated hemangiosarcoma, less than 2 years after surgical and other attempts failed to control this fast-spreading subcutaneous hemangiosarcoma.

metastasizing hemangioma, Stout (1943) said that the tumor "shows features which lead me to classify it as hemangioendothelioma and not simple benign hemangioma."

Kinkade (1949) reviewed the literature from 1934 to 1949 and called attention to the highly aggressive nature of the tumors he called angiosarcoma. He found that 45% of the tumors metastasized to regional lymph nodes and advanced the idea of regional node dissection for local control of the disease.

Grossly, hemangiosarcomas usually are solitary, firm, bulky tumors situated deep in soft tissues with hemorrhagic and cystic appearances.

Stout (1943), employing reticulin stain for microscopic studies of hemangiosarcomas, gave a classic description of hemangiosarcoma. He observed "first the formation of atypical endothelial cells in greater numbers than are required to line the vessels with a simple endothelial membrane, and second the formation of vascular tubes with a delicate framework of reticulin fibers and a marked tendency for their lumens to anastomose." The individual cells may appear polygonal, round, or fusiform. They may form several linings in well-formed vascular channels or appear in lumenless clusters, cell cords, or pseudorosettes.

Admittedly, the prognosis for hemangiosarcomas is dictated by their size and location rather than by their degree of differentiation (Table 6-5). In almost any of these tumors one can recognize a spectrum of microscopic changes ranging from a well-*differentiated angiomatous pattern to a poorly differentiated solid pattern* (Figs. 6-21, 6-22).

Because of the various morphologic patterns and bizarre cytomorphology of individual cells, hemangiosarcoma can be confused with other neoplasms (Fig. 6-23; Table 6-6). For differential diagnosis one may have to depend on the ultrastructural appearance of the tumor cells. Well-differentiated hemangiosarcomas have a number of features common with normal vessels. The tumor cells possess distinctive basal laminae, and there are numerous junctional complexes between adjacent cells. Moderate numbers of pinocytotic vesicles and fine filaments make the cytoplasms distinct. Occasionally, rod-shaped bodies, *Weibel-Palade bodies* (Fig. 6-1), with parallel striations similar to those in endothelial cells are found. It is disappointing, however, that these and other ultrastructural features are either partially or completely absent in hemangiosarcomas with spindle cell and undifferentiated patterns (Rosai et al, 1976; Waldo et al, 1977) (Fig. 6-24).

Hemangiosarcomas are the subject of numerous case reports and usually are reported under titles specifying anatomic sites or organs. Superficial hemangiosarcomas of the *head and neck* regions

TABLE 6-5. *Hemangiosarcoma*

	NO. OF CASES	MALE	FEMALE	MOST COMMON SITES	METASTASIS %	MORTALITY %
Stout (1943)	18	7	11	Skin	—	62
McCarthy and Pack (1950)	20	11	9	Subcutaneous tissue	45*	83
Hajdu (personal experience)	33	13	20	Head and thigh	81	79
Rosai et al (1976)	10	7	3	Skin of head and neck	50	—

*Metastasis to lymph node.

are known to be the disease of elderly males. They are commonly multifocal and appear clinically like hemorrhagic blisters. Because of their superficial, dermal location they are usually treated by surgical excision. About 75% of these tumors recur and roughly one third metastasize, usually to neck nodes and lung, and have a rapid progression usually less than 2 or 3 years (Caro and Stubenrauch, 1945; Reed et al, 1966; Farr et al, 1970; Nagashima et al, 1975; Rosai et al, 1976) (Fig. 6-25).

Bricklin and Rushton (1977) reported an angiosarcoma arising in a vein within the *radial nerve* and believed to be the second such case. So-called primary *endovascular angiosarcomas* must be considered rare, and without doubt most of the reported cases are papillary endothelial hyperplasia rather than sarcomas.

TABLE 6-6. *Microscopic Patterns of Growth of Hemangiosarcomas*

MICROSCOPIC PATTERNS		
WELL-DIFFERENTIATED ANGIOMATOUS	METAPLASTIC SPINDLE CELL	UNDIFFERENTIATED SOLID
Dilated vessels	Vascular slits	Lumenless clusters
Anastomosing sinusoids	Sheets	Cell cords
Hypertrophic endothelial cells	Elongated tumor cells	Polygonal tumor cells
Large nuclei	Slender nuclei	Prominent nuclei
Abundant cytoplasm	Small cytoplasm	Large cytoplasm
Giant cells	Blending into neighboring tissues	Cytoplasmic vacuoles
Intraluminal protrusions	RBC in stroma	Giant cells
RBC in lumens and stroma	Infiltrative and branching	Multicentric and infiltrative
Multicentric	No particular pattern with reticulin stain	No special pattern with reticulin stain
Tumor cells on luminal side with reticulin stain		
Differential Diagnosis	*Differential Diagnosis*	*Differential Diagnosis*
Hypertrophic hemangioma	Kaposi's sarcoma	Epithelioid sarcoma
A-V malformation	Monophasic tendosynovial sarcoma	Lymphangiosarcoma
Adenocarcinoma	Neurogenic sarcoma	Adenocarcinoma
Malignant melanoma	Spindle cell melanoma	Histiocytic lymphoma

Figure 6-20. A, Kaposi's sarcoma is a low-grade malignant neoplasm histologically and usually has a protracted clinical course.

It is composed of minute neoplastic capillary vessels, sheets of tightly packed oval or spindle cells, and extravasated red blood cells. The lumina of the capillary vessels are either obliterated or compressed by proliferating neoplastic endothelial cells. The cytoplasms and cytoplasmic processes are ill-defined. As it is seen in the left upper corner, solid nests of oval and spindle cells may dominate the field. In such a setting the only clue to the true identity of this neoplasm is the extravasated red blood cells (H & E, ×140).

B, Hemangiosarcoma of the breast. This is a high-grade malignant neoplasm. It is composed of branching and tortuous blood vessels lined by hypertrophic endothelial cells. The size of the blood vessels may vary from virtually lumenless cell clusters to dilated cavernous channels. In the lumen of the blood vessels red blood cells and detached endothelial cells are visible. The neoplastic capillary vessels are held together by a cellular network of reticular spindle cells. In this photograph there is only a solitary cluster of tubular or lobular epithelial cells, a remnant of mammary tissue, at the left upper corner (H & E, ×140).

C, Hemangiosarcoma. Histologically this neoplasm is a fully malignant lesion. The entire field is dominated by neoplastic blood vessels and an intricate network of slits and spaces lined by prominent cuboidal or polygonal endothelial cells. The cohesive linear arrangement of the neoplastic endothelial cells is interrupted by wide periodic gaps.

The intervascular stroma is minimal and broken-up by the omnipresent tortuous vascular channels (H & E, ×350).

D, Lymphangiosarcoma. This postmastectomy lymphangiosarcoma is composed of haphazardly arranged capillary vessels in dense fibroconnective tissue. The vessels range in size from minute practically lumenless cell nests to dilated cavernous lakes. The lining cells are pyknotic, protruding, and often bizarre.

The pattern of clustering and the diffuse infiltrative nature of these proliferating vessels in collagenous tissue attest to their aggressive and malignant nature (H & E, ×35).

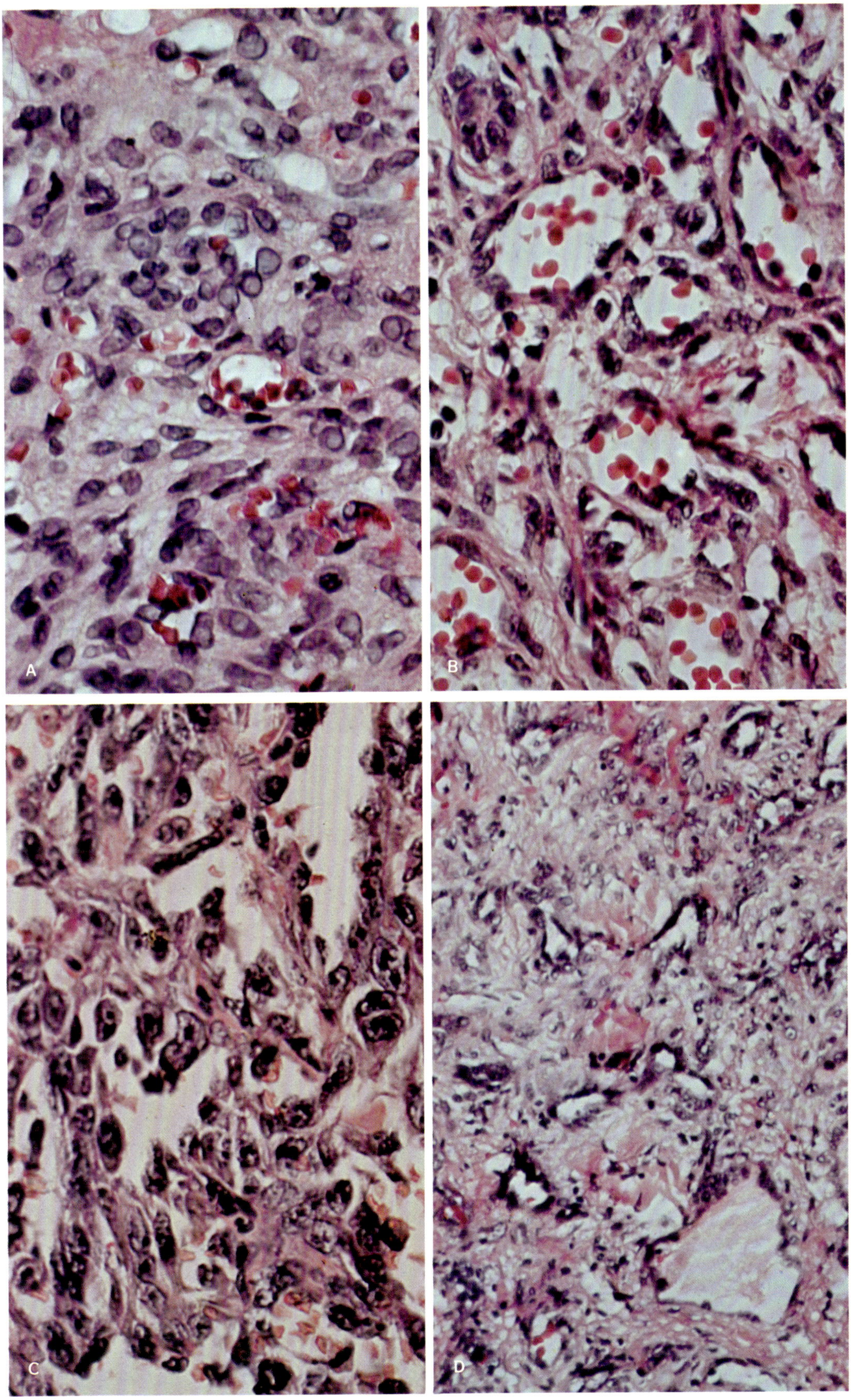

Figure 6-20.

Hemangiosarcoma of the *heart* comprises from 5 to 12% of all cardiac tumors. It is a rare entity and is rarely diagnosed antemortem. Crenshaw et al (1959) are credited with the first case that was diagnosed antemortem. It is almost invariably a fatal disease with massive metastasis to the lungs but rarely to other organs (Mahaim, 1945; Lange and Christiansen, 1947; Prichard, 1951; Rossi et al, 1976).

Examples of hemangiosarcoma *following irradiation* therapy have been reported (see Chapter 9).

Hemangiosarcoma of the *breast* is a distinct clinicopathologic entity. It is usually a disease of the young adult female. Despite its innocuous, well-differentiated appearance it has an ominous prognosis. The first authentic case of mammary hemangiosarcoma was reported by Borrmann in 1907. Since this report, primary mammary hemangiosarcomas have been the subject of numerous reports, among which the most important were written by McNalley et al, 1963; Steingaszner et al, 1965; Gulesserian and Lawton, 1969; Kessler and Kozenitsky, 1971; Saha et al, 1971; Beal, 1974. Dunegan et al, in 1976, published a review of 46 cases, together with 2 cases of their own, and emphasized that most of the mammary hemangiosarcomas are far advanced when diagnosed because of their insidious early manifestations. They metastasize through the blood stream, and the regional lymph nodes are rarely involved. It is not uncommon to see a fast downhill course and death in a matter of a few months after discovery of the primary disease (Fig. 6-26).

It is beyond the scope of this text to give a detailed account of hemangiosarcomas of the *spleen* or *liver*. Primary splenic angiosarcoma is a rare finding and in the majority of the cases it is diagnosed incidentally after rupture of the spleen.

Since Creech and Johnson, in 1974, reported the first cases of *angiosarcoma of the liver* in men working in polyvinyl chloride (PVC) plants, it has been shown in a number of reports that vinyl chloride causes hemangiosarcoma of the liver, not only in humans but also in experimental animals (Lee and Harry, 1974; Makk et al, 1976; Curran et al, 1977; Nicholson, 1977). It is also known since the original report of MacMahon and associates in 1947 that Thorotrast, which was used in the past as contrast material in diagnostic radiology, may produce hepatic hemangiosarcoma after a latent period of several decades. The epidemiology and the development of hepatic hemangioendothelioma induced by polyvinyl chloride, Thorotrast, and arsenic are the subject of two comprehensive review articles written by Brady et al (1977) and Popper et al (1978).

Primary hepatic angiosarcoma in patients without exposure to polyvinyl chloride, Thorotrast, and arsenic is equally rare. Our experience shows that less than 3% of primary hepatic tumors are hemangiosarcomas (Adams et al, 1972; Sussman et al, 1974).

At the time of selection of the best modality of treatment, it should be remembered that hemangiosarcomas can be multifocal and have a rather rapid growth and tendency for widespread metastasis to lungs, viscera, bones, and lymph nodes (Figs. 6-27, 6-28). At present, the generally accepted therapy is surgical excision when feasible. Response to radiation therapy is poor and not long lasting. Successful treatment of superficial hemangiosarcoma and Kaposi' sarcoma by carbon dioxide laser has been reported.

KAPOSI'S SARCOMA*

Kaposi, (see Chapter 1, Fig. 1-30) in 1872, gave the first account of what he called "multiple idiopathic pigmented sarcoma of the skin." Later he called it "multiple idiopathic hemorrhagic sarcoma" to distinguish it from other pigmented lesions such as malignant melanoma.

In his original article Kaposi gave a

* *Synonyms and related terms:* idiopathic hemorrhagic sarcoma, Kaposi's disease, angiosarcoma multiplex, acrosarcoma multiplex cutaneum, hemangioendothelioma cutaneum.

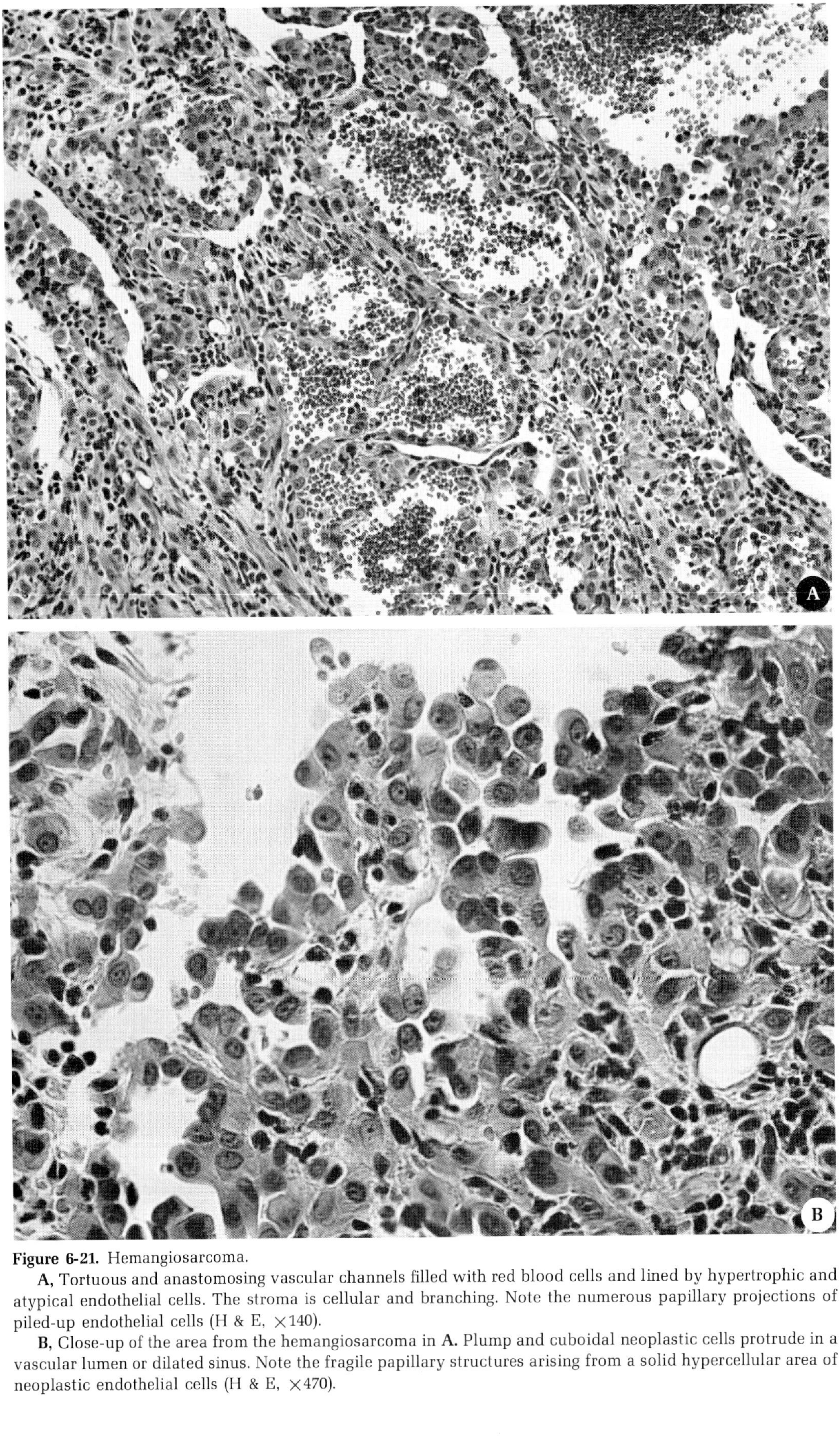

Figure 6-21. Hemangiosarcoma.

A, Tortuous and anastomosing vascular channels filled with red blood cells and lined by hypertrophic and atypical endothelial cells. The stroma is cellular and branching. Note the numerous papillary projections of piled-up endothelial cells (H & E, ×140).

B, Close-up of the area from the hemangiosarcoma in **A.** Plump and cuboidal neoplastic cells protrude in a vascular lumen or dilated sinus. Note the fragile papillary structures arising from a solid hypercellular area of neoplastic endothelial cells (H & E, ×470).

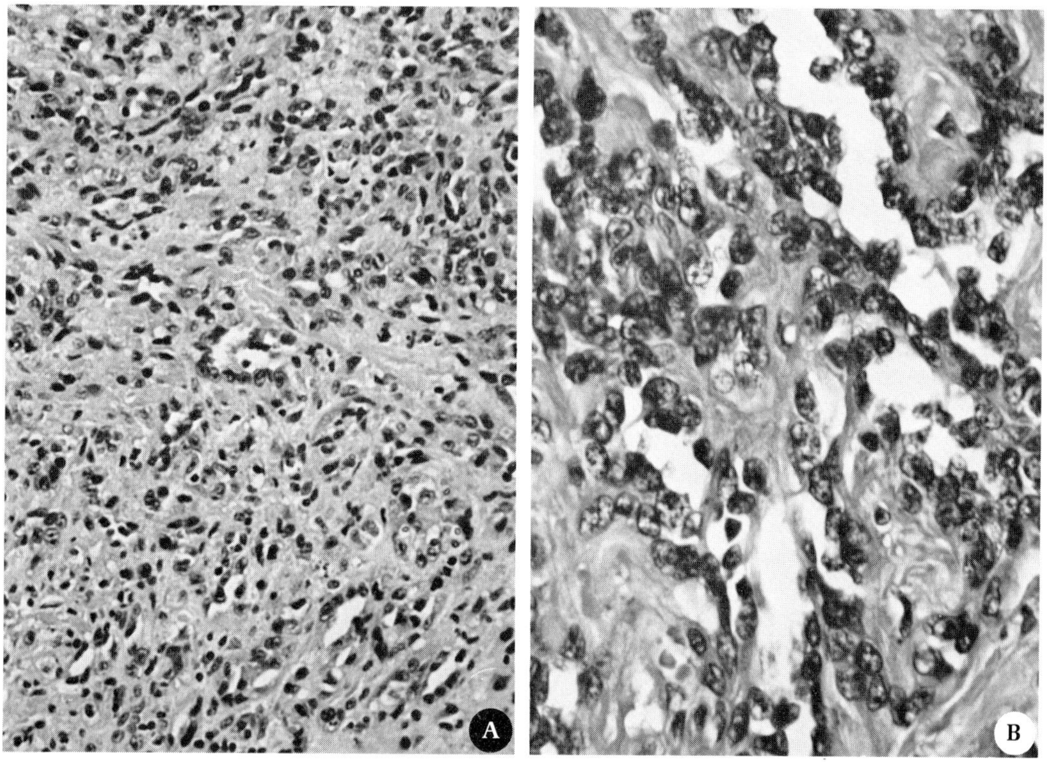

Figure 6-22. Hemangiosarcoma of the breast.

This tumor is composed of proliferating capillary vessels lined by atypical and cuboidal endothelial cells. There is a network of branching and intercommunication between neoplastic vessels. Note relatively sparse, cellular fibrous stroma. (**A,** H & E, ×140; **B,** H & E, ×350.)

classic description of the disease which was named after him:

"There develops on the skin, without known cause, either general or local, brown-red to blue-red nodules of the size of a grain of wheat, a pea or a hazelnut. Their surface is smooth, their consistency densely elastic and often they are swollen like a sponge filled with blood. Then the macules slowly coalesce into indurated plaques which appear symmetrically and from the extremities spread to the trunk and visceral organs as well as to lymph nodes" (Fig. 6-29).

Kaposi's sarcoma is admittedly more common than the literature would indicate. The etiology is unknown, but it is felt that prolonged lymphedema is a predisposing factor and it has been reported that many patients were employed in positions which kept them on their feet for long intervals. It has also been suggested that the widespread dissemination of Kaposi's sarcoma indicates the presence of some systemic cancerogen with special affinity for blood vessels. Taylor et al (1977) studied the growth kinetics of Kaposi's sarcoma and postulated that the progression and regression of the disease are determined by local vasomechanical factors and delayed hypersensitivity.

Kaposi's sarcoma has a worldwide distribution, but it has a racial propensity for male Jewish and Italian populations of Eastern Europe and Russia. It is also common in many parts of Africa and is the fifth most common malignant disease in Ugandan men. Because it is more common in the moist equatorial regions and rare on the upland plateau some environmental factors may have a role in its pathomechanism (Daview, 1962; Keen, 1962; Oettle, 1962).

Slavin et al (1970) and Templeton (1972) pointed out that the African form of

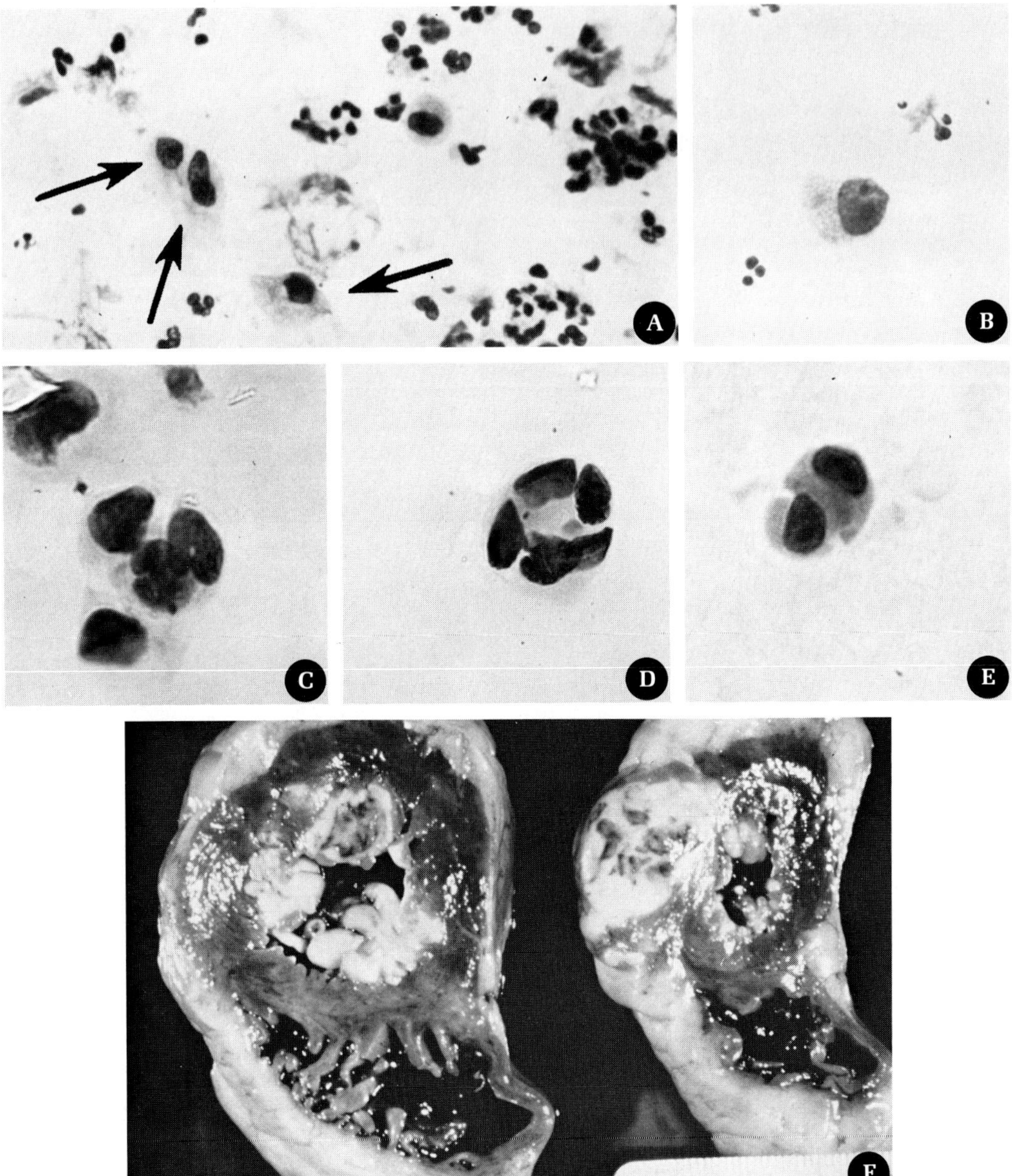

Figure 6-23. Exfoliated cells of hemangiosarcoma.

A and **B**, Smears prepared from sputum show isolated medium-sized round neoplastic cells with prominent nuclei and transparent cytoplasm (Pap stain, ×350).

C, **D**, and **E**, Clusters of malignant cells from pleural effusion. The cells form clusters which give the impression of glandular neoplastic cells. Note the dark nuclei and the ill-defined cytoplasm (Pap stain, ×450). (From Hajdu, S. I., and Hajdu, E. O.: Cytopathology of Sarcomas and Other Nonepithelial Malignant Tumors. Philadelphia, W. B. Saunders, 1976.)

F, Hemangiosarcoma from the head and neck area metastatic to the heart of a 10-year-old child. The left ventricle is almost completely filled with tumor.

Kaposi's sarcoma varies somewhat from the pattern of the disease in whites. In general, the patients are younger, lymph nodes and viscera are involved more commonly, and second neoplasms are less likely to develop than in whites.

Dorffel (1932) reviewed the literature up to 1931 and found 263 reported cases. He was the first to report a case of Kaposi's sarcoma not associated with known cutaneous lesions. There is little to add to the studies reported by McCarthy and Pack (1950) and O'Brien and Brasfield (1966) (Table 6-7). Interested readers may find it valuable to read Bluefarb's (1957) comprehensive monograph on Kaposi's sarcoma in which the history as well as the clinicopathology of the disease is summarized.

The exact cell of origin of Kaposi's sarcoma is still debated in the literature (Levan et al, 1972; Hardy et al, 1976; Taylor et al, 1977). Electron microscopic studies show without doubt that most of the cells resemble endothelial cells (Ramos et al, 1976; Gokel et al, 1976).

Histologically the appearance of Kaposi's sarcoma ranges from a mixed cellular to an anaplastic form according to the composition of cellular elements, preponderance of the vascular spaces, and degree of pleomorphism of the tumor cells. It seems that the microscopic appearance is related to the duration of the tumor and has no particular prognostic value. Classically most of the tumors are characterized by a mixture of spindle cells, vascular slits, and branching vascular channels. In most areas the stroma appears sparsely cellular and edematous and contains extravasated red blood cells. The tumor nodules of Kaposi's sarcoma can be fungating or infiltrating and there may be considerable pleomorphism and mitotic activity (Figs. 6-30, 6-31).

True metastasis does occur in Kaposi's sarcoma, but it is generally held that multifocal presentation is far more common than is reflected in the literature. There are numerous reported accounts of *visceral* (Tedeschi et al, 1947; Siegel et al, 1969), *nodal* (Ecklung and Valaitis, 1962; Lee and Moore, 1965; Ramos et al, 1976), *cardiac* (Choisser and Ramsey, 1939), *oral* (Gambardella, 1974), and *intracranial* (Rwomushana et al, 1975) Kaposi's sarcoma without apparent cutaneous lesions.

An interesting and puzzling feature of Kaposi's sarcomas is their frequent association with *malignant lymphoreticular neoplasms,* particularly with Hodgkin's disease. Cole and Crump in 1920 reported two cases of Kaposi's sarcoma complicated with lymphatic leukemia. Lane and Greenwood (1933) reported a patient who had mycosis fungoides and Kaposi's sarcoma and Mazzaferri and Penn (1968) reported the co-existence of Kaposi's sarcoma and multiple myeloma. By studying the case histories of patients with Kaposi's sarcoma O'Brien and Brasfield (1966) found that 18 of the 63 patients died of a

TABLE 6-7. ***Kaposi's Sarcoma***

	NO. OF CASES	MALE	FEMALE	AVG. AGE YR.	MOST COMMON SITES	ALIVE WITHOUT DISEASE %	MORTALITY %
McCarthy and Pack (1950)	36	33	3	57	Lower and upper extremities	17	28*
O'Brien and Brasfield (1966)	63	51	12	60	Lower and upper extremities	9	17

*Ranging from 2 to 20 years.

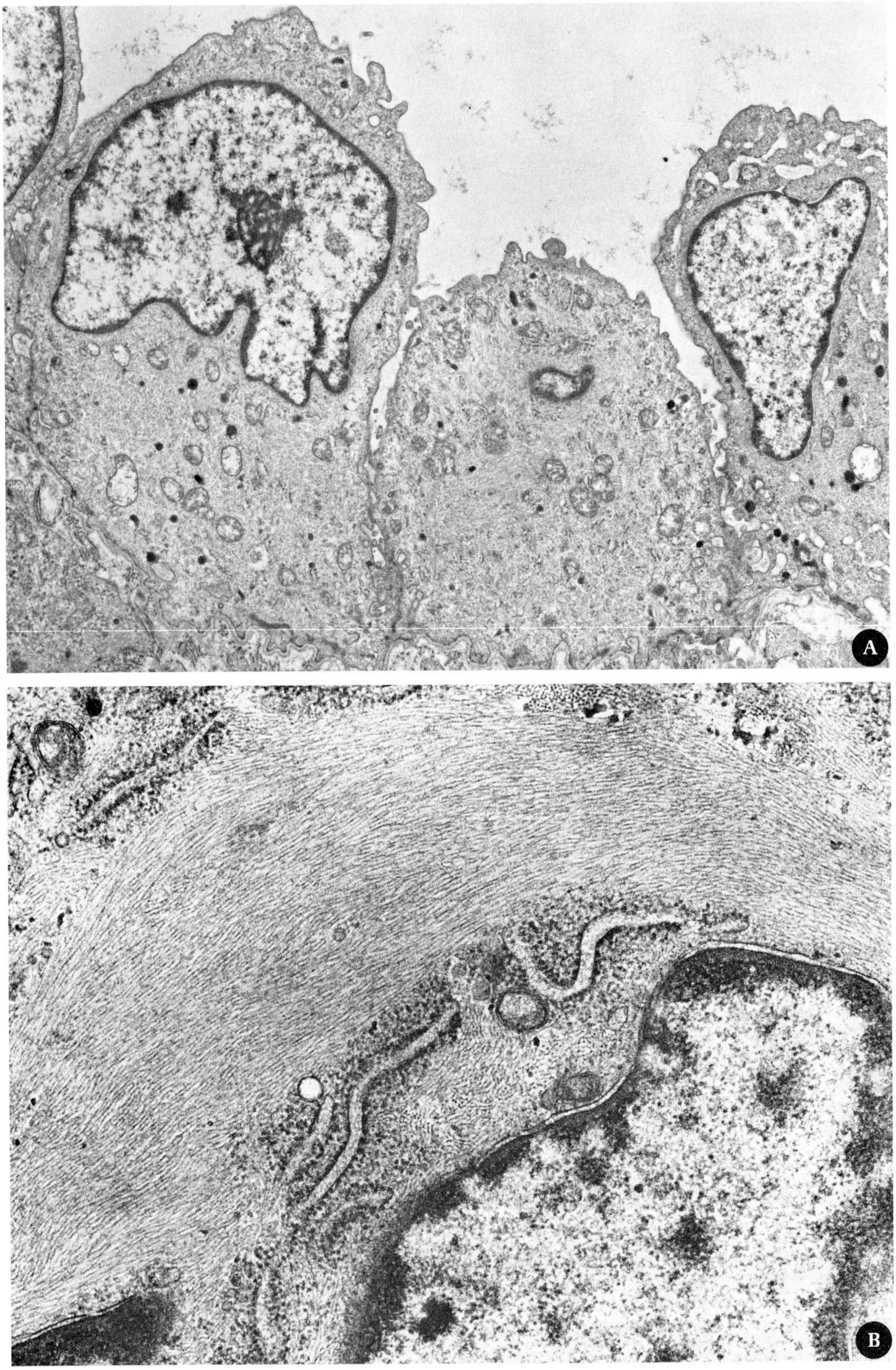

Figure 6-24. Hemangiosarcoma.

A, Neoplastic endothelial cells bulge into lumen. Note the cytoplasmic microfilaments, electron-dense lysosomes, and prominent basal lamina on the basal surfaces of the cells (×6,900).

B, Portion of neoplastic endothelial cell. Numerous microfilaments are seen in the cytoplasm (×8,000).

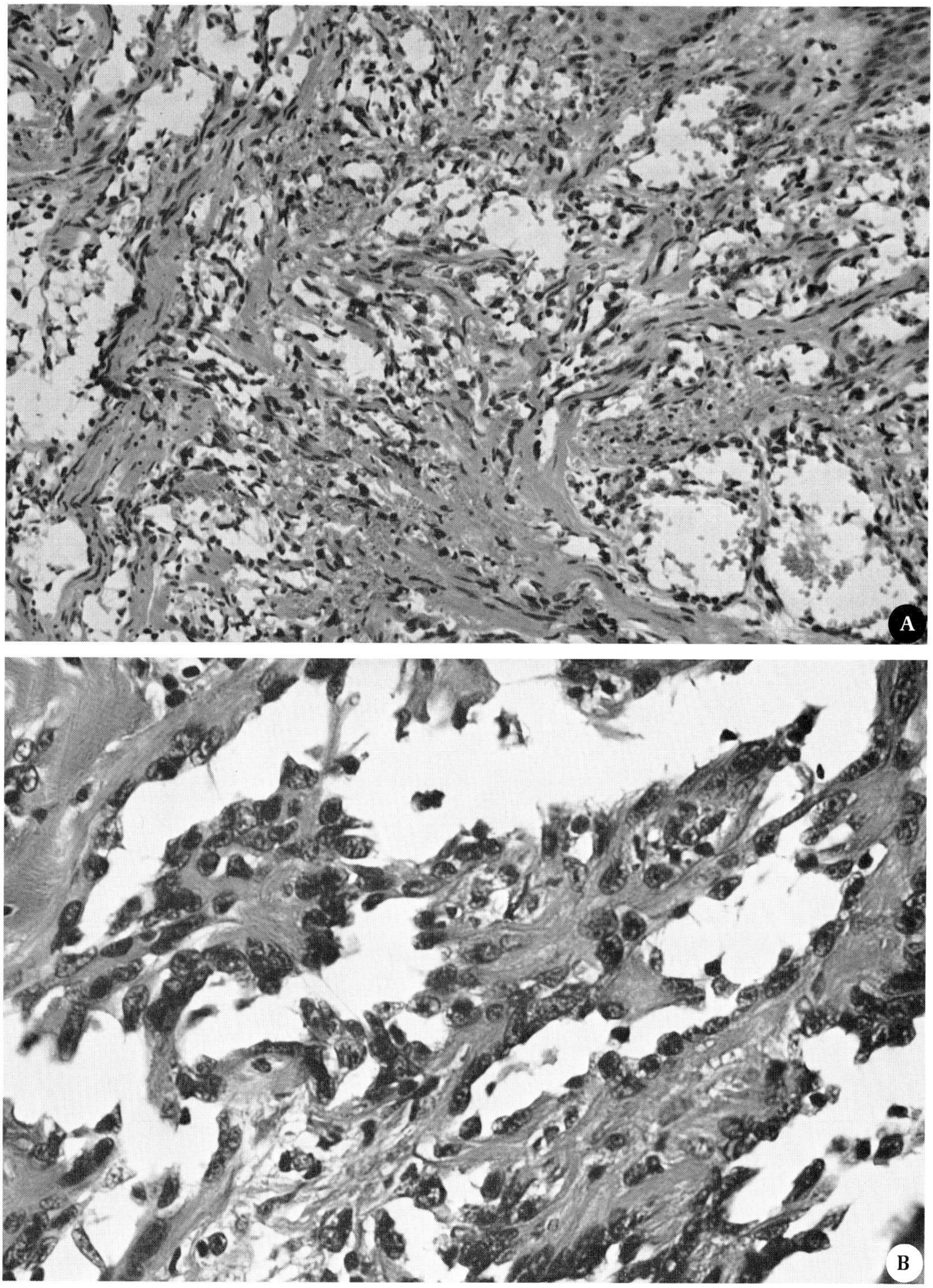

Figure 6-25. Hemangiosarcoma metastatic to the lung.

The tumor completely replaced the lung parenchyma. Note not only the proliferating neoplastic endothelial cells in vascular channels but also the reticular stroma with elongated spindle cells (**A,** H & E, ×140; **B,** H & E, ×350).

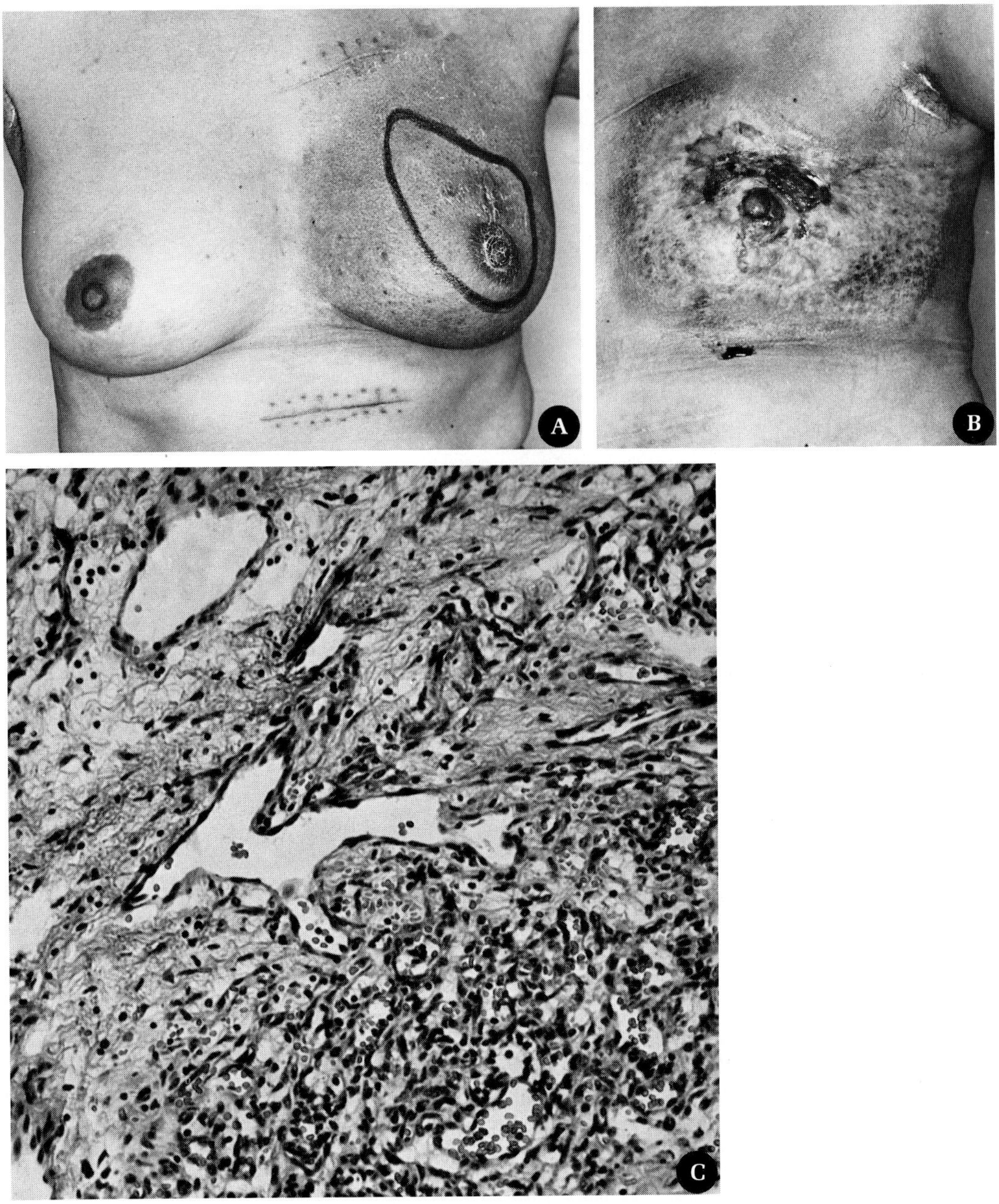

Figure 6-26. Hemangiosarcoma of the breast. Before **(A)** and after **(B)** radical treatment for local recurrences. **C,** Hypertrophic vascular channels of various sizes trapped in a stroma which is predominantly fibrous in nature. Note the branching and various sizes of neoplastic vessels (H & E, ×140).

second primary neoplasm and concluded that *the mortality from a second primary cancer was greater threat to life* (29%) *than the mortality from Kaposi's sarcoma* (17%). The most common second neoplasms in their series were Hodgkin's disease (5 patients), lymphosarcoma (3 patients), and carcinoma of the colon (3 patients).

It is postulated that both Kaposi's sarcoma and malignant lymphoreticular tumors are associated with deficient immune responsiveness. Hardy et al (1976) reported a case and cited 6 other cases in

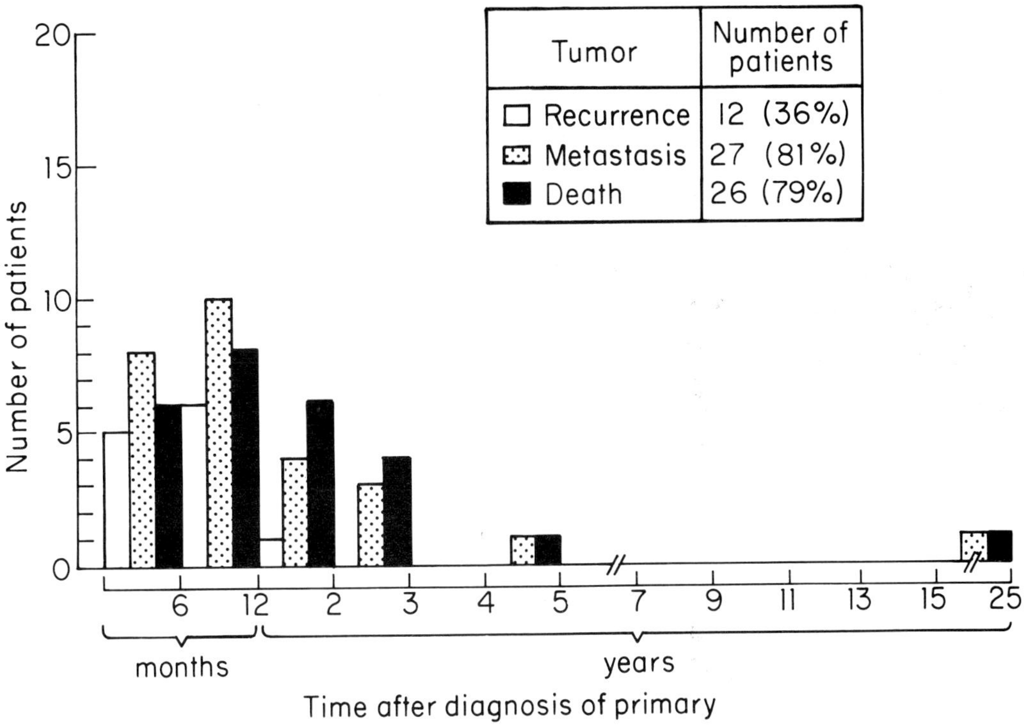

Figure 6-27. Rate of recurrence and metastasis of 33 hemangiosarcomas. Note the mortality of 79%. Most patients died within 3 years after diagnosis.

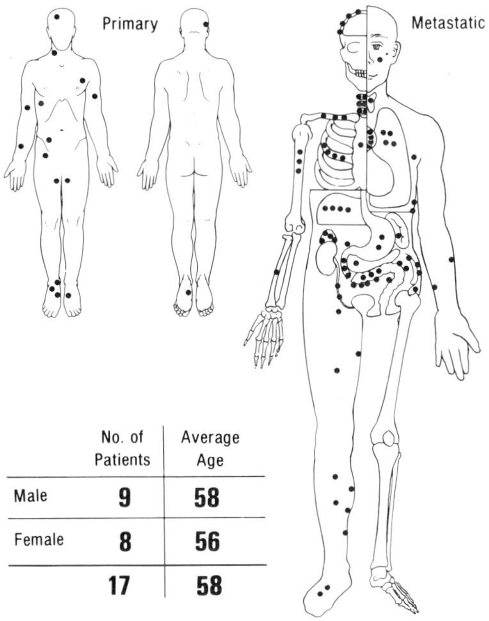

	No. of Patients	Average Age
Male	**9**	**58**
Female	**8**	**56**
	17	**58**

Figure 6-28. Anatomic distribution of metastatic tumors at autopsy. (See Appendix)

which Kaposi's sarcoma was discovered in recipients of renal allografts. The apparent cause-and-effect relationship is not blurred by the possibility that factors other than immunosuppression may also play a role in the development of cancer in transplant recipients, but it is worth noting the report of Klepp et al (1978). They found that Kaposi's sarcoma developed in 6 of 41 patients in their series following immunosuppressive medication for non-neoplastic conditions.

Irradiation therapy is regarded as the treatment of choice for most forms of Kaposi's sarcoma. Long-lasting remission has been reported, however, following treatment with actinomycin D.

Histologically, Kaposi's sarcoma rarely poses a diagnostic problem, but the mixed cellular phase of the disease may resemble *pyogenic granuloma*. However, in pyogenic granuloma there is a florid inflammatory component and the vascular components are inconspicuous.

Differentiation of Kaposi's sarcoma

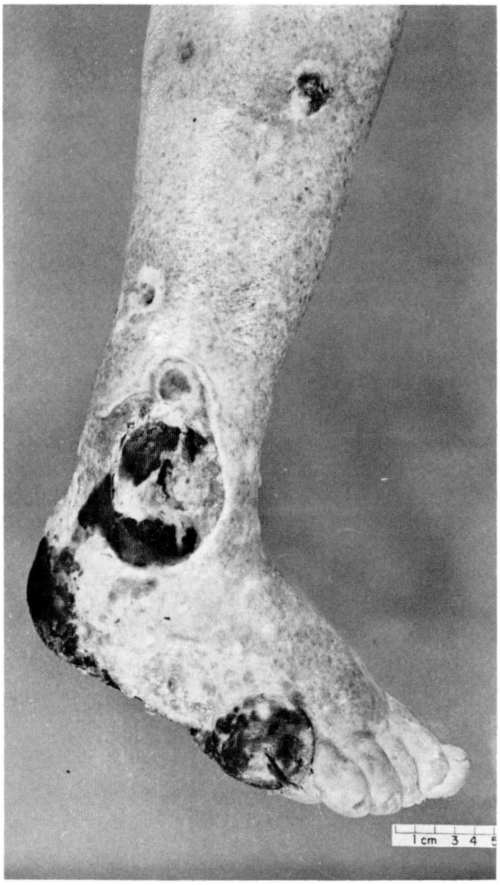

Figure 6-29. Recurrent and advanced Kaposi's sarcoma.

from *hemangiosarcoma* of the classic type should not pose any serious diagnostic problems. One must remember the clinical presentation while studying the microscopic appearance (Table 6-8).

HEMANGIOBLASTOMA*

Hemangioblastoma most commonly occurs in the cerebellum and is considered to be a familial disease in about 10% of the cases. Most of these tumors are localized globoid lesions and range in size from one centimeter to several centimeters.

Hemangioblastoma is distinguished from other vascular neoplasms by the *presence of a peculiar type of stromal cell between the vascular spaces lined by proliferating endothelial cells and pericytes.* According to Waldo et al (1977) and Kawamura et al (1973) the stromal cells are four times the size of pericytes, and their cytoplasms are filled with free ribosomes and randomly distributed fine microfilaments. Although the histogenesis of these cells is not known, it has been suggested that they originate from endothelial or pericytic cells (Kawamura et al, 1973). Another distinguishing feature of

* *Synonyms and related terms:* capillary hemangioblastoma, cerebellar hemangioblastoma, angioblastic meningioma, meningeal hemangiopericytoma.

TABLE 6-8. ***Comparison of Certain Clinicopathologic Features of Hemangiosarcoma and Kaposi's Sarcoma***

	HEMANGIOSARCOMA	KAPOSI'S SARCOMA
Race distribution	Not observed	Jewish, Italian
Age distribution	Younger than 40	Older than 40
Sex distribution	Equal	Male predominance
Most common site	Extremities	Extremities
Tissue site	Soft tissues	Skin
Number of tumors	Solitary	Multiple
Size	Bulky	Small
Lymphedema	No	Common
Growth	Rapid	Slow
Metastasis to lymph node	Common	Rare
Average survival	3 years	8 years
Mortality	85%	45%

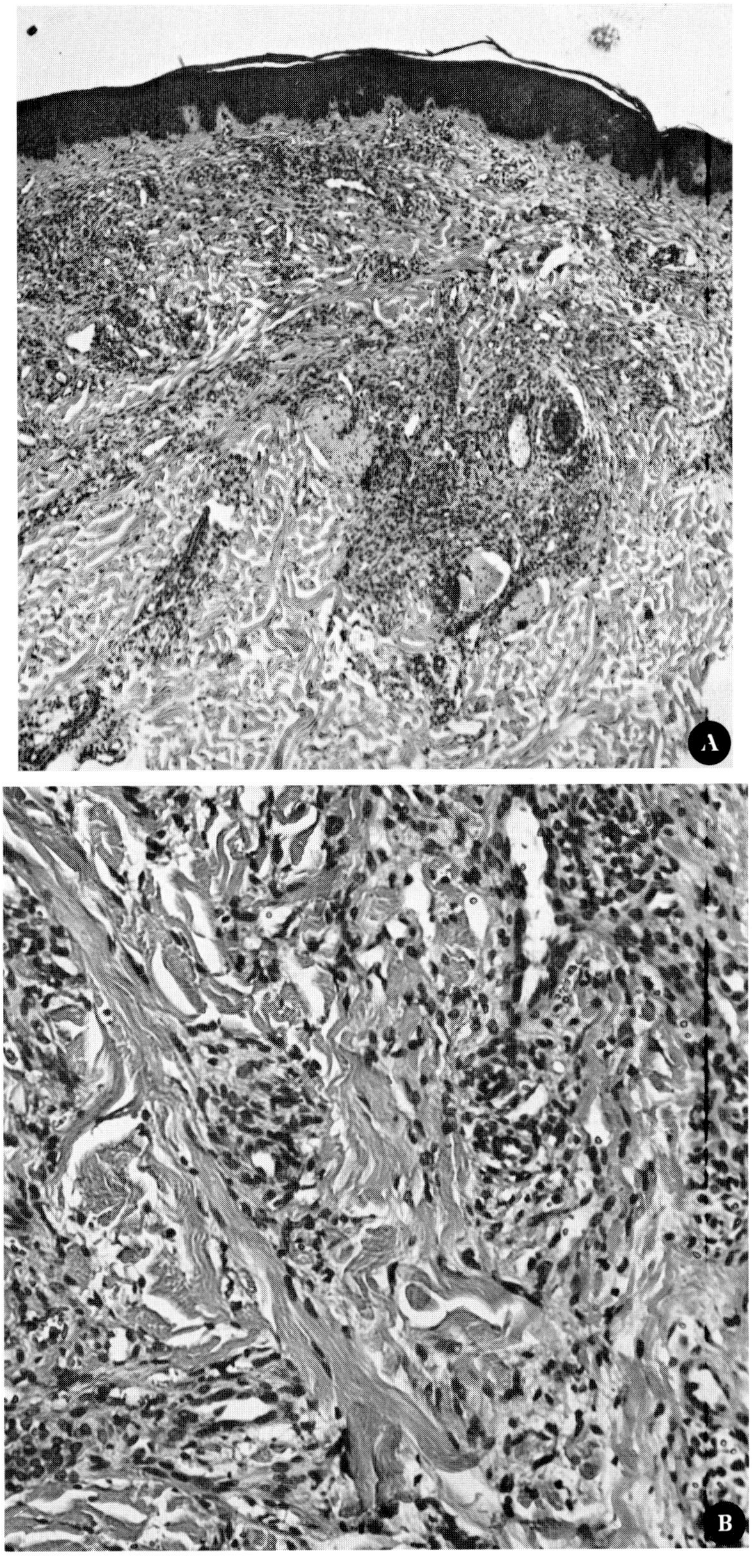

Figure 6-30. Kaposi's sarcoma of the skin.

Note the multifocal nests of minute capillary vessels and cuboidal or round cells. The tumor cells extend and form cords between collagenous fibers (**A,** H & E, ×35; **B,** H & E, ×85).

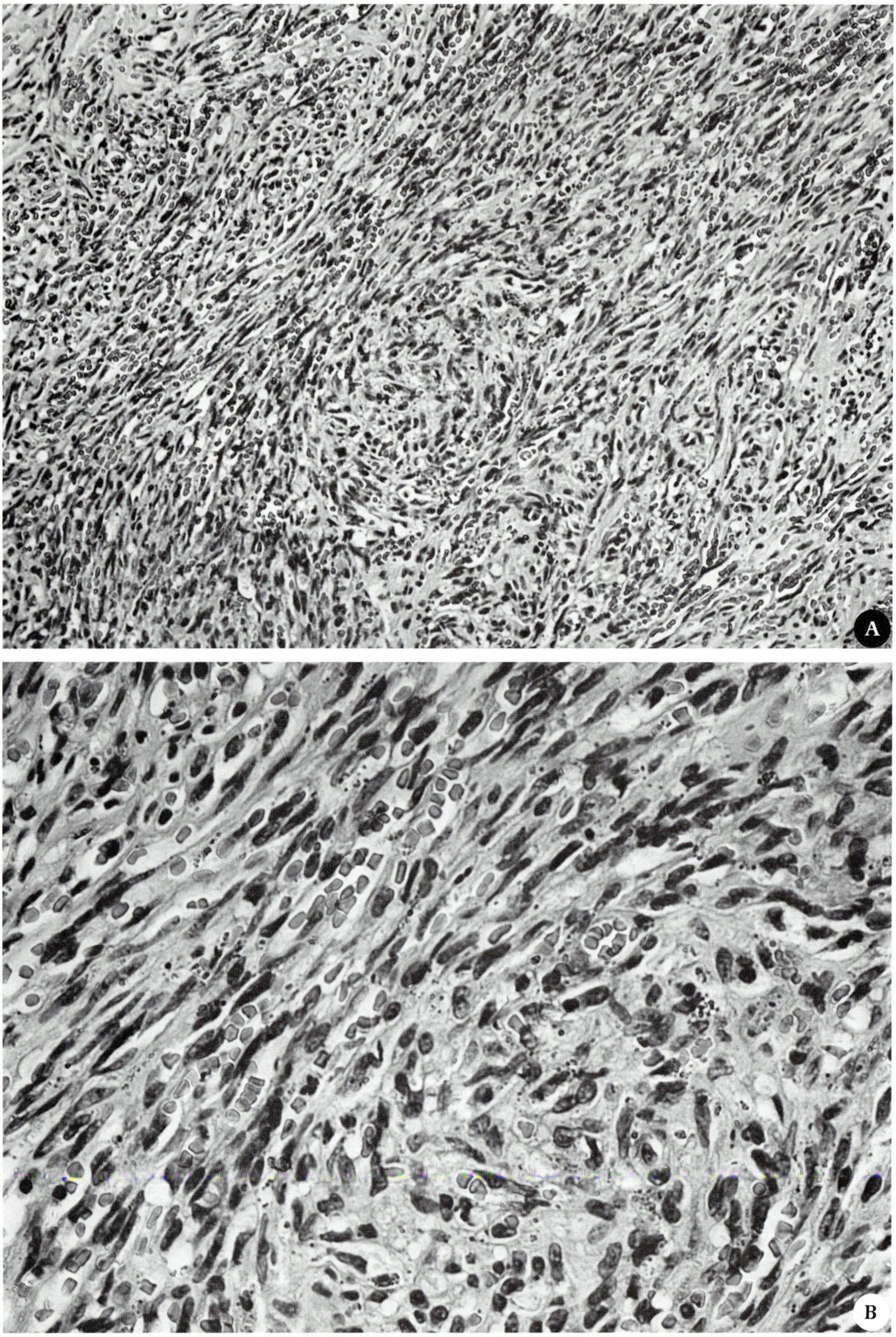

Figure 6-31. Kaposi's sarcoma, deeply invasive. Note the spindly tendency of the neoplastic slender cells and cords of red blood cells running along the neoplastic spindle cells (**A,** H & E, ×140; **B,** H & E, ×350).

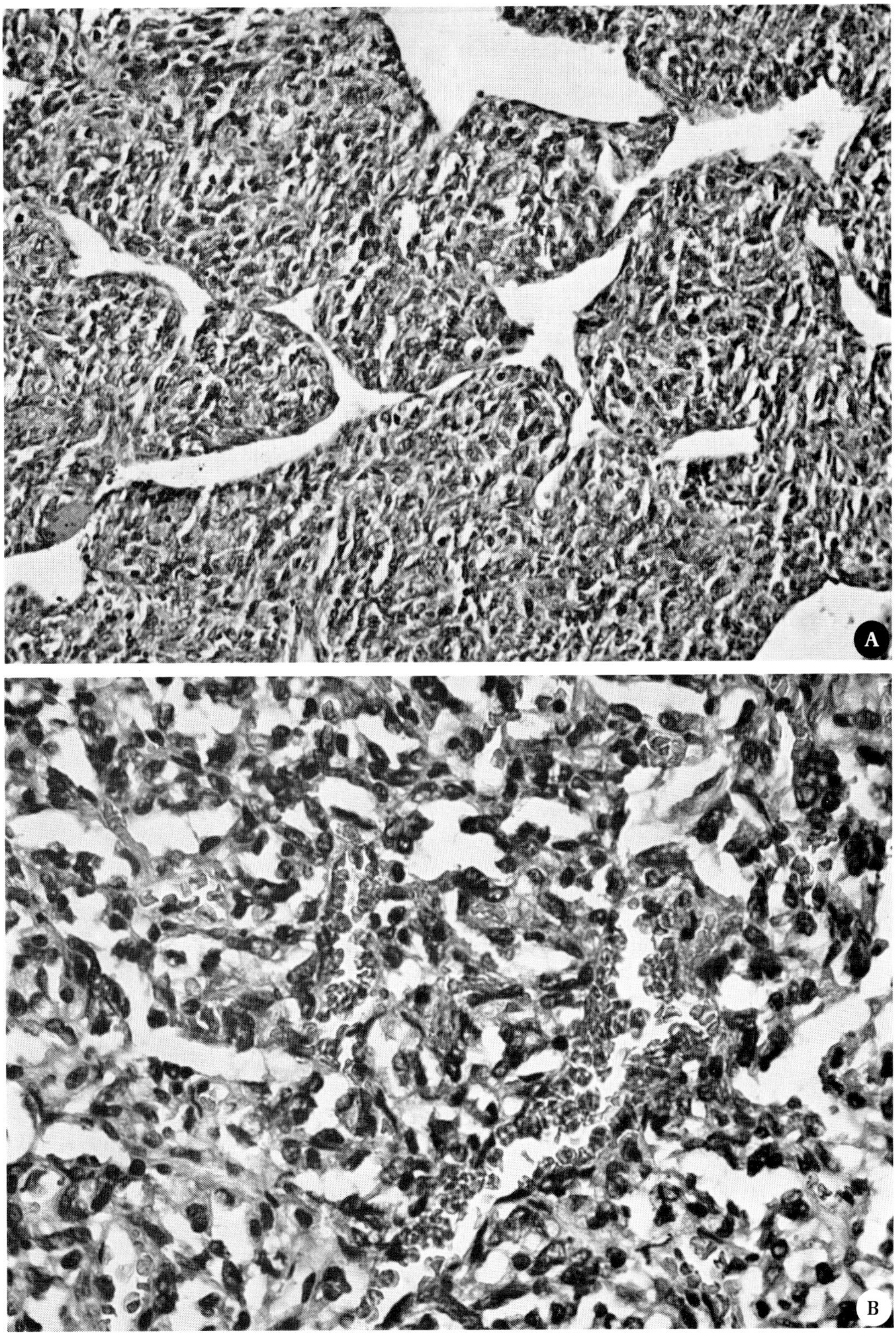

Figure 6-32. Hemangioblastoma of the cerebellum is composed of piled-up and proliferating neoplastic cells in arrangement resembling hemangiopericytoma. Branching and intercommunicating vascular channels are lined by plump endothelial cells and pericytic cells and are surrounded by small undifferentiated so-called stromal cells (**A,** H & E, ×140; **B,** H & E, ×350).

hemangioblastoma, when it is present, is foci of *extramedullary hematopoiesis.* Erythrocytosis which disappears after surgical excision of the lesion has been reported in more than 50% of the cases (Fig. 6-32).

In the differential diagnosis one should consider *meningeal hemangiopericytoma* (Pitkethy et al, 1970; Goellner et al, 1978).

Surgical treatment is effective in the majority of patients with hemangioblastomas, but rare instances of recurrences have been reported.

Tumors of Lymphatic Vessels

LYMPHANGIOMA

Lymphangiomas are benign neoplasms of lymphatic vessels and are far less common than hemangiomas. Despite their occasional appearance in late infancy and childhood they are congenital lesions. Rare instances of simultaneous occurrence of congenital lymphangiomas and hemangiomas have been reported, and it has been pointed out that such lesions may cause dystocia (Nelson and Gabbe, 1976).

Cystic hygroma is one of the best known forms of lymphangioma. Typically, it is found in the neck, but it may extend as far as pectoral or axillary regions (Fig. 6-33).

Capillary and *cavernous lymphangiomas* and *papillary endothelial hyperplasia* are usually discrete subcutaneous or submucosal lesions of various sizes. They are found most commonly in the head and neck areas, shoulder, pelvis, and the retroperitoneum. Not infrequently a number of small vesicles will fuse together and form the *lymphatic cyst* (Kalish et al, 1975; Cunningham and Winningham, 1972; Russo and Dewar, 1961). The cavernous and capillary lymphangiomas are composed of a conglomerate of dilated lymphatic vessels which freely communicate with adjacent normal lymphatic channels. The stroma of these lesions is cellular and dominated by elongated fibroblast-like cells. The papillary and cystic forms are usually sparsely cellular and the stroma is collagenous. Cunningham and Winningham (1972), who found 33 reported examples of retroperitoneal cystic lymphangiomas, stated that the majority of patients were more than 50 years old and most tumors were on the right side.

Lymphangiectasia, dilatation of the lymphatic vessels, of the small intestine is believed to play a cardinal role in the pathogenesis of the syndrome of infantile or childhood hypoproteinemia without proteinuria and with normal hepatic function (Walker-Smith et al, 1969). Lymphangiectasia of the intestines has been reported in association with widespread lymphatic abnormality resulting in chylothorax and lymphedema (Rienhoff et al, 1964; Laipply and Sherrick, 1958).

The treatment of lymphangiomas is surgical excision, if it is feasible, rather than irradiation or application of sclerosing solutions.

LYMPHANGIOMYOMA*

Lymphangiomyoma is a rare tumor manifested by proliferation of endothelial and smooth muscle cells of lymphatic channels. When this process affects more than one area, it is called *lymphangiomyomatosis.* Lymphangiomyoma is a rare acquired or congenital lesion which most commonly affects the abdominal and thoracic lymphatics and may cause *pulmonary insufficiency, chylothorax,* and episodes of *spontaneous pneumothorax.* Lymphangiomyoma as an entity was first recognized by Enterline and Roberts, in 1955; however, they erroneously called it lymphangiopericytoma.

Laipply and Sherrick (1958) were the first to call attention to the association of lymphangiomyomatosis and chylothorax. Cornog and Enterline (1966) found 14 reported cases of lymphangiomyoma in the literature to which they added 6 of their own. During the last decade a number of cases have been recorded in the literature,

**Synonyms and related terms:* lymphangiopericytoma, angiomyoma, angiomatous hyperplasia.

among which the most notable are those reported by Bush et al, 1969; Joliat et al, 1973; Wolff, 1973; Gray et al, 1975; Vazquez et al, 1976, and the review article by Corring et al in 1975.

Lymphangiomyomatosis affects women in the second to fourth decades. It has been postulated that lymphangiomyomatosis is a hamartomatous lesion. However, recent ultrastructural studies have demonstrated that immature myocytes, histologically similar to those in smooth muscle tumors, are the dominant elements in lymphangiomyomatous lesions irrespective of their location (Wolff, 1973; Vazquez et al, 1976). The pulmonary lesion begins generally in the third or fourth decade of life with hyperplasia of the smooth muscle of the lymphatics surrounding the bronchioli.

The prognosis for patients is variable. Some of the cases progress rapidly, whereas others remain stabilized for a long time.

A relationship between lymphangiomyomatosis and tuberous sclerosis has been described. In the majority of the cases reported no tuberous sclerosis was found, and the relationship between lymphangiomyomatosis and tuberous sclerosis remains controversial (Feldman et al, 1978; Kreisman et al, 1978).

Histologically, these lesions are composed of proliferating vascular channels showing heavy and tortuous walls. Microscopic diagnosis should not be difficult in technically adequate sections (Fig. 6-34).

LYMPHANGIOSARCOMA

In 1948, Stewart and Treves reported 6 cases of lymphangiosarcoma in lymphedematous arms following radical mastectomy for cancer of the breast (see Chapter 1, Figure 1-45). Martorell, in 1951, reported a patient in whom a lymphangiosarcoma occurred in a chronically lymphedematous extremity without evidence of antecedent tumor. Danese et al (1967) found 19 reported cases of lymphangiosarcoma arising in lymphedematous extremities. We recently reported a case of lymphangiosarcoma of a congenitally lymphedematous arm, in which we had the opportunity to follow the progression of the disease until death of the patient (Merrick et al, 1971) (Fig. 6-35).

Congenital lymphedema can be nonfamilial or familial (Milroy's disease). In these conditions the subcutaneous fat is replaced by lymphatic channels and fibrous tissue. Both endothelial as well as stromal elements proliferate and become more and more bizarre with age and duration of the lesion.

The origin of lymphangiosarcoma from the endothelial lining cells of lymphatic vessels is not universally accepted. A dual vascular-lymphatic origin of these tumors was reported by McConnell and Haslam in 1959. Salm (1963) suggested that some of the tumors reported as lymphangiosarcomas are actually metastases from antecedent carcinomas and said that mammary cancer cells are "using the dermal collagen fibers as a scaffolding."

Admittedly the *microscopic features of lymphangiosarcoma are not always sufficiently distinctive to separate it from hemangiosarcoma* or other neoplasms and one must consider the location and history of pre-existing chronic lymphedema. Especially if the tumor is undifferentiated, even the ultrastructural features are not specific, since in undifferentiated tumors the pinocytic vesicles and microfilaments as well as the intracellular lumina can be absent.

The pathomechanism of lymphangiosarcoma is poorly understood, but it is certain that long-standing *lymphedema* or *chronic lymph stasis* is an important and perhaps the sole etiologic factor. Lymphangiosarcoma with identical clinical and histologic appearance may appear as a sequel to congenital and acquired traumatic or parasitic lymphedema.

Clinically, the first sign of lymphangiosarcoma is the appearance of macular skin lesions which become confluent with areas of erosion and ulceration.

Since the original description of lymphangiosarcoma of a chronically edema-

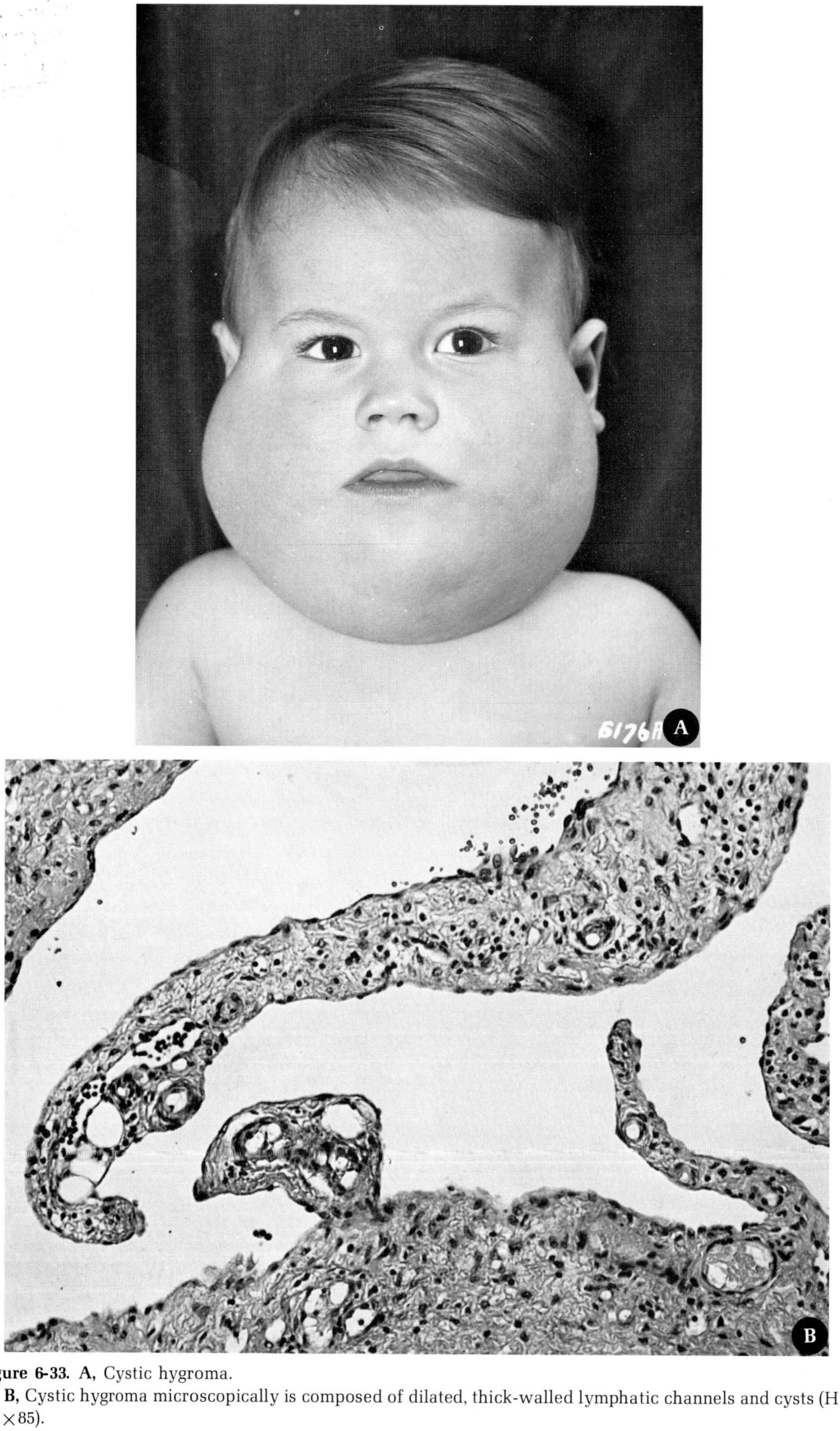

Figure 6-33. A, Cystic hygroma.

B, Cystic hygroma microscopically is composed of dilated, thick-walled lymphatic channels and cysts (H & E, ×85).

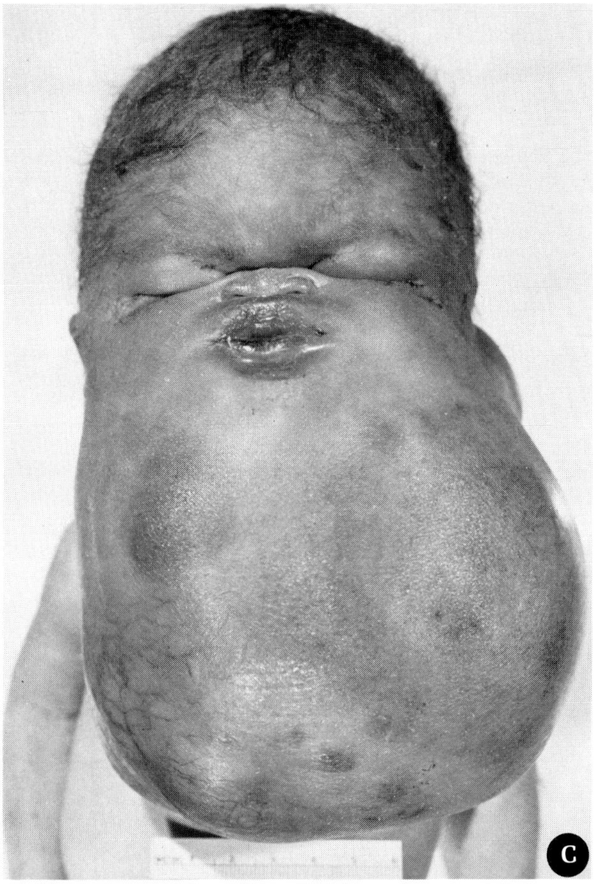

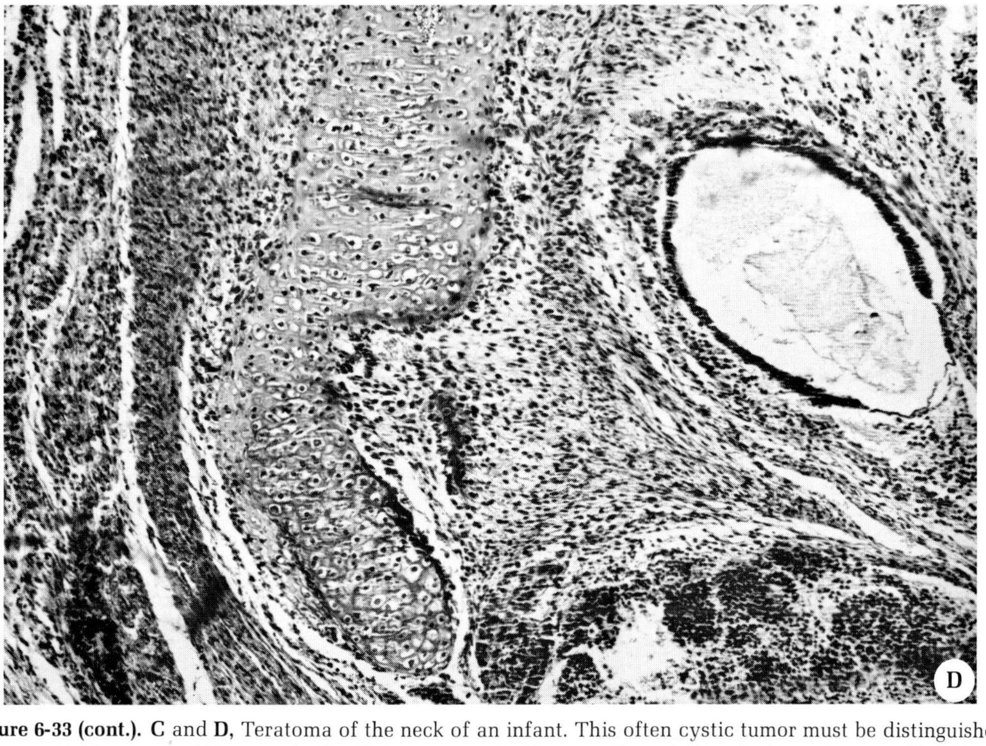

Figure 6-33 (cont.). C and **D,** Teratoma of the neck of an infant. This often cystic tumor must be distinguished from cystic hygroma. Microscopically, it is composed of mesenchymal chondroid and connective tissue elements, cystic spaces lined by epithelial cells, and undifferentiated neuroectodermal components (see right lower corner) (H & E, ×140).

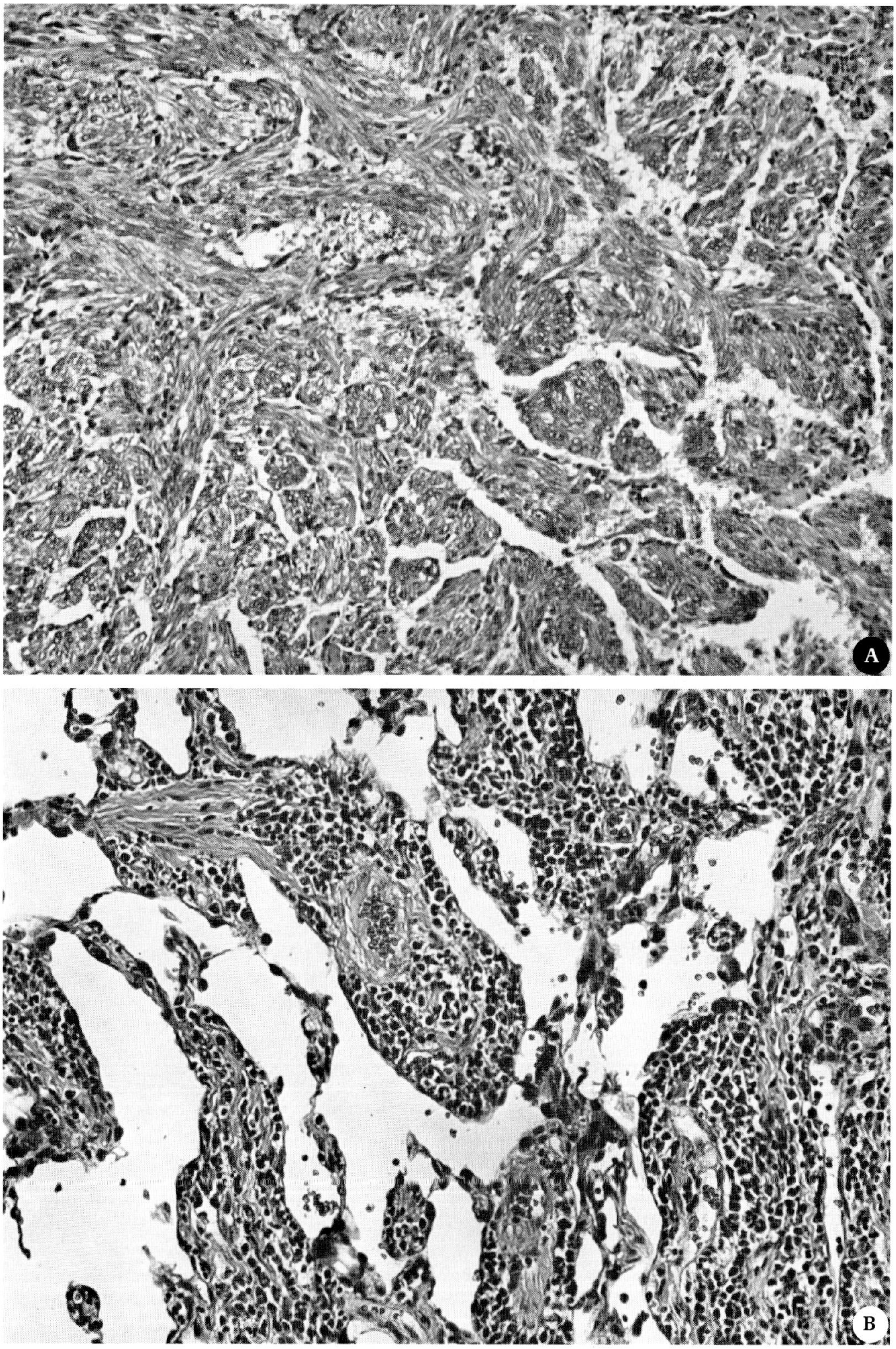

Figure 6-34. Lymphangiomyoma.

A, Lymphangiomyoma is composed of proliferating, spindly, smooth muscle cells and branching, empty-looking, lymphatic channels which often appear as nothing else than tissue slits (H & E, ×140).

B, Lympangiomyoma involving a lymph node. Here the branching vascular channels are more pronounced and the myocytic elements are less apparent (H & E, ×140).

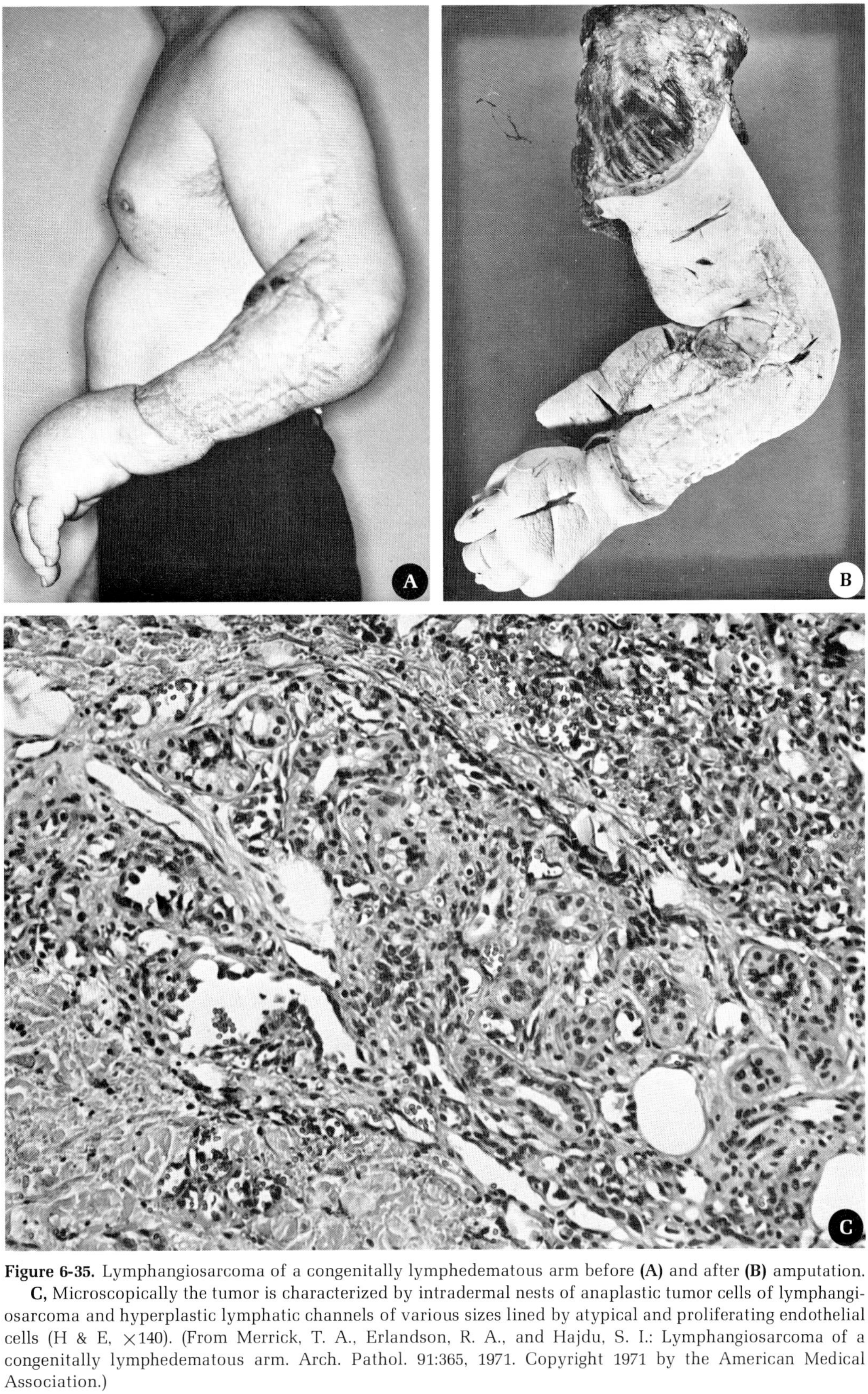

Figure 6-35. Lymphangiosarcoma of a congenitally lymphedematous arm before **(A)** and after **(B)** amputation. **C,** Microscopically the tumor is characterized by intradermal nests of anaplastic tumor cells of lymphangiosarcoma and hyperplastic lymphatic channels of various sizes lined by atypical and proliferating endothelial cells (H & E, ×140). (From Merrick, T. A., Erlandson, R. A., and Hajdu, S. I.: Lymphangiosarcoma of a congenitally lymphedematous arm. Arch. Pathol. 91:365, 1971. Copyright 1971 by the American Medical Association.)

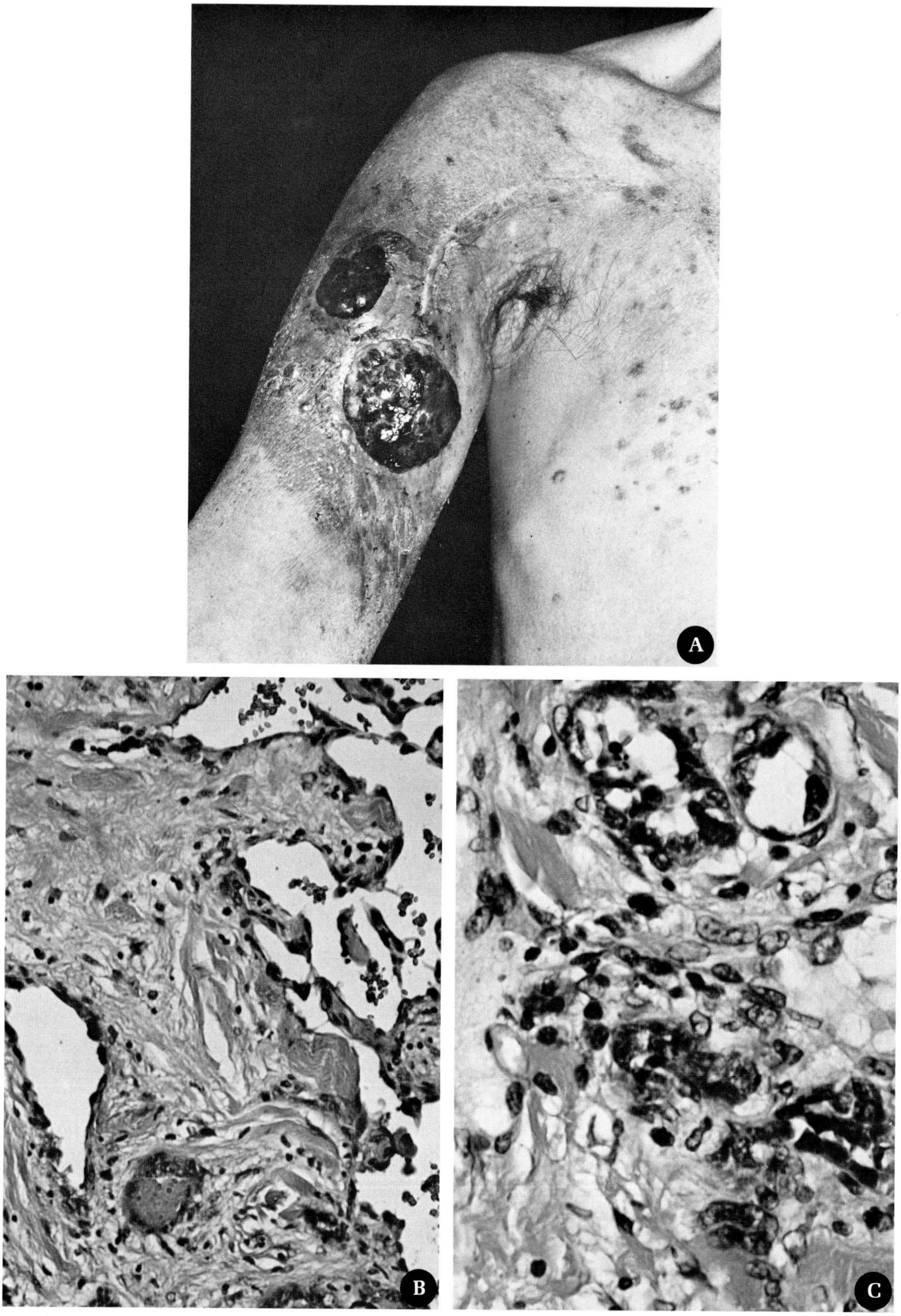

Figure 6-36. Postmastectomy lymphangiosarcoma.

A, This patient had a fast, progressive downhill course 15 years after initial therapy for mammary carcinoma.

B and **C,** Microscopic appearance of lymphangiosarcoma. Lymphatic channels of various sizes are lined by sparsely or tightly arranged endothelial cells. Note the numerous papillary projections and attempts of endothelial cells to form cell clusters and cell cords (**A,** H & E, ×140; **B,** H & E, ×350).

tous extremity by Stewart and Treves, in 1948, more than 200 histologically documented cases of lymphangiosarcoma of the upper extremity have been reported (Treves, 1957; Hermann, 1965; Eby et al, 1967; Woodward et al, 1972). Most lymphangiosarcomas of the upper extremity have occurred in patients with postmastectomy edema with an average duration of 10 years. Soon after the bluish papulous lesions appear, usually just above or below the antecubital fossa, the disease will spread over the extremity, to the chest wall and ultimately to the lungs and abdominal viscera (Fig. 6-36).

The results of treatment have been disappointing. According to Herrmann (1965) of the 71 patients he surveyed only 7% lived 5 or more years. In 1972, Woodward et al reviewed the end result of 162 reported cases and found that only 6% of the patients survived more than 5 years and 50% of the patients died within 19 months after treatment. It is felt that as an initial therapeutic attempt both external and internal irradiation should be used. If the sarcoma proves to be radioresistant, radical surgical therapy should be used.

Purely on the basis of histologic appearance, *Kaposi's sarcoma* and *hemangiosarcoma* should be considered in the differential diagnosis. Stewart and Treves pointed out the difficulties in differential diagnosis in their original report in 1948 by saying that "one of these new tumors had been subjected to biopsy and a report of Kaposi's sarcoma made."

REFERENCES

References are listed in chronological order in each category.

INTRODUCTION

Sabin, F. R.: Preliminary note on the differentiation of angioblasts and the method by which they produce blood-vessels, blood plasma and red blood cells as seen in the living chick. Anat. Rec. 13:199, 1917.

Rouviere, H.: Anatomy of the Human Lymphatic System. Ann Arbor, Michigan, Edwards Bros., 1938.

Kramer, H. E.: Electron microscope study of developing chick embryo aorta. J. Ultrastruct. Res. 4:420, 1960.

Movat, H. Z., and Fernando, N. V. P.: The fine structure of the terminal vascular bed. Exp. Mol. Pathol. 3:98, 1964.

Weibel, E. R., and Palade, G. E.: New cytoplasmic components in arterial endothelia. J. Cell Biol. 23:101, 1964.

Majno, G., Shea, S. M., and Leventhal, M.: Endothelial contraction induced by histamine type mediators. J. Cell Biol. 42:647, 1969.

Crocker, D. J., Murad, T. M., and Geer, J. C.: Role of the pericyte in wound healing. An ultrastructural study. Exp. Mol. Pathol. 13:51, 1970.

Sengel, A., and Stoebuer, P.: Golgi origin of tubular inclusions in endothelial cells. J. Cell Biol. 44:223, 1970.

Folkman, J.: Anti-angiogenesis: New concept for therapy of solid tumors. Ann. Surg. 175:409, 1972.

Becker, C. G., and Nachman, R. L.: Contractile proteins of endothelial cells, platelets and smooth muscle. Am. J. Pathol. 71:1, 1973.

Lewis, L. J., Hook, J. C., Maca, R. D., and Fry, G. L.: Replication of human endothelial cells in culture. Science 181:453, 1973.

Weber, K.: Ultrastructure of blood vessels in human granulation tissue. Arch. Dermatol. Forsch. 248:29, 1973.

Gabbiani, G., Badonnel, M. C., and Rona, G.: Cytoplasmic contractile apparatus in aortic endothelial cells of hypertensive rats. Lab. Invest. 32:227, 1975.

Handenschild, C. C., Zahniser, D., Folkman, J., and Klagsburn, M.: Human vascular endothelial cells in culture. Exp. Cell Res. 98:175, 1976.

Kelly, P. J., Suddith, R. L., Hutchinson, H. T., Werrback, K., and Haber, B.: Endothelial growth factor present in tissue culture of CNS tumor. J. Neurosurg. 44:343, 1976.

Toth, B., and Malick, L.: Scanning electron-microscopic study of the surface characteristics of neoplastic endothelial cells of blood vessels. J. Pathol. 118:59, 1976.

Macarak, E. J., Howard, B. V., and Kefalides, N. A.: Properties of calf endothelial cells in culture. Lab. Invest. 36:62, 1977.

Moore, A., Jaffe, E. A., Becker, C. G., and Nachman, R. L.: Myosin in cultured human endothelial cells. Br. J. Haematol. 35:71, 1977.

Wagenaar, S. Sc., and Wagenvoort, C. A.: Experimental production of longitudinal smooth muscle cells in the intima of muscular arteries. Lab. Invest. 39:370, 1978.

Wall, R. T., Harker, L. A., and Striker, G. E.: Human endothelial cell migration. Stimulation by a released platelet factor. Lab. Invest. 39:523, 1978.

NON-NEOPLASTIC LESIONS

Hunter, W.: Observations upon a particular species of aneurisms. Med. Obs. Soc. Phy. 2:350, 1762.

Lotzbeck, C.: Ein Fall von Schweissdrusengeschwulst an der Wange. Virchows Arch. [Pathol. Anat.] 16:160, 1859.

Babbington, B. G.: Hereditary epistaxis. Lancet 2:362, 1865.

Chiari, O.: Erfahrungen auf dem Gebiete der Hals-und-Nasen-Krankheiten. Vienna, Toepflitz and Deuticke, 1887.

Rendu, M.: Epistaxis repetees chez un sujet porteux de petits angiomes cutanes et muqueux. Bull. Mem. Soc. Med. Hop. Paris 13:731, 1896.

Ullmann, K.: Ueben einen Fall von multipler eruptiver Angiombildung im Gesichte. Arch. Dermatol. Syphil. 35:195, 1896.

Osler, W.: On a family form of recurring epistaxis, associated with multiple telangiectases of the skin and mucous membrane. Johns Hopkins Med. J. 12:333, 1901.

Hartzell, M. B.: Granuloma pyogenicum. J. Cutan. Dis. 22:520, 1904.

Weber, F. P.: Multiple hereditary developmental angiomata (telangiectases) of the skin and mucous membranes associated with recurring hemorrhages. Lancet 2:160, 1907.

Hanes, F. M.: Multiple hereditary telangiectases causing hemorrhage (hereditary hemorrhagic telangiectasia). Johns Hopkins Med. J. 20:63, 1909.

Symmers, D.: Primary hemangiolymphoma of the hemal nodes—An unusual variety of malignant tumor. Arch. Intern. Med. 28:467, 1921.

Goldstein, H. I.: Goldstein's heredofamilial angiomatosis with recurring familial hemorrhages (Rendu-Osler-Weber's disease). Arch. Intern. Med. 48:836, 1931.

Castleman, B.: Massachusetts General Hospital Case Records: Hyperplasia of mediastinal lymph nodes. N. Engl. J. Med. 250:26, 1954.

Lawton, R. L., Tidnick, R. T., and Brintmall, E. S.: A clinicopathologic study of multiple congenital A-V fistulae of the lower extremities. Angiology 8:161, 1957.

Harrison, E. G., and Bernatz, P. E.: Angiofollicular mediastinal lymph node hyperplasia resembling thymoma. Arch. Pathol. 75:284, 1963.

Kawada, A. K., Takahashi, H., and Anzai, T.: Eosinophilic folliculosis of the skin (Kimura's disease). Jpn. J. Dermitol. 76:61, 1965.

Tung, K. S. K., and McCormack, L. J.: Angiomatous lymphoid hamartoma. Cancer 20:525, 1967.

Hyman, A. B., Harris, H., and Brownstein, M. H.: Eccrine angiomatous hamartoma. N.Y. State J. Med. 68:2803, 1968.

Pinkus, H., and Rudner, E.: How we treat granuloma pyogenicum. Postgrad. Med. 45:270, 1969.

Wells, G. G. and Whimster, I. W.: Subcutaneous angiolymphoid hyperplasia with eosinophilia. Br. J. Derm. 81:1, 1969.

Wilson-Jones, E., and Bleehen, S. S.: Inflammatory angiomatous nodules with abnormal blood vessels occurring about the ears and scalp (pseudo or atypical pyogenic granuloma). Br. J. Dermatol. 81:804, 1969.

Angelopoulos, A. P.: Pyogenic granuloma of the oral cavity: statistical analysis of its clinical features. J. Oral Surg. 29:840, 1971.

Boxer, L. A., Boxer, G. J., Flair, R. C., Engstrom, P. F., and Brown, G. S.: Angiomatous lymphoid hamartoma associated with chronic anemia, hypoferremia and hypergammaglobulinemia. J. Pediatr. 81:66, 1972.

Hashimoto, K., and Pritzker, M. S.: Hereditary hemorrhagic telangiectasia. An electron microscopic study. Oral Surg. 34:751, 1972.

Reed, R. J., and Terazakis, N.: Subcutaneous angioblastic lymphoid hyperplasia with eosinophilia (Kimura's disease). Cancer 29:489, 1972.

Madata, J., Shane, J., and Scarlato, M.: Systemic endotheliomatosis. A case report. J. Clin. Pathol. 28:476, 1975.

Sussman, E. B., and Sternberg, S. S.: Hereditary hemorrhagic telangiectasia. Arch. Pathol. 99:95, 1975.

Lie, J. T., Daniel, F. J., and Mullerworth, M. H.: Epicardial tumorlike angiofibromatous proliferative lesion. An unusual complication of coronary bypass surgery. J. Thorac. Cardiovasc. Surg. 71:517, 1976.

Adams, H. P., Subbiah, B., and Bosch, E. P.: Neurologic aspects of hereditary hemorrhagic telangiectasia. Arch. Neurol. 34:101, 1977.

Eady, R. A. J., and Jones, E. W.: Pseudopyogenic granuloma. Enzyme histochemical and ultrastructural study. Hum. Pathol. 8:653, 1977.

Muller, J. Y., Michialov, T., Israel, V., and Bernard, J.: Maladie de Rendu-Osler dans une grande famille saharienne, 87 cas dans la meme famille. Nouv. Presse Med. 7:1723, 1978.

Lie, J. T.: Disseminated visceral giant cell arteritis. Histopathologic description and differentiation from other granulomatous vasculitides. Am. J. Clin. Pathol. 69:299, 1978.

Mullich, F. G., McAllister, H. A., Wagner, B. M.,

and Fenoglio, J. J.: Drug related vasculitis. Hum. Pathol. 10:313, 1979.

NEOPLASTIC LESIONS

Hey, W.: Practical Observation in Surgery. London, Cadell and Davies, 1803.

Eberth, C. J.: Von den Blutgefassen. *In* Edited by S. Stricker. Handbuch der Lehre von den Geweben des Menschen und der Thiere. Leipzig, Engelmann, 1871.

Kaposi, M.: Idipatisches multiples pigmentsarkom der Haut. Arch. Dermatol. Syph. 4:265, 1872.

Rouget, C.: Note sur le developpment de la tunique contractile des vaisseaux. C R Hebd. Seances Acad. Sci. 79:559, 1874.

Hoyer, H.: Uber umittelbare Einmundung kleinster Arterien in Gefassaste venosen Charakters. Arch. mikr. Anat. 13:603, 1877.

Kolaczek, J.: Uber das Angio-Sarkom. Dsch. Zr. Chir. 9:1; 889, 1878.

Langhans, T.: Pulsirende cavernose Geschwulst der Milz mit metastatischen Knoten in der leber. Virchows Arch. 75:273, 1879.

Maffucci, A.: Di un case di encondrome ed angioma multiple contribuzione alla genesi embrionale dei tumor. Movimento Medicaochirurgico 3:399, 1881.

Chandelux, A.: Recherches histologiques sur les tubercles souscutanes douloureux. Arch. Physiol. Normal Pathol. 2:9;639, 1882.

Koebner, H.: Krankenvorstellung (Idiopathisches multiples sarcoma haemorrhagicum der extremitaten). Arch. Dermat. Syphil. 23:119, 1891.

Bloodgood, J. C.: Haemangiomatous elephantiasis. Prog. Med. 4:154, 1903.

Borrmann, R.: Metastasenbildung bei histologisch gutartigen Geschwulsten. Beitr. Pathol. Anat. 40:372, 1907.

Mallory, F. B.: The results of the application of special histological methods to the study of tumors. J. Exp. Med. 10:575, 1908.

Dalla Favera, G. B.: Sarcoma idiop. mult. haemorrh. con special reguardo alle sue localizzaaioni viscerali. G. Ital. Mal. Vener. 51:144, 1910.

Jaques, D.: Inertion and seat of rhinopharyngeal fibromata. Ann. Otol. Rhinol. Laryngol. 20:881, 1911.

Denker, A.: Zur operativen Behandlung der typischen Nasenrachenfibrome. Z. Ohrenheilk. 64:1, 1912.

Konjetzny, G. E.: Zur pathologie der Angiome. Munch. Med. Wochenschr. 59:241, 1912.

Aschoff, L., and Kiyono, Y.: Zur Frage der grossen Mononuclären. Folia Hematol. 15: 383, 1913.

Ehrmann, W. B.: Ein eigenartiges Angioliposarkom der Niere. Frankfurt Z. Pathol. 15:51, 1914.

Shennan, T.: Histologically nonmalignant angioma with numerous metastases. J. Pathol. Bacteriol. 19:139, 1914.

Delevan, D. B.: The effect of radioactivity upon nasopharyngeal fibromas. Med. Rec., 1915.

Sherill, G., and Graves, F. S.: Hemangioendothelioblastoma of the stomach. Surg. Gynecol. Obstet. 20:443, 1915.

Barre, J. A.: Troubles sympathiques etendus et violents du membre superieur par tumeur du doigt; guerison. Rev. Neurol. 34:942, 1920.

Cole, H. N., and Crump, E. S.: Report of two cases of idiopathic hemorrhagic sarcoma (Kaposi), the first complicated with lymphatic leukemia. Arch. Dermat. Syphil. 11:283, 1920.

Ewing, J.: Neoplastic Diseases, 2nd ed. Philadelphia, W. B. Saunders Co., 1922.

Masson, P.: Hemangioendotheliome vegetant intravasculaire. Bull. Soc. Anat. 93:517, 1923.

Zimmerman, K. W.: Der Feinerg Bau der Blutkapillaren Ertwick-lungsgesch. Z. Anat. 68:20, 1923.

Barre, J. A., and Masson, P.: Etude anatomoclinique de certaines tumeurs sousungueales douloureuses (tumeurs du glomus neuro-myoarterial des extremites). Bull. Soc. Franc. Dermat. Syphil. 31:148, 1924.

Masson, P.: Le glomus neuromyo-arterial des regions tactiles et ses tumeurs. Lyon chir. 21:257, 1924.

Cushing, H., and Bailey, P.: Tumors Arising From the Blood Vessels of the Brain. Angiomatous Malformations and Hemangioblastomas. Springfield, Illinois, Charles C Thomas Company, 1928.

Wright, A. W.: Primary malignant hemangioma of the spleen with multiple liver metastases. Am. J. Pathol. 4:507, 1928.

Burman, M. S., and Milgram, J. E.: Haemangioma of tendon and tendon sheaths. Surg. Gynecol. Obstet. 50:397, 1930.

Cooper, T. V.: Case of "perithelioma" of fascial origin, with direct antecedent history of trauma. Lancet 2:1234, 1930.

Dorffel, J.: Histogenesis of multiple idiopathic hemorrhagic sarcoma of Kaposi. Arch. Dermat. Syphil. 26:608, 1932.

Jenkins, J. P., and Delaney, P. A.: Benign angiomatous tumors of skeletal muscle. Surg. Gynecol. Obstet. 55:464, 1932.

Lane, C. G. and Greenwood, A. M.: Lymphoblastoma (Mycosis Fungoides) and hemorrhagic sarcoma of Kaposi in the same person. Arch. Dermat. Syphil. 27:643, 1933.

Orsos, F.: Gefassprossgeschwulst (Gemmangioma). Beitr. Pathol. Anat. 93:121, 1934.

Popoff, N. W.: The digital vascular system with reference to the state of glomus in inflammation, arteriosclerotic gangrene, diabetic

gangrene, thrombo-angiitis obliterans and supernumerary digits in man. Arch. Pathol. 18:295, 1934.
Bailey, O. T.: The cutaneous glomus and its tumors—glomangiomas. Am. J. Pathol. 11:915, 1935.
Geschickter, C. F., and Keasbey, L. E.: Tumors of blood vessels. Am. J. Cancer 25:568, 1935.
Robinson, J. M., and Castleman, B.: Benign metastasizing hemangioma. Ann. Surg. 104:436, 1936.
Schmidt, H.: Zur Kenntnis des Gemmangioms und seiner Beziehungen zum Angiosarkom. Frankfurt Z. Pathol. 51:43, 1937.
Becker, W., and Thatcher, H. W.: Multiple idiopathic hemorrhagic sarcoma of Kaposi. J. Invest. Dermatol. 1:379, 1938.
Choisser, R. M., and Ramsey, E. M.: Angioreticuloendothelioma (Kaposi's disease) of the heart. Am. J. Pathol. 15:155, 1939.
Plaut, A.: Hemangio-endothelioma of lung. Two cases. Arch. Pathol. 29:517, 1940.
Watson, W. L., and McCarthy, W. D.: Blood and lymph vessel tumors: a report of 1,056 cases. Surg. Gynecol. Obstet. 71:569, 1940.
Vejlens, G.: Specific pulmonary alterations in tuberous sclerosis. Acta Pathol. Microbiol. Scand. 18:317, 1941.
Aegerter, E. E., and Peale, A. R.: Kaposi's sarcoma. A critical survey. Arch. Pathol. 34:413, 1942.
Murray, M. R., and Stout, A. P.: The glomus tumor: Investigation of its distribution and behavior, and the identity of its "epitheloid" cell. Am. J. Pathol. 18:183, 1942.
Stout, A. P., and Murray, M. R.: Hemangiopericytoma: A vascular tumor featuring Zimmerman's pericytes. Ann. Surg. 116:26, 1942.
Stout, A. P.: Hemangioendothelioma: a tumor of blood vessels featuring vascular endothelial cells. Ann. Surg. 118:445, 1943.
Mahaim, L.: Les tumeurs et les polyps du coeur. *In* Etude anatomoclinique. Paris, Masson, 1945.
Caro, M. R., and Stubenrauch, C. H.: Hemangioendothelioma of the skin. Arch. Dermatol. Syphil. 51:295, 1945.
Lange, H. F., and Christiansen, T.: Hemopericardium-angiosarcoma cordis. A case of primary heart tumor, diagnosed intra vitam. Acta Med. Scand. 127:107, 1947.
MacMahon, H. E., Murphy, A. S., and Bates, M. I.: Endothelial-cell sarcoma of the liver following Thorotrast injections. Am. J. Pathol. 23:585, 1947.
Tedeschi, C. G., Folsom, H. F., and Carnicelli, T. J.: Visceral Kaposi's disease. Arch. Pathol. 43:335, 1947.
Kuzman, J. F., and King, J. M.: Dyschondroplasia with hemangiomatosis (Maffucci syndrome) and teratoid tumor of the ovary. Arch. Pathol. 46:74, 1948.
Martin, H., Ehrlich, H. E., and Abels, J. C.: Juvenile nasopharyngeal angiofibroma. Ann. Surg. 127:153, 1948.
Stewart, F. W., and Treves, N.: Lymphangiosarcoma in postmastectomy lymphedema: A report of six cases in elephantiasis chirurgica. Cancer 1:64, 1948.
Kinkade, J. M.: Angiosarcoma: A review of the literature. Ann. Otol. Rhinol. 58:159, 1949.
Stout, A. P.: Hemangiopericytoma. A study of twenty-five new cases. Cancer 2:1027, 1949.
McCarthy, W. D., and Pack, G. T.: Malignant blood vessel tumor. A report of 56 cases of angiosarcoma and Kaposi's sarcoma. Surg. Gynecol. Obstet. 91:445, 1950.
Martorell, F.: Tumorigenic lymphedema. Angiology 2:386, 1951.
Prichard, R. W.: Tumors of the heart. Review of the subject and report of one hundred and fifty cases. Arch. Pathol. 31:98, 1951.
Stone, M. M., and Vincente, A. S.: Hemangioma intra-articular de la rodilla localizado en el menisco semilunar. Bol. Liga Cancer 26:27, 1951.
Bolck, F.: Die Endotheliome. Leipzig, 1952.
Fisher, E. R., Kaufman, N., and Mason, E. J.: Hemangiopericytoma histologic and tissue culture studies. Am. J. Pathol. 28:653, 1952.
Herrington, J. L.: Congenital angiomatous malformation involving the entire lower extremities. Surgery 34:759, 1953.
Stout, A. P.: Tumors of the soft tissues. Washington, D.C., Armed Forces Institute of Pathology, 1953.
Gorham, L. W., and Stout, A. P.: Hemangiomatosis and its relation to massive osteolysis. Trans. Assoc. Am. Physicians 67:302, 1954.
McCormack, L. J., and Gallivan, W. F.: Hemangiopericytoma. Cancer 7:595, 1954.
Sternberg, S. S.: Pathology of juvenile nasopharyngeal angiofibroma—A lesion of adolescent males. Cancer 7:15, 1954.
Bean, W. B.: Dyschondroplasia and hemangiomata (Maffucci's syndrome). Arch. Intern. Med. 95:767, 1955.
Enterline, H. T., and Roberts, B.: Lymphangiopericytoma. Cancer 8:582, 1955.
Southwick, H. E., and Slaughter, D. P.: Lymphangiosarcoma in post-mastectomy lymphedema. Five-year survival with irradiation treatment. Cancer 8:158, 1955.
Johnson, E. W., Ghormley, R. K., and Dockerty, M. B.: Hemangiomas of the extremities. Surg. Gynecol. Obstet. 102:531, 1956.
Landing, B. H., and Farber, S.: Tumors of the cardiovascular system. Atlas Tumor Pathol. (Washington) 3:7, 1956.
Bendeck, T. E., and Lichtenberg, F.: Cavernous hemangioma of striated muscle. Ann. Surg. 196:1011, 1957.
Bluefarb, S.: Kaposi's Sarcoma. Springfield, Illinois, Charles C Thomas Company, 1957.

Treves, N.: An evaluation of the etiological factors of lymphedema following radical mastectomy. An analysis of 1007 cases. Cancer 10:444, 1957.

Harma, R. A.: Nasopharyngeal angiofibroma. Acta Otolaryngol. 146:1, 1958.

Laipply, T. C., and Sherrick, J. C.: Intrathoracic angiomyomatous hyperplasia associated with chronic chylothorax. Lab. Invest. 7:378, 1958.

Oshner, S., and DeCamp, P. T.: Hemangiopericytoma of the lung. Ann. Rev. Tuber. 77:496, 1958.

Shurmond, T.: Hemangioendothelioma (angioplastic sarcoma). Br. J. Dermat. 70:132, 1958.

Crenshaw, J. F., Dowling, E. A., and Cresswell, W. F.: Primary hemangioendothelioma of the heart. Ann. Intern. Med. 50:1289, 1959.

Lampe, L., and Latourette, H. B.: The management of cavernous hemangiomas in infants. Pediatr. Clin. North Am. 6:511, 1959.

McConnell, E. M., and Haslam, P.: Angiosarcoma in postmastectomy lymphedema: A report of five cases and review of the literature. Br. J. Surg. 46:322, 1959.

Winer, L. H., and Levin, G. H.: Acquired vascular tumors of the skin in the adult. Arch. Dermatol. 79:17, 1959.

Dutz, W., and Stout, A. P.: Kaposi's sarcoma in infants and children. Cancer 13:684, 1960.

Fisher, J. R.: Hemangiopericytoma: A review of twenty cases. Can. Med. Assoc. J. 83:1136, 1960.

Kauffman, S. L., and Stout, A. P.: Hemangiopericytoma in children. Cancer 13:695, 1960.

Kauffman, S. L., and Stout, A. P.: Malignant hemangiopericytoma in infants and children. Cancer 14:1186, 1961.

Kohout, E., and Stout, A. P.: The glomus tumor in children. Cancer 14:555, 1961.

Russo, P. E., and Dewar, J. P.: Congenital lymphangioma. Am. J. Roentgenol. 85:726, 1961.

Daview, J. N. P.: Kaposi's sarcoma—A recent re-evaluation based on the disease in Africans. Acta Un. Int. Cancer 18:372, 1962.

Ecklung, R. E., and Valaitis, J.: Kaposi's sarcoma of lymph nodes. Arch. Pathol. 74:224, 1962.

Goidanich, J. G., and Campanacci, M.: Vascular hamartoma and infantile angioectatic osteohyperplasia of the extremities. J. Bone Joint Surg. 44A:815, 1962.

Keen, P.: Clinical features of Kaposi's sarcoma in South African Bantu. Acta Un. Int. Cancer 17:380–387, 1962.

Oettle, A. G.: Geographical and racial differences in the frequency of Kaposi's sarcoma—evidence of environmental or genetic causes. Acta Un. Int. Cancer 18:330, 1962.

Rice, J. S., and Fischer, D. S.: Blue rubber-bleb nevus syndrome. Arch. Dermatol. 86:503, 1962.

Taswell, H. F., Soule, E. H., and Conventry, M. B.: Lymphangiosarcoma arising in chronic lymphedematous extremities. J. Bone Joint Surg. 44A:277, 1962.

Barter, R. H., Letterman, G. S., and Schurter, M.: Hemangiomas in pregnancy. Am. J. Obstet. Gynecol. 87:625, 1963.

Bean, W. B., and Rather, J.: Universal angiomatosis. Arch. Intern. Med. 112:869, 1963.

Fink, H. E., and Oberman, H. A.: Hemangioendothelial cell sarcoma and hemangiopericytoma. Am. J. Roentgenol. 89:155, 1963.

Gorham, L. W.: Kaposi's sarcoma involving bone. Arch. Pathol. 76:465, 1963.

McNalley, M. C., Kelbe, D., Pryor, R., and Blount, S. G.: Angiosarcoma of the heart. Report of a case and review of the literature. Am. Heart J. 65:244, 1963.

Salm, R.: The nature of the so-called postmastectomy lymphangiosarcoma. J. Pathol. Bacteriol. 85:445, 1963.

Shugart, R. R., Soule, E. H., and Johnson, E. W.: Glomus tumor. Surg. Gynecol. Obstet. 117:334, 1963.

McCormack, L. J., and Gallivan, W. F.: Hemangiopericytoma. Cancer 17:595, 1964.

Rienhoff, W. F., Shellbey, W. M., and Cornell, W. P.: Lymphangiomatous malformation of thoracic duct associated with chylous pleural effusion. Ann. Surg. 159:180, 1964.

Cancilla, P. A., and Zimmerman, H. M.: The fine structure of a cerebellar hemangioblastoma. J. Neuropathol. Exp. Neurol. 24:621, 1965.

Cooper, A. G., and Bolande, R. P.: Multiple hemangiomas with cardiac hypertrophy. Pediatrics 35:28, 1965.

DeSilva Horta, J., Cayolla da Motta, L., Abbott, J. D., and Roriz, M. L.: Malignancy and other late effects following administration of Thorotrast. Lancet 2:201, 1965.

Gupta, R. K., Gilbert, E. F., and English, R. S.: Multiple painful glomus tumors of the skin. Arch. Dermatol. 92:670, 1965.

Hermann, J. B.: Lymphosarcoma of chronically edematous extremity. Surg. Gynecol. Obstet. 121:1107, 1965.

Lee, S. C. H., and Moore, O. S.: Kaposi's sarcoma of lymph nodes. Arch. Pathol. 80:651, 1965.

Meitner, E. R., and Pavur, J.: Uber einen Fall von Hemangiomatosis peritonei. Zentralb. Allg. Pathol. 107:28, 1965.

O'Brien, B., and Brasfield, R. D.: Hemangiopericytoma. Cancer 18:249, 1965.

Schock, J.: Die Elephantiasis der Extremitaten. Krankheitsbild Behandlung Z. Orthop. 99:361, 1965.

Steingaszner, L. C., Enzinger, F. M., and Taylor,

H. B.: Hemangiosarcoma of the breast. Cancer 18:352, 1965.

Cornog, J. L., and Enterline, H. T.: Lymphangiomyoma, a benign lesion of chyliferous lymphatics synonymous with lymphangiopericytoma. Cancer 19:1909, 1966.

Gray, G. F. Jr., Gonzalez-Licea, A., Hartmann, W. H., and Woods, A. C.: Angiosarcoma in lymphedema: An unusual case of Stewart-Treves syndrome. Bull. Johns Hopkins Hosp. 119:117, 1966.

O'Brien, P. H., and Brasfield, R. D.: Kaposi's sarcoma. Cancer 19:1497, 1966.

Reed, R. J., Palameque, F. E., Hairston, M. A., and Kremetz, E. T.: Lymphangiosarcoma of the scalp. Arch. Dermatol. 94:396, 1966.

Scott, W. P., and Voight, J. A.: Kaposi's sarcoma. Cancer 19:557, 1966.

Spiro, R. H., and McPeak, C. J.: On the so-called metastasizing leiomyoma. Cancer 19:546, 1966.

Svoboda, D. J., and Kirchner, F.: Ultrastructure of nasopharyngeal angiofibroma. Cancer 19:1949, 1966.

Baes, H.: Angiosarcoma in a chronic lymphedematous leg. Dermatology 134:331, 1967.

Danese, C. A., Grishman, E., Oh, C., and Dreiling, D. A.: Malignant vascular tumors of the lymphedematous extremity. Ann. Surg. 166:245, 1967.

Eby, C. S., Brennan, M. J., and Fine, G.: Lymphangiosarcoma. A lethal complication of chronic lymphedema. Arch. Surg. 94:223, 1967.

Prudden, J. F., and Worlarsky, E. R.: Lymphangiosarcoma of the thigh. Arch. Surg. 94:376, 1967.

Waddell, G. F.: A haemangioma involving tendons. J. Bone Joint Surg. 49B:138, 1967.

Davis, J.: Kaposi's sarcoma. N.Y. State J. Med. 68:2067, 1968.

Frack, M. D., Simon, L., and Dawson, B. H.: The lymphangiomatosis syndrome. Cancer 22:428, 1968.

Mazzaferri, E. L., and Penn, G. M.: Kaposi's sarcoma associated with multiple myeloma. Arch. Intern. Med. 122:521, 1968.

Murad, T. M., von Haam, E., and Murray, M. S. N.: Ultrastructure of a hemangiopericytoma and a glomus tumor. Cancer 22:1239, 1968.

Waiman, M.: Common hemangioma: to treat or not to treat. Postgrad. Med. 43:183, 1968.

Bredt, A. B., and Serpick, A. A.: Metastatic hemangiopericytoma treated with vincristine and Actinomycin D. Cancer 24:266, 1969.

Bush, J. K., McLean, R. L., and Sicker, H. O.: Diffuse lung disease due to lymphangiomyoma. Am. J. Med. 46:645, 1969.

Busk, K.: Hemangiopericytoma. Am. J. Surg. 35:351, 1969.

Dabska, M.: Malignant endovascular papillary angioendothelioma of the skin in childhood. Clinicopathologic study of six cases. Cancer 24:503, 1969.

Gulesserian, H. P., and Lawton, R. I.: Angiosarcoma of the breast. Cancer 24:1021, 1969.

Hajdu, S. I., and Foote, F. W.: Angiomyolipoma of the kidney: Report of 27 cases and review of the literature. J. Urol. 102:396, 1969.

Kuhn, C., and Rosai, J.: Tumors arising from pericytes—ultrastructure and organ culture of a case. Arch. Pathol. 88:653, 1969.

Mahnke, P. F.: Klassifikation, Histogenese und pathologische Anatomie der Hamangiome und Lymphangiome. Zr. Aerztl. Fortbild. 63:474, 1969.

Nemoto, T., Stubre, N., Gaeta, J., and Dao, T.: Pathogenesis of lymphangiosarcoma following mastectomy and irradiation. Surg. Gynecol. Obstet. 128:489, 1969.

Siegel, J. H., Janis, R., Alper, J. C., Schutte, H., Robbins, L., and Blaufox, M. D.: Disseminated visceral Kaposi's sarcoma. JAMA 207:143, 1969.

Tannovski, W. M., and Hashimoto, K.: Multiple glomus tumor. An ultrastructural study. J. Invest. Dermatol. 52:470, 1969.

Toker, C.: Glomangioma. An ultrastructural study. Cancer 23:487, 1969.

Tragus, E. T., and Wagner, D. E.: Current therapy for postmastectomy lymphangiosarcoma. Arch. Surg. 97:839, 1969.

Venkatachalam, M. A., and Greally, J. G.: Fine structure of glomus tumor: similarity of glomus cells to smooth muscle. Cancer 23:1176, 1969.

Walker-Smith, J. A., Rye, R. D. K., Soutter, G. B., and Kenrick, K. G.: Small intestinal lymphangioma. Arch. Dis. Child. 44:527, 1969.

Buckwinkel, K. D., and Diddams, J. A.: Hemangiopericytoma—Report of a case and comprehensive review of the literature. Cancer 25:896, 1970.

Farr, H. W., Carandang, C. M., and Huvos, A. G.: Malignant vascular tumors of the head and neck. Am. J. Surg. 120:501, 1970.

Finaly-Jones, L. R.: Lymphangiosarcoma of the thigh. Cancer 26:722, 1970.

Hall, R. M., and Odell, J. E.: An unusually large glomangioma simulating osteoarthritis of the hip. JAMA 214:1562, 1970.

Pitkethy, D. T., Hardman, J. M., Kempe, L. G., and Earle, K. M.: Angioblastic meningiomas, clinicopathologic study of 81 cases. J. Neurosurg. 32:539, 1970.

Slavin, S. G., Cameron, H. M., Forbes, C., and Mitchell, R. M.: Kaposi's sarcoma in East African children: Report of 51 cases. J. Pathol. 100:187, 1970.

Glaser, A., and Forster, P.: Das Lymphangiosarkom einer lymphodematosen Extremitat

(Stewart-Treves-Syndrom). Zentralbl. Chir. 96:584, 1971.

Goodman, T. F., and Abele, D. C.: Multiple glomus tumors. Arch. Dermatol. 103:11, 1971.

Harris, M.: Electron microscopy of a glomus tumor. J. Clin. Pathol. 24:520, 1971.

Hollmann, G., Hopner, F., and Daum, R.: Beitraf zur Klinik des Hamangiopericytoma. Langenbecks Arch. Chir. 330:128, 1971.

Kessler, E., and Kozenitzky, I. L.: Hemangiosarcoma of breast. J. Clin. Pathol. 24:530, 1971.

Merrick, T. A., Erlandson, R. A., and Hajdu, S. I.: Lymphangiosarcoma of a congenitally lymphedematous arm. Arch. Pathol. 91:365, 1971.

Mount, B. M., Hajdu, S. I., and Whitmore, W. F.: Retroperitoneal angiomyosarcoma. J. Urol. 106:837, 1971.

Saha, S. P., Thompson, R., and Still, R.: Angiosarcoma of the breast. South. Med. J. 64:1376, 1971.

Silverberg, S. G., Wilson, M. A., and Board, J. A.: Hemangiopericytoma of the uterus. An ultrastructure study. Am. J. Obstet. Gynecol. 110:397, 1971.

Adams, Y. G., Huvos, A. G., and Hajdu, S. I.: Malignant vascular tumors of liver. Ann. Surg. 173:375, 1972.

Allan, P. W., and Enzinger, F. M.: Hemangioma of skeletal muscle. Cancer 29:8, 1972.

Cunningham, J. J., and Winningham, D. C.: Retroperitoneal cystic lymphangioma presenting as an unusual pelvic mass. J. Urol. 108:717, 1972.

Davis, Z., Berliner, W. P., Weiland, L. H., and Clagett, O. T.: Primary pulmonary hemangiopericytoma. J. Thorac. Cardiovasc. Surg. 64:822, 1972.

English, G. M., Hemenway, W. G., and Cundy, R. L.: Surgical treatment of invasive angiofibroma. Arch. Otolaryngol. 96:312, 1972.

Grode, M. L.: Hemangiopericytoma of central nervous system. N.Y. State J. Med. 15:2557, 1972.

Levan, N. E., Korn, C. S., Booher, J., and Rounds, D. E.: Tissue culture of Kaposi's sarcoma. Arch. Dermatol. 106:37, 1972.

Templeton, A. C.: Studies in Kaposi's sarcoma. Cancer 30:854, 1972.

Woodward, A. H., Ivins, J. C., and Soule, E. H.: Lymphangiosarcoma arising in chronic lymphedematous extremities. Cancer 30: 652, 1972.

Fine, G., and Morales, A. R.: The ultrastructure of the "normal" human glomus apparatus of the nail bed. Am. J. Clin. Pathol. 60:131, 1973.

Joliat, G., Stalder, H., and Kapanci, Y.: Lymphangiomyomatosis: a clinico-anatomical entity. Cancer 31:455, 1973.

Kawamura, J., Garcia, J. H., and Kamijyo, Y.: Cerebellar hemangioblastoma: Histogenesis of stroma cells. Cancer 31:1528, 1973.

McSwain, B., Whitehead, W., and Bennett, L.: Angiosarcoma: report of three cases of postmastectomy lymphangiosarcoma and one of hemangiosarcoma. South. Med. J. 66:102, 1973.

Neel, H. B., Whicker, J. H., Devine, K. D., and Weiland, L. H.: Juvenile angiofibroma. Review of 120 cases. Am. J. Surg. 126:547, 1973.

Wolff, M.: Lymphangiomyoma—Clinicopathologic study and ultrastructural confirmation of its histogenesis. Cancer 31:988, 1973.

Beal, J. M.: Hemangiosarcoma of breast. Ill. Med. J. 146:39, 1974.

Creech, J. L., and Johnson, M. N.: Angiosarcoma of liver in the manufacture of polyvinyl chloride. J. Occup. Med. 16:150, 1974.

Gambardella, R. J.: Kaposi's sarcoma and its oral manifestations. Oral Surg. 38:591, 1974.

Gerner, R. E., Moore, G. E., and Pichren, J. W.: Hemangiopericytoma. Ann. Surg. 179:128, 1974.

Lee, F. I., and Harry, D. S.: Angiosarcoma of the liver in a vinyl-chloride worker. Lancet 2:1316, 1974.

Meade, J. B., Whitwell, F., Bickford, B. J., and Waddington, J. K. B.: Primary haemangiopericytoma of lung. Thorax 29:1, 1974.

Sussman, E. B., Nydick, I., and Gray, G. F.: Hemangioendothelial sarcoma of the liver and hemochromatosis. Arch. Pathol. 97:39, 1974.

Corring, B., Liebow, A. A., and Friedman, P. J.: Pulmonary lymphangiomyomatosis. Am. J. Pathol. 79:348, 1975.

Das, H. K., Sengupta, P., and Sarkar, S. K.: Angiofibroma of the nasopharynx. J. Indian Med. Assoc. 65:258, 1975.

Gray, S. R., Carrington, C. B., and Cornog, J. L.: Ureteral involvement and chyluria in lymphangiomatosis. Cancer 35:490, 1975.

Houston, W., Pontin, A., Kuhn, T., and Mambo, N.: Kaposi's sarcoma of the penis. Br. J. Urol. 47:315, 1975.

Kalish, M., Dorr, R., and Hoskins, P.: Retroperitoneal cystic lymphangioma. Urology 6:503, 1975.

Kaufman, S. D., and Scully, R. E.: Pericardial effusion and cutaneous hemangiomas. N. Engl. J. Med. 293:494, 1975.

Kermarec, J., and Varini, J. P.: Etude microscopique et ultrastructural d'une tumeur de Stewart-Treves. Archiv. Anat. Pathol. 23:193, 1975.

Kings, G. L. M.: Multifocal haemangiomatous malformation. A case report. Thorax 30:485, 1975.

Krishan, M., Panicker, C., and Thomas,

W. M. C.: Malignant pulmonary hemangiopericytoma. Aust. N. Z. J. Surg. 45:157, 1975.

McMaster, M. J., Soule, E. H., and Ivins, J. C.: Hemangiopericytoma. A clinicopathologic study and long-term follow-up of 60 patients. Cancer 36:2232, 1975.

Nagashima, C., Takahama, M., Nakayama, Y., and Asano, T.: Giant occipital hemangioendothelioma with thrombocytopenia, anemia and hypofibrinogenemia. Case report. J. Neurosurg. 43:74, 1975.

Rwomushana, R. J. W., Bailey, I. C., and Kyalwazi, S. K.: Kaposi's sarcoma of the brain. A case report with necropsy findings. Cancer 36:1127, 1975.

Salyer, W. R., and Salyer, D. C.: Intravascular angiomatosis. Development and distinction from angiosarcoma. Cancer 36:995, 1975.

Schow, S. R., Nespeca, J. A., Goyette, R. E., and Hunsuck, E. E.: Juvenile hemangioendothelioma. Report of case and review of the literature. J. Oral. Surg. 33:868, 1975.

Scott, M. B., Halpern, M., and Cosgrove, M. D.: Renal angiomyolipoma. Two varieties. Urology 6:768, 1975.

Wilbanks, G. D., Szymanska, Z., and Miller, A. W.: Pelvic hemangiopericytoma. Report of four patients and review of the literature. Am. J. Obstet. Gynecol. 123:555, 1975.

Bissada, N. K., and Redman, J. F.: Renal angiomyolipoma. South. Med. J. 69:205, 1976.

Bommer, G., Altenahr, E., Kuhnau, J., Jr., and Kloppel, G.: Ultrastructure of hemangiopericytoma associated with paraneoplastic hypoglycemia. Z. Krebsforsch. 85:231, 1976.

Boone, C. W., Takeichi, N., Paranjpe, M., and Gilden, R.: Vasoformative sarcomas arising from BABL/3T3 cells attached to solid substrates. Cancer Res. 36:1626, 1976.

Clearkin, K. P., and Enzinger, F. M.: Intravascular papillary endothelial hyperplasia. Cancer 38:1227, 1976.

Dunegan, L. J., Tobon, H., and Watson, C. G.: Angiosarcoma of the breast. A report of two cases and a review of the literature. Surgery 79:57, 1976.

Enzinger, F. M., and Smith, B. H.: Hemangiopericytoma. An analysis of 106 cases. Hum. Pathol. 7:61, 1976.

Feigin, I., Ransohoff, J., and Lieberman, A.: Sarcoma arising in oligodendroglioma of the brain. J. Neuropathol. Exp. Neurol. 35:679, 1976.

Gokel, J. M., Kurzl, R., and Hubner, G.: Fine structure and origin of Kaposi's sarcoma. Pathol. Eur. 11:45, 1976.

Hardy, M. A., Goldfarb, P., Levine, S., Dattner, A., Muggia, F. M., Levitt, S., and Weinstein, E.: De novo Kaposi's sarcoma in renal transplantation. Cancer 38:144, 1976.

Kuo, T., Sayers, P., and Rosai, J.: Masson's "vegetant intravascular hemangioendothelioma": A lesion often mistaken for angiosarcoma. Cancer 38:1227, 1976.

Kurrein, F.: Systemic angioendotheliomatosis with metastases. J. Clin. Pathol. 29:347, 1976.

Makk, L., Delmore, F., Creech, J. L., Ogdon, L. L., Fadell, E. H., Sungster, C. L., Clanton, J., Johnson, M. N., and Christopherson, W. M.: Clinical and morphologic features of hepatic angiosarcoma in vinyl chloride workers. Cancer 37:149, 1976.

Nelson, L. M., and Gabbe, S. G.: Massive hemangiomas and lymphangiomas causing dystocia. Am. J. Obstet. Gynecol. 126:1044, 1976.

Paik, H. H., and Komorowski, R.: Hemangiosarcoma of the abdominal wall following irradiation therapy of endometrial carcinoma. Am. J. Clin. Pathol. 66:810, 1976.

Ramos, C. V., Taylor, H. B., Hernandez, B. A., and Tucker, E. F.: Primary Kaposi's sarcoma of lymph nodes. Am. J. Clin. Pathol. 66:948, 1976.

Rosai, J., Sumner, H. W., Kostianovsky, M., and Perez-Mesa, C.: Angiosarcoma of the skin. A clinicopathologic and fine structural study. Hum. Pathol. 7:83, 1976.

Rossi, N. P., Kioschos, J. M., Aschenbrener, C. A., and Ehrenhaft, J. L.: Primary angiosarcoma of the heart. Cancer 37:891, 1976.

Vazquez, J. J., Fernandez-Cuervo, L., and Fidalgo, B.: Lymphangiomyomatosis. Cancer 37:2321, 1976.

Yadav, R. V. S., Sahariah, S., Mittal, V. K., and Banerjee, A. K.: Angiosarcoma of the male breast. Int. Surg. 61:463, 1976.

Brady, J., Liberatore, F., Harper, P., Greenwald, P., Burnett, W., Davies, J. N. P., Bishop, M., Polan, A., and Vianna, N.: Angiosarcoma of the liver: An epidemiologic study. J. Natl. Cancer Inst. 59:1383, 1977.

Bricklin, A. S., and Rushton, H. W.: Angiosarcoma of venous origin arising in radial nerve. Cancer 39:1556, 1977.

Curran, K. L., Kupchella, C. E., and Tamburro, C. H.: Urinary glycosaminoglycan patterns in angiosarcoma of the liver. Cancer 40:3050, 1977.

Eimoto, T.: Ultrastructure of an infantile hemangiopericytoma. Cancer 40:2161, 1977.

Langier, P., Olmos, L., Posternak, F., and Harms, M.: Angioendotheliome malin. Ann. Dermatol. Venerol. 104:557, 1977.

Mira, J. G., Chu, F. C., and Fortner, J. G.: The role of radiation therapy in the management of malignant hemangiopericytoma. Cancer 39:1254, 1977.

Nicholson, W. J.: Cancer following occupational exposure to asbestos and vinyl chloride. Cancer 39:1792, 1977.

Taxy, J. B.: Juvenile nasopharyngeal angiofibroma. Cancer 39:1044, 1977.

Taylor, J. F., Iversen, O. H., and Bjerknes, R.: Growth kinetics of Kaposi's sarcoma. Br. J. Cancer 35:470, 1977.

Waldo, E. D., Vuletin, J. C., and Kaye, G. I.: The ultrastructure of vascular tumors: Additional observations and a review of the literature. *In* Pathology Annual, Part 2. Edited by S. C. Sommers and P. P. Rosen. New York, Appleton-Century-Crofts, 1977.

Angervall, L., Kindblom, L-G., Nielsen, J. M., Stener, B., and Svendsen, P.: Hemangiopericytoma. A clinicopathologic augiographic and microangiographic study. Cancer 42:2412, 1978.

Biller, H. G.: Juvenile nasopharyngeal angiofibroma. Ann. Otol. Rhinol. Laryngol. 87:630, 1978.

Chaudhry, A. P., Montes, M., and Cohn, G. A.: Ultrastructure of cerebellar hemangioblastoma. Cancer 42:1834, 1978.

Feldman, P. S., Shneidman, D., and Kaplan, C.: Ultrastructure of infantile hemangioendothelioma of the liver. Cancer 42:521, 1978.

Goellner, J. R., Laws, E. R., Soule, E. H., and Okazaki, H.: Hemangiopericytoma of the meninges. Am. J. Clin. Pathol. 70:375, 1978.

Klepp, O., Dahl, O., and Stenwig, J. T.: Association of Kaposi's sarcoma and prior immunosuppressive therapy. A 5-year material of Kaposi's sarcoma in Norway. Cancer 42:2626, 1978.

Kreisman, H., Robitaille, Y., Dionne, G. P., and Palayew, M. J.: Lymphangiomyomatosis syndrome with hyperparathyroidism. Cancer 42:364, 1978.

Masin, M., and Masin, F.: Cytology of angiosarcoma of the breast. A case report. Acta Cytol. 22:162, 1978.

Popper, H., Thomas, L. B., Telles, N. C., Falk, H., and Selikoff, I. J.: Development of hepatic angiosarcoma in man induced by vinyl chloride, Thorotrast and Arsenic. Am. J. Pathol. 92:349, 1978.

Prioleau, P. G., and Santa Cruz, D. J.: Lymphangioma circumscriptum following radical mastectomy and radiation therapy. Cancer 42:1989, 1978.

Taxy, J. B., and Gray, S. R.: Cellular angiomas of infancy. An ultrastructural study of two cases. Cancer 43:2322, 1979.

chapter 7

Tumors of Peripheral Nerves

NON-NEOPLASTIC LESIONS
- ***Degeneration***
- ***Hypertrophy***
- ***Traumatic Neuroma***
  - Morton's Neuroma

NEOPLASTIC LESIONS
- ***Collagenous Schwannoma***
  - Neurofibroma
  - Neurofibromatosis
  - Angioneuroma
  - Plexiform Neuroma
  - Pacinian Neurofibroma
  - Glandular Schwannoma
  - Pleomorphic Schwannoma
  - Cystic Schwannoma
  - Neurofibrosarcoma
- ***Non-Collagenous Schwannoma***
  - Storiform Schwannoma
  - Epithelioid Schwannoma
  - Undifferentiated Schwannoma
- ***Neurogenic Sarcoma***
- ***Primitive Neuroectodermal Tumor***
- ***Neuroblastoma***
- ***Ganglioneuroblastoma***
- ***Ganglioneuroma***
- ***Paraganglioma***
  - Pheochromocytoma

THE peripheral nervous system is composed of *sensory neurons, motor neurons,* and *autonomic neurons* that are found outside of the central nervous system. The *Schwann cell,* the peripheral nervous system counterpart of the central nervous system oligodendrocyte, is a pluripotential supporting cell of the cell processes, axons, of peripheral nerves. *Undifferentiated neural crest cells* contribute most of the cells of the *nerve sheaths* and most of the *neuroblasts* and *chromaffin* or *paraganglionic cells* of the autonomic nervous system (Fig. 7-1) (Key and Retzius, 1876; Weston, 1970).

The division of the nervous system into *central* and *peripheral* parts is artificial and an oversimplification of a complex organ system. The embryonal neuroectoderm is the progenitor of most of the cells of the nervous system. Its differentiation into glial elements in the central nervous system and a complex of Schwann cells and perineurial cells enveloped in the peripheral apparatus does not exclude structural overlapping of the two systems. Raine (1976) observed that peripheral nervous system components can occur normally in the central nervous system and may be etiologically related to proliferation of peripheral nervous system elements frequently found in a number of central nervous system disorders, e.g., syringomyelia, tuberous sclerosis, and various gliomas.

The uncommon but distinct overlapping morphology of neoplastic nerve sheath cells (Schwann cells and perineurial cells) and nerve cells (neuroblasts and chromaffin cells), e.g., in ganglioneuromas, primitive neuroectodermal tumors, and so-called nevoid or epithelioid schwannomas indicates retention of embryonal potentials. The occasional occurrence of neuroblastoma with neurofibroma or malignant melanoma with neurofibroma in the same patient further underlines the intricate intermingling of nerve cells and supportive neural elements in the peripheral nervous system.

The *nerve trunks* of peripheral nerves are composed of *nerve fascicles* or *nerve*

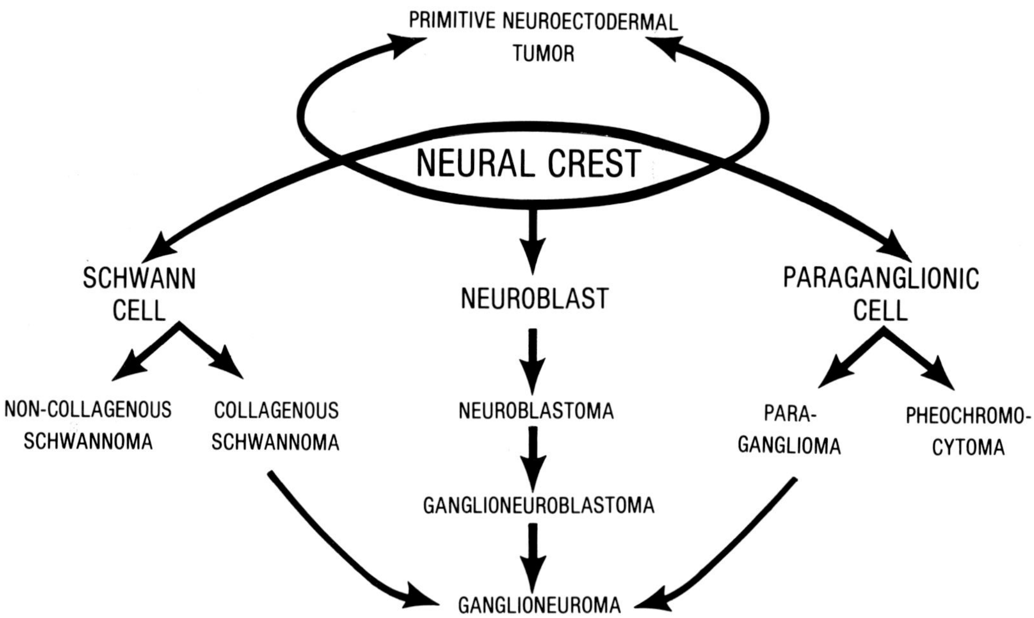

Figure 7-1. Schematic illustration of development and path of differentiation of neoplasms of the peripheral nervous system. Although an admixture of undifferentiated elements in the form of primitive neuroectodermal tumor is not uncommon, differentiated tumors rarely contain mixed elements.

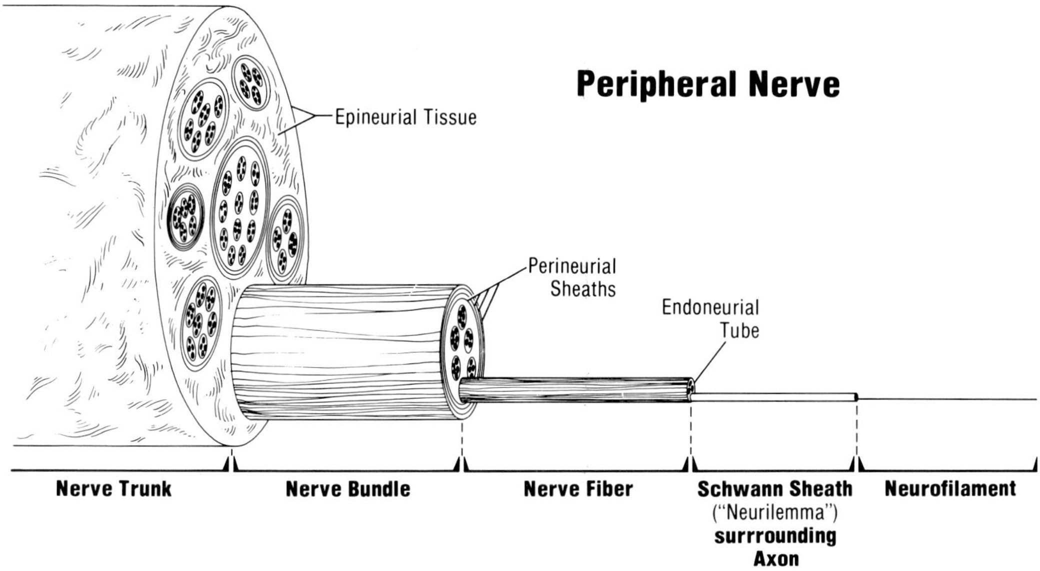

Figure 7-2. Cross section of a peripheral nerve trunk. Nerve bundles are held together by the epineurial fibroadipose tissue. The epineurium is separated from the endoneurium by the perineurial cells. Each axon is surrounded by a continuous network of Schwann cells in its entire length.

bundles. The nerve fascicles are held together by fibrovascular and fibroadipose tissues of the *epineurium.* Each individual fascicle is surrounded by a number of flattened, circularly oriented perineurial cells. The specialized nature of the concentrically arranged perineurial cell has been recorded in a number of reports (Thomas, 1963; Gamble and Eames, 1964; Cravioto, 1965; Waggener and Beggs, 1967) (Fig. 7-2).

The ultrastructure of perineurial cells shows the presence of well-developed basement membrane, pinocytotic vesicles, and cytoplasmic myofilaments within each cell. The cells are held together by tight junctions creating an almost impermeable perineural barrier. Cells of clearly fibroblastic nature can be seen to extend at irregular intervals between the perineurial cells. On the basis of ultrastructural studies it is evident that certain perineurial cells contain filaments similar to those observed in smooth muscle. The contractile property of perineurial cells is almost certainly responsible for the typical wavy or undulating appearance of peripheral nerves. According to Ross and Reith (1969) perineurial cells may also have the ability to retract or shorten the nerve, as needed, when sectioned or at the time of body movement.

Perineurial cells were originally described by Key and Retzius, in 1876, as endothelial-like cells. Santhaveerappa and Bourne (1966), who studied perineurial cells in various species of animals, including man, came to the conclusion that the multilayered perineurial membrane covering individual nerve fasciculi is composed of epithelial cells and is the direct continuation of the pia-arachnoid mater of the central nervous system (Fig. 7-5).

The *endoneurium* is a conglomerate of delicate fibroconnective tissue that occupies the space between nerve fibers and perineurial cells. The majority of the endoneurial cells are Schwann cells.

Schwann cells surround every axon, both myelinated and unmyelinated, in the peripheral nervous system and form the *axon-Schwann cell unit.* Schwann cells possess basement membrane, microfibrils, microtubules, mitochondria, membrane-bound granular or laminar perinuclear, so-called pi granules, clumps of glycogen, and an assortment of dense bodies. The role and function of Schwann cells is poorly understood, but they are considered *pluripotential primitive cells* which can multiply and proliferate like fibroblasts and assume phagocytic properties by converting into histiocytes. The endoneurium also contains a few haphazardly arranged fibroblasts, but most cells in the endoneurium are Schwann cells. After growing schwannomas in tissue culture, Murray and Stout, in 1942, observed that "Schwann cells can and do form collagen and reticulin." The distinction between Schwann cells and fibroblasts at light microscopic level is narrow. The characteristic bulging of Schwann cells is caused by the well-defined oval nuclei that are much wider than the narrow cytoplasmic ribbons containing them. The diameters of the nuclei of fibroblasts, on the other hand, are considerably smaller than those of Schwann cells (Fig. 7-3).

Since Harrison, in 1924, demonstrated the origin of Schwann cells from the neural crest, voluminous literature has accumulated on the role and nature of these cells. It has been shown that Schwann cells multiply after nerve injury (Romine et al, 1976). However, the precise nature of the trigger mechanism for Schwann cell proliferation remains to be known. The pluripotential nature of Schwann cells

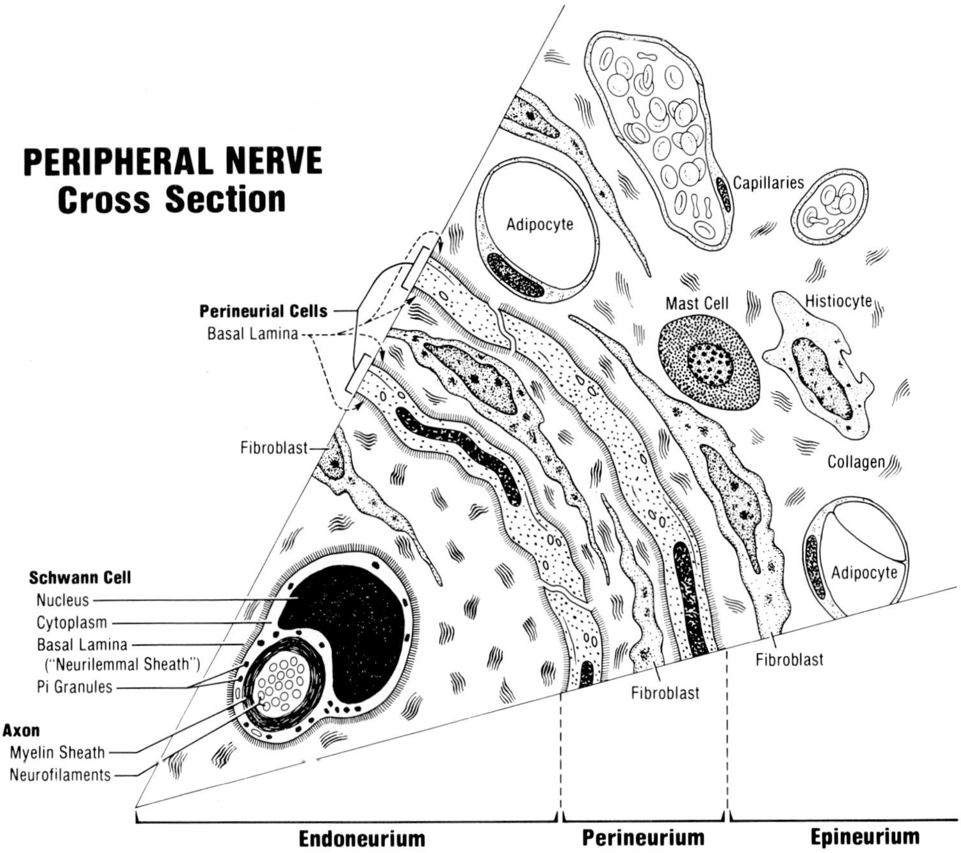

Figure 7-3. The endoneurium is a delicate layer of loosely arranged connective tissue surrounding each nerve fiber. The endoneurial tube contains the axon, Schwann cells, and myelin (in case of myelinated fibers). The neurilemma is nothing else than the basal lamina of Schwann cells and sheath of Plenck and Laidlow surrounding the Schwann cells. The perineurium is composed of several laminated and partly collagenous sheaths of perineurial cells and fibroblasts. Internally it is sharply demarcated from the endoneurium; however, externally it merges with the fibroadipose elements of the epineurium.

has been documented by many investigators (Cravioto, 1965; Sunderland, 1965; Ross, 1969; Church et al, 1973; Martin and Webster, 1973; Brown et al, 1976). The identification of ciliated Schwann cells by Bunge et al, in 1967, indicates that Schwann cells are able to assume forms and shapes of various mesenchymal cells, e.g., fibroblasts, myoblasts, chondroblasts, and osteoblasts but can also revert to a primitive neuroepithelial form.

NON-NEOPLASTIC LESIONS

The discussion of non-neoplastic lesions of peripheral nerves is not intended to be all inclusive or detailed. The literature on this topic is voluminous. Interested readers may find it useful to read some of the articles and books listed in the references at the end of the chapter, among which is the comprehensive text by Asbury and Johnson (1978).

DEGENERATION

Of the basic morphologic changes taking place in various neuropathies, only degeneration and hypertrophy of peripheral nerves will be considered. Although the three basic processes—*wallerian degeneration, segmental demyelination,* and *axonal degeneration*—have many common features, the pathomechanism in each process is quite different.

Wallerian degeneration, in most instances, is the result of transection of an axon. Almost immediately following laceration of the axon, perineurial cells and Schwann cells proliferate with alteration; later, the myelin sheath and axon are completely destroyed. Unmyelinated fibers appear to degenerate more rapidly and more extensively than myelinated nerve fibers. In due time histiocytes, macrophages, fibroblasts, and other reactive cells appear either by transformation of Schwann cells or from blood-borne mesenchymal cells (Thomas, 1964). If regeneration from the proximal stump does not take place, the myelin sheath and axoplasm will break up. The Schwann tubes shrink, and the nerve is replaced by connective tissue. In case of a motor nerve, the related muscle undergoes *denervation atrophy*. Singer and Steinberg (1972) believe that the Schwann cells are the agents responsible for the destruction of axons, as well as myelin sheaths, by invading the axoplasm.

During regeneration, however, proliferating Schwann cells, with generous complements of collagenous fibroblasts and perineurial cells, also provide guidance for axons. Regenerating axons that lose their way either disappear or convolute to form the so-called *traumatic neuroma*.

Degeneration of peripheral nerves by segmental demyelination can be induced by bacterial toxins, alcohol, and uremia, among other things, and malignant neoplasms. Demyelination has a random pattern and usually begins by detachment of myelin loops from the axolemma at the node of Ranvier. The process of remyelinization begins by elongation and convolution of the surface membrane of the Schwann cell about the axon. Related muscle may show disuse atrophy due to conduction block, but recovery is rapid and usually complete once the new myelin has been laid down (Kashef and Das Gupta, 1967; Lampert and Schochet, 1962; Warrell et al, 1968; Wisniewski et al, 1969; Dayan et al, 1970; Towfighi et al, 1976; Asbury, 1977).

Axonal degeneration means changes in the entire neuron by concomitant break down of myelin sheath and the axon. It can be induced by a number of metabolic derangements, e.g., vitamin deficiency, uremia, diabetes mellitus, amyloidosis, and malabsorption. The process of degeneration is centripetal and affects the largest myelinated nerve fibers first. Proliferation of Schwann cells begins simultaneously with axonal degeneration. Regeneration will take place eventually, but it is more protracted than in wallerian degeneration. It is perhaps important to point out that the exact pathomechanism of axonal degeneration has yet to be discovered, despite the fact that there are scores of substances and metabolic abnormalities known to be capable of inducing it (Table 7-1) (Eames and Lange, 1967; Dayan et al, 1970; Henson and Urich, 1970; Dyck et al, 1975; Asbury and Johnson, 1978).

HYPERTROPHY

Hypertrophy of peripheral nerves is a frequently encountered nonspecific change in a number of genetically determined and acquired neuropathies. It is caused by repeated episodes of segmental demyelination and remyelination coupled with hypertrophy and hyperplasia of Schwann cells and endoneurial fibroblasts resulting in an "onion bulb" appearance microscopically. In advanced cases, in addition, there is axonal degeneration, myxoid changes of the endoneurium, and vacuolation of endoneurial fibroblasts. As a rule, perineurial and epineurial elements do not participate in the process (Fig. 7-3).

Microscopically, the cross-sected nerve in hypertrophic neuropathy may resemble traumatic neuroma and solitary neuropathy from which it can be distinguished only with great difficulty (Weller and Das Gupta, 1968; Dyck and Lambert, 1970; Bray and Aguayo, 1974).

TRAUMATIC NEUROMA*

Neuromas are the result of laceration, amputation, or compression of a nerve. They are not neoplasms. They are the direct result of trauma-initiated *proliferation of the axon-Schwann cell unit.* The Schwann cell and its axon of the proximal stump grow in an effort to reattach to the proximal portion of the distal stump. In case the axon of the cut end of the nerve fails to fuse with the corresponding part of the distal stump, the axon will wander out into the soft tissues of the proximal stump, turn back on itself, and become tangled, thus producing a *conglomerate of axons, Schwann cells,* and *fibroblasts.* The haphazard growth of these elements at the amputation site or at the site of trauma will produce fusiform and multi-

* *Synonyms and related terms:* neuroma, amputation neuroma, hypertrophic neuroma, neurinoma, perineural fibroblastoma.

TABLE 7-1. ***Etiologic Classification of Peripheral Neuropathies***

CLASSIFICATION	EXAMPLES
Genetic	Hereditary sensory neuropathy, hypertrophic neuropathy, globoid cell leukodystrophy
Immune	Recurrent polyneuritis, serum sickness neuritis, idiopathic polyneuritis of Guillain-Barre
Metabolic	Nutritional, uremic, diabetic, dysproteinemic neuropathies
Toxic	Alcoholic, drug-induced, heavy metals induced neuropathies
Infectious	Leprosy, herpes, diphtheria
Ischemic	Vasculitis, arteriosclerosis, amyloidosis
Neoplastic	Primary or secondary tumors of peripheral nerves, carcinomas, sarcomas

nodular neuromas (Cieslak and Stout, 1946; Sunderland, 1968).

Although regenerating axons may be able to force their ways through dense fibrous tissue, the laminated perineurial sheath presents an impenetrable barrier to their growth. Therefore, the most reassuring way to prevent formation of neuroma is complete closure of the perineurial sheath of the severed nerve bundle. This will prevent migration of regenerating axons into the surrounding soft tissues where they are able to form neuromas (Verocay, 1908; Romine et al, 1976).

Grossly, traumatic neuromas are oval, gray-white, and rubbery firm. It is not uncommon to find a direct connection between the neuroma and adjacent nerves. They are prone to occur at or near the site of injury, but occasionally they may be found several centimeters proximal to the site of trauma (Cattell and St. Ville, 1961; Tuovinen et al, 1965) (Figs. 7-4, 7-5).

Morton's Neuroma. Morton's neuroma or so-called intermetatarsal neuroma or interdigital neuroma was first described by Morton in 1876. In his report of 12 cases he stated that "Under certain circumstances a bruising or pinching of the digital branches of the lateral plantar nerve between the fourth and fifth metatarsals may account for the neuralgia" and, of course, for the appearance of the neuroma. It is felt today that the Morton's neuroma can be found in any web space of the foot; however, it is found most commonly between the third and fourth toes and is the result of repeated compression severe enough to break up the myelin sheath and induce the proliferation of axons, Schwann cells, and perineurial elements (Hauser, 1971; Kite, 1966; King, 1946; Berlin, 1976).

Most traumatic neuromas are treated by surgical excision. The most effective way to eliminate them, however, is by applying preventive measures during surgery to isolate, retract, and seal off nerve bundles.

NEOPLASTIC LESIONS

The first clear description of a neurogenic tumor is in Bell's book, *Surgical Observations*, published in 1816. He described "a soft cancer in the centre of the popliteal nerve" and gave the following report: "On making a section of the tumour, it had much the appearance of a large ganglion on the tibial nerve: the fasciculi of the nerve could be traced only a little into its substance." Apparently the term *neuroma* was used by early writers indiscriminantly for all sorts of benign and malignant growths of nerve origin (Smith, 1849; Virchow, 1858).

A clearly malignant retroperitoneal tumor reported by Eberth in 1872 was almost surely a neurogenic neoplasm rather than a muscle neoplasm as he stated. Smith, in 1849, is credited with being the first to describe *multiple cutaneous neuromas*, and later Gerhardt, in 1878, reported his experience with multiple neuromas. A year later, Takacs, in 1879, while working in the Institute of von Recklinghausen, described multiple neuromas. These articles appeared years prior to the publication of a monograph on the same subject by von Recklinghausen in 1882.

Garre, in 1882, is credited with the first description of *malignant transformation* in a "neuroma," but it was a report by Hosoi, in 1931, that called attention to the potential danger of malignant transformation of neurofibromas in von Recklinghausen's disease.

Thoma, in 1896, described for the first time *Pacinian neurofibroma*, and sporadic reports appeared later (Prichard and Custer, 1952; Prose et al, 1957). Benda, in 1904, reported a case of *ganglioneuroma* of the vagus, and Barret and Cramer, in 1963, reporting on tumors of peripheral nerves, described ganglia of the peroneal nerve.

The first case of *intraneural angioma* was reported by Sato in 1913. Later,

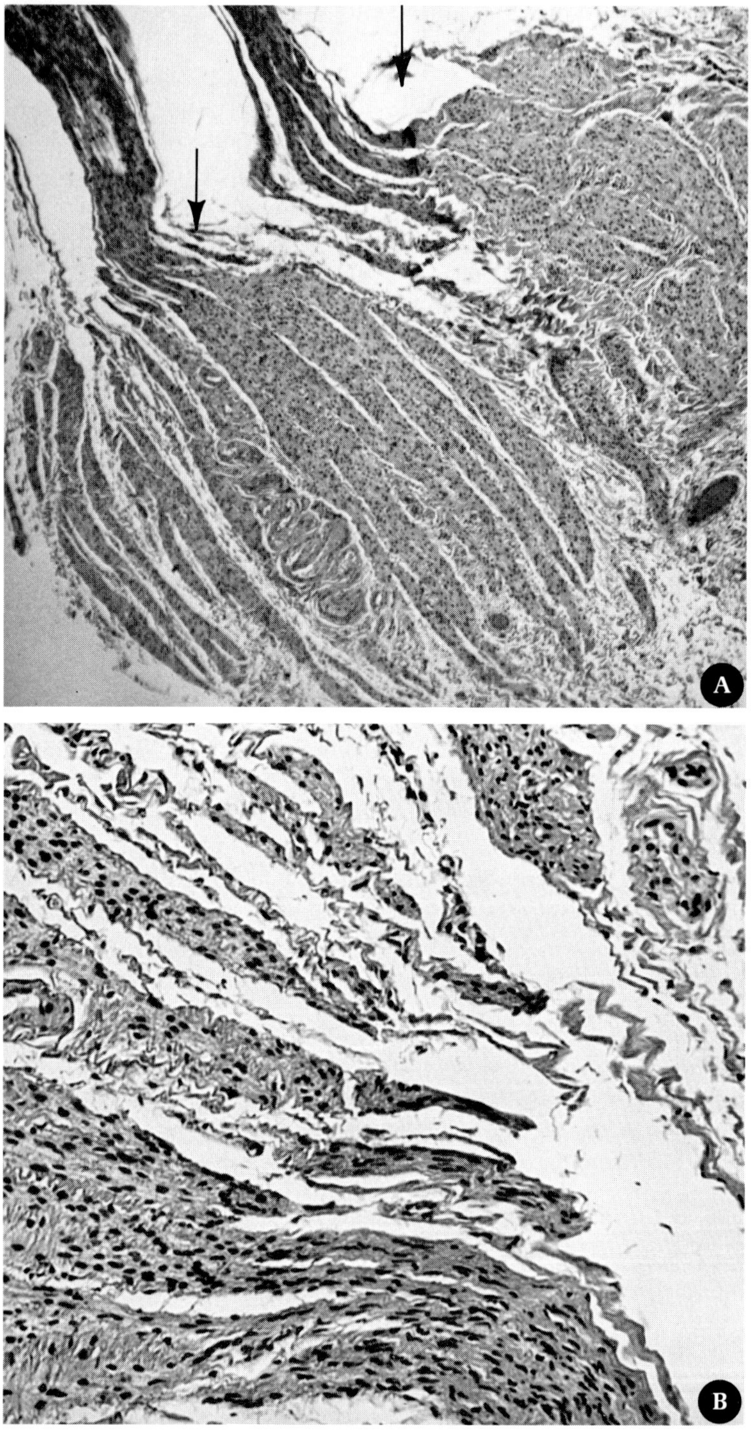

Figure 7-4. Traumatic neuroma. **A,** Note the lacerated nerves (arrows) from which the neuroma spreads out like a bristle from a broomstick (H & E, ×35). **B,** Edge of a neuroma. Schwann cells and perineurial cells are wrapped around the axons (H & E, ×140).

angiomas in combination with various nerve tumors were reported by a number of observers (Losli, 1952; Halpern and Currarino, 1965; Eckert, 1965; Cornell and Kirkendall, 1967; Greene et al, 1974). Nests of *ependymal cells, epithelioid,* or *frankly glandular epithelial cells* were reported occasionally (Lanford and Cohn, 1927; Cohn, 1928; Foraker, 1948). In more than a few reports on tumors of peripheral

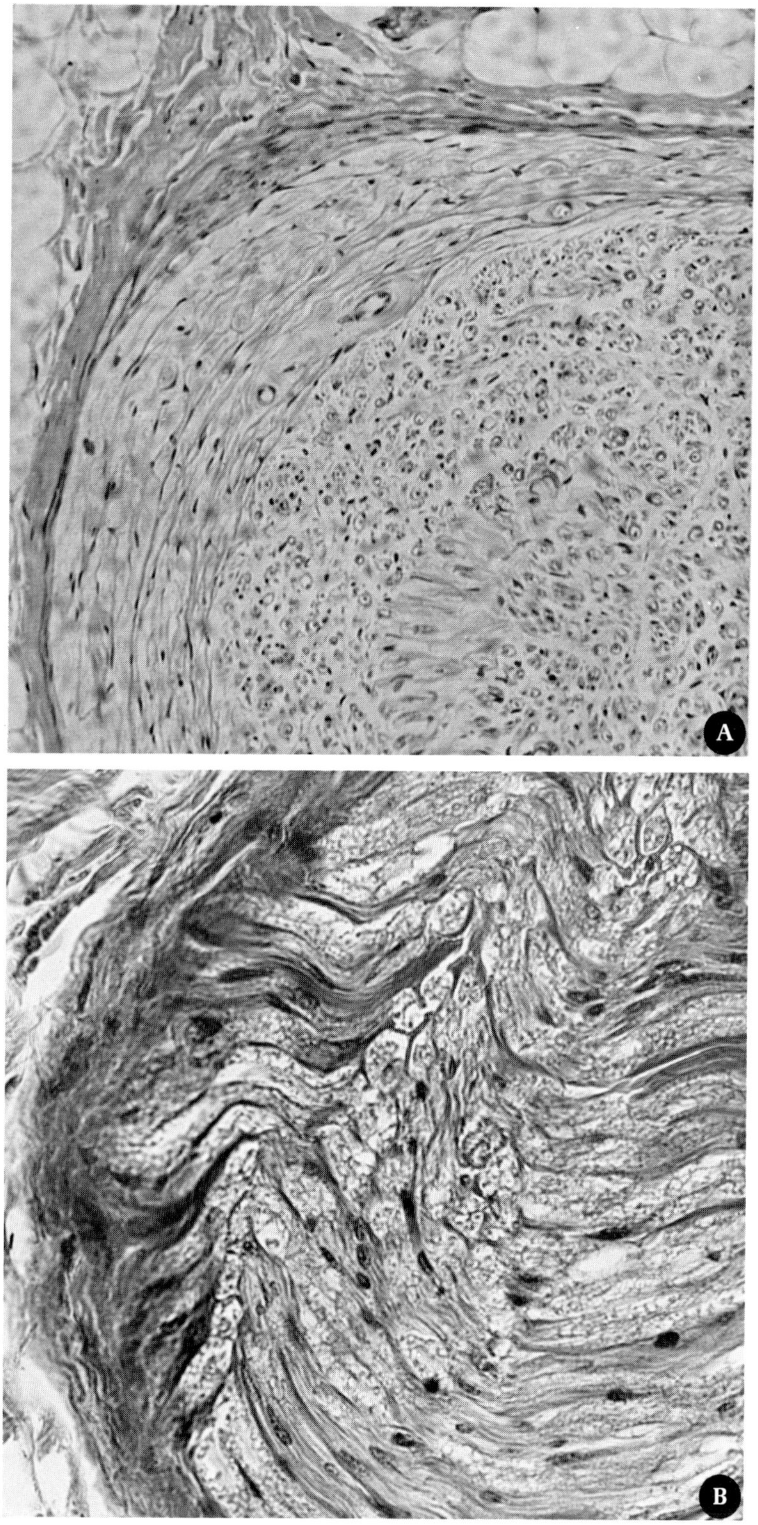

Figure 7-5. Cross section of a traumatized nerve. **A,** There is an abnormal proliferation of perineurial cells (H & E, ×140). **B,** Note the intimate intermingling of perineurial and Schwann cells (H & E, ×350).

nerves, reporters described *metaplastic elements* such as cartilage and bone. The most unique and perhaps the most significant heterotopic components found in nerve tumors are *rhabomyoblasts.* The first example of such a case was reported by Benenati in 1903; additional cases were recorded by Masson in 1938; Zimmerman et al, 1972; and Woodruff et al, 1973.

Verocay, in 1910, described the *bodies* that are named after him. In 1920, Antoni illustrated the palisading and arranged cells in peripheral nerve tumors and the loose myxofibrillar areas which are known today as *Antoni-A* and *Antoni-B* patterns (see Chapter 1).

Although Harrison, in 1924, demonstrated the origin of Schwann cells from the neural crest and foresightedly accepted the views of Nageotte (1922) that neuronal sheath cells, Schwann cells, and not neuroblasts are the source of so-called neuromas, various theories on the cellular origin of peripheral nerve tumors prevailed. As early as 1879, Takacs suggested that diffuse proliferation of the endoneurium is the structure of origin in neuroma. Masson (1932), Bailey and Herrmann (1938), and Ewing (1940) compared nerve tumors and nerve tissues microscopically and came to the conclusion that *benign as well as malignant nerve tumors originate from the sheath of Schwann.* Masson (1932) stated that "the pure connective tissue aspect (fibromatous, myxomatous) of certain neurinomas corresponds to special morphological modification of Schwann cells." Among the opposing views the most strongly held position is represented by Mallory (1914), Penfield (1932), and Cushing (1938) who believed that reticulin and collagen can be formed only by cells of mesodermal derivation. Thus peripheral nerve tumors must come from mesenchymal elements of the epineurium, perineurium, and endoneurium (Figs. 7-2, 7-3).

Murray and Stout (1940) demonstrated by in vitro studies that "Schwann cells can and do form collagen and reticulin" and authoritatively concluded in two subsequent studies in 1942 that Schwann cells and not fibroblasts are the origin of "nerve sheath tumors". Cravioto et al (1973) demonstrated in ethylnitrosourea-induced peripheral nerve tumors that the tumors are indeed made up of clearly identifiable Schwann cells, but *when the tumors become invasive, they lose their basement membrane and look much like altered fibroblasts.*

In reference to terminology, Stout, in 1935, adopted the terms *neurilemma* and *neurilemmal sheath* used by contemporary histologists to identify the outer membrane of Schwann cells and adjacent fibrillar structures (ultrastructural studies show that these correspond to the basement membrane of Schwann cells plus adjacent, mostly collagen, fibers, Fig. 7-3). He also coined the term *neurilemoma.* This term gained wide acceptance, owing to the prestige of its proponent, and even today it is part of our standard nomenclature despite common knowledge that the basal lamina of a cell cannot form a tumor (Fig. 7-3).

Schwannoma without doubt is the most appropriate term for tumors arising from so-called peripheral nerve sheaths, provided one can establish grossly, or at least microscopically, the source of origin of the neoplasm from a peripheral nerve or can identify in the tumor, microscopically, the so-called Schwannian features. Undoubtedly, Quick and Cutler, in 1927, and Stewart and Copeland, in 1931, recognized that although clinical and gross examination after surgical extirpation clearly reveals many neoplasms to be of nerve origin, none showed microscopic features commonly associated with schwannomas or neurofibrosarcomas. They called these tumors, tumors that originate from peripheral nerve but microscopically grow as fibrosarcomas or other forms of spindle and round cell sarcomas, neurogenic sarcomas. The term *neurogenic sarcoma* was used during the years in a number of publications (Maseritz, 1942; Godwin et al, 1950; Katz et al, 1971), but as a diagnostic term it is applied less frequently than it should be. Especially today when it is known that pluripotential cells, such as the Schwann cells and other endoneurial and perineurial cells, are capable of producing tumors which are predominantly one or another form of *fibrous histiocytoma, fibrosarcoma, leiomyosarcoma, liposarcoma,* or *rhabdomyosarcoma* and may also contain metaplastic elements such as cartilage and bone, the term *neurogenic sarcoma* seems to be reasonable to indicate common neurogenic histogenesis of a phenotypically diverse group of neoplasms.

Stewart and Copeland, in 1931, coined the term *malignant epithelioid schwannoma* for lesions which are more cellular than common schwannomas. They suggested that these lesions may bridge the gap between schwannoma or neurogenic sarcomas and malignant melanoma.

In an attempt to define certain recognizable morphologic patterns, in 1954, McCormack et al called attention to epithelioid schwannoma. Pung and Hirsch, in 1955, summarized their experience with *plexiform neurofibromatosis,* and Bednar, in 1957, described pigmented and nonpigmented *storiform neurofibromas.*

In 1965, Pineada called attention to the presence of *mast cells* in peripheral nerve tumors and Donohue et al reported radiation induced neurofibromata (see Chapter 9). Fisher and Vuzevski, in 1968, studied with the electron microscope the cells of origin of schwannomas, neurofibromas, and a group of closely related tumors.

We reported (Das Gupta et al, in 1969) a series of 303 cases of *benign solitary schwannomas* and pointed out the absence of stigmata of von Recklinghausen's disease and the lack of sarcomatous transformation. We also summarized our experience (Tang and Hajdu, in 1975) with 27 cases of primitive neuroectodermal tumors, which were reported under the title of "adult neuroblastomas."

COLLAGENOUS SCHWANNOMA

The classification of nerve tumors appears to be more confusing than it actually is because of the numerous synonyms and various concepts in regard to their histogenesis. Tumors of peripheral nerve may arise from three derivatives of the neural crest: *Schwann cells* (or nerve sheath cells), *neuroblasts,* and *paraganglionic cells* (or chromaffin cells) (Fig. 7-1).

Collagenous schwannomas as a group can be characterized best perhaps by their slender fibrillar and collagenous cells and frequent association with von Recklinghausen's disease. When they turn out to be malignant, they may assume a non-collagenous appearance (malignant fibrous histiocytoma or undifferentiated malignant schwannoma) or remain collagenous (neurofibrosarcoma or fibrosarcoma) (Fig. 7-1). For a discussion of malignant schwannomas or neurogenic sarcomas turn to page 455.

Neurofibroma. Perhaps the best known neurogenic tumor is the neurofibroma, which may occur singly without the stigmata of neurofibromatosis and commonly is referred to as *solitary schwannoma.* The literature on these entities is voluminous and numerous pertinent publications are listed in the bibliography.

Neurofibromatosis.* This chronic progressive hereditary disease is inherited as a mendelian dominant trait in more than 50% of the cases. Its hereditary nature was first recognized by Thomson in 1900. Neurofibromatosis is also called Recklinghausen's disease after von Recklinghausen who, in 1882, described multiple neurofibromatosis as a disease entity and discussed in detail its pathogenesis. Von Recklinghausen considered the tumors as fibromatous and used the term *neurofibroma* to express the nerve origin and the fibromatous nature. Chauffard, in 1889, describing pseudoxanthoma elasticum, also described the pigmentary changes (café-au-lait spots) associated with neurofibromata (Fig. 7-6).

Neurofibromatosis is classified among

* *Synonyms and related terms:* von Recklinghausen's disease, pigmented neurofibromatosis, cutaneous neurofibromata, neurofibroma, neuroma.

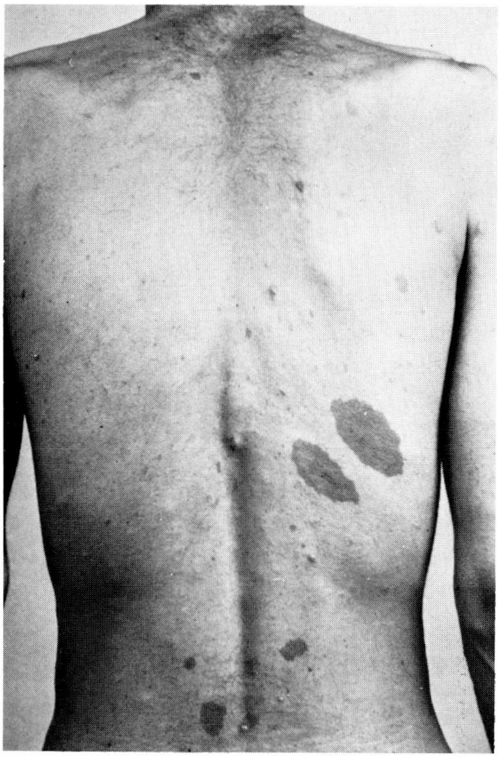

Figure 7-6. Neurofibromatosis (von Recklinghausen's disease) with cutaneous café-au-lait spots. (From Hajdu, S. I., and Hajdu, E. O.: Cytopathology of Sarcomas and Other Nonepithelial Malignant Tumors. Philadelphia, W. B. Saunders Co., 1976.)

the phakomatoses or neurocutaneous syndromes along with Sturge-Weber and von Hippel-Lindau disease, ataxia telangiectasia, and tuberous sclerosis. The etiology is unknown. According to Willis (1962), von Recklinghausen's disease is a hamartomatous disorder. It can affect any age, sex, race, or color. After a study of 110 patients, Brasfield (1972) reported that neurofibromatosis is most commonly diagnosed between ages of 30 and 40 and there is a slight female preponderance (Table 7-2). Cutaneous neurofibromas are most apparent on the trunk, head and neck areas, and the arms. Frequently neurofibromatosis manifests only by the appearance of café-au-lait spots or brownish, large, freckle-like discolorations. These cutaneous patches usually appear soon after birth and increase in size with age. Rare examples of *oral* (Baden et al, 1955; Hatziotis and Asprides, 1967), *vaginal* (Drescher and Herzog, 1961), *bladder* (Harvey and Tennant, 1934; Klerk and Campbell, 1954; Bitker et al, 1966) and *gastrointestinal* (Lukash et al, 1966) primary neurofibromas were reported. Multiple neurofibromas most commonly appear at puberty. Most of the tumors remain discrete for several years, but oth-

TABLE 7-2. ***Reported Studies of Benign Schwannomas***

	TOTAL NO. CASES	MALE	FEMALE	MOST COMMON SITES	RECKLING-HAUSEN'S DISEASE	MALIGNANT TRANSFORMATION
Cutler and Gross (1936)	20	—	—	Lower Extremity	—	—
Preston et al (1952)	61	61	—	Trunk Head and Neck	61	10
Oberman and Sullinger (1967)	31	17	14	Head and Neck	9	—
Das Gupta and Brasfield,* (1970)	303	172	131	Head and Neck Extremities	None	1
Brasfield† (1972)	110	56	54	Trunk Extremities	110	32

*All benign solitary schwannomas.
†All of the patients had von Recklinghausen's disease.

ers may become sessile or pedunculated. Some of these tumors, and as a rule one of the cutaneous neurofibromata, bursts into sudden growth after many years of quiescence and may reach enormous sizes in a short time (Figs. 7-7, 7-8). This is an alarming sign and in many cases is a sign of malignant transformation (see Neurogenic Sarcoma). However, such overgrowth rarely turns out to be benign so-called *elephantiasis neuromatosa,* with thickened, loose, and heavily pigmented skin which hangs in folds (Fig. 1-33).

In general, benign neurofibromas are well-circumscribed, but not encapsulated, globoid or fusiform rubbery firm masses. The cut surface is homogeneous and gray with a shiny semitranslucent appearance. In many instances, after careful dissection, a nerve or nerve fibers can be seen entering the tumor.

The precise histologic composition of neurofibromas and their cell of origin was a puzzle for a long time. In 1931, Stewart and Copeland stated, "the whole scope of von Recklinghausen's disease is not as yet defined, nor is there agreement as to the nature of cellular constituents making up the tumors which constitute the most prominent manifestation of the malady." Ultrastructural, histochemical, and cytologic studies have added to the better understanding of neurofibromas.

Microscopically, the typical neurofibroma is composed of elongated and fusiform cells, wrapped around axons or remnants of axons, and arranged in wavy thin fasicles. The cytoplasmic processes of these altered Schwann cells continue into delicate reticulin fibers and heavy collagenous fibers. Almost invariably a number of bizarre spindle cells, fibroblasts, are discernible among the proliferating Schwann cells. Once the endoneurial cells reach a certain density, the perineurial as well as some of the epineurial cells will begin to proliferate (Fig. 7-9).

Willis (1962) pointed out that the histologic distinction between collagen-producing Schwann cells of neuroectodermal origin and fibroblasts of mesenchymal origin may not be possible because Schwann cells and fibroblasts may form common blastomas in which the differentiation is determined not by their embryonal origin but by their relation with respect to each other and the axons. This theory at least partly explains the variable patterns seen in benign as well as malignant schwannomas. Endoneurial origin of collagen in von Recklinghausen's disease is supported by ultrastructural studies. Of the two different types of collagen (endoneurial and epineurial) usually present in nerve, the epineurial fibers are about twice as thick (500 to 700 Å in diameter) as the endoneurial collagenous fibers. According to Lassmann et al (1975), in von Recklinghausen's disease the endoneurial type of collagen predominates and is at least partly produced by the Schwann cells. The collagenous nature of these fibers is supported by their similarity to fibrous long-spacing collagen with "Luse bodies" which can be produced in vitro by adding acids to tropocollagen solutions (Luse et al, 1963).

Neurofibromatosis involving the *genitourinary tract* is rare. Since Gerhardt, in 1878, reported the first case, an additional three dozen cases have been recorded in the literature (Harvey and Tennant, 1934; Klerk and Campbell, 1954). According to Bitker et al (1966) the urinary bladder and more specifically the trigone is the most commonly involved site, but rare examples of intrascrotal and prostatic lesions are known. In about one third of the reported cases there was clear-cut evidence of von Recklinghausen's disease. According to Clark et al (1977) 15 cases of neurofibromatosis of the bladder have been reported in children, none of which showed malignant transformation.

Gastrointestinal involvement by neurofibromatosis is rarely documented in case reports (Lukash et al, 1966), but reported studies confirm the frequent scattering of neurofibromas throughout the gastrointestinal tract. Rare instances of

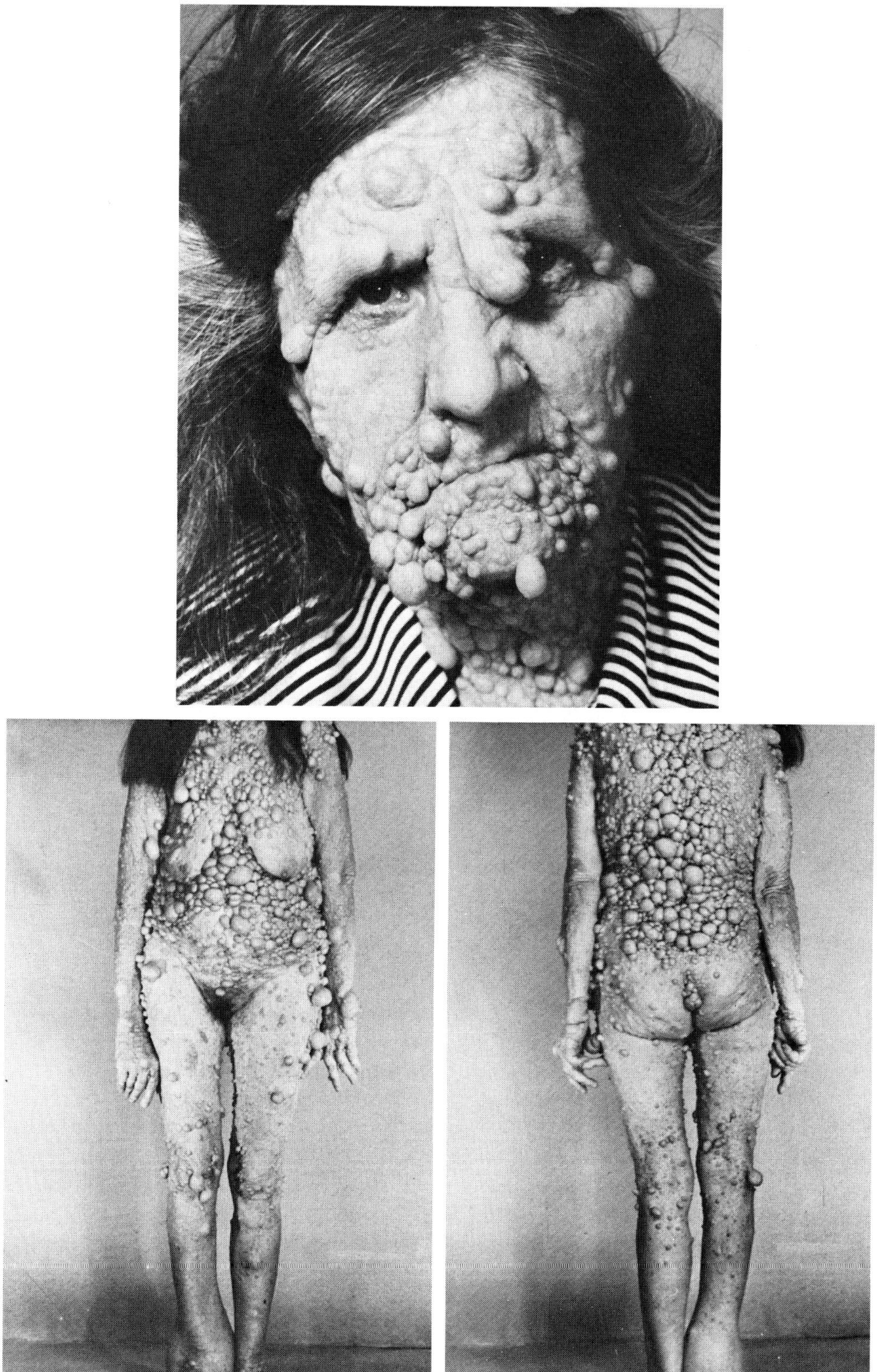

Figure 7-7. Neurofibromatosis with striking cutaneous manifestations in the form of multiple and various sizes of neurofibromas. (Courtesy of Lynch, H. T., et al.: Familial cancer syndromes: A survey. Cancer 39:1867, 1977.)

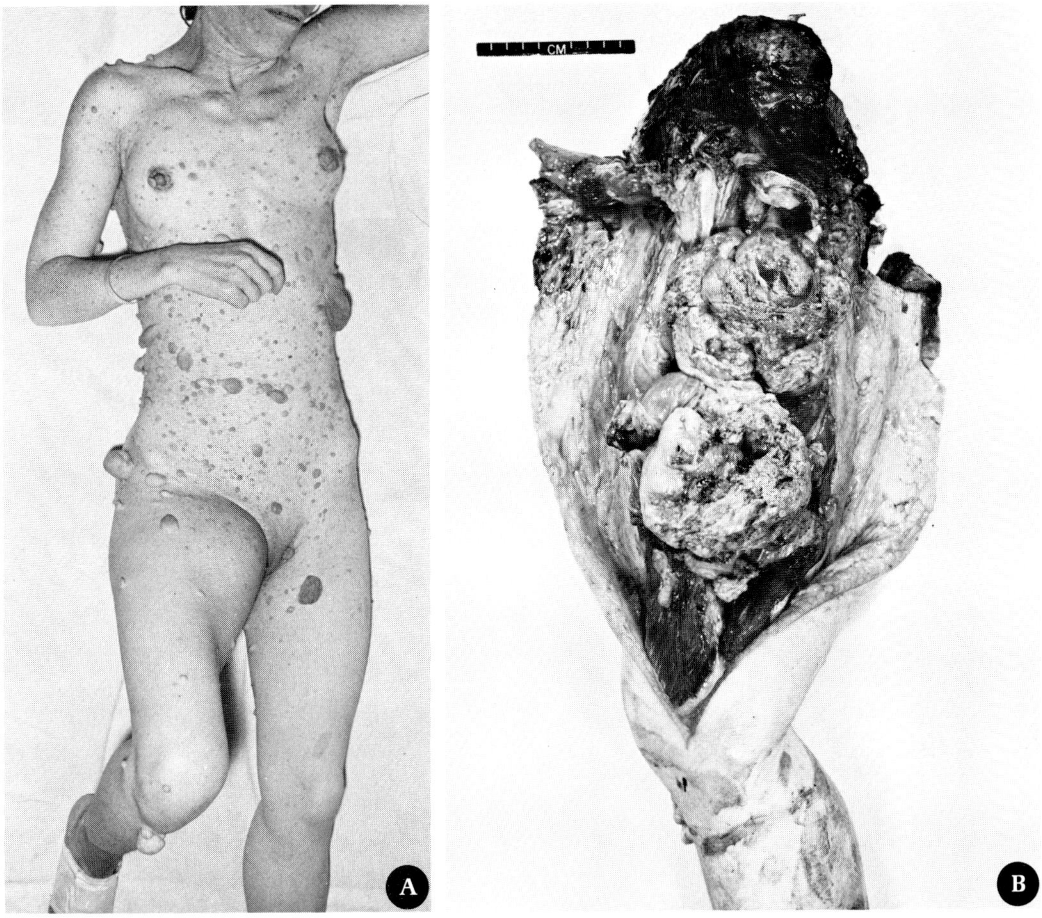

Figure 7-8. **A,** This 39-year-old woman had progressive neurofibromatosis from childhood. At age 38 a fast-growing mass appeared deep in the right thigh.

B, The tumor of the thigh was removed by hemipelvectomy and was classified histologically as neurofibrosarcoma. She died in less than a year with pulmonary metastases.

synchronously occurring leiomyomas, lipomas, and carcinoid tumors have been recorded.

In most reported series of *mediastinal tumors* the incidence of neurogenic tumors is between 25 and 30%, making it one of the most common mediastinal tumors. In spite of this, primary intrathoracic or mediastinal neurofibroma is rarely recorded in the literature (Godwin et al, 1950; Armstrong et al, 1972; Factor et al, 1976). When Schweisguth et al, in 1959, reviewed 68 cases of intrathoracic tumors in infants and children, they found no examples of schwannoma.

It is estimated that 1% of *head and neck tumors* are neuroectodermal in origin. In our experience (Das Gupta et al, 1969) 136 (45%) solitary schwannomas occurred in the head and neck regions, most commonly in the lateral neck. The incidence of intraoral schwannoma is given as 6.5% and the tongue is reported to be the most common site. This neoplasm may appear at any age (Baden et al, 1955; Hatziotis, 1967).

Laryngeal schwannomas are indeed rare neoplasms. El-Serafy in 1971 reviewed the literature and found only 89 reported cases. He noticed that the majority of the lesions originated from the aryepiglottic fold or from the false vocal cords.

Facial schwannomas are equally rare.

The first case was reported by Schmid, in 1930. Since then approximately 100 cases have been described in the literature. One of the largest series of 15 benign tumors and two malignant ones was reported by Conley and Janeka, in 1973. None of the benign lesions recurred after excision, but the two patients with malignant schwannoma died in a couple of years. After excision of neurofibromas, recurrence is the rule, but in many instances the "recurrence" is truly a new tumor arising from neighboring nerves.

Neurofibromatosis usually runs a benign course and in many instances is discovered as an incidental finding. However, according to reports (Preston et al, 1952; Brasfield, 1972) about 15 to 25% of the patients develop sarcomatous changes in usually one of the pre-existing masses (Fig. 7-8).

Among the many lesions that may be associated with von Recklinghausen's disease the most frequently mentioned are *scoliosis* and *erosion of bones* (Whiston, 1953), endocrine abnormalities such as *Frölich's syndrome* and *Addison's disease* and *endocrine tumors* (Champman et al, 1959; Williams and Pollack, 1966; Reubi, 1944; Bolande, 1970), *melanosis* and increased incidence of pigmented *moles* and *malignant melanoma* (Fox et al, 1964; Hoggins, 1975), *connective tissue neoplasms* (McCarrol, 1956; Lassman et al, 1975; Stay, 1977), and *mental disorders* (Preston et al, 1952). Rare instances of neurofibromatosis have also been described in association with *multiple lipomas, osteofibrosis, meningocele,* and *syringomyelia.*

Surgical extirpation of *solitary schwannomas* is facilitated by the fact that they are encapsulated and complete surgical removal can be done with ease. However, attempts should be made to keep essential nerve pathways intact by careful dissection. The microscopic pattern of solitary neurofibromas, properly called solitary collagenous schwannomas, is not significantly different from that of multiple neurofibromas of the von Recklinghausen's complex, but they are different in their rate of malignant transformation. Sarcomatous transformation in solitary schwannomas is so uncommon that we were able to find only one proven sarcomatous change in a series of 303 cases of solitary benign schwannomas (Das Gupta et al, 1969). Solitary benign schwannomas are slightly more common in females than in males and occur most commonly in the head and neck, upper extremity, trunk and lower extremity in this order of frequency (Table 7-3). No predilection of these tumors for the flexor surfaces of the extremities was noted. In our series 63% of the patients were between 30 and 60 years of age. Symptoms and signs of solitary schwannomas vary according to the anatomic sites; however, most patients present with a painless mass. Schwannomas can vary in size from a few millimeters to 20 cm, and the larger tumors may require sequential excisions. Of the 303 patients with benign solitary schwannomas 49 (16%) had either a synchronous or a metachronous malignant neoplasm apparently unrelated to peripheral nerves (Das Gupta et al, 1969).

The various patterns of growth of schwannomas which can be observed microscopically are influenced by size, loca-

TABLE 7-3. *Solitary Benign Schwannomas**

MOST COMMON SITES	NO. OF PATIENTS
Neck	60
Face	8
Oral cavity	31
Hand	20
Arm	13
Shoulder	10
Forearm	8
Trunk	26
Ankle	11
Knee	10
Mediastinum	20
Breast	8

*Modified from Das Gupta, T. K., Brasfield, R. D., Strong, E. W., and Hajdu, S. I.: Benign solitary schwannomas (neurilemmomas). Cancer 24:355, 1969.

tion, and duration of growth, predominance and degree of differentiation of cellular components, the amount of collagen production, invasiveness of the tumor, and number of lesions, whether solitary or multiple (see neurofibromatosis).

Microscopically, the solitary benign schwannomas are not significantly different from benign schwannomas of von Recklinghausen's disease except that they are of a less collagenous nature. Perhaps because they contain less collagen the classically arranged, Antoni-A and Antoni-B patterns can be seen more commonly than in tumors which are part of the von Recklinghausen's complex.

Classically, the *Antoni-A pattern* consists of compact and interwoven bundles of slender bipolar Schwann cells whose nuclei are characteristically aligned in rows or palisades between which the cell processes are fused into solid hyalinized cords and straight reticular fibers. Occasionally the Antoni-A pattern continues into a twisted, fern-like nodular arrangement, *Verocay bodies,* resembling tactile corpuscles. The *Antoni-B pattern* is much less distinct than the Antoni-A pattern. The Antoni-B pattern is basically a loosely arranged meshwork of myxomatous and fibrocellular tissues which almost invariably contain a generous complement of lymphocytes, histiocytes, and mast cells (Figs. 7-10, 7-11). (See also Chapter 1, Figure 1-40.)

Occasionally fine deposits of melanin can also be detected. Such lesions are commonly referred to as *pigmented schwannoma.*

There is a broad spectrum of microscopic patterns in collagenous schwannomas. The most common ones are *angioneuroma, plexiform neuroma, Pacinian neurofibroma, cystic schwannoma, pleomorphic schwannoma* and *glandular schwannoma.*

Angioneuroma. Dilated blood vessels with thickened hamartomatous hyaline walls, perivascular hyalin deposits, and fibrin thrombi are found sometimes in schwannomas. When such vascular components predominate in an otherwise schwannian background, it seems justified to call such lesions angioneuromas (Fig. 7-12). These hamartomatous blood vessels histogenetically resemble those in angiomyoma, angiomyolipoma (see Chapter 4), and angioglioma and give support to the theory that neurofibromas are hamartomatous lesions. Apparently, in angioneuromas, both neuroectodermal tissues and mesodermal angioblastic tissues proliferate in harmony and they are found frequently in association with von Recklinghausen's disease. Intraneurial *hemangiomas* have been reported (Losli, 1952), and Greene et al, in 1974, gave a concise summary of light and electron microscopic findings in arterial lesions associated with neurofibromatosis. They concluded that there is a marked increase in ground substance, fragmentation of elastic lamella, nodular aggregates of smooth muscle, and proliferation of fibrous tissue in the adventitia.

Plexiform Neuroma. These neuromas possess one of the most distinct microscopic growth patterns of schwannomas. The typical cirsoid or plexiform pattern is the result of the bizarre, distorted, and twisted arrangement of the axon, Schwann cells, and endoneurial fibroblasts somewhat *resembling traumatic neuroma* (Figs. 7-13, 7-4). Entire nerve trunks can be thickened, swollen, and beaded due to thickening of the perineurium and have the appearance of a "bag of worms." The stroma is sparsely vascular, but solitary dilated vessels are not uncommon findings. Usually there is delicate blending of myxoid and collagenous stromal elements. According to reports, less than 3% of plexiform neuromas undergo malignant transformation. In their comprehensive review of neurogenous tumors Stewart and Copeland (1931) discussed, among other things, the histogenesis and schwannian origin of plexiform neuromas. Their report has been updated by Pung and Hirsch, in 1955.

Pacinian Neurofibroma. This neurofi-

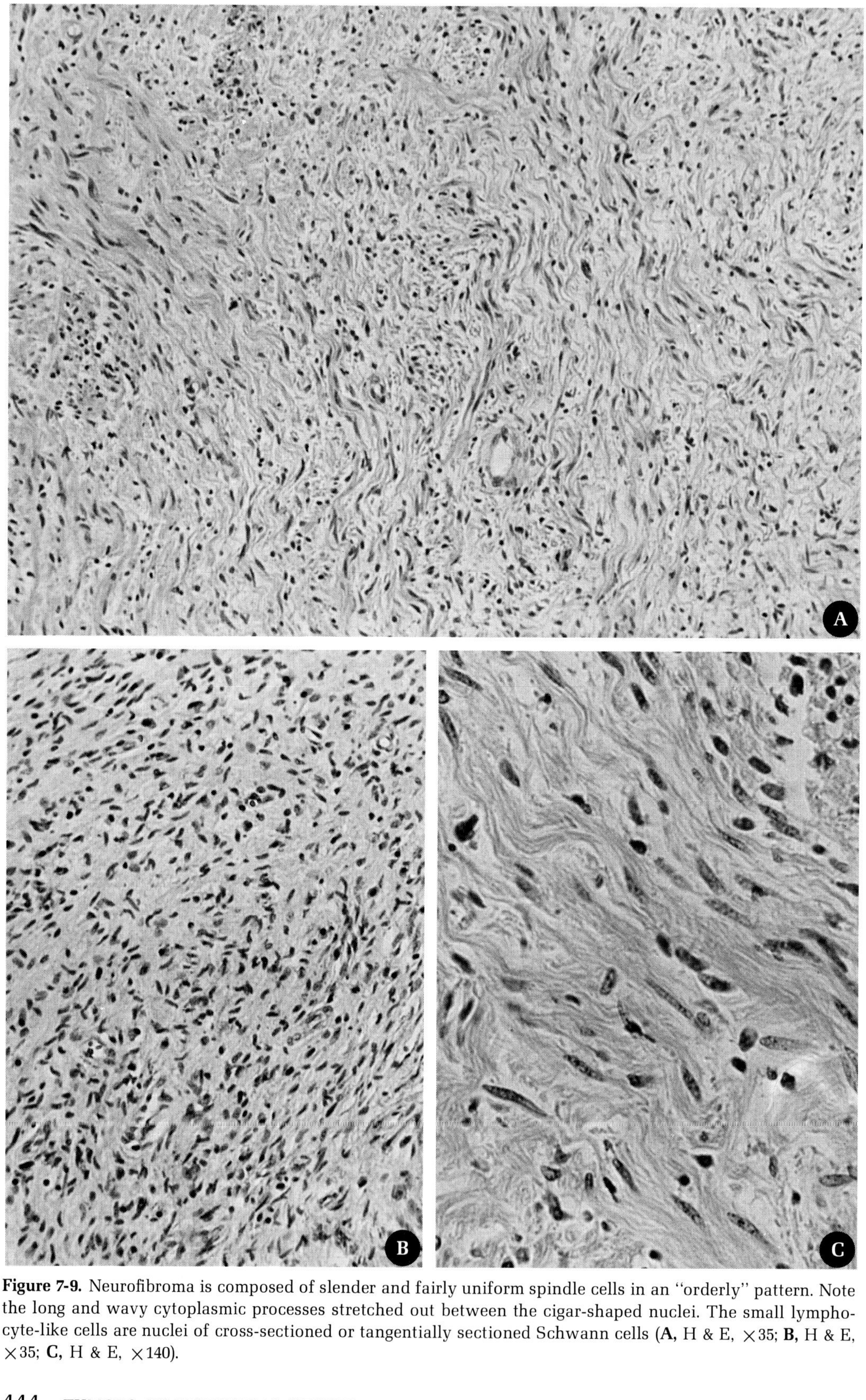

Figure 7-9. Neurofibroma is composed of slender and fairly uniform spindle cells in an "orderly" pattern. Note the long and wavy cytoplasmic processes stretched out between the cigar-shaped nuclei. The small lymphocyte-like cells are nuclei of cross-sectioned or tangentially sectioned Schwann cells (**A,** H & E, ×35; **B,** H & E, ×35; **C,** H & E, ×140).

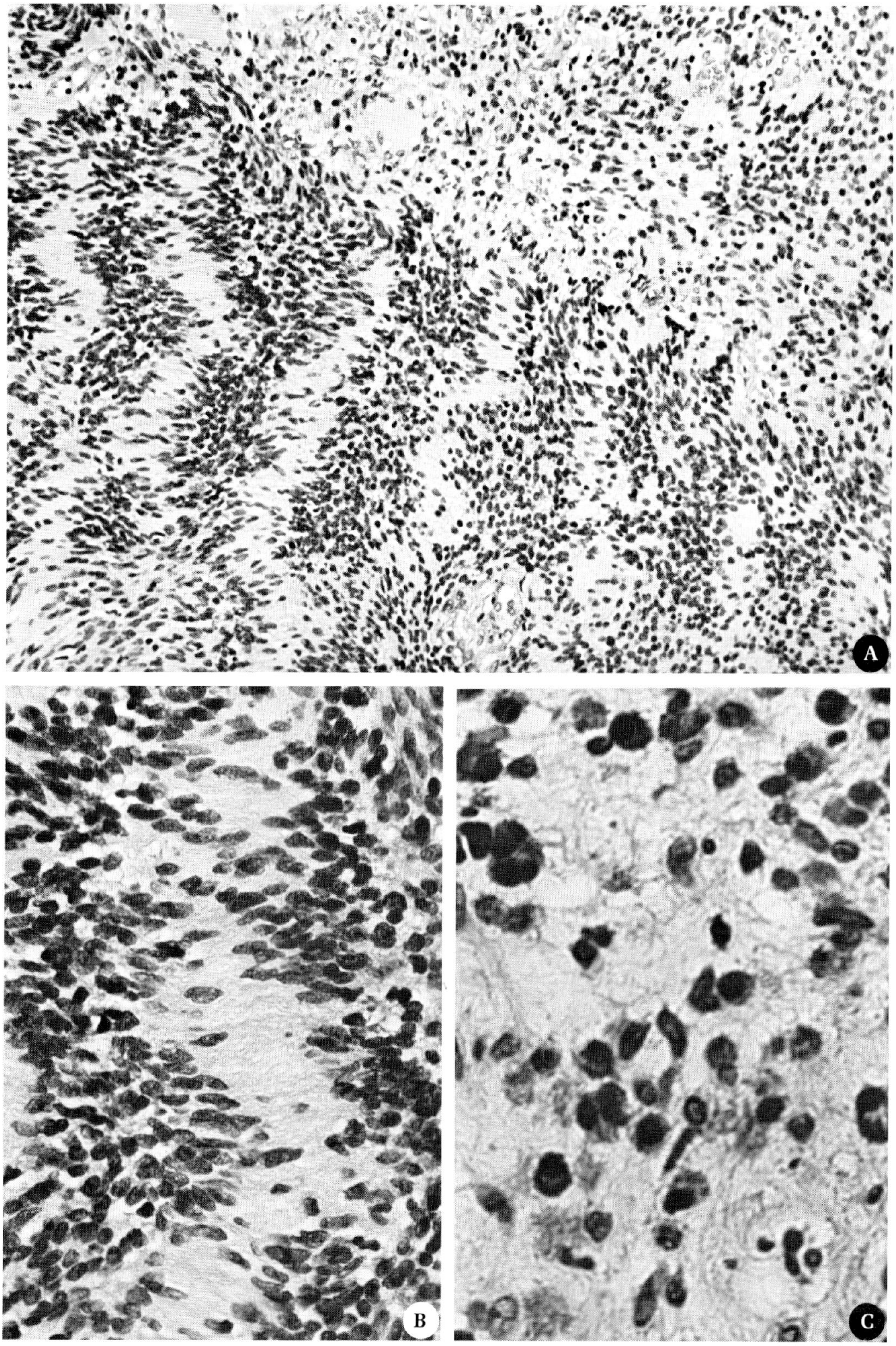

Figure 7-10. Neurofibroma with dual histologic pattern. **A,** Interdigitating Schwann cells in a side-by-side pattern of Antoni-A type (left half of picture). Note the merging of the wavy Antoni-A pattern with Antoni-B pattern (right upper corner) (H & E, ×85). **B,** Fibrillar processes and rows of nuclei of Schwann cells (H & E, ×140). **C,** Loosely patterned Schwann cells and a few granular cytoplasmic mast cells from an Antoni-B type area (H & E, ×350). (See also Chapter 1, Figure 1-40.)

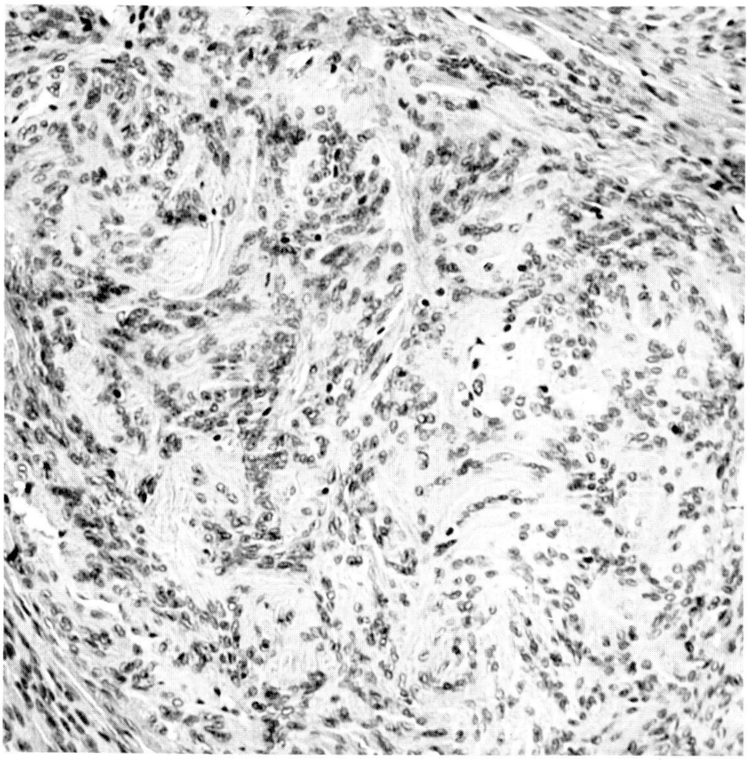

Figure 7-11. Neurofibroma showing a cross-sected and imperfect Antoni-A type area. Some of the cells are spreading out and forming less than perfect Verocay bodies (H & E, ×75).

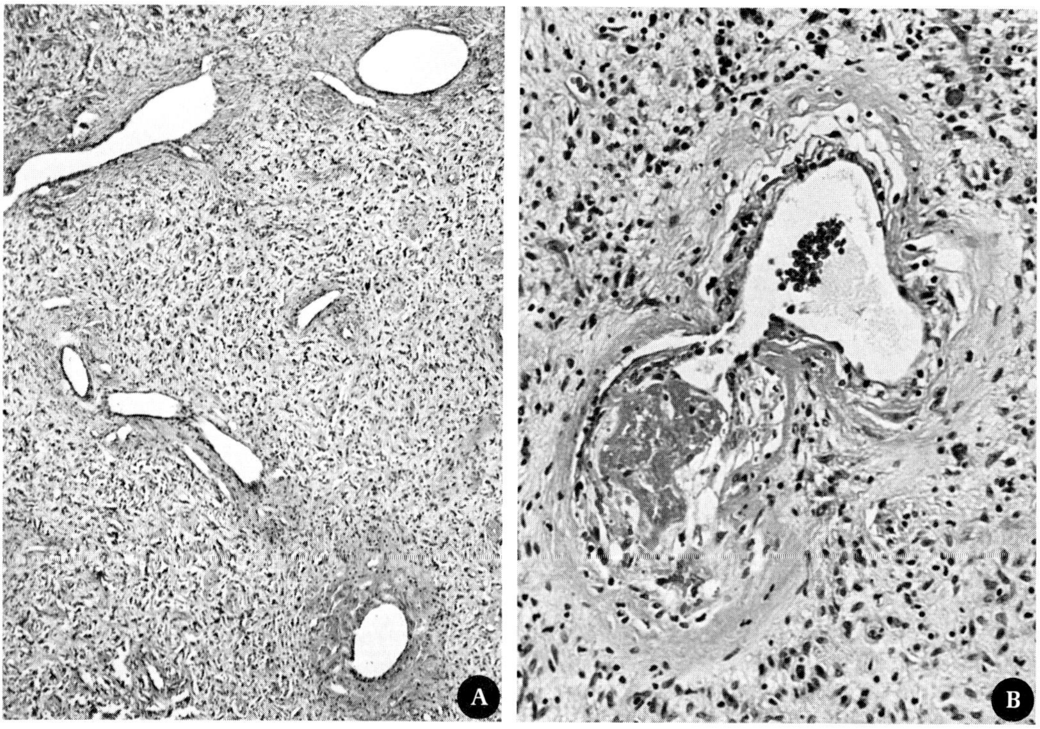

Figure 7-12. Angioneuroma. Hamartomatous thick-walled vessels in fibrillar and loosely arranged neurofibroma showing Antoni-B pattern. Note partial thrombosis of the vessel in **B** (**A,** H & E, ×35; **B,** H & E, ×85).

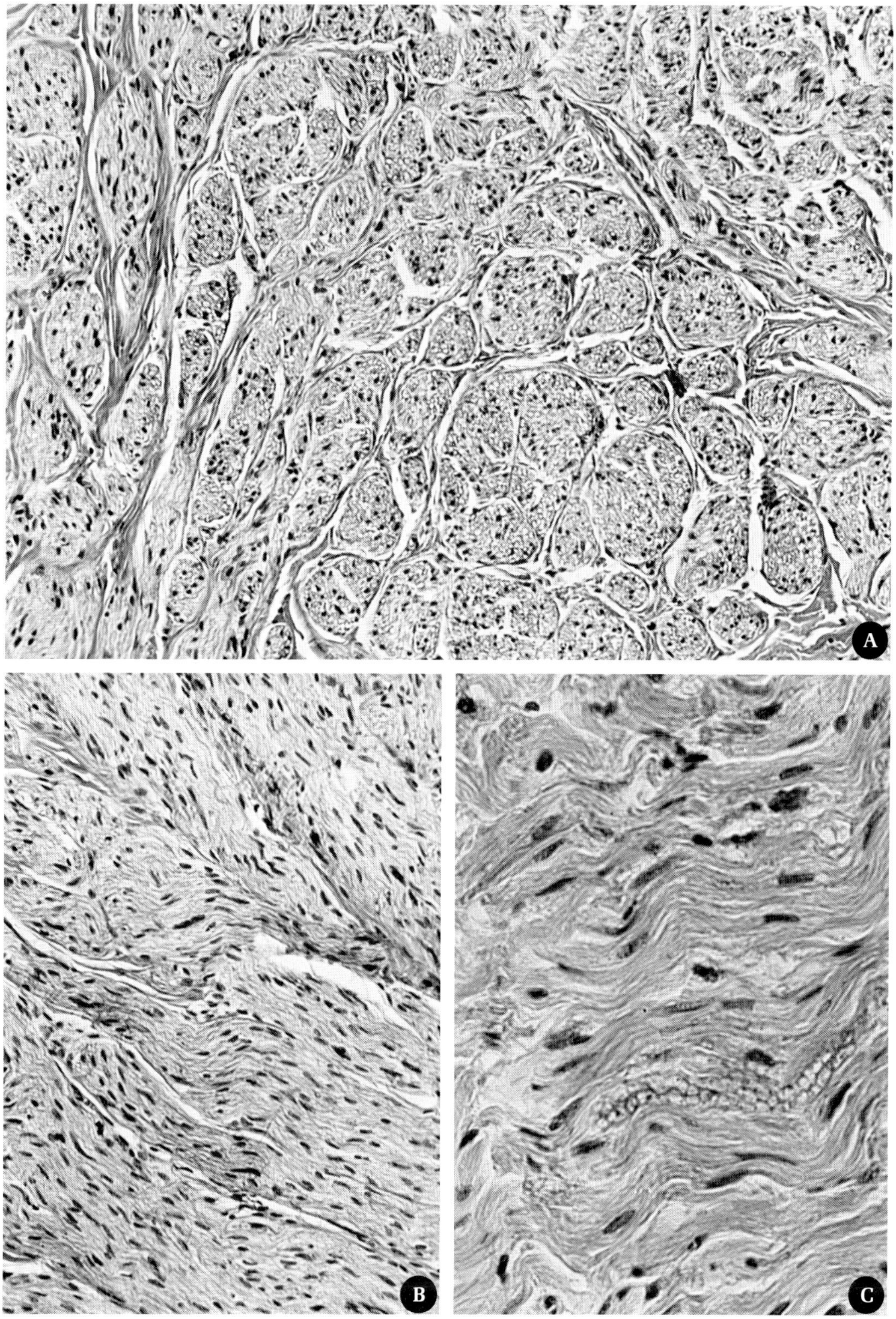

Figure 7-13. Plexiform neuroma showing trabecular and organoid arrangement of proliferating Schwann cells. **A,** Thin collagenous fibrous septae separate individual conglomerates of endoneurial elements (H & E, ×85). **B** and **C,** Tangential or side view shows the trabecular or fascicular pattern of wavy and tightly packed Schwann cells (**B,** H & E, ×85; **C,** H & E, ×140).

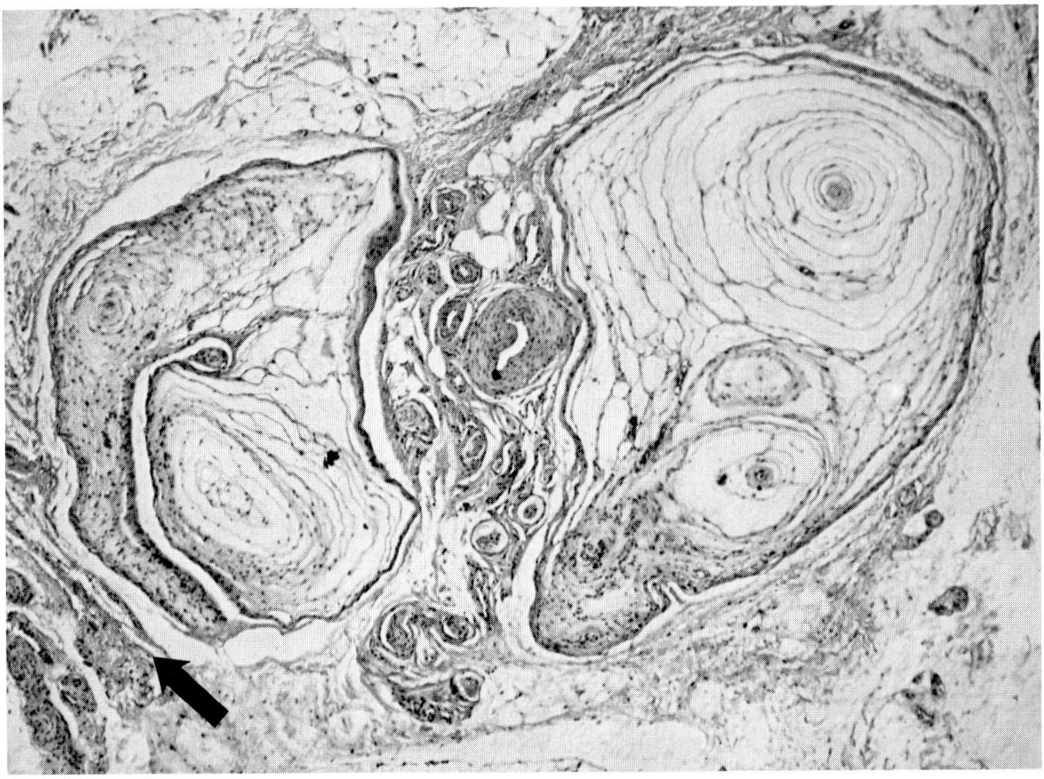

Figure 7-14. Pacinian neurofibroma from the hand of an adult male. Note the striking resemblance of these two giant structures to hypertrophic Pacinian corpuscles. The close relationship between the "onion ring" units and adjacent nerves is seen at the arrow (H & E, ×35).

broma was first described by Thoma in 1896. At rare intervals in the literature case reports have called attention to these uncommon tumors which resemble hypertrophic Pacinian corpuscles (Prichard and Custer, 1952; Prose et al, 1957). It is of interest that 6 of the 9 reported cases occurred either on the hand or on the foot. Grossly, they are small papular, slightly elevated, self-limited cutaneous tumors.

Histologically, the tumor nodule is partitioned by collagenous tissue into lobules. Each lobule contains several oval subunits resembling cellular Pacinian corpuscles with the typical onion ring appearance. The tumor cells range from oval to slender spindle forms and are embedded in a myxomatous or mucoid stroma (Fig. 7-14). The precise histogenesis of these lesions is unknown and the possibility that Pacinian neurofibroma is nothing else than a plexiform neuroma which underwent mucinous degeneration cannot be completely excluded.

Rare forms of solitary and superficial neurofibromas—so-called *molluscum fibrosum, liponeurofibroma,* and *nevoid neuroma*—are mentioned only for the sake of completeness (Fig. 7-15).

Glandular Schwannomas. These uncommon forms of atypical schwannomas deserve separate listing because of their unique morphology. Garre, in 1892, is credited with the description of the first case. Up to now the total number of recorded cases is 9 (Table 7-4). Age and sex distribution of the patients and anatomic and clinical presentation of the tumors do not appear different from those of schwannomas without glandular elements. Although the presence of nonciliated, *mostly mucinous glands* should be considered unique, in none of the reported cases were epithelial elements widespread. As a fact, in most of the cases they were chance findings in well-documented cellular schwannomas predominantly growing as neurofibromas associ-

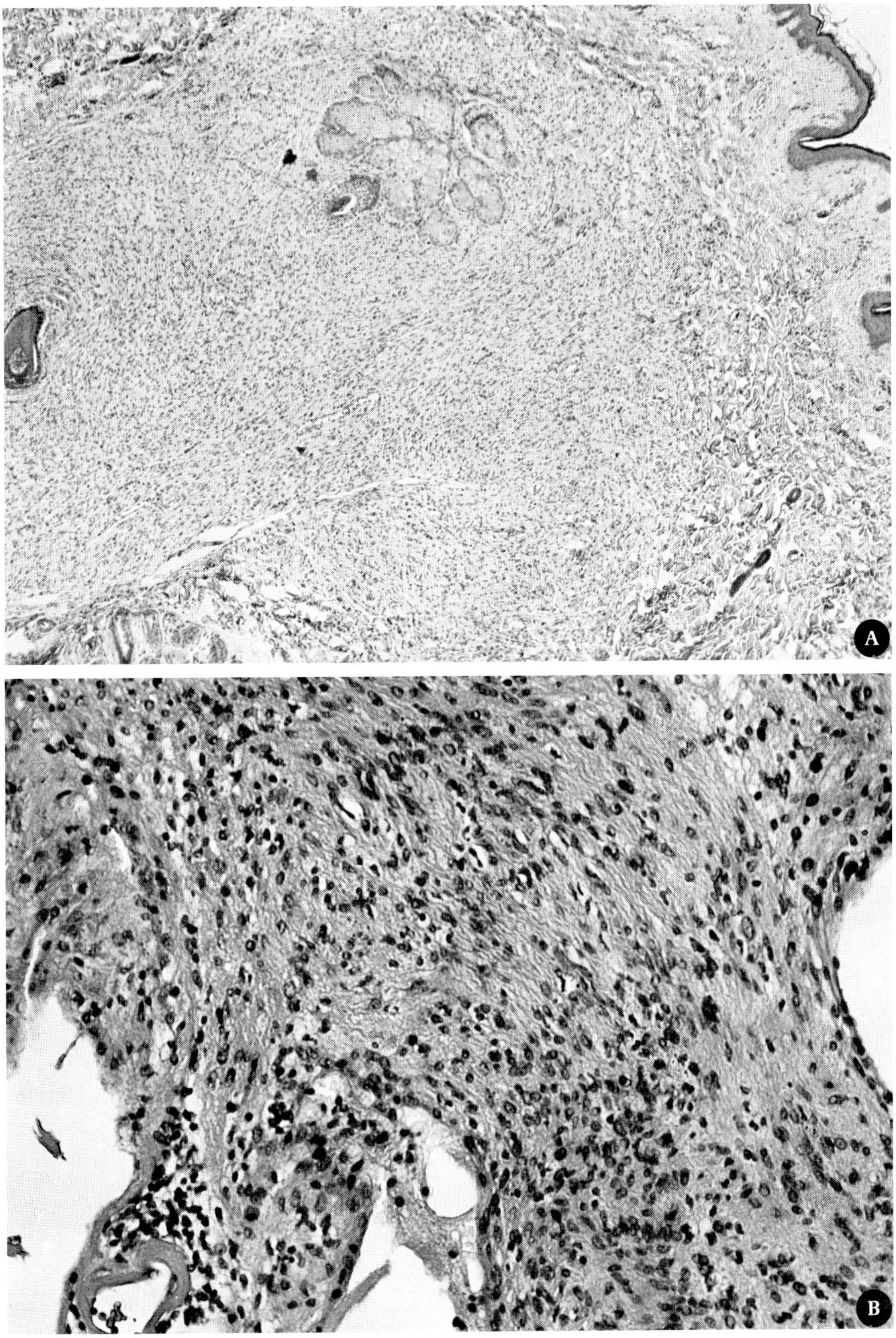

Figure 7-15. A, So-called molluscum fibrosum of the skin. Short oval, slender and uniform cells infiltrating the dermis in a defined area (H & E, ×35).

B, Benign cystic schwannoma. This lesion was present in the neck of a 40-year-old male for 5 years prior to excision. It is composed of fibrillar tumor cells in a partly pallisading pattern between cystic spaces and hamartomatous blood vessels (H & E, ×140).

TABLE 7-4. *Glandular Schwannomas*

	AGE	SEX	RECKLING-HAUSEN'S DISEASE	SITE AND TYPE OF TUMOR	RECURRENCE	FOLLOW-UP
Garre (1892)	31	F	Yes	Popliteal Space Neurofibrosarcoma	Yes	DcD, 6 mo.
Lanford and Cohn (1927)	35	M	Yes	Upper arm Neurofibrosarcoma	Yes	Alive, 4 yr.
Foraker (1948)	8	F	Yes	Brachial plexus Neurogenic sarcoma	Yes	DcD, 10 yr.
Woodruff (1976)	15	F	No	Perineum Nevoid schwannoma	Yes	Alive, 5 yr.
	15	F	Yes	Back Neurofibrosarcoma	No	Alive, 10 yr.
	27	M	No	Retroperitoneum Undiff. malignant schwannoma	—	DcD, 7 mo.
	32	F	Yes	Thigh Neurofibrosarcoma	Yes	DcD, 5 yr.
Hajdu, (unpublished)	46	F	No	Chest wall Benign glandular schwannoma	Yes	Alive, 3 yr.
	35	M	Yes	Retroperitoneum Neurofibrosarcoma	—	DcD, 1 yr.

DcD = died with disease.

ated with von Recklinghausen's disease (Fig. 7-16 A and B). Stewart and Copeland, in 1931, reported an epithelial-lined cyst within the obturator nerve in areas of neurofibroma and concluded that it is "some developmental nerve defect." It seems apparent that the epithelial components are expressions of the neuroectodermal nature of schwannomas and on their own possess no proven malignant potentials. *Whether tumors with such features should be considered benign or malignant must be decided, after considering clinical and pathologic findings, on the basis of cellular morphology and pattern of the spindle cell elements.* Even in such a limited number of cases, it is interesting to call attention to the ominous presence of von Recklinghausen's disease. Four of the 6 patients with glandular schwannoma associated with von Recklinghausen's disease died of the disease; on the other hand, only 1 of the 3 patients without stigmata of neurofibromatosis succumbed to the disease.

Pleomorphic and Cystic Schwannoma. It is not uncommon to find a few bizarre hyperchromatic mononucleated and multinucleated Schwann cells intermingled with other cells. Such lesions are occasionally referred to as *pleomorphic schwannoma.* So-called *cystic schwannomas* are the ones which contain spaces of varying sizes filled with semisolid proteinaceous material. (See Figure 7-15B.)

Neurofibrosarcoma. (See Neurogenic Sarcoma.)

NON-COLLAGENOUS SCHWANNOMA

Admittedly it is artificial and perhaps against common sense, from a histogenetic point of view, to divide schwannomas into collagenous and non-collagenous forms, but from the point of view of microscopic appearance I have found the subclassification of schwannomas analogous to the subdivision of fibrous tumors practical (see Chapter 2), since most of the neoplastic Schwann cells, functionally and morphologically, appear as facultative fibroblasts. Although we know that some of the neoplastic Schwann cells are capable of producing bands of collagen, whereas others do not, the factors controlling or influencing such functional activities are poorly understood. As a group, *non-collagenous schwannomas are characterized by their non-collagenous nature and their distinct storiform or epithelioid cellular appearance microscopically* (Table 7-5). They are rarely found in association with von Recklinghausen's disease and if they become malignant almost invariably will remain non-collagenous, malignant fibrous histiocytomas or undifferentiated malignant schwannomas.

Storiform Schwannoma. This so-called storiform neurofibroma, Bednar tumor, or melanotic neurofibroma is almost always a solitary, ill-defined neoplasm of the skin or subcutis. It may range from fractions of a centimeter to several centimeters in size. Most patients admit a slow but continuous growth of several months. There is often increased pigmentation of the overlying skin in the cross-sected tumor due to the presence of melanin. These neoplasms are mentioned in several reports on peripheral nerve tumors, but Bednar (1957) called attention to these neoplasms as a specific group. He described "the characteristic matting-like" or storiform or cartwheel pattern microscopically, which is most prominent near the center of the tumor; at the periphery the pattern of growth is a wavy, arranged pattern (Fig. 7-16C).

The Antoni-A pattern is commonly seen in storiform schwannomas. Occasionally the transition into hypertrophic nerve fiber is clearly visible. Masson first called attention to the storiform pattern in 1932, by saying that "the palisades that are found in schwannomas are derived from the sheath of Schwann." This pattern of growth of non-collagenous fibroblasts can be found, regardless of the histogenesis, in a number of non-collagenous fibrous tumors, e.g., in fibrous histiocytomas. The display of the storiform pattern, which is commonly seen in *dermatofibrosarcoma protuberans* (a fibroblastic fibrous histiocytoma, see Chapter 2) and *meningiomas* in peripheral nerve tumors, clearly indicates the facultative fibroblastic (histiocytic) potentials of Schwann cells. Admittedly, short of proof of origin from nerve it may be difficult to draw a distinction between *dermatofibrosarcoma protuberans,* which in most instances is almost certainly a non-collagenous fibroblastic growth of other than neurogenic origin, and storiform schwannoma. Both of these lesions most commonly occur in the trunk, and none of them is associated

TABLE 7-5. ***Comparison of Certain Clinicopathologic Features of Collagenous (Neurofibroma) and Non-collagenous Schwannomas***

COLLAGENOUS SCHWANNOMA	NON-COLLAGENOUS SCHWANNOMA
Solitary or multiple	Solitary
Not encapsulated	Encapsulated
Painful and tender	Asymptomatic
Occurs anywhere	Subcutaneous
Centripetal growth	Centrifugal growth
Nerve runs through tumor	Nerve runs in capsule
Homogeneous gray	Pleomorphic gray
Arranged spindle cells	Storiform pattern of cell
Collagenous bundles	Vascular stroma
Frequent mast cells	Rare mast cells
Malignant transformation common	Malignant transformation uncommon

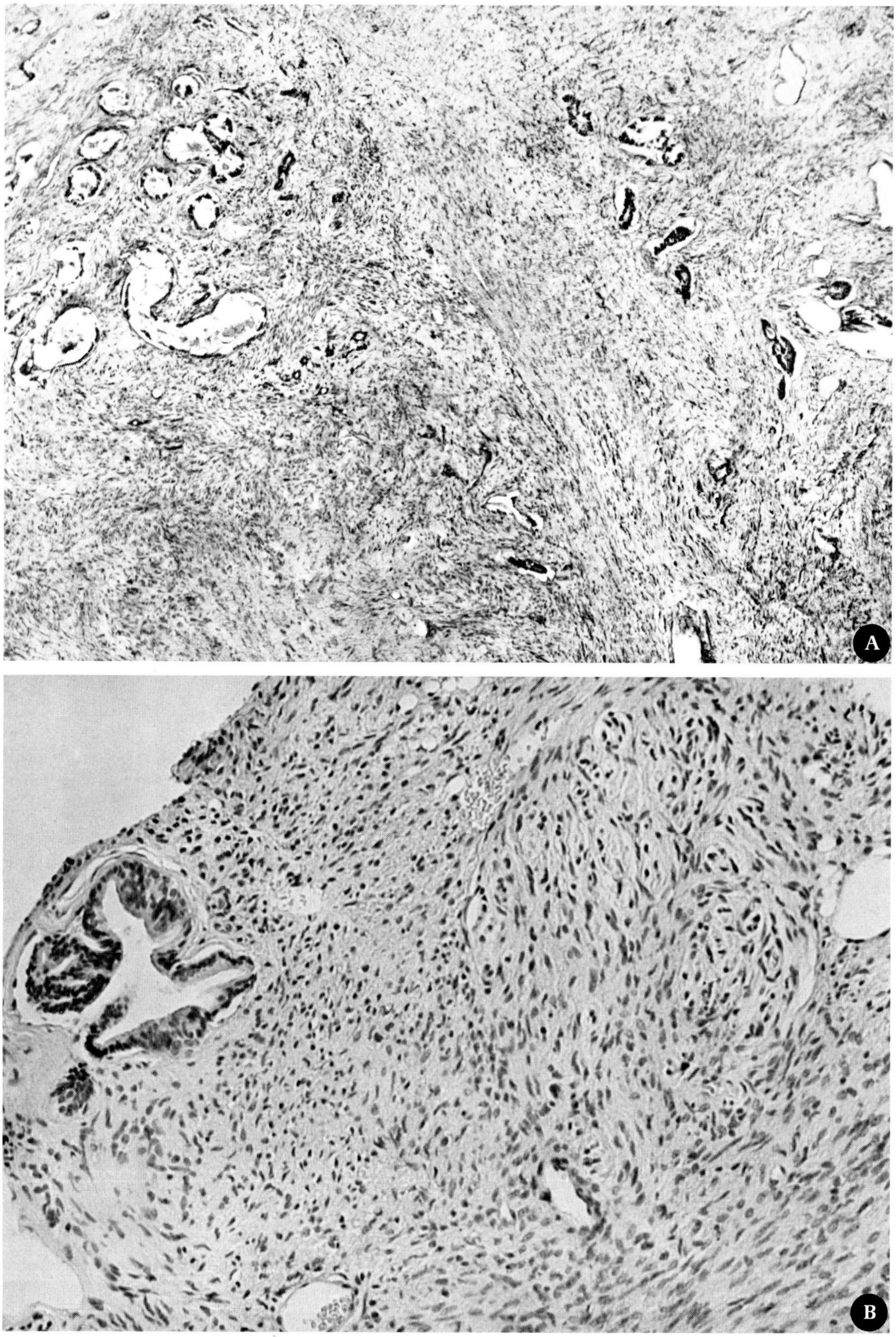

Figure 7-16. **A** and **B,** Benign glandular schwannoma showing well-defined glandular units composed of columnar epithelial cells. The glandular components appear distinct and localized to one or two areas in the tumor (**A,** H & E, ×35; **B,** H & E, ×85).

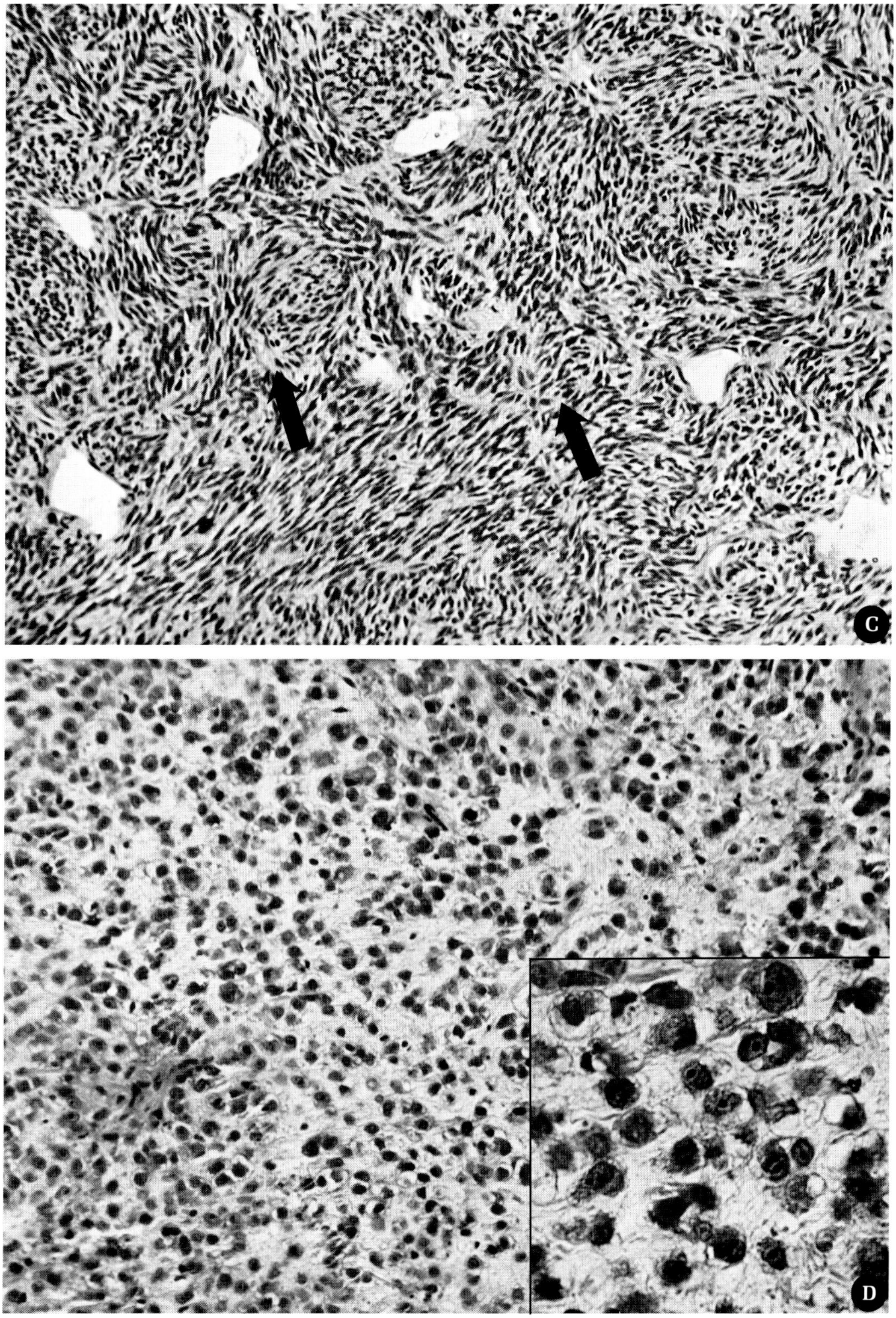

Figure 7-16 (cont.). C, Atypical storiform schwannoma with interdigitating subunits of Antoni-A pattern (arrows). The tumor is highly vascular; however, there is no particular affinity between blood vessels and tumor cells (H & E, ×140).

D, So-called benign nevoid schwannoma. Loosely arranged or cluster-forming oval and round cells with delicate fibrillar processes and prominent nuclei somewhat resembling melanocytes or tumor cells of primitive neuroectodermal tumor (H & E, ×140; inset, ×350).

with von Recklinghausen's disease. On the other hand, the differences are that storiform schwannoma may contain fine deposits of melanin, has no tendency to recur, does not reach large size, and no known instance of malignant transformation has been recorded. (For a discussion of dermatofibrosarcoma protuberans, see Chapter 2.)

Epithelioid Schwannoma. According to Stewart and Copeland (1931) *epithelioid schwannomas,* or so-called atypical nevoid schwannomas, bridge the gap between schwannomas, pigmented nevi, and malignant melanomas (Fig. 7-16D). Stewart and Copeland stated:

> We have observed tumors of deeper nerve trunks which looked like certain non-pigmented melanomas, yet did not run the clinical course of melanoma. . . . We have observed multiple tumors of the hands and legs which repeated biopsies convinced us fall in the melanoma group. Yet, the tumors are multiple, run a very chronic course and have not metastasized in a period of years.

These extremely rare neoplasms, by definition and microscopic appearance, in pure form, should be considered atypical cellular schwannomas with protracted clinical courses and low-grade malignant potentials. Epithelioid schwannomas may resemble well-differentiated *malignant melanomas,* atypical *cellular nevi,* and to a certain extent, *primitive neuroectodermal tumors,* and *clear cell sarcomas* (see Chapter 3) by virtue of clustering of the polyhedral and mostly round cells in arranged solid nests. For the sake of completeness, epithelioid schwannoma is listed here as a distinct morphologic entity; however, according to my personal experience, the epithelioid pattern is part of a spectrum and may be found in benign as well as malignant schwannomas, most commonly the ones which are unassociated with von Recklinghausen's disease.

Undoubtedly most of the melanin or melanosomes containing "clear cell sarcomas" are a clear cell form of epithelioid or nevoid schwannomas and their malignant potentials should be assessed by considering cellularity, size, site, and number of mitosis (see Chapter 1, Figures 1-55, 1-56, 1-57, and 1-58). These extremely rare neoplasms have been reported in the literature under various names (Millar, 1932; McCormack et al, 1954; Fox et al, 1964; Hoggins and Grundy, 1975; Dooling et al, 1977; Gelfand et al, 1977).

Undifferentiated Schwannoma. This is the so-called pluripotential schwannoma, and the term should be reserved for neurogenic neoplasms, benign or malignant, which arise from peripheral nerves and cannot be placed into any of the known categories on the basis of available material. Such neoplasms should be reviewed and reclassified as soon as additional material permits more precise classification.

Differential Diagnosis

The number of lesions from which benign schwannomas must be distinguished is almost limitless. The most commonly occurring lesions which may resemble benign schwannoma are *fibromatosis* (Chapter 2), *fibroma* (Chapter 2), *dermatofibrosarcoma protuberans* (Chapter 2), *leiomyoma* (Chapter 5), *angiomyoma* (Chapter 6), *angiomyolipoma* (Chapter 6), and *meningioma.* The chapters where the reader will find discussions of differential diagnostic features that are helpful in distinguishing such tumors from schwannomas are given in parentheses.

Of course, the reader should remember that precise histogenetic classification of schwannomas solely on the basis of microscopic appearance is an almost impossible task in many instances. Schwann cells are pluripotential cells and are capable of producing neoplasms which phenotypically or microscopically are identical with a number of soft tissue neoplasms of non-neurogenic origin.

NEUROGENIC SARCOMA*

The term *neurogenic sarcoma* is used in the sense it was conceived by Quick and Cutler (1927) and used by Stewart and Copeland (1931) as well as Oberman and Sullinger (1967). The term indicates a common histogenesis, nerve sheath origin, of a number of malignant neoplasms with a wide spectrum of microscopic appearance (Fig. 7-17). It is analogous in connotation to such terms as bronchogenic carcinoma or malignant germ cell tumor, all of which have a number of microscopic forms. The most commonly encountered and microscopically recognizable neurogenic sarcomas, all of which are known by a number of synonyms, are listed in Table 7-6.

As Stewart and Copeland (1931) observed, "the fully developed neurogenic sarcomas may be very *fibrous* or very *cellular*." When this observation was applied to a series of 91 cases of sarcomas which either were proven to arise from peripheral nerves or were found in association with von Recklinghausen's disease, a number of conclusions were analogous to those reached by D'Agostino et al, in 1963 (Figs. 7-18, 7-19).

The age of the patients at the time of diagnosis of sarcoma varied from 2 to 84 years, the average age being 39 years. Fifty-five of the patients were female and 36 male (Fig. 7-18). The most common primary sites were the back, neck, and axilla. No significant difference was noted among sexes in reference to primary site except that all 9 cases of primary neurogenic sarcomas of the buttock occurred in females (Fig. 7-19). If the anatomic site, age, sex, and survival are considered on the basis of whether the patients had neurofibromatosis or the neoplasms were solitary malignant schwannomas, there were significant differences between the two groups (Tables 7-7, Table 7-8).

It is important to point out not only the grave prognosis (97% mortality) of neurogenic sarcomas which originate in preexisting neurofibromas in association with von Recklinghausen's disease but also to call attention to the histologic differences of the two groups of neurogenic sarcomas, sarcomas with or without stigmata of von Recklinghausen's disease (Table 7-9, Figs. 7-20, 7-21, 7-22).

The majority of neurogenic sarcomas arising in association with neurofibromatosis were microscopically collagenous and contained heavy collagen type I fibers stainable with trichrome stain. Neurogenic sarcomas without stigmata of von Recklinghausen's disease, on the other hand, were almost all non-collagenous neoplasms or so-called malignant non-collagenous schwannomas (see Table 7-12).

Microscopically, the structural range of neurogenic sarcomas is great, ranging from high grade sarcoma to benign-looking schwannian areas. Occasionally, the various characteristic schwannian features are better expressed in recurrent and metastatic tumors than in the primary tumor (Figs. 7-23, color, to 7-27; Table 7-10). The histologic grade of the tumor, as expected in most soft tissue neoplasms, varies with the size of the tumor. Of the 17 patients who survived longer than 5 years without evidence of the disease, 4 of the 5 patients who presented with tumors larger than 5 cm had histologically high grade sarcoma. Of the remaining 12 tumors, all of which were smaller than 5 cm, there was only one microscopically high grade neoplasm (Table 7-11). (See also Chapter 1, Figure 1-59 and Table 1-15).

In general, histologic grade was assigned according to histologic pattern, based on cellularity and degree of differentiation. After consideration of the size and pattern neurogenic sarcomas that

**Synonyms and related terms:* malignant schwannoma, malignant neurilemoma, malignant neurogenous neoplasm, neurofibrosarcoma, malignant nerve tumor, malignant nerve sheath tumor, epithelioid schwannoma, peripheral nerve sarcoma, neurosarcoma, metaplastic malignant schwannoma, undifferentiated malignant schwannoma, Triton tumor, melanomatous schwannoma.

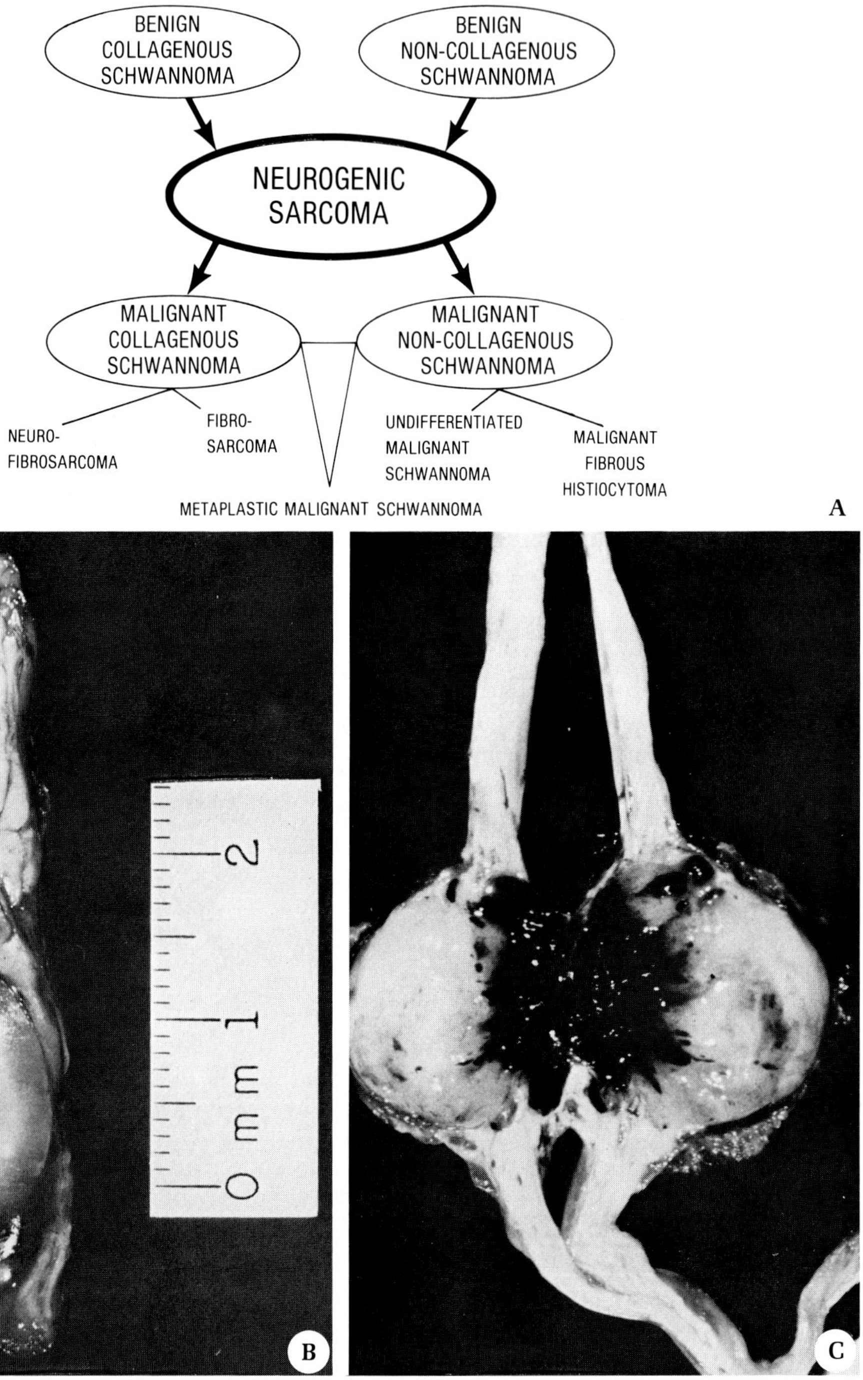

Figure 7-17. A, Neurogenic sarcoma as a term denotes malignant neoplasms which despite their diverse morphology all originate in peripheral nerves. Most of these neoplasms will retain some of the features that characterize schwannomas (see Table 7-5), will show clinicopathologic evidence of direct continuity with nerve or nerves, and can be identified as either a malignant collagenous schwannoma (neurofibrosarcoma) or a malignant non-collagenous schwannoma (undifferentiated malignant schwannoma). However, if the neurogenic origin cannot be established, either by gross or microscopic examination, most of these neoplasms should be classified according to histologic pattern, e.g., fibrosarcoma or malignant fibrous histiocytoma (see Table 7-12).

B, Solitary, benign non-collagenous schwannoma of the sciatic nerve.

C, Solitary, malignant collagenous schwannoma of the brachial plexus.

TABLE 7-6. ***Pattern of Growth and Differentiation of Neurogenic Sarcomas (Malignant Schwannomas)***

Neurofibrosarcoma
Desmoid tumor-like neurogenic sarcoma
Fibrosarcoma-like neurogenic sarcoma
Undifferentiated schwannoma
Fibrous histiocytoma-like neurogenic sarcoma
Clear cell sarcoma-like neurogenic sarcoma
Neurogenic sarcoma with elements of leiomyosarcoma
Neurogenic sarcoma with elements of rhabdomyosarcoma
Neurogenic sarcoma with chondroid or osseous elements
Neurogenic sarcoma with glandular elements
Neurogenic sarcoma with melanomatous elements

TABLE 7-7. ***Most Common Sites of Neurogenic Sarcoma***

ASSOCIATED WITH RECKLINGHAUSEN'S DISEASE			NO ASSOCIATION WITH RECKLINGHAUSEN'S DISEASE		
SITE	NO. PATIENTS	%	SITE	NO. PATIENTS	%
Back	7	19	Arm	8	15
Axilla	6	16	Neck	7	13
Thigh	6	16	Back	6	11
Neck	5	14	Buttock	6	11
Retroperitoneum	3	8	Head	5	9

TABLE 7-8. ***Neurogenic Sarcoma***

	RECKLINGHAUSEN'S DISEASE	
	WITH	WITHOUT
Number of patients		
Male	13	23
Female	24	31
Died with disease	36/37 (97%)	38/54 (70%)
Average age	34	42
Average time between:		
Diagnosis of von Recklinghausen's disease and diagnosis of sarcoma	15 yr.	—
Diagnosis of sarcoma and death	1 yr.	2.5 yr.

were growing as malignant schwannomas (neurofibrosarcoma, malignant epithelioid schwannoma, or undifferentiated malignant schwannoma) were graded on the basis of number of mitotic figures. Fewer than 5 mitoses/10 high-power microscopic field was required to classify a malignant tumor as low grade neoplasm. On the other hand, more than 5 mitoses/10 high-power field was the minimum to qualify a neurogenic sarcoma as high grade. Highly cellular and pleomorphic

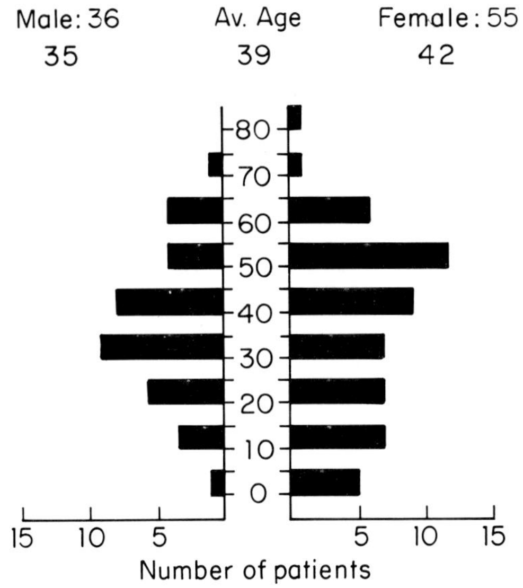

Figure 7-18. Age and sex distribution of 91 patients with neurogenic sarcoma including malignant collagenous and non-collagenous schwannomas (Hajdu, unpublished data).

neoplasms were considered high grade lesions, provided the mitotic count warranted such classification. On the other hand, tumors with moderate or scant cellularity despite focal pleomorphism were considered less than high grade, provided the mitotic count was less than that associated with high grade tumors (Figs. 7-28, 7-29).

Tumors classified as so-called malignant *metaplastic schwannomas* were graded after consideration of the histologic type and pattern of the metaplastic elements. For example, recognition of malignant embryonal or pleomorphic rhabdomyoblasts was considered sufficient to label a tumor as a high grade neoplasm, since the patients in 7 of 10 published cases and in 2 of 3 personal cases succumbed to the disease in less than one year on the average (Masson and Martin, 1938; D'Agostino et al, 1963; White, 1971; Woodruff et al, 1973, Karcioglu, et al, 1977) (Table 7-12; Figs. 7-30, 7-31).

Gore, in 1952, described a variety of unusual microscopic patterns in malignant nerve tumors, and Karcioglu et al, in 1977, emphasized the multipotential nature of migratory neural crest cells. Therefore, it should not be a surprise that neurogenic sarcomas, as seen in Table 7-12, may assume the microscopic appearance of rhabdomyosarcoma, fibrosarcoma, fibrous histiocytoma, or even liposarcoma. In view of these findings, perhaps it would not be impractical in reporting neurogenic sarcomas to list the various microscopic elements that were recognized.

Neurogenic sarcomas do not pose any particular *differential diagnostic problem* provided at least some of the microscopic *schwannian patterns* can be recognized (Table 7-5), or by careful gross dissection, the *neurogenic origin* can be established. And, of course, a history of von Recklinghausen's disease is important to consider. *Short of these findings, at the present time no laboratory technique would facilitate with certainty specific identification of neurogenic sarcomas.* However, the "geographic necrosis," slender, aligned spindle cells, blending of myxomatous and solid areas with occasional giant cells resembling bizarre ganglion cells, and rare vacuolated lipoblast-like forms should be considered as sug-

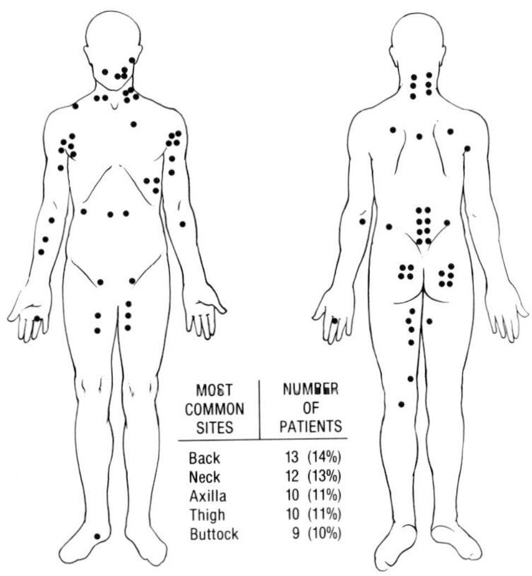

Figure 7-19. Schematic illustration of anatomic distribution of primary site of 91 neurogenic sarcomas treated at Memorial Sloan-Kettering Cancer Center.

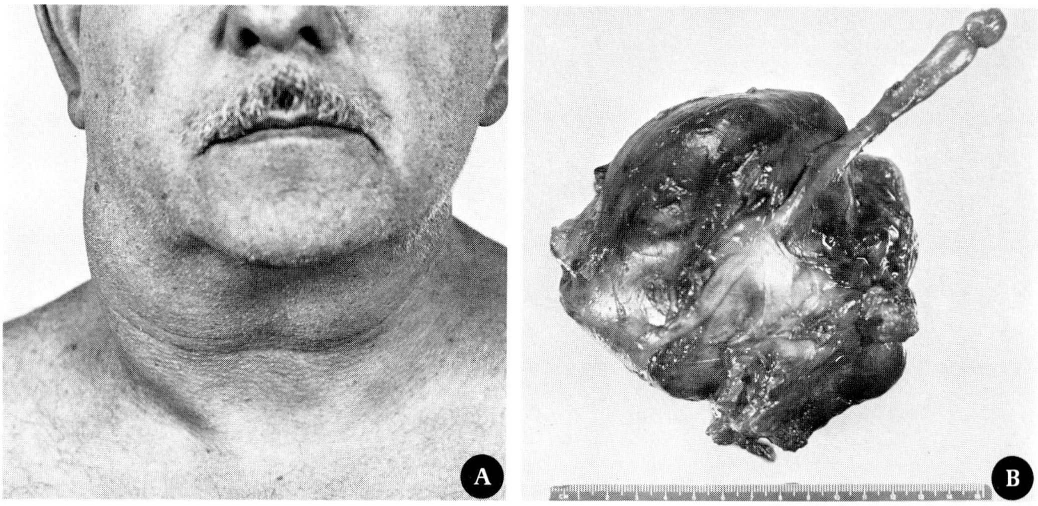

Figure 7-20. **A,** This 49-year-old man presented with a mass in the right neck. **B,** The tumor proved to be neurofibrosarcoma of the vagus nerve. It was removed with a clean margin, and the patient is alive without evidence of the disease more than 20 years after the operation.

gestive microscopic features that are of schwannian origin. On the other hand, considering the pluripotential nature of Schwann cells, it should not be surprising that undifferentiated spindle cell sarcomas of other nerve origin, e.g., certain forms of *leiomyosarcoma* (Chapter 5), *fibrosarcoma* (Chapter 2), or *monophasic synovial sarcoma* (Chapter 3) may mimic neurogenic sarcoma.

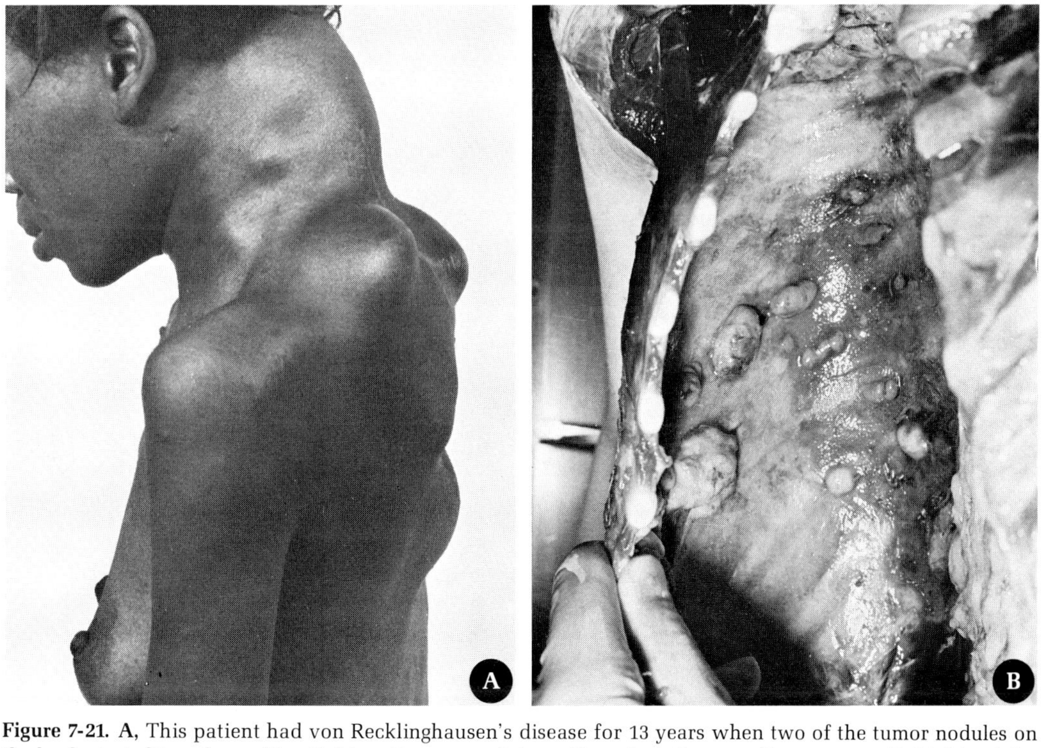

Figure 7-21. **A,** This patient had von Recklinghausen's disease for 13 years when two of the tumor nodules on the back started to enlarge. She died less than a year later with metastatic neurofibrosarcoma. **B,** Multinodular presentation of neurofibrosarcoma along the intercostal nerves.

TABLE 7-9. ***Pertinent Data of Patients Having Neurogenic Sarcoma and Recklinghausen's Disease****

NO. OF CASES	SEX	AGE AT DIAGNOSIS RECKLING-HAUSEN'S DISEASE YR.	MULTIPLE NEURO-FIBROMAS	CAFÉ-AU-LAIT SPOTS	TIME BETWEEN DIAGNOSIS OF NEUROFIBRO-MATOSIS AND NEUROGENIC SARCOMA, YR.	SITE OF NEURO-GENIC SARCOMA	TREAT-MENT	FOLLOW-UP
1	F	16	Yes	Yes	9	Flank	Exc.	2 yr. DcD
2	M	30	Yes	—	24	Thigh	Exc.	3 yr. DcD
3	M	12	Yes	Yes	17	Retroprt.	Exc.	1 yr. DcD
4	F	10	Yes	—	21	Back	Exc.	6 mo. DcD
5	M	4	Yes	Yes	20	Neck	Exc.	3 yr. DcD
6	F	39	Yes	—	2	Back	Exc.	1 yr. DcD
7	F	54	Yes	—	3	Axilla	Amp.	1 yr. DcD
8	M	—	Yes	—	—	Abdomen	Exc.	2 yr. DcD
9	F	9	Yes	—	17	Axilla	Exc.	1 yr. DcD
10	F	4	—	Yes	—	Buttock	Exc.	1 yr. DcD
11	F	20	Yes	—	19	Thigh	Exc.	2 yr. DcD
12	M	35	Yes	—	10	Back	Exc.	1 yr. DcD
13	F	8	Yes	Yes	13	Back	Exc.	1 yr. DcD
14	F	30	Yes	—	16	Thigh	Exc.	1 yr. DcD
15	M	Infant	Yes	Yes	15	Chest	Exc.	9 yr. DcD
16	F	6	Yes	Yes	4	Neck	Exc.	3 yr. DcD
17	M	—	Yes	—	—	Neck	Exc.	23 yr. NED
18	F	4	Yes	Yes	27	Neck	Exc.	13 yr. DcD
19	F	1	Yes	Yes	9	Neck	Exc.	1 yr. DcD
20	F	57	Yes	—	2	Buttock	Amp.	2 yr. DcD
21	F	Infant	Yes	Yes	3	Axilla	Exc.	2 yr. DcD
22	F	30	—	Yes	12	Abdomen	Exc.	1 yr. DcD
23	M	—	Yes	—	—	Foot	Exc.	2 yr. DcD
24	M	20	Yes	Yes	17	Neck	Exc.	6 mo. DcD
25	F	—	Yes	—	—	Thigh	Exc.	1 yr. DcD
26	F	18	Yes	Yes	15	Chest	Exc.	1 yr. DcD
27	F	Infant	Yes	Yes	49	Back	Exc.	2 yr. DcD
28	M	4	—	Yes	—	Retroprt.	Exc.	1 yr. DcD
29	M	—	Yes	—	20	Retroprt.	Exc.	4 yr. DcD
30	F	—	—	Yes	—	Pelvis	Exc.	6 mo. DcD
31	F	Infant	Yes	Yes	3	Axilla	Exc.	1 yr. DcD
32	F	2	Yes	Yes	11	Buttock	Exc.	1 yr. DcD
33	M	—	Yes	—	—	Thigh	Exc.	1 yr. DcD
34	M	10	Yes	—	21	Thigh	Amp.	1 yr. DcD
35	F	—	Yes	—	—	Axilla	Exc.	1 yr. DcD
36	F	13	Yes	—	39	Back	Exc.	1 yr. DcD
37	F	12	Yes	Yes	10	Back	Exc.	2 yr. DcD

*Unpublished data
Exc. = excision; Amp. = amputation; DcD = died with disease; NED = no evidence of disease.

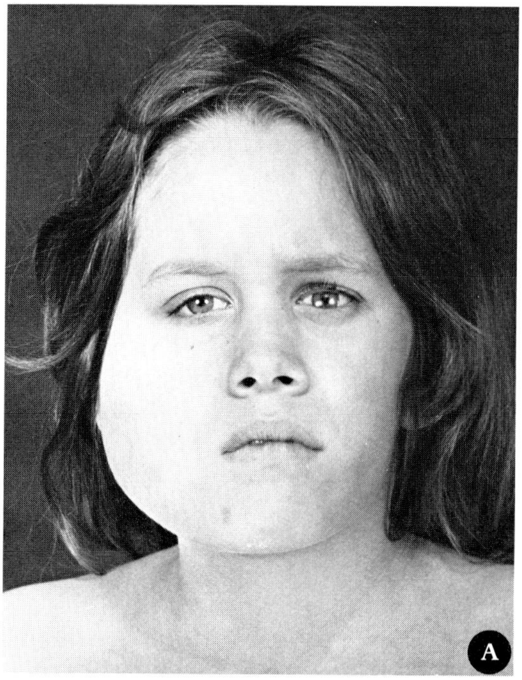

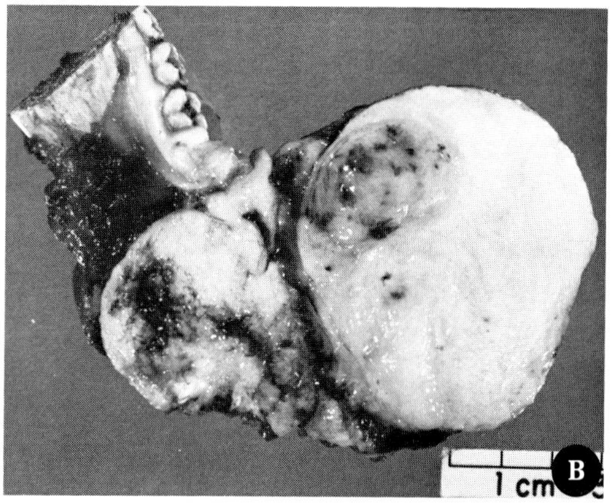

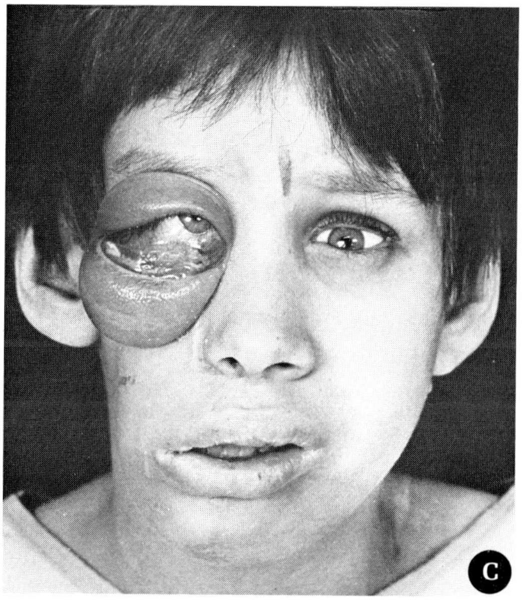

Figure 7-22. **A**, This 10-year-old girl presented with a fast-growing tumor of the right face. **B**, The bulky part of the tumor was removed by hemimandibulectomy and partial maxillectomy. Histologically the tumor was classified as poorly differentiated non-collagenous type of malignant schwannoma (see Figure 7-24). **C**, The patient succumbed to recurrent and metastatic disease 3 years after initial surgery.

PRIMITIVE NEUROECTODERMAL TUMOR*

Primitive neuroectodermal tumor or *peripheral neuroblastoma* or *neuroepithelioma* is a rare malignant neoplasm and is capable of metastasizing (Fig. 7-1). It usually occurs in the mediastinum, retroperitoneum, pelvis, trunk, or the extremities of young adults or adults. It is postulated that it represents a transition between arrested neoplastic Schwann cells, neuroblasts, and perhaps paraganglionic elements (Fig. 7-1). Bolande and Towler (1970) found ultrastructural

* *Synonyms and related terms:* adult neuroblastoma, malignant neuroepithelioma, peripheral medulloepithelioma, malignant epithelioid schwannoma, peripheral neuroblastoma, sympathogonioma.

Figure 7-23. Malignant collagenous schwannoma (or neurofibrosarcoma or collagenous neurogenic sarcoma). This neoplasm is composed of slender spindle cells with finely reticular cytoplasmic filaments extending at least in two directions from the cell body. Some of the filaments appear to be branching to adjacent cells. The nuclei are round pyknotic or elongated and cigar-shaped. The intimate blending of spindle and round cells is a feature of many neurogenic tumors. This neoplasm, despite its orderly and low-grade appearance, metastasized to regional and distant sites and caused the death of the patient.

B, Atypical benign and partly collagenous solitary schwannoma is composed of reticular oval and slender elongated tumor cells in a partly arranged pattern, the so-called tidal wave pattern. The tumor cells are tangled and twisted with heavy reticular cytoplasmic filaments. This tumor is sparsely cellular, and the tumor cells are widely separated by the partly collagenous intercellular matrix. Also notice the absence of necrosis and mitotic figures (H & E, ×140).

C, Malignant collagenous schwannoma (so-called neurofibrosarcoma or collagenous neurogenic sarcoma). This high-grade malignant tumor shows the combination of the characteristic punctate cells and slender cigar-shaped cells with long cytoplasmic filaments. It is difficult to tell at this magnification whether the punctate cells are oligondendrocyte-looking Schwann cells or lymphocytoid cells.

Note the sideway bulging of the cigar-shaped nuclei. Actually, in these slender neoplastic Schwann cells, the nuclei are wider than the cytoplasm. In neoplastic fibroblasts and myoblasts, usually the nuclei are shorter and the cytoplasm is much wider than those in Schwannian cells (H & E, ×350).

D, Low grade non-collagenous malignant schwannoma. The tumor cells have a disarranged or piled-up pattern without any particular feature suggestive of neurogenic origin, except for the gross presentation which clearly indicates that the primary site of origin of this tumor is in the sciatic nerve (H & E, ×350).

E, Malignant triton tumor (or "metaplastic" malignant schwannoma). The primary site of origin of this tumor was traced to the median nerve at the time of dissection. The tumor is composed of slender and pyknotic cigar-shaped neoplastic Schwannian cells and acidophilic round cells, rhabdomyoblasts, with nuclei eccentrically placed in the cytoplasm. Note a number of binucleated rhabdomyoblasts with nuclei arranged in horseshoe shape. The arrangement of the cells is relatively loose and the round cells are held together by the fine and spreading cytoplasmic filaments of the spindle cells (H & E, ×350).

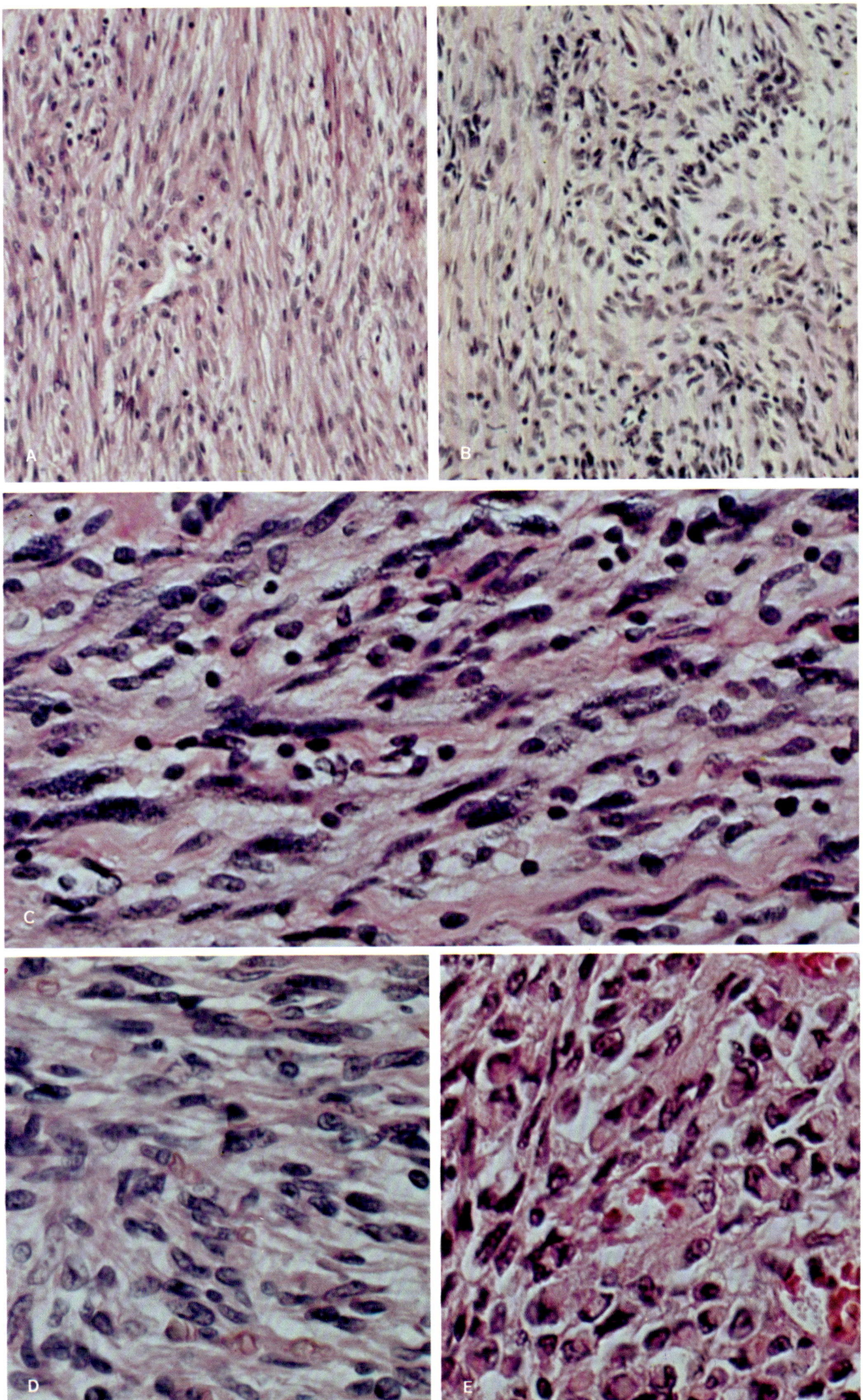

Figure 7-23.

TABLE 7-10. *Summary of Schwannian Features of Neurogenic Tumors*

	COLLAGENOUS SCHWANNOMA		NON-COLLAGENOUS SCHWANNOMA	
	BENIGN	MALIGNANT	BENIGN	MALIGNANT
Antoni A and B patterns	+	+−	++	−+
Interdigitating cell processes	+	+	++	+−
Periodic arrangement of nuclei	+−	−	++	+−
Tidal wave effect	−	−	++	−+
Geographic necrosis	−	−+	−	++
Slender cells	++	−+	+	−+
Mast cells	++	+	+−	+−
Lymphocytoid cells	++	+	+−	+−
Punctate cells	++	+	+−	+−
Collagen	++	+	−	−

++ = common; + = uncommon; +− = may be present; −+ = usually absent; − = absent.

TABLE 7-11. *Neurogenic Sarcoma*

	NO. OF CASES	MALE	FEMALE	MOST COMMON SITE	MORTALITY
Stewart and Copeland (1931)	27	20	7	Extremities Neck	82
Maseritz (1946)	192	96	96	Trunk Arms	
Vieta and Pack (1951)	31	18	13		
D'Agostino et al (1963)	21	12	9	Trunk Extremities	85
Hajdu (unpublished)	91	36	55	Back Neck	81

similarities between ganglioneuroma, neurofibroma, and neuroblastoma maturing into ganglioneurofibroma and suggested that neurofibromatosis may occasionally derive from neuroblastoma. On the other hand, in certain instances neuroblastoma may be the result of mutational abnormality of aberrantly migrating neural crest cells. Rarely it may appear as multifocal neoplasms and show striking gross resemblance to cellular schwannomas.

Recently I saw the microscopic slides of a case. The patient had had neuroblastoma of the right adrenal when she was one year old. After having no evidence of the disease for 16 years, she presented with retroperitoneal ganglioneuroma that transformed to malignant non-collagenous schwannoma in less than one year.

Stout, in 1918, described a neoplasm of the ulnar nerve, which he suggested resembled tumors of the retina. Verocay, as early as 1910, theorized that ganglion cells are the result of multiplication and differentiation of embryonal neurocytes and that the Schwann cell participated in the neoplastic process. During the past decade scattered case reports appeared in the literature (Monteiro et al, 1963; Buthker et al, 1964; Hutchinson et al, 1968; Langerkvist et al, 1969; Askin et al, 1979). Since our recent report (Tang and Hajdu, 1975) of 27 cases of neuroblastoma in adolescents and

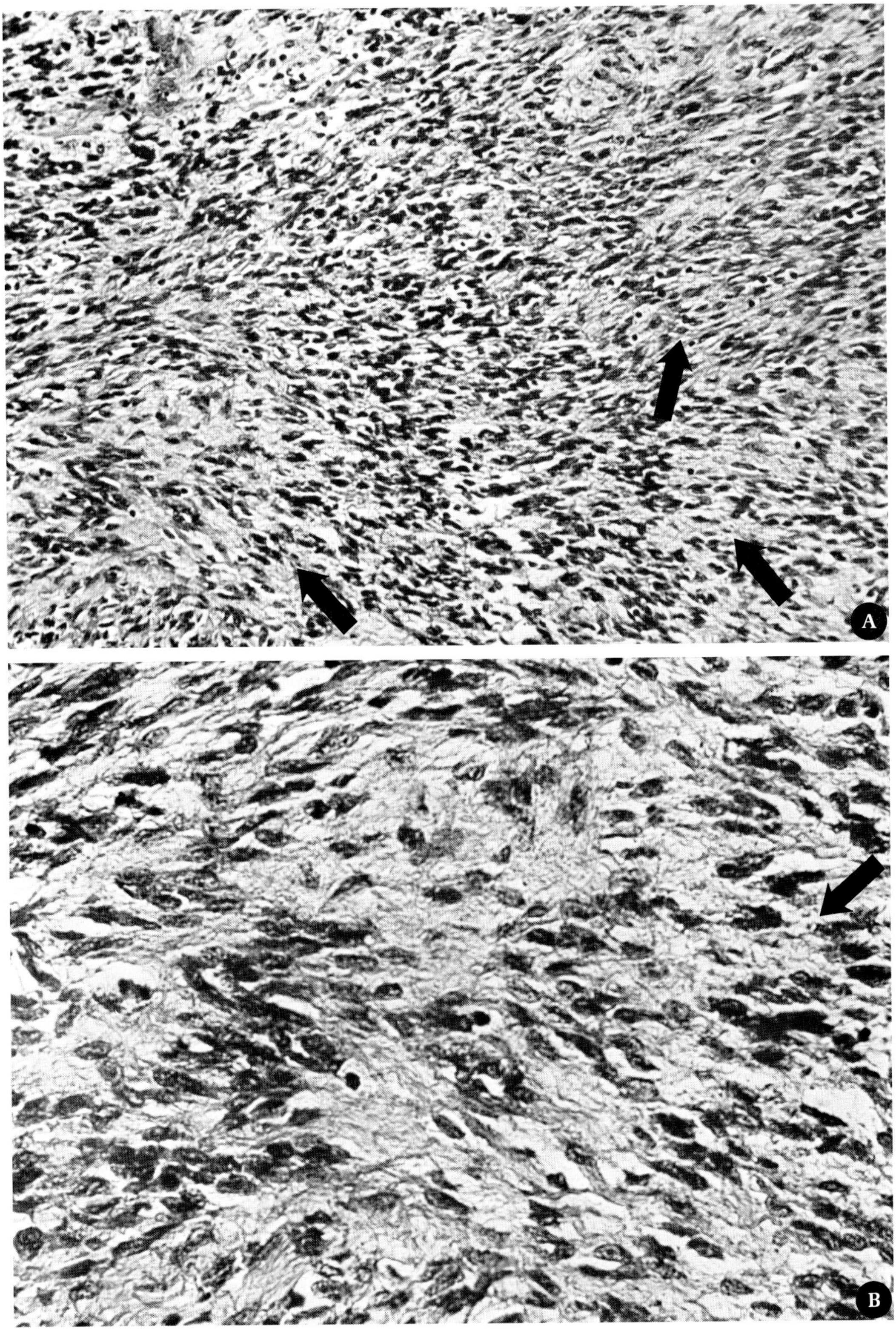

Figure 7-24. Undifferentiated malignant schwannoma (see Figure 7-23) predominantly growing as a non-collagenous spindle cell tumor. The tumor cells are fairly uniform spindle cells with long interdigitating fibrillar cell processes. Despite poor differentiation, the tumor cells attempt to form Antoni-A pattern (arrows). Note the occasional punctate, lymphocyte-like, nuclei of cross-sectioned Schwann cells and sparsity of mitotic figures (**A,** H & E, ×140; **B,** H & E, ×350).

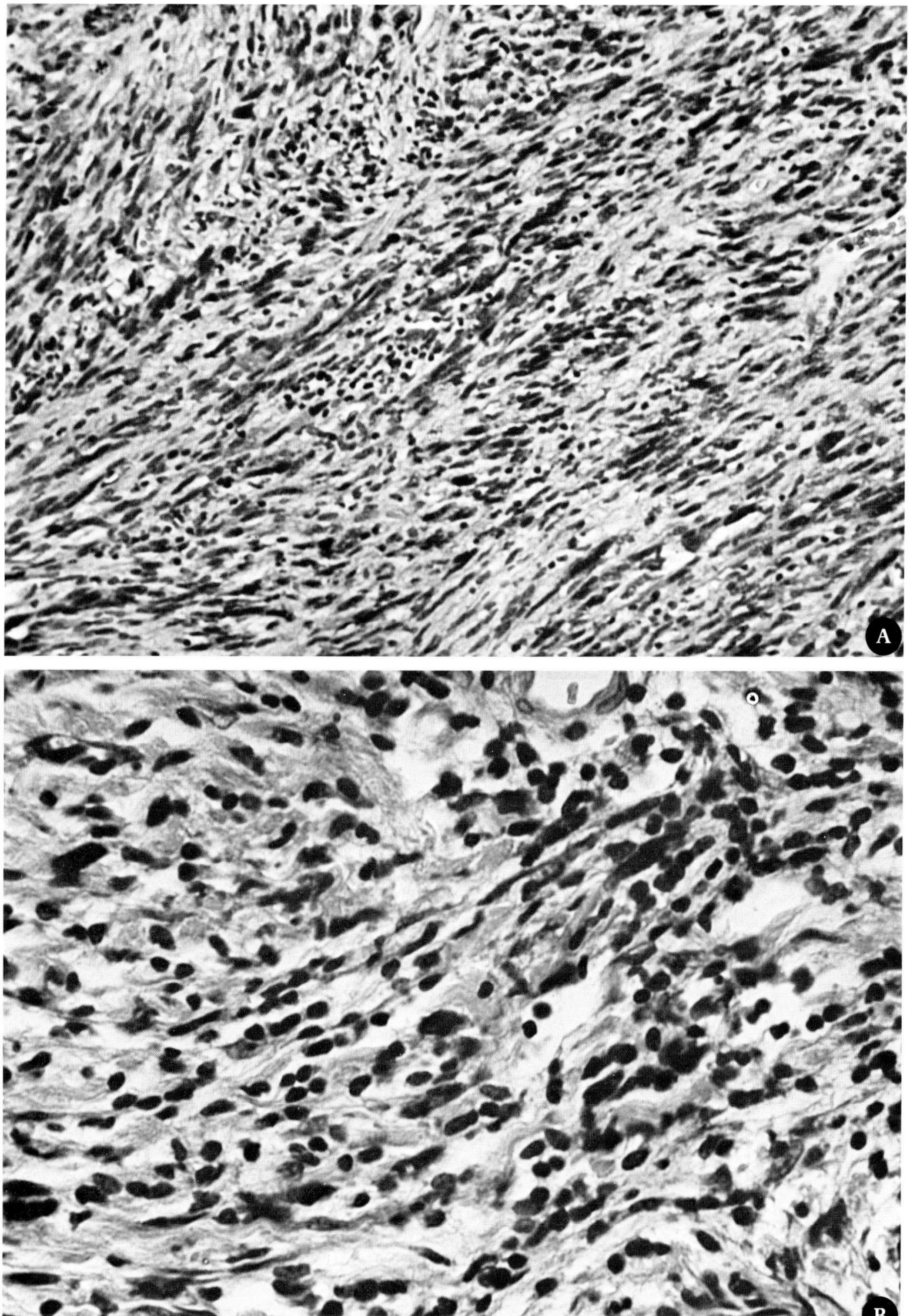

Figure 7-25. Undifferentiated malignant schwannoma showing marked variation in size of slender neoplastic cells. The tumor cells are tightly packed, and there is an intimate admixture of punctate (cross-sected) and spindly (parallel-cut) neoplastic Schwann cells (**A,** H & E, ×140; **B,** H & E, ×350).

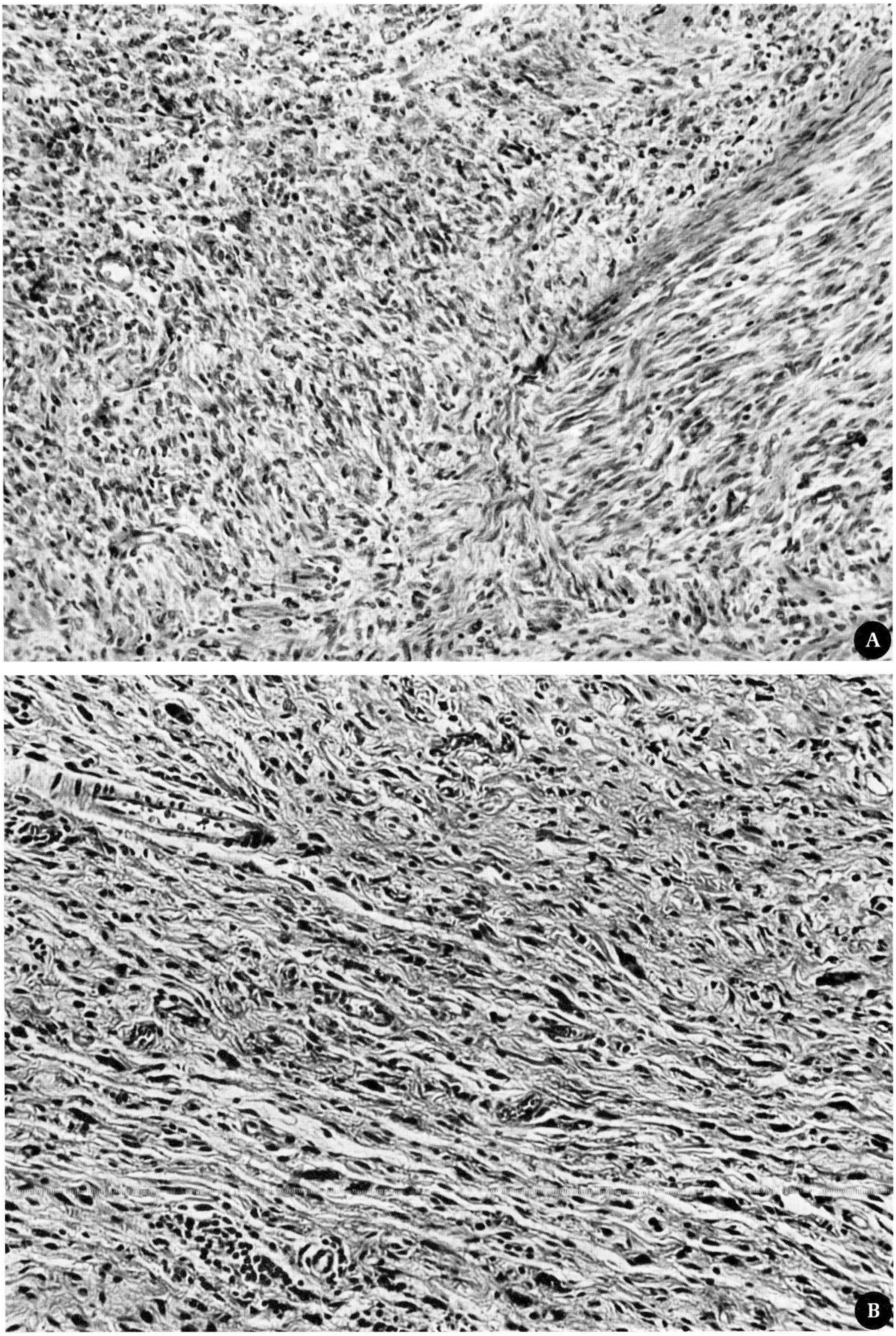

Figure 7-26. Neurofibrosarcoma showing distinct collagenous and thick fibrillar cell processes. The growth pattern is that of a malignant plexiform neuroma with well-outlined partitions between tightly packed bundles of neoplastic Schwann cells. There is an abortive attempt to form Antoni-A pattern **(A).** There is evidence of pleomorphism and mitotic figures, especially in **B.** (**A** and **B,** H & E, ×140).

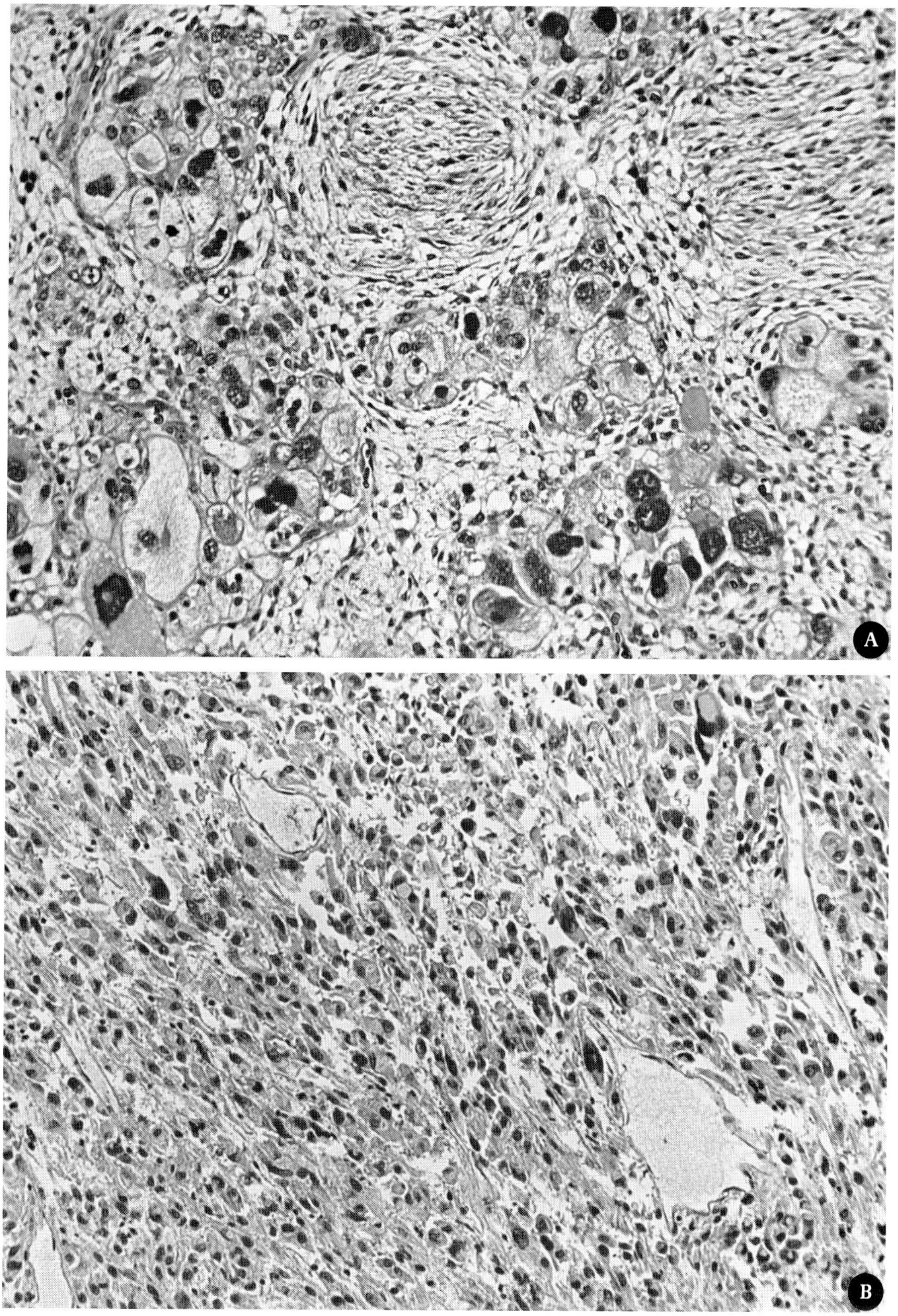

Figure 7-27. A, Undifferentiated malignant schwannoma showing large, bizarre mono- and multinucleated granular cytoplasmic cells in a clearly neurofibrillar or Schwannian background. The large cells show striking resemblance to pleomorphic paraganglionic (pheochromocytic) cells. Note the interdigitating delicate spindle cells (top and right upper corner) and the punctate small cells between the giant forms (H & E, ×140).

B, A pure culture of pleomorphic malignant rhabdomyoblasts found in an undifferentiated malignant schwannoma of the sciatic nerve (H & E, ×140).

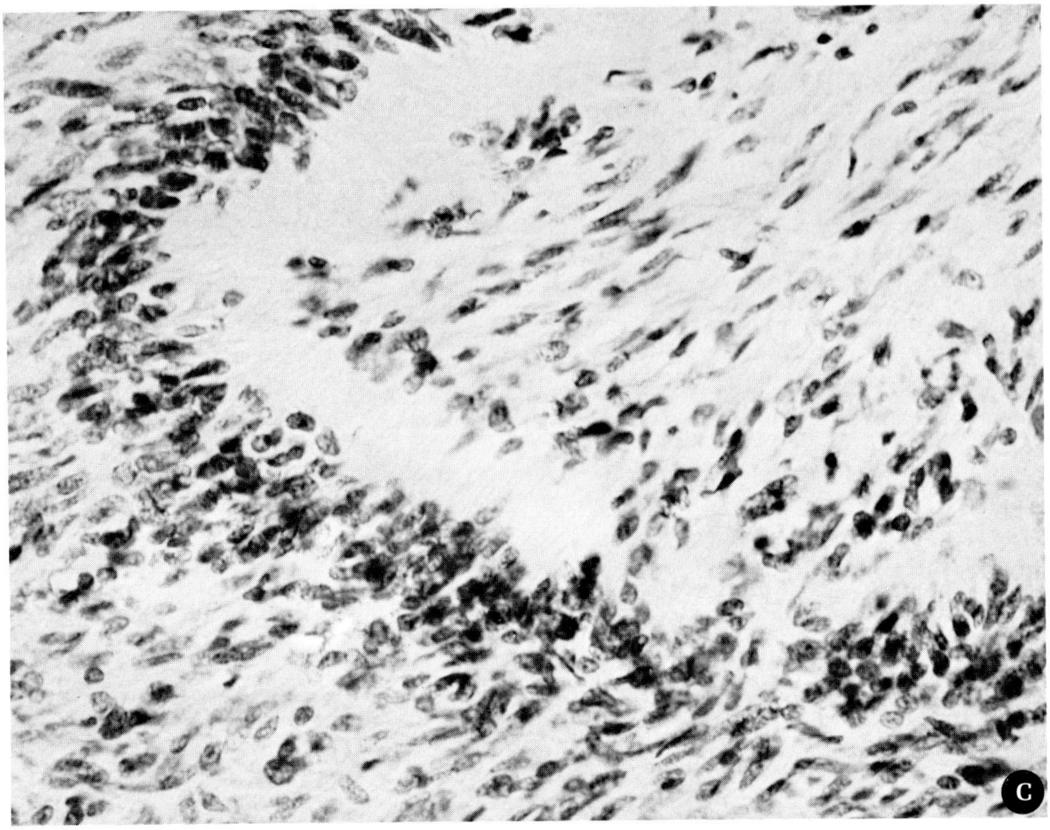

Figure 7-27 (cont.). C, Careful search in undifferentiated malignant schwannomas for schwannian features such as palisading of the tumor cells and geographic necrosis can be rewarding. Note the "tidal wave" palisade or pile-up of tumor cells at the edge of geographic necrosis (H & E, ×350).

adults, I had the opportunity to examine material from 4 additional cases which microscopically appeared to be primitive neuroectodermal tumors or so-called peripheral adult neuroblastomas, all of which were non-secretory and the values of catecholamine metabolites were within normal limits (Table 7-13).

Microscopically, these tumors are composed predominantly of fairly uniform round or oval cells arranged, in some areas, in rosettes or pseudorosettes around a central fibrillar lumen-like area that stains pale red with trichrome stain. Most of the cells, however, are in loosely arranged nests or cords in a sparsely vascular stroma. The mitotic rate is high and some of the tumor cells show tendency to be elongated with long-branching cytoplasmic filaments, which stain faintly positive, in focal areas with PAS before and after digestion with diastase (Fig. 7-32).

According to our experience, these neoplasms are locally invasive, highly destructive lesions with an unusually high tendency to metastasize. In our series the overall survival rate at one year was 67%, at 2 years 28%, and at 5 years or longer 13% (Table 7-12).

In the differential diagnosis *embryonal rhabdomysarcoma, Ewing's sarcoma,* and *hemangiopericytoma* should be considered. By the absence of acidophilic fibrillar cytoplasm, cross striation, highly vascular stroma, botryoid features, and positive PAS stain after diastase digestion, one can rule out embryonal rhabdomyosarcoma with certainty.

Hemangiopericytoma and Ewing's sar-

TABLE 7-12. ***Comparison of Microscopic Growth Pattern and Differentiation of Neurogenic Sarcomas***

	NUMBER OF CASES	
	ASSOCIATED WITH RECKLINGHAUSEN'S DISEASE	NO EVIDENCE OF RECKLINGHAUSEN'S DISEASE
Total number	37	54
Nerve origin, gross finding	12	34
Nerve origin, microscopic finding	25	20
Microscopic Growth Pattern		
Antoni A	11	4
Antoni B	20	37
Verocay body	2	—
Plexiform	21	20
Storiform	14	29
Pleomorphic	10	15
Angiomatous	6	1
Glandular	3	1
Epithelioid	1	16
Nevoid	—	6
Cystic	2	—
Dominant Pattern of Differentiation		
Neurofibrosarcoma	24	2
Desmoid tumor	1	—
Fibrosarcoma	8	6
Undifferentiated malignant schwannoma	2	14
Malignant fibrous histiocytoma*	1	26
Leiomyosarcoma	—	2
Rhabdomyosarcoma	1	2
Liposarcoma	—	1
Malignant mesenchymoma	—	1

*The pattern of malignant fibrous histiocytic growth was that of malignant fibroblastic fibrous histiocytoma (dermatofibrosarcoma protuberans) in 23 of the 26 cases. The remaining 3 tumors showed a mixture of histiocytic and pleomorphic fibrous histiocytic pattern.

TABLE 7-13. ***Primitive Neuroectodermal Tumors****

PRIMARY SITE	TOTAL NO. OF PATIENTS	NO. OF PATIENTS MALE	FEMALE	5-YR. FOLLOW-UP
Mediastinum	7	4	3	7 Died
Retroperitoneum	11	8	3	11 Died
Pelvis	5	2	3	5 Died
Neck	1	—	1	1 Alive
Trunk	3	1	2	2 Died 1 Alive
Extremity	4	3	1	2 Died 2 Alive
	31	18	13	

*Modified by permission from the New York State Journal of Medicine, copyright by the Medical Society of New York. Tang, C. K., and Hajdu, S. I.: Neuroblastoma in adolescence and adulthood. N.Y. State J. Med. 75:1434, 1975.

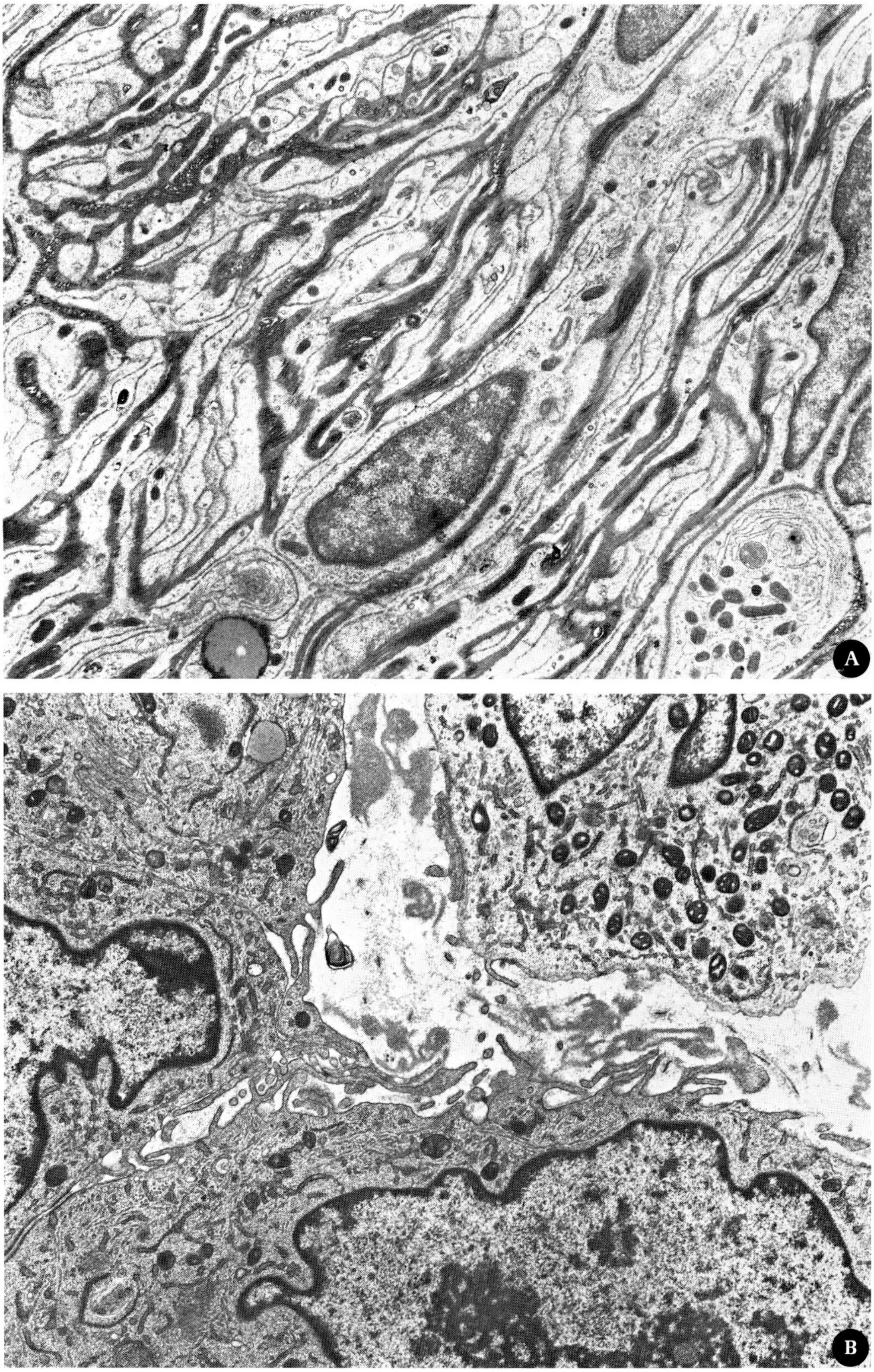

Figure 7-28. A, Ultrastructure of a benign schwannoma from an area of Antoni-A type tissue. Note the long complexly interdigitating cell processes surrounded by basal lamina and collagen fibrils (×4,800).

B, Neurofibrosarcoma associated with von Recklinghausen's disease. Fragments of basal lamina are seen in the space between the pleomorphic neoplastic cells (×8,800).

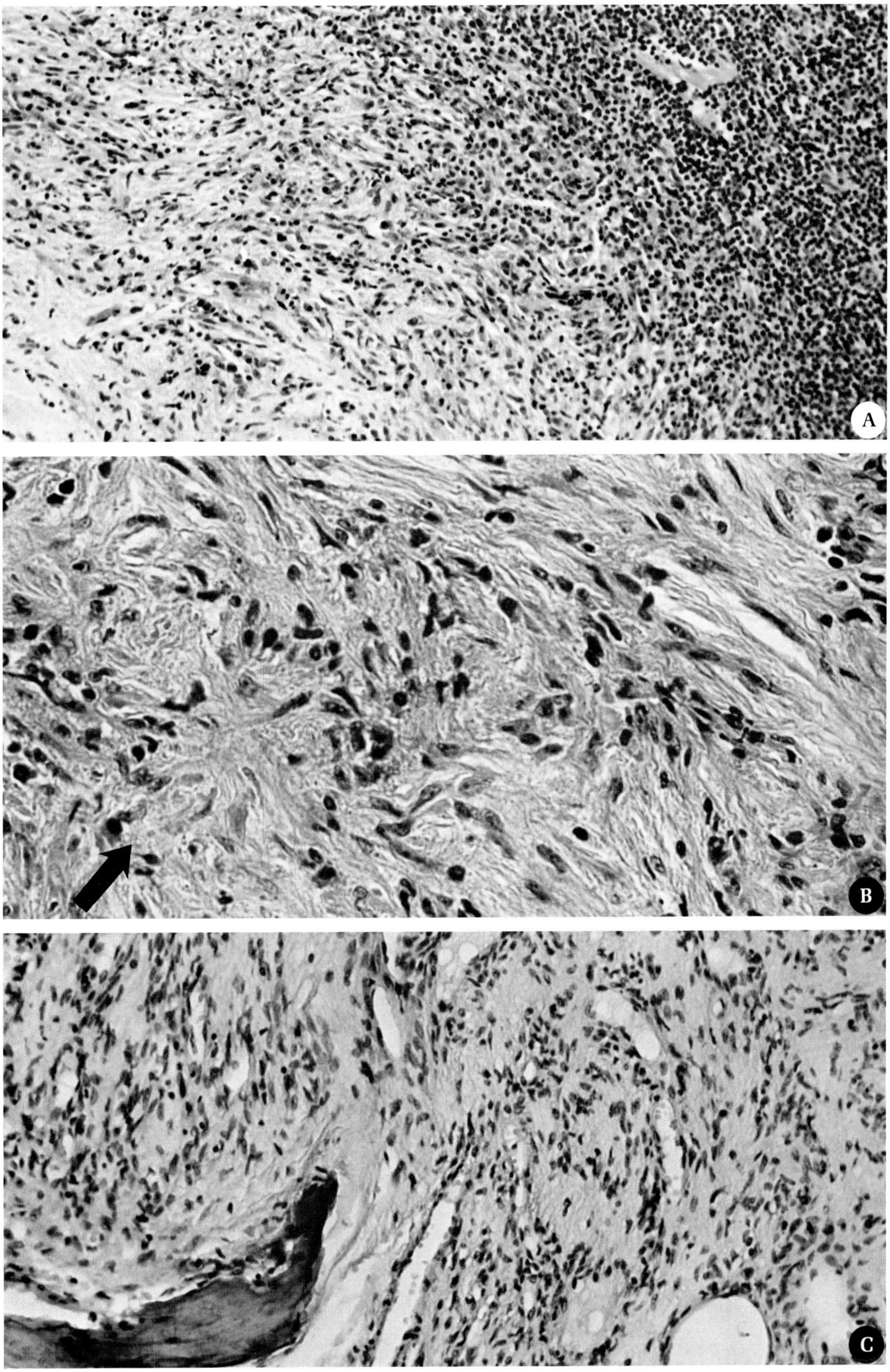

Figure 7-29. A and **B,** Neurofibrosarcoma metastatic to lymph node. The tumor cells are slender, collagenous, fibroblast-like spindle cells. Note the attempt to form a storiform pattern (arrow) (**A,** H & E, ×85; **B,** H & E, ×140).

C, Neurofibrosarcoma metastatic to bone. It is of interest that despite the fact that this is metastatic sarcoma the infiltrate does not look malignant histologically. I observed, in nude mice, similar "benign transformation" of fully malignant human schwannomas following subcutaneous grafting (H & E, ×85).

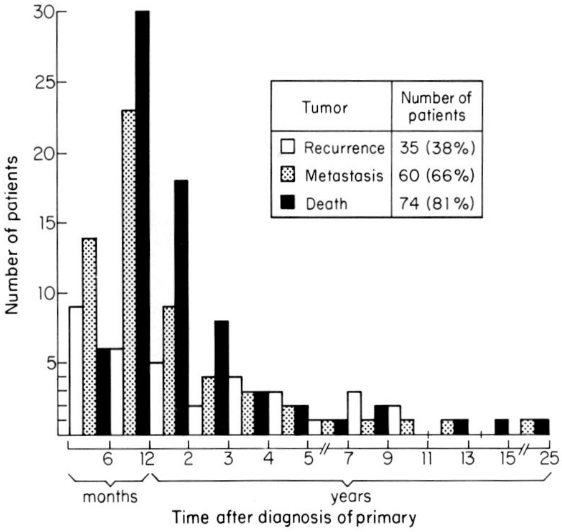

Figure 7-30. Number of recurrences, metastases, and time of death due to the spread of the tumor of 91 patients treated for neurogenic sarcoma at Memorial Sloan-Kettering Cancer Center.

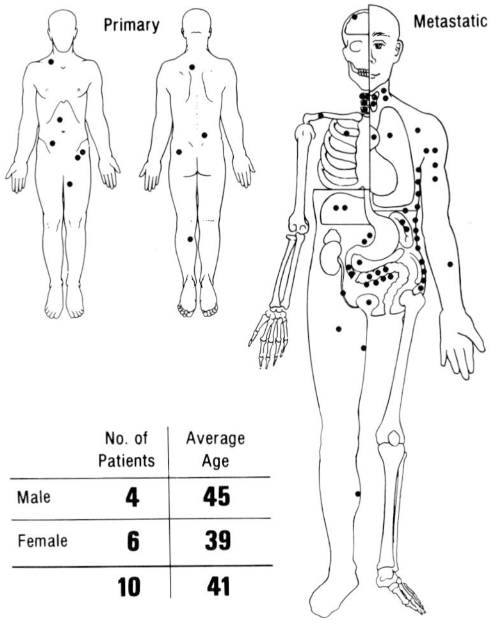

	No. of Patients	Average Age
Male	**4**	**45**
Female	**6**	**39**
	10	**41**

Figure 7-31. Primary and metastatic sites, as seen at the time of autopsy, of neurogenic sarcoma.

coma may be difficult to rule out with certainty on the basis of H & E stained slides. However, distinct perivascular arrangement of neoplastic pericytes can be easily demonstrated by reticulin stain in most hemangiopericytomas and occasionally abortive neurosecretory granules are detectable in primitive neuroectodermal tumors by ultrastructural examination (Figs. 7-33, 7-34).

NEUROBLASTOMA
GANGLIONEUROBLASTOMA
GANGLIONEUROMA
PARAGANGLIOMA

(These neoplasms are not considered in this text, since they are rarely confused with primary soft tissue neoplasms. Interested readers may find useful related references such as Hajdu and Hajdu, 1976.)

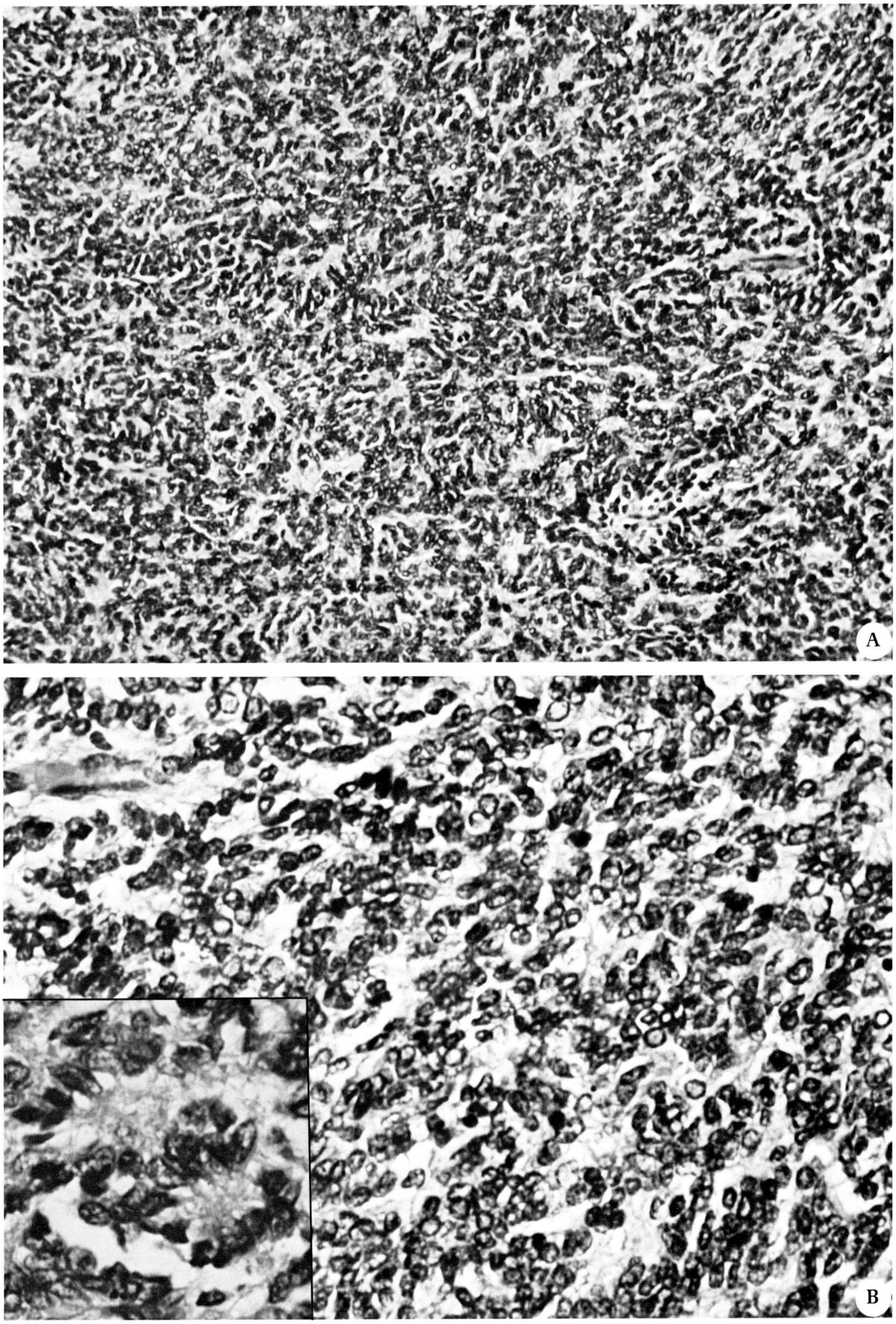

Figure 7-32. Primitive neuroectodermal tumor of the chest wall. The tumor cells are mostly round or oval cells with small, fibrillar or granular cytoplasm. There is a striking monotony and uniformity throughout the tumor. The tumor cells tend to join, by fusion of cell processes, into lumenless cell nests or pseudorosettes (see inset). There is frequent mitosis, but there is a conspicuous absence of blood vessels (**A,** H & E, ×85; **B,** H & E, ×140; inset, H & E, ×350).

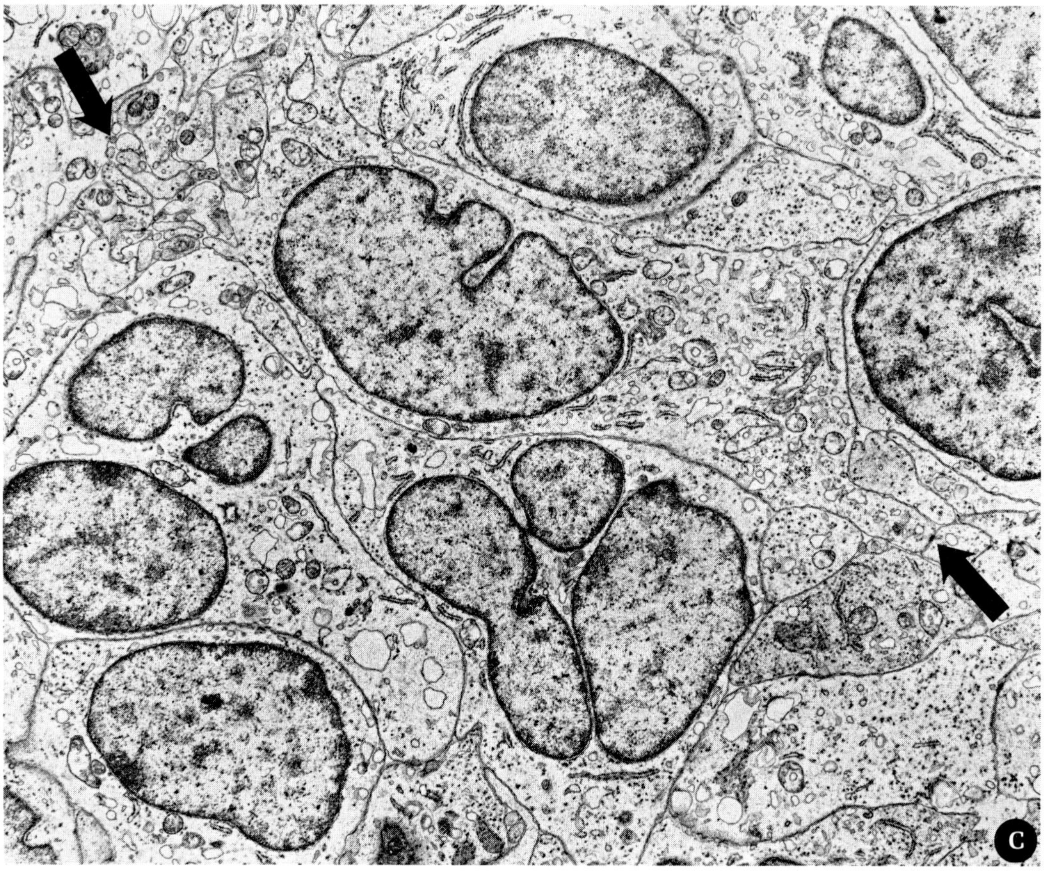

Figure 7-32 (cont.). C, Ultrastructure of primitive neuroectodermal tumor. Tightly packed spindle-shaped and ovoid cells are evident. Note the small dendritic processes (arrows) and occasional small desmosomes (arrow with tail) (×5,300).

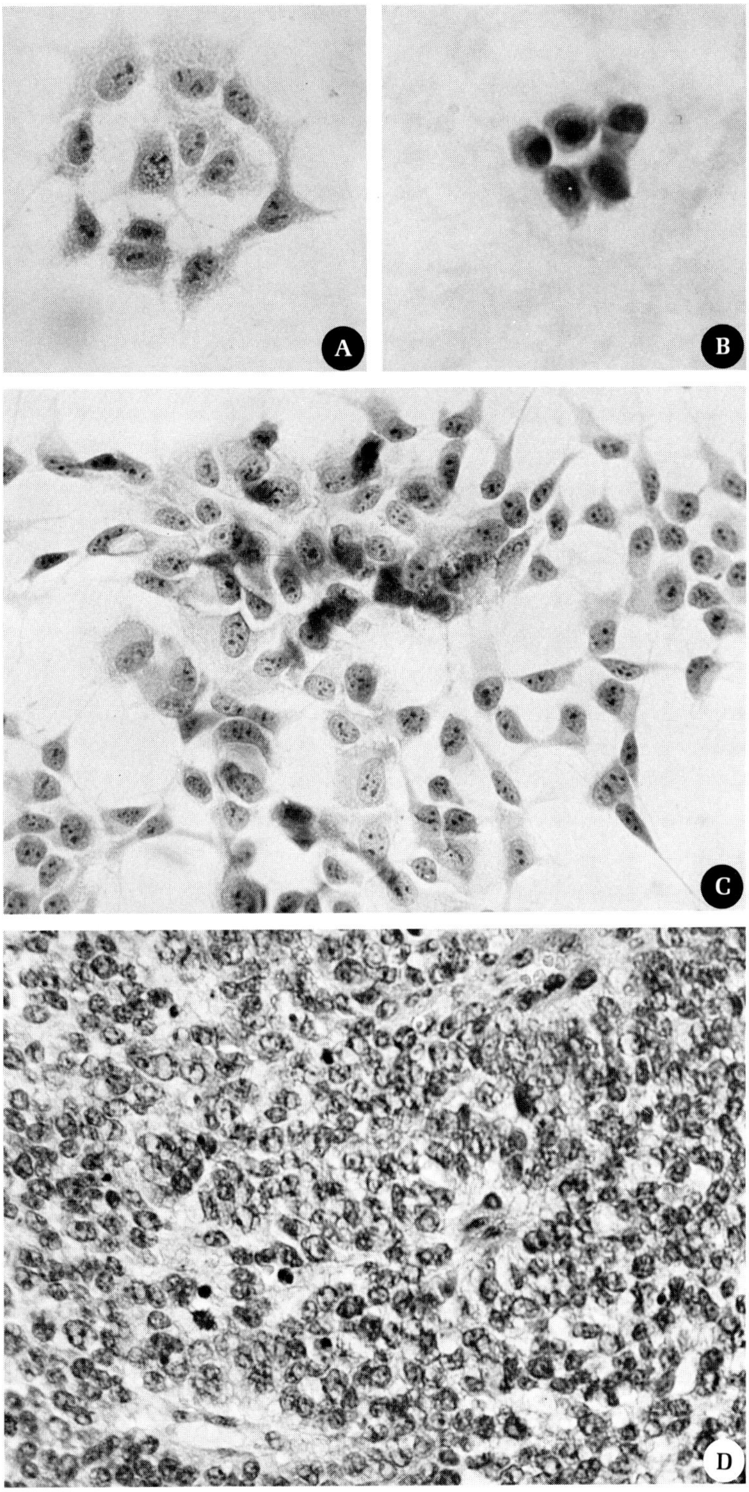

Figure 7-33. Neuroectodermal tumors such as neuroblastoma tend to form rosettes or pseudorosettes in monolayer tissue culture (**A** and **C**), as well as in cell suspension of trypsinized monolayer culture of neuroblastoma **(B)**. Tumor cells of human neuroblastoma, grown in tissue culture, following injection into nude mouse, grow with features of primitive neuroectodermal tumor **(D)**. (**A,** Pap stain, ×350; **B,** Pap stain, ×570; **C,** H & E, ×350; **D,** H & E, ×140). (**A** and **B** from Hajdu, S. I., and Hajdu, E. O.: Cytopathology of Sarcomas and Other Nonepithelial Malignant Tumors. Philadelphia, W. B. Saunders Co., 1976.)

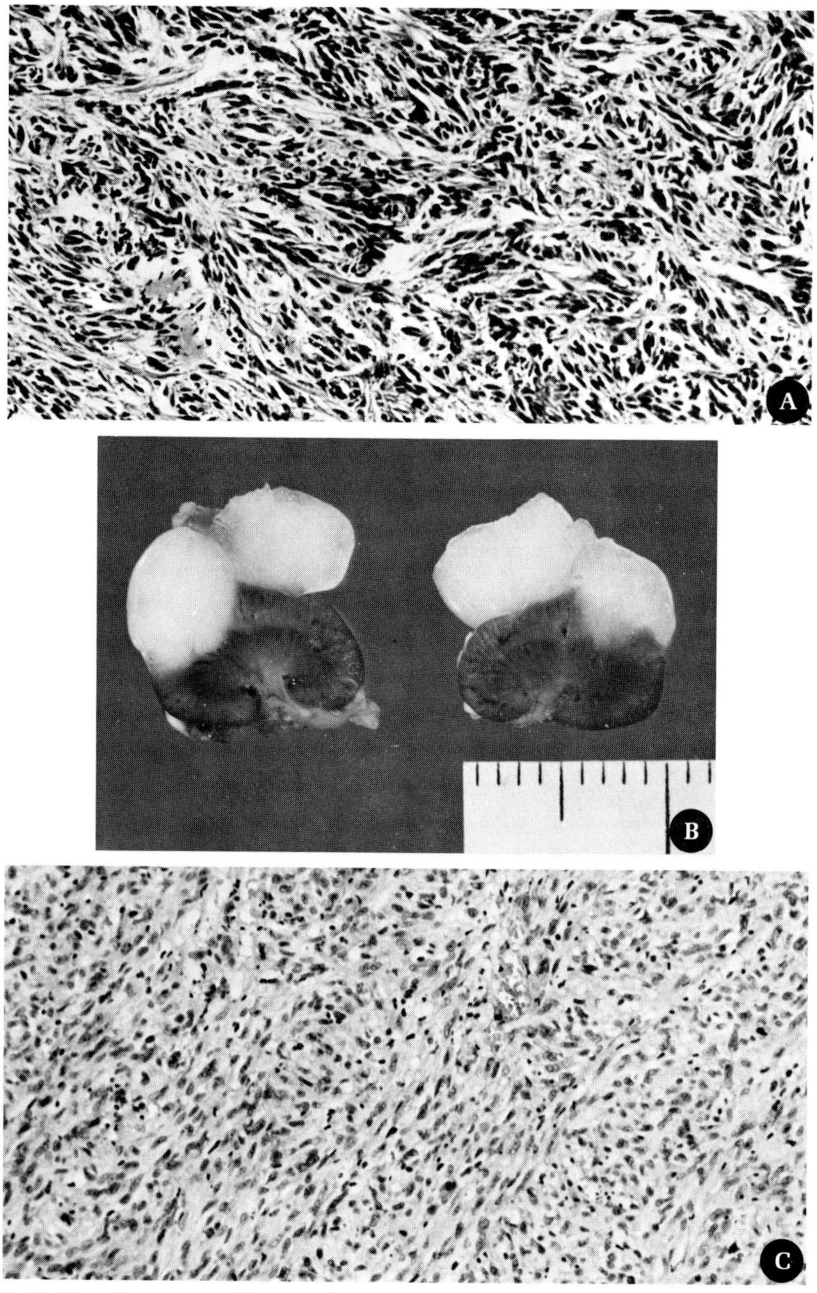

Figure 7-34. **A,** Partly collagenous malignant schwannoma excised from the patient (H & E, ×140). **B,** Tumor produced under renal capsule of nude mouse from injected cell suspension of patient's tumor. **C,** Undifferentiated malignant schwannoma excised from the kidney of nude mouse 3 weeks after subcapsular injection of the cell suspension. Note the spindle and punctate Schwann cells and compare it with Figure 7-25 (H & E, ×140).

REFERENCES

References are listed in chronological order in each category.

INTRODUCTION

Key, A., and Retzius, G.: Studien in der Anatomie des Nervensystem und des Bindegewebes. Stockholm, Samson and Wallin, 1876.

Harrison, R. G.: Neuroblasts versus sheath cell in the development of peripheral nerves. J. Comp. Neurol. 37:123, 1924.

Murray, M. R., and Stout, A. P.: Demonstration and formation of reticulin by schwannian tumor cells in vitro. Am. J. Pathol. 18:585, 1942.

Thomas, P. K.: The connective tissue of peripheral nerve: an electron microscope study. J. Anat. 97:35, 1963.

Gamble, H. J., and Eames, R. A.: An electron microscope study of the connective tissue of human peripheral nerve. J. Anat. 98:655, 1964.

Thomas, P. K., and Slatford, J.: Lamellar bodies in the cytoplasm of Schwann cells. J. Anat. 98:691, 1964.

Cravioto, H.: The role of Schwann cells in the development of human peripheral nerves. J. Ultrastruct. Res. 12:634, 1965.

Sunderland, S.: The connective tissues of peripheral nerves. Brain 88:841, 1965.

Cravioto, H.: The perineurium as a diffusion barrier. Ultrastructural correlates. Bull. Los Angeles Neurol. Soc. 31:196, 1966.

Santhaveerappa, T. R., and Bourne, G. H.: Perineurial epithelium: A new concept of its role in the integrity of the peripheral nervous system. Science 154:1464, 1966.

Bunge, M. B., Bunge, R. P., Peterson, E. R., and Murray, M. R.: A light and electron microscope study of long term organized clusters of rat dorsal root ganglia. J. Cell Biol. 32:439, 1967.

Burkel, W. E.: The histological fine structure of perineurium. Anat. Rec. 158:177, 1967.

Waggener, J. D., and Beggs, J.: The membranous coverings of neural tissues: an electron microscope study. J. Neuropathol. Exp. Neurol. 26:412, 1967.

Ross, M. H., and Reith, E. J.: Perineurium: evidence for contractile elements. Science 165:604, 1969.

Weston, J. A.: The Migration and Differentiation of Neural Crest Cells. *In* Advances in Morphogenesis. (Edited by M. Abercrombie, J. Brachet, and T. J. King. New York, Academic Press, 1970.

Olsson, Y., and Reese, T. S.: Permeability of vasa nervorum and perineurium in mouse sciatic nerve studied by fluorescence and electron microscopy. J. Neuropathol. Exp. Neurol. 30:105, 1971.

Church, R. L., Tanzer, M. L., and Pfeiffer, S. E.: Collagen and procollagen production by a clonal line of Schwann cells. Proc. Natl. Acad. Sci. USA 70:1943, 1973.

Martin, J. R., and Webster, H.: Mitotic Schwann cells in developing nerve: their changes in shape, fine structure and axon relationships. Dev. Biol. 32:417, 1973.

Brown, M. J., Pleasure, D. E., and Asbury, A. K.: Microdissection of peripheral nerve: collagen and lipid distribution with morphologic correlation. J. Neurol. Sci. 29:361, 1976.

Raine, C. S.: On the occurrence of Schwann cells within the normal central nervous system. J. Neurocytol. 5:371, 1976.

Romine, J. S., Bray, C. M., and Aguayo, A. J.: Schwann cell multiplication after crush injury of unmyelinated fibers. Arch. Neurol. 33:49, 1976.

NON-NEOPLASTIC LESIONS

Morton, T. C.: A peculiar and painful affection of the fourth metatarsophalangeal articulation. Am. J. Med. Sci. 71:37, 1876.

Verocay, J.: Multiple Geschwulste als Systemerkrankung am nervosen Apparate. Wien, W. Braumuller, 1908.

Cieslak, A. K., and Stout, A. P.: Traumatic and amputation neuromas. Arch. Surg. 53:646, 1946.

King, L. S.: Note on the pathology of Morton's metatarsalgia. Am. J. Clin. Pathol. 16:124, 1946.

Bartlett, M. J., and McDermott, W. V.: Amputation neuroma of the bile duct with obstructive jaundice. N. Engl. J Med. 251:213, 1954.

Cattell, R. B., and St. Ville, J.: Amputation neuromas of the bile duct with obstructive jaundice. Arch. Surg. 83:242, 1961.

Thomas, P. K.: Changes in the endoneurial sheaths of peripheral myelinated nerve fibers during wallerian degeneration. J. Anat. 98:175, 1964.

Gillesby, W. J., and Wu, K. H.: Amputation neuromas of vagus nerves. Am. J. Surg. 110:673, 1965.

Tuovinen, P. I., Alfthan, O., and Rusk, J.: Neuroma of the ureteral stump after nephrectomy: case report. J. Urol. 94:395, 1965.

Kite, J. H.: Morton's toe neuroma. South. Med. J. 59:21, 1966.

Eames, R. A., and Lange, L. S.: Clinical and pathological study of ischemic neuropathy. J. Neurol. Neurosurg. Psychiatry 30:215, 1967.

Kashef, R., and Das Gupta, T. K.: Segmental demyelination of peripheral nerves in the

presence of malignant tumors. Br. J. Cancer 21:411, 1967.
Johnson, R. T., and Richardson, E. P.: The neurologic manifestation of lupus erythematosus: a clinical-pathological study of 24 cases and review of the literature. Medicine 47:337, 1968.
Lampert, P. W., and Schochet, S. S.: Demyelination and remyelination in lead neuropathy: electron microscopic studies. J. Neuropathol. Exp. Neurol. 27:527, 1968.
Sunderland, S.: Nerve and Nerve Injuries. Baltimore, Williams & Wilkins, 1968.
Warrell, D. A., Godfrey, S., and Olsen, E. G. J.: Giant-cell arteritis with peripheral neuropathy. Lancet 1:100, 1968.
Weller, R. O., and Das Gupta, T. K.: Experimental hypertrophic neuropathy: an electron microscopic study. J. Neurol. Neurosurg. Psychiatry 31:31, 1968.
Wisniewski, H., and Terry, R. D.: Landry-Guillain-Barre syndrome: a primary demyelinating disease. Arch. Neurol. 21:269, 1969.
Dayan, A. D., Gardner-Thorpe, C., Down, P. F., and Gleadale, R. I.: Peripheral neuropathy in uremia. Neurology 20:649, 1970.
Dyck, P. J., and Lambert, E. H.: Polyneuropathy associated with hypothyroidism. J. Neuropathol. Exp. Neurol. 29:631, 1970.
Henson, R. A., and Urich, H.: Peripheral Neuropathy Associated with Malignant Disease. *In* Handbook of Clinical Neurology. Edited by P. J. Vinken and G. W. Bruyn. Amsterdam, North Holland Publishing Company, 1970.
Hauser, E. D. W.: Interdigital neuroma of the foot. Surg. Gynecol. Obstet. 133:265, 1971.
Davis, L. E., and Drachman, D. B.: Myeloma neuropathy: successful treatment of two patients and review of case. Arch. Neurol. 27:507, 1972.
McFarlin, D. E., Strober, W., and Waldmann, T. A.: Ataxia-telangiectasia. Medicine 51:281, 1972.
Singer, M., and Steinberg, M. C.: Wallerian degeneration: a re-evaluation based on transected and colchicine-poisoned nerves in the amphibian Triturus. Am. J. Anat. 133:51, 1972.
Asbury, A. K.: Renaut bodies: a forgotten endoneurial structure. J. Neuropathol. Exp. Neurol. 32:334, 1973.
Bray, G. M., and Aguayo, A. J.: Regeneration of peripheral unmyelineated axons. Rate of the axonal sprouts which develop after injury. J. Anat. 117:517, 1974.
Hawkes, C. H., Jefferson, J. M., Jones, E. L., and Smith, W. T.: Hypertrophic mononeuropathy. J. Neurol. Neurosurg. Psychiatry 37:76, 1974.
Whitaker, J. N., Falchuck, Z. M., Engel, W. K., Blaese, R. M., and Strober, W. H.: Hereditary sensory neuropathy: Association with increased synthesis of immunoglobulin A. Arch. Neurol. 30:359, 1974.
Behse, F., Buchthal, F., Carlsen, F., and Knappeis, G. G.: Unmyelinated fibers and Schwann cells of sural nerve in neuropathy. Brain 98:493, 1975.
Dyck, P. J., Thomas, P. K., and Lambert, E. H.: Peripheral Neuropathy. Philadelphia, W. B. Saunders Company, 1975.
Berlin, S. J.: Soft Somatic Tumors of the Foot: Diagnosis and Surgical Management. Mount Kisco, New York, Futura Publishing Company, 1976.
Romine, J. S., Bray, G. M., and Aguayo, A. J.: Schwann cell multiplication after crush injury of unmyelinated fibers. Arch. Neurol. 33:49, 1976.
Towfighi, J., Gonatas, N. K., Pleasure, D., Cooper, H. S., and McCree, L.: Glue sniffer's neuropathy. Neurology 26:238, 1976.
Asbury, A. K.: Proximal diabetic neuropathy. Ann. Neurol. 2:179, 1977.
Asbury, A. K., and Johnson, P. C.: Pathology of Peripheral Nerve. Philadelphia, W. B. Saunders Company, 1978.

NEOPLASTIC LESIONS

Bell, C.: Surgical Observations. London, Longman, 1816, p. 402.
Smith, R. W.: A Treatise on the Pathology, Diagnosis and Treatment of Neuroma. Dublin, Hodges and Smith, 1849.
Virchow, R.: Das wahre Neurom. Virchows Arch. [Pathol. Anat.] 13:256, 1858.
Eberth, C. J.: Myoma sarcomatodes renum. Virchows Arch. 55:518, 1872.
Gerhardt, C.: Zur Diagnostik multipler Neurombildung. Dtsch. Arch. Klin. Med. 21:268, 1878.
Takacs, A.: Ueber multiple Neurome. Virchows Arch. [Pathol. Anat.] 75:439, 1879.
von Recklinghausen, F. E.: Ueber die multiplen Fibrome der Haut und ihre Bezeihung zu den multiplen Neuromen. Berlin, Hirschwald, 1882.
Chauffard, A. M. E.: Xanthelasma dissemine et symmetrique, sans insuffisance hepatique. Bull. Mem. Soc. Med. Hosp. 6:412, 1889.
Garre, C.: Uber sekundar maligne Neurome. Beitr. Klin. Chir. 9:465, 1892.
Thoma, R.: Textbook of General Pathology and Pathological Anatomy. London, A & C Black, 1896.
Thomson, R.: On Neuroma and Neurofibromatosis. Edinburgh, Turnbull and Spears, 1900.
Benenati, U.: Uber einen fall von Rhabdomyom in einen verlagerten Hoden. Virchows Arch. 171:418, 1903.

Benda, C.: Ganglioneurome des N. vagus. Dtsch. Ges. Pathol. 7:266, 1904.
Verocay, J.: Zur Kenntnis der "Neurofibrome." Beitr. Pathol. Anat. Allg. Pathol. 48:1, 1910.
Sato, S.: Uber das cavernose Angiome des peripherischen Nerven-systems. Arch. Klin. Chir. 100:553, 1913.
Mallory, F. B.: The Principles of Pathologic Histology. Philadelphia, W. B. Saunders, 1914.
Stout, A. P.: A tumor of the ulnar nerve. Proc. N.Y. Pathol. Soc. 18:2, 1918.
Antoni, N. R. E.: Ueber Ruckenmarkstumoren und Neurofibrome. Munchen, J. F. Bergmann, 1920.
Berner, J.: Ein Fall von malignem Ganglioneurom. Beitr. Pathol. Anat. 70:203, 1922.
Nageotte, J.: L'organisation de la matiere dans ses rapports avec la vie. Etudes d'anatomie generale et de morphologie experimentale sur le tissue conjonctif et le nerf. Paris, F. Alcan, 1922.
Harrison, R. G.: Neuroblast versus sheath cell in the development of peripheral nerves. J. Comp. Neurol. 37:123, 1924.
Lanford, J. A., and Cohn, I.: Ependymal neoplasm of the median nerve with case report. South. Med. J. 20:273, 1927.
Quick, D., and Cutler, M.: Neurogenic sarcoma; clinical and pathological study. Ann. Surg. 86:810, 1927.
Cohn, I.: Epithelial neoplasms of the peripheral and cranial nerves; Report of three cases. Arch. Surg. 17:117, 1928.
Schmid, C.: Neurinom des N. Facialis. Zurich, Jahrensversommlung der Gesellschaft Schweizer Halsund Ohrenarzte., 1930.
Hosoi, K.: Multiple neurofibromatosis (von Recklinghausen's disease), with special reference to malignant transformation. Arch. Surg. 22:258, 1931.
Stewart, F. W., and Copeland, M. M.: Neurogenic sarcoma. Am. J. Cancer 15:1235, 1931.
Eichhoff, E.: Uber multiple periphere reine Neurinome. Arch. Klin. Chir. 170:246, 1932.
Masson, P.: Experimental and spontaneous schwannomas. Am. J. Pathol. 8:367, 1932.
Millar, W. G.: A malignant melanotic tumour of ganglion cells arising from a thoracic sympathetic ganglion. J. Pathol. Bacteriol. 35:351, 1932.
Penfield, W.: Tumors of the sheaths of the nervous system. Arch. Neurol. Psychiatr. 27:1298, 1932.
Harvey, D. F., and Tennant, R.: Primary neurogenic sarcoma of the bladder in an infant one month of age. Am. J. Pathol. 10:125, 1934.
Stout, A. P.: The peripheral manifestations of the specific nerve sheath tumor (neurilemoma). Am. J. Cancer 24:751, 1935.
Cutler, E. C., and Gross, R. E.: Neurofibroma and neurosarcoma of peripheral nerves, unassociated with von Recklinghausen's disease: a report of 25 cases. Arch. Surg. 33:733, 1936.
Rosenthal, D. B., and Willis, R. A.: The association of chromaffin tumors with neurofibromatosis. J. Pathol. Bacteriol. 42:599, 1936.
Bailey, P., and Herrmann, J. D.: The role of cells of Schwann in the formation of tumors of the peripheral nerves. Am. J. Pathol. 14:1, 1938.
Cushing, H., and Eisendrath, L.: Meningiomas: Their Classification, Regional Behavior, Life History and Surgical End Results. Baltimore, Thomas, 1938.
Masson, P., and Martin, J. F.: Rhabdomyomes der nerfs. Bull. Assoc. Fr. Cancer 27:751, 1938.
Ewing, J.: Neoplastic Diseases. A Treatise on Tumors, 4th ed. Philadelphia, W. B. Saunders, 1940.
Murray, M. R., and Stout, A. P.: Schwann cells versus fibroblast as the origin of the specific nerve sheath tumor: Observation upon normal nerve sheath and neurilemomas in vitro. Am. J. Pathol. 16:41, 1940.
Maseritz, I. H.: Neurogenic sarcoma. J. Bone Joint Surg. 24:586, 1942.
Murray, M. R., and Stout, A. P.: Characteristics of human Schwann cells in vitro. Anat. Rec. 84:275, 1942.
Murray, M. R., and Stout, A. P.: Demonstration and formation of reticulin by schwannian tumor cells in vitro. Am. J. Pathol. 18:585, 1942.
Ehrlich, H. E., and Martin, H.: Schwannomas (neurilemomas) in the head and neck. Surg. Gynecol. Obstet. 76:577, 1943.
Reubi, F.: Les vaisseaus et les glandes endocrines dans la neurofibromatose: le syndrome sympaticotonique dans le maladie de Recklinghausen. Schweiz. Z. Pathol. Bacteriol. 7:168, 1944.
Foraker, A. G.: Gland-like elements in a peripheral neurosarcoma. Cancer 1:286, 1948.
Saxen, E.: Tumors of the sheaths of the peripheral nerves. Acta Pathol. Microbiol. Scand. 79:(Suppl.), 1948.
Godwin, J. I., Watson, W. L., Pool, J. L., Cahan, W. G., and Nardiello, V. A.: Primary intrathoracic neurogenic tumors. J. Thorac. Surg. 20:169, 1950.
Martin, H., and Foote, F. W.: A third case of so-called retinal anlage tumor. Cancer 4:86, 1951.
Masson, P.: My conception of cellular nevi. Cancer 4:9, 1951.
Vieta, J. O., and Pack, G. T.: Malignant neurilemomas of peripheral nerves. Am. J. Surg. 82:416, 1951.

Gore, I.: Primary malignant tumors of nerve: Report of 8 cases. Cancer 5: 278, 1952.
Losli, E. J.: Intrinsic hemangiomas of the peripheral nerves. Arch. Pathol. 53:226, 1952.
Preston, F. W., Walsh, W. S., and Clarke, T. H.: Cutaneous neurofibromatosis. Clinical manifestations and incidence of sarcoma in 61 male patients. Arch. Surg. 64:813, 1952.
Prichard, R. W., and Custer, R. P.: Pacinian neurofibroma. Cancer 5:297, 1952.
Whiston, T. B.: Neurofibroma eroding carpales. J. Bone Joint Surg. 35B:260, 1953.
Klerk, J. N., and Campbell, W. A.: Neurofibromatosis of the bladder. J. Urol. 72:1167, 1954.
McCormack, L. J., Hazard, J. B., and Dickson, J. A.: Malignant epithelioid neurilemoma (schwannoma). Cancer 7:725, 1954.
Baden, E., Pierce, H. E., and Jackson, W. F.: Multiple neurofibromatosis with oral lesions. Oral Surg. 8:263, 1955.
Pung, S., and Hirsch, E. F.: Plexiform neurofibromatosis of the heart and neck. Arch. Pathol. 59:341, 1955.
Crowe, F. W., Schull, W. J., and Neel, J. V.: A Clinical, Pathological and Genetic Study of Multiple Neurofibromatosis. Springfield, Illinois, Charles C Thomas, 1956.
McCarrol, H. R.: Soft tissue neoplasms associated with congenital neurofibromatosis. J. Bone Joint Surg. 38A:717, 1956.
Bednar, B.: Storiform neurofibromas of the skin, pigmented and nonpigmented. Cancer 10:368, 1957.
Prose, P. H., Gherardo, G. J., and Coblez, A.: Pacinian neurofibroma. Arch. Dermatol. 76:65, 1957.
Economou, S. C., Southwick, H., and Slaughter, D. P.: Neurofibrosarcoma of cranial nerve origin. Arch. Surg. 77:271, 1958.
Champman, R. C., Kemp, V. E., and Taliaferro, J.: Pheochromocytoma associated with multiple neurofibromatosis and intracranial hemangioma. Am. J. Med. 26:883, 1959.
Schweisguth, O., Mathey, J., Renault, P., and Binet, J. P.: Intrathoracic neurogenic tumors in infants and children. Ann. Surg. 150:29, 1959.
Kragh, L. V., Soule, E. H., and Masson, J. K.: Benign and malignant neurilemomas of the head and neck. Surg. Gynecol. Obstet. 111:211, 1960.
Luse, S. A.: Electron microscope studies of brain tumor. J. Neurol. 10:881, 1960.
Drescher, H., and Herzog, W.: Uber Neurofibrome der Vulva und der Vagina. Zentralb. Gynaekol. 83:793, 1961.
Willis, R. A.: The Borderland of Embryology and Pathology. London, Butterworth, 1962.
Barret, R., and Cramer, F.: Tumors of the peripheral nerves and so called "ganglia" of the peroneal nerve. Clin. Orthop. 27:135, 1963.
D'Agostino, A. N., Soule, E. H., and Miller, R. H.: Primary malignant neoplasms of nerve (malignant neurilemomas) in patients without manifestation of multiple neurofibromatosis (von Recklinghausen's disease). Cancer 16:1003, 1963.
D'Agostino, A. N., Soule, E. H., and Miller, R. H.: Sarcomas of the peripheral nerves and somatic soft tissues associated with multiple neurofibromatosis (von Recklinghausen's disease). Cancer 16:1015, 1963.
Luse, S. A., Zopf, D., and Cox, J. W.: An electron microscope study of in vitro and in vivo long spacing collagen. Anat. Rec. 145:254, 1963.
Monteiro, C., DePaola, D., and Dias, L. P.: Primary neuroblastoma of the thigh in an adult. Rev. Bras. Cirug. 45:246, 1963.
Buthker, W., Feltkamp-Vroom, T., Groen, A. S. and Wieberdink, J.: Sympathicoblastoma in the anterior mediastinum. Dis. Chest 46:531, 1964.
Fox, H., Emery, J. L., Goodbody, R. A., and Yates, P. O.: Neurocutaneous melanosis. Arch. Dis. Child. 39:508, 1964.
Pineada, A.: Submicroscopic structure of acoustic tumors. Neurology 14:171, 1964.
Zobell, D. H.: Massive neurofibroma of the larynx. Laryngoscope 74:233, 1964.
Eckert, H.: Uber einen Fall von vaskularer Neurofibromatose der Lunge. Zentralbl. Pathol. 108:285, 1965.
Halpern, M., and Currarino, G.: Vascular lesions causing hypertension in neurofibromatosis. N. Engl. J. Med. 273:248, 1965.
Pineada, A.: Mast cells: their presence and ultrastructural characteristics in peripheral nerve tumors. Arch. Neurol. 13:372, 1965.
Bitker, M.: La neuro-fibromatose vesicale. J. Urol. Nephrol. 72:445, 1966.
Lukash, W. M., Morgan, R. I., Sennett, S. O., and Nielson, O. F.: Gastrointestinal neoplasms in von Recklinghausen's disease. Arch. Surg. 92:905, 1966.
Waggener, J. D.: Ultrastructure of benign peripheral nerve sheath tumors. Cancer 19:699, 1966.
Williams, E. D., and Pollack, D. J.: Multiple mucosal neuromata with endocrine tumor. J. Pathol. Bacteriol. 91:71, 1966.
Cornell, S. H., and Kirkendall, W. M.: Neurofibromatosis of the renal artery: an unusual cause of hypertension. Radiology 88:24, 1967.
Donohue, W. L., Jaffe, F. A., and Newcastle, N. B.: Radiation induced neurofibroma. Cancer 20:589, 1967.
Fawcett, K. J., and Dahlin, D. C.: Neurilem-

moma of bone. Am. J. Clin. Pathol. 47:759, 1967.

Hatziotis, J. C., and Asprides, H.: Neurilemmoma (schwannomas) of the oral cavity. Oral Surg. 24:510, 1967.

Oberman, H. A., and Sullinger, G.: Neurogenous tumors of the head and neck. Cancer 20:1992, 1967.

Fisher, E. R., and Vuzevski, V. D.: Cytogenesis of schwannoma (neurilemmoma) neurofibroma, dermatofibroma and dermatofibrosarcoma, as revealed by electron microscopy. Am. J. Clin. Pathol. 49:141, 1968.

Hutchinson, J. E., Nash, A. D., and McCord, C. W.: Neuroblastoma of the anterior mediastinum in an adult. J. Thorac. Cardiovasc. Surg. 56:147, 1968.

Rosenfeld, L., Graves, H., and Lawrence, R.: Primary neurogenic tumors of the lateral neck. Ann. Surg. 167:897, 1968.

Cravioto, H.: The ultrastructure of acoustic nerve tumors. Acta Neuropathol. (Berl.) 12:166, 1969.

Das Gupta, T. K., Brasfield, R. D., Strong, E. W., and Hajdu, S. I.: Benign solitary schwannomas (neurilemmomas). Cancer 24:355, 1969.

Herkin, J. C., and Reed, R. J.: Tumors of the peripheral nervous system. *In* Atlas of Tumor Pathology, second series, fasc. 3. Washington, D.C., A.F.I.P., 1969.

Lagerkvist, B., Ivermark, B., and Sylven, B.: Malignant neuroepithelioma in childhood, report of three cases. Acta Chir. Scand. 136:641, 1969.

Abell, M. R., Hart, W. R., and Olson, J. R.: Tumors of the peripheral nervous system. Hum. Pathol. 1:503, 1970.

Bolande, R. P., and Towler, W. F.: A possible relationship of neuroblastoma to von Recklinghausen's disease. Cancer 26:162, 1970.

Das Gupta, T. K., and Brasfield, R. D.: Solitary malignant schwannoma. Ann. Surg. 171:419, 1970.

Kramer, W.: Tumors of nerves. Handbook of Clinical Neurology. Amsterdam, North Holland Company, 1970.

El-Serafy, S.: Rare benign tumors of the larynx. J. Laryngol. Otol. 85:837, 1971.

Katz, A. D., Passy, V., and Kaplan, L.: Neurogenous neoplasms of major nerves of face and neck. Arch. Surg. 103:51, 1971.

Mennel, H. D., and Zulch, K. J.: Die Morphologie maligner Tumoren des peripheren Nerven. Zentralb. Neurochir. 32:11, 1971.

White, H. R.: Survival in malignant schwannoma. Cancer 27:720, 1971.

Armstrong, R. G., Lindberg, E. F., Troxler, G., Stanford, W., and Dooley, B. N.: Simultaneous excision of bilateral neurogenic tumors of the mediastinum. Chest 62:348, 1972.

Brasfield, R. D.: Von Recklinghausen's disease, a clinical-pathological study. Ann. Surg. 175:86, 1972.

Conley, J.: Neurogenic tumors of the head and neck. J. Otol. Laryngol. Soc. Amstr. 3:362, 1972.

Cravioto, H., Palekar, L., Weiss, E., and Bennett, K.: Experimental neurinoma in tissue culture. Acta. Neuropathol. 21:154, 1972.

Zimmerman, L. E., Font, R. L., and Anderson, S. R.: Rhabdomyosarcomatous differentiation in malignant intraocular medulloepitheliomas. Cancer 30:817, 1972.

Conley, J., and Janecka, I.: Neurilemmoma of the facial nerve. Plast. Reconstr. Surg. 52:55, 1973.

Cravioto, H., Weiss, J. F., Weiss, E. de C., Goebel, H. H., and Ransohoff, J.: Biological characteristics of peripheral nerve tumors induced by ethylnitrosourea. Acta Neuropathol. 23:265, 1973.

Ghosh, B. C., Ghosh, L., Huvos, A. G., and Fortner, J. G.: Malignant schwannoma. Cancer 31:184, 1973.

Woodruff, J. M., Chernik, N. L., Smith, M. C., Millett, W. B., and Foote, F. W.: Peripheral nerve tumors with rhabdomyosarcomatous differentiation (Malignant "Triton" tumors). Cancer 32:426, 1973.

Greene, J. F., Fitzwater, J. E., and Burgess, J.: Arterial lesions associated with neurofibromatosis. Am. J. Clin. Pathol. 62:481, 1974.

Schenkein, I., Bueker, E. D., Helson, L., Axelrod, F., and Dancis, J.: Increased nerve-growth-stimulating activity in disseminated neurofibromatosis. N. Engl. J. Med. 290:613, 1974.

Bowers, D. G., Jr.: The serious implications of multiple mucosal neuromata. Plast. Reconstr. Surg. 56:554, 1975.

Chandra, S., Jerva, M. J., and Clemis, J. D.: Ultrastructural characteristics of human neurilemmoma cell nuclei. Cancer Res. 35:2000, 1975.

Helson, L., Das Gupta, T. K., and Hajdu, S. I.: Human neuroblastomas in nude mice. Cancer Res. 35:2594, 1975.

Hoggins, G. S., and Grundy, M. C.: Melanotic neuroectodermal tumor of infancy. Report of a case. Oral Surg. 40:34, 1975.

Lassmann, H., Gebhart, W., and Stockinger, L.: The reaction of connective tissue fibers in the tumor of Recklinghausen's disease. Virchows Archiv. [Cell Pathol.] 19:167, 1975.

Tang, C. K., and Hajdu, S. I.: Neuroblastoma in adolescence and adulthood. N.Y. State J. Med. 75:1434, 1975.

Conley, F. K., Rubinstein, L. J., and Spence, A. M.: Studies on experimental malignant nerve sheath tumors maintained in tissue and organ culture systems. II. Electron microscopy observations. Acta Neuropathol. (Berl.) 34:293, 1976.

Factor, S., Turi, G., and Biempica, L.: Primary cardiac neurilemmoma. Cancer 37:883, 1976.

Hajdu, S. I., and Hajdu, E. O.: Cytopathology of Sarcomas and Other Nonepithelial Malignant Tumors. Philadelphia, W. B. Saunders Company, 1976.

Rubinstein, L. J., Conley, F. K., and Herman, M. M.: Studies on experimental malignant nerve sheath tumors maintained in tissue and organ culture systems. I. Light microscopy observations. Acta Neuropathol. (Berl.) 34:277, 1976.

Woodruff, J. M.: Peripheral nerve tumors showing glandular differentiation (Glandular schwannomas). Cancer 37:2399, 1976.

Clark, S. S., Marlett, M. M., Prudencio, R. F., and Das Gupta, T. K.: Neurofibromatosis of the bladder in children. J. Urol. 118:654, 1977.

Dooling, E. C., Chi, J. G., and Gilles, F. H.: Melanotic neuroectodermal tumor of infancy. Cancer 39:1535, 1977.

Gelfand, E. T., Taylor, R. F., Rao, S., Hendin, D., Akabutu, J., and Callaghan, J. C.: Melanotic malignant schwannoma of the right atrium. J. Thorac. Cardiovasc. Surg. 74:808, 1977.

Karcioglu, Z., Someren, A., and Mathes, S. J.: Ectomesenchymoma. A malignant tumor of migratory neural crest (Ectomesenchyme) remnants showing ganglionic, schwannian, melanocytic and rhabdomyoblastic differentiation. Cancer 39:2486, 1977.

Lynch, H. T., Guirgis, H. A., Lynch, P. M., Lynch, J. F., and Harris, R. E.: Familial cancer syndromes: A survey. Cancer 39:1867, 1977.

Ramzy, I.: Benign schwannoma: Demonstration of Verocay bodies using fine needle aspiration. Acta Cytol. 21:316, 1977.

Stay, E. J., and Vawter, G.: The relationship between nephroblastoma and neurofibromatosis (von Recklinghausen's disease). Cancer 32:2550, 1977.

Wirth, W. A., and Bray, C. B.: Intra-osseous neurilemoma. J. Bone Joint Surg. 59A:252, 1977.

Ashbury, A. K., and Johnson, P. C.: Pathology of Peripheral Nerve. Philadelphia, W. B. Saunders Company, 1978.

Askin, F. B., Rosai, J., Sibley, R. K., Dehner, L. P., and McAlister, W. H.: Malignant small cell tumor of the thoracopulmonary region in childhood. Cancer 43:2438, 1979.

chapter 8

Extraskeletal Bone Tumors

NON-NEOPLASTIC LESIONS

Chondroid Metaplasia
Osteoid Metaplasia
Myositis Ossificans

NEOPLASTIC LESIONS

Chondroma
Osteochondroma
Osteoma
Osteogenic Sarcoma
Chondrosarcoma
Ewing's Sarcoma

NON-NEOPLASTIC extraskeletal bone lesions may resemble neoplasms in their clinical and radiographic appearance. These lesions may also cause a considerable problem in differential diagnosis.

CHONDROID AND OSTEOID METAPLASIA

Schaffer in his book published in 1930 emphasized the close relationship of fibrous, adipose, and chondroid tissues, any of which may substitute for or replace any other under certain conditions. The occurrence in soft tissues of tumor-like masses containing metaplastic cartilage and bone has been recognized since Boneti (1700), who first called attention to it. However, it was Virchow, in 1863, who first publicized that cartilage as well as bone may arise by metaplasia from fibroblastic elements. He regarded chondroblasts and osteoblasts as modified fibroblasts.

Seidelin, in 1932, reported the occurrence of "chordoma-like round cells" in a liposarcoma lying between the pectoralis muscles (see Chapter 4). The presence of chondroid and bony tissues in an old hematoma at the site of trauma is not an unusual finding. Other examples of such metaplastic deposits of chondroid and osseous tissues are found at injection sites, blood vessel walls, and granulomas. The first case of an osseous tumor of the breast is recorded by Dyke in 1926. Busser (1929) described an osteochondroblastic "sarcoma" in a fibroadenoma of the breast.

In addition, metaplastic chondroid and osteoid tissues may occur in benign as well as in malignant neoplasms. Soft tissue tumors, especially the ones that are slowly growing or exposed to trauma, may contain foci of metaplastic cartilage and bone. Examples are leiomyomas, desmoid tumors, and neurofibromas. Such findings are not uncommon in tumors that have been incised or treated by irradiation (Table 8-1).

The mode of formation of metaplastic bone is similar to the formation of developing bone during intra- and extra-uterine life. It may form either directly from fibrous tissue or secondary to cartilage formation.

From the point of view of *differential diagnosis* chondroid and osteoid metaplasia rarely cause difficulty. Radiographically as well as histologically, the metaplastic changes present as ill-defined areas. The bony and the chondroid elements blend into the surrounding connective tissue and show all stages of transition from fibroblasts to mature chondrocytes and osteoids. Metaplastic bone is predominantly composed of well-formed, noncalcified lamellae of

TABLE 8-1. *Soft Tissue Sarcomas with Metaplastic Elements*

	TOTAL NO. CASES RECORDED	NO. CASES WITH METAPLASIA		
		CHONDROID	OSTEOID	BOTH
Embryonal rhabdomyosarcoma	95	0	2	0
Fibrosarcoma	160	2	4	6
Liposarcoma	142	0	1	8
Malignant fibrous histiocytoma	180	2	1	3
Tendosynovial sarcoma	151	2	0	4
Angiosarcoma	145	1	0	2
Pleomorphic rhabdomyosarcoma	125	1	4	0
Malignant schwannoma	142	0	1	3
Leiomyosarcoma	40	0	0	0
Other	70	2	1	2
	1250	10	14	28

bony substance edged by uniform and regularly arranged osteoids. Atypical and pleomorphic malignant osteoids and immature chondrocytes, characteristic components of osteogenic sarcoma and chondrosarcoma, are not seen in metaplastic lesions (Figs. 8-1, 8-2).

MYOSITIS OSSIFICANS

(See Chapter 5.)

NEOPLASTIC LESIONS

Neoplasms commonly seen in bones rarely occur in soft tissues. The only exception is the giant cell tumor which properly should be regarded as histiocytic fibrous histiocytoma. This entity is discussed in Chapters 2 and 3. As a rule, extraskeletal bone tumors should be diagnosed only when bone has been ruled out as the site of origin. Extreme caution is advised in diagnosis, especially in Ewing's sarcoma. Although extraskeletal Ewing's sarcoma may occur, it is also known that the intraskeletal primary lesion in disseminated Ewing's sarcoma may be so small that it can escape radiographic detection (Potozky and Fried, 1939).

CHONDROMA AND OSTEOCHONDROMA

Benign cartilagenous tumors of the soft tissues are uncommon. The first reference to chondromas of soft tissue was made by Paget in his book, *Lectures on Surgical Pathology,* in 1870. Chauvin and Roux, in 1920, reported a case of "fibrochondroma" of the foot apparently arising from the tendons of the fourth toe. *Synovial chondromatosis* (Chapter 3) is discussed in the literature more often than any other form of chondroid deposits. A case of fascial "enchondroma" was reported by Goldmann in 1928.

Although a few case reports of malignant transformation of chondroma to chondrosarcoma exist (Goldman and Lichtenstein, 1964; Mullins et al, 1965), most chondromas remain localized benign neoplasms, even after recurrences.

There are numerous case reports of extraskeletal chondroma, some of which are accounts of chondromas at unusual sites such as the *tongue, cheek, larynx* (Huizenga and Balogh, 1970), and *meninges* (Lynch and Uriburu, 1973). The most meaningful review articles are listed in Table 8-2.

Chondroma of soft tissues is a disease of adults and affects males as well as females most commonly during the fourth decade. The most common anatomic sites of chondromas are the hands and the feet. The majority of these tumors are less than 3 cm in size; however, occasional examples of larger tumors have been reported. The exact tissue of origin of chondroma often cannot be established, but their close association with tendon, tendon sheath, or joint capsule is mentioned in most reports.

The gross and microscopic appearances of extraskeletal chondromas are fairly characteristic and they rarely cause diagnostic difficulty. Most of these lesions are self-limited and "shell out" at operation. Microscopically, the majority of the tumors are composed of well-differentiated chondrocytes. There is little tendency of the tumor cells to form satellite nodules or exhibit cellular anaplasia. As a rule, these tumors are sparsely vascular, appear encapsulated, and may be partially calcified without evidence of necrosis. If there is any significant degree of ossification of chondrocytes, one may be justified to call such lesions *osteochondroma.*

Soft tissue chondromas, especially the ones near major joints or bursae, may be sparsely cellular and rich in myxoid stromal substance and may resemble *myxoma.* The myxoid material in chondromas, however, is sulfated mucopolysaccharides which stain positive with alcian blue stain before as well as after treatment of the sections with hyaluronidase. Myxomas, on the other hand, stain negative following depolymerization with hyaluronidase.

TABLE 8-2. *Chondroma of Soft Tissues*

	NO. CASES WITH FOLLOW-UP	AVG. AGE YR.	MOST COMMON SITE	RECURRENCE %	FOLLOW-UP
Murphy and Wilson (1958)	32	—	Hands	—	No evidence of disease
Dahlin and Salvador (1974)	68	—	Hands Feet	16	No evidence of disease
Chung and Enzinger (1978)	56	35	Hands Feet	25	No evidence of disease (54 patients); 2 patients died of unrelated cause
Hajdu (personal experience)	36	38	Hands Feet	15	No evidence of disease (30 patients); 6 patients died of carcinoma

The distinction between well-differentiated benign and malignant chondroid lesions is occasionally difficult and one must depend on clinical and radiographic findings, as well as microscopic appearance of individual tumors. Formation of satellite nodules, presence of binucleated and pleomorphic chondrocytes, evidence of increased vascularity, tendency to form lobules, and extension into surrounding soft tissues are signs of malignant changes and should be considered in light of available clinical and laboratory findings (Fig. 8-3).

OSTEOMA

It is generally accepted that formation of bone can take place anywhere in the body provided local tissue conditions permit such changes. True osteomas of soft tissues are rare and there are only a few cases reported in the literature (Kretschmer, 1938; Dietrich, 1940; Kautz, 1945; Cataldo et al, 1967).

Osteomas of the soft parts, in general, do not have sex predilection, with the exception of osteomas of the tongue which almost always occur in females. In most of the reported studies patients were in their 20's and 30's.

Most of the osteomas are solitary, self-limited lesions ranging in size from one centimeter to several centimeters. They are composed of a lamellated and circular conglomerate of mature bone. Calcification of the bony trabeculae is not uncommon and at the edge of the tumor, almost invariably, there is a rim of condensed fibrous connective tissue.

In reference to the pathogenesis of extraskeletal osteomas, several theories have been advanced, none of which explains satisfactorily the formation of these lesions. According to reports surgical excision assures definitive therapy.

OSTEOGENIC SARCOMA*

Since Boneti in 1700 described an "osteoma" of the mammary gland, innumerable case reports on extraskeletal osseous tumors have appeared. The earliest reports of tumors of soft parts that were histologically identical with osteogenic sarcoma of the bony skeleton are those by Jaidka (1919), Greenspan (1933), Mallory (1933), Broders (1934), Butler and Wooley (1936), and Haining and Poole (1936). Binkley and Stewart, in 1940, gave an interesting insight into the various theories in reference to the morphogenesis of extraskeletal osteogenic tumors and reported a case of osteogenic sarcoma in a 19-year-old male

* *Synonyms and related terms:* extraosseous osteogenic sarcoma, extraskeletal osteogenic sarcoma, osteosarcoma of soft tissues.

which they classified as a primary osteogenic sarcoma of the *pericardium.*

Primary osteogenic sarcoma of soft tissues is an extremely rare neoplasm. Since the early reports approximately 125 cases have been reported. Among the most important contributions are the articles listed in Table 8-3.

Extraskeletal osteogenic sarcoma is a disease of adults and occurs most commonly during the fifth and sixth decades. It has an almost equal sex distribution and the lower extremity, including the buttock, is the most common site of origin, followed by the upper extremity, including shoulder, and the trunk. Rarely, other sites such as the larynx may be the primary site (Dahm et al, 1978).

The size of these tumors usually varies from about 2 cm to 20 cm in maximum diameter. Most of the tumors are surrounded by dense fibroconnective tissue which makes surgical dissection difficult. The overlying skin is occasionally ulcerated. Radiographically, areas of ossification and sclerosis can be detected usually near the edge of the tumor (Figs. 8-4, 8-5).

The cut surfaces of extraskeletal osteogenic sarcomas usually display several combinations of color ranging from whitish-gray to yellowish-red. The central part of the majority of the tumors is cystic, whereas the periphery is firm and dense.

Microscopically, these tumors are composed of a fused conglomerate of neoplastic cells. The tumor cells are predominantly fusiform spindle cells with occasional giant cell forms. The arrangement of spindle cells is similar to that of fibrosarcomas. Although the degree of cellular pleomorphism and the number of tumor giant cells varies from field to field, cellular morphology is uniform throughout the tumor.

The number and size of epulis-type giant cells may vary from case to case and they are found most commonly adjacent to areas containing malignant osteoids. Areas of tumor necrosis and calcification are not uncommon; however, mitotic figures are infrequent. The single most important criterion for diagnosis of extraskeletal osteogenic sarcomas—the presence of malignant osteoids—is the same

TABLE 8-3. ***Extraskeletal Osteogenic Sarcoma***

					ANATOMIC SITES				
	NO. CASES	SEX M	SEX F	AVG. AGE	LOWER EXTREM. & BUTTOCK	UPPER EXTREM. & SHOULDER	TRUNK	OTHER	NO. PATIENTS ALIVE
Wilson (1941)	4	3	1	38	2	1	1	—	1
Fine and Stout (1956)	12	6	6	50	8	3	1	—	1
Das Gupta et al (1968)	9	2	7	48	6	1	1	1	2
Allan and Soule (1971)	26	14	12	47	18	6	2	—	5
Wurlitzer et al (1972)	9	4	5	57	7	—	2	—	0
Rao et al (1977)	8	4	4	59	5	3	—	—	2
Hajdu (personal experience)	21	11	10	55	14	7	—	—	5

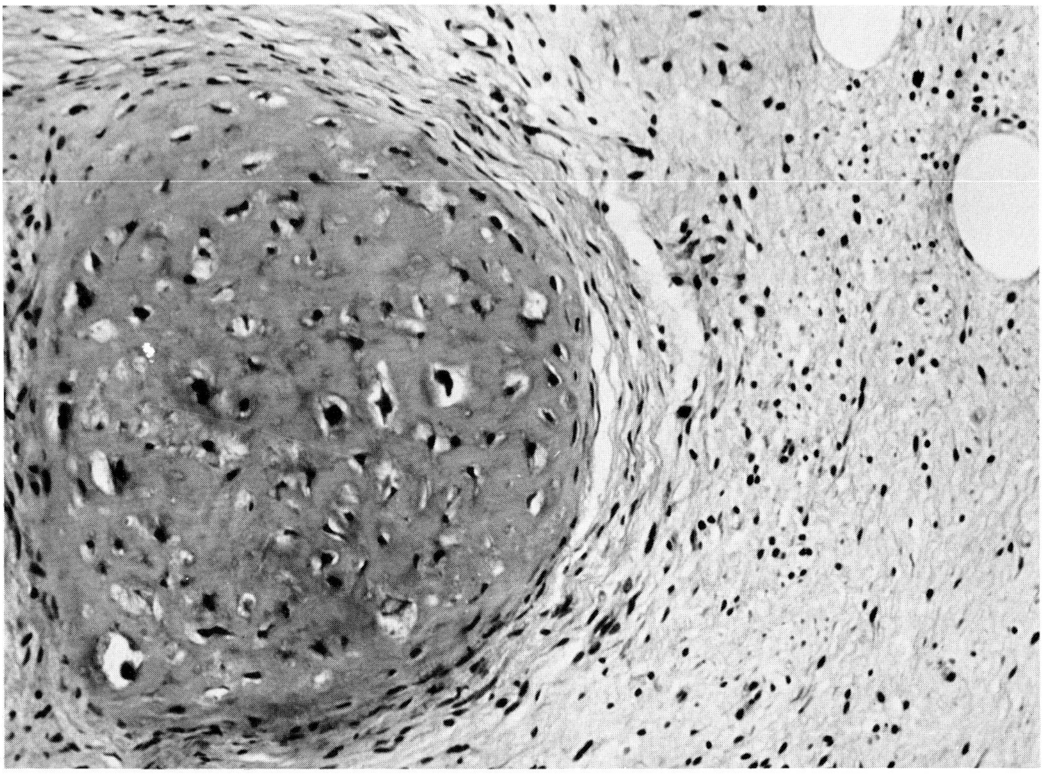

Figure 8-1. Chondroid metaplasia in a benign myxoid schwannoma (H & E, ×85).

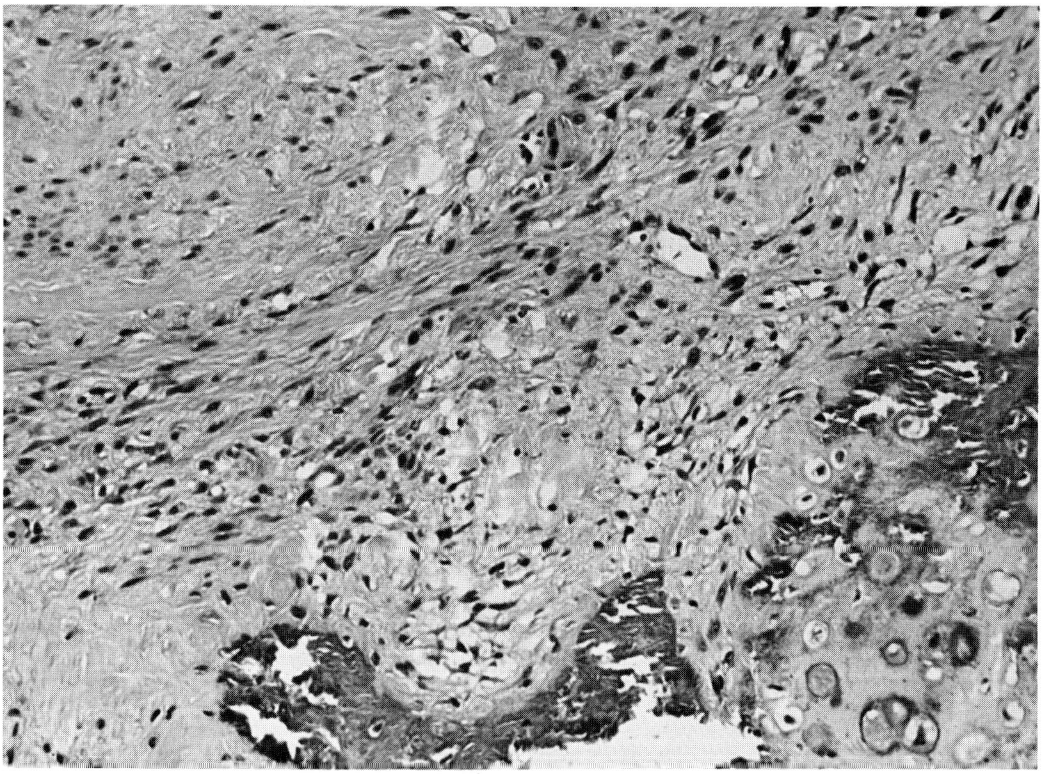

Figure 8-2. Metaplastic bone formation in a recurrent desmoid tumor (H & E, ×85).

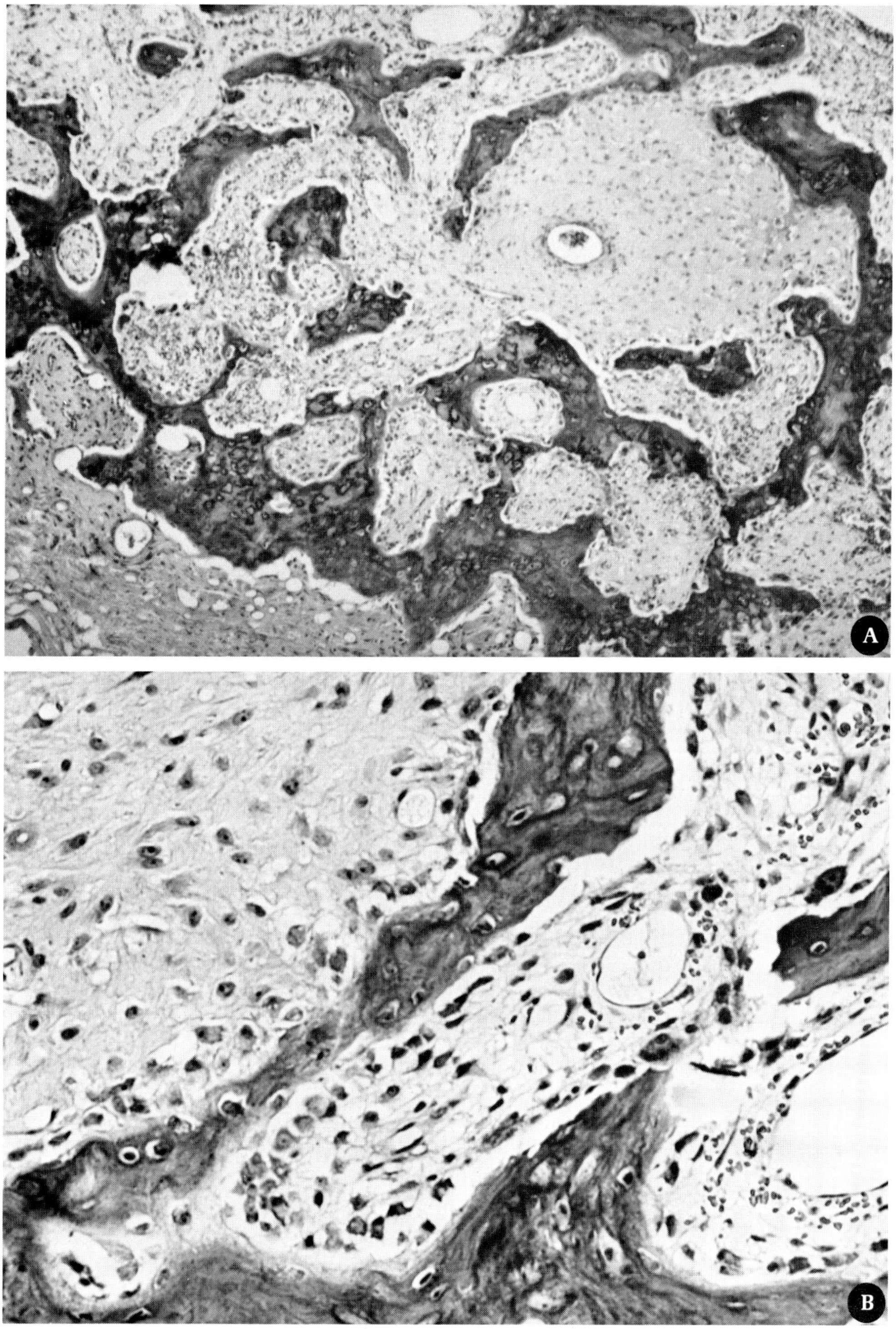

Figure 8-3. Osteochondroma in soft tissue of the thigh. This 10 cm ovoid mass was near the periosteum, but it was not attached to it. Adjacent skeletal muscles were compressed but uninvolved. Note an island of well-differentiated chrondrocytes and mature bone trabeculae (**A,** H & E, ×35; **B,** H & E, ×140).

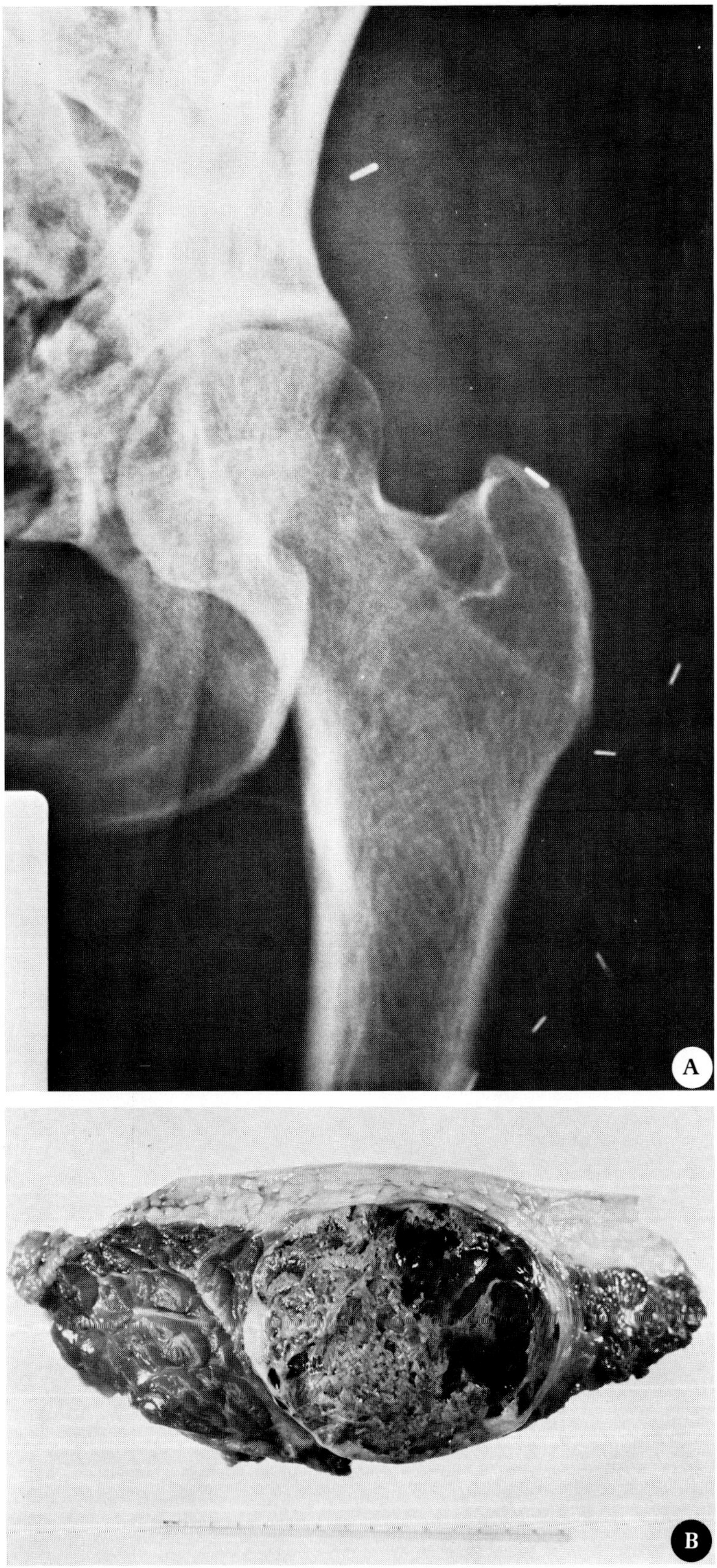

Figure 8-4. A, Extraskeletal osteogenic sarcoma of left buttock.

B, Surgical specimen after resection of the tumor. Note cystic and hemorrhagic areas and the dense pseudocapsule of the tumor.

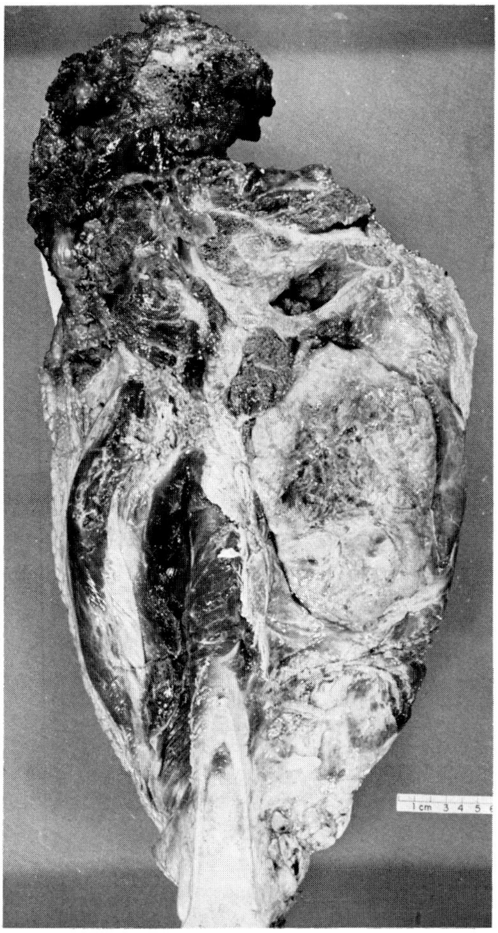

Figure 8-5. Large extraskeletal osteogenic sarcoma of the right thigh removed with clean surgical margins, by hemipelvectomy, from a 58-year-old man.

as that applied to intraosseous tumors (Figs. 8-6, 8-7).

Vascularity is not a marked feature of these tumors. Most of the intercellular spaces are filled by partly collagenous stroma and fibrillar cytoplasmic processes.

Osteogenic sarcomas have a tendency to infiltrate adjacent soft parts, and bones. As a rule, however, if adjacent bone shows radiographic evidence of involvement by the tumor, the sarcoma is more likely to be a primary bone tumor rather than a bone tumor of soft tissues. The association of elevated levels of *alkaline phosphatase,* in the absence of hepatic abnormality, with recurrence or metastasis of extraskeletal soft tissue sarcomas has been reported to be valuable in monitoring the progression of the disease (Das Gupta et al, 1968; Rao et al, 1978).

Extraskeletal osteogenic sarcomas, believed to be irradiation induced, have been reported (Auerbach et al, 1951; Boyer and Navin, 1965). Hasson et al (1975) reported a case of Thorotrast-induced extraskeletal osteogenic sarcoma of the neck.

Spontaneous transformation of myositis ossificans to osteogenic sarcoma have also been reported (Pack and Braund, 1942; Shanoff et al, 1967; Jarvi et al, 1968). Lee et al (1977) reported an extraosseous osteogenic sarcoma which developed 8 years following an intramuscular penicillin injection.

The histogenesis of extraosseous osteogenic sarcoma is not yet settled, but most observers agree with the concept first proposed by Virchow, in 1863, that "osteosarcoma is not necessarily a bone sarcoma". Ewing (1921) and Mallory (1933) adopted this view and advanced the idea that *chondroblasts and osteoblasts are modified fibroblasts and osteogenic sarcomas should be regarded as ossified fibrosarcomas.* After studying extraskeletal ossification, Binkley and Stewart, in 1940, came to the conclusion that the most important alteration leading to the assumption of the structure of osteogenic sarcoma was the laying down of dense hyaline tissue resulting in ischemia and the development of cavernous telangiectatic circulation favoring stasis and consequent anoxia. Furthermore, Brookes, in 1966, showed that in experimental animals elevation of carbon dioxide tension and maintenance of the pH between 6.8 and 7.2 with Po_2 of 40 mm Hg and Pco_2 of 50 mm Hg produced increased osteogenesis. Certainly, if one accepts the theory that bone is formed by metaplasia of connective tissue cells, most of the *multipotential primary bone sarcomas* (Hutter et al, 1966) and Stout's (1948) *mesenchymomas,* as well as Jacobson's (1977) *polyhistiomas,* can easily be placed at proper places in any subclassification scheme.

Once the diagnosis of extraskeletal os-

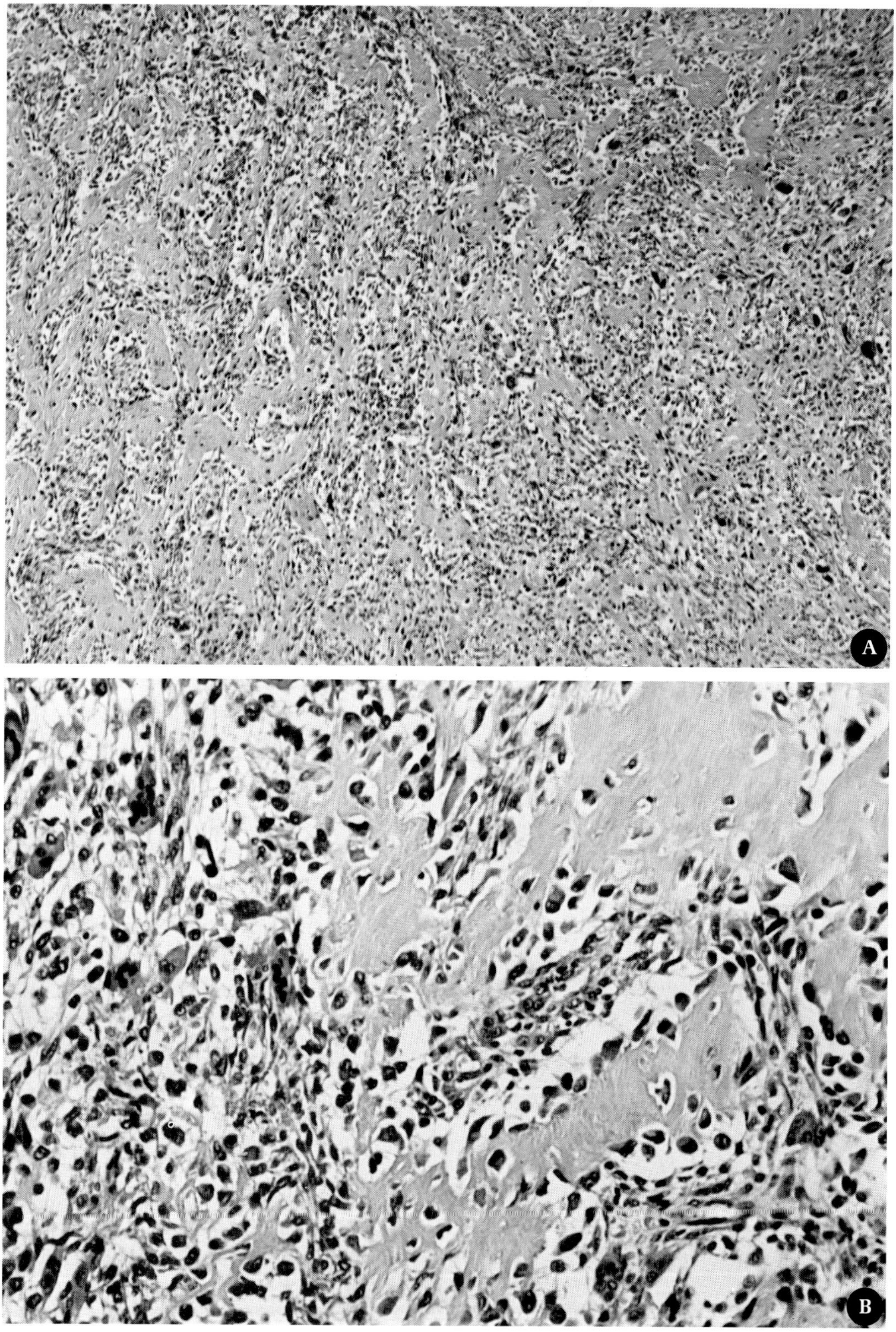

Figure 8-6. Extraskeletal osteogenic sarcoma.

A, Homogeneous growth pattern of tightly packed immature osteoids. There is no evidence of calcification or cartilagenous tissue (H & E, ×35).

B, The junction between trabeculae of immature osteoids and poorly differentiated mesenchymal stromal cells (H & E, ×140).

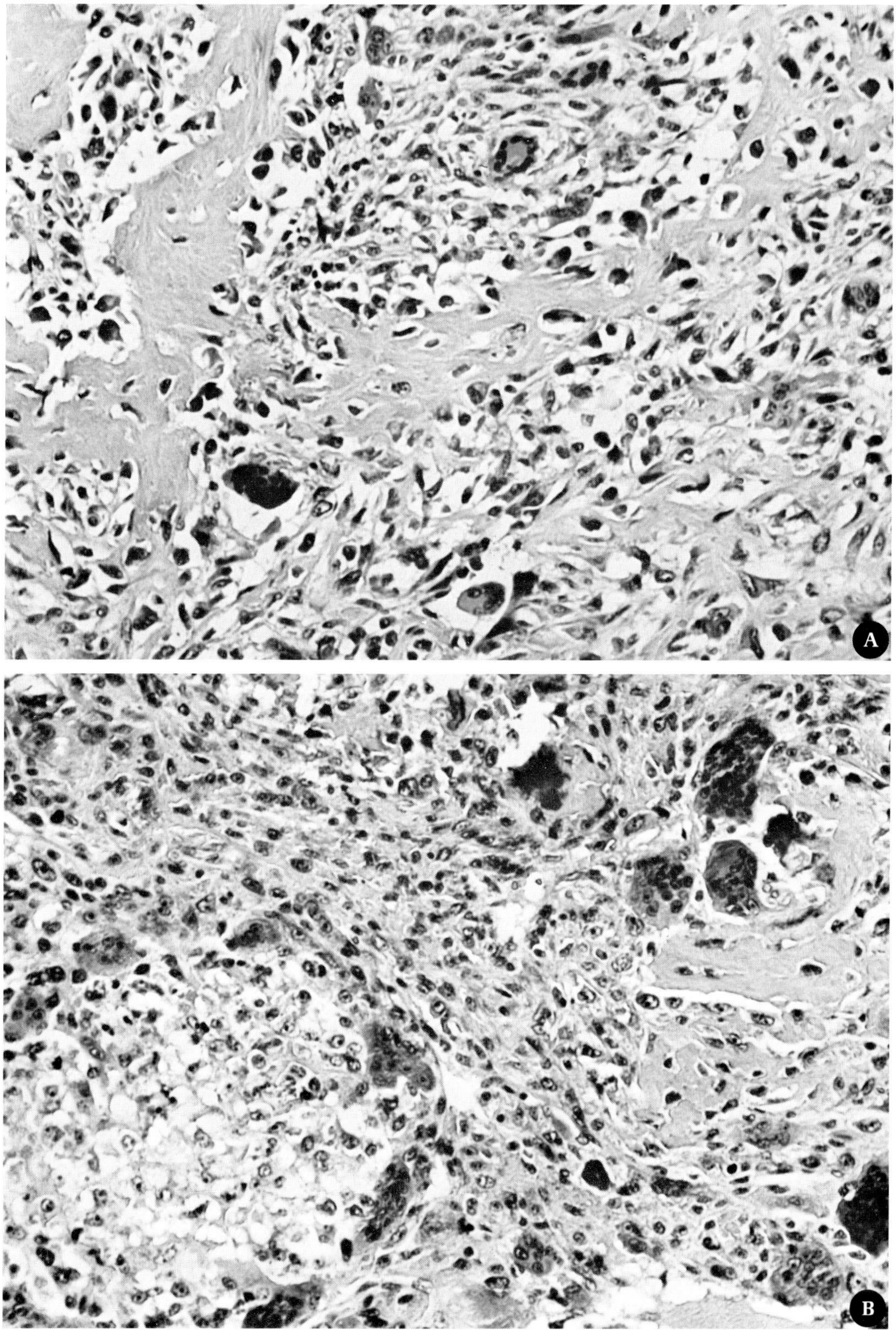

Figure 8-7. Extraskeletal osteogenic sarcoma.

A, Notice the delicate branching of immature osteoids and their close relationship to the neoplastic stromal elements (H & E, ×140).

B, A well-formed island of neoplastic chondrocytes (left lower corner) is ringed by multinucleated epulis-type giant cells. Other giant cells are scattered in the mesenchymal stroma and adjacent to neoplastic osteoids (H & E, ×140).

teogenic sarcoma is confirmed by tissue biopsy, the tumors should be widely excised with clean surgical margins. If this procedure is not feasible due to anatomic location or extent of the tumor, amputation should be done. Since the behavior of these tumors is comparable to that of skeletal osteogenic sarcomas, appropriate adjuvant chemotherapy should be initiated as soon as possible after tissue diagnosis in an effort to change the present dismal prognosis (Table 8-3).

Extraskeletal osteogenic sarcoma should be differentiated from *myositis ossificans* and *extraskeletal chondrosarcoma*. In osteogenic sarcoma, the neoplastic mesenchymal cells that are forming osteoid are in the periphery and are haphazardly arranged, whereas mature osteoid is located in the center of the tumor. This is in contrast to the orderly "zonal" deposit of mature and immature osteoids in myositis ossificans (see Chapter 5).

CHONDROSARCOMA*

The paucity of reports on extraskeletal chondrosarcoma indicates that it is a rare neoplasm. It may arise at any location; however, it is found most commonly in the extremities. Practically any form of mesenchymal tissues may be the site of origin of extraosseous chondrosarcoma: for example, *synovial tissue* (Goldman and Lichtenstein, 1964; King et al, 1967), *mammary tissue* (Busser, 1929), *scrotum* (Angervall et al, 1973), *lung* (Greenspan, 1933), *heart* (Muir and Seah, 1966), *pharynx* and *larynx* (Wirth and Shimkin, 1943; Huizenga and Balogh, 1970), *orbit* (Cardenas-Ramirez et al, 1971), *paravertebral areas* (Nezelof et al, 1965), and *intracranial region* (Raskind and Grant, 1966; Wu and Lapi, 1970; Scott et al, 1976; Scheithauer and Rubinstein, 1978). It may originate from malignant transformation of *synovial chondromatosis* (Goldman and Lichtenstein, 1964; Mullins et al, 1965; King et al, 1967) or *irradiated tissues* (Sears et al, 1967; Thompson and Entin, 1969) (see Chapter 9), but most commonly it is found without any significant antecedent history.

Although several case reports of extraskeletal chondrosarcoma were published (Caen, 1881; Busser, 1929; Greenspan, 1933; Mallory, 1933; Wilson, 1941; Wirth and Shimkin, 1943; Schaffer, 1952) prior to the article by Stout and Verner, in 1953, their article was the first to treat these tumors as a distinct entity. Stout and Verner discussed 7 extraskeletal chondrosarcomas and Kauffman and Stout (1963) reported 6 cases, all of which occurred in children. Subsequently, additional series have been reported (Table 8-4).

Extraskeletal chondrosarcoma affects males as well as females most commonly between 40 and 50 years of age. Characteristically, most of these tumors are far less aggressive in behavior than chondrosarcomas of bone. Our experience with these lesions is similar to that of others (Table 8-4).

Grossly, these neoplasms are usually bulky soft tissue masses measuring several centimeters in size and located in deep soft tissues. The lower extremities (including the buttock and groin) are the most commonly affected primary sites. The tumors usually appear as firm, ovoid, and lobulated circumscribed masses which can be easily separated from the surrounding tissues. The cut surface is lobulated and nodular with considerable variation in consistency and color, but the peripheral portions of the tumors are usually firm and whitish-gray and the central portion is soft and yellow (Figs. 8-8, 8-9).

Microscopically, chondrosarcomas may also vary in cellularity and degree of differentiation. The dominant elements are nests or foci of neoplastic chondrocytes at various stages of maturation, in myxoid or mucoid stroma (Fig. 8-10). Occasionally a considerable number of un-

**Synonyms and related terms:* mesenchymal chondrosarcoma, extraskeletal chondrosarcoma, chondrosarcoma of soft tissues, myxochondroid chondrosarcoma, undifferentiated chondrosarcoma, extraskeletal myxoid chondrosarcoma.

TABLE 8-4. *Extraskeletal Chondrosarcoma*

	NO. CASES	SEX M	SEX F	AVG. AGE	ANATOMIC SITES: LOWER EXTREMITY	UPPER EXTREMITY	TRUNK	OTHER	FOLLOW-UP*
Stout and Verner (1953)	7	7	—	41	5	2	—	—	1 died 1 alive, 3 yr. 4 Not followed
Kauffman and Stout† (1963)	6	2	4	5	3	1	1	1	3 died 3 alive
Goldenberg et al (1967)	7	3	4	47	6	1	—	—	1 died 4 alive 2 Not followed
Salvador et al‡ (1971)	9	4	5	41	3	—	2	4	2 died 3 alive 3 Not followed
Enzinger and Shiraki§ (1972)	34	22	12	49	29	5	—	—	4 died 20 alive 7 died without disease 5 Not followed
Hajdu (personal experience)	11	8	3	48	6	1	4	—	4 died 7 alive

*Follow-up ranges from days to years.
†Included patients under age 16 only.
‡Reported as mesenchymal chondrosarcoma.
§Reported as myxoid chondrosarcoma.

differentiated mesenchymal cells in the form of plump oval cells or slender spindle cells are found bordering cartilaginous islands and establishing direct continuity between chondrocytes and myxoid connective tissue elements. When these mesenchymal undifferentiated elements predominate, the tumors are usually referred to as *mesenchymal chondrosarcoma* (Dahlin and Henderson, 1962; Dowling, 1964; Chaves, 1965; Nezelof et al, 1965; Muir and Seah, 1966; Goldman, 1967; Gawlik, 1968; Salvador et al, 1971; Zimmerman, 1972; Guccion et al, 1973; Steiner et al, 1973; Mandelanakis, 1974; Pittman and Keller, 1974). If the tumor is rich in myxoid and mucoid substance, the tumors are usually called *myxoid chondrosarcoma* (Enzinger and Shiraki, 1972; Mehio and Ferenczy, 1978).

Mesenchymal chondrosarcoma, a rather unusual chondroid tumor, which was first described by Lichtenstein and Bernstein in 1959, may be intraosseous or extraosseous. Since the original description, approximately 65 well-documented cases have been reported (Table 8-4).

Classically, mesenchymal chondrosarcomas are composed mainly of two cell types: poorly differentiated mesenchymal cells and cells showing cartilaginous differentiation. The undifferentiated mesenchymal cells may display alveolar and perivascular arrangement, and the cartilaginous areas may show osteoid metaplasia and calcification. Steiner et al (1973) and Fu and Kay (1974) studied the ultrastructural features of mesenchymal chondrosarcoma and myxoid chondrosarcoma and confirmed the suggestion of Lichtenstein and Bernstein that the undifferentiated elements of mesenchymal chondrosarcoma are in fact "precartilage mesenchyme."

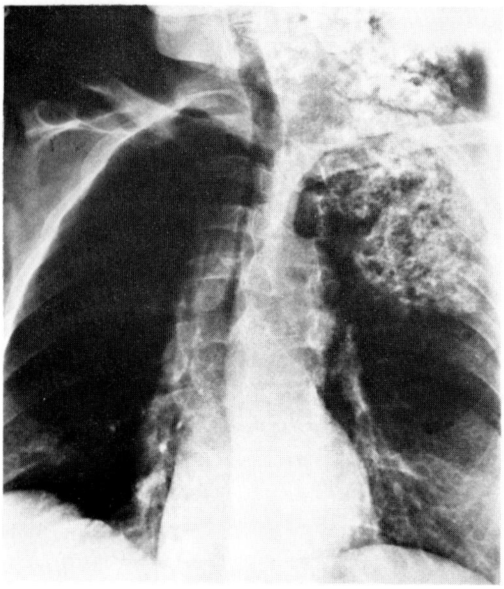

Figure 8-8. A 66-year-old female had a lump on the back for 20 years when suddenly the tumor started to grow. At the time of admission to the hospital there was a large tumor mass over the left scapula, with paravertebral extension without bone involvement. Surgical resection of this extraskeletal chondrosarcoma was attempted, but the patient died with pulmonary metastases in less than a year.

All available cytologic, histologic, histochemical, and ultrastructural studies indicate that Stout and Verner (1953) were right in saying that "extraskeletal chondrosarcomas show the histologic characteristics that are generally accepted as characterizing chondrosarcoma in bone." As in bone, extraskeletal chondrosarcomas can be divided into *mesenchymal, myxoid,* and *well-differentiated* forms (Figs. 8-11, 8-12, 8-13).

Differential Diagnosis and Treatment

In differential diagnosis, *myxoma* and *myxoid liposarcoma* should be considered. However, if cellular make-up, vascular pattern, and staining qualities of the mucoid substance of both of these tumors are carefully considered, there is only a remote chance that they are going to be confused with extraskeletal chondrosarcoma. For example, the mucoid ground substance of myxoma and liposarcoma contains hyaluronidase-sensitive mucopolysaccharide and is depolymerized by prior treatment with hyaluronidase. After such treatment, it does not stain with alcian blue or mucicarmine (see Chapter 4). The mucoid material in chondroid lesions contains sulfated glycosaminoglycans and is insensitive to prior treatment with hyalurondiase.

Chordoid sarcoma is a rare and unique form of chondromyxoid neoplasm which

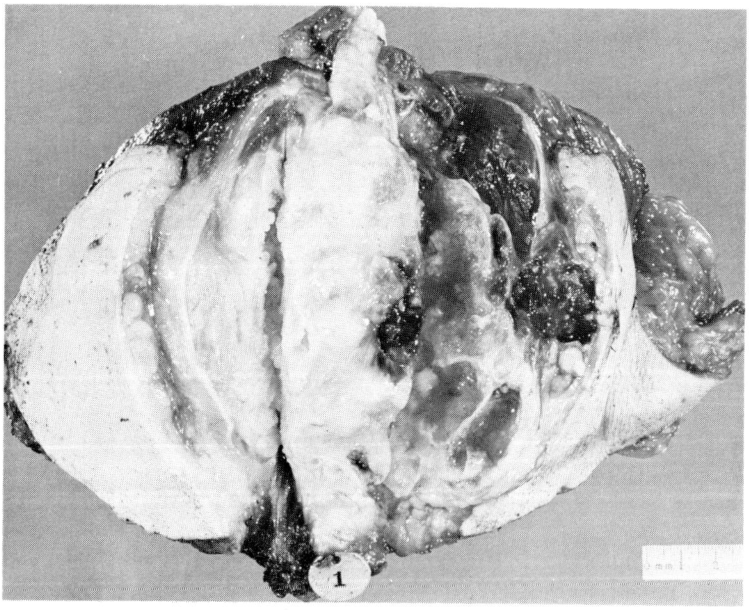

Figure 8-9. Extraskeletal chondrosarcoma resected from the anterior chest and abdominal walls.

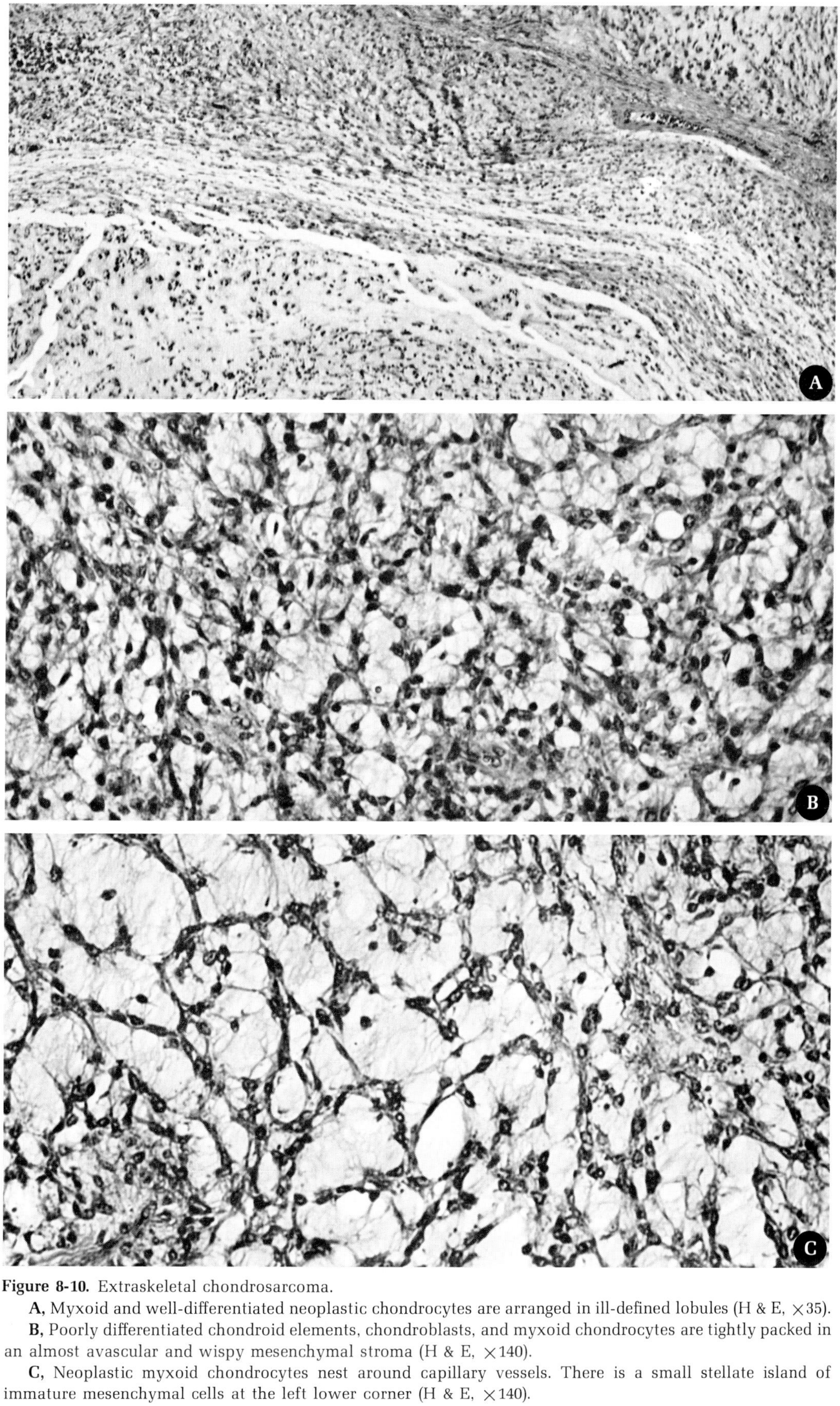

Figure 8-10. Extraskeletal chondrosarcoma.

A, Myxoid and well-differentiated neoplastic chondrocytes are arranged in ill-defined lobules (H & E, ×35).

B, Poorly differentiated chondroid elements, chondroblasts, and myxoid chondrocytes are tightly packed in an almost avascular and wispy mesenchymal stroma (H & E, ×140).

C, Neoplastic myxoid chondrocytes nest around capillary vessels. There is a small stellate island of immature mesenchymal cells at the left lower corner (H & E, ×140).

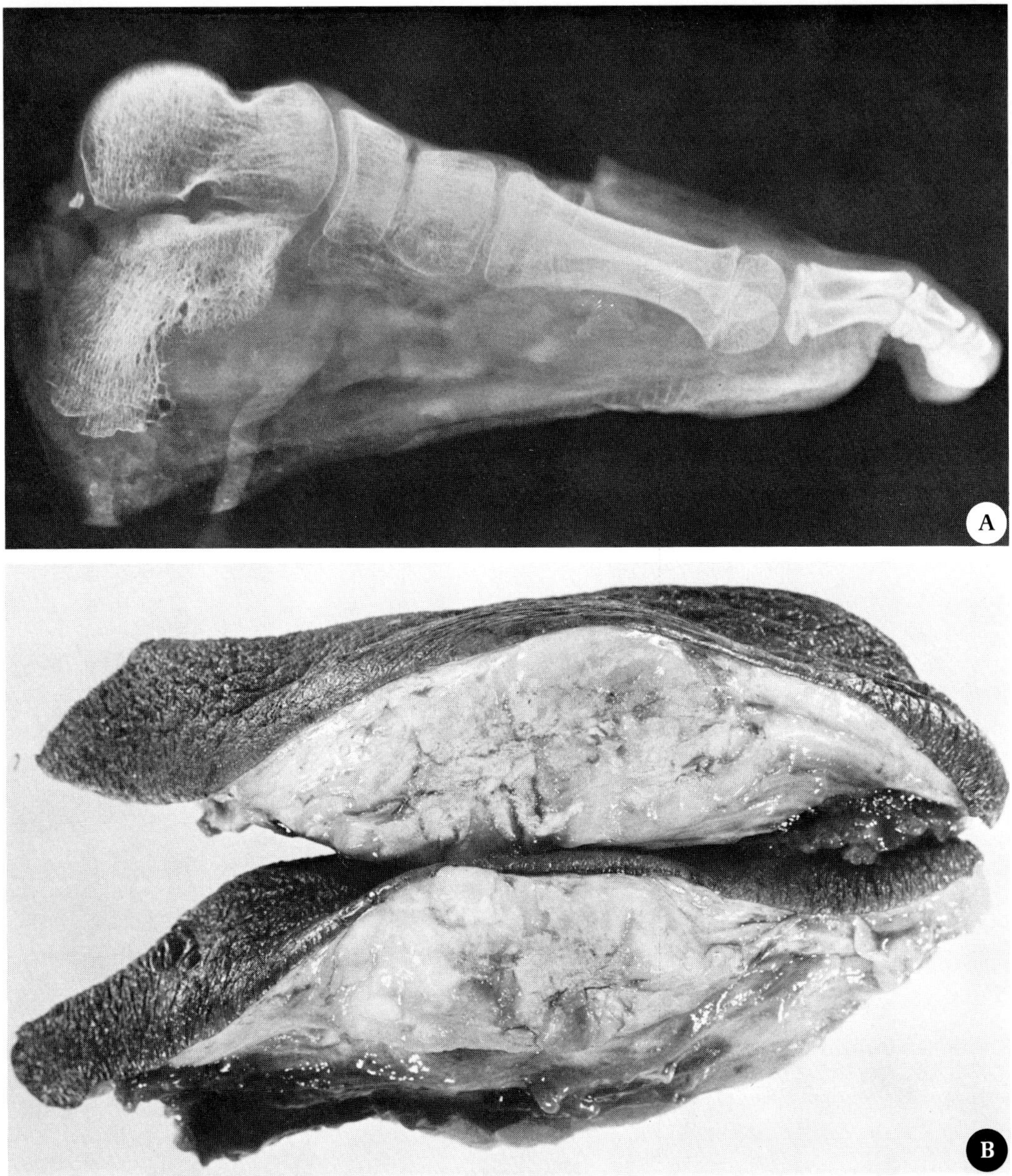

Figure 8-11. **A,** Mesenchymal chondrosarcoma of the plantar surface with erosion of the os calcis. **B,** Mesenchymal chondrosarcoma measuring 10 cm, excised from the anterior surface of the lower left leg.

may be a histogenetic link between tendosynovial sarcomas and extraskeletal chondrosarcomas (see Chapter 3).

It is generally agreed that the treatment of extraskeletal chondrosarcomas should be wide resection with clean margins. Amputation is indicated when the tumor recurs or when bone or other vital structures such as large vessels or nerves are invaded. The exact rate of recurrence and metastasis is difficult to assess on the basis of reported studies, but my estimate is that 14 of 50 patients (28%) with adequate follow-up succumbed to metastatic disease.

EWING'S SARCOMA

Ewing's tumor accounts for about 35% of malignant bone tumors in children. The peak incidence is in the second decade of

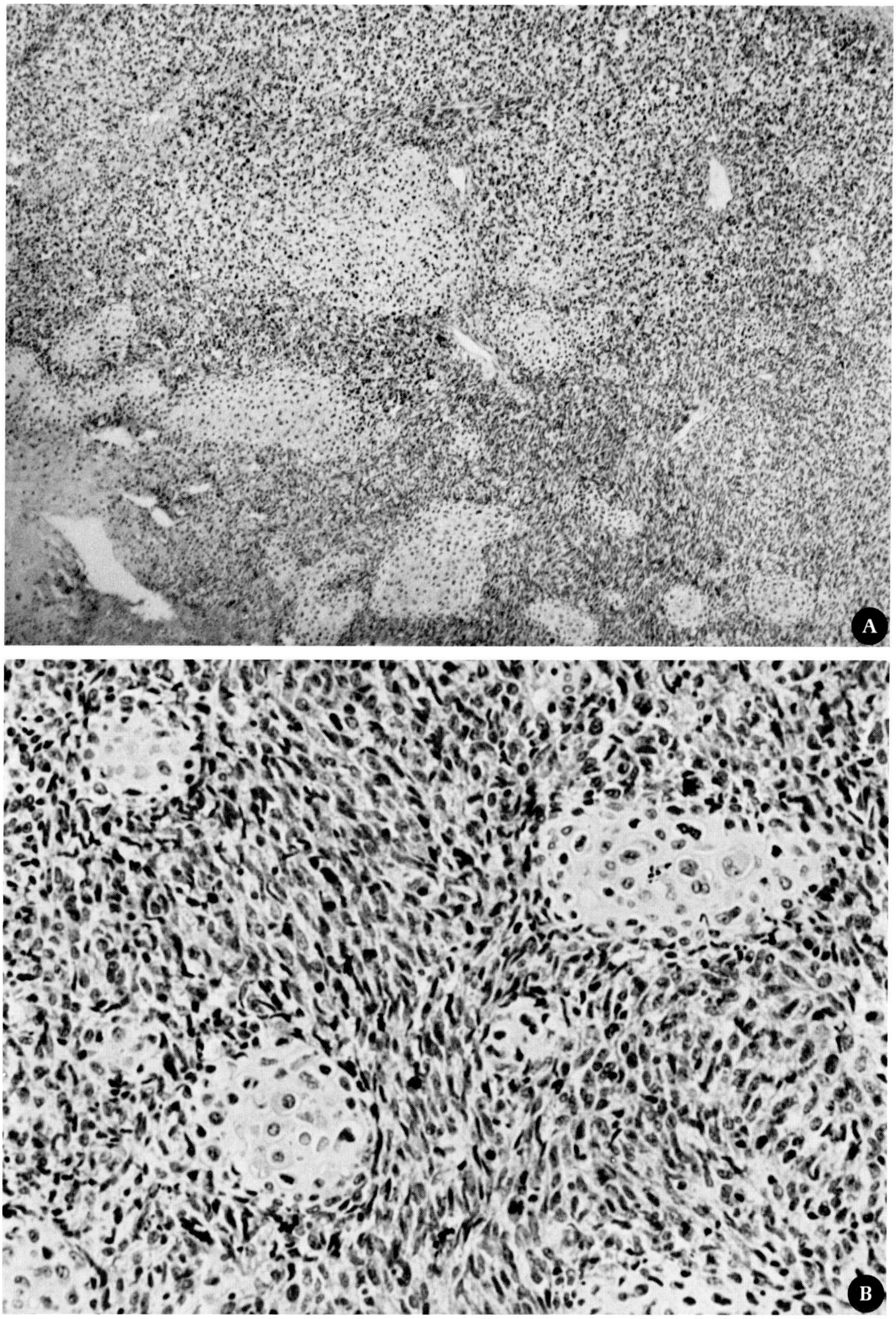

Figure 8-12. Mesenchymal chondrosarcoma.

A, Intimate blending of fairly homogeneous undifferentiated mesenchymal cells and islands of chondrocytes (H & E, ×35).

B, The majority of the mesenchymal cells are short spindle or oval cells with slender and limited cytoplasmic processes. They are tightly packed and show no particular pattern. There is conspicuous absence of blood vessels (H & E, ×140).

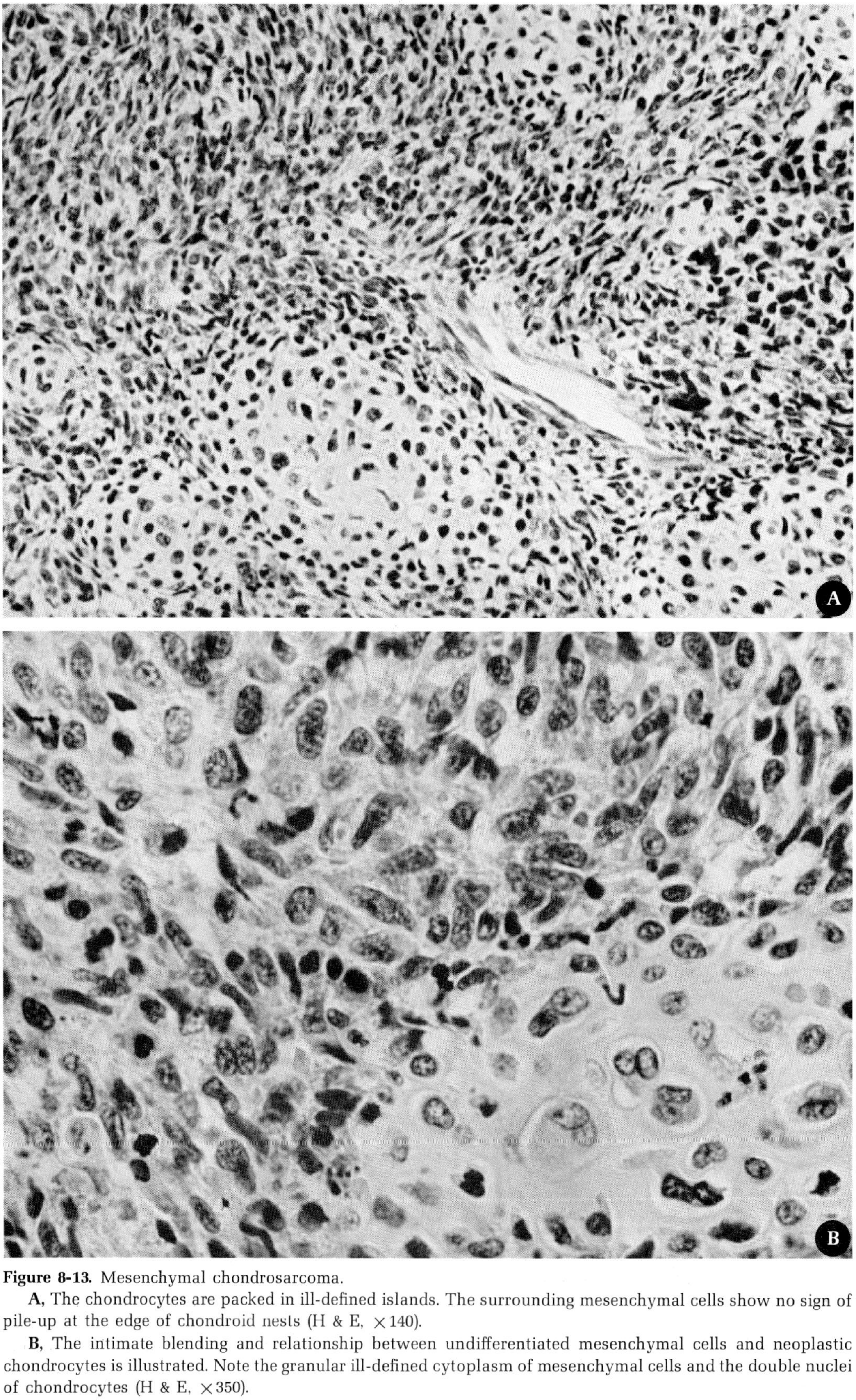

Figure 8-13. Mesenchymal chondrosarcoma.

A, The chondrocytes are packed in ill-defined islands. The surrounding mesenchymal cells show no sign of pile-up at the edge of chondroid nests (H & E, ×140).

B, The intimate blending and relationship between undifferentiated mesenchymal cells and neoplastic chondrocytes is illustrated. Note the granular ill-defined cytoplasm of mesenchymal cells and the double nuclei of chondrocytes (H & E, ×350).

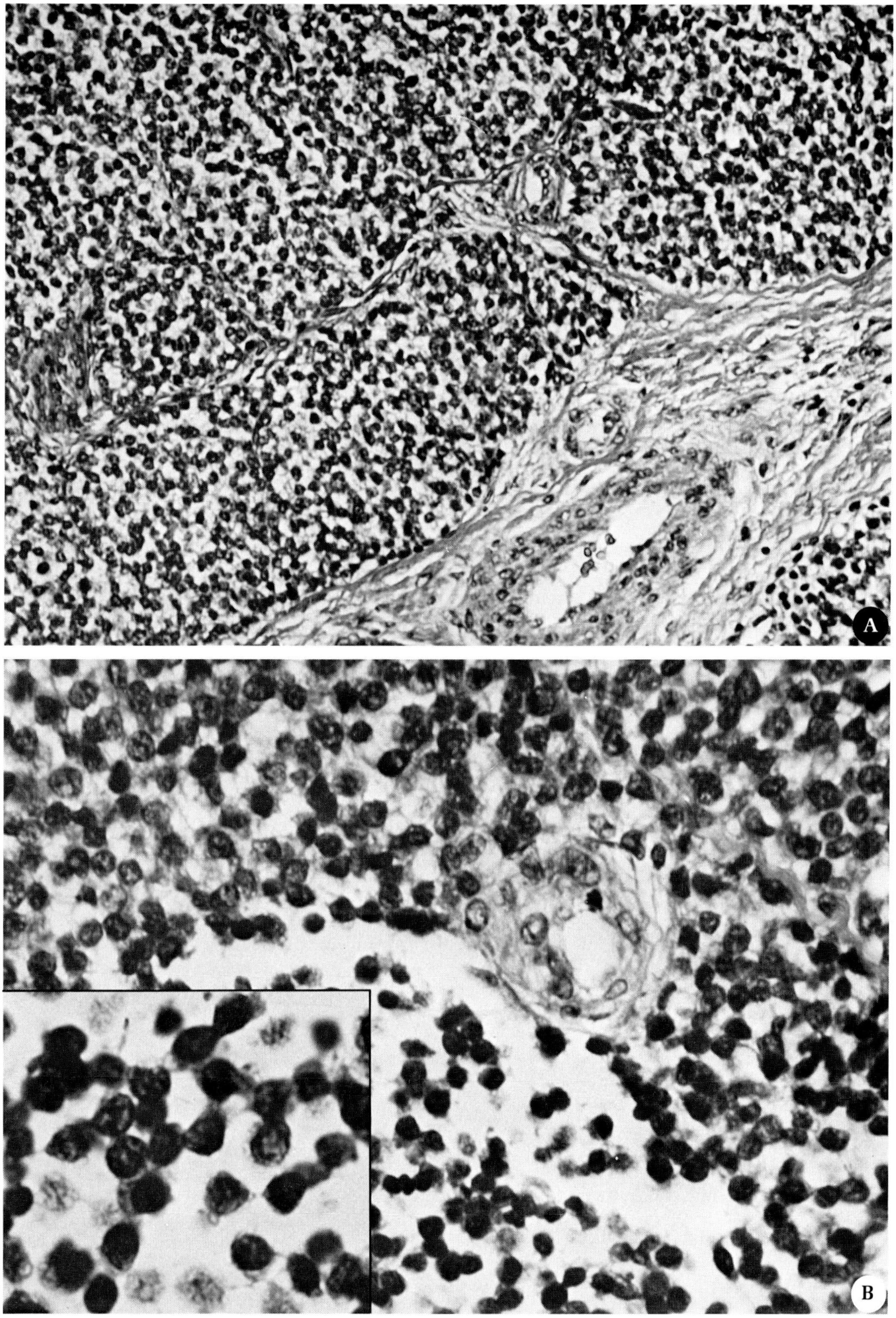

Figure 8-14. Extraskeletal Ewing's sarcoma.

Monomorphic, mostly round and dark, small cells are arranged in sheets in a richly vascular stroma. The cytoplasms of the tumor cells are small but sufficient enough to secure junction between adjacent cells. Many of the tumor cells are arranged about a central clearing, perhaps capillary lumen; others form well-defined pseudorosettes (see inset). (**A,** H & E, ×140; **B,** H & E, ×350; and inset, ×57.)

Figure 8-15. **A,** Extraskeletal osteogenic sarcoma is composed of partly sclerosing bone spicules, malignant osteoids, multinucleated epulis-type giant cells, and a fibrous histiocytic stroma.

The osteoids are either trapped in the bone spicules or bordering them with serrated indentations. The multinucleated giant cells blend intimately into the cellular and hypervascular stroma. The haphazard mixture of various mature and immature elements gives an unpredictable pattern from field to field (H & E, ×140).

B, Myxoid chondrosarcoma of soft tissue. This neoplasm is composed of two fields of uniform stellate cells separated by a fibrocollagenous band. The tumor cells are joined by fine cytoplasmic processes and clustered about minute capillary vessels.

The intercellular stroma is sparsely cellular and rich in myxoid mucopolysaccharide substance which stains positive with alcian blue before and after treatment with hyaluronate (H & E, ×140).

C, Mesenchymal chondrosarcoma of soft tissue. This neoplasm is composed of ill-defined islands of myxoid and mature chondrocytes. The center cells of such chondroid nests are vesicular and plump, well-differentiated chondrocytes. On the other hand, the cells at the edge of chondroid islands are small oval or spindle cells and resemble the surrounding non-chondroid mesenchymal tumor cells.

Neoplastic cells that are not part of the chondroid islands range in size from minute pyknotic forms with scanty cytoplasm to elongated cells with long reticular cytoplasmic filaments and cigar-shaped nuclei. The first appearance of transformed chondrocytes is indicated by the presence of myxochondroid lakes (see right upper corner) (H & E, ×350).

D, Extraskeletal Ewing's sarcoma is a poorly differentiated mesenchymal tumor which histologically resembles its intraskeletal counterpart. It is composed of uniform round or short oval cells in a sparsely reticular and vascular stroma. The cytoplasms of the tumor cells are so small that many of the nuclei appear naked. The tumor cells show no particular pattern of arrangement, but short cords and imperfect rosettes are seen throughout the tumor. Undoubtedly, the histologic diagnosis of this rare neoplasm should be made only after generous sampling of the tumor and full knowledge of the clinical history, as well as pertinent laboratory findings (H & E, ×350).

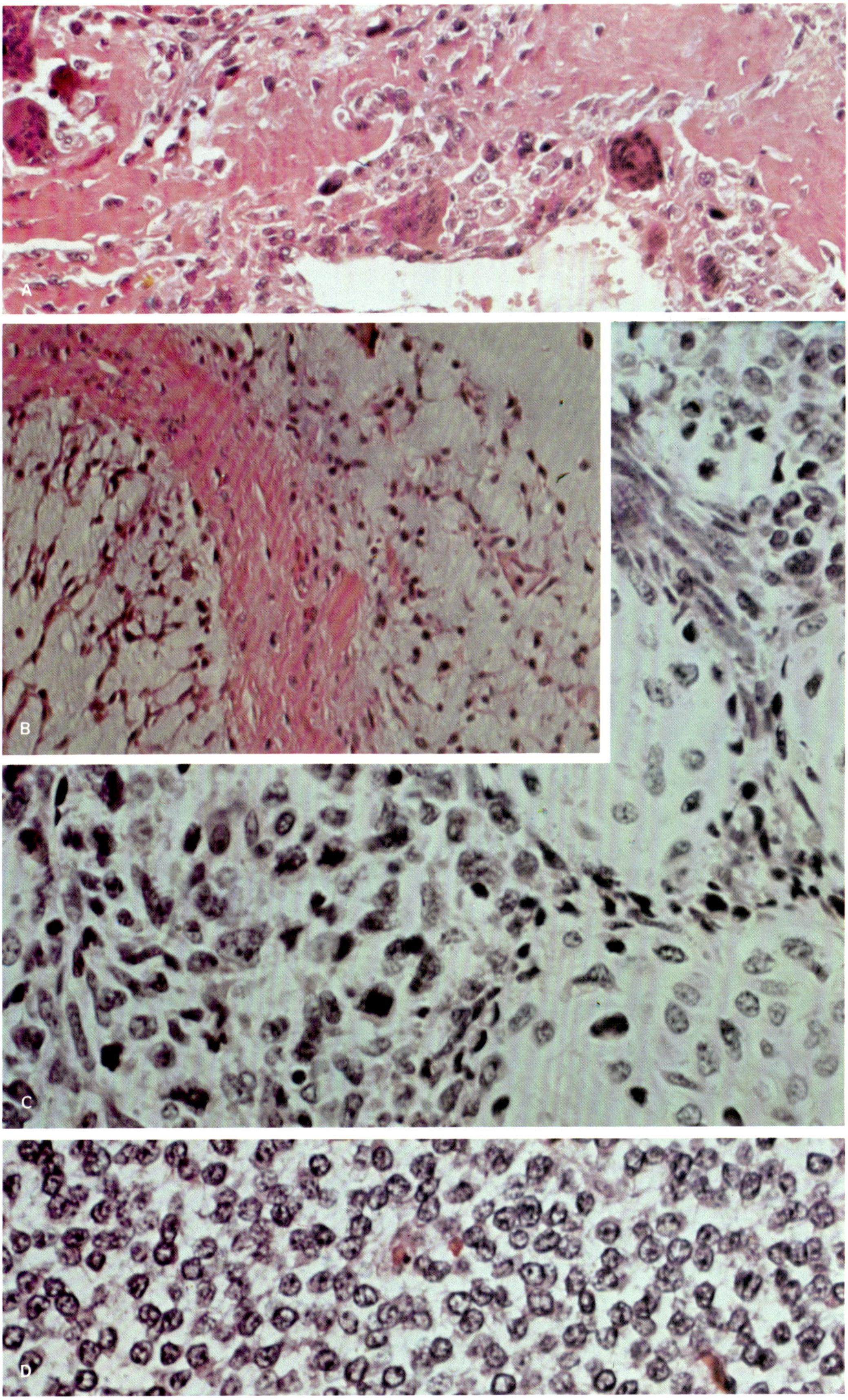

Figure 8-15.

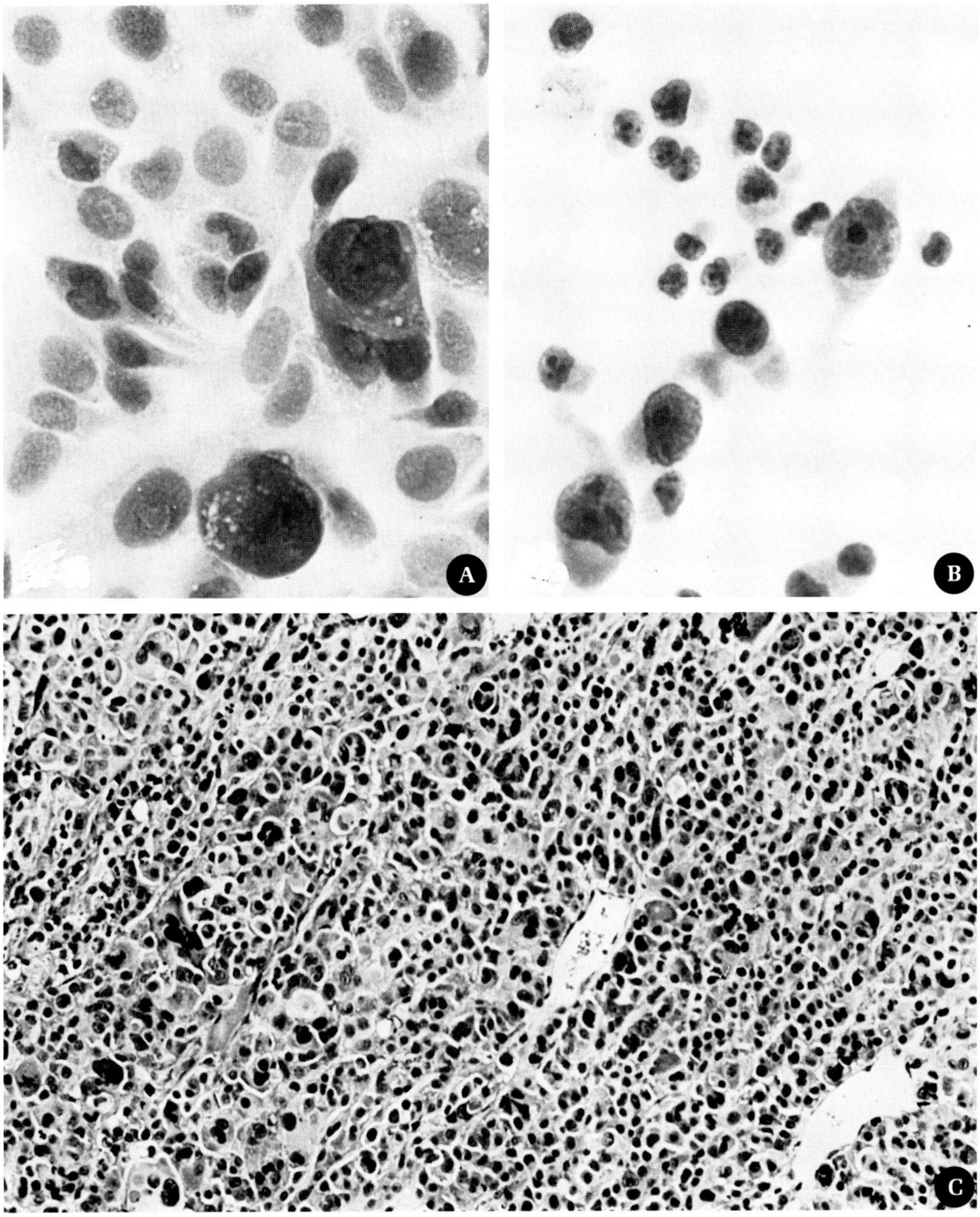

Figure 8-16. A, Osteogenic sarcoma in monolayer tissue culture (Pap stain, ×460).
B, Stained cell suspension of trypsinized monolayer culture of osteogenic sarcoma (Pap stain, ×460).
C, Human osteogenic sarcoma grown in subcutaneous tissue of nude mouse 4 weeks after injection of cell suspension prepared from tissue culture (H & E, ×140). (See Hajdu and Fogh, 1978.)

life. This neoplasm was first described by Ewing, in 1921, as a round cell neoplasm he called "diffuse endothelioma of bone." Recent electron microscopic, histochemical, ultrastructural, and heterotransplant studies indicate that Ewing's sarcoma is a primitive mesenchymal tumor and may arise from pluripotential mesenchymal cells, for example, pericytes. As such it may contribute to a number of malignant neoplasms, e.g., osteogenic sarcoma, mesenchymal chondrosarcoma, embryonal rhabdomyosarcoma, primitive neuroectodermal tumor, and hemangiopericytoma. At the earliest stage of differentiation, undifferentiated "small blue" mesenchymal cells often are arranged about blood vessels or form pseudorosettes (Kadin and Bensch, 1971; Hou-Jensen et al, 1972; Hajdu and Hajdu, 1976; Hajdu and Fogh, 1978; Mahoney et al, 1978).

Contrary to recent reports, extraskeletal neoplasms resembling Ewing's sarcoma have been reported in the past (Phemister, 1931; Poujol and Barone, 1937). In fact, Geschickter and Copeland, in 1936, were the first to introduce the term *Ewing tumor of soft parts.* Perhaps one of the best documented studies is that of Potozky and Fried, in 1939. They pointed out that in certain Ewing's sarcomas the extraskeletal part of the tumor can be so bulky and the intraosseous changes so minimal that radiographically they cannot be detected (see Chapter 1).

Due to a recent report on extraskeletal Ewing's sarcomas (Angervall and Enzinger, 1975) and reclassification of certain small cell tumors, e.g., embryonal rhabdomyosarcomas, the number of cases of extraosseous Ewing's sarcomas suddenly reached an epidemic proportion in certain laboratories. No doubt Ewing's sarcoma of soft parts exists; however, the diagnosis should be made histologically after diligent search has failed to establish the presence of intraosseous neoplasm and all available diagnostic techniques have been used to rule out other small cell neoplasms (Fig. 8-14). The prognosis is favorable following appropriate irradiation and chemotherapy.

In children, Ewing's sarcoma must be distinguished from *embryonal rhabdomyosarcoma* (Bale and Reye, 1975) (see Chapter 5), *neuroblastoma and leukemia* (Hajdu and Hajdu, 1976), and *malignant lymphoma* (Schajowicz, 1959) (see Chapter 9). In adults, *oat cell carcinoma* and other *small cell epithelial tumors, malignant lymphoma,* and *chloroma* (see Chapter 9) must be included in the differential diagnosis. The demonstration of diastase-sensitive glycogen in the cytoplasm of the tumor cells of Ewing's sarcoma may aid in the separation of this tumor from neuroblastoma and malignant lymphoma (Figs. 8-15, color, 8-16).

REFERENCES

References are listed in chronological order.

Boneti, T.: De ventris tumore, in Sepulchretum, sive anatoma practica excadaveribus morbo denatis, Vol. 3, Geneva, Cramer and Perachon, 1700, p. 522.

Virchow, R.: Die Krankhaften Geschwulste. Berlin, Hirschwald, 1863.

Paget, J.: Lectures on Surgical Pathology. London, Longmans, Green and Company, 1870.

Caen, E.: Chondroosteosarkom der weiblichen Brustdruse. Dtsch. Zr. Chir. 15:247, 1881.

Cahen, F.: Uber myositis ossificans. Dtsch. Zr. Chir. 31:372, 1891.

Jaidka, K. C.: Ossifying sarcoma of vastus externus. Br. Med. J. 2:379, 1919.

Chauvin et Roux: Fibro-chondrome de la girne tendineuse de l'extenseur du quatrieine orteil. Bull. Mem. Soc. Anat. Paris 90:75, 1920.

Ewing, J.: Diffuse endothelioma of bone. Proc. N.Y. Pathol. Soc. 21:17, 1921.

Dyke, S. C.: A bony tumor of the breast. Br. J. Surg. 14:232, 1926.

Goldman, D.: Die Enchondrome des unterhautzellewebes. Zentralbl. Chir. 55:2379, 1928.

Busser, F.: Sarcoma osteochondroblastique developpe aux depens d'un adenofibrome du sein. Ann. Anat. Pathol. 6:1247, 1929.

Schaffer, J.: *In* Handbuch der mikroskopischen Anatomie des Menschen. Edited by von Mollendorff. Berlin, J. Springer, 1929–1930.

Phemister, D. B.: Undifferentiated round-cell sarcoma. Ann. Surg. 93:125, 1931.

Seidelin, H.: Liposarcoma with chordoma-like cells. Acta Pathol. Microbiol. Scand. 9:289, 1932.

Greenspan, E. B.: Primary osteoid chondrosarcoma of the lung: report of case. Am. J. Cancer 18:603, 1933.

Mallory, T. B.: A group of metaplastic and neoplastic bone and cartilage containing tumors of the soft parts. Am. J. Pathol. 9:765, 1933.

Broders, A. C., and J. de J. Pemberton: Primary

osteogenic sarcoma of the thyroid gland. Surg. Gynecol. Obstet. 58:100, 1934.

Butler, F. E., and Wooley, I. M.: Osteogenic sarcoma arising from a calcified hematoma. Radiology 26:236, 1936.

Geschickter, C. F., and Copeland, M. M.: Tumors of Bone. New York American Journal of Cancer, 1936.

Haining, R. B., and Poole, P. E.: Osteoblastoma of the kidney histologically identical with osteogenic sarcoma. Arch. Pathol. 21:44, 1936.

Poujol, G., and Barone, R.: Un cas de sarcome primitif du coeur à forme infiltrante. Bull. Assoc. Franc. cancer 26:64, 1937.

Kretschmer, H. L.: Retroperitoneal pararenal osteoma. Surg. Gynecol. Obstet. 67:108, 1938.

Potozky, H., and Fried, J. R.: Ewing's tumor simulating sarcoma of soft-tissue origin. A clinical pathological and radiotherapeutic study of four cases. Am. J. Cancer 36:1, 1939.

Binkley, J. S., and Stewart, F. W.: Morphogenesis of extraskeletal osteogenic sarcoma and pseudo-osteosarcoma. Arch. Pathol. 29:42, 1940.

Dietrich, C.: Osteomatosis cutis. Arch. Dermatol. Syphil. 41:562, 1940.

Wilson, H.: Extraskeletal ossifying tumors. Ann. Surg. 113:95, 1941.

Pack, G. T., and Braund, R. R.: The development of sarcoma in myositis ossificans. JAMA 119:776, 1942.

Wirth, J. E., and Shimkin, M. B.: Chondrosarcoma of the nasopharynx simulating juvenile angiofibroma. Arch. Pathol. 36:83, 1943.

Kautz, F. G.: Capsular osteoma of the knee joint, report of four cases. Radiology 45:162, 1945.

Rottino, A., and Howley, C. P.: Osteoid sarcoma of the breast; a complication of fibroadenoma. Arch. Pathol. 40:44, 1945.

Stout, A. P.: Mesenchymoma, the mixed tissue of mesenchymal derivatives. Ann. Surg. 127:278, 1948.

Auerbach, O., Friedman, M., Weiss, L., and Amory, H. I.: Extraskeletal osteogenic sarcoma arising in irradiated tissue. Cancer 4:1095, 1951.

Schaffer, L. W.: Extraskeletal osteochondrosarcoma. Am. J. Surg. 18:739, 1952.

Stout, A. P., and Verner, E. W.: Chondrosarcoma of the extraskeletal soft tissues. Cancer 6:581, 1953.

Fine, G., and Stout, A. P.: Osteogenic sarcoma of the extraskeletal soft tissues. Cancer 9:1027, 1956.

Purser, D. W.: Extraskeletal osteochondromata. J. Bone Joint Surg. 38B:871, 1956.

Murphy, A. F., and Wilson, J. N.: Tendosynovial osteochondroma in the hand. J. Bone Joint Surg. 40A:1236, 1958.

Lichtenstein, L., and Bernstein, D.: Unusual benign and malignant chondroid tumors of bone. Cancer 12:1142, 1959.

Salm, R.: A case of primary osteogenic sarcoma of extraskeletal soft tissue. Br. J. Cancer 13:614, 1959.

Schajowicz, F.: Ewing's sarcoma and reticulum cell sarcoma of bone. With special reference to the histochemical demonstration of glycogen as an aid to differential diagnosis. J. Bone Joint Surg. 41A:349, 1959.

Godman, C. G., and Porter, K. R.: Chondrogenesis studied with the electron microscope. J. Biophys. Biochem. Cytol. 8:719, 1960.

Dahlin, D. C., and Henderson, E. D.: Mesenchymal chondrosarcoma. Cancer 15:410, 1962.

Kernohan, J. W., and Uihlein, A.: Sarcomas of the Brain. Springfield, Illinois, Charles C Thomas, 1962.

Kauffman, S. L., and Stout, A. P.: Extraskeletal osteogenic sarcomas and chondrosarcomas in children. Cancer 16:432, 1963.

Boer, W. C., de Oldhoff, J., and Stam, H. C.: Extraosseous ossifying sarcoma localized in the soft tissue. Arch. Chir. Neurol. 16:217, 1964.

Dowling, E. A.: Mesenchymal chondrosarcoma. J. Bone Joint Surg. 46A:747, 1964.

Goldman, R. L., and Lichtenstein, L.: Synovial chondrosarcoma. Cancer 17:1233, 1964.

Jussawalla, D. J., and Desai, J. G.: Primary osteogenic sarcoma arising in extraskeletal soft tissues of the neck. Br. J. Surg. 51:504, 1964.

Lichtenstein, L., and Goldman, R. L.: Cartilage tumors in soft tissues, particularly in the hand and foot. Cancer 17:1203, 1964.

Lowry, K., Jr., and Haynes, C. D.: Osteogenic sarcoma of extraskeletal soft tissues. A case report. Am. Surg. 30:97, 1964.

Boyer, C. W., Jr., and Navin, J. J.: Extraskeletal osteogenic sarcoma: A late complication of radiation therapy. Cancer 18:628, 1965.

Chaves, E.: Chondrosarcoma mesenquimal. Hospital 67:1217, 1965.

Gupta, D. N., and Aga, V.: Soft tissue osteogenic sarcoma (A case report). Indian J. Pathol. Bacteriol. 8:59, 1965.

Mullins, F., Berard, C., and Eisenberg, S. H.: Chondrosarcoma following synovial chondromatosis. Cancer 18:1180, 1965.

Nezelof, C., Mazabraud, A., and Meary, R.: Le chondrosarcome mesenchymateux; a propos d'un cas de localization pararachidienne. (Mesenchymal chondrosarcoma; on a case of paravertebral localization). Arch. Anat. Pathol. 13:26, 1965.

Rachman, R., and DiMasa, E. V.: Pelvic extraskeletal osteosarcoma associated with prostatic adenocarcinoma. Am. J. Clin. Pathol. 44:556, 1965.

Brookes, M.: The vascular factors in osteoarthritis. Surg. Gynecol. Obstet. 123:1255, 1966.

Hoffman, K., Fine, G., Ponka, J. L., and Welborn, J. K.: Extraskeletal osteogenic sarcoma: case report. Henry Ford Hosp. Med. Bull. 14:381, 1966.

Hutter, R. V. P., Foote, F. W., Francis, K. C., and Sherman, R. S.: Primary multipotential primary sarcoma of bone. Cancer 19:1, 1966.

Khoo, T. K., and Balachandran, N.: Osteogenic sarcoma of soft tissue. Singapore Med. J. 7:30, 1966.

Muir, C. S., and Seah, C. S.: Primary chondrosarcomatous mesenchymoma of the mitral valve. Thorax 21:254, 1966.

Raskind, R., and Grant, S.: Primary mesenchymal chondrosarcoma of the cerebrum: report of a case. J. Neurosurg. 24:676, 1966.

Cataldo, E., Shklar, G., and Meyer, I.: Osteoma of the tongue. Arch. Otolaryngol. 85:98, 1967.

Goldenberg, R. R., Cohen, P., and Steinlauf, P.: Chondrosarcoma of extraskeletal soft tissues: Report of seven cases and review of literature. J. Bone Joint Surg. 49A:1487, 1967.

Goldman, R. L.: Mesenchymal chondrosarcoma—A rare malignant chondroid tumor usually arising in bone—Case in soft tissue. Cancer 20:1494, 1967.

King, J. W., Spjut, H. J., Feehner, R. E., and Vanderpool, D. W.: Synovial chondrosarcoma of the knee joint. J. Bone Joint Surg. 49A:1389, 1967.

Korns, M. E.: Primary chondrosarcoma of extraskeletal soft tissue. Arch. Pathol. 83:13, 1967.

Sears, W. P., Tofft, M., and Cohen, J.: Post-irradiation mesenchymal chondrosarcoma. Pediatrics 40:254, 1967.

Shanoff, L. B., Spira, M., and Hardy, S. B.: Myositis ossificans: evolution to osteogenic sarcoma: Report of a histologically verified case. Am. J. Surg. 113:537, 1967.

DasGupta, T. K., Hajdu, S. I., and Foote, F. W.: Extraosseous osteogenic sarcoma. Ann. Surg. 168:1011, 1968.

Gawlik, Z.: Condrosarcoma mesenchymale (mesenchymal chondrosarcoma). Zakl. Anat. Pathol. 19:289, 1968.

Jarvi, O. H., Kvist, H. T. A., and Vainio, P. V.: Extraskeletal retroperitoneal osteosarcoma probably arising from myositis ossificans. Acta Pathol. Microbiol. Scand. 74:11, 1968.

Sheikh, M. A., and Koten, J. W.: A case of primary osteogenic sarcoma of connective tissue. East Afr. Med. J. 45:760, 1968.

Thompson, J. R., and Entin, S. D.: Primary extraskeletal chondrosarcoma. Cancer 23:936, 1969.

Ghadially, F. N., and Mehta, P. N.: Ultrastructure of osteogenic sarcoma. Cancer 25:1457, 1970.

Huizenga, C., and Balogh, K.: Cartilaginous tumors of the larynx. Cancer 26:201, 1970.

Wu, W. Q., and Lapi, A.: Primary non-skeletal intracranial cartilaginous neoplasms: Report of a chondroma and a mesenchymal chondrosarcoma. J. Neurol. Neurosurg. Psychiatry 33:469, 1970.

Allan, C. J., and Soule, E. H.: Osteogenic sarcoma of the somatic soft tissues—a clinicopathologic study of 26 cases and review of the literature. Cancer 27:1121, 1971.

Cardenas-Ramirez, L., Albores-Saavedra, J., and De Buen, S.: Mesenchymal chondrosarcoma of the orbit. Arch. Ophthalmol. 86:410, 1971.

Clark, W. E., Le Gros: The Tissues of the Body, 6th ed. Oxford, Clarendon Press, 1971.

Kadin, M. E., and Bensch, K. G.: On the origin of Ewing's tumor. Cancer 27:257, 1971.

Pavon, S. J., Bullough, P. G., and Marcove, R. C.: Mesenchymal chondrosarcoma—Medullary lesion of humerus. N.Y. State, J. Med. 71:1662, 1971.

Salvador, A. H., Beabout, J. W., and Dahlin, D. C.: Mesenchymal chondrosarcoma—Observations on 30 new cases. Cancer 28:605, 1971.

Enzinger, F. M., and Shiraki, M.: Extraskeletal myxoid chondrosarcoma. Hum. Pathol. 3:421, 1972.

Hou-Jensen, K., Priori, E., and Dmochowski, L.: Studies in the ultrastructure of Ewing's sarcoma of bone. Cancer 29:280, 1972.

Nishimura, H., Ishikawa, T., and Ishiko, T.: Extra-skeletal osteogenic sarcoma. A light microscopic and ultrastructural study of a case. Acta Pathol. Jpn. 22:195, 1972.

Wurlitzer, F., Ayala, A., and Romsdahl, M.: Extraosseous osteogenic sarcoma. Arch. Surg. 105:691, 1972.

Zimmerman, L. E.: Extraskeletal mesenchymal chondrosarcoma. Arch. Pathol. 95:336, 1972.

Angervall, L., Enerback, L., and Knutson, H.: Chondrosarcoma of soft tissue origin. Cancer 32:507, 1973.

Guccion, J. G., Font, R. L., Enzinger, F. M., and Zimmerman, L. E.: Extraskeletal mesenchymal chondrosarcoma. Arch. Pathol. 95:336, 1973.

Lynch, P. G., and Uriburu, E.: An intracranial cartilage-containing meningeal tumor. Case report. J. Neurosurg. 39:261, 1973.

Steiner, G. C., Mira, J. M., and Bullough, P. G.: Mesenchymal chondrosarcoma. A study of the ultrastructure. Cancer 32:926, 1973.

chapter 9

Miscellaneous Soft Tissue Tumors

MOST of the lesions discussed in this chapter are poorly defined from the histogenetic point of view (despite their well-known morphology). Some of the entities do not have any relation to each other, and they are included only for the sake of completeness of the text.

GRANULAR CELL TUMOR*

Despite the ubiquity and characteristic histologic features of granular cell tumor, or so-called granular cell myoblastoma, no unanimity exists as to its histogenesis. The first references to these lesions are the descriptions by Muller (1836) and Virchow (1854). However, the reader must be aware that in the past a number of benign, as well as malignant, lesions were called *rhabdomyoma* (Montpellier, 1929). In most publications, Abrikossoff (1926) is credited with the first description of this lesion, but the term *granular cell* was introduced by Diss, in 1927, in reporting a lesion of the anterior tongue in a 59-year-old patient.

The origin of granular cell tumors from *striated muscle,* as first proposed by Abrikossoff in 1926, was supported by many investigators on the basis of resemblance of the cells of granular cell tumor to myoblasts and their frequent and intimate association with altered skeletal muscle (Diss, 1927; Lattes, 1936; Murray, 1951; Christ and Ozzello, 1971). Stout and Lattes (1967) stated that "tissue culture studies show that the cellular outgrowth *in vitro* most nearly resembles striated muscle but does not account for the intracellular granules."

The origin of granular cell tumor *from nerve* has also been proposed by a number of investigators since Feyrter (1935) first proposed it (Fust and Custer, 1949; Pearse, 1950; Fisher and Wechsler, 1962; Magori and Szegvari, 1973). Pearse (1950) considered that granular cell tumors represented degeneration of perineurial and endoneurial fibroblasts. On the basis of ultrastructural and histochemical studies of five granular cell tumors Fisher and Wechsler (1962) concluded that the tumor cells were similar both morphologically and enzymatically to Schwann cells in traumatized nerve and proposed the designation of *granular cell schwannoma.* Leroux and Delarue, as early as 1939, proposed the concept that these lèsions are accumulated *reactive histiocytes* and not neoplasms, a view which received popularity in Europe (Azzopardi, 1956).

The morphologic similarity of cells of granular cell myoblastoma to elements of Gaucher's and Niemann-Pick diseases and their high concentration of acid phosphatase and esterase seem to support the histiocytic nature of these lesions. On the other hand, the well-documented examples of malignant transformation of granular cell myoblastomas may be considered as evidence in support of the neoplastic nature of these lesions (Ackerman and Phelps, 1946; Ross et al, 1952; Gamboa, 1955; Svejda and Horn, 1958; Usui et al, 1977). However, it may be argued that the so-called malignant granular cell myoblastomas are truly examples of an obscure and systemic storage disease.

So-called malignant granular cell myoblastomas must be considered even more carefully in light of the fact that up to 15% of benign granular cell lesions are multifocal (Klemperer, 1934; Meredith et al, 1958; Moscovic and Azar, 1967; Strong et al, 1970). Weitzner and Olsen (1968), for example, reported simultaneous occurrence of cutaneous and endobronchial lesions, and occasional instances of bone erosion have been noted in association with benign granular cell tumor.

Electron microscopic and histochemical observations support the concept that *granular cells are the product of a metabolic or other disturbance that may affect a variety of cells, including striated mus-*

* *Synonyms and related terms:* granular cell myoblastoma, Abrikossoff's tumor; granular cell neurofibroma, granular myoblastoma, myoblastoma, granular cell schwannoma, granular neuroma, lipid thesaurismosis.

cle cells, primitive mesenchymal cells, Schwann cells, perineurial cells, pericytes, and histiocytes. This view is also supported by observations that granular cytoplasmic changes similar to those seen in granular cell tumors have been seen in diverse neoplasms, e.g., schwannomas and tendosynovial tumors, and metabolic abnormalities (Fisher and Wechsler, 1962; Haisken and Langer, 1962; Christ and Ozzello, 1971; Sobel, 1974).

Several hundred examples of granular cell tumors have been reported in the literature. In most instances they are found in the submucosal and subcutaneous tissues and according to reports more than 50% of the tumors occur in the head and neck regions and have a special affinity for the tongue. Strong et al (1970) reviewed our experience with granular cell tumors at Memorial Sloan-Kettering Cancer Center (Fig. 9-1). They can occur in any age group but are relatively uncommon in children (Papageorgiou, 1967). In the series of Strong et al (1970) 69% of the patients were in their fourth to sixth decades, with the average age being 38 years.

Grossly, granular cell tumors usually measure 0.5 to 2.0 cm in diameter. They are firm, elevated, plaque-like or sessile and are not encapsulated. Symptoms will vary with the location and size of the lesion. Examples of granular cell tumors have been described to originate at unusual sites such as the *ear* (Horn and Stout, 1943), *esophagus* (Keshishian and Alford, 1964), *tracheobronchial tree* (Weitzner and Olsen, 1968; Valenstein and Thurer, 1978), *bile duct* (Coggins, 1952), *urinary bladder* (Ravich et al, 1945), and *female genitalia* (Wolfe and Mackles, 1963; Magori and Szegvari, 1973).

Microscopically, the cells in granular cell tumors vary in shape, but the predominant form is that of plump oval or globoid cells with occasional strap-like forms. The cytoplasm is abundant, staining eosinophilic or neutrophilic with hematoxylin and eosin stain, and contains distinctive granules which stain positive with PAS stain before and after diastase

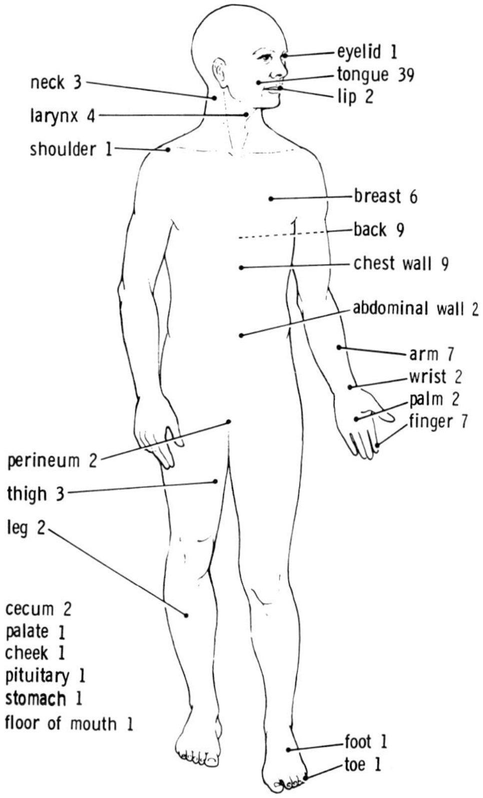

Figure 9-1. Anatomic distribution of 110 granular cell tumors (From Strong, E. W., McDivitt, R. W., and Brasfield, R. D.: Granular cell myoblastoma. Cancer 25:415, 1970).

digestion. Electron microscopy shows that most of the granules are phagolysosomes and other acid hydrolases. The cytoplasmic membrane is indistinct and blends into the background (Figs. 9-2, 9-3).

The nuclei are uniform in size and shape and eccentrically located in the cytoplasm. The cytologic appearance of individual cells can be assessed best in cytologic preparations (Naib, 1963; Sussman et al, 1973).

The cells adhere to each other and form sheets, nests, and clusters and frequently are surrounded by collagenous sheaths, as well as occasional fibroblasts. The granular cells may infiltrate or extend between tissue compartments to a considerable distance; however, any lesion that shows considerable pleomorphism and multinucleation and is larger than 5 cm and possesses branching and infiltrating cell cords

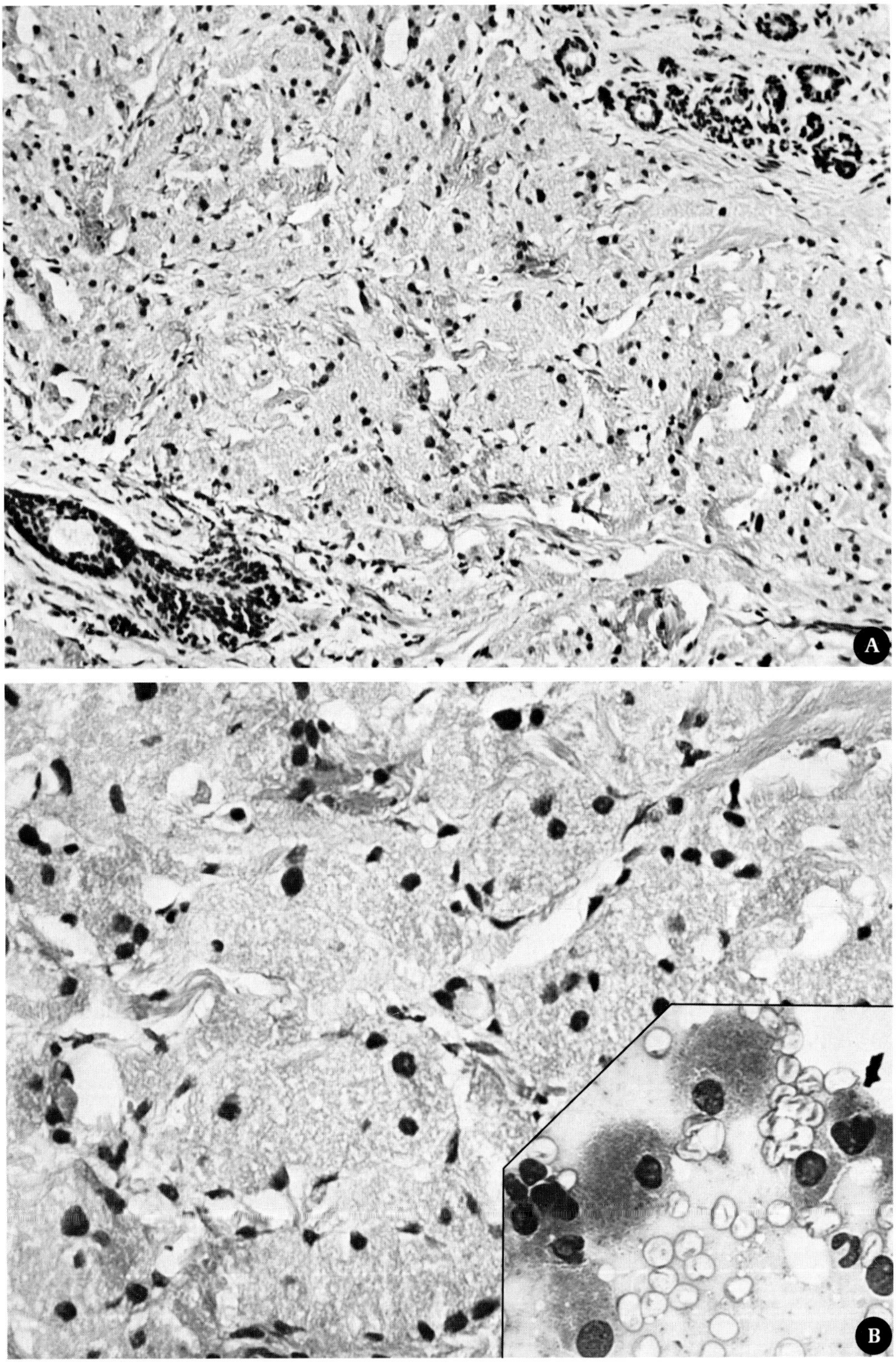

Figure 9-2. Benign granular cell tumor, so-called granular cell myoblastoma. This lesion is composed of well-defined and fairly uniform granular cells with pyknotic or vesicular solitary nuclei. The cells adhere to each other, but there is no particularly recognizable morphologic pattern except for the tendency to form loosely arranged cell cords at the edge of the lesion (**A,** H & E, ×140; **B,** H & E, ×350).

B (inset), Tumor cells of benign granular cell tumor as they appear in aspiration smear (H & E, ×570).

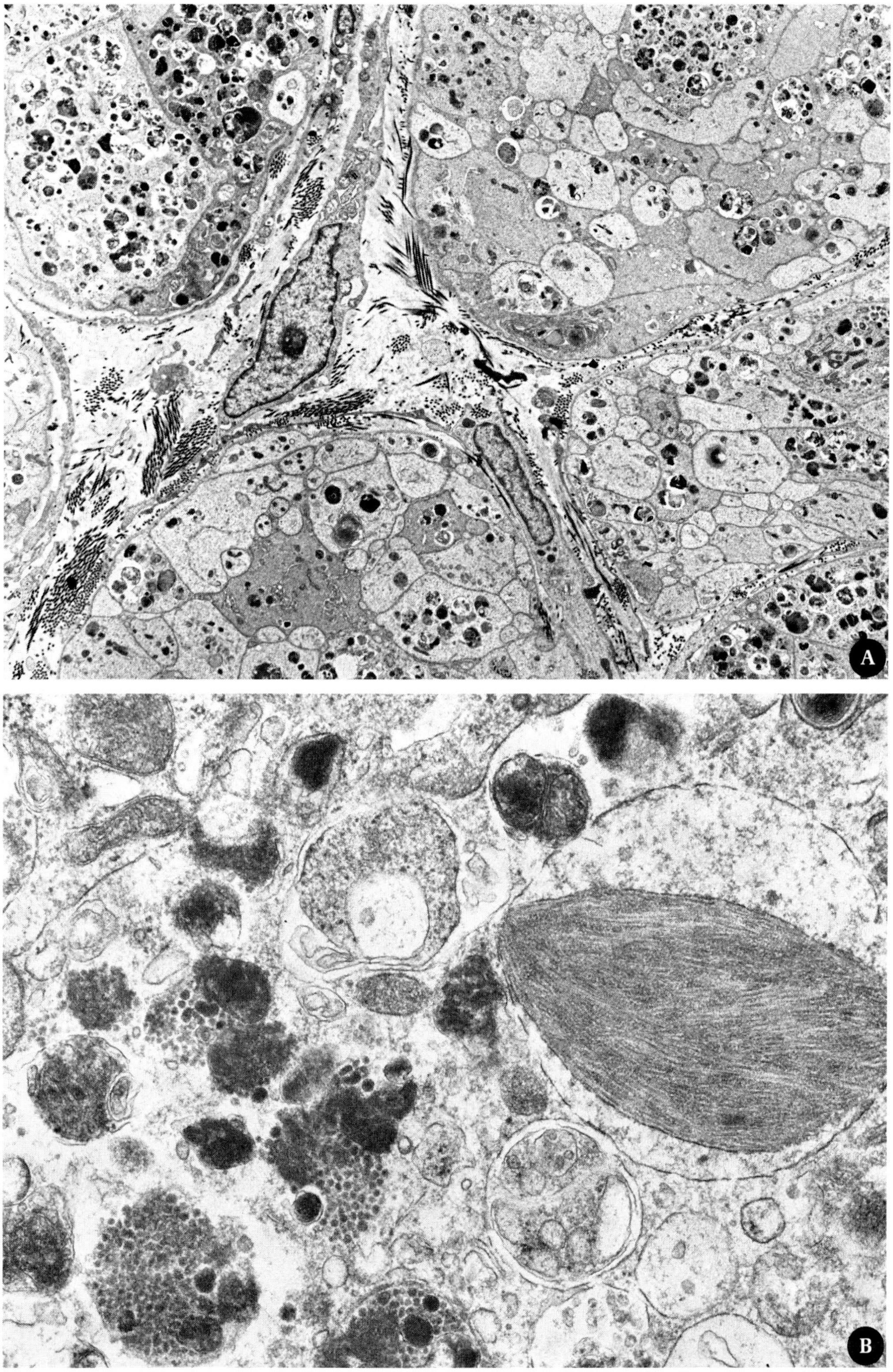

Figure 9-3. A, Benign granular cell tumor. Low power electron micrograph showing nests of granule containing cells resembling Schwann cells. Note the transsected axons surrounded by a fibrous stroma (×3,800).

B, Benign granular cell tumor. Portion of cytoplasm of a granular cell. Note the residual bodies and the large microtubule-containing angulate body (×29,000).

and satellite nodules at the periphery of the lesion should be considered locally troublesome and potentially malignant lesions.

Malignant variants of granular cell tumor do occur, but they are rare. Ravich et al, in 1945, are credited with the first description of a malignant granular cell tumor. Ross et al, in 1952, could find only 4 well-documented examples of malignant lesions in the literature, to which they added 3 new cases. At the present time, only 26 examples of malignant granular cell tumor or so-called granular cell myoblastoma have been reported in the literature (Table 9-1).

Every report mentions the difficulty in distinguishing histologically between the highly malignant lethal tumors and the ones with a benign course. It seems that large size of the tumor, larger than 5 cm, rapid growth with tendency to recur, and invasion into adjacent soft tissues, including lymphatic and blood vessels, are more reliable signs of malignant potentials than histologic or ultrastructural appearances. Despite occasional striking pleomorphism of the tumor cells in malignant lesions, mitotic figures are absent (Mackenzie, 1967; Strong et al, 1970; Al-Sarraf et al, 1971; Usui et al, 1977) (Fig. 9-4).

The differential diagnosis of granular cell tumors includes *alveolar soft part sarcoma, paraganglioma, rhabdomyoma* (see Chapter 5), and *rhabdomyoblastoma* (see Chapter 5).

ALVEOLAR SOFT PART SARCOMA*

Christopherson et al, in 1952, published 12 case reports of an unusual tumor from the files of the Pathology Department of Memorial Sloan-Kettering Cancer Center. They named it "alveolar soft part sarcoma." Christopherson et al acknowledged that tumors appearing identical to their alveolar soft part sarcomas were described and illustrated by others prior to 1952 (Klemperer, 1934; Horn and Stout, 1943; Ackerman and Phelps, 1946; Khanolkar, 1947) (see Chapter 1, Fig. 1-46).

Despite several attempts in the past to characterize this neoplasm, the histogenesis is still obscure (Fisher, 1956; Fassbender, 1960; Marshall and Horn, 1961; Lieberman et al, 1966; Shipkey et al, 1964). Shipkey et al, in 1964, studied alveolar soft part sarcomas by both light and electron microscopes and failed to find any of the characteristic structures that one expects to find in neoplasms of muscle or nerve. They also found that the ultrastructure of alveolar soft part sarcoma differed markedly from granular cell tumor, and in 9 of the 13 cases they studied they found protein-carbohydrate crystals. The crystals were seen in sections viewed with both the light and electron microscopes (see Chapter 1). Intracytoplasmic crystals in these tumors were first studied by Masson who described them in a letter addressed to Foote in 1950.

Ekfors et al (1979) reported that the crystals of alveolar soft part sarcoma are formed from intracytoplasmic, PAS-positive, dense granules. They also felt that because no monoamines were detected in the tumor cells by formaldehyde-induced fluorescence, alveolar soft part sarcoma is not of paraganglionic origin.

Fisher and Reidbord (1971) concluded after comparing the ultrastructural features of alveolar soft part sarcoma with those of granular cell tumors and alveolar rhabdomyosarcoma that alveolar soft part sarcoma can be classified best as a tumor of myogenic origin. It is also of note that Stout and Lattes as recently as 1967 discussed under one heading so-called malignant granular cell myoblastomas and alveolar soft part sarcomas.

Lieberman et al, in 1966, in an analysis of 53 cases on file at Memorial Sloan-Kettering Cancer Center summarized that

* *Synonyms and related terms:* granular cell myoblastoma with organoid structure.

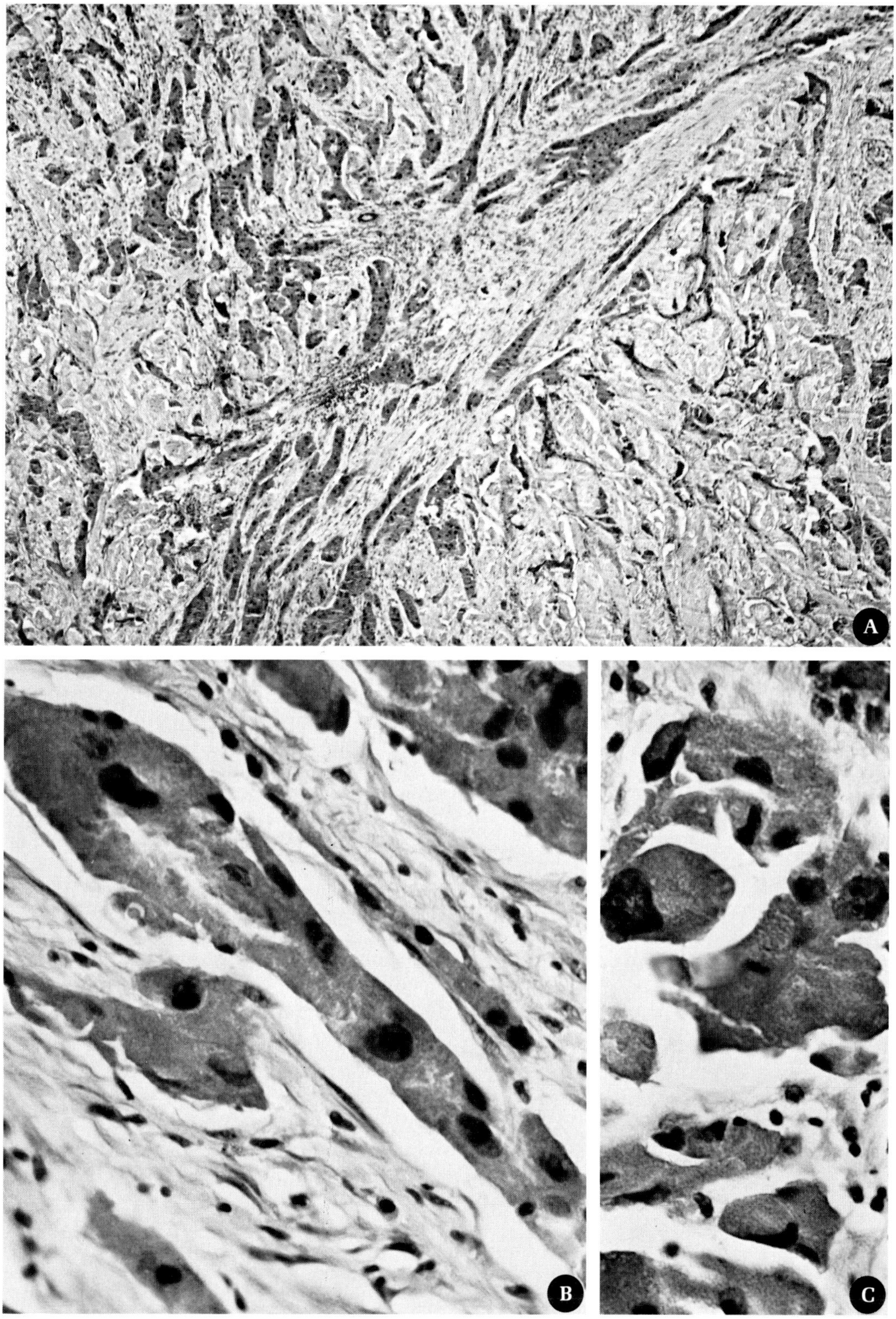

Figure 9-4. Malignant granular cell tumor.

A, Tightly packed cords of granular cells extend between tissue compartments, including perineurial and perivascular spaces. The slender and branching cords are often formed by the continuous lineup of single cells (H & E, ×85).

B and **C,** Tumor cells of malignant granular cell tumor show bizarre and pleomorphic granular cytoplasm and irregular pyknotic nuclei ranging in size from nuclei of lymphocytes to giant forms (H & E, ×350).

TABLE 9-1. ***Malignant Granular Cell Tumors***

REPORT	NO. OF CASES*	AGE YR.	SEX	SITE OF PRIMARY	THERAPY	RECURRENCE	METASTASIS	FOLLOW-UP
Ravich et al (1945)	1	31	M	Bladder	Exc.	—	To lungs, bones and liver	DcMD, 17 yr.
Powell (1946)	1	31	F	Trunk, multiple	Exc.	Multiple	To ovaries, 14 yr.; to esophagus and neck, 20 yr.	DcMD, 20 yr.
Dunnington (1948)	1	40	M	Orbit	Exc.	—	—	DcMD, 2 yr.
Ceelan (1949)	1	45	F	Arm, multiple	Exc.	—	To axilla and lung, 1 yr.	DcMD, 5 yr.
Ross et al (1952)	3	60	M	Lower back	Exc. Irrad.	2 mo.	To groin and lung, 2 yr.	Died, 3 yr.
		58	F	Leg	Exc.	8 mo. 3 yr.	To groin, 6 yr.; to brain, 8 yr.	DcMD, 8 yr.
		33	F	Thigh	Exc.	6 mo.	—	Alive, 14 yr.
Crawford and DeBakey (1953)	1	50	F	Breast	Exc.	—	To lung and liver	DcMD, 1 yr.
Gamboa (1955)	1	30	F	Thigh	Exc. Irrad.	—	To lung and groin	DcMD, 5 yr.
Busanny-Caspari and Hammar (1958)	1	40	M	Larynx	—	—	To cervical lymph nodes	Died, 2 yr.
Svejda and Horn (1958)	1	48	F	Groin	Exc. Irrad.	—	To lung and liver	DcMD, 4 yr.
Caby et al (1960)	1	40	F	Thigh	Exc.	—	To groin	Died, 13 yr.
Hunter and Dewar (1960)	1	75	F	Colon	Exc.	—	—	Alive, 15 mo.
Obiditsh-Mayer and Salzer-Kuntschik, (1961)	1	23	F	Esophagus	—	—	To mediastinal lymph nodes	Died, post-op.

Kreig (1962)	1	64	F	Upper arm	Partial Exc.	—	To lung, liver, and axilla, 10 mo.	DcMD, 14 mo.
Nitze (1966)	1	66	M	Buccal mucosa	Exc.	—	To retro-orbit	DcMD, 18 mo.
Mackenzie (1967)	1	82	F	Lower back	Exc.	2 yr.	To axilla and groin, 2 yr.	DcMD, 3 yr.
McCabe and Harman (1969)	1	60	M	Tongue	Exc.	—	To neck	Died
Al-Sarraf et al (1971)	1	35	M	Buttock	Exc.	18 mo.	To groin, 18 mo.	Alive, with dis.
Kuchemann (1971)	1	38	F	Shoulder	Exc.	—	To axilla	—
Magori and Szegvari (1973)	1	49	F	Vulva	Exc.	—	To groin, 4 mo.	Alive, 1 yr.
Cadotte (1974)	1	60	F	Thigh	Irrad.	—	—	DcMD, 9 mo.
Haustein (1974)	1	73	F	Head	—	—	To chest, lymph nodes, spleen	DcMD
Usui et al (1977)	1	34	F	Upper arm	Exc.	3 mo.	To axilla, 3 mo.; to lung, 4 mo.	DcMD, 7 mo.
Hajdu (unpublished)	1	42	F	Lower back	Exc.	6 mo. and 9 mo.	—	Alive with recurrence, 2 yr.

Exc. = excision; Irrad. = irradiation; DcMD = died with metastatic disease.

*An additional case was reported by Madhavan et al (1974).

these tumors are found more often in females and most of the tumors are diagnosed during the third and fourth decades. Most of the alveolar soft part sarcomas involve the extremities, but abdominal wall and retroperitoneal primary sites are not uncommon (Figs. 9-5, 9-6).

Microscopically, the most prominent features of alveolar soft part sarcomas are the uniform pattern and their similarity to each other (Fig. 9-7). There are many endothelial-lined vascular channels and septa. In sections stained with silver, the septa are seen to separate alveolar groups and vascular channels. No reticulin fibers separate the individual cells.

Cells are arranged in a pseudoalveolar, or organoid, fashion, either in compact groups of four or five to perhaps fifty cells or in peripheral rows with central spaces devoid of organized structure. According to Christopherson et al (1956), the latter arrangement may lead to an erroneous diagnosis. These investigators further reported:

"The component cell is large, oval to polyhedral, usually with distinct cell boundaries. The abundant cytoplasm takes a light eosinophilic hue in hematoxylin and eosin preparations. It stains light brown with both Masson trichrome and phosphotungstic acid hematoxylin. The cytoplasm is finely granular or reticulated with occasional vacuoles that usually do not stain with mucicarmine, osmic acid, or Sudan stains, although in degenerated areas some of the vacuoles are sudanophilic. In a single instance in which stains for glycogen were done, small amounts were demonstrated in a finely granular distribution throughout many of the cells. The cytoplasm is never as deeply acidophilic as that in classical rhabdomyosarcoma nor is there any suggestion of striations, or elongated, ribbon-like cells suggestive of known types of muscle tumors. The coarse granularity characteristic of myoblastoma is not present, although the similarity of individual cells to those found in myoblastomas is admittedly great. An eccentrically placed vesicular nucleus containing one or more distinct nucleoli is usually present. As a rule, there is minimal variation in the nuclei, although an occasional cell is binucleated and larger than usual, and a few nuclei are hyperchromatic. Mitoses are usually present but never in great numbers. Variations in cytology appear to be more related to degeneration than to activity."

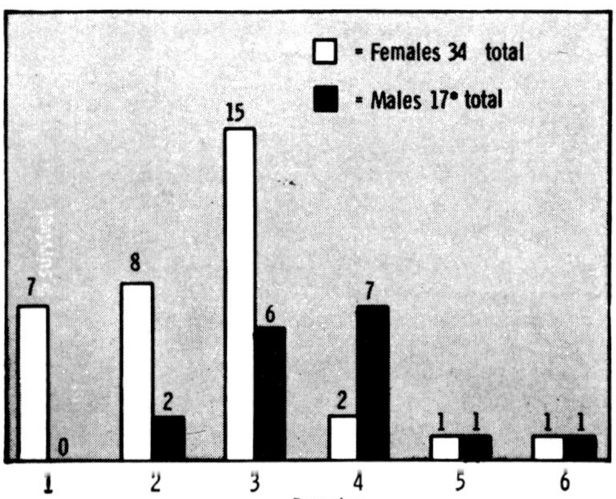

Figure 9-5. Age and sex distribution of 51 patients diagnosed to have alveolar soft-part sarcomas. Two patients of unknown age are not included. (Courtesy of Lieberman, P., Foote, F. W., Stewart, F. W., and Berg, J. W.: Alveolar soft-part sarcoma. JAMA 198:1047, 1966. Copyright 1966 by the American Medical Association.)

The survival data analyzed by Lieberman et al (1966) show that 59% of the patients survived for 5 years and 47% of the patients were alive at the tenth anniversary of the primary diagnosis. These authors pointed out, however, that metastatic lesions developed in 6 patients, 10 or more years after primary therapy (Fig. 9-8).

Because of the protracted course of the disease conservative, limb-saving surgical measures are the judicious treatment.

MALIGNANT LYMPHORETICULAR NEOPLASMS

Malignant lymphomas rarely present as soft tissue neoplasms without evidence of nodal disease. Poorly differentiated lymphocytic lymphoma and histiocytic lymphoma, however, may appear occasionally for a considerable period of time as soft tissue neoplasms.

Cytologically, the tumor cells are similar to those commonly seen in the nodal form of the disease, but their arranged pattern and tendency to be oval or spindle-shaped may cause a dilemma in diagnosis. In case of doubt, after all essential laboratory work-up, including lymphangiography, has been done, one may find it advantageous to perform immunofluorescent and ultrastructural studies. We have found that cytologic assessment of the tumor cells in aspiration or imprint smears can be informative because most genuine, non-lymphoreticular neoplasms appear in smear preparation in cohesive cell clusters, whereas lymphoreticular neoplasms, without exception, are in noncohesive single cell patterns (Hajdu and Hajdu, 1976) (Fig. 9-9).

*Granulocytic sarcoma** is a rare extramedullary variant of acute granulocytic leukemia. The term *granulocytic sarcoma,* first proposed by Rappaport in 1966, is more appropriate than *chloroma,* introduced by King in 1853, because the distinctive pigmentation is often absent. Usually the soft tissue mass appears several months before the disseminated disease.

Burns, in 1811, is credited with the description of the first case, and Turk, in 1903, established the relationship between chloroma and granulocytic leukemia. Since then, virtually all cases of granulocytic sarcomas have been demonstrated to be associated with either granulocytic or monocytic leukemia (Ross, 1955; Wiernik and Serpick, 1970; Muss and Moloney, 1973; Cavdar et al, 1978).

The most common site of granulocytic sarcoma is the subperiosteal region of bones, especially in the orbital and chest wall areas. Tumors unrelated to bone are far less common. Granulocytic sarcoma is a disease of children and young adults and the overall survival of patients with granulocytic sarcoma is similar to that of patients with acute granulocytic leukemia. Frequent differentiation of the leukemia toward the myelomonocytic form has

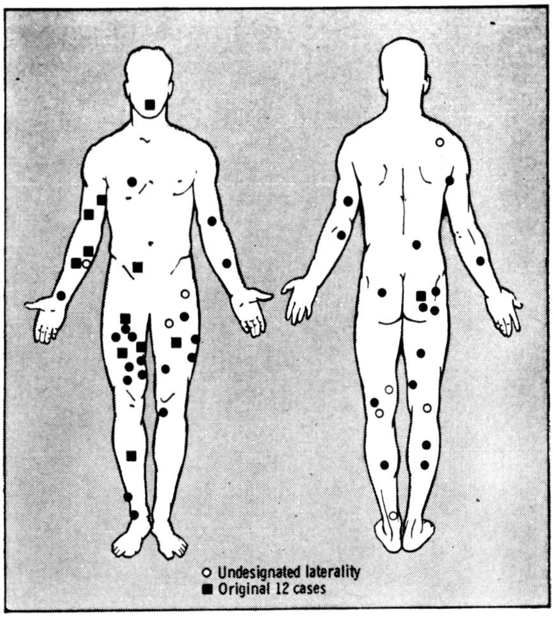

Figure 9-6. Anatomic distribution of the 12 original cases of alveolar soft-part sarcoma reported by Christopherson et al. in 1952 and 41 additional cases. (Courtesy of Lieberman, P., Foote, F. W., Stewart, F. W., and Berg, J. W.: Alveolar soft-part sarcoma. JAMA 198:1047, 1966. Copyright 1966 by the American Medical Association.)

been observed among children in Africa and Japan (Cavdar et al, 1978).

Grossly, granulocytic sarcomas usually appear green in white light and often fluoresce red with ultraviolet light. The green color tends to fade upon exposure to air but can be temporarily restored in fresh tissue by soaking the tissue in glycerin or in case of formalin-fixed tissue by placing the section in hydrogen peroxide. Schultz and Rosenthal (1959) came to the conclusion that the peculiar green color is due to crystalline myeloperoxidase which has a red fluorescence under ultraviolet light.

Granulocytic sarcoma is composed of relatively uniform cells resembling the neoplastic cells of a number of other neoplasms, e.g., histiocytic lymphoma (see Chapter 6), embryonal rhabdomyosarcoma (see Chapter 5), Ewing's sarcoma (see Chapter 8), eosinophilic granuloma, and primitive neuroectodermal tumor. The definite diagnosis must be based on the identification of neoplastic granulo-

* *Synonyms and related terms:* chloroma, myeloblastic sarcoma, chloroleukemia.

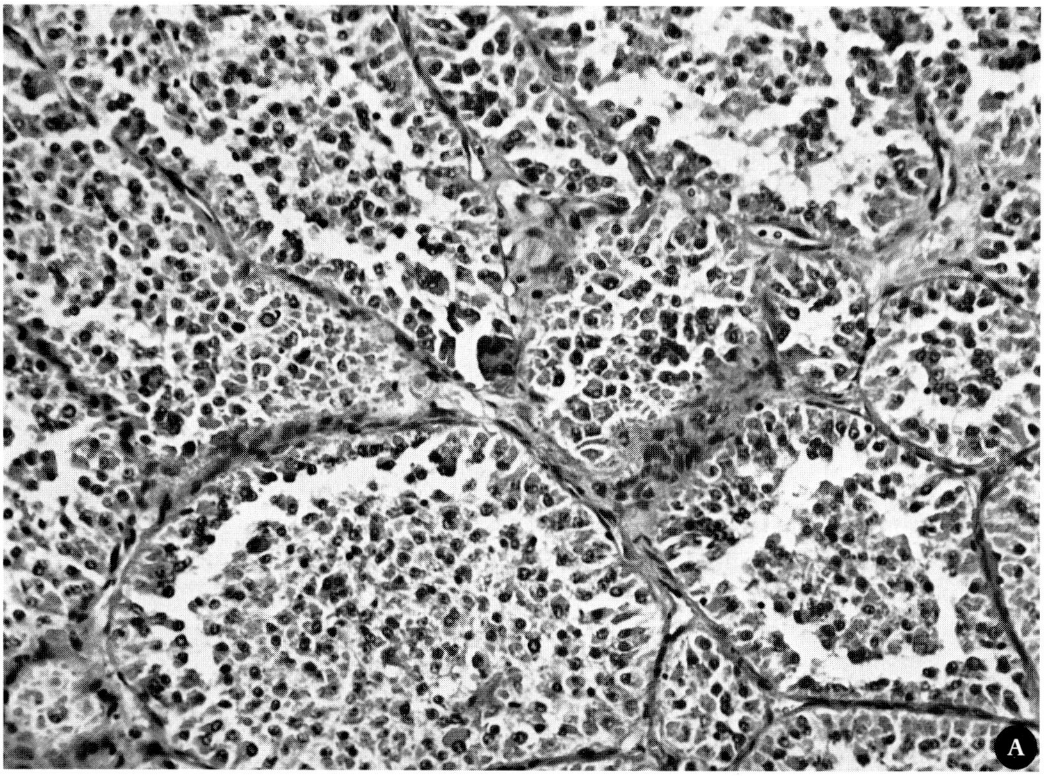

Figure 9-7. Alveolar soft-part sarcoma. This tumor is composed of large polygonal cells having granular cytoplasm and large vesicular nuclei. The tumor cells may range in size from medium-sized mononuclear cuboidal forms to binucleated or multinucleated giant cells.

Most of the tumor cells are arranged in distinct alveolar pattern and fill the reticulovascular frame by alignment of the neoplastic cells along tissue septae. Notice the bizarre mitotic figures (**A,** H & E, ×85; **B,** H & E, ×140; **C,** H & E, ×350). (See ultrastructure, Chapter 1, Figure 1-49.)

cytic cells in the bone marrow and peripheral blood. Also, demonstration of the intracytoplasmic granules, either by electron microscopy or by enzyme chemical stain, may facilitate proper diagnosis even in the aleukemic phase of the disease. Optimal results can be obtained by staining imprint smears with Giemsa stain along with special esterase, peroxidase, or other histochemical stains (Muss and Moloney, 1973). Simple imprint or aspiration smears are often useful in distinguishing neoplastic cells of granulocytic sarcoma from rhabdomyoblasts, neuroblasts, and tumor cells of Ewing's sarcoma. From the point of view of differentiational diagnosis it is also important to point out the frequent epidural and perineural localization of granulocytic tumors (Fig. 9-10).

*Plasmacytoma** of soft tissues is a rare but distinct neoplasm. In a literature review in 1963 Fruhling and Chadli observed that 13% of all plasma cell tumors are extramedullary. The majority occur in the upper airways (Gordon and Walker, 1944; Stout and Kenney, 1949; Ewing and Foote, 1952; Dharamadhack et al, 1965, Herskovic et al, 1965; Bahadori and Liebow, 1973; Buell et al, 1976; Baroni et al, 1977).

Castro et al (1973) of Memorial Sloan-Kettering Cancer Center reported 24 cases of plasmacytomas arising in the head and neck region. These represented 6% of 420 plasmacytomas of all sites. They also re-

**Synonyms and related terms:* extramedullary plasmacytoma, plasma cell myeloma of soft tissues, extraskeletal plasma cell myeloma.

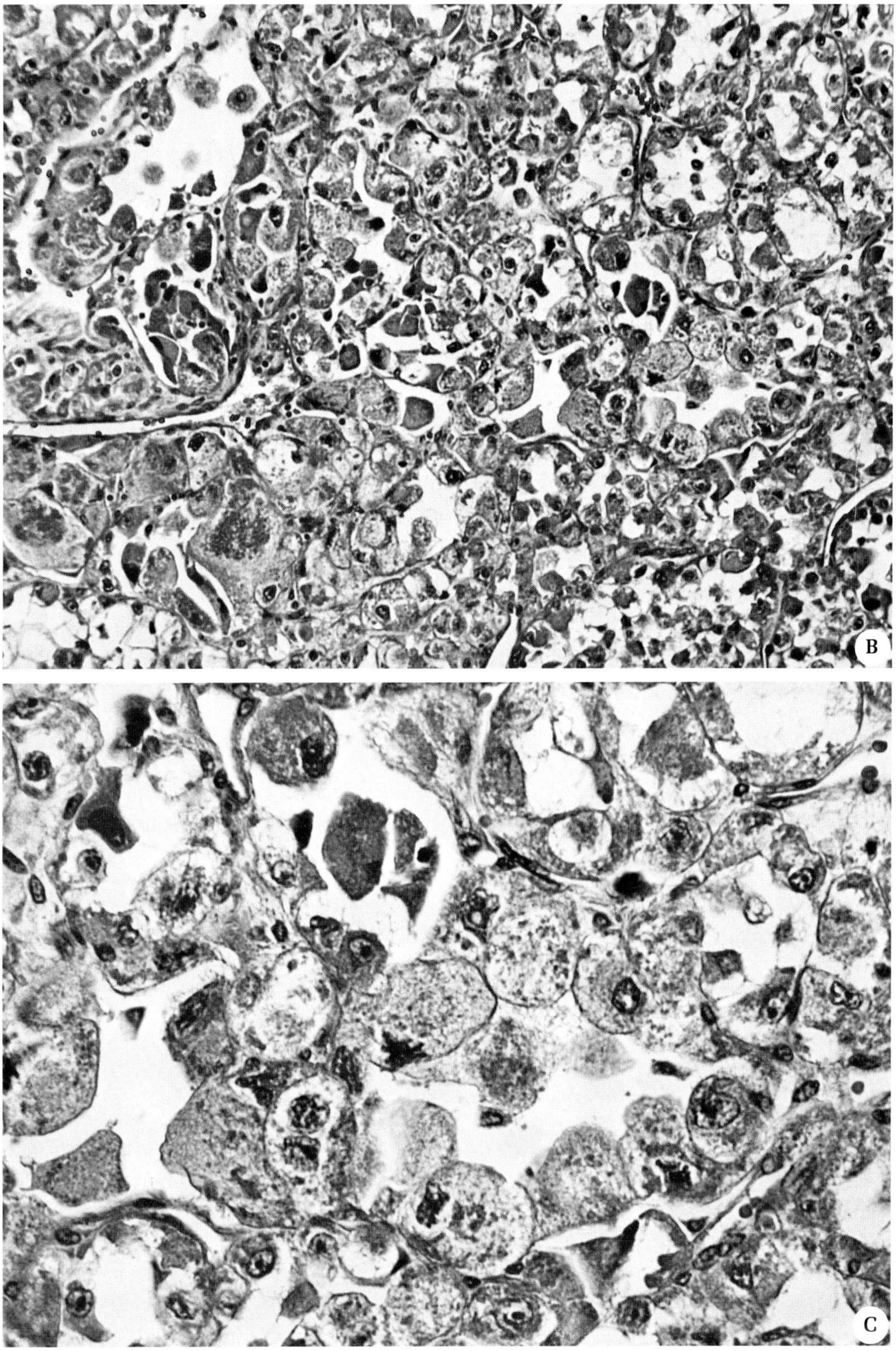

Figure 9-7 (continued).

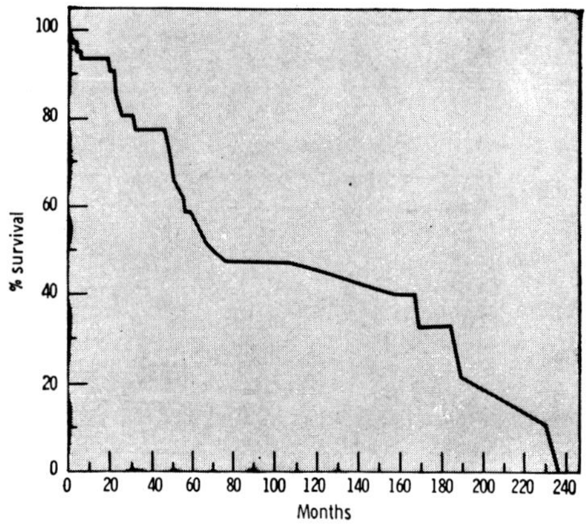

Figure 9-8. Cumulative survival of 46 patients with alveolar soft-part sarcoma. (Courtesy of Lieberman, P., Foote, F. W., Stewart, F. W., and Berg, J. W.: Alveolar soft-part sarcoma. JAMA 198:1048, 1966. Copyright 1966 by the American Medical Association.)

viewed the literature and found 192 reported cases of plasmacytomas arising in the head and neck region. Apparently the nasal cavity, paranasal sinuses, and nasopharynx are the most common sites.

Extramedullary plasma cell tumors may occur anywhere in the body. Gaston et al (1969) reported 2 cases of primary plasmacytoma of lymph nodes. Nielson et al (1972) reported a colonic primary plasmacytoma and recently Doss (1978) published a case report of simultaneous plasmacytomas of the vagina and vulva.

There are no valid criteria for prognosis in extraskeletal plasmacytoma, and the survival of patients seems to depend on the site and extent of the tumor. There is general agreement in the literature that about 45% of the patients with plasmacytoma of soft tissues which does not involve the respiratory tract survive for 5 years; only 20% of the patients with plasmacytoma of the airways survive for 5 years.

Wiltshaw (1976), after reviewing the natural history of extramedullary plasmacytoma, emphasized that most of the tumors recur locally prior to dissemination. Plasmacytomas which eventually lead to the patient's death usually show a multifocal pattern of spread which includes soft tissues as well as the skeletal system.

There is no agreement in the literature regarding the treatment of extramedullary plasmacytomas, but long-term survivals were reported following irradiation as well as local surgical treatment.

POSTIRRADIATION SARCOMA

The occurrence of lymphangiosarcoma in the upper extremity and chest wall as a long-term complication of radical mastectomy has become well-known since its first description by Stewart and Treves in 1948. Other tumors that may develop following therapeutic irradiation or incidental irradiation include various epithelial tumors (Curtin et al, 1977, Duffy and Fitzgerald, 1950; Rachmaninoff et al, 1961; Wanebo et al, 1966; Janower and Niettinen, 1971; Curtin et al, 1977), *lymphoreticular neoplasms* (Bisbee and Thoeny, 1975; Archer, 1977), and particularly *bone neoplasms* (Martland, 1931; Wilson and Brunschwig, 1937; Cahan et al, 1948; Boyer et al, 1965; Sears et al, 1967; Tefft et al, 1968; Modan et al, 1974; Meadows et al, 1975).

It is less well-known that radiation often affects not only the bone and parenchymal and lymphoreticular organs but also fibroconnective and other soft tissues. The alarming figures reported by Tefft et al (1968) indicate that all patients given irradiation therapy must be considered candidates for postradiation tumors, including soft tissue sarcomas.

Malignant fibrous tumors of soft parts have been reported by Pettit et al, 1954; Schwartz and Rothstein, 1968; and Oberman and Oneal, 1970.

Since Warren and Sommer, in 1936, described the first case of *fibrosarcoma* developing after irradiation for carcinoma of the breast a number of additional cases have been reported.

Angiosarcomas have been induced by various chemical carcinogens. Thorotrast and polyvinyl chloride are associated with angiosarcoma of the liver.

Angiosarcoma of the abdominal wall following therapeutic irradiation has been reported (Calman and Cowdell, 1959; Legerlotz, 1962; McSwain et al, 1973; Paik and Komorowski, 1976). March (1966) reported a case of angiosarcoma of the face following radiation therapy.

Meyer et al (1978) reported a case of *meningioma* and *schwannoma* in a patient who had undergone Thorotrast myelography 33 years previously. Donohue et al (1967) reported 2 cases of *neurofibroma* occurring as a late complication of radiation therapy. One of the tumors occurred 13 and the other 11 years after extensive irradiation.

An *extraskeletal osteogenic sarcoma* as a late complication of radiation therapy was reported by Boyer and Navin in 1965. Recently, Urano et al (1979) reported development of osteogenic and soft tissue sarcomas in 41 of 67 mice, on the average within 490 days, after radiation therapy of a mouse mammary carcinoma.

Our experience, at Memorial Sloan-Kettering Cancer Center, with postirradiation soft tissue sarcomas is summarized in Table 9-2. According to histologic type the tumors were malignant fibrous histiocytoma (4 cases), desmoid tumor (4 cases), fibrosarcoma (5 cases), tendosynovial sarcoma (1 case), myosarcoma (3 cases), angiosarcoma (3 cases), neurogenic sarcoma (4 cases), and undifferentiated sarcoma (5 cases) (Figs. 9-11, 9-12, 9-13). On the average, 65% of the patients died with metastatic disease in less than 2 years, and only 9 patients are alive without evidence of the disease, including all 4 patients who had desmoid tumor. The patients received irradiation for various conditions, and on the average more than 10 years elapsed between the time of irradiation therapy and the diagnosis of the soft tissue sarcoma (Table 9-2).

At the present time, the oncogenic potential of chemotherapeutic agents is uncertain, but many of the drugs in use for the treatment of lymphoreticular neoplasms are known oncogens in laboratory animals (Harris, 1976). Also, one should consider the oncogenic effect of various immunosuppressive medications. At present immunodeficiency with altered immunosurveillance is one of the most attractive hypotheses for the pathogenesis of induced tumors (Penn, 1976).

It is apparent that as more patients survive because of effective use of irradiation and chemotherapeutic agents the appearance of induced neoplasms in humans will increase. The paradox of irradiation cancers is the long period of precancerous changes in the tissues which may last for years or decades; yet once the cancer appears there is a fast downhill course with a high rate of metastasis and mortality. It is hoped that one day the better understanding of the formation of these predictably dangerous, induced neoplasms will shed some light on the formation of other neoplasms (Fig. 9-14).

MESENCHYMOMA

The term *mesenchymoma* was used in the past to describe different types of connective tissue tumors (Klein, 1932; Cellina, 1932; Gilmour, 1943). The term *mesenchymoma* as employed by Ewing and Harrison (1935) and Stout (1948) means tumors composed of two or more distinctly different mesodermal elements, but tumors in which one of the two elements is fibroblastic or the histologically diverse components are metaplastic should not be considered mesenchymomas.

During the last 20 years, as knowledge concerning soft tissue neoplasms has accumulated and criteria, as well as the histogenesis of various soft tissue neoplasms, have been better defined, the use of the term *mesenchymoma* (benign or malignant) has become unnecessary. Practically all soft tissue tumors contain a spectrum of mesenchymal elements at various stages of differentiation, but any given tumor should be classified on the basis of the highest grade and most differentiated histologic elements. For example, if an area of hemangiosarcoma is identified microscopically in a tumor, the tumor should be classified as hemangiosarcoma despite the fact that the bulky part of the tumor looks fibroblastic, lipoblastic, or

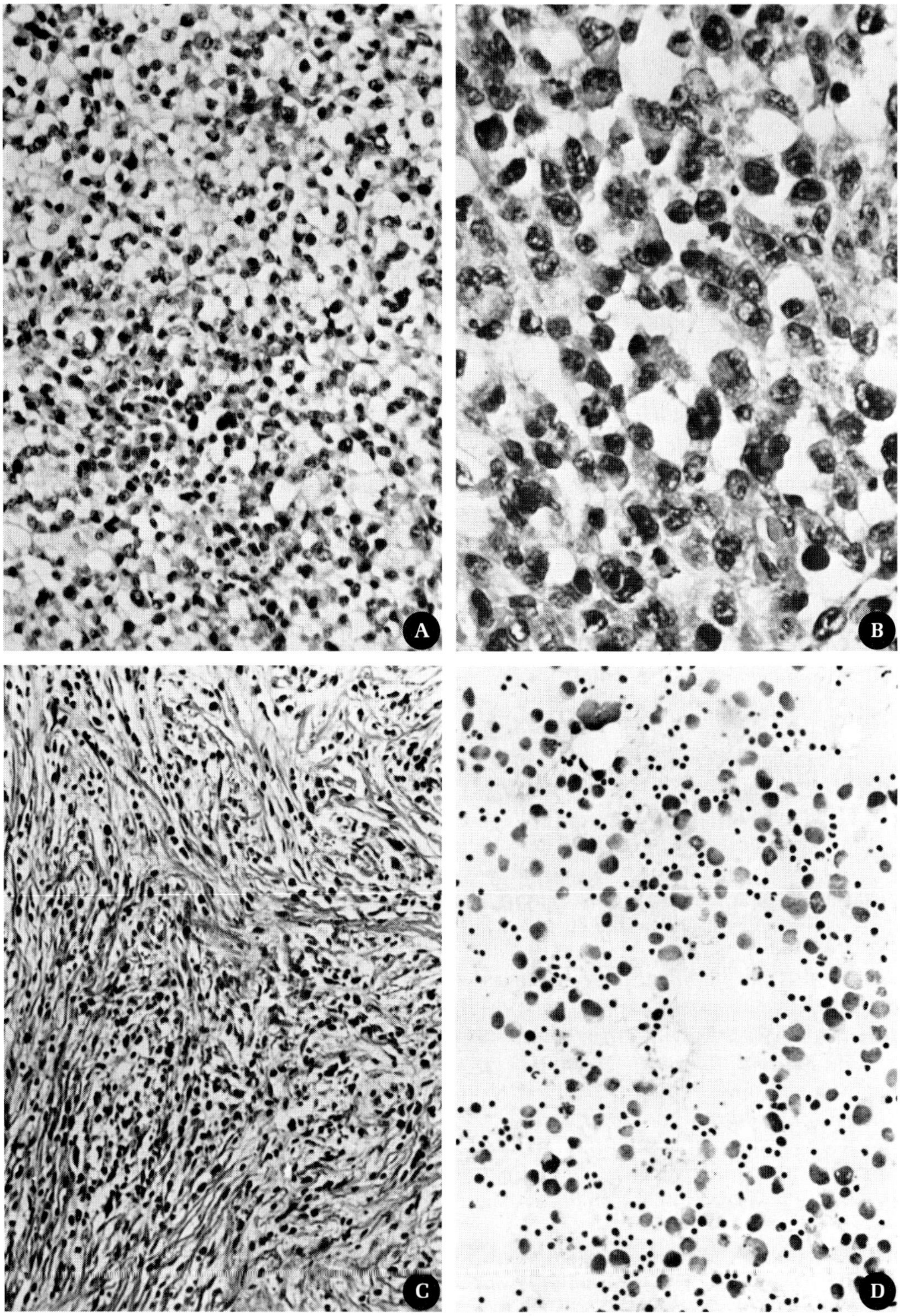

Figure 9-9. A and **B,** Poorly differentiated histiocytic lymphoma presented as a solitary mass of inner thigh. Note the oval, occasionally spindle shape of the tumor cells. The vacuoles are remnants of stromal tissue compartments, and the cohesive pattern of single cells is created by the reticular framework of the host tissue. (**A,** H & E, ×85; **B,** H & E, ×250.)

C and **D,** Hodgkins' disease presents as a chest wall lesion.

C, Small lymphoreticular neoplastic cells cluster between fibrocollagenous elements which are either remnants of the host tissue or part of the neoplastic proliferation (H & E, ×85).

D, An imprint smear prepared from the cross-sected tumor. Fairly characteristic spread of isolated, non-cohesive neoplastic lymphoreticular cells is seen (H & E, ×85).

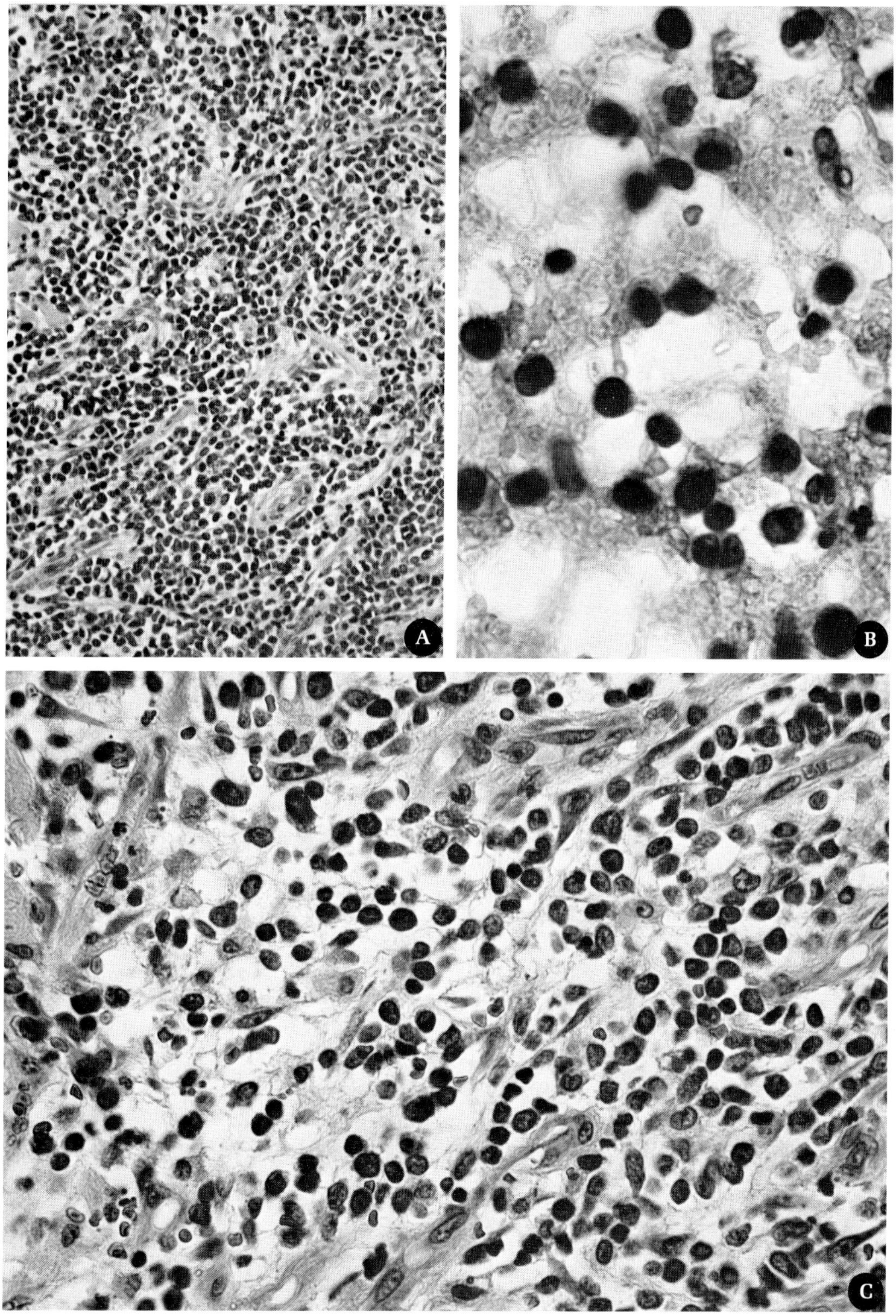

Figure 9-10. Granulocytic sarcoma of the chest wall. Uniform round or slightly oval cells in a loose, noncohesive arrangement. The fibrovascular stroma may align the granulocytes in cords or clusters. Imprint smear **(B)** shows that the tumor cells are uniform round cells with minimal cytoplasms and there is no cohesion between the tumor cells (**A,** H & E, ×85; **B,** H & E, ×570; **C,** H & E, ×350).

TABLE 9-2. *Postirradiation Soft Tissue Sarcomas*

	AGE AT DIAGNOSIS	SEX	RADIATION THERAPY	AMOUNT RADIATION (r)	POSTIRRADIATION SARCOMA	INTERVAL BETWEEN IRRADIATION AND POSTIRRADIATION SARCOMA, Yr.	FOLLOW-UP
1	49	F	Hodgkin's disease, right axilla	3600	Malignant fibroblastic fibrous histiocytoma, rt. chest wall	5	DcMD, 6 mo.
2	41	F	Malignant lymphoma, right axilla	—	Malignant fibroblastic fibrous histiocytoma, rt. shoulder	25	NED, 2 yr.
3	30	F	Histiocytic lymphoma, left axilla	2200	Malignant pleomorphic fibrous histiocytoma, lt. shoulder	9	NED, 1 yr.
4	61	M	Seminoma of testis	3200	Malignant histiocytic fibrous histiocytoma	20	DcMD, 2 yr,
5	38	M	Hodgkin's disease, right axilla	3000	Desmoid tumor, rt. chest wall	9	NED
6	40	F	Chondrosarcoma, left shoulder	—	Desmoid tumor, lt. chest wall	3	NED, 16 yr.
7	61	F	Cancer, right breast	—	Desmoid tumor, rt. chest wall	35	NED, 4 yr.
8	63	M	Left hand	—	Desmoid tumor, lt. hand	15	NED, 11 yr.
9	57	M	Carcinoma of lung	3800	Fibrosarcoma, chest wall	3	NED, 1 yr.
10	62	F	Uterine carcinoma	—	Fibrosarcoma, pelvis	11	DcMD
11	71	F	Carcinoma, right breast	—	Fibrosarcoma, rt. arm	41	DcMD, 1 yr.
12	54	F	Carcinoma, right breast	4000	Fibrosarcoma, rt. arm	10	DcMD, breast, 2 yr.
13	56	F	Carcinoma, right breast	2200	Fibrosarcoma	6	DcMD, 2 yr.

14	48	M	Malignant lymphoma	5000	Tendosynovial sarcoma, lt. shoulder	13	DcMD
15	14	M	Mediastinum	3000	Embryonal rhabdomyosarcoma, chest wall	8	—
16	52	M	Carcinoma, larynx	—	Pleomorphic rhabdomyosarcoma	20	DcMD, 5 yr.
17	48	F	Epidermoid carcinoma, cervix	—	Leiomyosarcoma, buttock	10	Alive with metas. tumor, 1 yr.
18	62	M	Carcinoma, right pelvis	—	Hemangiosarcoma, abdominal wall (Fig. 9-12)	55	DcMD, 4 yr.
19	56	F	Carcinoma, right breast	3000	Lymphangiosarcoma, rt. upper arm	11	DcMD, 3 yr.
20	30	F	Angioma, thigh	—	Hemangiosarcoma	15	DcMD, 2 yr.
21	46	M	Carcinoma, right neck	—	Neurofibrosarcoma	9	NED, 22 yr.
22	60	F	Menorrhagia	—	Malignant schwannoma, buttock	24	DcMD, 3 yr.
23	46	M	Malignant lymphoma	—	Neurogenic sarcoma, back	13	DcMD, 2 yr.
24	29	F	Hodgkin's disease	3200	Malignant schwannoma	8	—
25	59	F	Carcinoma, right breast	2000	Undifferentiated sarcoma, chest wall	13	Alive with metas. tumor, 1 yr.
26	44	M	Hodgkin's disease, mediastinum	3200	Undifferentiated sarcoma, chest wall	7	NED, 1 yr.
27	21	M	Hodgkin's disease, mediastinum	4200	Undifferentiated sarcoma, chest wall	6	DcMD, 1 yr.
28	32	F	Desmoid tumor, right face	4300	Undifferentiated sarcoma, face	11	DcMD, 2 yr.
29	65	F	Carcinoma, gall bladder	—	Undifferentiated sarcoma, back	13	Alive with metas. dis., 10 mo.

DcMD = died with metastatic disease; NED = no evidence of disease.

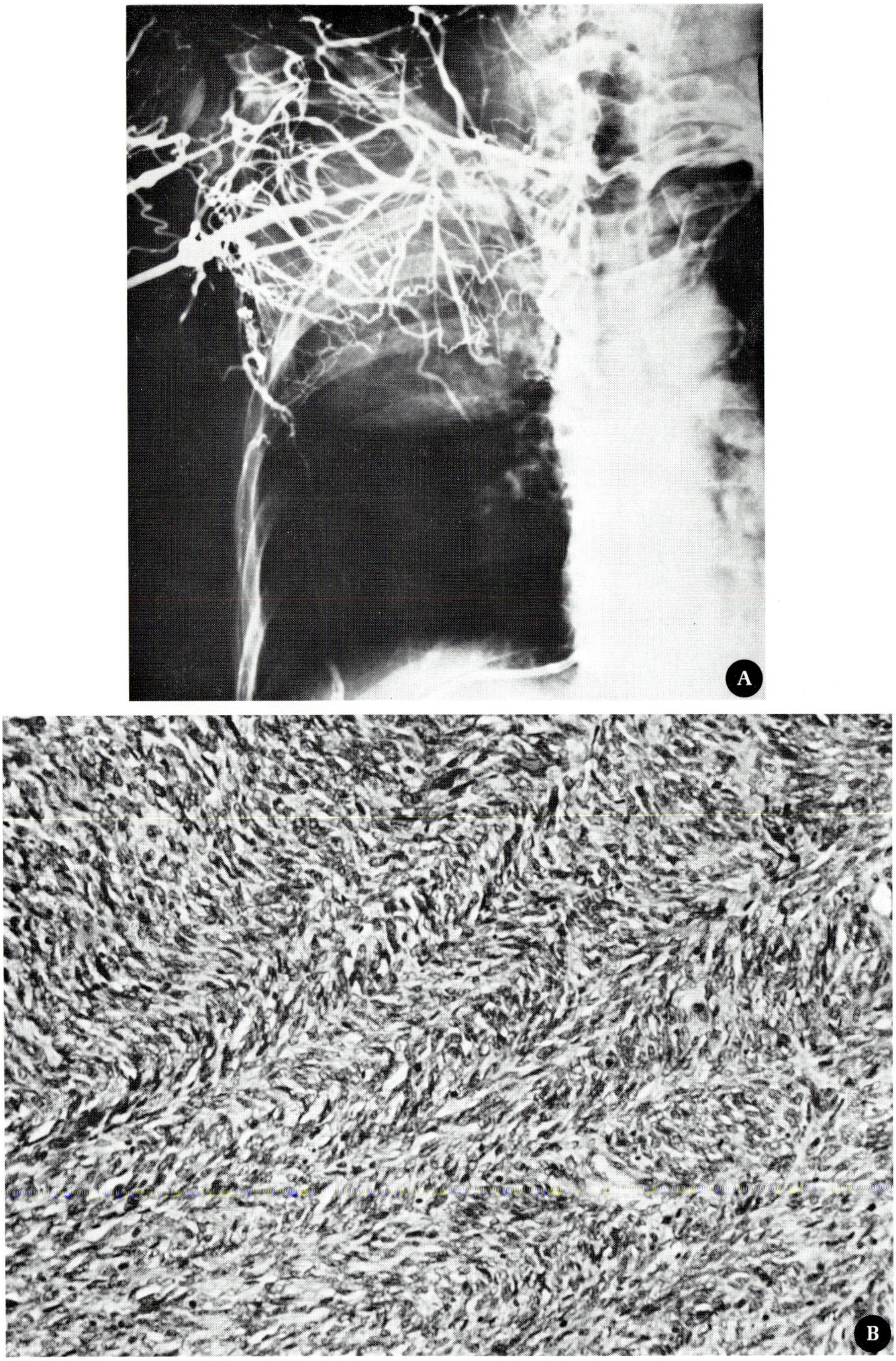

Figure 9-11. Postirradiation fibrosarcoma of the right shoulder. **A,** The tumor is highly vascular with numerous anastomosing branches.

B, Microscopically the tumor is composed of partly collagenous fibroblasts arranged in the characteristic herringbone pattern (H & E, ×140).

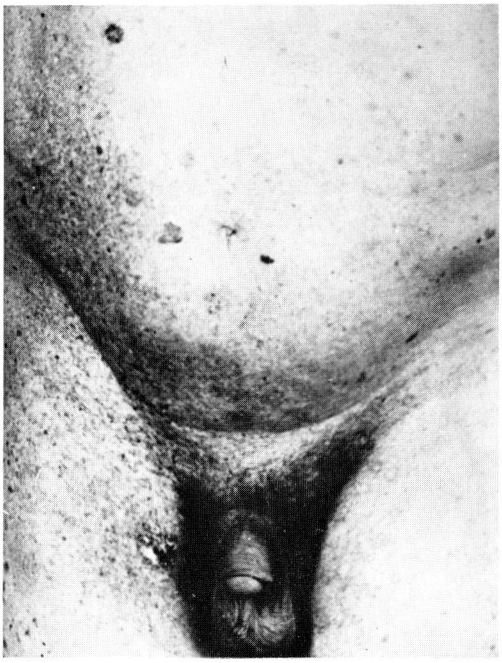

Figure 9-12. Multifocal postirradiation hemangiosarcoma of the abdominal wall 55 years after irradiation for "tuberculous osteomyelitis."

myoblastic. Adopting this principle makes the use of the term *mesenchymoma* unnecessary. However, if one is unable to decide which one of the recognized histologic elements should be used for classification purposes, it is perhaps appropriate, at least for the time being, to list all pertinent elements. Such classification is analogous to the classification of germ cell tumors, e.g., "malignant soft tissue tumor composed of fibrosarcomatous, liposarcomatous, and myosarcomatous elements." (See Chapter 1, Fig. 1-59 and Table 1-15 in reference to Grading and Staging).

UNDIFFERENTIATED SOFT TISSUE NEOPLASMS

Undoubtedly a tumor may defy all attempts at proper classification. After all available clinical and laboratory techniques have failed to supply a clue to the exact nature of a soft tissue neoplasm, the tumor should be classified as an undifferentiated soft tissue neoplasm or primitive mesenchymal tumor. In addition, the pathologist's report should indicate whether, on the basis of microscopic appearance (see Chapter 1), the lesion is considered to be benign or malignant.

According to my experience, and the experience of the staff at Memorial Sloan-Kettering Cancer Center, less than 5% of the soft tissue neoplasms are so undifferentiated that, even after generous sampling, subclassification remains unwarranted. It should also be remembered that practically any soft tissue tumor may, at a certain stage of growth, be capable of forming a stellate or storiform pattern. It would be a mistake to classify such tumors as fibrous histiocytomas and not search for the identity of the tumor, just as it would be wrong to call poorly differentiated carcinomas "undifferentiated carcinoma" and give up attempts to specify whether the tumor is epidermoid or glandular in origin.

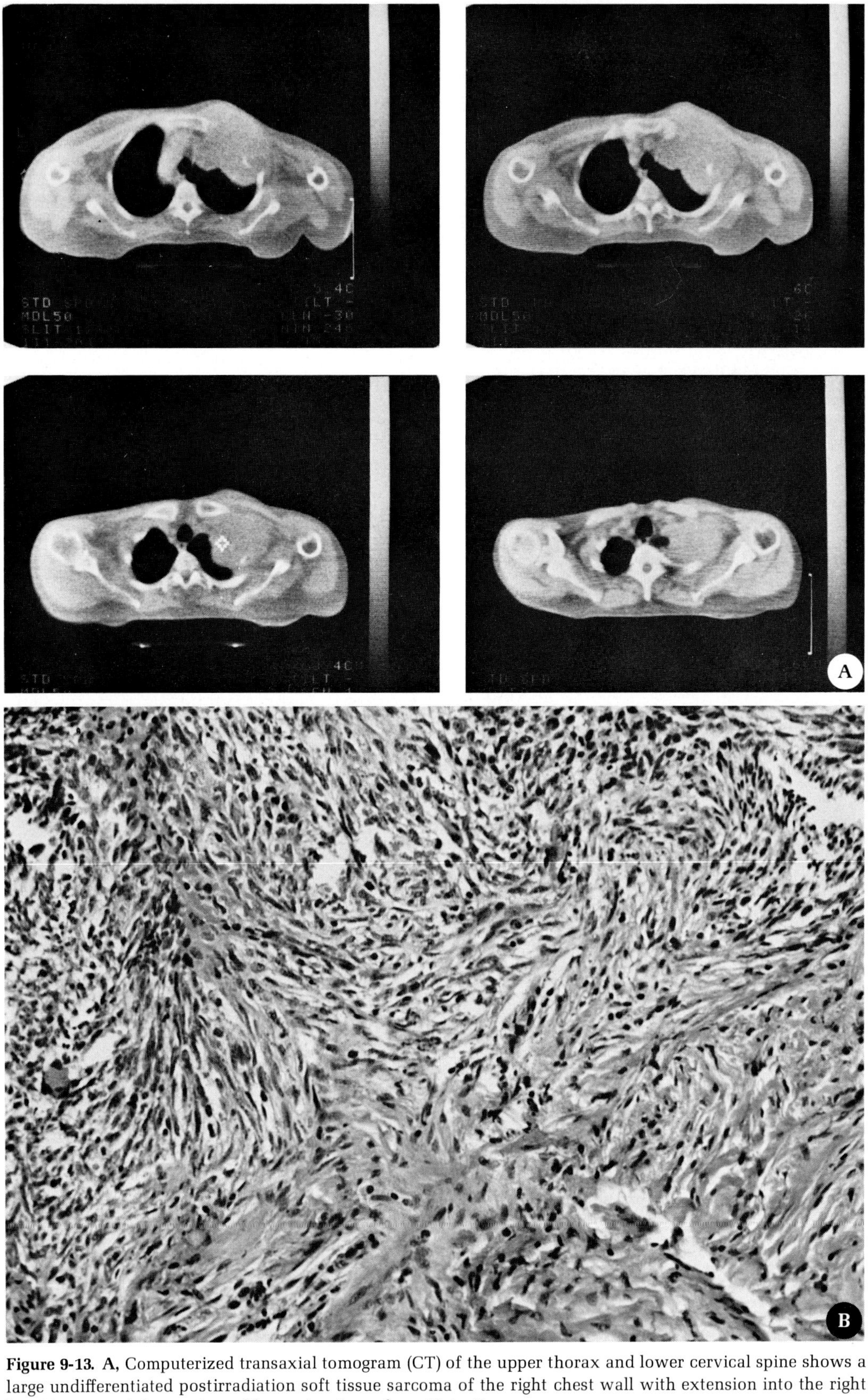

Figure 9-13. A, Computerized transaxial tomogram (CT) of the upper thorax and lower cervical spine shows a large undifferentiated postirradiation soft tissue sarcoma of the right chest wall with extension into the right hemithorax and destruction of bony structures from T_1 to T_5.

B, Undifferentiated postirradiation soft tissue sarcoma composed of a mixture of elongaged spindle cells with slender reticular and collagenous cytoplasmic processes and small round and oval undifferentiated cells in a sparsely vascular background (H & E, ×140).

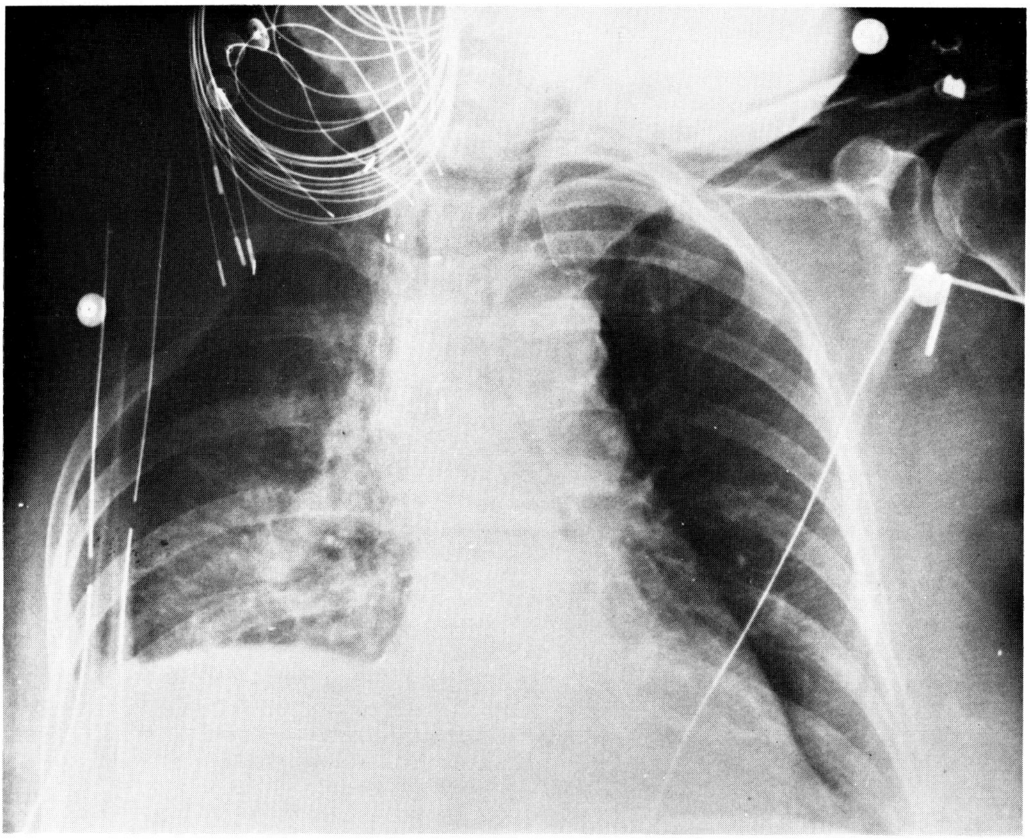

Figure 9-14. Ir-192 seeds were afterloaded through plastic tubes into tumor-bearing areas following resection of the right arm in continuity with the entire scapula, clavicle, and segment of the 1st, 2nd, 3rd, and 4th ribs for undifferentiated postirradiation sarcoma (see Fig. 9-13 and Appendix).

REFERENCES

References are listed in chronological order.

Burns, A.: Observation on the Surgical Anatomy of the Head and Neck. Edinburgh, Bryce, 1811.

Muller, J.: Jahresbericht uber die Fortschritte der anatomischphysiologischen Wissenschaften im Jahre 1835. 4. Pathologische Anatomie. Arch. Anat. Physiol. Med. 3:175, 1836.

King, A.: Case of chloroma. Monthly J. Med. Sci. 7:97, 1853.

Virchow, R.: Ueber Makroglossie und pathologische Neubildung quergerstreifter Muskelfasern. Arch. Path. Anat. Physiol. 7:126, 1854.

Turk, W.: Acute myeloide Leukamie mit Grunfarbung der Knochenmarks. Mitt. Geselbach Med. Kinderhk. 2:39, 1903.

Abrikossoff, A. L.: Uber Myome Ausgehend von der Guergstreiften Willkuslichen Muskulatur. Virchows Arch. [Pathol. Anat.] 260:215, 1926.

Diss, A.: Un nouveau type de tumeur musculaire; le rhabdomyome granulocellulaire. Bull. Assoc. Franc. Cancer 16:862, 1927.

Montpellier, J.: Les rhabdomyomes. Caracteres genereux et varietes anatomo-clinique. Bull. Assoc. Franc. Cancer 18:538, 1929.

Martland, H. S.: The occurrence of malignancy in radio-active persons; a general review of data gathered in the study of radium dial painters, with special reference to the occurrence of osteogenic sarcoma and the inter-relationship of certain blood diseases. Am. J. Cancer 15:2435, 1931.

Cellina, M.: I tumori mesenchimali del fegato. Arch. Ital. Anat. Istol. Patol. 3:609, 1932.

Klein, W.: Mesenchymoma. J. Med. Soc. N.J. 29:774, 1932.

Klemperer, P.: Myoblastoma of striated muscle. Am. J. Cancer 20:324, 1934.

Ewing, M. R., and Harrison, C. V.: Mesenchymoma. Br. J. Surg. 44:408, 1935.
Feyrter, F.: Ueber eine eigenartige Geschwulstform des Nervengewebes im menschlichen Verdauungsschlauch. Virch. Arch. [Pathol. Anat.] 295:480, 1935.
Lattes, R.: Mioblastoma and elementi granulosi della lingua. Arch. Sci. Med. 61:590, 1936.
Warren, S., and Sommer, G. N.: Fibrosarcoma of soft parts with special reference to recurrence and metastasis. Arch. Surg. 33:425, 1936.
Wilson, H., and Brunschwig, A.: Irradiation sarcoma. Surgery 2:607, 1937.
Leroux, R., and Delarue, J.: Sur trois cas de tumeurs a cellules granuleuses de la cavite buccale. Bull. Assoc. Franc. Cancer 28:427, 1939.
Tarr, L., and Ferris, H. W.: Multiple myeloma associated with nodular deposits of amyloid in the muscles and joints with Bence Jones proteinuria. Arch. Intern. Med. 64:820, 1939.
Hellwig, C. A.: Extramedullary plasma cell tumors as observed in various locations. Arch. Pathol. 36:95, 1942.
Gilmour, J. R.: A recurrent tumor of mesenchyme in an adult. J. Pathol. Bacteriol. 55:495, 1943.
Horn, R. C., and Stout, A. P.: Granular cell myoblastoma. Surg. Gynecol. Obstet. 76:315, 1943.
Gordon, J., and Walker, C.: Plasmacytoma of the lung. Arch. Pathol. 37:222, 1944.
Ravich, A., Stout, A. P., and Ravich, R. A.: Malignant granular cell myoblastoma involving the urinary bladder. Ann. Surg. 121:361, 1945.
Ackerman, L. V., and Phelps, C. R.: Malignant granular cell myoblastoma of the gluteal region. Surgery 20:511, 1946.
Haagensen, C. D., and Stout, A. P.: Granular cell myoblastoma of the mammary gland. Ann. Surg. 124:218, 1946.
Powell, E. B.: Granular cell myoblastoma. Arch. Pathol. 42:517, 1946.
Khanolkar, J. R.: Granular cell myoblastoma. Am. J. Pathol. 23:721, 1947.
Cahan, W. G., Woodward, H. Q., Higinbotham, N. L., Stewart, F. W., and Coley, B. L.: Sarcoma arising in irradiated bone: Report of eleven cases. Cancer 1:3, 1948.
Dunnington, J. H.: Granular cell myoblastoma of the orbit. Arch. Ophthalmol. 40:14, 1948.
Stewart, F. W., and Treves, N.: Lymphangiosarcoma in post-mastectomy lymphedema: A report of six cases in elephantiasis chirugica. Cancer 1:64, 1948.
Stout, A. P.: Mesenchymoma, the mixed tumor of mesenchymal derivatives. Ann. Surg. 127:278, 1948.
Ceelan, W.: Uber die Natur der sog. Myoblasten-myome. Zentralbl. Allg. Pathol. 85:289, 1949.
Fust, J. A., and Custer, R. P.: On the neurogenesis of so-called granular cell myoblastoma. Am. J. Clin. Pathol. 19:522, 1949.
Stout, A. P., and Kenney, F. R.: Primary plasma-cell tumors of the upper air passages and oral cavity. Cancer 2:261, 1949.
Duffy, B. J., and Fitzgerald, P. J.: Cancer of the thyroid in children. A report of 28 cases. J. Clin. Endocrinol. Metab. 10:1296, 1950.
Hyde, W. R., White, J. E., and Stout, A. P.: Mesenchymoma of the mesentery. Cancer 3:653, 1950.
Pearse, A. G. E.: The histogenesis of granular-cell myoblastoma (? granular-cell perineurial fibroblastoma). J. Pathol. Bacteriol. 62:351, 1950.
Huneman, M. W., and Lehman, M. L.: Mediastinal mesenchymoma masquerading as liposarcoma. Cancer 4:692, 1951.
Murray, M. R.: Cultural characteristics of three granular cell myoblastomas. Cancer 4:857, 1951.
Symmers, W. St. C., and Nangle, E. J.: An unusual recurring tumor formed of connective tissue of embryonic type, so-called mesenchymoma. J. Pathol. Bacteriol. 63:419, 1951.
Christopherson, W. M., Foote, F. W., and Stewart, F. W.: Alveolar soft part sarcomas; structurally characteristic tumors of uncertain histogenesis. Cancer 5:100, 1952.
Coggins, R. P.: Granular cell myoblastoma of common bile duct. Arch. Pathol. 54:398, 1952.
Ewing, M. R., and Foote, F. W.: Plasma cell tumors of the mouth and upper air passages. Cancer 5:499, 1952.
Ross, R. C., Miller, T. R., and Foote, F. W.: Malignant granular-cell myoblastoma. Cancer 5:112, 1952.
Crawford, E. S., and deBakey, M. E.: Granular cell myoblastoma. Two unusual cases. Cancer 6:786, 1953.
Pack, G. T., and Lisa, J. R.: Mesenchymoma. Surgery 35:277, 1954.
Pettit, V. D., Chamness, J. T., and Ackerman, L. V.: Fibromatosis and fibrosarcoma following irradiation therapy. Cancer 7:149, 1954.
Gamboa, L. G.: Malignant granular cell myoblastoma. Arch. Pathol. 60:663, 1955.
Ross, R. R.: Chloroma and chloroleukemia. Am. J. Med. 18:671, 1955.
Azzopardi, J. G.: Histogenesis of granular cell myoblastoma. J. Pathol. Bacteriol. 71:85, 1956.
Dolin, S., and Dewar, J. P.: Extramedullary plasmacytoma. Am. J. Pathol. 32:83, 1956.

Ewing, M. R., and Harrison, C. V.: Mesenchymoma. Br. J. Surg. 44:408, 1956.
Fisher, E. R.: Histochemical observations on an alveolar soft part sarcoma with reference to histogenesis. Am. J. Pathol. 32:721, 1956.
Masson, P.: Tumeurs humaines, histologie, diagnostics et techniques, 2nd ed. Paris, Libraire Maloine, 1956, p. 213.
Boquein, Y., Kerneis, J. P., Hervouet, D., and LeForestier, H. L.: Un cas de mesenchymome retroperitoneal. Arch. Mal. Appar. Dig. 46: suppl., 971, 1957.
Hamperl, H., and Lattes, R.: A study of the argyrophilia of nonchromaffin paragangliomas and granular cell myoblastoma. Cancer 10:408, 1957.
Busanny-Caspari, W., and Hammar, C. H.: Zur Malignitat der sogenanarten Myoblastenmyome. Z. Allg. Pathol. 98:401, 1958.
Meredith, J. M., Kay, S., and Bosher, L. H.: Case of granular cell myoblastoma (organoid type) involving arm, lung and brain, with twenty-years survival. J. Thorac. Surg. 35:80, 1958.
Svejda, J., and Horn, V.: A disseminated granular-cell pseudotumor; so-called metastasizing granular cell myoblastoma. J. Pathol. Bacteriol. 76:343, 1958.
Calnan, J., and Cowdell, R. H.: Lymphangioendothelioma of the anterior abdominal wall: Report of a case. Br. J. Surg. 375, 1959.
Schultz, Z., and Rosenthal, S.: Iron inactivation and myeloperoxidase. J. Biol. Chem. 234:2486, 1959.
Caby, F., Duperrat, B., and Ecochard, J. C.: Un cas de tumeur d'Abrikossoff a evolution maligne. Mem. Acad. Chir. 86:585, 1960.
Fassbender, H. C.: Das alveolare Myoblastensarkom der Skelett-muskulatur. Oncologia 13:184, 1960.
Hunter, D. T., and Dewar, J. P.: Malignant granular cell myoblastoma. Report of a case and review of literature. Am. Surg. 26:554, 1960.
Marshall, R. B., and Horn, R. C.: Nonchromaffin paraganglioma. Cancer 14:779, 1961.
Nash, A., and Stout, A. P.: Malignant mesenchymomas in children. Cancer 14:524, 1961.
Obiditsch-Mayer, I., and Salzer-Kuntschik, M.: Malignes gekorntzelliges Neurom sogenannartes Myoblastenmyom des Oesophagus. Beitr. Pathol. Anat. 125:357, 1961.
Rachmaninoff, N., McDonald, J. R., and Cook, J. C.: Sarcoma-like tumors of the skin following irradiation. Am. J. Clin. Pathol. 36:427, 1961.
Fisher, E. R., and Wechsler, H.: Granular cell myoblastoma—misnomer; electron microscopic and histochemical evidence concerning its Schwann cell derivation and nature (granular cell schwannoma). Cancer 15:936, 1962.
Haisken, W., and Langer, E.: Die submikroskopische structure des sog. Frankfurt. Z. Pathol. 71:600, 1962.
Kreig, A. F.: Malignant granular cell myoblastoma—A case report. Arch. Pathol. 74:251, 1962.
LeBer, M. S., and Stout, A. P.: Benign mesenchymomas in children. Cancer 15:598, 1962.
Legerlotz, C.: Strahleninduziertes malignes Haemangioblastom. Zentralbl. Allg. Pathol. 104:58, 1962.
Aboulker, P., Ronjeau, J., and Nebut, M.: Mesenchymome retroperitoneal. Arch. Anat. Pathol. 11:257, 1963.
Fruhling, L., and Chadli, A.: Le sarcome plasmocytaire extrasquelettigue. Ann. Anat. Pathol. 8:317, 1963.
Naib, M., and Goldstein, H. G.: Exfoliative cytology of a case of bronchial granular cell myoblastoma. Dis. Chest 42:645, 1963.
Wolfe, S. A., and Mackles, A.: Uncommon myogenic tumors of the female genital tract. Obstet. Gynecol. 22:199, 1963.
Helmus, C.: Extramedullary plasmacytoma of the head and neck. Laryngoscope 74:553, 1964.
Keshishian, J. M., and Alford, T. C.: Granular cell myoblastoma of the esophagus. Am. Surg. 30:263, 1964.
Shipkey, F. H., Lieberman, P. H., Foote, F. W., and Stewart, F. W.: Ultrastructure of alveolar soft part sarcoma. Cancer 17:821, 1964.
Boyer, C. W., and Navin, J. J.: Extraskeletal osteogenic sarcoma: A late complication of radiation therapy. Cancer 18:628, 1965.
Dharamadhack, A., Chatikavanij, K., and Pacharee, P.: Extramedullary plasmacytoma of the lung. Lancet 85:163, 1965.
Herskovic, T., Andersen, J. A., and Bayzd, E. D.: Intrathoracic plasmacytomas. Presentation of 21 cases and review of literature. Dis. Chest 47:1, 1965.
Lieberman, P., Foote, F. W., Stewart, F. W., and Berg, J. W.: Alveolar soft-part sarcoma. JAMA 198:1047, 1966.
March, K.: Zur Frage des Lymphangioendotheliomas. Arch. Klin. Exp. Dermatol. 226:318, 1966.
Nitze, H.: Das sogenannte Myoblastenmyom und seine maligne Verlaufsform. Z. Laryngol. Rhinol. Otol. 45:740, 1966.
Rappaport, H.: Atlas of Tumor Pathology. Sec. III Fascicle 8. Washington, D.C., Armed Forces Institute of Pathology, 1966.
Wanebo, C., Johnson, K., Sato, K., and Thorslung, T. W.: Breast cancer after expo-

sure to the atomic bombings of Hiroshima and Nagasaki. N. Engl. J. Med. 279:667, 1966.
Donohue, W. L., Jaffe, F. A., and Rewcastle, N. B.: Radiation-induced neurofibromata. Cancer 20:589, 1967.
Mackenzie, D. H.: Malignant granular cell myoblastoma. J. Clin. Pathol. 20:739, 1967.
Moscovic, E. A., and Azar, H. A.: Multiple granular cell tumors (Myoblastomas). Cancer 20:2032, 1967.
Papageorgiou, S., Litt, J. Z., and Pomeranz, J. R.: Multiple granular cell myoblastoma in children. Arch. Dermatol. 96:168, 1967.
Sears, W. P., Tofft, M., and Cohen, J.: Post-irradiation mesenchymal chondrosarcoma. Pediatrics 40:254, 1967.
Stout, A. P., and Lattes, R.: Tumors of the soft tissue. *In* Atlas of Tumor Pathology, 2nd series. Washington, D.C., Armed Forces Institute of Pathology, 1967.
Arkin, C. R., and Ward, L. R.: Multiple myeloma with amyloid in synovium. Postgrad. Med. 44:86, 1968.
Martinelli, C., and Rulli, M. A.: Primary plasmacytoma of soft tissue. Oral Surg. 25:607, 1968.
Schwartz, E. E., and Rothstein, J. D.: Fibrosarcoma following radiation therapy. JAMA 203:296–298, 1968.
Tefft, M., Vawter, G. F., and Mitus, A.: Second primary neoplasms in children. Am. J. Roentgenol. 103:800, 1968.
Weitzner, S., and Olsen, J. F.: Granular cell myoblastoma of the bronchus. Am. Rev. Resp. Dis. 97:923, 1968.
Furey, J. G., Barett, D. L., and Seibert, R. H.: Alveolar soft-part sarcoma. Report of a case presenting as a sacral bone tumor. J. Bone Joint Surg. 51A:185, 1969.
Gaston, E. A., Dollinger, M. R., Strong, E. W., and Hajdu, S. I.: Primary plasmacytoma of lymph nodes. Lymphology 2:7, 1969.
McCabe, M. M., and Harman, J. W.: Malignant myoblastoma. J. Ir. Med. Assoc. 62:284, 1969.
Pascoe, H. R., and Dorfman, R. F.: Extramedullary plasmacytoma of the submaxillary gland. Am. J. Clin. Pathol. 51:501, 1969.
Thomas, W. O., Harris, H. H., and Enden, J. A.: Postirradiation malignant neoplasm of the uterine fundus. Am. J. Obstet. Gynecol. 104:209, 1969.
Zaslow, L., and Staub, R. T.: Amyloidosis associated with an extramedullary plasmacytoma. South. Med. J. 62:443, 1969.
Gane, N. F. C., Lindup, R., Strikland, P., and Bennett, M. H.: Radiation induced fibrosarcoma. Br. J. Cancer 24:705, 1970.
Garancis, J. G., Komorowski, R. A., and Kuzman, J. F.: Granular cell myoblastoma. Cancer 25:542, 1970.
Hatfield, P. M., and Schultz, M. D.: Postirradiation sarcoma, including 5 cases after x-ray therapy of breast carcinoma. Radiology 96:593, 1970.
Oberman, H. A., and Oneal, R. M.: Fibrosarcoma of the chest wall following resection and irradiation of carcinoma of the breast. Am. J. Clin. Pathol. 53:407, 1970.
Paunier, J. P., and Candayis, G.: Sarcoma developing after radiotherapy. Radiol. Clin. Biol. 36:249, 1970.
Strong, E. W., McDivitt, R. W., and Brasfield, R. D.: Granular cell myoblastoma. Cancer 25:415, 1970.
Wiernik, P. H., and Serpick, A. A.: Granulocytic sarcoma (Chloroma). Blood 35:361, 1970.
Al-Sarraf, M., Loud, A. V., and Vaitkevicius, V. K.: Malignant granular cell tumor. Histochemical and electron microscopic study. Arch. Pathol. 91:550, 1971.
Christ, M. L., and Ozzello, L.: Myogenous origin of a granular cell tumor of the urinary bladder. Am. J. Clin. Pathol. 56:736, 1971.
Fisher, E. R., and Reidbord, H.: Electron microscopic evidence suggesting myogenous derivation of so-called alveolar soft-part sarcoma. Cancer 24:150, 1971.
Janower, M., and Niettinen, O.: Neoplasms after childhood irradiation of the thymus gland. JAMA 213:753, 1971.
Kuchemann, K.: Malignes granulases Neurom (Granularzellmyoblastom). Zentralbl. Allg. Pathol. 114:426, 1971.
Sharma, T. C., Huvos, A. G., and Grabstald, H.: Retroperitoneal malignant mesenchymoma. J. Urol. 106:60, 1971.
Nielsen, S. M., Shenken, J. R., and Cawley, L. P.: Primary colonic plasmacytoma. Cancer 30:261, 1972.
Bahadori, M., and Liebow, A. A.: Plasma cell granulomas of the lung. Cancer 31:191, 1973.
Castro, E. B., Lewis, J. S., and Strong, E. W.: Plasmacytoma of paranasal sinuses and nasal cavity. Arch. Otolaryngol. 97:326, 1973.
Magori, A., and Szegvari, M.: Rezidivierender und metastasierender Abrikossoff tumor der vulva. Zentralbl. Allg. Pathol. 117:265, 1973.
Mason, T. E., Dmare, R. S., and Margolis, C. I.: Granulocytic sarcoma (chloroma), two years preceding myelogenous leukemia. Cancer 31:423, 1973.
McSwain, B., Whitehead, W., and Bennett, L.: Angiosarcoma. South. Med. J. 66:102, 1973.
Muss, H. B., and Moloney, W. C.: Chloroma and other myoblastic tumors. Blood 42:721, 1973.
Sussman, E. B., Hajdu, S. I., and Gray, G. F.: Granular cell myoblastoma of the breast. Am. J. Surg. 126:669, 1973.

Cadotte, M.: Malignant granular cell myoblastoma. Cancer 33:1417, 1974.

Haustein, U. F.: Malignes metastasierendes Granularzellmyoblastom Abrikosow mit symptomatischez Dermatomyositis. Dermatol. Monatsschr. 160:318, 1974.

Madhavan, M., Aurora, A. L., and Sen, S. B.: Malignant granular cell myoblastoma—report of a case. Indian J. Cancer 11:360, 1974.

Modan, B., Mart, H. I., Baidatz, D., and Steinitz, R.: Radiation induced head and neck tumors. Lancet 1:277, 1974.

Sobel, H. J., and Marquet, E.: Granular cells and granular cell lesions. *In* Pathology Annual. Edited by S. C. Sommers. New York, Appleton-Century-Crofts, 1974.

Bisbee, A. C., and Thoeny, R. H.: Malignant lymphoma of the thyroid following irradiation. Cancer 35:1296, 1975.

Hasson, J., Hartman, K. S., Milikow, E., and Mittelman, J. A.: The Thorotrast-induced extraskeletal osteosarcoma of the cervical region. Report of a case. Cancer 36:1827, 1975.

Meadows, A. T., D'Angio, G. J., Evans, A. E., Harris, C. C., Miller, R. W., and Mike, V.: Oncogenesis and other late effects of cancer treatment in children. Radiology 114:175, 1975.

Buell, R., Wang, N. S., Seemayer, T. A., and Ahmed, M. N.: Endobronchial plasma cell granuloma (xanthoma pseudotumor). A light and electron microscopic study. Hum. Pathol. 7:411, 1976.

Hajdu, S. I., Espinosa, M. H., and Robbins, G. F.: Recurrent cystosarcoma phyllodes: a clinicopathologic study of 32 cases. Cancer 38:1402, 1976.

Hajdu, S. I., and Hajdu, E. O.: Cytopathology of Sarcomas and Other Nonepithelial Malignant Tumors. Philadelphia, W. B. Saunders Company, 1976.

Harris, C.: The carcinogenicity of anticancer drugs: A hazard in man. Cancer 37:1014, 1976.

Paik, H. H., and Komorowski, A.: Hemangiosarcoma of the abdominal wall following irradiation therapy of endometrial carcinoma. Am J. Clin. Pathol. 66:810, 1976.

Penn, I.: Second malignant neoplasms associated with immunosuppressive medications. Cancer 37:1024, 1976.

Wiltshaw, E.: The natural history of extramedullary plasmacytoma and its relation to solitary myeloma of bone and myelomatosis. Medicine 55:217, 1976.

Adam, Y. G., and Reif, R. R.: Radiation induced fibrosarcoma following treatment of breast cancer. Surgery 81:421, 1977.

Archer, V. E.: Occupational exposure to radiation as a cancer hazard. Cancer 39:1802, 1977.

Baroni, C. D., Mineo, T. C., Ricci, C., Guarino, S., and Mandelli, F.: Solitary secretory plasmacytoma of the lung in a 14 year old boy. Cancer 40:2329, 1977.

Curtin, C. T.: McHeffy, B., and Kolarsick, A. J.: Thyroid and breast cancer following childhood radiation. Cancer 40:2911, 1977.

Usui, M., Ishii, S., Yamawaki, S., Sasaki, T., Minami, A., and Hizawa, K.: Malignant granular cell tumor of the radial nerve. Cancer 39:1547, 1977.

Cavdar, A. O., Arcasoy, A., Babacan, E., Gozdasoglu, S., Topuz, U., and Fraumeni, J. F.: Ocular granulocytic sarcoma (chloroma) with acute myelomonocytic leukemia in Turkish children. Cancer 41:1606, 1978.

Doss, L. L.: Simultaneous extramedullary plasmacytomas of the vagina and vulva. Cancer 41:2468, 1978.

Meyer, M. W., Powell, H. C., Wagner, M., and Niwayama, G.: Thorotrast induced adhesive arachnoiditis associated with meningioma and schwannoma. Hum. Pathol. 9:366, 1978.

Uehara, H.: Cytology of alveolar soft part sarcoma. Acta Cytol. 22:191, 1978.

Udoji, W. C., and Frigy, A. F.: Cytoplasmic fibrils in plasma cells of a solitary myeloma. Am. J. Clin. Pathol. 70:836, 1978.

Valenstein, S. L., and Thurer, R. J.: Granular cell myoblastoma of the bronchus. Case report and literature review. J. Thorac. Cardiovasc. Surg. 76:465, 1978.

Ekfors, T. O., Kalimo, H., Rantakokko, V., Latvala, M., and Parvinen, M.: Alveolar soft part sarcoma. A report of two cases with some histochemical and ultrastructural observations. Cancer 43:1672, 1979.

Urano, M., Koike, S., and O'Hara, K.: Secondary malignant neoplasms following radiotherapy of a mouse mammary carcinoma. Cancer 43:151, 1979.

appendix A

Recent Trends in Treatment of Soft Tissue Sarcomas

MAN H. SHIU, M.D.
Assistant Attending Surgeon
GORDON B. MAGILL, M.D.
Associate Attending, Solid Tumor Service
SEYMOUR HOPFAN, M.D.
Assistant Attending Radiation Therapist
Memorial Sloan-Kettering Cancer Center
New York, New York

The therapeutic approach to soft tissue sarcomas has changed considerably during the last 10 years, but debate over the most effective treatment of local and metastatic tumors continues in the literature. As in the past, surgical treatment is considered by most authorities as the main form of therapy for primary soft tissue tumors.

EXCISION

During the early decades of this century *simple excision* or enucleation was the usual method of treating a soft tissue sarcoma. The literature is replete with accounts of rapid recurrences of tumor at the site of excision following such treatment. As pathologists pointed out that this neoplasm possessed a false capsule and that tumor cells were present not only in this capsule but also outside its confines, surgeons began to carry out *wide excisions*. Despite this change, disconcertingly high local recurrence rates from 30% to over 60% continued to be reported from various centers (Fine et al, 1973). Disillusioned with such results, many surgeons turned to amputation as the primary treatment of all soft part sarcomas arising in an extremity.

MONOBLOC SOFT PART RESECTION

Cognizant of the infiltrative nature of soft tissue sarcomas and their usual origin and spread within musculofascial structures, Bowden and Booher described in 1958 the technique of *monobloc soft part resection* for sarcomas of soft somatic tissues. This technique is eminently suitable for the majority of tumors in the fleshy parts of the trunk and extremity and has since been adopted by most surgeons experienced in the management of these neoplasms. The risk of spilling or leaving behind tumor cells can be substantially minimized by dissecting at a distance and maintaining an intact barrier of one or more musculofascial layers enveloping gross or suspected tumor tissue. In a series of 75 previously untreated sarcomas of the thigh treated by such monobloc resection at Memorial Sloan-

Kettering Cancer Center, tumors recurred locally in only 11 patients, a recurrence rate of 15% (Shiu et al, 1975).

Sarcomas in the distal non-fleshy parts of an extremity and those approximate to major neurovascular structures, bones, or joints pose special anatomic problems which militate against the proper execution of a monobloc resection. With such tumors it is often difficult to obtain a wide margin of resection with one or more tissue barriers. In the series of lower extremity sarcomas referred to previously, most of the recurrences developed after resecting tumor close to either the femoral vessels in the groin or the popliteal neurovascular bundle adjacent to the knee. Tumors can recur locally in such anatomic settings even though microscopic examination of the resection margins fails to demonstrate tumor.

Sarcomas recurring at the site of previous resection may be the result of iatrogenesis. Viable tumor may have been implanted in multiple fascial layers that were traversed during dissection in the skin incision, as well as in drain tracks. High local recurrence rates can be expected in these circumstances. For tumors recurring after previous attempts at resection, the recurrence rate was as high as 44% in 158 cases treated by radical monobloc resection, despite every effort to obtain wide margins and to reexcise the previous scars and drain tracks.

AMPUTATION

Because of the high risk of local recurrence *amputation* is an obvious alternative for treatment of sarcomas of an extremity. For many years, amputation has also been regarded as absolutely indicated for sarcomas directly involving major blood vessel, nerve, bone, or joint. Recurrence in the amputation stump should be rare if the surgeon chooses a sufficiently high level of amputation or exarticulation and remembers that any muscle or aponeurotic structure contiguous with the area of sarcoma may harbor microscopic nests of tumor. This precaution usually requires exarticulation at a level of one joint or more proximal to the neoplasm. There were 10 stump recurrences in 139 exarticulative and amputative procedures in one series of lower extremity sarcomas, mostly in instances where hemipelvectomy should have been performed instead of hip-joint disarticulation or thigh amputation for tumors of the inguinal or thigh regions. Despite the low risk of local recurrence, treatment by amputation does not offer any significant improvement in survival, for the prognosis of patients with sarcoma is mainly governed by the size, site, and histologic grade of the neoplasm which is expressed in stages, see Chapter 1, Fig. 1-59 and Table 1-15 (Shiu et al, 1975; Russell et al, 1977).

REGIONAL LYMPH NODE RESECTION

The question of *regional lymph node dissection* is often raised in the management of soft tissue sarcoma, particularly with tendosynovial and embryonal rhabdomyosarcomas which sometimes develop metastases in regional lymph nodes. Prophylactic lymphadenectomy has not been found to have any therapeutic value (Shiu et al, 1979; Weingard and Rosenberg, 1978; Hajdu et al, 1979). If a biopsy of a grossly enlarged lymph node shows metastases, the node should be extirpated, preferably en bloc with the primary sarcoma. Unfortunately, lymphatic metastasis usually signals advanced uncontrollable disease, so that patients are seldom salvaged by lymphadenectomy, even though its palliative value must be recognized.

FUNCTION-SAVING METHODS

The high recurrence rate of certain tumors of the extremities and the failure of amputative procedures to offer improved survival rates have prompted the development of innovative function-saving methods of treatment, all aimed at reducing the risk of local recurrence with maximal conservation of limb function. Extending the scope of soft part resection can often avert the need for amputation. Thus, involvement of a major blood vessel is no longer an absolute indication for amputation, for the affected segment of vessel can be resected en bloc with the neoplasm. Resection is followed by appropriate vascular reconstruction. Simultaneous excision of the femoral artery and vein, with grafting of both vessels, has been carried out successfully at the time of monobloc muscle group resection for sarcoma, resulting in excellent limb function and prolonged survival. Portions of bone, joint, or major nerve can also be resected as necessary with the sarcoma, as long as reasonable function can be restored by means of reconstructive, prosthetic, or other rehabilitative measures. Eilber et al (1979) reported that it is technically possible to resect the hemipelvis and maintain a viable extremity. The addition of these techniques where indicated to the standard monobloc resection of sarcoma improves the monobloc method of dissection, because intact fascial barriers remain with the neoplasm to be extirpated. Such techniques should not increase the risk of local recurrence if properly applied and therefore deserve increased application by surgical teams skilled in these procedures (Fortner et al, 1977).

Whenever possible, function-saving monobloc muscle group or soft part resections should be performed. With deeply infiltrative sarcomas, when major neurovascular or skeletal structures have been invaded to such an extent that their simultaneous excision would preclude successful reconstruction or rehabilitation, extirpation by *high exarticulation* should be regarded as a wise decision. Attempts to dissect out these sarcomas would usually either violate or spill tumor and leave behind fragments of microscopic or macroscopic disease. Local recurrence is a certainty if adjunctive radiation therapy or regional chemotherapy fails.

ADJUNCTS TO SURGICAL PROCEDURES

High-dose postoperative radiation therapy to the tumor-bearing field is an adjunctive method of treatment that may be applied when the risk of local tumor recurrence is high. Because considerable evidence has been adduced in recent years to support the belief that minute deposits of soft tissue sarcomas can be controlled by high radiation doses, Suit et al (1973), Lindberg (1976), and others have advocated simple limited excision of sarcomas followed by radiation therapy.

Similarly, *isolation-perfusion chemotherapy* or the delivery of *intra-arterial infusion chemotherapy* to the extremity bearing a sarcoma has been used before or after surgical excision, in the belief that the need for amputation can be obviated and the frequency of local recurrence can be diminished (McBride, 1974).

Historically soft tissue sarcomas usually are referred to as radioresistant; however, it has been shown recently that some soft tissue sarcomas are radioresponsive (Suit et al, 1973; Lindberg, 1976). McNeer et al (1968) concluded that *preoperative irradiation* followed by surgical excision is the preferred method of treatment for sarcomas of the soft parts. They advised a dose of 4,000 rads for four weeks before operation. The clinical response of 42 of 58 of patients (72%) treated preoperatively was good and the tumor was completely destroyed in 33% of the patients so treated.

Radiotherapy has an important role in the primary management of soft tissue sarcomas. Despite innovations in technique and equipment, local recurrences are encountered after seemingly adequate resection and radiation. Questions about optimal timing of radiotherapy in relation to surgery and chemotherapy, methods of dosage fractionation, and sensitivity of individual tissue types remain to be answered. At Memorial Hospital, we are investigating the use of high-dose irradiation of the tumor bed by immediate postoperative application of radioactive seeds. From 1975 to 1976, we treated 16 patients in this relatively unique fashion. After the usual wide excision of the primary tumor had been carried out, e.g., muscle group excision, the tumor bed was implanted with plastic tubes at the time of excision or reexcision of the tumor. The ends of these geometrically placed tubes came out through normal skin and were *after-loaded with Ir-192*. In each case 6,000 rads were delivered to a plane of tissue 0.5 cm from the plane of the iridium (see Fig. 9-14). Four weeks later, 4,000 rads of external irradiation, or the biologic equivalent, was applied to a wide field, including the implanted area.

This modality of treatment to deliver a high dose of irradiation to restricted volumes of tissue is felt to diminish the chance of local recurrence, make amputation unnecessary, and improve survival. Preliminary data are being evaluated and are encouraging.

The medical management of soft part sarcomas was generally disappointing prior to the advent of adriamycin (Edland, 1967; Cupps et al, 1969). Since the advent of this agent soft part sarcomas have fallen into the category of moderately responsive solid tumors (Gottlieb et al, 1972; Jaffe et al, 1973; Haskell et al, 1974; Tan et al, 1975; Magill et al, 1977). During the past 5 years various combinations of chemotherapy using adriamycin as one of the main drugs, with and without immunotherapy, have been under study at Memorial Sloan-Kettering Cancer Center (Table A-1). The preliminary results are promising and we are beginning to see some pattern of responses that may help us in future protocols. For example, liposarcomas, embryonal rhabdomyosarcoma, and apparently fibrosarcomas appear to respond more consistently than malignant schwannomas and malignant fibrous histiocytomas.

In terms of the relative efficacy of various agents, certainly adriamycin is number one for the soft part sarcomas in general. Because of the limitations of dosage relating to cardiac toxicity, as well as to the development of resistant tumor clones, other agents are needed with adriamycin. The relative roles of cyclophosphamide (Cytoxan), dimethyl triazenoimidazole carboxamide (DTIC), high dose methotrexate, and the nitrosoureas are still not clear.

TABLE A-1. ***Chemotherapy of Soft Tissue Sarcomas***

	MAV*			OMAD†			ALOMAD‡ (S-4)			CYOMAD§ (S-7)			TOTAL		
	#A	RESP	%	#A	RESP	%	#A	RESP	%	#A	RESP	%	#A	RESP	%
Malignant fibrous histiocytoma	–	–	–	–	–	–	2	0	0	–	–	–	2	0	0
Fibrosarcoma	1	0	–	5	2	40	1	1	100	3	1	33	10	4	40
Tendosynovial sarcoma	1	1	100	7	2	29	5	1	20	3	2	67	16	6	37
Liposarcoma	3	2	66	7	4	57	7	3	43	3	1	33	20	10	50
Rhabdomyosarcoma	6	2	33	3	2	66	2	1	50	–	–	–	11	5	45
Leiomyosarcoma	11	5	45	10	4	40	16	5	31	16	3	19	53	17	32
Hemangiosarcoma	–	–	–	–	–	–	2	0	0	1	0	0	3	0	0
Hemangiopericytoma	–	–	–	–	–	–	2	1	50	2	0	0	4	1	25
Malignant schwannoma	–	–	–	1	0	0	3	1	33	–	–	–	4	1	25
Alveolar soft part sarcoma	–	–	–	–	–	–	1	0	0	1	0	0	2	0	0

*MAV = MeCCNU, adriamycin, and vincristine.
†OMAD = vincristine, methotrexate, adriamycin, and actinomycin D.
‡ALOMAD = OMAD plus DTIC and chlorambucil.
§CYOMAD = vincristine, methotrexate, adriamycin, DTIC, and cyclophosphamide.

Immunotherapy in the form of MBV (mixed bacterial vaccines) has also been under study, but to date no significant benefit has been demonstrated. Among the new chemotherapeutic agents that have been given limited trials, neither PZF (Pyrazofurin) nor DVA (Vindesine) have demonstrated useful effects.

Postoperative adjuvant therapy in certain soft part sarcomas has been undergoing evaluation for the past several years with the S-4 protocol (ALOMAD). According to this protocol, a six-drug combination is used: *day one,* vincristine and methotrexate; *day two,* DTIC and adriamycin followed by leukovorin rescue; *days 15 to 29 and 57 to 71,* chlorambucil; *days 22 and 64,* actinomycin; and *day 43,* adriamycin. As noted in Table A-1 it appears to have been of some benefit. It is too early to say whether this is merely a temporary benefit or whether there may be some actual permanent gain, but preliminary results suggest that adjuvant chemotherapy is useful at least in prolonging the disease-free interval after operation (Sordillo et al, 1979).

Although preliminary results of adjuvant techniques appear promising, long-term experience in a large number of patients is still awaited. The unpredictable sensitivity of a given soft tissue sarcoma to radiation therapy or chemotherapy must remain worrisome to those who utilize these adjunctive modalities, particularly when standard methods of monobloc wide resection are not used to extirpate the neoplasm.

Until the efficacy and limitations of these and other adjunctive methods are fully defined by further clinical trial, proper surgical extirpation of soft tissue neoplasms according to established tenets of cancer surgery would seem to be the most appropriate choice of therapy.

Clinicians must strive to offer a patient with primary or locally recurrent sarcoma the most anatomically adequate en bloc resection consistent with functional preservation, and to apply the most effective method of adjunctive local therapy when the risk of local recurrence is high. Ablation of clinically occult distant micrometastases is becoming a clinical reality, and postoperative systemic chemotherapy should prove to be an important part of the treatment process for sarcomas with high metastatic potential. Resection of pulmonary metastases also has proven therapeutic merit and must be considered in suitable patients. It is hoped that with improvements in the components of such multimodal therapy in the future the devastating frequency of local recurrence and distant metastases currently experienced will be minimized.

SELECTED REFERENCES ON THERAPY

References are listed in chronological order.

Bowden, L., and Booher, R. J.: The principles and techniques of resection of soft parts for sarcoma. Surgery 44:963, 1958.

Perry, H., and Chu, F.: Radiation therapy in the palliative management of soft tissue sarcomas. Cancer 15:179, 1962.

Edland, R. W.: Embryonal rhabdomyosarcoma. Five-year survival of a patient treated by radiation and chemotherapy. Am. J. Roentgenol. 99:400, 1967.

Cantin, J., McNeer, G. P., Chu, F., and Booher, R. J.: The pattern of local recurrence after treatment of soft tissue sarcoma. Ann. Surg. 168:47, 1968.

Das Gupta, T. K., Hajdu, S. I., and Foote, F. W.: Extraosseous osteogenic sarcoma. Ann. Surg. 168:1011, 1968.

McNeer, G. P., Cantin, J., Chu, F., and Nickson, J. J.: Effectiveness of radiation therapy in the management of sarcoma of the soft somatic tissues. Cancer 22:391, 1968.

Cupps, R. E., Ahmann, D. C., and Soule, E. H.: Treatment of pulmonary metastatic disease with radiation therapy and adjuvant actinomycin D. Cancer 24:719, 1969.

Das Gupta, T. K., Brasfield, R. D., Strong, E. W., and Hajdu, S. I.: Benign solitary schwannomas. Cancer 24:355, 1969.

Spittle, M. F., Newton, K. A., and Mackenzie, D. H.: Liposarcoma. A review of 60 cases. Br. J. Cancer 24:696, 1970.

Salvador, A. H., Beabout, J. W., and Dahlin, D. C.: Mesenchymal chondrosarcoma—observations on 30 new cases. Cancer 28:605, 1971.

Feldman, P. S., and Kyriakos, M.: Pulmonary resection for metastatic sarcoma. J. Thorac. Cardiovasc. Surg. 64:784, 1972.
Gottlieb, J. A., Baker, L. H., Quagliana, J. M., Luce, J. K., Whitecar, J. P., Sinkovics, J. G., Rivkin, S. E., Brownlee, R., and Frei, E.: Chemotherapy of sarcomas with a combination of adriamycin and dimethyl triazeno imidazole carboxamide. Cancer 30:1632, 1972.
Castro, E. B., Hajdu, S. I., and Fortner, J. G.: Surgical therapy of fibrosarcoma of extremities. Arch. Surg. 107:284, 1973.
Fine, G., Ohorodnik, J. M., and Horn, R. C., Jr.: Soft tissue sarcomas: Their clinical behavior and course and influencing factors. *In* Seventh National Cancer Conference Proceedings. Philadelphia, J. B. Lippincott Co., 1973, pp. 873–882.
Jaffe, N., Filler, R. M., Farber, S., Traggis, D. G., Vawter, G. F., Tefft, M., and Murray, J. E.: Rhabdomyosarcoma in children. Improved outlook with multidisciplinary approach. Am. J. Surg. 125:482, 1973.
Kinne, D. W., Chu, F. C. H., Huvos, A. G., Yagoda, A., and Fortner, J. G.: Treatment of primary and recurrent retroperitoneal liposarcoma. Cancer 31:53, 1973.
Suit, H. D., Russell, W. O., and Martin, R. G.: Management of patients with sarcoma of soft tissue in an extremity. Cancer 31:1247, 1973.
Wanebo, H. J., Shah, J., Knapper, W., Hajdu, S. I., and Booher, R.: Reappraisal of surgical management of sarcoma of the buttock. Cancer 31:97, 1973.
Haskell, C. M., Silverstein, M. J., Rangell, D. M., Hunt, J. S., Sparks, F. C., and Morton, D. L.: Multimodality cancer therapy in man: A pilot study of adriamycin by arterial infusion. Cancer 33:1485, 1974.
Lee, S. M., Hajdu, S. I., and Exelby, P. R.: Synovial sarcoma in children. Surg. Gynecol. Obstet. 138:701, 1974.
Martini, N., Bains, M. S., Huvos, A. G., and Beattie, E. J.: Surgical treatment of metastatic sarcoma to the lung. Surg. Clin. North Am. 54:841, 1974.
McBride, C. M.: Sarcoma of the limbs: Results of adjuvant chemotherapy using isolation perfusion. Arch. Surg. 109:304, 1974.
McMaster, M. J., Soule, E. H., and Ivins, J. C.: Hemangiopericytoma. A clinicopathologic study and long-term follow-up of 60 patients. Cancer 36:2232, 1975.
Shiu, M. H., Castro, E. B., Hajdu, S. I., and Fortner, J. G.: Surgical treatment of 297 soft tissue sarcomas of the lower extremity. Ann. Surg. 182:597, 1975.
Shiu, M. H., Chu, F., Castro, E. B., Hajdu, S. I., and Fortner, J. G.: The results of surgical and radiation therapy in the treatment of liposarcoma arising in the extremity. Am. J. Roentgenol. 123:577, 1975.
Tan, C., Rosen, G., Ghavimi, F., Haghbin, M., Helson, L., Wollner, N., and Murphy, M. L.: Adriamycin in pediatric malignancies. Cancer Chemotherap. Rep. 6:259, 1975.
Lindberg, R. D.: Soft tissue sarcoma. Curr. Probl. Cancer 1:4, 1976.
Morton, D. L., Eilber, F. R., Towsend, C. M., Grant, T. T., Mirra, J., and Weisenburger, T. H.: Limb salvage from a multidisciplinary treatment approach for skeletal and soft tissue sarcomas of the extremity. Ann. Surg. 184:268, 1976.
Fortner, J. G., Kim, D. K., and Shiu, M. H.: Limb-preserving vascular surgery for malignant tumors of the lower extremity. Arch. Surg. 112:391, 1977.
Hajdu, S. I., Shiu, M. H., and Fortner, J. G.: Tendosynovial sarcoma. A clinicopathological study of 136 cases. Cancer 39:1201, 1977.
Magill, G. B., Golbey, R. B., and Krakoff, I. H.: Chemotherapy combinations in adult sarcomas. Proc. Am. Soc. Clin. Oncol. 18:264, 1977.
Russell, W. O., Cohen, J., Enzinger, F., Hajdu, S. I., Heise, H., Martin, R. G., Meissner, W., Miller, W. T., Schmitz, R. L., and Suit, H. D.: A clinical and pathological staging system for soft tissue sarcomas. Cancer 40:1562, 1977.
Weingard, D. N., and Rosenberg, S. A.: Early lymphatic spread of osteogenic and soft tissue sarcomas. Surgery 84:231, 1978.
Wong, P. P., and Yagoda, A.: Chemotherapy of malignant hemangiopericytoma. Cancer 41:1256, 1978.
Eilber, F. R., Grant, T. T., Sakai, D., and Morton, D. L.: Internal hemipelvectomy. Excision of the hemipelvis with limb preservation. Cancer 43:806, 1979.
Shiu, M. H., McCormack, P. M., Hajdu, S. I., and Fortner, J. G.: Surgical treatment of tendosynovial sarcoma. Cancer 43:889, 1979.
Hajdu, S. I., Erlandson, R. A., and Fortner, J. G.: Histologic classification of liposarcomas (in press).
Sordillo, P., Magill, G. B., Howard, J., and Golbey, R. B.: Adjuvant chemotherapy in adult soft part sarcomas with "ALOMAD" (in press).

appendix B

Differential Diagnosis of Soft Tissue Tumors

	TABLE
Age and Sex Prevalence	B-1, B-2, B-3, B-4, B-5
Size	B-6
Site	B-7, Figures B-1 and B-2; B-8, B-9, B-10
Histologic Morphology	B-11, B-12, B-13, B-14, B-15, B-16
Special Stains	B-17
Ultrastructure	B-18
Computerized Differential Diagnosis	B-19
Autopsy Findings	B-20, B-21, B-22, B-23
References	

TABLE B-1. *Average Age and Sex Prevalance of Patients with Benign Soft Tissue Tumors*

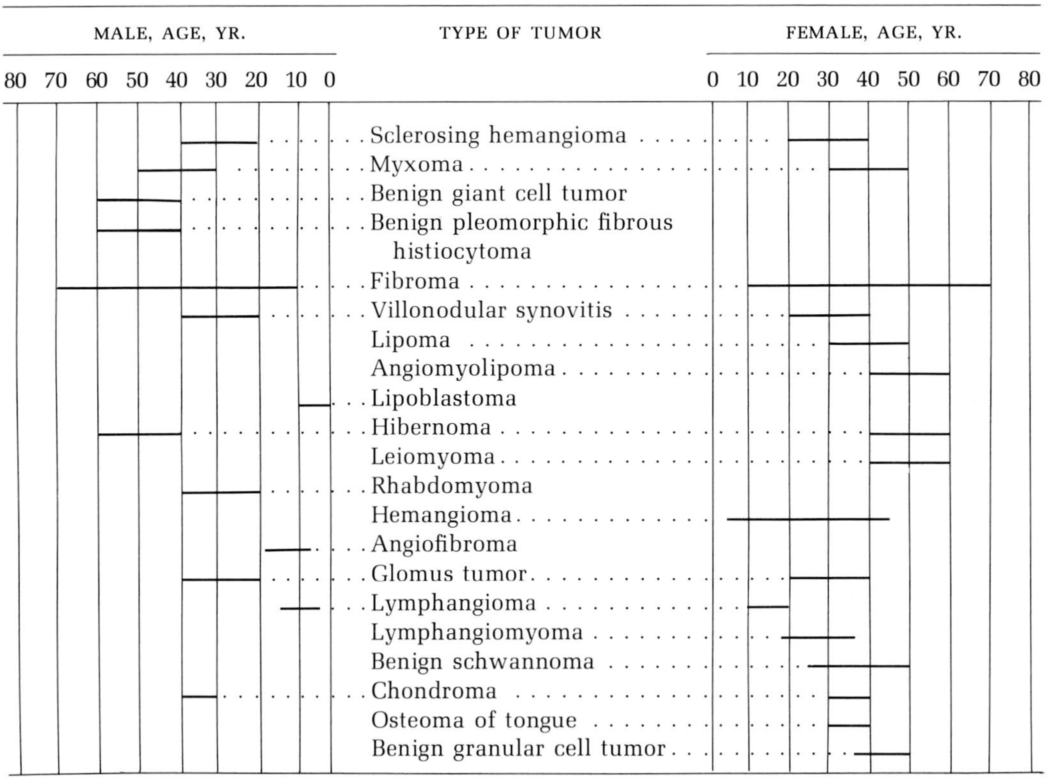

TABLE B-2. *Average Age and Sex Prevalance of Patients with Malignant Soft Tissue Tumors*

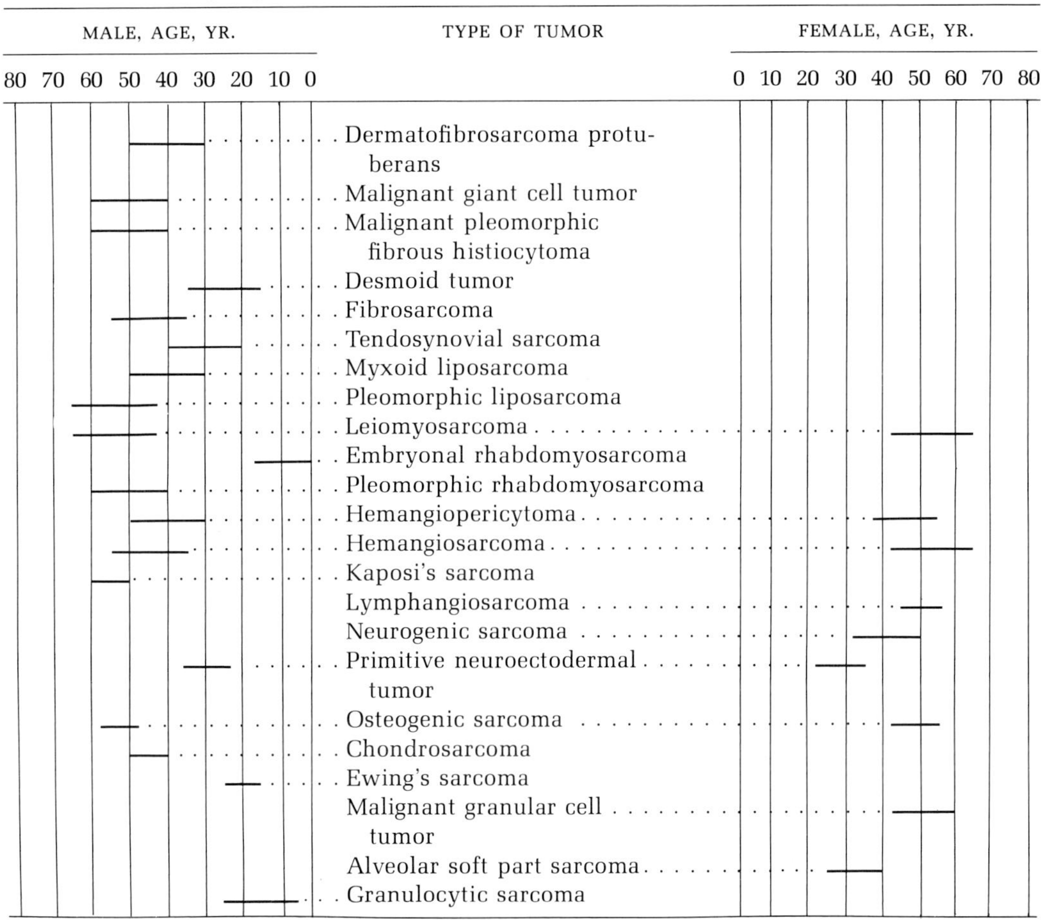

TABLE B-3. *The Most Common Primary Soft Tissue Tumors*

BENIGN	AGE	MALIGNANT
Lipoblastoma Angiofibroma Hemangioma Lymphangioma	0–20	Embryonal rhabdomyosarcoma Ewing's sarcoma
Sclerosing hemangioma Fibroma Villonodular synovitis Rhabdomyoma Hemangioma Glomus tumor Lymphangiomyoma Benign schwannoma	20–40	Desmoid tumor Tendosynovial sarcoma Primitive neuroectodermal tumor Alveolar soft part sarcoma
Myxoma Benign giant cell tumor Benign pleomorphic fibrous histiocytoma Fibroma Lipoma Angiomyolipoma Hibernoma Leiomyoma Benign granular cell tumor	40–60	Malignant fibrous histiocytoma Fibrosarcoma Liposarcoma Leiomyosarcoma Pleomorphic rhabdomyosarcoma Hemangiopericytoma Hemangiosarcoma Kaposi's sarcoma Lymphangiosarcoma Neurogenic sarcoma Osteogenic sarcoma Chondrosarcoma Malignant granular cell tumor

TABLE B-4. *Sex Prevalance of Benign Soft Tissue Tumors*

MALE	FEMALE
Benign giant cell tumor	Lipoma
Benign pleomorphic fibrous histiocytoma	Angiomyolipoma
Lipoblastoma	Leiomyoma
Rhabdomyoma	Hemangioma
Angiofibroma	Lymphangiomyoma
	Benign schwannoma
	Osteoma of tongue
	Benign granular cell tumor

TABLE B-5. *Sex Prevalance of Malignant Soft Tissue Tumors*

MALE	FEMALE
Malignant fibrous histiocytoma	Lymphangiosarcoma
Fibrosarcoma	Neurogenic sarcoma
Tendosynovial sarcoma	Malignant granular cell tumor
Liposarcoma	Alveolar soft part sarcoma
Rhabdomyosarcoma	
Kaposi's sarcoma	
Osteogenic sarcoma	
Chondrosarcoma	

TABLE B-6. *Size of Soft Tissue Sarcomas**

USUALLY SMALL (LESS THAN 5 cm)	USUALLY BULKY (MORE THAN 10 cm)
Epithelioid sarcoma	Dermatofibrosarcoma protuberans
Clear cell sarcoma	Malignant giant cell tumor
Chordoid sarcoma	Desmoid tumor
Hemangiosarcoma	Liposarcoma
Kaposi's sarcoma	Pleomorphic rhabdomyosarcoma
Lymphangiosarcoma	Primitive neuroectodermal tumor

*See also Chapter 1, Figure 1-59 and Table 1-15.

TABLE B-7. *The Most Common Sites of Benign Soft Tissue Tumors*

	HEAD & NECK	EXTREMITIES		TRUNK
		UPPER	LOWER	
Sclerosing hemangioma	+	++		
Myxoma		+	++	
Benign giant cell tumor		++	+	
Benign pleomorphic fibrous histiocytoma	+	++[1]		
Fibroma		++		+
Lipoma		+		++
Lipoblastoma			+	++
Hibernoma	+			++[2]
Rhabdomyoma	++			+
Angiofibroma	++			+
Glomus tumor		++[3]	+[3]	
Lymphangioma	++	+	+	
Chondroma		++[3]	+[3]	
Benign schwannoma	+			++
Benign granular cell tumor	++			+

+ = common; ++ = most common.
[1]Shoulder.
[2]Back.
[3]Fingers or toes.

TABLE B-8. *The Most Common Sites of Malignant Soft Tissue Tumors*

	HEAD & NECK	EXTREMITIES UPPER	LOWER	TRUNK
Dermatofibrosarcoma protuberans		+[1]		++
Malignant giant cell tumor		+[1]	++[2]	
Malignant pleomorphic fibrous histiocytoma		+[1]	++[2]	
Desmoid tumor	+	++[3]	++[3]	+
Fibrosarcoma		+[3]	++[3]	
Tendosynovial sarcoma		+	++	
Liposarcoma		+	++[4]	
Embryonal rhabdomyosarcoma	+		++	
Pleomorphic rhabdomyosarcoma		+	++[4]	
Hemangiosarcoma	+			++
Kaposi's sarcoma		+[5]	++[5]	
Hemangiopericytoma			++	+
Lymphangiosarcoma	+	++		
Osteogenic sarcoma		+	++	
Chondrosarcoma		+	++	
Ewing's sarcoma			++[4]	+
Malignant granular cell tumor	+		++	+
Alveolar soft part sarcoma		+	++[4]	

+ = common; ++ = most common.
[1]Shoulder.
[2]Buttock.
[3]Proximal part.
[4]Thigh.
[5]Distal part.

TABLE B-9. *The Most Common Superficial Tumors**

- Sclerosing hemangioma
- Dermatofibrosarcoma protuberans
- Fibroma
- Epithelioid sarcoma
- Lipoma
- Lipoblastoma
- Hibernoma
- Rhabdomyoma
- Hemangioma
- Angiofibroma
- Lymphangioma
- Kaposi's sarcoma
- Lymphangiosarcoma
- Neurofibroma

*See Chapter 1, Figure 1-59 and Table 1-15.

TABLE B-10. *The Most Common Multifocal Tumors*

- Epithelioid sarcoma
- Lipoblastoma
- Leiomyoma
- Hemangioma
- Lymphangiosarcoma
- Kaposi's sarcoma
- Neurofibroma
- Chondroma

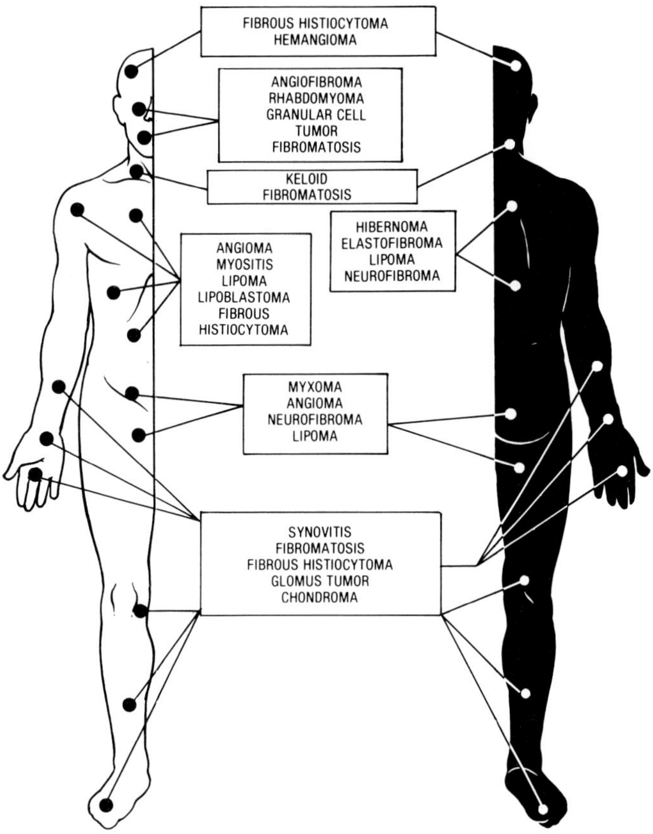

Figure B-1. The most common sites of certain benign soft tissue neoplasms and tumor-like lesions.

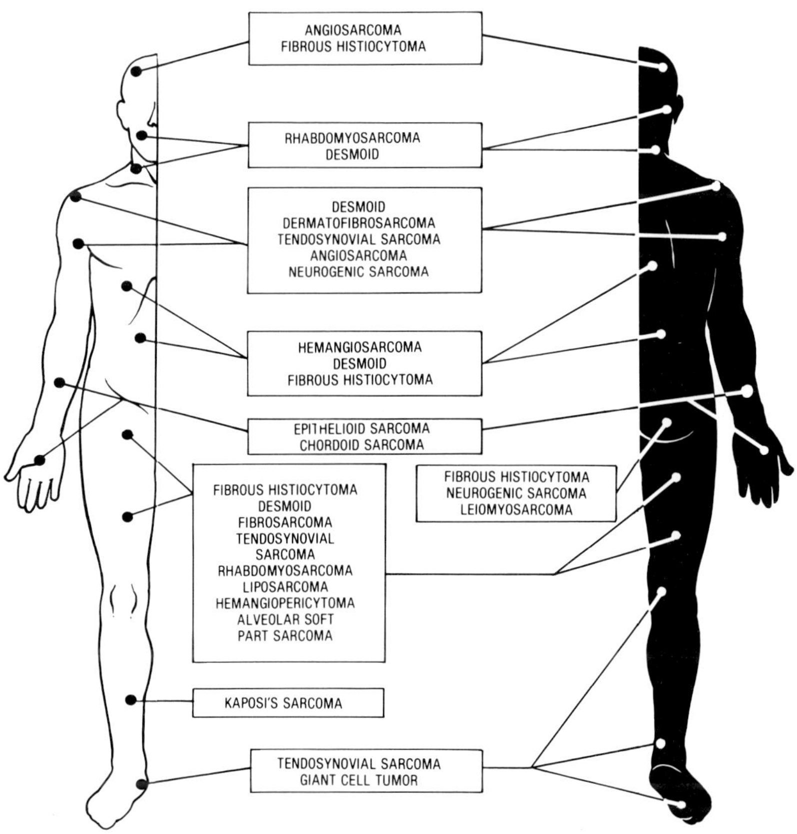

Figure B-2. Site predilection of certain malignant soft tissue tumors.

TABLE B-11. ***Histologic Morphology of Soft Tissue Sarcomas***

	CELL TYPE				
	SPINDLE	OVAL	ROUND	PLEOMORPHIC	GIANT
Malignant fibroblastic fibrous histiocytoma	++	+	-+	-	-
Malignant histiocytic fibrous histiocytoma	+	++	+	+	++
Malignant pleomorphic fibrous histiocytoma	+	+	+	++	++
Desmoid tumor	++	+	-	+-	-
Fibroblastic fibrosarcoma	++	-	-	-	-
Pleomorphic fibrosarcoma	+	+	-	++	++
Monophasic tendosynovial sarcoma, spindle cell type	++	+	-	-	-
Biphasic tendosynovial sarcoma	+	+	+	-	-
Tendosynovial sarcoma, monophasic pseudoglandular type	-	+	+	-	-
Epithelioid sarcoma	+-	++	+	-	-
Clear cell sarcoma	-	+	++	-	+-
Chordoid sarcoma	-	+	+	-	-
Well-differentiated liposarcoma	-	+	++	+-	-
Myxoid liposarcoma	+-	+	+-	-	-
Fibroblastic liposarcoma	++	+	-	-	-
Lipoblastic liposarcoma	-	+	++	-	-
Pleomorphic liposarcoma	+	+	+	++	++
Leiomyosarcoma	++	+	-	+-	+-
Leiomyoblastoma	-	+	++	+	+-
Embryonal rhabdomyosarcoma	+	++	+	-	-
Rhabdomyoblastoma	-	+	++	-+	++
Pleomorphic rhabdomyosarcoma	+	+	+	++	++
Hemangiopericytoma	+	++	+	-	-
Hemangiosarcoma	-	+	++	++	+
Kaposi's sarcoma	++	+	-+	-	-
Lymphangiosarcoma	-+	+	++	++	+-
Malignant non-collagenous schwannoma	++	+	-+	-	-
Malignant collagenous schwannoma	++	+	-	+	+-
Primitive neuroectodermal tumor	-	++	++	-	-
Malignant granular cell tumor	-	-	+	++	+-
Alveolar soft part sarcoma	-	-	+	++	+-
Granulocytic sarcoma	-	-	++	-	-

++ = most common; + = common; +- = may occur; -+ = usually absent; - = absent.

STROMA					
MYXOID	RETICULAR	FIBROUS	VASCULAR	NECROTIC	GROWTH PATTERN
+-	++	-+	-	-	Storiform, arranged
-	++	-+	+	+	Mixed
-	++	-+	-	+	Pleomorphic
-	+	++	-	-	Spreading
-	+	++	-	-	Herringbone, monomorphic
-	+-	++	-	+	Pleomorphic
-	++	-	+	-	Streaming, monomorphic
+-	++	-	+	+	Biphasic
-	+	-	+	+	Pseudoglandular
+-	++	+-	+-	+	Epithelioid
-	+	-	+	+-	Monomorphic
++	+	-	+	+	Stellate
+-	+	-	+-	-	Lipoma-like
++	+	-	++	-	Stellate, vascular
+-	++	+-	++	-	Storiform, vascular
-	++	-	+	+-	Epithelioid, vascular
+-	++	+-	+	++	Pleomorphic
+-	+	-	-+	+-	Streaming
+-	+	-	+	+	Mixed
+-	+	-	++	+-	Monomorphic
-	+	-	+	+-	Globoid
-	+	+-	-+	+	Pleomorphic
-+	++	-	++	+-	Pericytic
-	+	+-	++	++	Intravascular
+-	++	-+	++	++	Streaming, vascular
-	+	-+	++	+	Intravascular
+	++	-	-	+-	Arranged
+-	+	++	-	+-	Spreading, arranged
-	++	-	+	-+	Rosetting
-	+	-	+	-	Globoid
-	++	-	+	+	Alveolar
-	-	-	+	+	Mosaic

TABLE B-12. ***Predominantly Spindle Cell Soft Tissue Sarcomas***

Malignant fibroblastic fibrous histiocytoma
Desmoid tumor
Fibroblastic fibrosarcoma
Tendosynovial sarcoma, monophasic spindle cell type
Fibroblastic liposarcoma
Leiomyosarcoma
Kaposi's sarcoma
Malignant schwannoma

TABLE B-13. ***Predominantly Oval Cell Soft Tissue Sarcomas***

Malignant histiocytic fibrous histiocytoma
Epithelioid sarcoma
Embryonal rhabdomyosarcoma
Hemangiopericytoma
Primitive neuroectodermal tumor

TABLE B-14. ***Predominantly Round Cell Soft Tissue Sarcomas***

Clear cell sarcoma
Well-differentiated liposarcoma
Lipoblastic liposarcoma
Leiomyoblastoma
Rhabdomyoblastoma
Hemangiosarcoma
Lymphangiosarcoma
Malignant granular cell tumor
Alveolar soft part sarcoma
Granulocytic sarcoma

TABLE B-15. ***Predominantly Pleomorphic Soft Tissue Sarcomas***

Malignant histiocytic fibrous histocytoma
Malignant pleomorphic fibrous histiocytoma
Pleomorphic fibrosarcoma
Pleomorphic liposarcoma
Pleomorphic rhabdomyosarcoma
Hemangiosarcoma
Lymphangiosarcoma
Alveolar soft part sarcoma

TABLE B-16. ***Predominantly Giant Cell Soft Tissue Sarcomas***

Malignant histiocytic fibrous histiocytoma
Malignant pleomorphic fibrous histiocytoma
Pleomorphic liposarcoma
Rhabdomyoblastoma
Pleomorphic rhabdomyosarcoma

TABLE B-17. *Special Stains of Soft Tissue Sarcomas**

TUMOR	PAS	PAS WITH DIASTASE	ALCIAN BLUE	ALCIAN BLUE WITH HYALURONIDASE	FAT STAIN	MUCICARMINE	RETICULIN STAIN	TRICHROME STAIN	PTAH	HISTOCHEMICAL STAINS
Myxoma	+	−	+	−	−+	+−	+	−	−	
Histiocytic fibrous histioctyoma	+	−	−+	−	−+.	−	+	−	−	Esterases
Fibrosarcoma	+−	−	−	−	−	−	+	+	−	
Biphasic tendosynovial sarcoma	+	−	−+	−	−	+−	+	−	−	
Chordoid sarcoma	+	+−	+	+−	−+	−	+	−	−	
Liposarcoma	+−	−	+	−	+	−	+	−	−	
Myosarcoma	+	−	−	−	−	−	+	−	+	ATP-ase Myosin
Hemangiosarcoma	+−	−	−	−	−	−	+	−	−	ATP-ase 5-Nucleotidase, Alkaline phosphatase
Schwannoma	+−	+−	+−	+−	−	+−	+	+−	+−	
Osteogenic sarcoma	+	+−	+−	+−	+−	−	+−	+−	−	Alkaline phosphatase
Chondrosarcoma	+	+	+	+	−	−	−+	−	−	Alkaline phosphatase
Ewing's sarcoma	+	−	−	−	−	−	−+	−	−	
Granular cell tumor	+	+	−	−	−	−	+	−	+	
Alveolar soft part sarcoma	+	+	−	−	−	−+	+	−	+	

*See References and individual chapters.

++ = most common; + = common; +− = may occur; −+ = usually absent; − = absent.

TABLE B-18. ***Ultrastructural Features of Soft Tissue Sarcomas****

TUMOR	FEATURES
Malignant fibrous histiocytoma	Extensive RER, free polyribosomes, Golgi complexes, cytoplasmic vacuoles, glycogen-like particles, dense bodies, abundant lysosomes, cytoplasmic filopodia
Fibrosarcoma	Prominent RER, richly collagenous stroma
Tendosynovial sarcoma	Junctional complexes, microvilli-lined lumina, absence of basement membrane, fibroblast-like cells prominent in RER and glycogen, phagocytic epithelioid cells containing sparse RER
Liposarcoma	Intracytoplasmic lipid droplets, glycogen, compressed cytoplasmic organelles
Leiomyosarcoma	Myofibrils with associated pinocytotic vesicles, arranged cytoplasmic actin filaments, basement membranes, dense plaques, dense bodies
Rhabdomyosarcoma	Thick and thin myofilaments and myofibrils
Hemangiopericytoma	Cytoplasmic microfibrils, pinocytotic vesicles, glycogen, basement membrane or fragments of basement membrane
Hemangiosarcoma	Cytoplasmic microfibrils, pinocytotic vesicles, basement membrane, tight junctions, Weibel-Palade bodies
Malignant schwannoma	Long interdigitating cytoplasmic processes, intact or fragmented basement membrane, long-spaced collagen, remnants of "pi" granules, microtubules, clumps of glycogen, occasional dense bodies
Alveolar soft part sarcoma	Intracytoplasmic granules and crystals

*See References and individual chapters.
RER = rough endoplasmic reticulum.

TABLE B-19. *Computerized Differential Diagnosis of Soft Tissue Tumors*

NUMERICAL LISTING	DIFFERENTIAL DIAGNOSIS* (For type of tumor see numerical listing in left column.)
1. Myxoma	2-10-11-15-31-41-fasciitis
2. Malignant fibroblastic fibrous histiocytoma	9-17-19-21-27-41-42
3. Benign giant cell tumor	4-5-26-49-reparative granuloma
4. Malignant giant cell tumor	3-9-26-49-reparative granuloma
5. Benign pleomorphic fibrous histiocytoma	3-6-13-18
6. Malignant pleomorphic fibrous histio-cytoma	4-5-9-18-21-25-41-47-49
7. Fibroma	1-2-8-11-17-19-33-43-fibromatosis
8. Desmoid tumor	7-9-19-21-33-43-fibromatosis
9. Fibrosarcoma	2-4-5-8-17-21-27-43-44-49
10. Lipoblastoma	1-7-15-24
11. Sclerosing lipoma	1-7-17-33-fat necrosis, fasciitis
12. Angiolipoma	1-32-33-35
13. Pleomorphic lipoma	5-6-11-18-lipogranuloma, fat necrosis
14. Well-differentiated liposarcoma	11-13-15-fat necrosis
15. Myxoid liposarcoma	1-10-31-41
16. Lipoblastic liposarcoma	4-10-15-20-24-29-30-37-41-45-50
17. Fibroblastic liposarcoma	1-2-9-15-21-27-33-37-41
18. Pleomorphic liposarcoma	6-9-13-21-25
19. Leiomyoma	7-8-21-33-43
20. Leiomyoblastoma	4-16-21-23-27-29-30-34-41-42
21. Leiomyosarcoma	4-6-9-18-25-42
22. Rhabdomyoma	23-46-proliferative myositis
23. Rhabdomyoblastoma	23-24-25-46-47
24. Embryonal rhabdomyosarcoma	16-17-23-29-37-42-50
25. Pleomorphic rhabdomyosarcoma	6-9-18-21-23-38
26. Villonodular synovitis	3-4-5-synovitis
27. Tendosynovial sarcoma, monophasic spindle cell type	2-9-17-21-37-42
28. Biphasic tendosynovial sarcoma	42-44-skin adnexal tumor
29. Epithelioid sarcoma	16-30-fasciitis, granuloma, fibromatosis
30. Clear cell sarcoma	16-20-29-nevoid schwannoma, melanoma
31. Chordoid sarcoma	1-15-mesenchymal chondrosarcoma
32. Hemangioma	35-angioneuroma
33. Angiofibroma	7-12-19-32
34. Glomus tumor	32-37
35. Lymphangioma	32-36-40
36. Lymphangiomyoma	19-35-37
37. Hemangiopericytoma	27-28-34-36-38-40-50
38. Hemangiosarcoma	37-39-40
39. Kaposi's sarcoma	37-38-40-pyogenic granuloma
40. Lymphangiosarcoma	35-36-37-38
41. Benign non-collagenous schwannoma	2-16-19-20-sclerosing hemangioma
42. Malignant non-collagenous schwannoma	2-6-17-19-20-21-24-27-28-29
43. Benign collagenous schwannoma	7-8-9-19
44. Malignant collagenous schwannoma	9-21-28
45. Primitive neuroectodermal tumor	24-37-50-neuroblastoma, lymphoma
46. Benign granular cell tumor	22-23-47-proliferative myositis
47. Malignant granular cell tumor	21-22-23-25-46-48-paraganglioma
48. Alveolar soft part sarcoma	47-adenocarcinoma, skin adnexal tumor
49. Extraskeletal osteogenic sarcoma	4-6-9-25-myositis ossificans
50. Extraskeletal Ewing's sarcoma	16-24-37-45-neuroblastoma, lymphoma

*See also individual chapters.

TABLE B-20. *Most Common Metastatic Sites of 294 Soft Tissue Sarcomas at Autopsy*

HISTOLOGIC TYPE	SITES OF METASTASIS
Malignant fibrous tumors	Lung, bone, lymph node, intestine, liver
Tendosynovial sarcoma	Lung, chest wall, diaphragm, bone, lymph node
Liposarcoma	Lymph node, intestine, lung, liver, chest wall
Embryonal rhabdomyosarcoma	Bone, lymph node, lung, intestine, liver
Pleomorphic rhabdomyosarcoma	Lung, kidney, heart, lymph node, liver
Leiomyosarcoma	Intestine, lung, lymph node, liver, kidney
Angiosarcoma	Bone, skin, lymph node, intestine, liver
Malignant schwannoma	Skin, lymph node, intestine, retroperitoneum, chest wall

TABLE B-21. *Local Autopsy Findings in 294 Patients with Soft Tissue Sarcomas*

HISTOLOGIC TYPE	LOCAL RECURRENCE (%)	METASTASIS TO REGIONAL LYMPH NODE (%)	VASCULAR INVASION (%)	INVASION OF BONE (%)
Malignant fibrous histiocytoma	50	5	15	5
Fibrosarcoma	40	2	5	10
Tendosynovial sarcoma	60	15	10	2
Liposarcoma	50	20	35	2
Embryonal rhabdomyosarcoma	40	45	10	2
Pleomorphic rhabdomyosarcoma	25	2	35	5
Angiosarcoma	30	15	–	10
Malignant schwannoma	20	0	0	0

TABLE B-22. ***The Most Common Metastatic Soft Tissue Sarcomas at Autopsy***

SITES OF METASTASES	HISTOLOGIC TYPES
Brain	Embryonal rhabdomyosarcoma Liposarcoma Malignant fibrous tumors
Lung	Tendosynovial sarcoma Pleomorphic rhabdomyosarcoma Embryonal rhabdomyosarcoma
Heart	Pleomorphic rhabdomyosarcoma Embryonal rhabdomyosarcoma Malignant fibrous tumors
Thyroid	Leiomyosarcoma Schwannoma Pleomorphic rhabdomyosarcoma
Liver	Embryonal rhabdomyosarcoma Liposarcoma Pleomorphic rhabdomyosarcoma
Pancreas	Embryonal rhabdomyosarcoma Liposarcoma Leiomyosarcoma
Kidney	Pleomorphic rhabdomyosarcoma Leiomyosarcoma Embryonal rhabdomyosarcoma
Spleen	Embryonal rhabdomyosarcoma Leiomyosarcoma Schwannoma
Adrenal	Embryonal rhabdomyosarcoma Pleomorphic rhabdomyosarcoma Angiosarcoma
Skull	Angiosarcoma Embryonal rhabdomyosarcoma Malignant fibrous tumors
Sternum	Embryonal rhabdomyosarcoma Liposarcoma Angiosarcoma
Rib	Embryonal rhabdomyosarcoma Angiosarcoma Tendosynovial sarcoma
Chest Wall	Tendosynovial sarcoma Liposarcoma Schwannoma
Skin	Angiosarcoma Schwannoma Malignant fibrous tumors

TABLE B-23. *Most Common Metastatic Sites of 169 Soft Tissue Sarcomas*

ANATOMIC SITE	NO. OF PATIENTS	%
Lung	114	67
Lymph nodes	102	60
Bone	100	59
Intestine	71	42
Liver	48	28
Skin	37	22
Chest wall	33	20
Adrenal	31	18
Heart	30	18
Kidney	30	18
Diaphragm	27	16
Pancreas	23	14
Retroperitoneum	22	13
Brain	21	12
Soft tissue	20	12
Pelvis	18	11

SELECTED REFERENCES ON SPECIAL STAINS

Mallory, F. B., and Parker, F.: Reticulum. Am. J. Pathol. 3:515, 1927

Fisher, E. R.: Histochemical observation on an alveolar soft part sarcoma with reference to histogenesis. Am. J. Pathol. 32:721, 1956.

Hamperl, H., and Lattes, R.: A study of argyrophilia of nonchromaffin paragangliomas and granular cell myoblastoma. Cancer 10:408, 1957.

Lever, J. D., and Ford, E. H. R.: Histological, histochemical and electron microscopic observation on synovial membrane. Anat. Rec. 132:525, 1958.

Winslow, D. J., and Enzinger, F. M.: Hyaluronidase sensitive acid mucopolysaccharides in liposarcomas. Am. J. Pathol. 37:497, 1960.

Delaunay, A., and Bazin, S.: Mucopolysaccharides, collagen, and nonfibrillar proteins in inflammation. Int. Rev. Conn. Tiss. Res. 2:301, 1964.

Elizalde, A., and Korman, S.: Cytochemical studies of glycogen, neutral mucopolysaccharides and fat in malignant tissues. Cancer 21:1061, 1968.

Fine, G., and Horn, R. C.: Soft tissue tumors: Aids in differential diagnosis. *In* Pathology Annual Edited by S. C. Sommers. New York, Appleton-Century-Crofts, 1969, p. 211.

Engel, W. K., Bishop, D. W., and Cunningham, G. G.: Tubular aggregates in type II muscle fibers: Ultrastructural and histochemical correlation. J. Ultrastr. Rec. 31:507, 1970.

Van de Velde, R. L., and Brown, B. A.: A modified Bodian Protargol stain for identification of striated muscle elements. Am. J. Clin. Pathol. 54:768, 1970.

Mori, M., Murakami, M., Hirose, I., and Shimozato, T.: Histochemical studies of myxoma of the jaw. J. Oral Surg. 33:529, 1975.

Filipe, M. I., and Mackenzie, D. H.: Histochemical characteristics of mucosubstances in three soft tissue tumours. J. Pathol. 118:17, 1976.

Sarnat, H. B., deMello, D. E., and Siddiqui, S. Y.: Diagnostic value of histochemistry in embryonal rhabdomyosarcoma. Am. J. Surg. Pathol. 3:177, 1979.

SELECTED REFERENCES ON ULTRASTRUCTURE OF SOFT TISSUE TUMORS

Luse, S. A.: A synovial sarcoma studied by electron microscopy. Cancer 13:312, 1960.

Scarpelli, D. G., and Greider, M. H.: A correlative cytochemical and electron microscopic study of a liposarcoma. Cancer 15:776, 1962.

Price, H. M.: The skeletal muscle fibre in the light of electron microscopic studies. Am. J. Med. 35:589, 1963.

Cancilla, P. A., and Zimmerman, H. M.: The fine structure of a cerebellar hemangioblastoma. J. Neuropathol. Exp. Neurol. 24:621, 1965.

Pineada, A.: Mast cells: their presence and ultrastructural characteristics in peripheral nerve tumors. Arch. Neurol. 13:372, 1965.

Norton, W. L., and Ziff, M.: Electron microscopic observations on the rheumatoid synovial membrane. Arthritis Rheum. 9:589, 1966.

Ross, R., and Greenless, T. K.: Electron microscopy: Attachment sites between connective tissue cells. Science 153:997, 1966.

Fisher, E. R., and Vuzevski, V. D.: Cytogenesis of schwannoma, neurofibroma, dermatofibroma and dermatofibrosarcoma as revealed by electron microscopy. Am. J. Clin. Pathol. 49:141, 1968.

Murad, T. M., von Haam, E., and Murray, M. S. N.: Ultrastructure of a hemangiopericytoma and a glomus tumor. Cancer 22:1239, 1968.

Cornog, J. L.: The ultrastructure of leiomyoblastoma. Arch. Pathol. 87:404, 1969.

Ghadially, F. N., and Mehta, P. N.: Ultrastructure of osteogenic sarcoma. Cancer 25:1457, 1970.

Gonzales-Crussi, F.: Ultrastructure of congenital fibrosarcoma. Cancer 26:1289, 1970.

Horvat, B. L., Caines, M., and Fisher, E. R.: The ultrastructure of rhabdomyosarcoma. Am. J. Clin. Pathol. 53:555, 1970.

Al-Sarraf, M., Loud, A. V., and Vaitkevicius, V. K.: Malignant granular cell tumor. Histochemical and electron microscopic study. Arch. Pathol. 91:550, 1971.

Merkow, L. P., Frich, J. C., Jr., Sliskin, M., Kyreages, C. G., and Pardo, M.: Ultrastructure of a fibroxanthosarcoma. Cancer 28:372, 1971.

Boram, L. H., Erlandson, R. A., and Hajdu, S. I.: Mesodermal mixed tumors of the uterus. Cancer 30:1295, 1972.

Gabbiani, G., Fu, Y. S., Gordon, I., Kaye, G. I., Lattes, R., and Magno, G.: Epithelioid sarcoma. A light and electron microscopic study suggesting synovial origin. Cancer 30:486, 1972.

Gabbiani, G., and Majno, G.: Dupuytren's contracture: fibroblast contraction? An ultrastructural study. Am. J. Pathol. 66:131, 1972.

Hajdu, S. I., Erlandson, R. A., and Paglia, M. A.: Light and electron microscopic studies of a gastric leiomyoblastoma. Arch. Pathol. 93:36, 1972.

Hou-Jensen, K., Priori, E., and Smochowski, L.: Studies in the ultrastructure of Ewing's sarcoma of bone. Cancer 29:280, 1972.

Kahn, L. B.: Malignant giant cell tumor of tendon sheath. Ultrastructural study and review of the literature. Arch. Pathol. 95:203, 1973.

Kalderon, A. E., and Fethiere, W.: Fine structure of two liposarcomas. Lab. Invest. 28:60, 1973.

Carstens, P. H. B., and Schrodt, G. R.: Ultrastructure of sclerosing hemangioma. Am. J. Pathol. 77:377, 1974.

Cervos-Navarro, J., and Matakas, F.: The ultrastructure of reticulin. Acta Neuropathol. Suppl. 6:137, 1975.

Chandra, S., Jerva, D. K., and Clemis, J. D.: Ultrastructural characteristics of human neurilemmoma cell nuclei. Cancer Res. 35:2000, 1975.

Morales, A. R., Fine, G., Pardo, V., and Horn, R. C.: Ultrastructure of smooth muscle tumors with a consideration of the possible relationship of glomangiomas, hemangiopericytomas and cardiac myxomas. *In* Pathology Annual (Edited by S. C. Sommers), New York, Appleton-Century-Crofts, 1975.

Stiller, D., and Katenkamp, D.: Cellular features in desmoid fibromatosis and well-differentiated fibrosarcomas. An electron microscopic study. Virchows Arch. [Pathol. Anat.] 369:155, 1975.

Battifora, H.: Spindle cell carcinoma. Ultrastructural evidence of squamous origin and collagen production of the tumor cells. Cancer 37:2275, 1976.

Flenker, H.: Myxoid liposarcoma. Light and electron microscopic investigation. Virchows Arch. [Pathol. Anat.] 371:171, 1976.

Gokel, J. M., Kurzl, R., and Hubner, G.: Fine structure and origin of Kaposi's sarcoma. Pathol. Eur. 11:45, 1976.

Gould, V. E., Jao, W.: Comparative ultrastructure of hibernomas and myxoid and pleomorphic liposarcomas. Lab. Invest. 34:316, 1976.

Hajdu, S. I., and Hajdu, E. O.: Cytopathology of Sarcomas and Other Nonepithelial Malignant Tumors. Philadelphia, W. B. Saunders, 1976.

Rosai, J., Summer, H. W., Kostianovsky, M., and Perez-Mesa, C.: Angiosarcoma of the skin. A clinicopathologic and fine structural study. Hum. Pathol. 7:83, 1976.

Weiss, S. W.: Ultrastructure of the so-called "chordoid sarcoma." Cancer 37:300, 1976.

Alguacil-Garcia, A., Unni, K. K., and Goellner, J. R.: Malignant giant cell tumor of soft parts. An ultrastructural study of four cases. Cancer 20:244, 1977.

Patchefsky, A. S., Soriano, R., and Kostianovsky, M.: Epithelioid sarcoma. Ultrastructural similarity to nodular synovitis. Cancer 143, 1977.

Taxy, J. B., and Battifora, H.: Malignant fibrous histiocytomas: An electron microscopic study. Cancer 40:254, 1977.

Desai, U., Ramos, C. V., and Taylor, H. B.: Ultrastructural observations in pleomorphic liposarcoma. Cancer 42:1248, 1978.

Feldman, P. S.: A comparative study including ultrastructure of intramuscular myxoma and myxoid liposarcoma. Cancer 43:512, 1979.

Kindblom, L. G., and Save-Soderbergh, J.: The ultrastructure of liposarcoma. Acta Pathol. Microbiol. Scand., Section A 87:109, 1979.

Reddick, R. L., Michelitch, H., and Triches, T. J.: Malignant soft tissue tumors (malignant fibrous histiocytoma, pleomorphic liposarcoma and pleomorphic rhabdomyosarcoma: An electron microscopic study. Hum. Pathol. 10:327, 1979.

Tomec, R., Ahmad, I., Fu, Y. S., and Jaffe, S.: Malignant hemangioendothelioma (angiosarcoma) of the salivary gland. Cancer 43:1664, 1979.

Hajdu, S. I., Erlandson, R. A., and Fortner, J. G.: Classification and histologic grading of liposarcomas (in press).

appendix C

Review and Self-Assessment Questions (Key to Answers at the end of text)

1. *One of the following tumors is extremely rare in children:*
   - A Desmoid tumor
   - B Tendosynovial sarcoma
   - C Lipoblastoma
   - D Liposarcoma
   - E Neurofibroma
2. *The ultrastructure of the following tumors is fairly characteristic except:*
   - A Pleomorphic rhabdomyosarcoma
   - B Leiomyosarcoma
   - C Granular cell myoblastoma
   - D Malignant schwannoma
   - E Alveolar soft part sarcoma
3. *The epulis type of multinucleated giant cells is commonly seen in all of the following lesions except:*
   - A Reparative granuloma
   - B Giant cell tumor
   - C Pleomorphic liposarcoma
   - D Osteogenic sarcoma
   - E Villonodular synovitis
4. *The statement "cells come from cells" is credited to:*
   - A Papanicolaou
   - B Ewing
   - C Virchow
   - D Rokitansky
   - E J. Muller
5. *As a rule, none of the following tumors exfoliates pleomorphic cells except:*
   - A Leiomyoblastoma
   - B Ewing's sarcoma
   - C Lipoblastoma
   - D Dermatofibrosarcoma
   - E Kaposi's sarcoma

6. *All of the following statements are true except:*
A Immobilization facilitates the development of collagenous rather than cellular fibrous growths.
B Chondrocytes in tissue culture inhibit growth of endothelial cells.
C Ultrastructurally tumor cells of Kaposi's sarcoma resemble angiosarcoma.
D Pericytes are found around blood vessels as well as around lymphatic vessels.
E Sarcomere is a functional as well as a morphologic unit of skeletal muscle.

7. *Which of these tumors has the best prognosis:*
A Hemangiopericytoma
B Lipoblastic liposarcoma
C Fibroblastic liposarcoma
D Epithelioid sarcoma
E Extraskeletal chondrosarcoma

8. *One of the following statements is not true:*
A The anatomic distribution of lipomas and liposarcomas is identical.
B Dermatofibrosarcoma protuberans is found most commonly in the trunk and shoulder.
C Fibromatoses are more common in the distal part of the extremities than in the proximal.
D Fibrous histiocytomas, in general, do not stain positive with trichrome stain.
E Fibrosarcomas stain positive with trichrome stain.

9. *One of the following tumors is more radiosensitive than any of the others:*
A Myxoid liposarcoma
B Pleomorphic rhabdomyosarcoma
C Fibroblastic fibrous histiocytoma
D Monophasic synovial sarcoma
E Leiomyoblastoma

10. *One of the following statements is not true:*
A In general, in liposarcomas there is an inverse relationship between the amount of cytoplasmic fat globules and the grade of malignancy.
B Lipoblasts and foam cells are common in lipoblastic liposarcoma.
C Microscopically, lipoblastic liposarcoma may resemble histiocytic lymphoma.
D Spindle cells and stellate cells are prominent features of pleomorphic liposarcoma.
E Recurrent or metastatic liposarcomas may be so anaplastic that it is often difficult to identify them as liposarcomas.

11. *All of the following statements about nodular fasciitis are true except:*
A It is a disease of young adults.
B The majority involve the superficial fascia.
C It is common in the lower extremity.
D It can be very myxoid in appearance.
E It stains negative with trichrome stain.

12. *All statements are true except:*
A Mediastinal fibromatosis was described by Ormonds.
B "Calcifying aponeurotic fibroma" was first described by Keasbey.
C "Subdermal fibrous tumor of childhood" was originally described by Reye.
D Inclusion-like structures were described in digital fibromatosis.
E Myositis proliferans was first described by Kern.

13. *All of the following are correct except:*
A Steatopygia is a sign of distinction in certain cultures.
B Piezogenic papules are lipomas of the foot.
C Dercum's disease is commonly associated with psychic abnormality.
D Exogenous paraffin hydrocarbons are common findings in lipogranuloma of male genitalia.
E Dystrophia adiposogenitalis is also known as Frölich's syndrome.

14. *One of the following statements is not true:*

A Recurrent and metastatic liposarcomas tend to be less differentiated than the primary liposarcomas.

B Tumors of adipose tissue are more common in the head and neck area than are tumors of fibrous tissues.

C The most common site of liposarcoma is the thigh.

D Liposarcoma metastasizes to the brain more commonly than most of the other soft tissue sarcomas.

E Patients with myxoid liposarcoma are younger than those with pleomorphic liposarcoma.

15. *All of these are true except:*

A Myxoid liposarcoma is composed of preadipocytes and adipocytes.

B Tumor cells of pleomorphic liposarcoma may contain so-called hyalin globules.

C The terms *lipoblastic liposarcoma* and *round cell liposarcoma* are synonyms.

D It is possible that some of the well-differentiated liposarcomas are actually lipomas that turned malignant.

E Most of the retroperitoneal lipoid lesions are either benign or low-grade malignant tumors.

16. *There is a female preponderance in all of the following conditions except one:*

A Synovial cyst

B Well-differentiated lipoma

C Schwannoma

D Villonodular synovitis

E Synovial sarcoma

17. *One of the following statements is not true:*

A Epithelioid sarcoma readily metastasizes to lymph nodes.

B Malignant fibrous histiocytoma metastasizes more commonly to lymph nodes than fibrosarcoma.

C Liposarcoma has a tendency to metastasize to lymph nodes.

D Dermatofibrosarcoma protuberans does not have a tendency to metastasize to lymph nodes.

E Desmoid tumors may metastasize.

18. *All of the following are true except:*

A Alveolar soft part sarcoma is more common in males than in females.

B Giant cell tumor of a tendon sheath is more common in females than in males.

C Schwannoma is more common in females than in males.

D Lipomas are more common in females than in males.

E Synovial sarcoma is more common in males than in females.

19. *All are true except one:*

A Ganglions are found predominantly in females.

B The synovium is composed of type A and type B cells.

C Giant cell tumors of tendon sheath occur most frequently in males.

D Arborescent lipoma is a tendosynovial lipoma.

E The term *benign synovioma* should not be used.

20. *All of the following are true except:*

A Montpellier introduced the term *alveolaire sarcoma* in 1929.

B The term *leiomyoblastoma* was first used by Bartkowiak, in 1936.

C The term *embryonal rhabdomyosarcoma* was first used by Stobbe and Dargeon, in 1950.

D Veratti, in 1902, described the sarcoplasmic reticulum.

E The striation of skeletal muscle was first noted by Leeuwenhoeck, in 1721.

21. *All of the following statements are true except:*

A Actin filaments are present in smooth muscle as well as in striated muscle.
B Myosin filaments are the so-called thick or anisotropic filaments.
C Type I muscle fibers are more common in humans than type II fibers.
D The band pattern of myofibrils is caused by the arrangement of the myofilaments.
E Skein-like filaments are precursors of myofilaments.

22. *The following tumors have a female preponderance except:*

A Metastasizing leiomyoma
B Peritoneal leiomyomatosis
C Intravascular leiomyoma
D Uterine leiomyosarcoma
E Oral leiomyosarcoma

23. *All statements are true except:*

A Myogenic tumors may arise in bone.
B The tumor nodules in peritoneal leiomyomatosis are composed of decidual tissue.
C Intravenous leiomyomatosis means smooth muscle growth beyond the confines of the uterus.
D The clarity of the cytoplasm in leiomyoblastomas is caused by poor fixation.
E The rectum is more commonly the site of smooth muscle tumors than the ascending colon.

24. *All of the following statements are true except:*

A Keloids have a predilection for the abdomen and shoulder.
B Fasciitis has a preponderance to the forearm.
C The most common site of elastofibroma is the back.
D Digital fibromatosis is found most commonly on the extensor surface.
E Palmar fibromatosis is often bilateral.

25. *All of these statements are true except:*

A Type III collagen fibers stain positive with reticulum stain.
B Protocollagen is synthesized on ribosomes.
C Phosphofructokinase is a source of energy for fibroblasts during collagen synthesis.
D All fibroblasts are able to synthesize collagen as well as hyaluronate.
E In many collagen diseases the major abnormalities are in the composition of the ground substance.

26. *Both type A and type B cells are involved in the synthesis of hyaluronate.*

A False
B True

27. *The concentration of non-protein nitrogen, uric acid, and glucose is equal in synovial fluid and serum.*

A False
B True

28. *The function of adipose cells includes lipogenesis, lipid deposition, mobilization of lipid, and maintenance of stored lipid.*

A False
B True

29. *A high concentration of acid phosphatase and esterase is a feature of histiocytes.*

A False
B True

30. *Granular cell myoblastoma or granular cell tumor should be considered a lesion which may arise from a variety of cells.*

A False
B True

31. *The presence of intracytoplasmic granules distinguishes malignant granulocytes from the benign ones.*
A False
B True

32. *Synovial cysts decrease in size on motion of the joint.*
A False
B True

33. *Intraosseous synovial cysts are subchondral in location.*
A False
B True

34. *Synovial cysts are more common in females than in males.*
A False
B True

35. *Tumor cells of lymphoreticular tumors in smears appear as isolated cells, and the cells of Ewing's sarcoma, as well as embryonal rhabdomyosarcoma, are in clusters.*
A False
B True

36. *Pleomorphic fibrosarcoma and osteogenic sarcoma are strikingly similar in an aspiration smear.*
A False
B True

37. *Cross-striation is a common feature of embryonal rhabdomyoblasts.*
A False
B True

38. *Tumor cells of benign and malignant mesenchymal tumors can be easily distinguished with the electron microscope.*
A False
B True

39. *The majority of patients with tuberous sclerosis have renal angiomyolipoma.*
A False
B True

40. *Myxoma is a distinct clinicopathologic entity without relation to myxoid fibrous histiocytoma or myxoid adipose tumors.*
A False
B True

41. *Anchoring filaments are found in lymphatic vessels.*
A False
B True

42. *Pericytes may detach and become histiocytic or ameboid.*
A False
B True

43. *Weibel-Palade bodies are found in leiomyoblasts.*
A False
B True

44. *Perivascular fibroblasts are called "veil" cells.*
A False
B True

45. *Lymphatic capillaries do not have pericytes.*
A False
B True

46. *Palmar fibromatosis is almost exclusively a disease of white males.*
A False
B True

47. *Asteroid bodies are fragmented intracytoplasmic collagen fibrils.*
A False
B True

48. *Endothelial cells are activated in tissue culture by serum growth factor.*
A False
B True

49. *There is a well-expressed branching capillary network in both myxoid and fibroblastic liposarcomas.*
A False
B True

50. *Most of the malignant schwannomas possess specific microscopic features.*
A False
B True

51. *All of the following statements are true except:*
A Segmental demyelination may be caused by malignant neoplasms.
B Axonal degeneration means breakdown of the axon without changes in the myelin sheath.
C Traumatic neuroma is a conglomerate of proliferating axons, Schwann cells, and fibroblasts.
D From the histogenetic point of view there is no such tumor as the neurilemoma.
E Malignant transformation of solitary benign schwannomas is rare.

52. *All of the following are more common in females than in males except:*
A Synovial cyst
B Lipoma
C Kimura's disease
D Hemangioma
E Lipoblastoma

53. *All of the following are more common in males than in females except:*
A Osteoma of the tongue
B Rhabdomyoma
C Synovial chondromatosis
D Keloid
E Myositis proliferans

54. *All of the following are found most commonly during the fourth and fifth decades except:*
A Hemangiopericytoma
B Chondroma of soft tissues
C Dermatofibrosarcoma protuberans
D Desmoid tumor
E Lipoma

55. *All of these are true except:*
A There are multinucleated giant cells in myositis proliferans.
B Rhabdomyoma is predominantly a disease of adult females.
C Osteoma of the tongue is a disease of adult females.
D Embryonal rhabdomyosarcoma of the bile ducts has a predilection for females.
E Rhabdomyoblastoma is a malignant tumor.

56. *All statements are true except:*

A Subcutaneous fat necrosis can be found in association with pancreatitis.
B One route of fat synthesis is by reversed beta-oxidation.
C Endothelial cells of venules contain few lysosomes.
D "Veil" cells are perivascular fibroblasts.
E Endothelial cells contain actomyosin.

57. *All of these statements are true except:*

A Confluent endothelial cells in vitro respond to serum growth factors.
B There is a functional relationship between endothelial cells and platelets.
C Angioblastic lymphoid hyperplasia commonly occurs on the face.
D "Blue rubber-bleb nevus syndrome" means angiomatosis.
E Glomus cells have intracytoplasmic myofilaments.

58. *All statements are true except:*

A Malignant granular cell tumor is predominantly a disease of females.
B In older patients malignant granular cell tumor occurs more frequently than alveolar soft part sarcoma.
C Alveolar soft part sarcoma is more common in males than in females.
D Benign granular cell tumor is more common in females than in males.
E Granulocytic sarcoma is a disease of children and young adults.

59. *None of the following statements is true except:*

A Histologic grading of soft tissue tumors must be done on the basis of mitotic count.
B Staging of soft tissue sarcomas must be done by clinicians.
C The site of the tumor has no influence on prognosis.
D Low-grade bulky tumors may be more aggressive neoplasms than small high-grade tumors.
E Age does not influence prognosis.

Match by association

60. *Asteroid bodies*	A No basement membrane
61. *Russell bodies*	B Endothelial cells
62. *Döhle's bodies*	C Leukocytes
63. *Weibel-Pallade bodies*	D Absolute alcohol
64. *Anitsckow cells*	E Plasma cells
65. *Synovial cells*	F Giant cells
66. *Synovial A cells*	G Myocytes
67. *Urate crystals*	H Phagocytic and have filopodia
68. *Cytochrome pigment*	I Brown fat
69. *Positive mucin clot*	J Traumatic arthritis

Match by association:

70. *Milroy's disease*	A Congenital lymphedema
71. *Kimura's disease*	B Corpora cavernosa
72. *Ormond's disease*	C Keloid
73. *Peyronie's disease*	D Liposarcoma
74. *Alibert's disease*	E Retroperitoneal fibromatosis
75. *Dercum's disease*	F Adiposis dolorosa
76. *Unna's Lochkern*	G Granular cell tumor
77. *Abrikossoff's tumor*	H Neuroma
78. *Madelung's*	I Fat neck
79. *Morton's*	J Angioblastic lymphoid hyperplasia

Match by association:

80. *Piezogenic papules*	A Fat necrosis
81. *Protocollagen synthesis*	B Ribosomes
82. *Type I fibers*	C Myotonic dystrophy

83. *Thin filaments* D Fat synthesis
84. *Glycosaminoglycan* E No mitosis
85. *Reversed beta-oxidation* F Schwann cells
86. *G_2 phase* G The longest phase
87. *G_1 phase* H RNA synthesis
88. *Out of phase* I Hyaluronic acid
89. *Pi granules* J Tropomyosin

90. *Lipoma has a female preponderance and liposarcoma a male preponderance.*
A False
B True

91. *Keloids as well as fibromatoses are more common in blacks than in whites.*
A False
B True

92. *Pericytes and Schwann cells are pluripotential cells.*
A False
B True

93. *Schwann cells and perineurial cells have basal laminae.*
A False
B True

94. *Neurilemoma is a tumor arising from the neurilema.*
A False
B True

95. *Both lipomas and angiomyolipomas are observed most frequently in females.*
A False
B True

96. *The lower extremities are the most common sites of lipomas and liposarcomas.*
A False
B True

97. *Dystrophia adiposogenitalis was first described by Fröhlich in 1901.*
A False
B True

98. *Renal angiomyolipoma is a common finding in patients with tuberous sclerosis.*
A False
B True

99. *The mucinous stroma in myxoid liposarcomas is rich in hyaluronic acid and is removable by prior treatment of tissue sections with hyaluronidase.*
A False
B True

100. *Most of the synovial sarcomas arise from tendon sheaths and bursae and not from articular surfaces.*
A False
B True

101. *Extraskeletal Ewing's sarcomas have been reported prior to 1940.*
A False
B True

102. *The difference between vascular and lymphatic capillaries is that the latter do not possess pericytes.*
A False
B True

103. *Erythrophagocytosis is a distinctive feature of neoplastic cells of Kaposi's sarcoma.*
A False
B True

104. *There is a close morphologic and developmental relationship between fibroblasts and pericytes.*
A False
B True

105. *Extramedullary hematopoiesis is a distinguishing feature of hemangioblastoma.*
A False
B True

106. *Primitive neuroectodermal tumor is a disease of children.*
A False
B True

107. *Bednar described pigmented neurofibromas, in 1957, and Chauffard described café-au-lait spots in 1889.*
A False
B True

108. *Lichtenstein reported the first case of extraskeletal osteogenic sarcoma.*
A False
B True

109. *Freke, in 1740, reported the first case of myositis ossificans and Munchmeyer, in 1869, coined the term* myositis ossificans.
A False
B True

110. *Berard, in 1894, coined the term* embryonal rhabdomyosarcoma; *and Montpellier, in 1929, introduced the term* alveolare rhabdomyosarcoma.
A False
B True

111. *The term* leiomyoblastoma *was introduced by Bartkowiak, in 1936; Jaffe, in 1926, coined the term* lipoblastoma.
A False
B True

112. *All of the following tumors are characterized as spindle cell tumors except:*
A Fibrosarcoma
B Fibroblastic fibrous histiocytoma
C Neurofibrosarcoma
D Chordoid sarcoma
E Fibroblastic liposarcoma

113. *All of these tumors are characterized as round cell tumors except:*
A Rhabdomyoblastoma
B Leiomyoblastoma
C Nevoid schwannoma
D Hemangioblastoma
E Histiocytic fibrous histiocytoma

114. *All of these are characterized as pleomorphic tumors except:*
A High grade fibrosarcoma
B Pleomorphic fibrous histiocytoma
C Extraskeletal osteogenic sarcoma
D Mesenchymal chondrosarcoma
E High grade collagenous schwannoma

115. *All of these are considered to be small cell tumors except:*
- A Clear cell sarcoma
- B Ewing's sarcoma
- C Embryonal rhabdomyosarcoma
- D Botryoid sarcoma
- E Lipoblastic liposarcoma

116. *All of these are high grade tumors except:*
- A Hemangiosarcoma
- B Rhabdomyosarcoma
- C Pleomorphic fibrous histiocytoma
- D Primitive neuroectodermal tumor
- E Pleomorphic liposarcoma

117. *These are all low grade malignant tumors except:*
- A Desmoid tumor
- B Fibroblastic liposarcoma
- C Alveolar soft part sarcoma
- D Dermatofibrosarcoma protuberans
- E Chordoid sarcoma

118. *All statements are true except:*
- A Fibrous histiocytomas should be considered embryonal or undifferentiated forms of fibroblastic tumors.
- B It is known that the rich capillary network plays a role in the histogenesis of myxoid and fibroblastic liposarcomas.
- C The arrangement of the tumor cells in chordoma and alveolar soft part sarcoma are distinctly different.
- D The presence of basal lamina facilitates collagen formation.
- E The first microscopic atlas of pathology was printed in France.

119. *None of the following is true except:*
- A At the time of diagnosis of well-differentiated liposarcoma one should concentrate on the perivascular areas.
- B Fibroblastic liposarcomas possess a rich capillary network.
- C Desmoid tumors are composed of tight bundles of slender fibroblasts.
- D Ewing's sarcoma of soft tissue is a specific and differentiated neoplasm.
- E High mitotic count in soft tissue tumors invariably indicates poor prognosis.

Match by association

120. *Stout, in 1935*	A First used the term *chordoid sarcoma*
121. *Stewart, in 1948*	B First cases of postradiation fibrosarcoma
122. *Woringer, in 1931*	C Coined the term *elastofibroma*
123. *Warren and Sommer, in 1936*	D First used the term *glomus tumor*
124. *Jarvi and Saxen, in 1961*	E First described villonodular synovitis
125. *Quick and Cutler, in 1927*	F First description of clear cell sarcoma
126. *Barre and Masson, in 1924*	G Devised the term *hemangioendothelioma*
127. *Phemister, in 1931*	H Introduced grading of sarcoma
128. *Chassaignac, in 1859*	I Coined the term *neurilemoma*
129. *Mallory, in 1908*	J Introduced the term *histiocytoma*

130. *All statements are true except:*
- A In general, recurrent and metastatic tumors are less differentiated than the primary neoplasm.
- B At the time of staging of soft tissue tumors, size, site, and histologic grade should be considered.
- C Storiform and stellate patterns may be seen in tumors other than fibrous histiocytomas.

D Whether a histiocytic fibrous histiocytoma is malignant should be decided by considering the stromal cells.
E Epulis-type and Touton giant cells are the product of amitotic division.

131. *In general, for the treatment of soft tissue sarcomas the best chemotherapeutic agent is:*
A Adriamycin
B Cyclophosphamide
C Actinomycin D
D DTIC
E Vincristine

132. *All of the following statements are true except:*
A Vascular or bone invasion necessitate amputation.
B The recurrence rate is about 15% after monobloc muscle group resection.
C In case of proximal thigh sarcomas hip joint disarticulation or hemipelvectomy may be indicated to prevent local recurrence.
F Ir-192 is used in treatment of soft tissue sarcomas.
E In case of biopsy, if an excisional biopsy cannot be done, a generous incisional biopsy is required.

133. *These statements are true, except:*
A Type A synovial cells are phagocytic and contain pi granules.
B Type B synovial cells contain prominent RER and secrete hyaluronate.
C Schwann cells have basement membrane and microfibrils and contain clumps of glycogen and dense bodies.
D Schwannian features include interdigitating fibrillar cell processes and periodic arrangement of nuclei.
E Fragmented basal lamina may be seen in malignant schwannoma.

134. *All statements are true except:*
A Lymphangiomyoma is the disease of young adult females.
B Angiomyolipoma is predominantly found in adult females.
C Desmoid tumor is seen predominantly in middle-aged males.
D Granulocytic sarcoma is predominantly the disease of young males.
E Kaposi's sarcoma is rare in females.

135. *All statements are true except:*
A Rhabdomyoma is most common in the head and neck areas.
B Dermatofibrosarcoma protuberans is commonly seen in the extremities.
C The most common site of liposarcoma is the thigh.
D Lipomas are most commonly seen in the back and upper chest.
E Benign granular cell tumors are most common in the head and neck regions.

136. *All statements are true except:*
A The 5-year survival of patients having myxoid liposarcoma is better than 85%.
B The 5-year survival of patients with alveolar soft part sarcoma is less than 50%.
C The 5-year survival of patients with tendosynovial sarcoma, monophasic spindle cell type is less than 30%.
D The 5-year mortality of patients with neurogenic sarcoma associated with von Recklinghausen's disease is above 90%.
E The mortality with desmoid tumor and dermatofibrosarcoma protuberans is about 10%.

137. *All statements are true except:*
A The majority of liposarcomas arising in lipoma are myxoid liposarcoma.
B Retroperitoneal liposarcomas are almost always myxoid liposarcomas.
C Alveolar rhabdomyosarcoma is a poorly defined entity.
D Fibrous histiocytoma may arise in a schwannoma.
E Tendosynovial clear cell sarcoma is a rare tumor and does not contain melanin.

138. *None of the following statements is true except:*

A Tumor necrosis has no bearing on histologic grade.
B The presence of inflammatory cells indicates high histologic grade.
C High mitotic count always indicates high histologic grade.
D Fibrous tumors in children are less aggressive than those in adults.
E Vascularity of soft tissue tumors does not influence prognosis.

139. *All statements about the ultrastructure are true except:*

A Leiomyosarcoma is characterized by dense plaques and dense bodies.
B Thick and thin myofilaments are found in rhabdomyosarcoma.
C Fragmented basement membrane and pi granules are seen in hemangiosarcoma.
D Cytoplasmic filopodia, extensive RER, abundant lysosomes, and polyribosomes characterize fibrous histiocytomas.
E Interdigitating cytoplasmic processes, microtubules, dense bodies, and clumps of glycogen are features of schwannomas.

140. *All statements are true except:*

A Myxoid liposarcoma stains positive with alcian blue after hyaluronidase digestion.
B Osteogenic sarcoma is alkaline phosphatase positive.
C Rhabdomyosarcoma is ATP-ase positive.
D Endothelial cells stain positive with PAS.
E The intracytoplasmic granules in alveolar soft part sarcoma are PAS positive before and after diastase digestion.

Match by association:

141. *Schwannoma*	A Mast cells
142. *Myxoid liposarcoma*	B 80% 10-year survival
143. *Desmoid tumor*	C CTT density about 90
144. *Undifferentiated sarcoma*	D Under age 10
145. *Tendosynovial sarcoma*	E Postirradiation sarcoma
146. *Lipoblastoma*	F Mucicarmine positive
147. *Granular cell tumor*	G Unknown in malignant form
148. *Hibernoma*	H Head and neck
149. *Rhabdomyoblastoma*	I Teratoma
150. *Kaposi's sarcoma*	J Hodgkin's disease

ANSWERS TO REVIEW AND SELF-ASSESSMENT QUESTIONS

1. D	26. B	51. B	76. D	101. B	126. D
2. D	27. B	52. E	77. G	102. B	127. F
3. C	28. B	53. A	78. I	103. B	128. E
4. C	29. B	54. D	79. H	104. B	129. G
5. A	30. B	55. B	80. A	105. B	130. E
6. D	31. A	56. C	81. B	106. A	131. A
7. E	32. A	57. A	82. C	107. B	132. A
8. A	33. B	58. C	83. J	108. A	133. A
9. A	34. B	59. D	84. I	109. B	134. C
10. D	35. B	60. F	85. D	110. B	135. B
11. C	36. B	61. E	86. H	111. B	136. B
12. A	37. A	62. C	87. G	112. D	137. B
13. B	38. A	63. B	88. E	113. D	138. D
14. B	39. A	64. G	89. F	114. D	139. C
15. E	40. A	65. A	90. B	115. A	140. A
16. E	41. B	66. H	91. A	116. C	141. A
17. C	42. B	67. D	92. B	117. B	142. B
18. A	43. A	68. I	93. B	118. C	143. C
19. C	44. B	69. J	94. A	119. B	144. E
20. C	45. B	70. A	95. B	120. I	145. F
21. C	46. B	71. J	96. A	121. A	146. D
22. E	47. B	72. E	97. A	122. J	147. H
23. B	48. A	73. B	98. A	123. B	148. G
24. A	49. B	74. C	99. B	124. C	149. I
25. D	50. A	75. F	100. B	125. H	150. J

index

Page numbers in *italics* refer to major entries; page numbers followed by f refer to illustrations; page numbers followed by t refer to tables.